P9-BAV-200

KARY LIBRARY
VERMONT COLLEGE
6 COLLEGE STREET
MONTPELIER, VT 05602

WITHDRAWN

WITHDRAWN

Please remember that this is a library book,
and that it belongs only temporarily to each
person who uses it. Be considerate. Do
not write in this, or any, library book.

CONTEMPORARY INTELLECTUAL ASSESSMENT

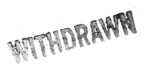

CONTEMPORARY INTELLECTUAL ASSESSMENT

CONTEMPORARY
INTELLECTUAL ASSESSMENT

Theories, Tests, and Issues

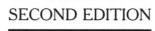

SECOND EDITION

Edited by

DAWN P. FLANAGAN
PATTI L. HARRISON

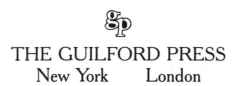

THE GUILFORD PRESS
New York   London

153.93
C761
2005

65,00

© 2005 The Guilford Press
A Division of Guilford Publications, Inc.
72 Spring Street, New York, NY 10012
www.guilford.com

All rights reserved

No part of this book may be reproduced, translated, stored in a retrieval system, or transmitted, in any form or by any means, electronic, mechanical, photocopying, microfilming, recording, or otherwise, without written permission from the Publisher.

Printed in the United States of America

This book is printed on acid-free paper.

Last digit is print number: 9 8 7 6 5 4 3

Library of Congress Cataloging-in-Publication Data

Contemporary intellectual assessment: theories, tests, and issues / edited by Dawn P. Flanagan and Patti L. Harrison.—2nd ed.
    p. cm.
  Includes bibliographical references and index.
  ISBN 1-59385-125-1
  1. Intelligence tests. I. Flanagan, Dawn P. II. Harrison, Patti L.
  BF431.C66 2005
  153.9′3—dc22

                                                                    2004016931

About the Editors

Dawn P. Flanagan, PhD, is Professor of Psychology at St. John's University in New York. She writes and conducts research on such topics as the structure of intelligence, psychoeducational assessment, learning disabilities evaluation and diagnosis, and professional issues in school psychology. Dr. Flanagan's articles and chapters on these topics appear in school and clinical psychology journals and books. She is senior author of *The Wechsler Intelligence Scales and Gf-Gc Theory: A Contemporary Approach to Interpretation, Essentials of Cross-Battery Assessment, The Achievement Test Desk Reference (ATDR): Comprehensive Assessment of Learning Disabilities, Diagnosing Learning Disability in Adulthood,* and *Essentials of WISC-IV Assessment*; coauthor of *The Intelligence Test Desk Reference (ITDR): Gf-Gc Cross-Battery Assessment* and *Essentials of WJ III Cognitive Assessment*; and coeditor of *Clinical Use and Interpretation of the WJ III.* Dr. Flanagan is a Fellow of the American Psychological Association and Diplomate of the American Board of Psychological Specialties, as well as a past recipient of the APA's Lightner Whitmer Award.

Patti L. Harrison, PhD, is Professor in the School Psychology Program and Associate Dean of the Graduate School at the University of Alabama. She has conducted research on intelligence, adaptive behavior, and preschool assessment. Dr. Harrison's articles and chapters on assessment topics appear in school and clinical psychology and special education journals and texts, and she has presented over 100 refereed and invited presentations on these topics at conferences of professional organizations in psychology and education. She was Editor of *School Psychology Review* and has been an editorial board member for several school psychology and related journals, including *School Psychology Quarterly,* the *Journal of School Psychology,* the *Journal of Psychoeducational Assessment,* the *American Journal on Mental Retardation,* and *Diagnostique.*

Contributors

Vincent C. Alfonso, PhD, Graduate School of Education, Fordham University, New York, New York

Michelle S. Athanasiou, PhD, Department of Professional Psychology, University of Northern Colorado, Greeley, Colorado

Nayena Blankson, MA, Department of Psychology, University of Southern California, Los Angeles, California

Bruce A. Bracken, PhD, School of Education, College of William and Mary, Williamsburg, Virginia

Jeffery P. Braden, PhD, Department of Psychology, North Carolina State University, Raleigh, North Carolina

Rachel Brown-Chidsey, PhD, Department of School Psychology, University of Southern Maine, Gorham, Maine

John B. Carroll, PhD, (deceased) Department of Psychology, University of North Carolina, Chapel Hill, North Carolina

Jie-Qi Chen, PhD, Erikson Institute, Chicago, Illinois

V. Susan Dahinten, PhD, RN, School of Nursing, University of British Columbia, Vancouver, British Columbia, Canada

J. P. Das, PhD, Department of Educational Psychology, University of Alberta, Edmonton, Alberta, Canada

Felicia A. Dixon, PhD, Department of Educational Psychology, Ball State University, Muncie, Indiana

Agnieszka M. Dynda, MS, Department of Psychology, St. John's University, Jamaica, New York

Colin D. Elliott, PhD, Gevirtz Graduate School of Education, University of California, Santa Barbara, California

Dawn P. Flanagan, PhD, Department of Psychology, St. John's University, Jamaica, New York

Randy G. Floyd, PhD, Department of Psychology, University of Memphis, Memphis, Tennessee

Laurie Ford, PhD, Department of Educational and Counseling Psychology, University of British Columbia, Vancouver, British Columbia, Canada

Howard Gardner, PhD, Mind, Brain, and Education Program, Harvard Graduate School of Education, Cambridge, Massachusetts

Joseph J. Glutting, PhD, School of Education, University of Delaware, Newark, Delaware

John L. Horn, PhD, Department of Psychology, University of Southern California, Los Angeles, California

Randy W. Kamphaus, PhD, Department of Educational Psychology, University of Georgia, Athens, Georgia

Alan S. Kaufman, PhD, Child Study Center, Yale University School of Medicine, New Haven, Connecticut

James C. Kaufman, PhD, Department of Psychology and Human Development, California State University, San Bernardino, California

Nadeen L. Kaufman, EdD, Child Study Center, Yale University School of Medicine, New Haven, Connecticut

Jennie Kaufman-Singer, PhD, Parole Outpatient Clinic, California Department of Corrections, Sacramento, California

Timothy Z. Keith, PhD, Department of Educational Psychology, University of Texas at Austin, Austin, Texas

Sangwon Kim, MA, Department of Educational Psychology, University of Georgia, Athens, Georgia

Jennifer T. Mascolo, PsyD, Department of Psychology, St. John's University, Jamaica, New York

Nancy Mather, PhD, Department of Special Education, Rehabilitation, and School Psychology, University of Arizona, Tucson, Arizona

R. Steve McCallum, PhD, Department of Education Psychology and Counseling, University of Tennessee, Knoxville, Tennessee

Kevin S. McGrew, PhD, Institute for Applied Psychometrics, St. Cloud, Minnesota

David E. McIntosh, PhD, Department of Education Psychology, Ball State University, Muncie, Indiana

Jack A. Naglieri, PhD, Department of Psychology, George Mason University, Fairfax, Virginia

Bradley C. Niebling, PhD, Heartland Area Education Agency 11, Johnston, Iowa

Salvador Hector Ochoa, PhD, Department of Educational Psychology, Texas A&M University, College Station, Texas

Samuel O. Ortiz, PhD, Department of Psychology, St. John's University, Jamaica, New York

Mark Pomplun, PhD, Riverside Publishing, Itasca, Illinois

Suzan Radwan, MSEd, Graduate School of Education, Fordham University, New York, New York

Cecil R. Reynolds, PhD, Department of Educational Psychology, Texas A&M University, College Station, Texas

Gale H. Roid, PhD, Department of Psychology, Washington State University, Vancouver, Washington

Ellen W. Rowe, MA, Department of Educational Psychology, University of Georgia, Athens, Georgia

Frederick A. Schrank, PhD, Woodcock–Muñoz Foundation, Olympia, Washington

Robert J. Sternberg, PhD, Department of Psychology, Yale University, New Haven, Connecticut

David S. Tulsky, PhD, Kessler Medical Rehabilitation Research and Education Corporation, West Orange, New Jersey

John D. Wasserman, PhD, Department of Psychology, George Mason University, Fairfax, Virginia

Marley W. Watkins, PhD, Departments of Education and School Psychology and Special Education, Penn State University, University Park, Pennsylvania

Larry Weiss, PhD, The Psychological Corporation, San Antonio, Texas

Barbara J. Wendling, MA, consultant, Dallas, Texas

Anne Pierce Winsor, PhD, Department of Educational Psychology, University of Georgia, Athens, Georgia

Eric A. Youngstrom, PhD, Department of Psychology, Case Western Reserve University, Cleveland, Ohio

Jianjun Zhu, PhD, The Psychological Corporation, San Antonio, Texas

Preface

The history of intelligence testing has been well documented from the early period of mental measurement to present-day conceptions of the structure of intelligence and its operationalization. The foundations of psychometric theory and practice were established in the late 1800s and set the stage for the ensuing enterprise in the measurement of human cognitive abilities. The technology of intelligence testing was apparent in the early 1900s, when Binet and Simon developed a test that adequately distinguished children with mental retardation from children with normal intellectual capabilities, and was well entrenched when the Wechsler–Bellevue was published in the late 1930s. In subsequent decades, significant refinements and advances in intelligence testing technology were made, and the concept of individual differences was a constant focus of scientific inquiry.

Although several definitions and theories have been offered in recent decades, the nature of intelligence, cognition, and competence continues to be elusive. Perhaps the most popular definition was that offered by Wechsler in 1958. According to Wechsler, intelligence is "the aggregate or global capacity of the individual to act purposefully, to think rationally and to deal effectively with his environment" (p. 7). It is on this conception of intelligence that the original Wechsler tests were built. Because for decades the Wechsler batteries were the dominant intelligence tests in the field of psychology, were found to measure global intelligence validly, and for many years were largely without rival, they assumed "number one" status and remain in that position today. As such, Wechsler's (1958) definition of intelligence continues to guide and influence the present-day practice of intelligence testing.

In light of theoretical and empirical advances in cognitive psychology, however, it is clear that earlier editions of the Wechsler tests were not based on the most dependable and current evidence of science, and that overreliance on these instruments served to widen the gap between intelligence testing and cognitive science. During the 1980s and 1990s, new intelligence tests were developed to be more consistent with contemporary research and theoretical models of the structure of cognitive abilities. Since the publication of the first edition of *Contemporary Intellectual Assessment: Theories, Tests, and Issues* in 1997, there has been tremendous growth in intelligence theory and measurement of cognitive constructs. Importantly, since 1997, numerous new instruments have been developed and existing instruments have been revised. The authors and publishers of all these instruments have relied on recent theory and research to develop subtests, to analyze validity data, and to organize frameworks for interpretation and use of test results.

Recent tests that use contemporary psychometric theory as their foundation include the Kaufman Assessment Battery for Children, Second Edition; the Stanford–Binet Intelligence Scales, Fifth Edition; the Woodcock–Johnson Psycho-Educational Battery, Third Edition;

the Cognitive Assessment System; the Universal Nonverbal Intelligence Test; and the Reynolds Intellectual Assessment Scales. It is noteworthy that even the most recent revisions of the Wechsler scales (including the Wechsler Intelligence Scale for Children—Fourth Edition, the Wechsler Preschool and Primary Scale of Intelligence—Third Edition, and the Wechsler Adult Intelligence Scale—Third Edition) reflect contemporary theory and research to a greater extent than their predecessors, although they remain atheoretical.

The information presented in this text on modern intelligence theory and assessment technology suggests that clinicians should be familiar with the many approaches to assessing intelligence that are now available. In order for the field of intellectual assessment to continue to advance, clinicians should use instruments that operationalize empirically supported theories of intelligence, and should employ assessment techniques that are designed to measure the broad array of cognitive abilities represented in current theory. It is only through a broader measurement of intelligence, grounded in a well-validated theory of the nature of human cognitive abilities, that professionals can gain a better understanding of the relationship between intelligence and important outcome criteria (e.g., school achievement, occupational success) and can continue to narrow the gap between the professional practice of intelligence testing and advances in cognitive psychology.

PURPOSE AND OBJECTIVES

The purpose of the second edition of this book is to provide a comprehensive conceptual and practical overview of current theories of intelligence and measures of cognitive ability. This text summarizes the latest research in the field of intellectual assessment and includes comprehensive treatment of critical issues that should be considered when the use of intelligence tests is warranted (e.g., nondiscriminatory assessment, utility of subtest profile analysis, use of cross-battery methods, diagnosis of learning disability). The three primary objectives of this book are as follows: (1) to present in-depth descriptions of prominent theories of intelligence, tests of cognitive abilities, and issues related to the use of intelligence tests with special populations (e.g., individuals with disabilities, individuals from culturally and linguistically diverse backgrounds); (2) to provide important information about the validity of contemporary intelligence tests; and (3) to demonstrate the utility of a well-validated theoretical foundation for developing intelligence tests and interpretive approaches, and for guiding research and practice. The ultimate goal of this book is to provide professionals with the knowledge necessary to use the latest intelligence batteries effectively.

ORGANIZATION AND THEME

This book consists of 29 chapters, organized into six parts. Part I, "The Origins of Intellectual Assessment," traces the historical roots of test conceptualization, development, and interpretation up to the present day. Part II, "Contemporary and Emerging Theoretical Perspectives," introduces recently revised and emerging theories of intelligence, with updates of several models presented in the first edition of this text. These theories are described in terms of (1) how they reflect recent advances in psychometrics, neuropsychology, and cognitive psychology; (2) what empirical evidence supports them; and (3) how they have been operationalized. The theories presented in Part II represent a significant departure from traditional views and conceptualizations of the structure of intelligence, and they provide a viable foundation for building more broad-based and culturally sensitive intelligence batteries.

Part III, "Contemporary and Emerging Interpretive Approaches," a section not found in the first edition, includes chapters about the latest research and models for interpretation and use of intelligence test results. Topics include application of a cross-battery approach to interpretation based on the Cattell–Horn–Carroll theory, information-processing approaches, interpretation that promotes nondiscriminatory assessment, and issues related to the common practice of profile analysis. Part III concludes with a chapter of primary importance in the assessment of children: linking intellectual assessment with academic interventions.

Part IV, "New and Revised Intelligence Batteries," includes comprehensive chapters on the latest intelligence batteries and their utility in understanding the cognitive capabilities of individuals from toddlerhood through adulthood. Part V, "Use of Intelligence Tests in Different Populations," is another new section for the second edition. Part V's chapters address a number of the populations with whom individual intelligence tests are typically used, including children with learning disabilities, individuals from diverse backgrounds, and individuals with whom a nonverbal test should be used.

Part VI, "Emerging Issues and New Directions in Intellectual Assessment," focuses mainly on issues related to the validity of intelligence batteries. Part VI also includes an important chapter on the implications of intellectual assessment in a standards-based educational reform environment. Suggestions and recommendations regarding the appropriate use of intelligence tests, as well as future research directions, are provided throughout this section of the book.

Practitioners, university trainers, researchers, undergraduate and graduate students, and other professionals in psychology and education will find this book interesting and useful. It would be appropriate as a primary text in any graduate (or advanced undergraduate) course or seminar on cognitive psychology, clinical or psychoeducational assessment, or measurement and psychometric theory.

ACKNOWLEDGMENTS

We wish to thank the individuals who have contributed to or assisted in the preparation of this book. We are extremely appreciative of the chapter authors' significant contributions. It has been a rewarding experience to work with a dedicated group of people who are nationally recognized authorities in their respective areas. The contributions of Chris Jennison, Chris Coughlin, and the rest of the staff at The Guilford Press are also gratefully acknowledged. Their expertise, and their pleasant and cooperative working style, made this project an enjoyable and productive endeavor.

D. P. F.
P. L. H.

REFERENCE

Wechsler, D. (1958). *The measurement and appraisal of adult intelligence* (4th ed.). Baltimore: Williams & Wilkins.

Contents

VI. Emerging Issues and New Directions in Intellectual Assessment   579

CONTEMPORARY INTELLECTUAL ASSESSMENT

The Origins
of Intellectual Assessment

Part I of this textbook consists of two chapters that describe the historical and theoretical origins of intellectual assessment. In the first chapter, "A History of Intelligence Assessment," John D. Wasserman and David S. Tulsky trace the history of intelligence tests from the latter part of the 19th century to the present day. In particular, they explore the increased interest in intelligence and its measurement in the early 20th century, with special emphasis on the work of Alfred Binet and David Wechsler. In Chapter 2, "A History of Intelligence Test Interpretation," Randy W. Kamphaus, Anne Pierce Winsor, Ellen W. Rowe, and Sangwon Kim provide a historical account of dominant methods of test interpretation designed to quantify a general level of intelligence, clinical and psychometric approaches to interpreting profiles of cognitive performance, and a theory-based approach to test interpretation. The discussion of these approaches provides readers with an understanding of how current practices evolved, as well as a basis for improving contemporary approaches to test interpretation. Overall, the chapters included in Part I trace the historical roots of test conceptualization, development, and interpretation to modern times, providing the necessary foundation from which to understand and elucidate the contemporary and emerging theories, tests, and issues in the field of intellectual assessment that are presented in subsequent sections of this volume.

1

A History of Intelligence Assessment

JOHN D. WASSERMAN
DAVID S. TULSKY

... we borrow from biology the following comparison; the primordial biological element is the cell; in grouping themselves, cells form the tissues; tissues in their turn form the organs. In the same way one might say that the intellectual functions of memory, attention, judgment, etc., correspond to the cells; combining themselves, they form something analogous to a tissue. What corresponds to the organ is our scheme of thought, because, like the organ, this scheme has a function.
—BINET AND SIMON (1909/1916, pp. 152–153)

By the end of his life, Alfred Binet (1857–1911) had arrived at a conceptual model of intelligence that in many ways resembles contemporary models of cognition. Binet's framework is, in many ways, a predecessor to the hierarchically organized contemporary models that have been advanced by John Carroll (1993) Horn and Cattell (1966) Binet termed his model of intelligence a *scheme of thought,* and he alluded to a model with three hierarchical levels of cognition: (1) a superordinate factor of general intelligence (which he called *judgment* or *adaptation* in various writings); (2) 4 lower-order elementary cognitive processes (*comprehension, inventiveness, direction,* and *criticism*); and (3) as many as 10 first-order intellectual faculties (*memory, imagery, imagination, attention, comprehension, suggestibility, aesthetic sentiment, moral sentiment, muscular force and strength of will or persistence,* and *coordination skills and*

quick visual judgments (Binet & Henri, 1895/1973). His work and ideas were truly revolutionary at the time. Factor analysis, which in contemporary practice is commonly used to develop models, did not exist at the time Binet was developing his model. However, Binet provided thorough description of the model's structural features and explicitly described different levels of analysis. Complex functions were placed at higher levels; simpler and narrower functions were placed at lower levels; and both of these were topped by a single, complex unitary function to which all others were subordinated (Binet & Simon, 1909/1916). Despite his best efforts, Binet was never able to design a test that could disentangle individual faculties, and his success with the Binet–Simon intelligence scales was largely due to his abandonment of faculty psychology (a theory positing that the mind consists of separate "faculties" of powers) in favor of a more dynamic psychology, involving tasks requiring the participation of many cognitive functions whose separate roles are not distinguished (e.g., Terman, 1916). The development of a hierarchical cognitive model tapping discrete human abilities would remain for others to develop decades later.

Binet's work is perhaps the most striking example of how the early pioneers of cognitive testing were at the forefront of some of the most important debates about the definition of intelligence and how best to measure it. In fact, the debatable topics continue to be relevant to this day, and the diversity of opinions about the construct of intelligence can be seen in the diversity of topics and ideas expressed throughout this book. Toward the end of the chapter, "contemporary" theories and measurement strategies are presented as recurrent themes in the evolution of cognitive testing.

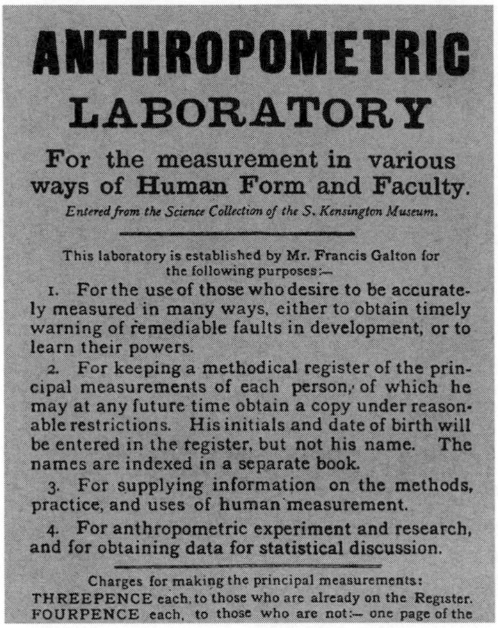

ANTECEDENTS TO CONTEMPORARY INTELLIGENCE TESTING

The use of objective techniques in efforts to measure intelligence began with the efforts of Francis Galton (1822–1911). He first described the concept of intelligence tests in 1865, and his stated objective was to create "a system of competitive examinations" (p. 165) that would be used to identify individuals most likely to produce talented offspring. Galton eventually created a series of tests (many requiring specialized mechanical instruments) that could be taken by the members of the general public for threepence in his Anthopometric Laboratory at the London International Health Exhibition and, after the exhibition closed, at the South Kensington Museum (see Figure 1.1). From 1884 to 1890, a total of 9,337 individuals completed the tests in what could be described as the first large-scale standardized collection of data for psychological tests. Galton's tests changed over time, but it included measures of physical characteristics (e.g., height, weight, head size, and arm span), sensory acuity (vision, audition, olfaction), motor strength, reaction time (to visual and auditory stimuli), and visual judgments (line bisection and estimating an angle) (Galton, 1869, 1883, 1888). Of the

FIGURE 1.1. An advertisement for Francis Galton's Anthropometric Laboratory. From Pearson (1914).

tests and measures utilized by Galton, only one originally created by Jacobs (1887) remains in the psychologist's armamentarium: digit span. (Figure 1.2 provides additional facts about Galton.)

James McKeen Cattell (1860–1944) is generally credited with coining the term *mental tests*. He was strongly influenced by Galton; after completing his doctorate in experimental psychology with Wilhelm Wundt, Cattell arranged for a 2–year research fellowship at Cambridge University, where he worked in Galton's laboratory. In 1890, Cattell published a test battery in his paper "Mental Tests and Measurements," including many of Galton's tests, as well as some adapted from Fechner and Wundt. Cattell's tests were intended for use with college students "to determine the condition and progress of students [and] the relative value of different courses of study" (Cattell, 1893, cited in Sokal, 1987, p. 32); he did not otherwise have specific objectives for the battery, because he expected the value and implications of test results to be self-evident. Galton expressed support for Cattell's testing battery:

- Galton was a cousin of Charles Darwin and sought to apply to humans the same principles described in *On the Origin of Species* (Darwin, 1859).
- This work eventually gave birth to a misguided but influential movement known as *eugenics.*
- Galton is best remembered for his efforts to demonstrate that *eminence*, which he equated with intelligence, runs in families.
- Galton never offered a formal definition of *intelligence* and incorrectly believed that variation in intelligence could be reflected by measuring sensory acuity: "The only information that reaches us concerning outward events appears to pass through the avenue of our senses; and the more perceptible our senses are of difference, the larger the field upon which our judgment and intellect can act" (1883, p. 19).

FIGURE 1.2. Additional facts about Francis Galton.

It is to obtain a general knowledge of the capacities of a man by sinking shafts, as it were, at a few critical points. In order to ascertain the best points for the purpose, the sets of measures should be compared with an independent estimate of the man's powers. We thus may learn which of the measures are the most instructive. (Quoted in Cattell, 1890, p. 380)

Like Galton, Cattell and Farrand (1896) designed these tests to focus more on "measurement of the body and of the senses" than on "the higher mental processes" (pp. 622–623). The Cattell battery consisted of 10 basic tests:

- *Dynamometer pressure*: An index of strength, measured by the maximum pressure for each hand.
- *Rate of hand movement*: An index of motor speed, measuring the quickest possible movement of the right hand and arm from rest through 50 centimeters.
- *Two-point sensation thresholds*: A measure of fine sensory discrimination, involving the minimum discriminable separation distance of two points on the skin.
- *Pressure causing pain*: A sensory test, measuring the minimal degree of pressure applied from a hard rubber instrument before pain is reported.
- *Least noticeable difference in weight*: A perceptual judgment task, measuring the lowest difference threshold at which the weights of two wooden boxes can be discriminated.
- *Reaction time for sound*: A reaction time task, measuring the time elapsed between an auditory stimulus and a voluntary motor response.
- *Time for naming colors*: A speed task, measuring the time required to name 10 colors.
- *Bisection of a line*: A perceptual judgment task, determining the accuracy with which the midpoint of a 50-centimeter rule may be identified.
- *Judgment of 10 seconds of time*: A perceptual judgment task, measuring the accuracy with which an interval of 10 seconds can be estimated.
- *Number of letters repeated on one hearing*: An immediate memory span task, measuring the maximum number of letters that can be repeated immediately after auditory presentation.

These were supplemented by a more comprehensive series of 50 tests—33 of which measured different forms of sensory acuity and discrimination (sight, hearing, taste and smell, touch and temperature); 7 of which measured reaction time for simple and complex decisions; 7 of which measured mental intensity and extensity; and 3 of which measured motor abilities.

Upon his return to the United States, Cattell became a professor of psychology at the University of Pennsylvania, moving shortly thereafter to Columbia University. As part of accepting the faculty position at Columbia, Cattell arranged for the examination of every incoming student at Columbia College's School of Arts and School of Mines, and he aggressively promoted the potential value of his testing program, even though the effectiveness of the program had not been demonstrated. This testing program came to an end, however, when one of Cattell's graduate students, Clark Wissler, used the then-new statistic of correlation coefficients to examine the correlations between Cattell's tests and student grades for over 300 undergraduates (Wissler, 1901). The results showed negligible correlations between Cattell's laboratory tests and overall academic performance,

as well as negligible intercorrelations between the laboratory tests, indicating that
the tests had little relationship to each other
or to academic achievement. At the same
time, the correlations between assigned grades
in various college classes, however, were substantially higher than any correlations of the
tests with grades.

Thus Cattell's ambitious testing program,
combined with Wissler's psychometric evaluation, served to change the face of psychology and IQ testing. (Figure 1.3 provides
some facts about Cattell's subsequent career.) Sokal (1987) wrote: "Wissler's analysis
struck most psychologists as definitive, and
with it [Wissler's publication of his disserta-
tion], anthropometric mental testing, as a
movement, died" (p. 38). With the end of the
era of so-called "brass psychology" and
"anthropometric testing," alternative methods for evaluating intelligence were needed.
Such an alternative had been gaining momentum in France in the early 1900s.

- Cattell would continue to own and edit some
  leading scientific journals.
- Cattell continued to build Columbia University's
  department of psychology until he was
  ignominiously dismissed from Columbia in 1917
  for public opposition to the draft, as well as
  long-standing conflicts with the university
  administration.
- By all accounts, the years immediately
  following the dismissal from Columbia were
  difficult for Cattell, and he withdrew to his home
  for some 2 years.
- Cattell bounded back in 1921, founding The
  Psychological Corporation in New York with his
  former colleagues at Columbia, Edward L.
  Thorndike and Robert S. Woodworth.
  - The offices were held by leading
    psychologists of the day (Thorndike was
    voted chairman of the board, and vice-
    presidents were Walter Dill Scott and Lewis
    Terman).
  - The mission of The Psychological
    Corporation was to provide applied
    psychological services.
  - Cattell had difficulty identifying revenue
    streams for the fledgling company, and soon
    after its inception, it was struggling financially.
    As a result, Cattell resigned in 1926 (to be
    succeeded by Walter Van Dyke Bingham).

FIGURE 1.3. Additional facts about James
McKeen Cattell.

BINET AND THE FIRST MODERN INTELLIGENCE TESTS

Modern intelligence testing can be most
properly considered to begin with the work
of Alfred Binet, who may justifiably be
called the father of cognitive and intellectual assessment. A brilliant, versatile, and
imaginative talent, he authored nearly 300
articles, books, plays, and tests during his
career. Yet the experiences that drove him
were his failures—including withdrawal
from medical school after an emotional
breakdown, and a humiliating recantation
of published research on hypnosis that was
compromised by demand effects. Binet was
self-taught in psychology and had few students and no academic affiliations, failing
to obtain any of the three French profes-
sorships for which he applied. Binet did
not attend professional conferences, leaving
the first intelligence scale to be presented
by Théodore Simon alone at the 1905 International Congress of Psychology in
Rome. In a 1901 letter, he wrote to a
friend: "I educated myself all alone, without any teachers; I have arrived at my present scientific situation by the sole force of
my fists; *no one*, you understand, no one,
has ever helped me" (cited in Wolf, 1973,
p. 23; emphasis in original).

It may be argued that his institutional independence enabled him to challenge many
of the conventions of the day. Binet was a remarkably innovative thinker and came up
with several novel ideas. He anticipated developments in psychology, and several of his
ideas are as important today as when he first
wrote about them. Though he didn't have
the prestige of a university professorship and
tended to be a loner, not attending conferences where he could share his ideas with his
colleagues, he found a very effective means
of professional dissemination. In 1895, Binet
founded the first French journal of psychology, *L'Année Psychologique*, and many of
his milestone writings were first published in
this journal.

Binet had keen observational skills and developed many of his ideas after studying the
behavior and problem-solving methods of
his daughters, Alice and Madeleine, and
their friends. In 1890, he published his first
three articles on the study of individual differences; in these papers, his observations of

his daughters were both insightful and detailed. The beginnings of his greatest contribution, however, came in the second volume of *L'Année Psychologique* in 1895, when he collaborated with Victor Henri (1872–1940) to outline a project for developing a test of intelligence that would differentiate a number of independent higher-order mental faculties. Binet and Henri recognized the limitations of the sensory and motor assessment procedures of Galton and Cattell:

> If one looks at the series of experiments that have been made—the *mental tests*, as the English say—one is astonished by the considerable place reserved to the sensations and simple processes, and by the little attention lent to superior processes, which some [experimenters] neglect completely ... (Binet & Henri, 1895/1973, p. 426)

After several years of research, Binet concluded that several critical faculties could not be purely, separately, and efficiently measured (Binet & Simon, 1905a/1916, 1905b/1916). Investigations in the United States (e.g., Sharp, 1899) also challenged support for the differentiation of mental faculties. Eventually Binet abandoned the effort to measure each faculty separately and purely, and decided to use complex tasks that might be influenced by+ several mental faculties at once. In his book *L'Étude Expérimentale de l'Intelligence,* Binet (1903) used the term *intelligence* to refer to the sum total of the higher mental processes, although he sought measures to differentiate cognitive faculties until the end of his life.

In the fall of 1904, the French Minister of Public Instruction responded to the inability of children with mental retardation to benefit from France's universal education laws. The minister appointed a commission to study problems with the education of such children in Paris, and Binet, who was an educational activist and leader of the La Société Libre pour l'Étude Psychologique de l'Enfant (Free Society for the Psychological Study of the Child), was appointed to the commission. La Société had originally been founded to give teachers and school administrators an opportunity to discuss problems of education and to be active in collaborative research. Binet's appointment to the commission was hardly an accident, since members

of La Société had been principal advocates with the ministry on behalf of school children. Eventually the commission, which had grown to 16 members, recommended that children who did not benefit from education, teaching, or discipline should receive a "medico-pedagogical examination" before being removed from primary schools, and that such children, if educable, should be placed in special classes. However, the commission did not offer any substance for the examination. Binet, having thought about intelligence for nearly a decade, saw the need; together with a new collaborator, Théodore Simon, he undertook the task of developing a reliable diagnostic system to identify children with mental retardation.

The first Binet–Simon Scale was completed in 1905 and was intended to be efficient and practical: "We have aimed to make all our tests simple, rapid, convenient, precise, heterogeneous, holding the subject in continued contact with the experimenter, and bearing principally upon the faculty of judgment" (Binet & Simon, 1905a/1916). The scale consisted of 30 items, which were scored on a pass–fail basis. The scale included several important innovations that would be followed by subsequent measurers of intelligence. Items were ranked in order of difficulty and accompanied by careful instructions for administration. Binet and Simon also utilized the concept of age-graded norms pioneered by Damaye (1903, as cited in Wolf, 1973). The use of developmental age scales permits an individual's *mental age* to be defined by reference to the age level of the individual tasks that an individual can complete.

The 1905 scale was revised in 1908 (Binet & Simon, 1908/1916) and again in 1911 (Binet & Simon, 1911/1916). By the completion of the 1911 edition, Binet's scales were extended through adulthood and were balanced with five items at each age level. The scales included procedures assessing language (e.g., receptive naming and expressive naming to visual confrontation, sentence repetition, and definitions of familiar objects), auditory processing (e.g., word rhyming), visual processing (e.g., rapid discrimination of lines, drawing what a folded paper with a piece cut out would look like if unfolded), learning and memory (e.g., repeating prose passages, repeating phrases and sentences of increasing length, drawing two designs from memory, recalling the names of pictured objects, and repeating numbers), and judgment and problem solving (e.g., answering problems of social and practical comprehension, giving distinctions between abstract terms).

Although many scholars in the United States were introduced to the Binet–Simon Scales through *L'Année Psychologique*, they became widely known after Henry H. Goddard, director of research at the Training School for the Retarded in Vineland, New Jersey, arranged for his assistant Elizabeth Kite to translate the 1908 scale. Impressed by its effectiveness in yielding scores in accord with experienced clinicians, Goddard distributed 22,000 copies and 88,000 answer blanks of the translated test by 1915. Within a few years, the tests had changed the landscape for mental testing throughout the world. By 1939 (which was the year the Wechsler–Bellevue Scale was published), there were some 77 available adaptations and translations of the Binet–Simon Scales (Hildreth, 1939). The top-ranked instrument among psychologists was the Stanford–Binet, which was adapted and developed by Lewis Terman at Stanford University. Interestingly enough, Théodore Simon claimed that Binet gave Terman the rights to publish an American revision of the Binet–Simon scale "for a token of one dollar" (quoted in Wolf, 1973, p. 35).

ARMY MENTAL TESTING DURING WORLD WAR I

Psychological testing was experiencing considerable growth in the years immediately prior to World War I, due to the dissemination of Binet's work (Binet & Simon, 1905a/1916, 1908/1916, 1911/1916) and American adaptations by Robert M. Yerkes (Yerkes, Bridges, & Hardwick, 1915) and Lewis M. Terman (1916), among others. However, historians have suggested that the contribution of the war to the growth of psychological testing may have been greater than psychology's contribution to military decision making (e.g., Reed, 1987). The origins of the Army mental tests lay in the ambitious initiatives of Robert M. Yerkes, then president of the American Psychological As-

sociation (APA). Von Mayrhauser (1987) notes that Yerkes used the wartime circumstances to assert "near-dictatorial power within the profession" (p. 135). On April 6, 1917, the day of the U.S. declaration of war, Yerkes initiated a special APA session to discuss the contributions that psychology could make to the war effort. Just 15 days later, a special meeting of the APA council (Yerkes, Walter Dill Scott, Walter V. Bingham, Knight Dunlap, Roswell Angier, APA secretary Herbert Langfeld, and former APA president Raymond Dodge) was convened in Philadelphia, Pennsylvania. This meeting was characterized by some discord (Scott and Bingham walked out before its end), but resulted in the appointment of 12 APA committees, with Yerkes naming himself as chairman of the committee charged with developing proposals for the psychological testing of army recruits. A group of leading American psychologists appointed by Yerkes (Bingham, H. H. Goddard, Thomas M. Haines, Lewis M. Terman, F. L. Wells, and Guy M. Whipple) planned the tests in Vineland, New Jersey over the span of several weeks from May to June; based upon their recommendations, Yerkes assembled a staff of 40 psychologists who created the Army Alpha and Army Beta tests. Nearly half of the Army tests came from the work of Arthur S. Otis. As a graduate student under the direction of Lewis Terman, Otis had adapted the Stanford–Binet tests for group administration, and Terman readily shared this new methodology with the psychologists on the committee (Yerkes, 1921). Several pilot studies were conducted over the next months, and the committee was expanded to include many leaders in psychology (e.g., Otis, Robert S. Woodworth, E. K. Strong, L. L. Thurstone, and E. L. Thorndike, who became chief statistician). After an official testing trial was conducted with some 85,000 men, official permission was granted in January 1918 for all Army recruits to be tested. A total of 350 enlisted men were trained as psychological examiners in the School for Military Psychology at Camp Greenleaf, Georgia, and approximately 1.7 million men had been tested with the Army mental tests by the time the armistice was signed in November 1918 (Yoakum & Yerkes, 1920, p. 12).

E. G. Boring, who reported to Camp

Greenleaf as a captain in February 1918, described the experience as formative:

> We lived in barracks, piled out for reveillé, stood inspection, drilled and were drilled, studied testing procedures, and were ordered to many irrelevant lectures. As soon as I discovered that everyone else resembled me in never accomplishing the impossible, my neuroses left me, and I had a grand time, with new health created by new exercise and many good friendships formed with colleagues under these intimate conditions of living. (1961, p. 30)

Somewhat more cynically, Arthur Otis recalled that at Camp Greenleaf "we had to learn how to salute and make beds and how to pick up cigarette butts" (see Lennon, 1985).

The Army mental tests consisted of two separate tests, both group-administered. The Army Alpha was intended for examinees who were fluent in English and able to read and write, whereas the Army Beta was a performance scale intended for examinees who had inadequate mastery of English and who were illiterate. According to Yoakum and Yerkes (1920), "Examinations Alpha and Beta are so constructed and administered as to minimize the handicap of men who because of foreign birth or lack or education are little skilled in the use of English" (p. 17). Examination Alpha consisted of eight subtests, and examination Beta consisted of seven subtests (see Table 1.1). Alpha was typically administered to men who could read newspapers and write letters home in

English, with at least a fourth-grade education and 5 years of residency in the United States (Yerkes, 1921, p. 76). Beta was typically administered with pantomimed directions to groups as large as 60. Reports of intelligence ratings were made within 24 hours and entered on service records and qualification cards. Boring (1961) described the process: "You went down the line saying 'You read American newspaper? No read American newspaper?'—separating them in that crude manner into those who could read English and take the Alpha examination and those who must rely for instructions on the pantomime of the Beta examination" (p. 30).

The success of the Army mental tests launched the advent of widespread testing in schools, colleges, industry, and the military, which advanced the field of psychology. It was a public relations triumph, although its actual contribution to recruit selection was modest (Boring, 1957; Camfield, 1970; Kevles, 1968). Moreover, it generated a large database that formed the basis of numerous studies and books over the next decade. Finally, the concentrated testing effort brought together psychologists from all over the United States. Terman (1932/1961) expressed appreciation for "the opportunity they [the Army] gave me to become acquainted with nearly all of the leading psychologists of America" (p. 325). In the words of Kevles, "the wide use of the examinations during the war had dramatized intelligence testing and made the practice respectable. Gone were the public's prewar wariness and ignorance of measuring intelligence" (1968, p. 581).

TABLE 1.1. Subtests in the Army Alpha and Beta Tests

Army Alpha	Army Beta
Oral Directions	Mazes[b]
Memory for Digits[a]	Cube Analysis
Disarranged Sentences	X-O Series
Arithmetical Problems[a]	Digit–Symbol[a]
Information[a]	Number Checking
Synonym–Antonym	Picture Completion[a]
Practical Judgment[a]	Geometric Construction
Number Series Completion	
Analogies	
Number Comparison	

Note. [a]Subtests that would be adapted by Wechsler for the Wechsler–Bellevue.
[b]Subtests that would be adapted by Wechsler for the Children's Version.

Terman, Wechsler, and 20th-Century Intelligence Testing

When World War I ended, the members of the committee that developed the Army mental tests, as well as some prominent examiners in the war, sought civilian applications of the tests and the testing program. Their work following the war would have a profound impact upon clinical and psychoeducational testing for years to come. The tests were declassified, and many of the Army psychologists quickly adapted the tests or simply "repackaged" the test items as commercial products (see Table 1.2), which were immediately successful.

TABLE 1.2. Published Tests in the 1920s and 1930s Modeled after the Army Alpha Test

Test title	Date	Author(s)	Comments and reference(s)
Group Intelligence Scale	1918	Arthur S. Otis	Otis's method for group administration of the Binet–Simon tests of intelligence was adopted by the World War I APA committee and influenced the Army Alpha and Beta. Published by World Book Company and sold over a half million copies in its first 6 months. Survived in various forms to the present day. References: Otis (1918a, 1918b, 1918c).
Terman Group Test of Mental Ability	1919	Lewis Terman	Sold over 500,000 copies per year through the 1920s. Reference: Terman (1920)
National Intelligence Tests	1920	M. E. Haggerty, L. M. Terman, E. L. Thorndike, G. M. Whipple, and R. M. Yerkes	Published by World Book Company and sold 200,000 copies in the first 6 months. References: Haggerty et al. (1920), Whipple (1921), and Terman and Whitmire (1921).
Revision of the Army Alpha Examination, Form A, Form B	1925, 1935	Else O. Bregman	References: Bregman (1925, 1935).
Scholastic Aptitude Tests (SAT) of the College Entrance Examination Board	1926	C. C. Brigham	The SAT have survived to this day (though the current tests have evolved considerably from the original Army Alpha based exam). References: Brigham (1935), Lemann (1995).
Michigan Modification of the Army Alpha Test	1928	H. F. Adams et al.	Personality test based upon the army tests. Reference: Adams et al. (1928).
Abbreviated Army Alpha Test	1931	G. Hendrickson	Reference: Hendrickson (1931).
"Scrambled" or modified Carnegie adaption of the Army Alpha Examination	1931	Bureau of Personnel Research, Carnegie Institute of Technology, Pittsburgh, PA	Reference: Ford (1931).
Revised Alpha Examination, Form 5, Form 7	1932	Fred L. Wells	Published by The Psychological Corporation, 1932–1933. Reference: Wells (1932).
Revised Alpha Examination, Form 6, Short Form	1933	C. R. Atwell and Fred L. Wells	Short form of the Alpha test for high school, college, and adults. Published by The Psychological Corporation. Reference: Atwell and Wells (1933).
Revised Beta Examination	1934	C. E. Kellogg and N. W. Morton	Published by The Psychological Corporation. The Beta has survived to this day. Most recently revised in 1999 as the "Beta-III." Reference: Kellogg and Merton (1934).
Revision of the Army Alpha Examination	1938	J. P. Guilford	Revision of the Army Alpha just prior to World War II. Yields three primary factors. Reference: Guilford (1938).
Revision of the American Army Alpha Test	1932	N. M. Hales	Australian adaptation of the Army Alpha. Reference: Hales (1932).

With these publications, the developers of the Army Alpha and Beta tests soon became commercial test "authors"—in other words, the first generation of testing scholar-entrepreneurs. More importantly, these publications enabled the Army test battery (e.g., Alpha, Beta, and Individualized tests) to quickly dominate psychological and psycho-educational assessment fields, and ultimately became the basis of modern-day test batteries.

Terman, the Stanford–Binet, and the Birth of the Testing Industry

No single American was more important in the birth of the intelligence testing industry than Lewis M. Terman. Terman developed the most successful American version of the Binet–Simon Scales, but he was also responsible for training Arthur Otis and bringing Otis's group intelligence methodology to the committee responsible for developing the Army mental tests. In addition to Arthur Otis, Terman was responsible for training numerous individuals who helped lead the testing field (e.g., Samuel Kohs, who collected the first normative sample on the color cube Design Block test, and Florence Goodenough, author of the Draw-a-Person Test).

Having authored the Stanford Revision of the Binet–Simon tests, Terman was well versed in test publishing; following the war, he published the Stanford Achievement Test (Terman, 1923) and the Metropolitan Achievement Test (Terman, 1933). Moreover, Terman helped Otis publish the Group Intelligence Scale that Otis (1918a, 1918b, 1918c) had developed as his dissertation project. Otis also published the Otis Mental Ability Test (Otis, 1936) and eventually became the World Book Company's editor of psychological and educational tests. The World Book Company merged with Harcourt, Brace in 1960 and was combined with The Psychological Corporation in 1976.

Having followed Binet's work since 1901 and 1902 (Fancher, 1985), Terman saw ways to improve upon this work. Terman had been a high school teacher and principal who obtained his PhD in psychology at Clark University under G. Stanley Hall. His 1906 dissertation, *Genius and Stupidity: A Study of the Intellectual Processes of Seven*

"Bright" and Seven "Stupid" Boys, was based upon testing procedures that independently resembled those developed by Binet and Simon. The dissertation included eight categorical domains of testing procedures: *invention and creative imagination, logical processes, mathematical ability, language mastery, interpretation of fables, game-playing (chess) rules and strategies, memory,* and *motor skill.* Terman's dissertation proved essential to his later work.

Terman noted some limitations of Binet's work, including the tendency of some items to overestimate mental age for young children and to underestimate mental age for older children. By 1912, he had eliminated some items and added others while testing several hundred children to improve the Binet–Simon procedures. By 1916, he had made more improvements and tested more than 2,300 individuals from early childhood through midadolescence. These improvements were published as the Stanford Revision and Extension of the Binet–Simon Scale by the Houghton Mifflin Company. Terman was not the only author of a U.S. translation or adaptation of the Binet–Simon Scales (see editions by Drummond, 1914; Herring, 1922; Kuhlmann, 1922; Melville, 1917; Town, 1915), but his version is the only one to survive to the present time—a tribute to his scientific approach, methodological rigor, and collection of the leading normative sample (for its period). Upon its publication, the Stanford–Binet rapidly became the leading measure in the field and the standard against which other intelligence tests were measured (Fancher, 1985).

As Minton (1988) has reported, the Stanford–Binet offered several advantages over other intelligence tests: (1) It was the most thorough and extensive revision of the Binet–Simon Scales; (2) the standardization procedure was the most ambitious and rigorous of its time; (3) its comprehensive examiner's guide made it easy to teach and learn; and (4) its use of the *intelligence quotient* (IQ) became the new standard for intelligence tests. Terman had adapted Stern's (1912/1914) concept to yield an IQ, which was computed by dividing mental age by chronological age.

Within two decades of its publication, the Stanford–Binet was the leading instrument for intellectual assessment. It had been translated into several languages and was available internationally. Terman recognized, however, that there were problems with the 1916 scale; he felt that the scale had been inadequately standardized, had insufficient floor and ceiling, spanned too narrow an age range, and contained some individual test items that lacked validity (see Minton, 1988). He also considered the absence of an alternate form to be a severe limitation, making the test susceptible to the effects of coaching. Using grants from Stanford University and assisted by Maud Merrill as codirector of the project, he worked for 7 years to create a revision, which was entitled the New Revised Stanford–Binet Tests of Intelligence (Terman & Merrill, 1937) and published by the Houghton Mifflin Company. The 1937 revision created two alternate forms (Form L for Lewis, and Form M for Maud), each with 129 items. Form L bore the stronger resemblance to the original Stanford–Binet. The estimation of abilities for adults and preschoolers was improved, with greater weighting of nonverbal tasks for young children and diminished emphasis on rote memory for the higher ages. Scoring was objectified, and directions for administration were clarified. High reliability coefficients were reported. A new standardization sample of 3,200 native-born white participants between the ages of 1½ and 18 were included, with efforts to improve the geographical and socioeconomic distribution.

The 1937 edition was well received and continued to be the standard for intellectual assessment. Some problems remained, including its failure to assess separate abilities, its unsuitability for gifted adults (due to a low ceiling for adults), and the inefficiency of the all-or-none scoring system. The presence of German-made toys as manipulatives became controversial in the years leading up to World War II, and eventually the relevant test items had to be deleted because replacement toys could not be located.

Since Terman's death in 1956, the test has been revised four additional times. Maud Merrill assumed most responsibility for the third revision, creating the Stanford–Binet Intelligence Scale, Form L-M (Terman & Merrill, 1960), in which she merged the two alternate forms by selecting the most discriminating items from the 1937 versions. With Maud Merrill's retirement, Robert L.

Thorndike was selected to head up a renorming study of the Stanford–Binet Form L-M in 1972. A fourth edition was later published (Thorndike, Hagen, & Sattler, 1986), and, very recently, a fifth edition has appeared (Roid, 2003; see Roid & Pomplun, Chapter 15, this volume).

Wechsler's Clinical and Practical Perspectives

Beginning in the 1950s and 1960s, the Stanford–Binet was supplanted as the most widely used intelligence test by the Wechsler intelligence scales (Lubin, Wallis, & Paine, 1971), and the practice of intellectual assessment in the second half of the 20th century may arguably have been most strongly influenced by the work of David Wechsler (1896–1981). Surveys of psychological test usage in the decades after his death show that Wechsler's intelligence tests continue to dominate intellectual assessment among school psychologists, clinical psychologists, and neuropsychologists (Archer, Maruish, Imhof, & Piotrowski, 1991; Butler, Retzlaff, & Vanderploeg, 1991; Camara, Nathan, & Puente, 2000; Harrison, Kaufman, Hickman, & Kaufman, 1988; Lees-Haley, Smith, Williams, & Dunn, 1996; Piotrowski & Keller, 1989; Watkins, Campbell, & McGregor, 1988; Wilson & Reschly, 1996).

The origins of Wechsler's subtests and items can be found in the Army test battery and other tests that were developed in the early 1900s. Surprisingly few of the items or tasks were novel or original (see Boake, 2002; Frank, 1983; Tulsky, Chiaravalloti, Palmer, & Chelune, 2003; Tulsky, Saklofske, & Zhu, 2003), and it appears that Wechsler's strength was not in writing and developing items. Instead, Wechsler was a master at synthesizing tests and materials that were already in existence. He created the Wechsler–Bellevue Scale in 1939 by borrowing from existing material (Wechsler, 1939b). The Wechsler–Bellevue would soon become the most widely used test of intelligence, surpassing the Stanford–Binet. The test was almost instantly popular (as documented by the positive reviews published at the time of its release–see Boake, 2002; Buros, 1941, 1949; Tulsky, 2003). Its popularity was based upon (1) the dearth of tests available for adults; (2) the integration of Verbal and Performance tests into a single battery; (3) the "conorming" of tests that were commonly used in practice; (4) a "state-of-the-art" normative sample (for the time); and (5) an emphasis on psychometric rigor, which included the introduction of a superior type of composite score (the deviation IQ, which quickly became the standard in the field).

Wechsler was well positioned to make this contribution to the field, and the Wechsler scales can easily be traced to his early educational and professional experiences. Wechsler was introduced to most of the procedures that would eventually find a home in his intelligence and memory scales as a graduate student at Columbia University (with faculty members including James McKeen Cattell, Edward L. Thorndike, and Robert S. Woodworth) and as an Army psychological examiner in World War I. As part of a student detachment from the military, Wechsler attended the University of London in 1919, where he spent some 3 months working with Charles E. Spearman. From 1925 to 1927, he would work for The Psychological Corporation in New York, conducting research and developing tests (e.g., his tests for taxicab drivers; Wechsler, 1926). Finally, Wechsler sought training from several of the leading clinicians of his day, including Augusta F. Bronner and William Healy at the Judge Baker Foundation in Boston and Anna Freud at the Vienna Psychoanalytic Institute (for 3 months in 1932). By virtue of his education and training, Wechsler should properly be remembered as one of the first scientist-clinicians in psychology.

Wechsler's introduction of the Wechsler–Bellevue Intelligence Scale (Wechsler, 1939a, 1939b) was followed by the Wechsler Intelligence Scale for Children (WISC; Wechsler, 1949), the Wechsler Adult Intelligence Scale (WAIS; Wechsler, 1955), and the Wechsler Preschool and Primary Scale of Intelligence (WPPSI; Wechsler, 1967). His innovations in psychological assessment were to make assessment practical and to align clinical practice with psychometrically rigorous test development. He observed the preferences of practitioners to administer separate Verbal and Performance scales, and responded by packaging both types in a single, practical, and conormed battery of tests. Wechsler did not believe that the division of his intelligence scales into Verbal and Performance

subtests tapped separate dimensions of intelligence; rather, he felt that this dichotomy was diagnostically useful (e.g., Wechsler, 1967). In essence, the Verbal and Performance scales constituted different ways to assess *g*. Late in his life, Wechsler described the Verbal and Performance scales (as well as the various subtests) as "different 'languages' . . . which may be easier or harder for different subjects" and represent ways to communicate with a person (Wechsler, 1974, p. 5). Wechsler is also cocredited (with Arthur Otis) for the development and implementation of the deviation IQ, which permitted rankings of performance relative to individuals of the same age group and which solved the limitations of Stern's IQ (100 times mental age in months divided by chronological age). For detailed discussion of the current versions of the Wechsler scales, see Tulsky, Saklofske, and Zhu (2003) and Zhu and Weiss (Chapter 14, this volume).

Wechsler directly or indirected influenced most contemporary intelligence test authors. For example, Richard W. Woodcock left jobs in a sawmill and butcher shop for a position at the Veterans' Testing Bureau after becoming inspired to study psychology by reading Wechsler's (1939a) *The Measurement of Adult Intelligence*. Alan S. Kaufman worked directly with Wechsler on the WISC-R during his employment at The Psychological Corporation from 1968 to 1974. Later at the University of Georgia, Kaufman extended Wechsler's influence to a group of his own graduate students, including Bruce Bracken, Jack Cummings, Patti Harrison, Randy Kamphaus, Jack Naglieri, Cecil Reynolds, and R. Steve McCallum, all of whom would become leading contemporary test authors.

RECURRENT THEMES IN THE HISTORY OF INTELLIGENCE ASSESSMENT

Issues of Definition

During a videotaped interview (Wechsler, 1975), David Wechsler recalled one of the first major efforts to reach a concensus on the definition and conceptualization of intelligence (Henmon et al., 1921; Thorndike et al., 1921). Wechsler commented that right from the start, it was difficult for the leaders in the field to come up with an acceptable definition of the term *intelligence*. He said:

> The definition of intelligence goes way back . . . to . . . the famous conference or symposium from 1921 by the then leading members of the profession (Thorndike, Thurstone, Terman . . . there were about 14). The interesting thing was that there were 14 different definitions . . . so people got scared off (from studying intelligence). Well, I wasn't scared. It just proved to me that intelligence was a multisomething [rather than being] one thing. Depending upon your area of interest or specialization you favored one or another definitions. The anthropologist favored . . . the concept "to adapt" and one of the earliest definitions was "a person's capacity to adapt to the environment." Well that is one aspect . . . but adaptation was an overappreciated area . . . there are a great many other ways [in which intelligence manifests itself]. . . . If you were an educator . . . children who have good intelligence will learn faster . . . so that to an educator . . . learning is important. . . . I say to you that they are all right but not a single one of them suffices. In presenting a definition . . . it has to be accepted by your peers. (Wechsler, 1975)

Wechsler's comments are as lively today as they were when he gave the interview or as they were when the 1921 symposium papers were published. Over 100 years of debate have failed to lead to a consensus definition of this core psychological construct.

The term *intelligence* comes from the Latin *intelligere*, meaning *to understand*. The first psychology text known to use the term *intelligence* was Herbert Spencer's (1855/1885) *The Principles of Psychology*, which treated intelligence as a biological characteristic that evolved through adaptation of organisms to their environments ("the adjustment of internal to external relations"). Several of the early pioneers in intelligence followed this emphasis on adaptation. Binet wrote on intelligence and adaptation from several perspectives in his career, concluding that "intelligence serves in the discovery of truth. But the conception is still too narrow; and we return to our favorite theory; the intelligence marks itself by the best possible adaptation of the individual to his environment" (Binet & Simon, 1911/1916, pp. 300–301). In 1912, William Stern, who proposed the use of IQ (a ratio of mental age to chronological age) to facilitate comparison between children, defined intelligence as "a general capacity of an individual consciously to adjust his thinking to new requirements . . . a general mental adaptability to new problems and conditions of life" (Stern, 1912/1914, p. 21). As we will see, David Wechsler retained the element of adaptation in his earliest definition. Robert J. Sternberg, perhaps the most prolific of contemporary intelligence theorists, defines intelligence in everyday life as "the purposive adaptation to, selection of, and shaping of real-world environments relevant to one's life and abilities" (Sternberg, 1988, p. 65).

At the same time, scholars have disagreed on many aspects of the construct of *intelligence*. Binet, who never produced a formal definition of the term, wrote about the central and superordinate role of *judgment* at the end of his career:

> In intelligence there is a fundamental faculty, the alteration or the lack of which is of the utmost importance for practical life. This faculty is judgment, otherwise called good sense, practical sense, initiative, the faculty of adapting one's self to circumstances. To judge well, to comprehend well, to reason well, these are the essential activities of intelligence. A person may be a moron or an imbecile if he is lacking in judgment; but with good judgment he can never be either. (Binet & Simon, 1905a/1916, pp. 42–43)

There was little unity regarding the nature or construct of intelligence throughout most of these early years, and this lack of unity was highlighted in the symposium described by Wechsler (1975) and published in the *Journal of Educational Psychology* in 1921. A list of the various definitions offered in those papers (Henmon et al., 1921; Thorndike et al., 1921) is presented in Table 1.3. Wechsler was not the only one to comment about the variety of definitions that emerged from the symposium. Charles E. Spearman (1927) exclaimed:

> Chaos itself can go no further! The disagreement between different testers—indeed, even the doctrine and the practice of the selfsame tester—has reached its apogee. If they still tolerate each other's proceedings, this is only rendered possible by the ostrich-like policy of not looking facts in the face. In truth, "intelligence" has become a mere vocal sound, a word with so many meanings that it finally has none. (p. 14)

TABLE 1.3. Definitions of Intelligence

Author	Definition
Colvin	Ability to learn or having learned to adjust oneself to the environment.
Dearborn	The capacity to learn or profit by experience.
Freeman	Sensory capacity, capacity for perceptual recognition, quickness, range or flexibility of association, facility and imagination, span of attention, quickness or alertness in response.
Haggerty	Sensation, perception, association, memory, imagination, discrimination, judgment, and reasoning.
Henmon	" . . . the capacity for knowledge and the knowledge possessed" (Henmon et al., 1921, p. 195).
Peterson	A biological mechanism by which the effects of a complexity of stimuli are brought together and given a somewhat unified effect in behavior.
Pintner	" . . . the ability of the individual to adapt himself adequately to relatively new situations in life. It seems to include the capacity for getting along well in all sorts of situations" (Thorndike et al., 1921, p. 139).
Terman	" . . . the capacity to form concepts to relate in diverse ways, and to grasp their significance. An individual is intelligent in proportion as he is able to carry on abstract thinking" (Thorndike et al., 1921, p. 128).
Thorndike	" . . . the power of good responses from the point of view of truth or fact . . . " (Thorndike et al., 1921, p. 124).
Thurstone	"(a) the capacity to inhibit an instinctive adjustment, (b) the capacity to redefine the inhibited instantive adjustment in light of imaginally experienced trial and error, (c) the volitional capacity to realize the modified instinctive adjustment into overt behavior to the advantage of the individual as social animal" (Henmon et al., 1921, pp. 201–202).
Woodrow	" . . . the capacity to acquire capacity" (Henmon et al., 1921, p. 207).

Note. In 1921, the editors of the *Journal of Educational Psychology* asked 17 leading investigators to define intelligence. Although their views were highly divergent, there was a frequent emphasis on adaptation to new situations.

Perhaps the most widely referenced and enduring definition of intelligence comes from David Wechsler (1939a):

> Intelligence is the aggregate or global capacity of the individual to act purposefully, to think rationally and to deal effectively with his environment. It is global because it characterizes the individual's behavior as a whole; it is an aggregate because it is composed of elements or abilities which, though not entirely independent, are qualitatively differentiable. (p. 3)

It is unclear why this definition became so widely known. It may have become so popular because it was associated with the Wechsler intelligence scales, because it may have been one of the better syntheses of work by leading scholars of the era, or because it was the definition advanced in *The Measurement of Adult Intelligence* (which was a leading textbook for almost 40 years). Despite their familiarity with this definition, psychologists today are no closer to reaching a consensus over the definition of the construct. A follow-up to the 1921 symposium was published by Sternberg and Detterman (1986) with 25 "contemporary" contributors, and again there was a failure to reach a consensus on the topic. Jensen (1998) recommended that psychologists "drop the ill-fated word from our scientific vocabulary, or use it only in quotes, to remind ourselves that it is not only scientifically unsatisfactory but wholly unnecessary" (p. 49). The reader can simply review all of the definitions published in this current book to see how little agreement there is about the nature of the construct of intelligence.

The General or *g* Factor

In 1904, a graduate student named Charles E. Spearman (1863–1945) published a seminal paper entitled " 'General Intelligence,' Objectively Determined and Measured," which constituted the first major effort to develop a theory of intelligence with empirical underpinnings. Spearman's discovery of the *g* factor has remained durable and constitutes "one of the most central phenomena in all of behavioral science, with broad explanatory powers" (Jensen, 1998, p. xii). The paper was almost instantly controversial, and it spawned scholarly debates with E. L. Thorndike and Godfrey Thomson that would span decades. Spearman would devote the rest of his career to elaboration and defense of the theory, authoring *The Nature of Intelligence and the Principles of Cognition* (1923), *The Abilities of Man: Their Nature and Measurement* (1927) and *Human Ability: A Continuation of "The Abilities of Man"* (Spearman & Wynn Jones, 1951).

Spearman (1904) asserted that "all branches of intellectual activity have in common one fundamental function (or group of functions)" (p. 284), which he later described using concepts from physics as "the amount of a general mental energy" (Spearman, 1927, p. 137). The *g* factor is a mathematically derived general factor, stemming from the shared variance that saturates batteries of cognitive/intelligence tests. Jensen (1998) summarizes the literature showing that correlates of *g* include scholastic performance, reaction time, success in training programs, job performance in a wide range of occupations, occupational status, earned income, socially significant creativity in the arts and sciences, and biologically anchored variables (e.g., average evoked potential and some physical characteristics in families).

Spearman's theory was originally called *two-factor theory* (Spearman, 1904), because it dichotomized variance into the general factor *g* (common variance, shared across measures) and specific factors *s* (test or subtest variance, unique to measures). Spearman originally conceptualized *s* as specific test-related factors, and he staunchly rejected endeavors to divide mental activity

into compartments (i.e., the separate faculties) that accounted for significant variance (i.e., transcended test-specific variance). Over time, however, he grudgingly acknowledged the existence of group factors that were shared between groups of tests but independent from the variance due to the general factor *g*:

> Overlapping specific factors have since often been spoken of as "group factors." They may be defined as those which occur in more than one but less than all of any given set of abilities. Thus they indicate no particular characters in any of the abilities themselves, but only some kinship between those which happen to be taken together in a set. Any element whatever in the specific factor of an ability will be turned into a group factor, if this ability is included in the same set with some other ability which also contains this element. The most that can be said is that some elements have a broader range than others, and therefore are more likely to play the part of group factors. (Spearman, 1927, p. 82)

Throughout the 20th century, the major researchers in intelligence were unable to ignore the concept of *g*. For instance, Binet (1905a/1916), who was publicly critical of Spearman, implicitly accepted the role of a general factor in his intelligence test. Likewise, Wechsler (1939a), who often favored the interpretation of subtests and specific abilities, wrote that Spearman's theory and its proofs constitute "one of the great discoveries of psychology" (p. 6); he also noted that "the only thing we can ask of an intelligence scale is that it measures sufficient portions of intelligence to enable us to use it as a fairly reliable index of the individual's global capacity" (p. 11). Even the most ardent critics of Spearman's work seem unable to totally dismiss the existence of a general factor. With the notable exceptions of John L. Horn (e.g., Horn & Noll, 1997; see also Horn & Blankson, Chapter 3, this volume) and Raymond B. Cattell (Cattell, 1987; see also McGrew, Chapter 8, this volume), most contemporary modelers of intelligence retain a *g* factor. For instance, several researchers have presented evidence that *g* is essentially reasoning ability and is synonymous with a broad fluid reasoning ability factor (Carroll, 1993; Cronbach, 1984; Gustaffson, 1988; Undheim, 1981a, 1981b). Others (e.g., Kyllonen & Chrystal, 1990) have suggested that *g* may be working memory capacity, which they argue drives reasoning ability. Still others have concluded that *g* is directly related to neural efficiency (Eysenck, 1986a, 1986b; Vernon, 1987) or mental complexity (e.g., Larson, Merritt, & Williams, 1988; Marshalek, Lohman, & Snow, 1983).

In contemporary models, variance in intelligence test performance may be partitioned into several different categories, depending upon the number of hierarchical levels in the model: *common variance*, which is attributable to a general ability factor (*g*) shared among subtests; *group factor variance*, which is shared among clusters of subtests; attributable to broad ability factors; *subtest-specific variance*, which is unique to a subtest; and *error variance*, which is due to poor subtest precision and reliability.

This "partitioning" and the categorization of intelligence are what lie at the heart of the challenge to Spearman's theory. Are there multiple forms of intelligence? Spearman's seminal 1904 paper, as well as his subsequent work, has been at the center of some of the most interesting and spirited academic debates (and alternate theories are presented in the following section). Some individuals have pointed out that the original 1904 paper contained computational errors (Fancher, 1985). Others have pointed out that Spearman was prone to hyperbole (e.g., his assertion that his results were "almost fatal to experimental psychology as a profitable branch of science" [1904, p. 284]). Still others have published papers disproving major elements of his work. Yet the importance of *g* versus multiple factors is an issue that is still being hotly disputed today—so much so, that Tulsky, Saklofske, and Ricker (2003) have pointed out that "this debate is just as relevant today as it was years ago" (p. 17).

Factor Theory and More Complex Structures of Intelligence

As described above, Spearman dichotomized test-related variance into general and specific variance, and he long resisted acknowledging that some variance in test performance could be accounted for by cognitive factors that are distinct from the general factor but that transcend test-specific variance. Critics of Spearman's position included Edward L. Thorndike, whom he debated for some 15 years beginning in 1909, and Godfrey

Thomson, who began a two-decade series of exchanges with Spearman in 1916. Accounts of the scholarship behind these rivalries are available in Thorndike with Lohman (1990) and Brody (1992).

However, many of the challenges to Spearman's model came about with the statistical advances at the beginning of the 20th century. In a landmark challenge to Spearman's theory, Truman Kelley used partial correlational techniques to remove the general factor from a dataset and uncover evidence of group factors, as detailed in his 1928 book, *Crossroads in the Mind of Man*. Moreover, a newer, more elegant family of multivariate techniques known as *factor analysis* held the promise to identify the fundamental dimensions underlying measures of intelligence and thereby to reveal its true structure. Louis L. Thurstone (1887–1955) was at the forefront of this research; beginning in the mid-1930s, his challenges to general ability and use of factor-analytic techniques helped set a foundation for the contemporary views of multiple-factor models of intelligence that are still interpreted today.

In this section, we describe the history of multifactor models of cognitive ability, as well as contemporary thinking in the factor-derived structures of cognitive ability. Multiple-factor models of intelligence hold that human cognitive abilities may be empirically divided into a number of distinct but related core dimensions. In its contemporary form, these models are dependent upon such techniques as exploratory and confirmatory factor analysis.

Thurstone's Factor Derivations

Thurstone developed the technique of multiple-factor analysis, which permitted him to analyze correlation matrices and extract separate ability factors that were largely unrelated to each other. He used the principle of simple structure to define factors (i.e., to maximize the loading of each test on one or more factors and to result in zero loadings of the test on remaining factors, while maintaining the orthogonality of all the factors). In 1934, Thurstone obtained scores on 56 tests (in a 15–hour test battery) from a sample of 240 university students. He conducted a centroid factor analysis and obtained 13 factors, seven of which were interpreted and termed *primary mental abilities*:

spatial visualization, perceptual speed, numerical facility, verbal comprehension, associative memory, word fluency, and *reasoning.* Thurstone (1938a) did not find evidence of Spearman's g in his factor analyses: "As far as we can determine at present, the tests that have been supposed to be saturated with the general common factor divide their variance among primary factors that are not present in all the tests. We cannot report any general common factor in the battery of fifty-six tests that have been analyzed in the present study" (p. ix). Cattell (1987) described the reaction among psychologists to this investigation as "a psychological earthquake" (p. 30) for overthrowing the dominance of the general intelligence factor. Thurstone (1936a, 1936b, 1936c, 1938b) recommended that each individual should be described in terms of a profile of mental abilities instead of a single index of intelligence. Spearman (1939a, 1939b) challenged Thurstone's findings, reanalyzing the data and extracting g as the major factor, along with small group factors for verbal, spatial, number, and memory abilities. Later Thurstone developed higher-order factor-analytic techniques, and by 1947, he was willing to admit the possible existence of Spearman's g at a higher-order level.

Cattell and Horn's Fluid and Crystallized Abilities

Raymond B. Cattell developed factor-analysis-based theories of both intelligence *and* personality that are influential to this day. Cattell completed his PhD in 1929 at University College, London, under the direction of Charles Spearman, and was deeply involved with and influenced by Spearman's factor-analytic work. In 1937, Cattell joined E. L. Thorndike's research staff at Columbia University, where he worked closely with adherents of the opposing multiple-factor models of intelligence. Cattell introduced his theory of intelligence in a 1941 APA convention presentation; briefly put, he suggested that Spearman's g was not enough (Cattell, 1941). Instead, Cattell maintained that there were two separate general factors, g_f (fluid ability, or fluid intelligence) and g_c (crystallized ability, or crystallized intelligence). (In most present-day publications, these are given as Gf and Gc.)

Fluid ability has been described by Cattell (1963, 1971) and Horn (1976) as a facility in reasoning, particularly where adaptation to new situations is required and crystallized learning assemblies are of little use. In general, ability is considered to be fluid when it takes different forms or utilizes different cognitive skill sets according to the demands of the problem requiring solution. For Cattell, fluid ability is the most essential general-capacity factor, setting an upper limit on the possible acquisition of knowledge and crystallized skills.

Crystallized intelligence refers to accessible stores of knowledge and the ability to acquire further knowledge via familiar learning strategies. It is typically measured by recitation of factual information, word knowledge, quantitative skills, and language comprehension tasks, because these include the domains of knowledge that are culturally valued and educationally relevant in the Western world (Cattell, 1941, 1963, 1971, 1987; Horn & Cattell, 1966). In the 1960s, Cattell and his student John L. Horn expanded the number of ability factors from two to five (adding *visualization, retrieval capacity,* and *cognitive speed*; Horn & Cattell, 1966); in the 1990s, Horn expanded the model even further, to nine ability factors (e.g., Horn & Noll, 1997). Horn's revisions to the theory are discussed in Chapter 3 of this book, and, though steeped in rich history, offer a contemporary view of intelligence.

Important Intermediate Structures: Vernon, Guilford, and Gustafsson

In a hierarchical factorial model, P. E. Vernon (1961) defined a superordinate g factor and two lower-order factors, which he called v:ed (verbal–educational ability) and k:m (mechanical–spatial ability). The v:ed is subdivided into verbal and numerical, while k:m is subdivided into space ability, manual ability, and mechanical information.

In his structure-of-intellect theory, Guilford (1967) rejected a verbal–nonverbal distinction by proposing four categories in the content of intellect: *figural, symbolic, semantic,* and *behavioral.* Guilford noted: "Historically, there seems to have been a belief that a psychological operation is the same whether it is performed with verbal–meaningful information or with visual–

figural information . . . . Extensive factor-analytical results have proved wrong the belief that the same ability is involved regardless of the kind of information with which we deal" (p. 61).

In 1984, Gustafsson proposed an integrated hierachical model of intelligence. At the highest level is *g* (general intelligence); at the next level are two broad factors "reflecting the ability to deal with verbal and figural information, respectively." These factors are labelled *crystallized intelligence* (dealing with verbal information) and *general visualization* (dealing with figural information), although fluid intelligence is noted as a second-order factor that is identical to the third-order *g* factor.

Carroll's Three-Stratum Model

John B. Carroll (1993 and Chapter 4, this volume) has proposed a hierachically organized three-stratum (three-level) model of human cognitive abilities based upon his meta-analyses of 461 separate test-based datasets. Carroll's 1993 book, *Human Cognitive Abilities: A Survey of Factor-Analytic Studies*, is often cited for its thoroughness and encyclopedic nature; perhaps because of this, it is lauded as a seminal publication among proponents of multiple factors of intelligence. The meta-analytic study took decades to complete. The study drew from data in 461 existing studies dating back 50 years or more, selecting datasets that included representation of known or postulated factors. It involved systematically performing factor analyses on the datasets, whereupon each factor was given a tentative name reflecting its likely interpretation. The factors were then sorted into broad domains or classes, according to preconceptualized categories. These classifications formed the basis for the three-stratum model.

Carroll's (1993) three-stratum model is graphically represented in Chapter 4 (see Figure 4.1). It includes a third-order factor of general intelligence, 8 or more second-order broad-ability factors, and as many as 65 first-order narrow-ability factors (subsequent researchers have identified even more). The *stratum* (or level, or hierarchical order) at which a factor is placed refers to the degree of generality over its constituent cognitive abilities, so general ability appears in the

highest stratum as a function of its broadness and generality, whereas very specific and narrow factors are placed at the lowest stratum. At the highest-order or third stratum, Carroll found evidence for a factor of general intelligence that dominates factors of variables involved in performing reasoning tasks. In other words, the *g* factor is essentially synonymous with the fluid intelligence factor. At the second stratum, a number of broad-ability factors were identified, listed in Figure 4.1 in descending strength of association with the general factor. Finally, the first-stratum narrow-ability factors defining each broad second-stratum factor are listed in descending order according to their factor salience (i.e., from higher to lower, according to their frequency of occurrence across the datasets and their average factor pattern coefficients).

REFERENCES

Adams, H. F., Furniss, L., & Debow, L. A. (1928). Personality as revealed by mental test scores and by school grades. *Journal of Applied Psychology, 12,* 261–277.

Archer, R. P., Maruish, M., Imhof, E. A., & Piotrowski, C. (1991). Psychological test usage with adolescent clients: 1990 survey findings. *Professional Psychology: Research and Practice, 22*(3), 247–252.

Atwell, C. R., & Wells, F. L. (1933). Army Alpha revised—Short form. *Personnel Journal, 12,* 160–165.

Binet, A. (1903). *L'étude expérimentale de l'intelligence.* Paris: C. Reinwald & Schleicher.

Binet, A., & Henri, V. (1895). La psychologie individuelle. *L'Année Psychologique, 2,* 411–465.

Binet, A., & Simon, T. (1916). New methods for the diagnosis of the intellectual level of subnormals. In *The development of intelligence in children* (E. S. Kite, Trans.). Baltimore: Williams & Wilkins. (Original work published 1905a)

Binet, A., & Simon, T. (1916). Upon the necessity of establishing a scientific diagnosis of inferior states of intelligence. In *The development of intelligence in children* (E. S. Kite, Trans.). Baltimore: Williams & Wilkins. (Original work published 1905b)

Binet, A., & Simon, T. (1916). The development of intelligence in the child. In *The development of intelligence in children* (E. S. Kite, Trans.). Baltimore: Williams & Wilkins. (Original work published 1908)

Binet, A., & Simon, T. (1916). The intelligence of the feeble-minded. In *Intelligence of the feeble-minded* (E. S. Kite, Trans.). Baltimore: Williams & Wilkins. (Original work published 1909)

Binet, A., & Simon, T. (1916). New investigation upon the measure of the intellectual level among school children. In *The development of intelligence in children* (E. S. Kite, Trans.). Baltimore: Williams & Wilkins. (Original work published 1911)

Boake, C. (2002). From the Binet–Simon to the Wechsler–Bellevue: Tracing the history of intelligence testing. *Journal of Clinical and Experimental Neuropsychology, 24*(3), 383–405.

Boring, E. (1957). *History of experimental psychology* (2nd ed.). New York: Appleton-Century-Crofts.

Boring, E. G. (1961). *Psychologist at large: An autobiography and selected essays of a distinguished psychologist.* New York: Basic Books.

Bregman, E. O. (1925, 1935). *Revision of the Army Alpha Examination, Form A, Form B.* New York: Psychological Corporation.

Brigham, C. C. (1935). *Examining fellowship applicants.* Princeton, NJ: Princeton University Press.

Brody, N. (1992). *Intelligence* (2nd ed.). San Diego, CA: Academic Press.

Buros, O. K. (Ed.). (1941). *The 1940 mental measurements yearbook.* Highland Park, NJ: Gryphon Press

Buros, O. (1949). *The third mental measurements yearbook.* Highland Park, NJ: Gryphon Press.

Butler, M., Retzlaff, P., & Vanderploeg, R. (1991). Neuropsychological test usage. *Professional Psychology: Research and Practice, 22,* 510–512.

Camara, W. J., Nathan, J. S., & Puente, A, E. (2000). Psychological test usage: Implications in professional psychology. *Professional Psychology: Research and Practice, 31,* 141–154.

Camfield, T. M. (1970). *Psychologists at war: The history of American psychologists and the First World War.* Unpublished doctoral dissertation.

Carroll, J. B. (1993). *Human cognitive abilities: A survey of factor analytic studies.* New York: Cambridge University Press.

Cattell, J. M. (1890). Mental tests and measurements. *Mind, 15,* 373–381.

Cattell, J. M., & Farrand, L. (1896). Physical and mental measurements of the students of Columbia University. *Psychological Review, 3,* 618–648.

Cattell, R. B. (1941). Some theoretical issues in adult intelligence testing. *Psychological Bulletin, 38,* 592.

Cattell, R. B. (1963). Theory of fluid and crystallized intelligence: A critical experiment. *Journal of Educational Psychology, 54,* 1–22.

Cattell, R. B. (1971). *Abilities: Their structure, growth, and action.* Boston: Houghton Mifflin.

Cattell, R. B. (1987). *Intelligence: Its structure, growth, and action.* New York: North-Holland.

Cronback, L. J. (1984). *Essentials of psychological testing* (4th ed.). New York: Harper & Row.

Darwin, C. (1859). *On the origin of species.* New York: Appleton.

Drummond, W. B. (1914). *Mentally defective children.* New York: Longmans, Green.

Eysenck, H. J. (1986a). Inspection time and intelligence: A historical introduction. *Personality and Individual Differences, 7,* 603–607.

Eysenck, H. J. (1986b). Toward a new model of intelligence. *Personality and Individual Differences, 7,* 731–736.

Fancher, R. E. (1985). *The intelligence men: Makers of the IQ controversy.* New York: Norton.

Ford, A. (1931). *Group experiments in elementary psychology.* New York: Macmillan.

Frank, G. (1983). *The Wechsler enterprise: An assessment of the development, structure, and use of the Wechsler tests of intelligence.* Oxford: Pergamon Press.

Galton, F. (1865). Hereditary talent and character. *Macmillan's Magazine, 12,* 157–166, 318–327.

Galton, F. (1869). *Hereditary genius: An inquiry into its laws and consequences.* London: Macmillan.

Galton, F. (1883). *Inquiries into human faculty and its development.* London: Macmillan.

Galton, F. (1888). Co-relations and their measurement, chiefly from anthropometric data. *Proceedings of the Royal Society, London, 45,* 135–145.

Guilford, J. P. (1938). A new revision of the Army Alpha examination. *Journal of Applied Psychology, 22,* 239–246.

Guilford, J. P. (1967). *The nature of human intelligence.* New York: McGraw-Hill.

Gustaffson, J. E. (1988). Hierarchical models of individual differences in cognitive abilities. In R. J. Sternberg (Ed.), *Advances in the psychology of human intelligence* (Vol 4, pp. 35–71). Hillsdale, NJ: Erlbaum.

Haggerty, M. E., Terman, L. M., Thorndike, E. L., Whipple, G. M., & Yerkes, R. M. (1920). *National Intelligence Tests, Scale A–Scale B.* Yonkers, NY: World.

Harrison, P. L., Kaufman, A. S., Hickman, J. A., & Kaufman, N. L. (1988). A survey of tests used for adult assessment. *Journal of Psychoeducational Assessment, 6*(3), 188–198.

Haines, T. H. (1916). Mental measurements of the blind. *Psychological Monographs, 21*(1, Whole No. 89).

Hales, N. M. (1932). *An advanced test of general intelligence.* Melbourne, Australia: Melbourne University Press.

Hendrickson, G. (1931). An abbreviation of the Army Alpha. *School and Society, 33,* 467–468.

Henmon, V. A. C., Peterson, J., Thurstone, L. L., Woodrow, H., Dearborn, W. F., & Haggerty, M. E. (1921). Intelligence and its measurement: A symposium. *Journal of Educational Psychology, 12*(4), 195–216.

Herring, J. P. (1922). *Herring Revision of the Binet–Simon Tests: Examination manual, Form A.* Yonkers, NY: World Book.

Hildreth, G. (1939). *Bibliography of mental tests and measurements* (2nd ed.). New York: Psychological Corporation.

Horn, J. L. (1976). Human abilities: A review of research and theory in the early 1970s. *Annual Review of Psychology, 27,* 437–485.

Horn, J. L., & Cattell, R. B (1966). Refinement and test of the theory of fluid and crystallized general intelligences. *Journal of Educational Psychology, 57*(5) 253–270.

Horn, J. L., & Noll, J. (1997). Human cognitive capabilities: G_f-G_c theory. In D. P. Flanagan, J. L. Genshaft, & P. L. Harrison (Eds.), *Contemporary intellectual assessment: Theories, tests, and issues* (pp. 53–91). New York: Guilford Press.

Jacobs, J. (1887). Experiments on "prehension." *Mind, 12,* 75–79.

Jensen, A. R. (1998). *The g factor: The science of mental ability.* Westport, CT: Praeger.

Kelley, T. L. (1928). *Crossroads in the mind of man.* Stanford, CA: Stanford University Press.

Kellogg, C. E., & Morton, N. W. (1934). Revised Beta Examination. *Personnel Journal, 13,* 94–100.

Kevles, D. J. (1968). Testing the Army's intelligence: Psychologists and the military in World War I. *Journal of American History, 55,* 565–581.

Kuhlman, F. (1922). *Handbook of mental tests: A further revision and extension of the Binet–Simon Scale.* Baltimore: Warwick & York.

Kyllonen, P. C., & Chrystal, R. E. (1990). Reasoning ability is (little more than) working memory capacity?! *Intelligence, 14,* 389–433.

Larson, G. E., Merritt, C. R., & Williams, S. E. (1988). Information processing and intelligence: Some implications of task complexity. *Intelligence, 12,* 131–147.

Lees-Haley, P. R., Smith, H. H., Williams, C. W., & Dunn, J. T. (1996). Forensic neuropsychological test usage: An empirical survey. *Archives of Clinical Neuropsychology, 11,* 45–51.

Lemann, N. (1999). *The big test: The secret history of American meritocracy.* New York: Farrar, Straus & Giroux.

Lennon, R. T. (1985). Group tests of intelligence. In B. B. Wolman (Ed.), *Handbook of intelligence: Themes, measurements, and applications.* New York: Wiley.

Lubin, B., Wallis, R. R., & Paine, C. (1971). Patterns of psychological test usage in the United States: 1935–1969. *Professional Psychology: Research and Practice, 2,* 70–74.

Marshalek, B., Lohman, D. F., & Snow, R. E. (1983). The complexity continuum in the radix and hierarchical models of intelligence. *Intelligence, 7,* 107–127.

Melville, N. J. (1917). *Standard method of testing juvenile mentality by the Binet–Simon Scale with the original questions, pictures, and drawings.* Philadelphia: Lippincott.

Minton, H. L. (1988). *Lewis M. Terman: Pioneer in psychological testing.* New York: New York University Press.

Otis, A. S. (1918a). An absolute point scale for the group measurement of intelligence: Part I. *Journal of Educational Psychology, 9,* 239–261.

Otis, A. S. (1918b). An absolute point scale for the group measurement of intelligence: Part II. *Journal of Educational Psychology, 9,* 323–348.

Otis, A. S. (1918c). *Otis Group Intelligence Scale, Advanced Examination.* Yonkers, NY: World Book.

Otis, A. S. (1936). *Mental Ability Test.* Yonkers, NY: World Book.

Pearson, K. (1914). *The life, letters and labours of Francis Galton: Vol. 2. Researchers of middle life.* Cambridge, UK: Cambridge University Press.

Piotrowski, C., & Keller, J. W. (1989). Psychological testing in outpatient mental health facilities: A national study. *Professional Psychology: Research and Practice, 20*(6), 423–425.

Reed, J. (1987). Robert M. Yerkes and the mental testing movement. In M. M. Sokal (Ed.), *Psychological testing and American society: 1890–1930* (pp. 75–94). New Brunswick, NJ: Rutgers University Press.

Roid, G. (2003). *Stanford–Binet Intelligence Scales, Fifth Edition.* Itasca, IL: Riverside.

Sharp, S. E. (1899). Individual psychology: A study in psychological method. *American Journal of Psychology, 10,* 329–391.

Sokal, M. M. (1987). James McKeen Cattell and mental anthropometry: Nineteenth-century science and reform and the origins of psychological testing. In M. M. Sokal (Ed.), *Psychological testing and American society: 1890–1930* (pp. 21–45). New Brunswick, NJ: Rutgers University Press.

Spearman, C. (1904). "General intelligence," objectively determined and measured. *American Journal of Psychology, 15,* 201–293.

Spearman, C. (1923). *The nature of intelligence and the principles of cognition.* London: Macmillan.

Spearman, C. (1927). *The abilities of man: Their nature and measurement.* New York: Macmillan

Spearman, C. (1939a). The factorial analysis of ability. II. Determination of factors. *British Journal of Psychology, 30,* 78–83.

Spearman, C. (1939b). Thurstone's work re-worked. *Journal of Educational Psychology, 30,* 1–16.

Spearman, C., & Wynn Jones, L. (1950). *Human ability: A continuation of "the abilities of man."* London: Macmillan.

Spencer, J. (1885). *The principles of psychology.* New York: S. Appelton (Original work published 1855)

Stern, W. (1914). *The psychological methods of testing intelligence* (Educational Psychology Monographs, No. 13; G. M. Whipple, Trans.). Baltimore: Warwick& York. (Original work published 1912)

Sternberg, R. J. (1988). *The triarchic mind: A new theory of human intelligence.* New York: Viking.

Sternberg., R. J., & Detterman, D. K. (1986). *What is intelligence?: Contemporary viewpoints on its nature and definition.* Norwood, NJ: Ablex.

Terman, L. M. (1916). *The measurement of intelligence.* Boston: Houghton Mifflin.

Terman, L. M. (1920). *The Terman Group Test of Mental Ability.* Yonkers-on-Hudson, NY: World Book Company.

Terman, L. M. (1923). *Stanford Achievement Test.* Yonkers, NY: World Book.

Terman, L. M. (1933). *Metropolitan Achievement Test.* Yonkers, NY: World Book.

Terman, L. M. (1961). Trails to psychology. In C. Murchison (Ed.), *A history of psychology in autobiography* (Vol. 2. pp.). New York: Russell & Russell. (Original work published 1932)

Terman L. M., & Merrill, M. A. (1937). *Measuring in-*

telligence: A guide to the administration of the new revised Stanford–Binet tests of intelligence. Boston: Houghton Mifflin.

Terman, L. M., & Merrill, M. A. (1960). *Stanford–Binet Intelligence Scale: Manual for the Third Revision, Form L-M*, Boston: Houghton Mifflin.

Terman, L. M., & Whitmire, E. D. (1921). Age and grade norms for the National Intelligence Tests, Scales A and B. *Journal of Educational Research, 3*, 124–132.

Thorndike, E. L., et al. (1921). Intelligence and its measurement: A symposium. *Journal of Educational Psychology, 12*, 123–147.

Thorndike, R. L., Hagen, E. P., & Sattler, J. M. (1986). *The Stanford–Binet Intelligence Scale: Fourth Edition guide for administering and scoring*. Chicago. Riverside.

Thorndike, R. M. (with Lohman, D. F.). (1990). *A Century of ability testing*. Chicago: Riverside Publishing Company.

Thurston, L. L. (1936a). The factorial isolation of primary abilities. *Psychometrika, 1*, 175–182.

Thurston, L. L. (1936b). The isolation of seven primary abilities. *Psychological Bulletin, 33*, 780–781.

Thurston, L. L. (1936c). A new conception of intelligence. *Educational Record, 17*, 441–450.

Thurstone, L. L. (1938a). The absolute zero in intelligence measurement. *Psychological Review, 35*, 175–197.

Thurston, L. L. (1938b). *Primary Mental Abilities: Psychometric Monographs No. 1*. Chicago: University of Chicago Press.

Town, C. H. (1915). *A method of measuring the development of the intelligence of young children* (3rd ed.). Chicago: Chicago Medical Book.

Tulsky, D. S. (2003). Reviews and promotional material for the Wechsler–Bellevue and Wechsler Memory Scale. In D. S. Tulsky et al. (Eds.), *Clinical interpretation of the WAIS-III and WMS-III* (pp. 579–602). San Diego, CA: Academic Press.

Tulsky, D. S., Chiaravalloti, N. D., Palmer, B., & Chelune, G. J. (2003). The Wechsler Memory Scale—Third Edition: A new perspective. In D. S. Tulsky et al. (Eds.), *Clinical interpretation of the WAIS-III and WMS-III* (pp. 93–139). San Diego, CA: Academic Press.

Tulsky, D. S., Saklofske, D. H., & Ricker, J. H. (2003). Historical overview of intelligence and memory: Factors influencing the Wechsler scales. In D. S. Tulsky et al. (Eds.), *Clinical interpretation of the WAIS-III and WMS-III* (pp. 7–41). San Diego, CA: Academic Press.

Tulsky, D. S., Saklofske, D. H., & Zhu, J. (2003). Revising a standard: An Evaluation of the origin and development of the WAIS-III. In D. S. Tulsky et al. (Eds.), *Clinical interpretation of the WAIS-III and WMS-III* (pp. 43–92). San Diego, CA: Academic Press.

Undheim, J. O. (1981a). On intelligence: II. A neo-Spearman model to replace Cattell's theory of fluid and crystallized intelligence. *Scandiavian Journal of Psychology, 22*(3), 181–187.

Undheim, J. O. (1981b). On Intelligence: IV. Toward a restoration of general intelligence. *Scandinavian Journal of Psychology, 22*(4), 251–265.

Vernon, P. A. (1987). *Speed of information-processing and intelligence*. Norwood, NJ: Ablex.

Vernon, P. E. (1961). *The measurement of abilities* (2nd ed.). Oxford: Philosophical Library.

Von Mayrhauser, R. T. (1987). The manager, the medic, and the mediator: The clash of professional psychological styles and the wartime origins of group mental testing. In M. M. Sokal (Ed.), *Psychological testing and American society: 1890–1930* (pp. 128–157). New Brunswick, NJ: Rutgers University Press.

Watkins, C. E., Campbell, V. L., & McGregor, P. (1988). Counseling psychologists' uses of and opinions about psychological tests: A contemporary perspective. *Counseling Psychologist, 16*(3), 476–486.

Wechsler, D. (1926). Tests for taxicab drivers. *Journal of Personnel Research, 5*, 24–30.

Wechsler, D. (1939a). *The measurement of adult intelligence*. Baltimore: Williams & Wilkins.

Wechsler, D. (1939b). *Wechsler–Bellevue Intelligence Scale*. New York: Psychological Corporation.

Wechsler, D. (1949). *The Wechsler Intelligence Scale for Children*. New York: Psychological Corporation.

Wechsler, D. (1955). *Wechsler Adult Intelligence Scale*. New York: Psychological Corporation.

Wechsler, D. (1967). *Wechsler Preschool and Primary Scale of Intelligence*. New York: Psychological Corporation.

Wechsler, D. (1974). *Wechsler Intelligence Scale for Children—Revised manual*. New York: Psychological Corporation.

Wechsler, D. (1975). Intelligence defined and undefined: A relativistic appraisal. *American Psychologist, 30*, 135–139.

Wells, F. L. (1932). Army Alpha—revised. *Personnel Journal, 10*, 411–417.

Whipple, G. M. (1921). The National Intelligence Tests. *Journal of Educational Research, 4*, 16–31.

Wilson, M. S., & Reschly, D. J. (1996). Assessment in school psychology training and practice. *School Psychology Review, 25*, 9–23.

Wissler, C. (1901). The correlation of mental and physical tests. *Psychological Review, 3*(Monograph Suppl. 16).

Wolf, T. (1973). *Alfred Binet*. Chicago: University of Chicago Press.

Yerkes, R. M. (1921). *Psychological examining in the United States Army* (Memoirs of the National Academy of Sciences, Vol. 15). Washington, DC: Government Printing Office.

Yerkes, R. M., Bridges, J. W., & Hardwick, R. S. (1915). *A point scale for measuring mental ability*. Baltimore: Warwick & York.

Yoakum, C. S., & Yerkes, R. M. (1920). *Army mental tests*. New York: Holt.

2

A History of Intelligence Test Interpretation

RANDY W. KAMPHAUS
ANNE PIERCE WINSOR
ELLEN W. ROWE
SANGWON KIM

Formal methods of intelligence test interpretation emerged subsequent to Binet's creation of the first successful intelligence scale (Kamphaus, 2001). These first methods, sometimes referred to colloquially as the "dipstick approach" to intelligence test use and interpretation, attempted primarily to quantify a general level of intelligence. With the introduction of subtest scores to clinical tests and the emergence of group tests measuring different abilities, *clinical profile analysis* replaced the "dipstick approach" as the dominant heuristic for intelligence test interpretation. *Psychometric profile analysis* soon followed. However, as measurement approaches to intelligence test interpretation developed, psychometric problems with profile analysis surfaced. Today, as the gap between intelligence theory and test development narrows substantially, test interpretation is becoming easier, clearer, and more accurate.

Our presentation of interpretation approaches is necessarily incomplete. We focus exclusively on a historical account of dominant methods of intelligence test interpretation. Fortunately, there is much to be learned from such an overview. As E. G. Boring (1929) wisely observed in the case of the experimental psychologist, "Without such [historical] knowledge he sees the present in dis-

torted perspective, he mistakes old facts and old views for new, and he remains unable to evaluate the significance of new movements and methods" (p. vii).

QUANTIFICATION OF A GENERAL LEVEL: THE FIRST WAVE

The process of analyzing human abilities has intrigued scientists for centuries. Indeed, some method for analyzing people's abilities has existed since the Chinese, more than 2,000 years ago, instituted civil service exams and formulated a system to classify individuals according to their abilities. Their system provided a means of associating ability with a profession in a way that also met the needs of society (French & Hale, 1990).

Early work in interpretation of intelligence tests focused extensively on classification of individuals into groups. Early classification provided a way to organize individuals into specified groups based on scores obtained on intelligence tests—an organization that was dependent on the acceptance of intelligence tests by laypersons as well as by professionals. Today, professionals in the fields of psychology and education benefit from the use of well-researched and objective instruments that were derived through periods of investigation and development. The following discussion is a brief description of some of the early work leading to the development of instrumentation.

The Work of Early Investigators

At the beginning of the 20th century, practitioners in the fields of psychology and education were beginning to feel the compelling influence of Alfred Binet and his colleagues in France. Binet's studies of the mental qualities of children for school placement led to the first genuinely successful method for classifying persons with respect to their cognitive abilities (Goodenough, 1949). Binet and Théodore Simon's development of the first empirical and practical intelligence test for applied use in the classification of students represented a technological breakthrough in the field of intelligence assessment. The first Binet–Simon scale (Binet & Simon, 1905) would lead to future scales and, according to Anastasi (1988), an overall increase in the use of intelligence tests for a variety of purposes.

Binet's efforts reflected his great interest in certain forms of cognitive activity. These included the abilities related to thinking and reasoning, the development and application of strategies for complex problem solving, and the use of adaptation of abilities for success in novel experiences (Pintner, 1923). His work appeared to stem from an interest in the complex cognitive processes of children and would eventually lead to a series of popular instruments, most recently represented in the Stanford–Binet Intelligence Scales, Fifth Edition (SB5; Roid, 2003).

At the same time, scientists such as James McKeen Cattell in the United States were conducting equally important work of a different kind. Cattell's investigations frequently focused on measures of perception and motor skills. Although different in scope and purpose from that of Binet and Simon, Cattell's work would ultimately have a profound effect on the popularization and use of intelligence tests (Pintner, 1923). Cattell's experimentation resulted in the appointment of a special committee whose members, with the assistance of the American Psychological Association, were charged with developing a series of mental ability tests for use in the classification and guidance of college students (Goodenough, 1949). The development of these tests placed great emphasis on the need for standardized procedures.

Procedures for standardization were introduced with the idea that the measurements associated with an individual would be even more informative when compared to the measurements of another person in the same age group who was administered the same test under the same conditions (Pintner, 1923). Indeed, the conditions of test administration must be controlled for everyone if the goal is scientific interpretation of the test data (Anastasi, 1988). Some of the earliest attempts at scientific test interpretation, used before and during World War II, included the classification of individuals into groups based on their test scores and defined by descriptive terminology.

Classification Schemes

The first well-documented efforts at intelligence test interpretation emphasized the assignment to a descriptive classification based on an overall intelligence test composite score. This practice seemed a reasonable first step, given that (1) the dominant scale of the day, the Stanford–Binet (Stanford Revisions and Extension of the Binet–Simon Scale [Terman, 1916] or the Revised Stanford–Binet [Terman & Merrill, 1937]), yielded only a global score; and (2) Spearman's (1927) general intelligence theory emphasized the preeminence of an underlying *mental energy*.

According to Goodenough (1949), the identification of mental ability was regarded as a purely physical/medical issue until the beginning of the 20th century. Wechsler (1944) made a similar statement, noting that the vocabulary of choice included medical–legal terms such as *idiot*, *imbecile*, and *moron*. Levine and Marks (1928, p. 131) provided an example of a classification system incorporating these terms (see Table 2.1).

This classification system used descriptive terms that were evaluative and pejorative (especially when employed in the vernacular), leading to abuse of the terms. In addition, the many category levels contained bands of scores with different score ranges. The top and bottom three levels comprised bands of 24 score points each, while those in the middle, from *borderline* to *very bright*,

TABLE 2.1. The Levine and Marks Intelligence Test Score Classification System

Level	Range in IQ
Idiots	0–24
Imbeciles	25–49
Morons	50–74
Borderline	75–84
Dull	85–94
Average	95–104
Bright	105–114
Very bright	115–124
Superior	125–149
Very superior	150–174
Precocious	175 or above

comprised bands of 9 points each. Although the band comprising the *average* range was not far from our present conceptions of *average* (except for this example's upper limit), the use of numerous uneven levels was potentially confusing to the layperson.

Wechsler (1944) introduced another classification scheme that attempted to formulate categories according to a specific structural rationale. Specifically, the system proposed by Wechsler was based on a definition of intelligence levels related to statistical frequencies, in which each classification level was based on a range of intelligence scores lying specified distances from the mean (Wechsler, 1944). In an effort to move away from somewhat arbitrary qualities, his classification scheme incorporated estimates of the prevalence of certain intelligence levels in the United States at that time (see Table 2.2).

Wechsler's system is notable for bands of IQ limits that are somewhat closer to those we use at the present time. Both the Levine and Marks (1928) and the Wechsler (1944) schemes provide a glimpse at procedures used in early attempts at test interpretation.

TABLE 2.2. Wechsler's Intelligence Classification According to IQ

Classification	IQ limits	% included
Defective	65 and below	2.2
Borderline	66–79	6.7
Dull normal	80–90	16.1
Average	91–110	50.0
Bright normal	111–119	16.1
Superior	120–127	6.7
Very superior	128 and over	2.2

In the period since World War II, both scientists and practitioners have moved to a less evaluative vocabulary that incorporates parallel terminology around the mean, such as *above average* and *below average* (Kamphaus, 2001).

Considerations for Interpretation Using Classification Systems

The structure of classification systems appears to be more stable today than in the past. Previously, practitioners often applied Terman's classification system, originally developed for interpretation of the Stanford–Binet, in their interpretation of many different tests that measured a variety of different abilities (Wechsler, 1944). Fortunately, many test batteries today provide their own classification schemes within the test manual, providing an opportunity to choose among appropriate tests and interpret the results accordingly. In addition, these classification systems are often based on deviation from a mean of 100, providing consistency across most intelligence tests and allowing comparison of an individual's performance on them. Clearly, we have made progress regarding the use of classification schemes in the evaluation of human abilities.

Calculation of intelligence test scores, or IQs, became a common way of describing an individual's cognitive ability. However, test score calculation is only the first step in the interpretive process, and this has been the case since the early days of testing (Goodenough, 1949). Although scores may fall neatly into classification categories, additional data should be considered when clinicians are discussing an individual's abilities. For example, individuals in the population who are assessed to have below-average intellectual abilities do not necessarily manifest the same degree of retardation and, in fact, may demonstrate considerable variability in capabilities (Goodenough, 1949). In a similar statement, Wechsler (1958) noted that an advantage to the use of scores in the classification process is to keep clinicians from forgetting that intelligence tests are completely relative and, moreover, do not assess absolute quantities.

These concerns of Goodenough and Wechsler have influenced intelligence test interpretation for many years. Clinicians continue to use classification schemes based on global IQ scores for diagnosis and interpretation, and the concerns of Goodenough and Wechsler are alive today. With the understanding that global IQ scores represent the most robust estimate of ability, they are frequently used in the diagnosis of mental retardation, giftedness, learning disabilities, and other conditions. Still, we caution that global cutoff scores may not always be appropriate or adequate for the decisions typically made on the basis of intelligence test scores (Kaufman, 1990). In addition to the intelligence test data, clinicians must examine any further data related to an individual's cognitive functioning.

CLINICAL PROFILE ANALYSIS: THE SECOND WAVE

Rapaport, Gill, and Schafer's (1945–1946) seminal work has exerted a profound influence on intelligence test interpretation to the present day. These authors, recognizing an opportunity provided by the publication of the Wechsler–Bellevue Scale (Wechsler, 1939), advocated interpretation of the newly introduced subtest scores to achieve a more thorough understanding of an individual's cognitive skills; in addition, they extended intelligence test interpretation to include psychiatric diagnoses.

Profiles of Subtest Scores

Rapaport and colleagues (1945–1946) espoused a new perspective in the interpretation of intelligence tests, focusing on the shape of subtest score profiles in addition to an overall general level of intellectual functioning. Whereas the pre-World War II psychologist was primarily dependent on the Binet scales and the determination of a general level of cognitive attainment, the post-Rapaport and colleagues psychologist became equally concerned with the shape of a person's profile of subtest scores. Specifically, patterns of high and low subtest scores could presumably reveal diagnostic and psychotherapeutic considerations:

> In our opinion, one can most fully exploit intelligence tests neither by stating merely that the

patient was poor on some and good on other subtests, nor by trying to connect directly the impairments of certain subtest scores with certain clinical-nosological categories; but rather only by attempting to understand and describe the psychological functions whose impairment or change brings about the impairment of scores. . . . Every subtest score—especially the relationship of every subtest score to the other subtest scores—has a multitude of determinants. If we are able to establish the main psychological function underlying the achievement, then we can hope to construct a complex psychodynamic and structural picture out of the interrelationships of these achievements and impairments of functions . . . (Rapaport et al., 1945–1946, p. 106)

The Rapaport and colleagues (1945–1946) system had five major emphases, the first of which involved interpretation of item responses. The second emphasis involved comparing a subject's item responses within subtests. Differential responding to the same item type (e.g., Information subtest items assessing U.S. vs. international knowledge) was thought to be of some diagnostic significance. The third emphasis suggested that meaningful interpretations could be based on within-subject comparisons of subtest scores. They introduced the practice of deriving diagnostic information from comparisons between Verbal and Performance scales, the fourth interpretive emphasis. The authors suggested, for example, that a specific Verbal–Performance profile could be diagnostic of depression (Rapaport et al., 1945–1946, p. 68). The fifth and final emphasis involved the comparison of intelligence test findings to other test findings. In this regard, they noted, "Thus, a badly impaired intelligence test achievement has a different diagnostic implication if the Rorschach test indicates a rich endowment or a poor endowment" (p. 68).

The work of Rapaport and colleagues (1945–1946) was a considerable developmental landmark due to its scope. It provided diagnostic suggestions at each interpretive level for a variety of adult psychiatric populations. Furthermore, their work introduced an interpretive focus on intraindividual differences—a focus that at times took preeminence over interindividual comparison in clinical work with clients.

In addition to the breadth of their approach, the structure of the Rapaport et al. (1945–1946) method gave clinicians a logical, step-by-step method for assessing impairment of function and for making specific diagnostic hypotheses. These authors directed clinicians to calculate a mean subtest score that could be used for identifying intraindividual strengths and weaknesses, and they gave desired difference score values for determining significant subtest fluctuations from the mean subtest score. The case of so-called "simple schizophrenia" (see Table 2.3) provides an example of the specificity of the diagnostic considerations that could be gleaned from a subtest profile.

Because of its thorough and clinically oriented approach, Rapaport and colleagues' (1945–1946) work provided a popular structure for training post-World War II clinical psychologists in the interpretation of intelligence test scores (i.e., the Wechsler–Bellevue Scale). Today, some clinicians still address the shape of intelligence test results in their interpretation (Kamphaus, 2001).

Verbal–Performance Differences and Subtest Profiles

Wechsler (1944) reinforced the practice of profile analysis by advocating a method of interpretation that also placed a premium on shape over a general level, with particular emphasis on subtest profiles and Verbal–Performance differences (scatter). His interpretive method is highlighted in a case exam-

TABLE 2.3. Diagnostic Considerations for the Case of "Simple Schizophrenia"

Subtest	Considerations
Vocabulary	Many misses on relatively easy items, especially if harder items are passed
	Relatively low weighted scores
	Parallel lowering of both the mean of the Verbal subtest scores (excluding Digit Span and Arithmetic) and the Vocabulary score
Information	Two or more misses on the easy items
	Relatively well-retained score 2 or more points above
	Vocabulary
Comprehension	Complete failure on any (especially more than one) of the seven easy items
	Weighted score 3 or more points below the Vocabulary score (or below the mean of the other Verbal subtests: Information, Similarities, and Vocabulary)
	Great positive Comprehension scatter (2 or more points superior to Vocabulary) is not to be expected
Similarities	Failure on easy items
	Weighted score 3 points below Vocabulary
Picture Arrangement	Tends to show a special impairment of Picture Arrangement in comparison to the other Performance subtests
Picture Completion	Weighted score of 7 or less
Object Assembly	Performance relatively strong
Block Design	No significant impairment from Vocabulary level
	Tends to be above the Performance mean
Digit Symbol	May show some impairment, but some "bland schizophrenics" may perform well

TABLE 2.4. Wechsler's Case Example for "Adolescent Psychopaths"

Subtest	Standard score
Comprehension	11
Arithmetic	6
Information	10
Digits	6
Similarities	5
Picture Arrangement	12
Picture Completion	10
Block Design	15
Object Assembly	16
Digit Symbol	12
Verbal IQ (VIQ)	90
Performance IQ (PIQ)	123

ple presented as a set of results for what he called "adolescent psychopaths" (see Table 2.4).

It is noteworthy that Wechsler did not provide a Full Scale IQ (FSIQ) for this case example, focusing instead on shape rather than level. Wechsler (1944) offered the following interpretation of this "psychopathic" profile of scores:

> White, male, age 15, 8th grade. Continuous history of stealing, incorrigibility and running away. Several admissions to Bellevue Hospital, the last one after suicide attempt. While on wards persistently created disturbances, broke rules, fought with other boys and continuously tried to evade ordinary duties. Psychopathic patterning: Performance higher than Verbal, low Similarities, low Arithmetic, sum of Picture Arrangement plus Object Assembly greater than sum of scores on Blocks and Picture Completion. (p. 164)

This case exemplifies the second wave of intelligence test interpretation. This second wave was more sophisticated than the first, in that it suggested that intelligence test interpretation should involve more than mere designation of a general level of intelligence. However, methodological problems existed, eliciting one central question about these approaches: How do we know that these various subtest profiles accurately differentiate between clinical samples, and thus demonstrate diagnostic utility? The next wave sought to answer this salient question by applying measurement science to the process of intelligence test interpretation.

PSYCHOMETRIC PROFILE ANALYSIS: THE THIRD WAVE

The availability of computers and statistical software packages provided researchers of the 1960s and 1970s greater opportunity to assess the validity of various interpretive methods and the psychometric properties of popular scales. Two research traditions—*factor analysis* and *psychometric profile analysis*—have had a profound effect on intelligence test interpretation.

Factor Analysis

Cohen's (1959) seminal investigation addressed the second wave of intelligence test interpretation by questioning the empirical basis of the intuitively based "clinical" methods of profile analysis. He conducted one of the first comprehensive factor analyses of the standardization sample for the Wechsler Intelligence Scale for Children (WISC; Wechsler, 1949), analyzing the results for 200 children from three age groups of the sample. Initially, five factors emerged: Factor A, labeled Verbal Comprehension I; Factor B, Perceptual Organization; Factor C, Freedom from Distractibility; Factor D, Verbal Comprehension II; and Factor E, quasi-specific. Cohen (1959) chose not to interpret the fourth and fifth factors, subsuming their loadings and subtests under the first three factors. Hence the common three-factor structure of the WISC was established as the de facto standard for conceptualizing the factor structure of the Wechsler scales. Eventually, Kaufman (1979) provided a systematic method for utilizing the three factor scores of the WISC-R (Wechsler, 1974) to interpret the scales as an alternative to interpreting the VIQ and PIQs, calling into question the common clinical practice of interpreting the Verbal and Performance scores as if they were measures of valid constructs. Cohen's labels for the first three factors were retained as names for the Index scores through the third revision of the Wechsler Intelligence Scale for Children (WISC-III; Wechsler, 1991). In addition, Cohen's study popularized the Freedom from Distractibility label for the controversial third factor (Kamphaus, 2001).

Cohen (1959) also popularized the consideration of subtest specificity prior to making subtest score interpretations. Investigation of the measurement properties of the subtests was crucial, as Cohen noted:

> A body of doctrine has come down in the clinical use of the Wechsler scales, which involves a rationale in which the specific intellective and psychodynamic trait-measurement functions are assigned to each of the subtests (e.g., Rapaport et al., 1945–1946). Implicit in this rationale lies the assumption that a substantial part of a test's variance is associated with these specific measurement functions. (p. 289)

According to Cohen (1959), *subtest specificity* refers to the computation of the amount of subtest variance that is reliable (not error) and specific to the subtest. Put another way, a subtest's reliability coefficient represents both reliable specific and shared variance. When shared variance is removed, a clinician may be surprised to discover that little reliable specific variance remains to support interpretation. Typically, the clinician may draw a diagnostic or other conclusion based on a subtest with a reliability estimate of .80, feeling confident of the interpretation. However, Cohen cautioned that this coefficient may be illusory, because the clinician's interpretation assumes that the subtest is measuring an ability that is only measured by this subtest of the battery. The subtest specificity value for this same subtest may be rather poor if it shares considerable variance with other subtests. In fact, its subtest specificity value may be lower than its error variance (20).

Cohen (1959) concluded that few of the WISC subtests could attribute one-third or more of their variance to subtest specific variance—a finding that has been replicated for subsequent revisions of the WISC (Kamphaus, 2001; Kaufman, 1979). Cohen pointedly concluded that adherents to the "clinical" rationales would find no support

in the factor-analytic studies of the Wechsler scales (p. 290). Moreover, he singled out many of the subtests for criticism; in the case of the Coding subtest, he concluded that Coding scores, when considered in isolation, were of limited utility (p. 295).

This important study set the stage for a major shift in intelligence test interpretation—that is, movement toward an emphasis on test interpretation supported by measurement science. Hallmarks of this approach are exemplified in Cohen's work, including the following:

1. Renewed emphasis on interpretation of the FSIQ (harkening back to the first wave), as a large second-order factor accounts for much of the variance of the Wechsler scales.
2. Reconfiguration of the Wechsler scales, proposing the three factor scores as alternatives or supplements to interpretation of the Verbal and Performance scales.
3. Deemphasis on individual subtest interpretation, due to limited subtest reliable specific variance (specificity).

Kaufman's Psychometric Approach

Further evidence of the influence of measurement science on intelligence test interpretation and the problems associated with profile analysis can be found in an influential book by Kaufman (1979), *Intelligent Testing with the WISC-R*. He provided a logically appealing and systematic method for WISC-R interpretation that was rooted in sound measurement theory. He created a hierarchy for WISC-R interpretation, which emphasized interpretive conclusions drawn from the most reliable and valid scores yielded by the WISC-R (see Table 2.5).

Although such interpretive methods remained "clinical," in the sense that interpre-

TABLE 2.5. Kaufman's Hierarchy for WISC-R Interpretation

Source of conclusion	Definition	Reliability	Validity
Composite scores	Wechsler IQs	Good	Good
Shared subtest scores	Two or more subtests combined to draw a conclusion	Good	Fair to poor
Single subtest scores	A single subtest score	Fair	Poor

tation of a child's assessment results was still dependent on the child's unique profile of results (Anastasi, 1988), the reliance on measurement science for the interpretive process created new standards for assessment practice. Application of such methods required knowledge of the basic psychometric properties of an instrument, and consequently required greater psychometric expertise on the part of the clinician.

These measurement-based interpretive options contrasted sharply with the "clinical" method espoused by Rapaport and colleagues (1945–1946)—an approach that elevated subtest scores and item responses (presumably the most unreliable and invalid scores and indicators) to prominence in the interpretive process. The measurement science approach, however, was unable to conquer some lingering validity problems.

Diagnostic and Validity Problems

Publication of the Wechsler scales and their associated subtest scores created the opportunity for clinicians to analyze score profiles, as opposed to merely gauging an overall intellectual level from one composite score. Rapaport and colleagues (1945–1946) popularized this method, which they labeled *scatter analysis*:

> Scatter is the pattern or configuration formed by the distribution of the weighted subtest scores on an intelligence test . . . the definition of scatter as a configuration or pattern of all the subtest scores implies that the final meaning of the relationship of any two scores, or of any single score to the central tendency of all the scores, is derived from the total pattern. (p. 75)

However, Rapaport and colleagues (1945–1946) began to identify problems with profile analysis of scatter early in their research efforts. In one instance, they expressed their frustration with the Wechsler scales as a tool for profile analysis, observing that "the standardization of the [Wechsler–Bellevue] left a great deal to be desired so that the average scattergrams of normal college students, Kansas highway patrolmen . . . and applicants to the Meninger School of Psychiatry . . . all deviated from a straight line in just about the same ways" (p. 161).

Bannatyne (1974) constructed one of the more widely used recategorizations of the WISC subtests into presumably more meaningful profiles (see Table 2.6). Matheson, Mueller, and Short (1984) studied the validity of Bannatyne's recategorization of the WISC-R, using a multiple-group factor analysis procedure with three age ranges of the WISC-R and data from the WISC-R standardization sample. They found that the four categories had high reliabilities, but problems with validity. For example, the Acquired Knowledge category had sufficiently high reliabilities, but it was not independent of the other three categories, particularly Conceptualization. As a result, Matheson and colleagues (1984) advised that the Acquired Knowledge category not be interpreted as a unique entity; instead, the Acquired Knowledge and Conceptualization categories were best interpreted as one measure of verbal intelligence, which was more consistent with the factor-analytic research on the WISC-R and other intelligence test batteries.

Similarly, Kaufman (1979) expressed considerable misgivings, based on a review of research designed to show links between particular profiles of subtest scores and child diagnostic categories (although he too had provided detailed advice for conducting profile analysis). Kaufman noted that the profiles proved to be far less than diagnostic:

> The apparent trends in the profiles of individuals in a given exceptional category can sometimes provide one piece of evidence to be

TABLE 2.6. Bannatyne's Recategorization of WISC Subtests

Spatial	Conceptualization	Sequencing	Acquired Knowledge
Block Design	Vocabulary	Digit Span	Information
Object Assembly	Similarities	Coding	Arithmetic
Picture Completion	Comprehension	Arithmetic	Vocabulary
		Picture Arrangement	

weighed in the diagnostic process. When there is ample support for a diagnosis from many diverse background, behavioral, test-related (and in some cases medical) criteria, the emergence of a reasonably characteristic profile can be treated as one ingredient in the overall stack of evidence. However, the lack of a characteristic profile should not be considered as disconfirming evidence. In addition, no characteristic profile, in and of itself, should ever be used as the primary basis of a diagnostic decision. We do not even know how many normal youngsters display similar WISC-R profiles. Furthermore . . . the extreme similarity in the relative strengths and weaknesses of the typical profiles for mentally retarded, reading-disabled, and learning-disabled children renders differential diagnosis based primarily on WISC-R subtest patterns a veritable impossibility. (pp. 204–205)

Profile analysis was intended to identify intraindividual strengths and weaknesses—a process known as *ipsative interpretation*. In an ipsative interpretation, the individual client was used as his or her own normative standard, as opposed to making comparisons to the national normative sample. However, such seemingly intuitive practices as comparing individual subtest scores to the unique mean subtest score and comparing pairs of subtest scores are fraught with measurement problems. The clinical interpretation literature often fails to mention the poor reliability of a *difference score* (i.e., the difference between two subtest scores). Anastasi (1985) has reminded clinicians that the standard error of the difference between two scores is larger than the standard error of measurement of the two scores being compared. Thus interpretation of a 3- or 5-point difference between two subtest scores becomes less dependable for hypothesis generation or making conclusions about an individual's cognitive abilities. Another often-cited problem with ipsative interpretation is that the correlations among subtests are positive and often high, suggesting that individual subtests provide little differential information about a child's cognitive skills (Anastasi, 1985). Furthermore, McDermott, Fantuzzo, Glutting, Watkins, and Baggaley (1992), studying the internal and external validity of subtest strengths and weaknesses, found these measures to be wholly inferior to basic norm-referenced information.

Thus the long-standing practice of using profile analysis to draw conclusions about intraindividual strengths and weaknesses did not fare well in numerous empirical tests of its application. Even with empirical support, the lack of validity support for profile analysis remained unsolved (Kamphaus, 2001). Measurement problems remained, many of which were endemic to the type of measure used (e.g., variations on the Wechsler tradition). These indicated the need for the fourth wave, wherein theory and measurement science became intermingled with practice considerations to enhance the meaningfulness of interpretation.

APPLYING THEORY TO INTELLIGENCE TESTS: THE FOURTH WAVE

Merging Research, Theory, and Intelligence Testing

Kaufman (1979) was among the first to cogently argue the case that intelligence tests' lack of theoretical clarity and support constituted a critical issue of validity. He proposed reorganizing subtests into clusters that conformed to theories of intelligence, thus allowing the clinician to produce more meaningful conclusions. The fourth wave has addressed intelligence test validity through the development of contemporary instruments founded in theory, and through integration of test results with multiple sources of information—hypothesis validation, as well as testing of rival hypotheses (Kamphaus, 2001).

Test Design for Interpretation

The history of intelligence test interpretation has been characterized by a disjuncture between the design of the tests and inferences made from those tests. A test, after all, should be designed a priori with a strong theoretical foundation, and supported by considerable validity evidence in order to measure a particular construct or set of constructs (and *only* those constructs). Prior to the 1990s, the interpretive process was conducted by clinicians who sometimes applied relatively subjective clinical acumen in the absence of empirically supported theoretical bases to interpret scores for their consumers.

For more valid and reliable interpretation of intelligence tests, instrument improvement would now need to focus on constructing tests designed to measure a delimited and well-defined set of intelligence-related constructs.

During the second half of the 20th century, several theories on the structure of intelligence were introduced, promoting a shift to seeking theoretical support for the content of intelligence tests. Among the most significant theories have been Carroll's three-stratum theory of cognitive abilities, the Horn–Cattell fluid–crystallized (Gf-Gc) theory, the Luria–Das model of information processing, Gardner's multiple intelligences, and Sternberg's triarchic theory of intelligence (see Chapters 4–8 of the present volume for reviews). Two popular theoretical models of intelligence have the primary distinction of fostering this shift. First, the factor-analytic work of Raymond Cattell and John Horn (Horn & Cattell, 1966) describes an expanded theory founded on Cattell's (1943) constructs of *fluid intelligence* (Gf) and *crystallized intelligence* (Gc). Cattell described fluid intelligence as representing reasoning and the ability to solve novel problems, whereas crystallized intelligence was thought to constitute abilities influenced by acculturation, schooling, and language development. This fluid–crystallized distinction was supported by Horn (1988), who delineated additional contributing abilities such as visual–spatial ability, short-term memory, processing speed, and long-term retrieval. Subsequent to this research was John Carroll's (1993) integration of findings from more than 460 factor-analytic investigations that led to the development of his three-stratum theory of intelligence. The three strata are organized by generality. Stratum III, the apex of the framework, consists of one construct only—general intelligence or *g*, the general factor that has been identified in numerous investigations as accounting for the major portion of variance assessed by intelligence test batteries. Stratum II contains eight broad cognitive abilities contributing to the general factor *g*, and is very similar to Gf-Gc abilities as described by Horn. Carroll's model proposes numerous narrow (specific) factors subsumed in stratum I. The two models are sometimes used together and are referred to in concert as the *Cattell–Horn–Carroll* (CHC) model of intelligence (see Chapters 4–8 in this volume).

Theory and Design Combined

Most modern intelligence tests are based in part or whole on a few widely accepted theories of intelligence—theories built upon and consistent with decades of factor-analytic studies of intelligence test batteries (Kamphaus, 2001).

The commonality of theoretical development is demonstrated in the following brief descriptions of several widely used tests, many of which have been newly published or revised over the past few years. All are examples of a greater emphasis on theory-based test design. The intelligence tests are described in great detail in individual chapters in this book.

Among contemporary intelligence tests, the Woodcock–Johnson III (WJ III; Woodcock, McGrew, & Mather, 2001) is the instrument most closely aligned with the Cattell–Horn (Cattell, 1943; Horn, 1988; Horn & Cattell, 1966) and Carroll (1993) theories of intelligence. According to the WJ III technical manual (McGrew & Woodcock, 2001), Cattell and Horn's Gf-Gc theory was the theoretical foundation for the Woodcock–Johnson Psycho-Educational Battery—Revised (WJ-R; Woodcock & Johnson, 1989). Four years after publication of the WJ-R, Carroll's (1993) text was published; professionals interested in theories of intelligence began to think in terms of a combination or extension of theories, the CHC theory of cognitive abilities (McGrew & Woodcock, 2001). CHC theory, in turn, served as the blueprint for the WJ III. The WJ III developers designed their instrument to broadly measure seven of the eight stratum II factors from CHC theory, providing the following cognitive cluster scores: Comprehension–Knowledge (crystallized intelligence), Long-Term Retrieval, Visual–Spatial Thinking, Auditory Processing, Fluid Reasoning (fluid intelligence), Processing Speed, and Short-Term Memory. Moreover, individual subtests are intended to measure several narrow abilities from stratum I. Finally, the General Intellectual Ability score serves as a measure of overall *g*, representing stratum III.

Similarly, the newly revised SB5 (Roid, 2003) is based on the CHC model of intelligence. The SB5 can be considered a five-factor model, in that it includes five of the broad stratum II factors having the highest loadings on *g*: Fluid Reasoning (fluid intelligence), Knowledge (crystallized knowledge), Quantitative Reasoning (quantitative knowledge), Visual–Spatial Processing (visual processing), and Working Memory (short-term memory). Among these factors, Visual–Spatial Processing is new to this revision—an attempt to enrich the nonverbal measures of the SB5, aiding in the identification of children with spatial talents and deficits. Moreover, the SB5 is constructed to provide a strong nonverbal IQ by creating nonverbal measures for all five factors.

The Wechsler Intelligence Scale for Children—Fourth Edition (WISC-IV; Wechsler, 2003) also emphasizes a stratified approach by replacing the VIQ and PIQ dichotomy with the four factor-based index scores that were supplemental in previous editions. The Index scores have been retitled to more accurately reflect the new theoretical structure, as well as new subtests introduced in this version. For example, the Perceptual Organization Index from the WISC-III has evolved into the Perceptual Reasoning Index, with new subtests designed to assess fluid reasoning abilities while reducing the effects of timed performance and motor skills. The controversial Freedom from Distractibility Index has become the Working Memory Index, reflecting research demonstrating working memory's essential role in fluid reasoning, learning, and achievement (Fry & Hale, 1996). Ten subtests contribute to the four Index scores, which in turn contribute to the FSIQ; however, the primary focus of interpretation is on the Index scores.

The Differential Ability Scales (DAS; Elliott, 1990a) battery is based upon a hierarchical model of cognitive abilities as well, although not upon a unique theory of human abilities. Rather, it was created to represent various theoretical viewpoints. Calling this "a deliberately eclectic approach," Elliott (1990b) has explained two reasons for this direction. First, considering the controversy surrounding human intelligence, reliance on a single theory may be unnecessarily narrow. Second, noting that clinicians are often eclectic in their choice of theory, Elliott has tried to accommodate various theoretical stances. The DAS provides three levels of interpreta-

tion: the composite General Cognitive Ability (GCA), cluster, and subtest. Some of the subtests cluster into groups, and these groups intercorrelate and yield psychometric *g*. Adopting various theories allows the interpretation of scores at each level. However, score interpretation can be different from age range to age range, because cognitive abilities become differentiated as children mature. Consistent with this developmental consideration, the DAS generates unique scores for each age group. For children below 3 years and 6 months (3:6) old, there are only subtest scores and GCA; between ages 3:6 and 5:11, the subtests produce both GCA and the two cluster scores of Verbal Ability and Nonverbal Ability; for ages 6:0–17:11, the Spatial Ability cluster is added for a total of three cluster scores in addition to the GCA.

The newly developed Reynolds Intellectual Assessment Scales (RIAS; Reynolds & Kamphaus, 2003) exemplifies this movement to design intelligence tests on current theory and research as well as for ease of interpretation. The following paragraphs use the RIAS to demonstrate a theoretical approach that supports modem intelligence test construction and interpretation.

The factor-analytic work of Carroll (1993) informed the creation of the RIAS by demonstrating that many of the latent traits assessed by intelligence test were test battery independent. The RIAS focuses on the assessment of stratum III and stratum II abilities from Carroll's three-stratum theory. The RIAS is designed to assess four important aspects of intelligence: general intelligence (stratum Ill), verbal intelligence (stratum II, "Crystallized Abilities"), nonverbal intelligence (stratum II, "Visualization/Spatial Abilities"), and memory (stratum II, "Working Memory, Short-Term Memory, or Learning"). These four constructs are assessed by combinations of the six RIAS subtests.

Although most contemporary tests of intelligence seek to measure at least some of the components from the extended Gf-Gc (Horn & Cattell, 1968) and the three-stratum (Carroll, 1993) models of intelligence, some tests based on different theories of intelligence are available. An example of an intelligence theory not aligned with Carroll's model is the *planning, attention, simultaneous, and successive* (PASS; Das,

Naglieri, & Kirby, 1994) theory of cognitive functioning. The PASS theory is founded in Luria's (1966) neuropsychological model of integrated intellectual functioning, and a description of the PASS theory is presented by Naglieri and Das in Chapter 7 of this volume.

Naglieri and Das (1990) argue that traditional models of intelligence and means of assessing intelligence are limited. From the PASS theory's focus on cognitive processes, Naglieri and Das (1997) have created the Cognitive Assessment System (CAS). The PASS theory and the CAS offer an expansion of the more traditional conceptualizations of intelligence. Moreover, the CAS is a prime example of an instrument guided by theory in both development and interpretation. The four CAS scales were designed to measure the four constructs central to the theory. Hence the composite scales are labeled Planning, Attention, Simultaneous, and Successive. For those who subscribe to a Gf-Gc theory or a more traditional approach to the assessment of intelligence, the interpretation of results from the CAS may seem awkward or difficult. For example, most intelligence tests include a verbal scale or a scale designed to measure crystallized intelligence. The CAS has no such scale. On the other hand, interpretation of the CAS flows directly from the theory on which it was based.

The effects of basing intelligence tests on the confluence of theory and research findings are at least threefold. First, test-specific training is of less value. Once a psychologist knows these theories, which are marked by numerous similarities, he or she can interpret most modern intelligence, tests with confidence. In other words, it is now important for a clinician to understand the constructs of intelligence, as opposed to receiving specific "Wechsler" or "Binet" training. Second, pre- and postprofessional training priority shifts to sufficient knowledge of theories of intelligence that inform modern test construction and interpretation. Third, as intelligence tests seek to measure similar core constructs, they increasingly resemble commodities. A psychologist's decision to use a particular test may be based not so much on differences in validity as on differences in preference; intelligence test selection will now include issues of administration time, availability of scoring software, packaging, price, and other convenience-oriented considerations.

Theory and Hypothesis Validation

To address the meager reliability and validity of score profiles, Kamphaus (2001) suggests an integrative method of interpretation that has two central premises. First, intelligence test results can only be interpreted meaningfully in the context of other assessment results (e.g., clinical findings, background information, and other sources of quantitative and qualitative information). Second, all interpretations made should be supported by research evidence and theory. Presumably, these two premises should mitigate against uniform interpretations that do not possess validity for a particular case (i.e., standard interpretations that are applied to case data but are at odds with information unique to an individual), as well as against interpretations that are refuted by research findings (i.e., interpretations that are based on clinical evidence but contradicted by research findings).

Failure to integrate intelligence test results with other case data can yield flawed interpretations. Matarazzo (1990) gives the following example from a neuropsychological evaluation in which the clinician failed to integrate test results with background information:

> There is little that is more humbling to a practitioner who uses the highest one or two Wechsler subtest scores as the only index of a patient's "premorbid" level of intellectual functioning and who therefore interprets concurrently obtained lower subtest scores as indexes of clear "impairment" and who is then shown by the opposing attorney elementary and high school transcripts that contain several global IQ scores, each of which were at the same low IQ levels as are suggested by currently obtained lowest Wechsler subtest scaled scores. (p. 1003)

To protect against such failures to integrate information, Kamphaus (2001) advises the intelligence test user to establish a standard for integrating intelligence test results with other findings. He suggests a standard of at least two pieces of corroborating evidence for each test interpretation made. Such a standard "forces" the examiner to carefully consider other findings and information prior to offering conclusions. A clinician, for example, may calculate a WISC-IV FSIQ score of 84 (below average) for a young girl and conclude that she possesses below-average intelligence. Even this seemingly obvious conclusion should be corroborated by two external sources of information. If the majority of the child's achievement scores fall into this range and her teacher reports that the child seems to be progressing more slowly than the majority of the children in her class, the conclusion of below-average intelligence has been corroborated by two sources of information external to the WISC-IV. On the other hand, if this child has previously been diagnosed with an anxiety disorder, and if both her academic achievement scores and her progress as reported by her teacher are average, the veracity of the WISC-IV scores may be in question. If she also appears highly anxious and agitated during the assessment session, the obtained scores may be even more questionable.

The requirement of research (i.e., validity) support for test-based interpretation is virtually mandatory in light of the publication of the *Standards for Educational and Psychological Testing* (American Educational Research Association, American Psychological Association, & National Council on Measurement in Education, 1999) and the increased expectations of consumers for assessment accuracy (Kamphaus, 2001). Clinical "impressions" of examiners, although salient, are no longer adequate for supporting interpretations of a child's intelligence scores (Matarazzo, 1990). Consider again the example above in which the young girl obtains a WISC-IV FSIQ score of 84. Let us assume that she has been independently found to have persistent problems with school achievement. Given the data showing the positive relationship between intelligence and achievement scores, the results seem consistent with the research literature and lend support to the interpretation of below-average intelligence. Should it become necessary to support the conclusion of below-average intelligence, the clinician could give testimony citing studies supporting the correlational relationship between intelligence and achievement test scores (Matarazzo, 1990).

TESTING RIVAL HYPOTHESES

There is some research to suggest that clinicians routinely tend to overestimate the accuracy of their conclusions. There is virtually no evidence to suggest that clinicians underestimate the amount of confidence that they have in their conclusions (Dawes, 1995). Therefore, intelligence test users should check the accuracy of their inferences by challenging them with alternative inferences.

A clinician may conclude, for example, that a client has a personal strength in verbal intelligence relative to nonverbal. An alternative hypothesis is that this inference is merely due to chance. A clinician may then use test manual discrepancy score tables to determine whether the difference between the two standard scores is likely to be reliable (i.e., statistically significant) and therefore not attributable to chance. Even if a difference is reliable, however, it may not be a "clinically meaningful" difference if it is a common occurrence in the population. Most intelligence test manuals also allow the user to test the additional hypothesis that the verbal–nonverbal score inference is reliable, but too small to be of clinical value for diagnosis or intervention, by determining the frequency of the score difference in the population. If a difference is also rare in the population, the original hypothesis (that the verbal and nonverbal difference reflects a real difference in the individual's cognitive abilities) provides a better explanation than the alternative rival hypothesis (that the verbal–nonverbal difference is not of importance) for understanding the examinee's cognitive performances.

Knowledge of theory is important above and beyond research findings, as theory allows the clinician to do a better job of conceptualizing an individual's scores. Clearer conceptualization of a child's cognitive status, for example, allows the clinician to better explain the child's test results to parents, teachers, colleagues, and other consumers of the test findings. Parents will often want to know the etiology of the child's scores. They will question, "Is it my fault for not reading to her?" or "Did he inherit this problem? My father had the same problems in school." Without adequate theoretical knowledge, clinicians will find themselves unprepared to give reasonable answers to such questions.

CONCLUSION

In this chapter, we have presented several overarching historical approaches to the interpretation of intelligence tests. For heuristic purposes, these approaches are portrayed as though they were entirely separate in their inception, development, and limitations. In the reality of clinical practice, however, much overlap exists. Moreover, aspects of each of these approaches continue to date. For example, since Spearman's (1927) publication of findings in support of a central ability underlying performance on multiple tasks, clinicians typically have interpreted a single general intelligence score. Most intelligence tests yield a general ability score, and research continues to provide evidence for the role of a general ability or g factor (McDermott & Glutting, 1997). In Carroll's (1993) hierarchical theory, g remains at the apex of the model. Therefore, the ongoing practice of interpreting this factor seems warranted, and elements of what we describe as the first wave remain. At the same time, clinicians continue to consider an individual's profile of scores. For the most part, the days of making psychiatric diagnoses or predictions of psychiatric symptoms on the basis of intelligence test scores as Rapaport and his colleagues (1945–1946) suggested are past, but profiles are still discussed—that is, in terms of ability profiles related to achievement or educational outcomes. Furthermore, as was the case in what we describe as the third wave, results from psychometric analyses still inform and guide our interpretations. Now, however, they are also integrated into broad descriptions and theories of intelligence. Carroll's theory is the result of factor-analytic research, and writers have labeled many of the dominant theories of intelligence as *psychometric* in their approach (Neisser et al., 1996). Thus we see the progress in the area of intellectual assessment and interpretation as an evolution, rather than a series of disjointed starts and stops. This evolution has culminated in the integration of empirical research, theory development, and test design, resulting in more accurate and meaningful test interpretation.

What Will Be the Fifth Wave of Intelligence Test Interpretation?

Of course, the substance and direction of the next wave in intelligence test interpretation remain unknown. What seems safe to predict is that ongoing educational reform and public policy mandates will continue to shape intellectual assessment and their associated interpretations. The influence of educational needs and public policy were present when the first formal intelligence tests were introduced over a century ago, and their influence has not abated in subsequent years. This becomes a particularly salient issue today, as legislators at the federal level are involved in discussions regarding the definitions of learning disabilities and other special education service categories. Should substantive changes occur, they are very likely to have an impact on use and interpretation of intelligence test results.

We hypothesize that the next wave will focus on the publication of new tests with stronger evidence of content validity; if the ultimate purpose of intelligence testing is to sample behavior representing a construct and then draw inferences about that construct, the process of interpretation is limited by the clarity of the construct(s) being measured. It may also be time to apply a broader concept of *content validity* to intelligence test interpretation (e.g., Flanagan & McGrew, 1997). Cronbach (1971) suggested such an expansion of the term more than three decades ago, observing:

> Whether the operations that finally constitute the test correspond to the specified universe is the question of content validity. It is so common in education to identify "content" with the subject matter of the curriculum that the broader application of the word here must be stressed. (p. 452)

As intelligence tests incorporate current research-based theories of intelligence into their design, psychological interpretations will become more reliable and valid. This trend will be modified as changes occur in intelligence-testing technology, fostered by breakthrough theories (e.g., neurological). Although it is difficult to draw inferences about the vast and somewhat undefined "universe" of cognitive functioning, it is also *de rigueur*. Psychologists make such interpretations about the complex universe of human behavior and functioning on a daily basis. The emergence of tests that better measure well-defined constructs will allow psychologists to provide better services to their clients than were possible even a decade ago.

ACKNOWLEDGMENTS

We would like to express our gratitude to Martha D. Petoskey and Anna W. Morgan for their contributions to the first edition of this chapter.

REFERENCES

American Educational Research Association, American Psychological Association, and National Council on Measurement in Education. (1999). *Standards for educational and psychological testing.* Washington, DC: American Educational Research Association.

Anastasi, A. (1985). Interpreting results from multiscore batteries. *Journal of Counseling and Development, 64,* 84–86.

Anastasi, A. (1988). *Psychological testing* (6th ed.). New York: Macmillan.

Bannatyne, A. (1974). Diagnosis: A note on recategorization of the WISC scale scores. *Journal of Learning Disabilities, 7,* 272–274.

Binet, A., & Simon, T. (1905). Methodes nouvelles pour le diagnostic du niveau intellectuel des anormaux [A new method for the diagnosis of the intellectual level of abnormal persons]. *L'Année Psychologique, 11,* 191–244.

Boring, E. G. (1929). *A history of experimental psychology.* New York: Century.

Carroll, J. B. (1993). *Human cognitive abilities: A survey of factor-analytic studies.* New York: Cambridge University Press.

Cattell, R. B. (1943). The measurement of adult intelligence. *Psychological Bulletin, 40,* 153–193.

Cohen, J. (1959). The factorial structure of the WISC at ages 7–6, 10–6, and 13–6. *Journal of Consulting Psychology, 23,* 285–299.

Cronbach, L. J. (1971). Test validation. In R. L. Thorndike (Ed.), *Educational measurement* (2nd ed., pp. 443–506). Washington, DC: American Council on Education.

Das, J. P., Naglieri, J. A., & Kirby, J. R. (1994). *Assessment of cognitive processes: The PASS theory of intelligence.* Needham Heights, MA: Allyn & Bacon.

Dawes, R. M. (1995). Standards of practice. In S. C. Hayes, V. M. Vollette, R. M. Dawes, & K. E. Grady (Eds.), *Scientific standards of psychological practice: Issues and recommendations* (pp. 31–43). Reno, NV: Context Press.

Elliott, C. D. (1990a). *Differential Ability Scales.* San Antonio, TX: Psychological Corporation.

Elliott, C. D. (1990b). *Differential Ability Scales: Introductory and technical handbook.* San Antonio, TX: Psychological Corporation.

Flanagan, D. P., & McGrew, K. S. (1997). A cross-battery approach to assessing and interpreting cognitive abilities: Narrowing the gap between practice and cognitive science. In D. P. Flanagan, J. L. Genshaft, & P. L. Harrison (Eds.), *Contemporary intellectual assessment: Theories, tests, and issues* (pp. 314–325). New York: Guilford Press.

French, J. L., & Hale, R. L. (1990). A history of the development of psychological and educational testing. In C. R. Reynolds & R. W. Kamphaus (Eds.), *Handbook of psychological and educational assessment of children* (pp. 3–28). New York: Guilford Press.

Fry, A. F., & Hale, S. (1996). Processing speed, working memory and fluid intelligence: Evidence for a developmental cascade. *Psychological Science, 7*(4), 237–241.

Goodenough, F. L. (1949). *Mental testing: Its history, principles, and applications.* New York: Rinehart.

Horn, J. L. (1988). Thinking about human abilities. In J. R. Nesselroade & R. B. Cattell (Eds.), *Handbook of multivariate psychology* (2nd ed., pp. 645–865). New York: Academic Press.

Horn, J. L., & Cattell, R. B. (1966). Refinement and test of the theory of fluid and crystallized general intelligences. *Journal of Educational Psychology, 57,* 253–270.

Kamphaus, R. W. (2001). *Clinical assessment of children's intelligence.* Needham Heights, MA: Allyn & Bacon.

Kaufman, A. S. (1979). *Intelligent testing with the WISC-R.* New York: Wiley-Interscience.

Kaufman, A. S. (1990). *Assessing adolescent and adult intelligence.* Needham Heights, MA: Allyn & Bacon.

Levine, A. J., & Marks, L. (1928). *Testing intelligence and achievement.* New York: Macmillan.

Luria, A. R. (1966). *Human brain and higher psychological processes.* New York: Harper & Row.

Matarazzo, J. D. (1990). Psychological assessment versus psychological testing?: Validation from Binet to the school, clinic, and courtroom. *American Psychologist, 45*(9), 999–1017.

Matheson, D. W., Mueller, H. H., & Short, R. H. (1984). The validity of Bannatyne's acquired knowledge category as a separate construct. *Journal of Psychoeducational Assessment, 2,* 279–291.

McDermott, P. A., Fantuzzo, J. W., Glutting, J. J., Watkins, M. W., & Baggaley, A. R. (1992). Illusions of meaning in the ipsative assessment of children's ability. *Journal of Special Education, 25,* 504–526.

McDermott, P. A., & Glutting, J. J. (1997). Informing stylistic learning behavior, disposition, and achievement through ability subtests—or, more illusion of meaning? *School Psychology Review, 26*(2), 163–176.

McGrew, K. S., & Woodcock, R. W. (2001). *Woodcock–Johnson III technical manual.* Itasca, IL: Riverside.

Naglieri, J. A., & Das, J. P. (1990). Planning, attention, simultaneous, and successive (PASS) cognitive processes as a model for intelligence. *Journal of Psychoeducational Assessment, 8*, 303–337.

Naglieri, J. A., & Das, J. P. (1997). *Das–Naglieri Cognitive Assessment System*. Itasca, IL: Riverside.

Neisser, U., Boodoo, G., Bouchard, T. J., Boykin, A. W., Brody, N., Ceci, S. J., et al. (1996). Intelligence: Knowns and unknowns. *American Psychologist, 51*, 77–101.

Pintner, R. (1923). *Intelligence testing*. New York: Holt, Rinehart & Winston.

Rapaport, D., Gil, M., & Schafer, R. (1945–1946). *Diagnostic psychological testing* (2 vols.) Chicago: Year Book Medical.

Reynolds, C. R., & Kamphaus, R. W. (2003). *Reynolds Intellectual Assessment Scales*. Lutz, FL: Psychological Assessment Resources.

Roid, G. H. (2003). *Stanford–Binet Intelligence Scales, Fifth Edition*. Itasca, IL: Riverside.

Spearman, C. (1927). *The abilities of man*. New York: Macmillan.

Terman, L. M. (1916). *The measurement of intelligence: An explanation and a complete guide for the use of the Stanford revision and extensions of the Binet–Simon Scale*. Boston: Houghton Mifflin.

Terman, L. M., & Merrill, M. A. (1937). *Measuring intelligence: A guide to the administration of the new Revised Stanford–Binet Tests of Intelligence*. Boston: Houghton Mifflin.

Wechsler, D. (1939). *The measurement of adult intelligence*. Baltimore: Williams & Wilkins.

Wechsler, D. (1944). *The measurement of adult intelligence* (3rd ed.). Baltimore: Williams & Wilkins.

Wechsler, D. (1949). *Wechsler Intelligence Scale for Children*. San Antonio, TX: Psychological Corporation.

Wechsler, D. (1958). *The measurement and appraisal of adult intelligence* (4th ed.). Baltimore: Williams & Wilkins.

Wechsler, D. (1974). *Wechsler Intelligence Scale for Children—Revised*. New York: Psychological Corporation.

Wechsler, D. (1991). *Wechsler Intelligence Scale for Children—Third edition*. San Antonio, TX: Psychological Corporation.

Woodcock, R. W., & Johnson, M. B. (1989). *Woodcock–Johnson Psycho-Educational Battery—Revised*. Allen, TX: DLM Teaching Resources.

Woodcock, R. W., McGrew, K. S., & Mather, N. (2001). *Woodcock–Johnson III*. Itasca, IL: Riverside.

II

Contemporary and Emerging Theoretical Perspectives

Part II of this textbook includes several chapters focusing on major theories of intelligence. Most of the chapters described in this section were authored or coauthored by the individuals who developed these theories and are updated versions of chapters that appeared in the first edition (1997) of this textbook. A comprehensive description of each theory is provided, focusing specifically on its historical origins, as well as the rationale and impetus for its development and modifications made to the theory since the publication of the first edition. In addition, the component parts and empirical support for each theory are enumerated, along with a discussion of the mechanisms through which the model has been operationalized.

The first chapter in this section of the book (Chapter 3) is "Foundations for Better Understanding of Cognitive Abilities," coauthored by John L. Horn and Nayena Blankson. This chapter provides a historical overview of the development and refinement of and validity for structural theories of intelligence, beginning with Spearman's functional unity theory of general ability and ending with the Gf-Gc theory of multiple intelligences. Chapter 4 is a reprint of a chapter from the 1997 edition of the textbook—"The Three-Stratum Theory of Cognitive Abilities," by the late John B. Carroll. Carroll summarized his development of the three-stratum theory and described his review of the factor-analytic research on the structure of cognitive abilities, which encompassed nearly all of the more important and classic factor-analytic studies collected over a period of nearly six decades.

A theory that encompasses many distinct intelligences is Gardner's theory of multiple intelligences (or MI theory). This theory is described by Jie-Qi Chen and Howard Gardner in Chapter 5, "Assessment Based on Multiple-Intelligences Theory." Another expanded theory of intelligence is presented in Chapter 6, "The Triarchic Theory of Successful Intelligence," by Robert J. Sternberg. In this chapter, Sternberg focuses on the abilities needed for successful intelligence and presents his three interrelated subtheories of intelligence (componential, experiential, and contextual) within an updated framework. Still another alternative to traditional theoretical conceptions of intelligence is presented by Jack A. Naglieri and J. P. Das in Chapter 7, "Planning, Attention, Simultaneous, Successive Theory: A Revision of the Concept of Intelligence." Naglieri and Das have based their definition of the components of human intelligence on the work of A. R. Luria, whose research identified functional aspects of brain structures.

Part II culminates with "The Cattell–Horn–Carroll Theory of Cognitive Abilities: Past, Present, and Future" (Chapter 8), by Kevin S. McGrew. In this chapter, McGrew presents a synthesized Carroll and Horn–Cattell Gf-Gc framework.
McGrew's chapter represents a much-needed "bridge" between the theoretical
and empirical research and the practice of assessing and interpreting human cognitive abilities.

The theories presented in Part II represent significant departures from traditional views and conceptualizations of the structure of intelligence. Although the
theories included in this section have undergone varying degrees of empirical validation, they all represent viable foundations from which to develop and interpret measures of intelligence—measures that may lead to greater insights into the
nature, structure, and neurobiological substrates of cognitive functioning, and
that may be more appropriate for assessing the cognitive abilities of individuals
with learning difficulties and disabilities and from culturally, linguistically, and
ethnically diverse backgrounds.

3

Foundations for Better Understanding of Cognitive Abilities

JOHN L. HORN
NAYENA BLANKSON

PURPOSES AND PROVISOS

The extended theory of fluid and crystallized (Gf and Gc) cognitive abilities is wrong, of course, even though it may be the best account we currently have of the organization and development of abilities thought to be indicative of human intelligence. All scientific theory is wrong. It is the job of science to improve theory. That requires identifying what is wrong with it and finding out how to change it to make it more nearly correct. That is what we try to do in this chapter. First, we lay out the current theory. Then we indicate major things that we think are wrong with it. We end by suggesting some lines of research that may lead to improvement of the theory.

In laying out the theory, we speak of what we think we know. We say that something is known if there is evidence to support the claim that it is known. Since such evidence is never fully adequate or complete, we do not imply that what we say "is known" is really (*really*) known to be true. We do not provide full critiques to indicate why what we say is not necessarily true, but we provide provisos and cautions, and put research in a context such that major limitations can be seen.

Among the provisos are some we can point to immediately in this introduction.

First, because we depend on developmental evidence to a considerable extent, we point out that research on the development of human abilities is seriously lacking in major features of design required for strong inference about cause and effect. None of the research employs a controlled, manipulative (experimental) design in which age, genes, gender, or any of a host of other quite relevant independent variables are randomly assigned. Such design is, of course, impossible in studies of human development. But the fact that it is impossible doesn't correct for its lack. The design is weak. Many relevant independent variables, including age, are confounded. Effects cannot be isolated. For this reason, what we say "is known" can only be a judgment call.

A second major proviso stems from the fact that most of the research we refer to as indicating "what is known about development" is cross-sectional. This means that usually we are referring to findings of age differences, not findings of age changes. Age differences may suggest age changes, but they do not establish them. Yet, we speak of such differences in ways that imply that they indicate age changes. Our statements of "what is known" are judgments based on such incomplete evidence.

A third proviso stems from the fact that almost all the results we review are derived from averages calculated across measures, not on changes within individuals. This is no less true of the findings from repeated-measures longitudinal research than of the findings from cross-sectional research. It means that the evidence is not directly indicative of change within persons.

This is a rather subtle point, often not well recognized. It is worthwhile to take a moment to consider it in more detail. To do this, look at a simple example that illustrates the problem.

Suppose $N1$ people increase in an ability by $k1$ units from age $A1$ to $A2$, while $N2$ people decrease $k2$ in this ability over the same age period; assume no error. If $N1 = N2$ and $k1 = k2$, the net effect of averaging the measures at $A1$ and $A2$ is zero, which fosters the clearly wrong conclusion that there is no change. Yet this is the kind of finding on which we base our statements about what is known. Averages at different ages or times of measurement are the findings. Findings such as that of this example are regarded as indicating "no aging change." The correct conclusion is that some people have increased in the ability, while other people have decreased.

In this simple, balanced example, it is easy to see that the conclusion is incorrect. But the incorrectness of this conclusion is no less true when it is not so easily seen—as when $N1$ and $N2$ and $k1$ and $k2$ are not perfectly balanced. If there are more $N1$ people than $N2$ people, for example, and $k1$ and $k2$ are equal, then the incorrect conclusion is that the ability has increased from $A1$ to $A2$. On the other hand, if $N1$ equals $N2$ but $k2$ is larger than $k1$, the incorrect conclusion is that the ability has decreased from $A1$ to $A2$. Every other possible combination of these N's and k's is also incorrect. Most important, none of the results directly indicate what is true (assuming no error)—namely, that some people have increased in the ability and others have decreased. In regard to what is lawfully happening, it is not a matter of averaging over those who improve by $k1$ amounts and those who decline by $k2$ amounts. It's a matter of whether there is nonchance improvement and/or decline—and if so, by how much, over how long, and (most important) in relation to what variables that might indicate why. Indeed, it takes only one individual's reliable improvement in some function to disprove a generalization based on averages that the function necessarily declines.

In general, then, as we report "what is known," readers should remain aware that what we say is known may not be true. But readers should also remain aware that what we say is known may be true. The evidence of averages for groupings of individuals *may* indicate processes of age changes within individuals. The fact that such findings do not necessarily indicate such changes does not prove the opposite. Indeed, the findings provide a basis for reasonable judgments. We judge (with provisos) that most likely the averages indicate what we say is known.

What is known about human cognitive capabilities derives primarily from two kinds of research: (1) *structural research* (studies of the covariation patterns among tests designed to indicate basic features of human intelligence) and (2) *developmental research* (studies designed to indicate the ways in which cognitive capabilities develop over age). Our own particular understanding of development has derived primarily from the study of adults, but we use some evidence from research on children as well. We also use bits of evidence derived from research on genetic, neural, academic, and occupational correlates of abilities and their development.

EVIDENCE OF STRUCTURAL ORGANIZATION

The accumulated results from over 100 years of research on covariations among tests, tasks, and paradigms designed to identify fundamental features of human intelligence indicate no fewer than 87 distinct, different elementary capacities. Almost entirely, the covariation model has been one of linear relationship—and to a major extent and in the final analyses, this work has been based on a common-factor, simple-structure factor-analytic model. Thus the implicit theory has been that relationships indicating order among abilities are linear, and that a relatively small number of separate, independently distributed (although often interrelated) basic capacities account for the myriad of individual differences in abilities that thus far have been observed and measured. The findings of this research and the resulting structural theory are working assumptions—first approximations to the description and organization of human cognitive capacities.

The 80-some abilities indicated in this work are regarded as first-order factors among tests. They are often referred to as *primary mental abilities*. There are likely to be many more such elementary capacities, but this is the number indicated thus far by structural evidence (Carroll, 1993; Horn, 1991).

The same kind of factor-analytic evidence on which the theory of primary abilities is based has also indicated some eight (or nine) broader, second-order factors among the primary factors.[1] Rather full descriptions of these abilities are given in Carroll (1993), Flanagan, Genshaft, and Harrison (1997), McGrew (1994), McGrew and Flanagan (1998), McGrew, Werder, and Woodcock (1991), and elsewhere in the current volume. Here we indicate the nature of these abilities and the relationships between first-order and second-order abilities in Table 3.1, with descriptions of primary abilities under headings of the second-order ability with which each primary ability is most closely associated.

Most of what is known about the development of abilities, and most theories about the nature of human intelligence, pertain to the second-order abilities. These can be described briefly as follows:

Acculturation knowledge (Gc), measured in tests indicating breadth and depth of knowledge of the language, concepts, and information of the dominant culture.

Fluid reasoning (Gf), measured in tasks requiring reasoning. It indicates capacities for identifying relationships, comprehending implications, and drawing inferences within content that is either novel or equally familiar to all.

Short-term apprehension and retrieval (SAR), also referred to as *short-term memory (Gsm)* and *working memory.* It is measured in a variety of tasks that require one to maintain awareness of elements of an immediate situation (i.e., the span of a minute or so).

Fluency of retrieval from long-term storage (TSR), also labeled *long-term memory (Glm).* It is measured in tasks indicating consolidation for storage and tasks that require retrieval through association of information stored minutes, hours, weeks, and years before.

Processing speed (Gs), although involved in almost all intellectual tasks, it is measured most purely in rapid scanning and comparisons in intellectually simple tasks in which almost all people would get the right answer if the task were not highly speeded.

Visual processing (Gv), measured in tasks involving visual closure and constancy, as well as fluency in recognizing the way objects appear in space as they are rotated and flip-flopped in various ways.

Auditory processing (Ga), measured in tasks that involve perception of sound patterns under distraction or distortion, maintaining awareness of order and rhythm among sounds, and comprehending elements of groups of sounds.

Quantitative knowledge (Gq), measured in tasks requiring understanding and application of the concepts and skills of mathematics.

The structural evidence indicating that the primary abilities are parts of these distinct higher-order common factors has been obtained in samples that differ in gender, level of education, ethnicity, nationality, language, and historical period. The higher-order abilities account for the reliable individual-differences variability measured in conglomerate IQ tests and neuropsychological batteries. What is known about IQ, and what is referred to as Spearman's *g*, are known analytically in terms of the second-order abilities of which IQ and *g* are composed.

The higher-order abilities are positively correlated, but independent. Independence is indicated in a first instance by structural evidence: A best-weighted linear combination of any set of seven of the second-order abilities does not account for the reliable covariance among the elements of the eighth such ability.[2] More fundamentally, independence is indicated by evidence of distinct construct validities—that is, the evidence that measures representing different factors have different relationships with a variety of other variables (principally age, but also variables of neurology, behavioral genetics, and school and occupational performance).

TABLE 3.1. Primary Abilities Described under Headings Indicating Second-Order Abilities

Primary ability label		Description
Gv: Visualization and spatial orientation abilities		
Vi	Visualization	Mentally manipulate forms to "see" how they would look under altered conditions
S	Spatial orientation	Visually imagine parts out of place and put them in place (e.g., solve jigsaw puzzles)
Cs	Speed of closure	Identify Gestalt when parts of the whole are missing—Gestalt closure
Cf	Flexibility of closure	Find a particular figure embedded within distracting lines and figures
Ss	Spatial planning	Survey a spatial field to find a path through it (e.g., pencil mazes)
Xa	Figural flexibility	Try out possible arrangements of visual pattern to find one that satisfies conditions
Le	Length estimation	Estimate length of distances between points
DFI	Figural fluency	Produce different figures, using the lines of a stimulus figure
DFS	Seeing illusions	Report illusions in such tests as the Muller–Lyer, Sanders, and Poggendorf
Ga: Abilities of listening and hearing		
ACV	Auditory comprehend	Demonstrate understanding of oral communications
TT	Temporal tracking	Demonstrate understanding of sequencing in sounds (e.g., reorder sets of tones)
AR	Auditory relations	Demonstrate understanding of relations among tones (e.g., identify notes of a chord)
TP	Identify tone patterns	Show awareness of differences in arrangements of tones
RYY	Judging rhythms	Identify and continue a beat
AMS	Auditory span memory	Immediately recall a set of notes played once
DS	Hear distorted speech	Show understanding of speech that has been distorted in different ways
Gc: Acculturational knowledge abilities		
V	Verbal comprehension	Demonstrate understanding of words, sentences, paragraphs
Se	Seeing problems	Suggest ways to deal with problems (e.g., fix a toaster)
Rs	Syllogistic reasoning	Given stated premises, draw logical conclusions even when nonsensical
VSI	Verbal closure	Show comprehension of sentences when parts are missing—verbal Gestalt
CBI	Behavioral relations	Judge interaction between persons to estimate how one feels about a situation
Mk	Mechanical knowledge	Identify tools, equipment, principles for solving mechanical problems
Vi	General information	Indicate understanding of a wide range of information
Gf: Abilities of reasoning under novel conditions		
I	Inductive reasoning	Indicate a principle of relationships among elements
R	General reasoning	Find solutions to verbal problems
CFR	Figural relations	Solve problems of relationships among figures
CMR	Semantic relations	Demonstrate awareness of relationships among pieces of information
CSC	Semantic classification	Show how symbols do not belong in class of several symbols
CFC	Concept formation	Given several examples of a concept, identify new instances
SAR: Abilities of short-term apprehension and retrieval		
Ma	Associate memory	When presented with one element of associated pair, recall the other element
Ms	Span memory	Immediately recall sets of elements after one presentation
Mm	Meaningful memory	Immediately recall items of a meaningfully related set
MMC	Chunking memory	Immediately recall elements by categories in which they are classified
MSS	Memory for order	Immediately recall the position of an element within a set of elements
DRM	Disrupted memory	Recall last word in previous sentence after being presented with other sentences

(continued)

TABLE 3.1. *(continued)*

Primary ability label		Description
TSR: Abilities of long-term storage and retrieval		
DLR	Delayed retrieval	Recall material learned hours before
DMT	Originality	Produce clever expressions or interpretations (e.g., story plots)
DMC	Spontaneous flexibility	Produce diverse functions and classifications (e.g., uses of a pencil)
Fi	Ideational fluency	Produce ideas about a stated condition (e.g., lady holding a baby)
Fe	Expression fluency	Produce different ways of saying much the same thing
Fa	Association fluency	Produce words similar in meaning to a given word
Gs: Speed of thinking abilities		
P	Perceptual speed	Quickly distinguish similar but different visual patterns
CDS	Correct decision speed	Quickly find or state correct answers to easy problems
FWS	Flexible writing speed	Quickly copy printed mixed upper- and lower-case letters and words
Gq: Quantitative mathematical abilities		
CMI	Estimation	Indicate information required to solve mathematical problems
Ni	Number facility	Do basic operations of arithmetic quickly and accurately
CMS	Algebraic reasoning	Find solutions for problems that can be framed algebraically

This indication of structural organization of human abilities is referred to as *extended Gf-Gc theory*. This theory was derived in the first instance from Spearman's (1927) theory of a general, common *g* factor pervading all cognitive capabilities. It was modified notably by Thurstone's (1938, 1947) theory of some six or seven primary mental abilities. It was then altered by Cattell's (1941, 1957, 1971) recognition that while the Thurstone primary abilities were positively correlated and this positive manifold might indicate Spearman's *g*, still the general factor did not describe the evidence; there had to be at least two independent and broad common factors—Gf and Gc—because some of the abilities thought to indicate the *g* factor were associated in quite different ways with neurological damage and aging in adulthood. The extended theory then grew out of Cattell's theory, as evidence accumulated to indicate that two broad abilities did not represent relationships for visual, auditory, and basic memory functions. Abilities in these domains, too, were associated in notably different ways with genetic, environmental, biological, and developmental variables. The two-factor theory had to be extended to a theory of several dimensions, as suggested by the listings above and in Table 3.1.

The broad abilities appear to represent behavioral organizations founded in neural structures and functions. The abilities are realized through a myriad of learning and bio-logical/genetic influences operating over the course of a lifetime. Although there are suggestions that some of the abilities are somewhat more related to genetic determinants than are others, the broad patterns do not define a clean distinction between genetic and environmental determinants. Each broad ability involves learning, and is manifested as a consequence of many factors that can affect learning over years of development. Similarly, each ability is affected by genetic factors, as these can be expressed at different times throughout development. More detailed and scholarly accounts of the structural evidence are provided in Carroll (1993), Cattell (1971), Detterman (1993), Flanagan and colleagues (1997), Horn (1998), Masanaga and Horn (2000), McArdle, Hamagami, Meredith, and Bradway (2001), McArdle and Woodcock (1998), McGrew (1994), McGrew and Flanagan (1998), McGrew and colleagues (1991), and Perfect and Maylor (2000).

DEVELOPMENTAL EVIDENCE

The structural evidence indicates what is associated with what. The developmental evidence indicates what is correlated with age.[3] The structural evidence—showing how abilities indicate distinct factors—has informed the design of developmental research aimed at identifying how abilities relate to age.

Variables that correlate to indicate a factor should relate to age in a manner indicating that they represent the same function or process. Similarly, the evidence indicating how different abilities correlate with age has informed the design of structural studies. Variables that change together over age should correlate to indicate the same factor. To the extent that variables both correlate to indicate the same factor and change together to indicate the same function, the two lines of evidence converge to provide evidence of cognitive processes. For the most part, this is the kind of evidence that has produced extended Gf-Gc theory. To a lesser extent, the theory is based on evidence derived from studies of behavioral-genetic and neurological relationships.

The second-order abilities of structural research are positively correlated. This suggests that there must be some higher-order organization among them. It is widely believed that this higher-order organization must be Spearman's g, or something very like it (Jensen, 1998). It turns out, however, that this is not a good explanation of the evidence. The interrelationships among the second-order abilities and their relationships with indicators of development and neurological functioning do not indicate a single factor. Rather, they suggest something along the following lines:

1. *Vulnerable abilities.* Gf, SAR, and Gs constitute a cluster of abilities to which much of Spearman's theory does indeed apply—in particular, his descriptions of capacities for apprehension and the eduction of relations and correlates. The abilities of this cluster are interrelated and associated in much the same way with variables indicating neurological, genetic, and aging effects.

2. *Expertise abilities.* Gc, TSR, and Gq constitute a cluster of abilities that correspond to the outcomes specified in the investment hypothesis of Cattell's theory of fluid and crystallized intelligence. It turns out that what Cattell described in investment theory is largely the same as what is described as the development of expertise in cognitive capabilities (which can be distinguished from various other kinds of expertise and from expertise in general). An important new twist on this integration of

theory is recognition of new abilities in this cluster that in some ways parallel the abilities of the vulnerable cluster, but are developmentally independent of the vulnerable abilities. These new abilities differ from the vulnerable abilities not only in terms of structural relationships, but also in terms of their relationships to learning and socialization determinants. It is hypothesized that they have different relationships, also, with neurological, genetic, and aging influences.

3. *Sensory-perceptual abilities.* Mainly, the evidence in this case indicates that the abilities defining Gv and Ga are distinct from the other two clusters. They have some of the qualities of the vulnerable abilities, but they also have qualities of the expertise abilities; their relationships do not put them clearly in either class. More than this, they are closely linked to sensory modalities and appear to represent particular characteristics, strengths, and weaknesses of these modalities.

Most of the developmental evidence of which we speak derives from studies of adulthood. To a very considerable extent, this research has been directed at describing declines, and the findings consistent with this view are for the abilities of Gf, Gs, and SAR. Almost incidentally, the research directed at identifying adulthood declines has adduced evidence of age-related improvements and maintenance of some abilities; the findings in this case are primarily in respect to the abilities of Gc, TSR, and Gq. The aging curves for the sensory-perceptual abilities generally fall between those for the vulnerable and expertise abilities—not declining as early, as regularly, or as much as the former, and not improving as consistently or as much as the latter. Also, the declines often can be linked directly to declines in a sensory modality or damage to a particular function of the neural system.

The research producing the developmental evidence has been both cross-sectional and longitudinal. Although these two kinds of research have different strengths and weaknesses, and control for and reveal different kinds of influences, in studies of abilities they have most often led to very similar conclusions (Schaie, 1996). The results differ somewhat in detail—the average age at which plateaus and declines in development are reached,[4] for example—but as concerns which abilities decline and which improve and the general phases of development through which such changes occur, the evidence of repeated-measures longitudinal and cross-sectional research is essentially the same. In the following section, we summarize this evidence within an explanatory framework.

Research of the future should probably be directed at understanding abilities that are maintained or that improve with age in adulthood, and our thought is that expertise abilities in particular should be most carefully studied. To provide perspective for this view, we first review evidence on abilities that do not decline, or decline little and late in adulthood, and then consider the more extensive evidence and theory pertaining to aging decline.

Capabilities for Which There Is Little or No Aging Decline

The results indicating improvement and maintenance of abilities has come largely from the same studies in which evidence of aging decline was sought and found. The two most prominent kinds of abilities for which there is replicated evidence of improvement in adulthood are those of Gc (indicating breadth of knowledge of the dominant culture) and those of TSR (indicating fluency in retrieval of information from this store of knowledge).

Gc: Knowledge

The abilities of Gc are often referred to in efforts to specify what is most important about human intelligence. They are indicative of the intelligence of a culture, inculcated into individuals through systematic influences of acculturation. The range of such abilities is large. No particular battery of tests is known to sample the entire range. The sum of the achievement tests of the Woodcock–Johnson Psycho-Educational Battery—Revised (WJ-R) has probably provided the most nearly representative measure. The Verbal IQ of the Wechsler Adult Intelligence Scales (WAIS) has been a commonly used estimate. Indicators of the factor are measures of vocabulary, esoteric analogies, listening comprehension,

and knowledge in the sciences, social studies, and humanities. Such measures correlate substantially with socioeconomic status, amount and quality of education, and other indicators of acculturation.

On average, through most of adulthood, there is increase with age in Gc knowledge (e.g., Botwinick, 1978; Cattell, 1971; Harwood & Naylor, 1971; Horn, 1998; Horn & Cattell, 1967; Horn & Hofer, 1992; Kaufman, 1990; Rabbitt & Abson, 1991; Schaie, 1996; Stankov & Horn, 1980; Woodcock, 1995). Results from some studies suggest improvement into the 80s (e.g., Harwood & Naylor, 1971, for WAIS Information, Comprehension, and Vocabulary). Such declines as are indicated show up in the averages late in adulthood—age 70 and beyond—and are small (Schaie, 1996). If differences in years of formal education are statistically controlled for, the increment of Gc with advancing age is increased (Horn, 1989; Kaufman, 1990).

TSR: Tertiary Storage and Retrieval

Two different kinds of measures indicate TSR abilities. Both kinds of indicators involve encoding and consolidation of information in long-term storage, and both involve fluency of retrieval from that storage. The parameters of association that characterize encoding and consolidation also characterize retrieval (Bower, 1972, 1975; Estes, 1974).

The first kind of test to identify TSR involves retrieval through association over periods of time that range from a few minutes to a few hours or longer. The time lapse must be sufficient to ensure that consolidation occurs, for this is what distinguishes these measures from indicators of SAR. For example, if a paired-associates test were to be used to measure the factor, recall would need to be obtained at least 5 minutes after presentation of the stimuli; if recall were obtained immediately after presentation, the test would measure SAR.

The second kind of test indicates associations among pieces of information that would have been consolidated and stored in a system of categories (as described by Broadbent, 1966) in the distant past, not just a few hours earlier. In a word association test, for example, an individual provides words similar in meaning to a given word. The person accesses an association category of information and pulls information from that category into a response mode.

Tests to measure TSR may be given under time limits, but these limits must be generous, so that subjects have time to drain association categories. If given under highly speeded conditions, the tests will measure cognitive speed (Gs), not TSR.

The retrieval of TSR is from the knowledge store of Gc, but facility in retrieval is independent of measures of Gc—independent in the sense that the correlation between TSR and Gc is well below their respective internal consistencies, and in the sense that they have different patterns of correlations with other variables.

For TSR abilities, as for Gc, the research results usually indicate improvement or no age differences throughout most of adulthood (Horn, 1968; Horn & Cattell, 1967; Horn & Noll, 1994; Schaie, 1996; Stankov & Horn, 1980; Woodcock, 1995).

Abilities That Decline with Age

Research on human abilities initially focused on infancy and childhood development and was directed at identifying abilities that characterize the intelligence of the human species. Research on adults focused from the start on abilities that, it was feared, declined with age in adulthood, and the abilities considered were those that had been identified in research on children. This research did not seek to identify abilities that characterize the intelligence of adults. That focus shifted a bit with the discovery that some of the abilities identified in childhood research improved with age in adulthood. In recent years the emphasis has shifted somewhat yet again, with recognition that cognitive expertise emerges in adulthood. Even today, however, the predominant view of human intelligence is that it is something that develops primarily only in childhood and declines with age in adulthood. The predominant view is that human intelligence is best characterized by the vulnerable abilities—Gf, SAR, and Gs.

The term *vulnerable* to characterize the Gf, SAR, and Gs abilities was adopted largely because the averages for these abilities were found to decrease with age in ad-

ulthood and to decline irreversibly with deleterious neurological and physiological changes—such as those that occur when high fever persists, or blood pressure drops to low levels, or anoxia is induced (as by alcoholic inebriation), or parts of the brain are infected or damaged (as by stroke). When it was found that in the same persons in whom vulnerable abilities declined, there were other abilities that improved (as in the case of adulthood aging) or either did not decline or the decline was reversible (as in the case of brain damage), the term *maintained* was coined to characterize these abilities—largely those of Gc, TSR, and Gq. What the research findings indicate is that when there is damage to particular parts of the brain (as in stroke), these abilities either do not decline (depending on the ability and where the damage is), or if there is decline, it is relatively small and does not persist. Thus the terms *vulnerable* and *maintained* signal a finding that in groups of people in whom some abilities decline, other abilities do not, and still other abilities improve. Though we must keep in mind that the findings are for averages, the suggestion is that within each of us some abilities are declining, others are being maintained, and some are improving. We have some reasonable ideas about "what" the vulnerable and maintained abilities are; we have less clear ideas about "why."

The findings are consistent in indicating that Gf, SAR, and Gs abilities are interrelated in a manner that calls for them to be considered together: Over most of the period of adulthood and in respect to many malfunctions of the central nervous system, there is decline in all three classes of abilities. Some notable differences, however, distinguish the three vulnerable abilities from one another.

Gf: Fluid Reasoning

The age-related decline in the Gf abilities is seen with measures of syllogisms and concept formation (McGrew et al., 1991); in reasoning with metaphors and analogies (Salthouse, 1987; Salthouse, Kausler, & Saults, 1990); with measures of comprehending series, as in letter series, figural series, and number series (Noll & Horn, 1998; Salthouse et al., 1990); and with measures of mental rotation, figural relations, matrices, and topology (Cattell, 1979). In each case, the decline is indicated most clearly if the elements of the test problems are novel—such that no advantage is given to people with more knowledge of the culture, more information, or better vocabulary.

The Gf abilities represent a kind of opposite to the Gc abilities: Whereas measures of Gc indicate the extent to which the knowledge of the culture has been incorporated by the individual, measures of Gf indicate abilities that depend minimally on knowledge of the culture.

But the feature that most clearly distinguishes the Gf abilities from the other vulnerable abilities is reasoning. All of the measures that most clearly define the Gf factor require, in one sense or another, reasoning. This is not to say that other measures do not fall on the factor, but it is to say that those other measures fall on other factors and are not the sine qua non of Gf. This will be seen more clearly as we consider how other abilities can account for some but not all of the reliable developmental changes in Gf.

SAR: Short-Term Memory

Memory is one of the most thoroughly studied constructs in psychology. There are many varieties of memory. The SAR factor indicates covariability among most of the many rather distinct kinds of short-term memory. This is the form of memory that has been most intensively studied in psychology.

There are two principal features of short-term memory. One is that it is memory over retrieval and recognition periods of less than 2 minutes. Retrieval and recognition over longer periods of time bring in other factors (largely the TSR factor), which we discuss later. The second feature is that it is memory for largely unrelated material; that is, most people usually do not have a logical system for organizing of—or making sense out of—the elements to be remembered. We have more to say about this later, too, particularly when we discuss expertise.

Over and above these two distinguishing characteristics of SAR, there is considerable heterogeneity among the various different short-term memory indicators of the factor. The different indicators have somewhat different relations to age in adulthood, for ex- ample, and thus are indicative of different aspects of a short-term memory function. It's as if SAR were an organ—say, analogous to the heart—in which different parts are more and less susceptible to the ravages of age. It is rather as if the right auricle of the heart were more susceptible than the left auricle to damages produced by coarctation of the aorta (which, indeed, is true).

Clang Memory

One notable way in which these different indicators of short-term memory are distinguished is in respect to the period of time over which retrieval or recognition is required. Characterized in this way, short-term memory ranges from apprehension (retrieval after milliseconds) (Sperling, 1960) to very short-term memory (recency), to somewhat longer short-term memory (primacy), to short-term span memory (retrieval after as much as a minute), and to what we have referred to above as not being short-term, and not indicating the SAR factor at all, but rather intermediate-term memory (retrieval after 2–10 minutes) and long-term memory (Atkinson & Shiffrin, 1968; Waugh & Norman, 1965—retrieval after hours, days, weeks, months, years). The intermediate-term and long-term kinds of memory indicate TSR, not SAR. The TSR factor does not decline with age in adulthood. Its correlates with other variables are generally different from those of SAR.

Recency and primacy are serial-position memory functions. These have been studied in considerable detail (Glanzer & Cunitz, 1966). *Recency* is memory for the last elements in a string of elements presented over time. It dissipates quickly; if there is delay of as much as 20 seconds, it is usually absent in most people. *Primacy* is memory for the first elements in a string of elements (retention being somewhat longer—30 seconds). Primacy seems to be an early indication of the consolidation that can lead to long-term memory. There is some aging decline in both recency and primacy, but the decline is small.

The total forward memory span encompasses both primacy and recency, and also the memory for elements in between the first and the last elements in a string. This component of SAR is often referred to as indicating a "magical number seven plus or minus two"

(Miller, 1956). Most of us are able to remember only about seven things that we do not organize (i.e., unrelated things). But there are individual differences in this: Some can remember up to about nine unrelated things; others can remember only as many as five such things. The aging decline of this memory is small, too, but somewhat larger than the decline for either primacy or recency (Craik, 1977; Craik & Trehub, 1982; Horn, Donaldson, & Engstrom, 1981).

Short-Term Working Memory

Backward memory span helps define SAR, but is also often a prominent indicator of Gf. A backward span memory test requires recall of a string of elements in the reverse of the order in which they were presented (e.g., recall of a telephone number in the reverse of the order in which it would be dialed). The average span for such memory is about five elements, plus or minus two. Age-related differences in backward span memory are substantial and in this respect notably different from age-related differences in forward span memory. Not only is the age-related decline for this memory much larger than the decline for forward span memory, but also it is more correlated with the aging decline of Gf.

Backward span memory is one of several operational definitions of *short-term working* memory (STWM; Baddeley, 1993, 1994; Carpenter & Just, 1989; Stankov, 1988). STWM is an ability to hold information in the span of immediate apprehension while doing other cognitive things, such as converting the order of things into a different order (as in backward span), searching for particular symbols, or solving problems. Another operational definition of STWM that illustrates this characteristic is a test that requires one to remember the last word in each sentence as one reads a passage of several sentences under directions to be prepared to answer questions about the passage; the measure of STWM is the number of last words recalled.

Indicators of STWM are dual-factor measures, as much related to Gf as they are to SAR. As noted, they also have larger (absolute-value) negative relationships to age (Craik, 1977; Craik & Trehub, 1982; Salthouse, 1991; Schaie, 1996).

An Exception: Expertise Wide-Span Memory (EWSM)

This is a form of short-term memory that is not indicative of SAR and that appears to increase, not decline, over much of adulthood (Ericsson & Kintsch, 1995; Masanaga & Horn, 2000, 2001). In some respects EWSM appears to be operationally the same as STWM (or even forward span memory); it is memory for a set of what can appear to be quite unrelated elements. There is a crucial difference, however: In EWSM the elements that can appear to be quite unrelated (and are quite unrelated for some people) can be seen to be related by an expert. For example, chess pieces arranged on a chessboard can seem to be quite unrelated to one who is not expert in understanding chess, but to a chess expert there can be relationships in the configuration of such pieces. Such relationships enable the expert to remember many more than merely seven plus or minus two pieces and their locations.[5] Also, such memories can be retained by experts (to varying degrees for varying levels of expertise) for much longer than a minute or two. In blindfold chess, for example, the expert retains memory for many more than seven elements for much more than 2 minutes.

Thus EWSM does not meet the two criteria for defining SAR abilities that decline with age—namely, the criterion of short time between presentation and retrieval, and the criterion of no basis for organizing or making sense of the to-be-remembered elements. This suggests that EWSM will not be among the vulnerable abilities that irreversibly decline with age and neural damage. Indeed, evidence from recent studies suggests that if efforts to maintain expertise continue to be made in adulthood, there is no aging decline in EWSM. We return to a consideration of this matter in a later section of this chapter, when we discuss expertise in some detail.

Summary of Evidence on SAR

Thus what we know about aging in relation to short-term apprehension and retrieval memory (SAR) is that decline is small for measures that primarily require retention over very short periods of time (i.e., measures that are largely indicative of apprehension). There are virtually no age differences for memory measured with the Sperling (1960) paradigm. The retention in this case is for a few milliseconds, but the span is relatively large—9 to 16 elements. As the amount of time one must retain a memory and the span of memory are increased, the negative relation between age and the measure of SAR increases (Cavanaugh, 1997; Charness, 1991; Craik & Trehub, 1982; Ericsson & Delaney, 1996; Gathercole, 1994; Kaufman, 1990; Salthouse, 1991; Schaie, 1996). As long as the memory measure is not a measure of working memory, however, the correlation with age never becomes terribly large: It is less than .25 for measures of reasonable reliability over an age range from young (in the 20s) to old (in the 70s) adulthood. Also, such a memory measure is not much involved in the reasoning of Gf and does not account for much of the aging decline in Gf. As a measure of SAR takes on the character of working memory, however, the relationship of the measure to age becomes substantial—$r = .35$ and up for backward span measures of approximately the same reliability as forward span measures and over the same spread of ages—and the measure relates more to Gf and to the aging decline in Gf.

What we also know is that it is not simply the short period of presentation of elements to be remembered that defines the SAR factor; it is that coupled with the condition that the retriever has no organization system with which to make sense of the elements. When there is a system for making sense out of the presented elements, and the retriever knows and can use that system, the resulting memory is not particularly short term, nor is the span limited to seven plus or minus two. Decline with age in adulthood and decline with neurological damage may not occur, or may not occur irreversibly, with such memory. There is need for further evidence on this point.

The elements of short-term memory tasks are presented one after another under speeded conditions. It may be that speed of apprehension is partially responsible for correlations of SAR measures with other variables. To bring this possibility more fully into focus, let us turn now to a consideration of the rather complex matter of cognitive speed as it relates to aging in adulthood.

Gs: Cognitive Speed—A Link to General Factor Theories?

Most tests of cognitive abilities involve speed in one form or another—speed of apprehending, speed of decision, speed of reacting, movement speed, speed of thinking, and generally speed of behaving. Usually these different kinds of speed are mixed (confounded) in a given measure. There are positive intercorrelations among measures that are in varying degrees confounded in this manner. Generally, measures that are regarded as indicating primarily only speed per se (what we refer to as *chronometric measures*, such as reaction time and perceptual speed [Gs] correlate positively with measures of cognitive capabilities that are not regarded as defined primarily by speed of performance (what we refer to as *cognitive capacity measures*). But there is confounding: The cognitive capacity measures require one or more of the elementary forms of speed mentioned above.

Chronometric measures have often been found to be negatively correlated with age in adulthood. There has been a great amount of research documenting these relationships and aimed at understanding just how speed is involved in human cognitive capability and aging (Birren, 1974; Botwinick, 1978; Eysenck, 1987; Hertzog, 1989; Jensen, 1987; Nettelbeck, 1994; Salthouse, 1985, 1991; Schaie, 1990).

Salthouse (1985, 1991) has provided comprehensive reviews of the evidence showing positive interrelationships among measures of speediness and negative correlation with age. The chronometric tasks that indicate these relationships are varied—copying digits, crossing off letters, comparing numbers, picking up coins, zipping a garment, unwrapping Band-Aids, using a fork, dialing a telephone number, sorting cards, digit–symbol substitution, movement time, trail making, and various measures of simple and complex reaction time. In studies in which young and old subjects were provided opportunity to practice complex reaction time tasks, practice did not eliminate the age differences, and no noteworthy age × practice interactions were found (Madden & Nebes, 1980; Salthouse & Somberg, 1982).

These kinds of findings have spawned a theory that slowing, particularly cognitive slowing, is a general feature of aging in adulthood (Birren, 1974; Kausler, 1990; Salthouse, 1985, 1991, 1992, 1993, 1994). This evidence has also been cited in support of a theory that there is a general factor of cognitive capabilities (e.g., Eysenck, 1987; Jensen, 1982, 1987, 1993; Spearman, 1927). That is, Spearman had proposed that neural speed is the underlying function governing central processes of g (his concept of general intelligence), and investigators such as Eysenck and Jensen (among many others), citing the evidence relating chronometric measures to cognitive capacity measures, have regarded the evidence as supportive of Spearman's theory. Salthouse (1985, 1991), coming at the matter primarily from the perspective of age relationships, has proposed that speed of information processing, reflecting speed of transmission in the neural system, is the essence of general intelligence.

These investigators bring a great deal of information to the table in coming to these conclusions. Still, we think that in the end they come to wrong conclusions. The evidence, when all of it is considered, does not indicate one common factor of g, the essence of which is cognitive speed. Indeed, evidence of this kind does not support a theory of one general factor of intelligence, a theory of one general factor of cognitive speed, or a theory of one general factor of aging.

The basic argument for these theories of a general factor is that the intercorrelations among reliable variables measuring that which is said to be general are all positive. One problem with this argument is that not all such intercorrelations are positive. But that's not the principal problem.[6] The problem is that even if the correlations were all positive, that evidence is not sufficient to establish a general common factor. Many, many variables are positively correlated, but that fact does not indicate one cause, or only one influence operating or only one common factor (Horn, 1989, 2002; Thomson, 1916; Thurstone, 1947).

Research Examining Evidence for a Theory of g

Let us consider, first, structural evidence pertaining to a theory of g. This evidence indicates that many variables related to human brain function are positively correlated, both as seen within any given person and as seen in measures of individual differences. Indeed, there are many variables associated more generally with human body function that are positively correlated, and correlated with variables related to brain function. More than this, many variables of personality are positively intercorrelated and correlated with measures of brain and body functions. Indeed, positive intercorrelations are ubiquitous among between-person measures of various aspects of human function. Most of the measures of individual differences—everything from morality to simple reaction time—can (with reflection) be fitted within a quadrant of positive intercorrelations.

Thus, if the only requirement for a g factor are positive intercorrelations among variables, then many variables that are not abilities and not indicative of intelligence must be accepted as indicating that factor: It would be defined by a huge variety of questionnaire measures of temperament, attitudes, beliefs, values, motives, and indicators of social and ethnic classifications, as well as ability variables. Such a broad definition of a factor does not indicate the nature of human intelligence.

Spearman, both from the start (Spearman, 1904) and as his theory fully developed (Spearman, 1927), required more than simply positive intercorrelations to support his theory of g. The model to test the theory required that not only should the variables of g correlate positively; they should correlate with that common factor *alone* (i.e., they should correlate with no other common factor). Also, the different variables of a battery designed to provide evidence of the g factor should comprehensively represent the capabilities regarded as indicative of human intelligence. The basic capabilities were described as capacity for apprehension, capacity for eduction of relationships, and capacity for eduction of correlates. These were expected to reflect speed of neural processing and to be manifested in capabilities measured with cognitive tests designed to indicate human intelligence.

Thus, to provide evidence of the g factor, an investigator would need to assemble a battery of variables that together comprehensively represented human intelligence, and each variable considered on its own would have to uniquely indicate an aspect of *g*, and could not at all indicate any other common factor. The model is demanding, but it's testable. That's a beauty of Spearman's theory.

Indeed, the theory has been tested quite a number of times. There have been direct tests, in which very careful attention was given to selecting one and only one test to represent the capacities specified in the theory (Alexander, 1935; Brown & Stephenson, 1933; Burt, 1909; 1949; El Kousey, 1935; Horn, 1965, 1989; Rimoldi, 1948; Spearman, 1927, 1939). And there have been indirect tests, in which comprehensive batteries of cognitive tests hypothesized to be indicative of intelligence were submitted to common-factor analysis, and evidence of one common factor was sought at one level or another (e.g., Carroll, 1993; Cohen, 1959; Guilford, 1956; Gustafsson, 1984; Jackson, 1960; McArdle & Woodcock, 1998; Saunders, 1959; Stephenson, 1931; Thurstone, 1938; Vernon, 1950). The results from these various analyses are clear in indicating that one common factor will not suffice to represent the intercorrelations among all variables that represent the abilities thought to be indicative of human intelligence. In the direct tests, it is found that one common factor will not reproduce the intercorrelations. In the indirect tests, it is found that while one factor at a second or third order is indicated, it either is not a one-and-only one common factor or is identical to a factor that is separate from other factors at a lower level (e.g., in Gustafsson, 1984, results).

The common factor that was separate from other factors at the second order and identical with a factor identified at the third order in Gustafsson's (1984) study was interpreted as Gf. This factor corresponds most closely to the construct Spearman described. It has been shown that it is possible to assemble indicators of this factor (reasoning, concentration, working memory, careful apprehension, and comparison speed) that very nearly satisfy the conditions of the Spearman model: one and only one common factor (uncorrelated uniquenesses) that accounts for the variable intercorrelations (Horn, 1991, 1998). This Gf factor does not, however, account for the intercorrelations for other variables that are indicative of human intelligence—in particular, variables indicative of Gc, TSR, Ga, and Gv.

The structural evidence thus does not support a theory of *g*. The developmental evidence is even less supportive. In general, construct validation evidence is counter to a theory that human intelligence is organized in accordance with one common principle or influence. The evidence from several sources points in the direction of several distinct kinds of factors.

Many of the tests that have indicated adulthood aging decline of Gf are administered under time-limited, speeded conditions. This accounts in part for the age-related relationship usually found between Gf and Gs. However, when the confounding of cognitive speed and cognitive capability measures is reduced to a minimum (it is probably never eliminated entirely), the correlations between the two kinds of measures are not reduced to near-chance levels. Nonzero relationships remain for measures of Gs with measures of Gf and SAR (Horn et al., 1981; Horn & Noll, 1994). The relationships for simple (one-choice) reaction time measures become near zero (chance-like), but for two-choice and several-choice reaction time measures the correlation is clearly above that expected by chance.

The more any speeded measure involves complexity—in particular, the more a chronometric measure involves complexity—the higher the correlation is with other cognitive measures and with age. Simple reaction time, in which one reacts as quickly as possible to a single stimulus, correlates at a low level ($r <$ .20) with most measures regarded as indicating some aspect of cognitive ability. For complex reaction time, in which one reacts as quickly as possible to one or another of several stimuli, the correlations with cognitive ability measures increase systematically with increases in the number of different stimuli and patterns of stimuli one needs to take into account before reacting (Jensen, 1987).

The aging decline in Gf can be clearly identified with tests that minimize speed of performance—provided (and this is important) that the tests have a high ceiling of difficulty in the sample of people under investigation, and thus that score on the test is a measure of the level of difficulty of the problems solved, not a measure of the speed of obtaining solutions (Horn, 1994; Horn et al., 1981; Noll & Horn, 1998).

Research Examining Evidence for a General Factor of Cognitive Speed

The structural evidence does not support this theory. Carroll (1993) has done a comprehensive review of the research bearing on this point. He found replicated evidence for factors of movement time, reaction time, correct decision speed (CDS), incorrect decision speed, perceptual speed (Gs), short-time retrieval speed, and fluency/speed of retrieval from long-term memory (TSR). Several different lines of evidence suggest that these factors do not relate to each other or to other variables in a manner that indicates a measure of one process of cognitive speed or one process of aging.

First, one line of evidence indicates that the Gs factor correlates negatively with age and positively with Gf and SAR, both of which decline with age, while moderately speeded retrieval tests (i.e.,TSR) correlate positively with Gs and other speeded measures, but not negatively, with age. TSR also relates positively to Gc, which correlates positively, not negatively, with age. The TSR measures of speed thus have notably different correlations with age and other variables than do other Gs measures.

Second, the evidence of Walsh's (1982) careful studies of speed of visual perception shows that speed measures indicating peripheral functions (at the level of each eye—optic neural processing) correlate at only a near-zero (chance-like) level with speed measures indicating central nervous system functioning, although each of these two unrelated kinds of measures correlates negatively and substantially with age in adulthood. The aging decline in one kind of factor is not indicative of the decline in the other. It appears that just as hair turning gray and going bald are related to aging but are quite separate processes, so declines in peripheral processing speed and central processing speed are related to aging but are separate processes.

Third, although chronometric measures have often been found to relate positively to cognitive capacity measures (when these are confounded with speed), such relationships are found to sink to zero in homogeneous samples—people of the same age and education level. In particular, highly speeded simple-decision tests correlate at the chance level, or even negatively, with low-speed tests

that require solving of complex intellectual problems (Guilford, 1964). Thus, cognitive speed and cognitive capability are not positively related; they are negatively related when cognitive capability is measured in terms of the difficulty of the problems solved. Speed in solving problems is not intrinsically indicative of the complexity of the problems one is able to solve.

Capacity for Sustaining Attention: The Link between Cognitive Speed and Vulnerable Abilities

The evidence now suggests that the kind of cognitive speed that relates to decline of vulnerable abilities is a capacity for focusing and maintaining attention, not speed per se. This leads to a conclusion that cognitive speed measures relate to cognitive capability and aging primarily because they require focused attention, not because they require speed. This is indicated by evidence that chronometric measures relate to unspeeded measures of capacity for focusing and maintaining attention. In part-correlation analyses, it is shown that the unspeeded measures of attention account for most of the aging decline in speeded measures and for most of the relationship between cognitive speed and cognitive capacities. The evidence adds up as follows.

First, measures of behaving as quickly as possible correlate substantially with measures of behaving as slowly as possible (Botwinick & Storandt, 1997). Second, these two kinds of measures correlate substantially (negatively) with age in adulthood, and both correlate substantially with cognitive capacity measures that decline with age in adulthood. Next, when the slowness measures are partialed from the speediness measures, the resulting residualized speediness correlates only very modestly with age, and at a chance level with the cognitive capacity measures (of Gf) that decline with age in adulthood (Horn et al., 1981; Noll & Horn, 1998). The slowness measures also correlate substantially with other indicators of maintaining attention. Behaving slowly requires that one focus and maintain attention on a task. Conclusion: Focusing and maintaining attention appears to be an aspect of the capacity for apprehension that Spearman described as a major feature of g (see also Baddeley, 1993;

Carroll, 1993; Cunningham & Tomer, 1990; Hertzog, 1989; Horn, 1968, 1998, 2002; Horn et al., 1981; Hundal & Horn, 1977; Madden, 1983; Noll & Horn, 1998; Salthouse, 1991; Walsh, 1982).

The evidence thus suggests that the relationships of chronometric measures to age and to cognitive capacity is not due primarily to speed per se, but to the fact that speeded measures require focused and sustained attention. It is not cognitive speed that is at the core of cognitive capability; it is a capacity for focusing and maintaining attention. This is required in speedy performance, and it is required in solving complex problems. It accounts for the correlation between these two kinds of measures. This capacity declines with age in adulthood.

Age-related declines have been found for other sustained-attention tasks. Measures of vigilance, for example (in which subjects must detect a stimulus change imbedded in an otherwise invariant sequence of the stimuli), decline with age (Kausler, 1990; McDowd & Birren, 1990). Age-related declines have been found for divided-attention and selective-attention tasks (Bors & Forrin, 1995; Horn et al., 1981; Horn & Noll, 1994; Madden, 1983; McDowd & Birren, 1990; McDowd & Craik, 1988; Plude & Hoyer, 1985; Rabbitt, 1965; Salthouse, 1991; Wickens, Braune, & Stokes, 1987). When separate measures of concentration (slow tracing) and divided attention are partialed separately and together from measures of working memory, it is found that each independently accounts for some, but not all, of the aging decline in working memory.

Older adults perform more poorly than their younger counterparts on the Stroop test, a measure of resisting interference (Cohn, Dustman, & Bradford, 1984), and on distracted visual search tasks (Madden, 1983; Plude & Hoyer, 1985; Rabbitt, 1965). Hasher and Zacks (1988) suggest that aging decline in cognitive capability is due to distractibility and susceptibility to perceptual interference. These investigators found that the manifest retrieval problems of older adults were attributable to inability to keep irrelevant information from obscuring relevant information. Horn and colleagues (1981) also found that measures of eschewing irrelevancies in concept formation were

related to measures of short-term memory, working memory, and Gf, and accounted for some of the age differences in these measures. All of these measures require concentration to maintain focused attention on a task. Hasher and Zacks concluded that a basic process in working memory is one of maintaining attention. Baddeley (1993) argued that working memory can be described as *working attention*.

It is concluded from a number of these partialing studies that Gf (which so resembles Spearman's *g*) involves processes of (1) gaining awareness of information (attention) and (2) holding different aspects of information in the span of awareness (working memory), both of which are dependent on (3) a capacity for maintaining concentration. Capacity for concentration may be dependent on *neural recruitment* (i.e., synchronous firing of many neurons in patterns that correspond to the patterns of abilities involved in solving a complex problem). If neurons of a neural recruitment pattern are lost, the synchrony and hence the efficiency of the firing pattern are reduced. Grossly, this is seen in the decline of Gf, SAR, and Gs.

AN EMERGING THEORY OF HUMAN INTELLIGENCE: ABILITIES OF EXPERTISE

The results we have just reviewed provide some glimmerings of the nature of human intelligence. But these are only glimmerings; some important things are missing.

The picture is one of aging decline, but decline doesn't characterize everyday observations of adult intelligence. These observations are of adult who do most of the work of maintaining and advancing the culture—people who are the intellectual leaders in science, politics, business, and academics, people who raise children and are regarded as smarter than their teenagers and young adults. This picture is one of maturing adults functioning at ever-higher intellectual levels. Granted that the research results for Gc and TSR are consistent with this view, they seem insufficient to describe the thinking of high-functioning adults. There is reason to question whether the description of human intelligence that is provided by the extant research is accurate.

Inadequacies of Current Theory

Indeed, there are problems with the tests that are assumed to indicate human intelligence. Consider the tests defining Gc, the factor that does indeed show intelligence improving in adulthood. This factor should be a measure of the breadth and depth of cultural knowledge, but the tests that define the factor (e.g., vocabulary, information, and analogies) measure only surface knowledge, not depth of knowledge, and the knowledge sampled by these tests is narrow relative to the broad and diverse range of the knowledge of a culture.

The fundamental problem is that the tests thus far identified as indicating Gc measure only introductory, dilettante knowledge of a culture. They don't measure the depth of knowledge, or the knowledge that is most difficult to acquire. Difficult reasoning is not measured in the factor. This can be seen in esoteric analogies, a test used to estimate a reasoning aspect of Gc. The items of such a test sample understanding of relationships in several areas of knowledge, but the reasoning involved in the relationships of each area is simple, as in an item of the form "*Annual* is to *perennial* as *deciduous* is to _____." If one has a cursory knowledge of botany or horticulture, completing the analogy is simple; it doesn't take much reasoning. The variance of the analogies test thus mainly indicates the extent to which one has such introductory knowledge in several areas of scholarship. It does not represent ability in dealing with difficult abstractions in reasoning in any area. But difficult reasoning is what is called for in the work of a scientist, legislator, engineer, or plumber. Difficult reasoning is called for in measures of intelligence.

Thus, in-depth knowledge and in-depth reasoning are not assessed in current measures of Gc. A dilettante, flitting over many areas of knowledge, will score higher on the measure than a person who has developed truly profound understanding in an area of knowledge. It is the latter individual, not the dilettante, who is most likely to make significant contributions to the culture and to be judged as highly intelligent. Such a person is otherwise referred to as an *expert*. An expert best exemplifies the capabilities that indicate the nature and limits of human intelligence.

Defining Intelligence in Terms of Expertise

After childhood, adolescence, and young adulthood, people continue to think and solve problems, but usually (to an ever-larger extent as development proceeds) this thinking is directed to solving novel problems in fields of work. Adults develop abilities that help them to become expert. They come to understand a great deal about some things, to the detriment of increasing understanding other things. They neglect the work of maintaining and improving previously developed abilities that are not presently relevant for developing expertise. Thus the intelligence of maturing adults becomes manifested in abilities of expertise more and more as development proceeds.

We conclude that (1) the measures currently used to estimate intelligence probably do not assess all the important abilities of human intelligence; (2) abilities that come to fruition in adulthood represent the quintessential expression of human intellectual capacity; (3) these abilities are abilities of expertise; and (4) the principal problems of research for describing these abilities are problems of identifying areas of expertise, designing measures of the abilities of expertise in these areas, and obtaining samples of people who can represent the variation needed to demonstrate the presence and range of expertise abilities.

Expertise Abilities of Intelligence

Intellectual expertise depends on effective application of a large amount of knowledge in reasoning to cope with novel problems. The abilities exemplified in different domains of expertise are indicative of human intelligence. The levels of complexities in reasoning resolved in expressions of expertise are comparable to the levels of complexities resolved in expressions of Gf abilities, and the problems solved often appear to be novel.

In contrast to the reasoning that characterizes Gf, which is largely inductive, the reasoning involved in exercise of expertise is largely knowledge-based and deductive. This is seen in descriptions of the thinking in several areas of expertise—in chess, financial planning, and medical diagnosis (Charness,

1981a, 1981b, 1991; de Groot, 1978; Ericsson, 1996; Walsh & Hershey, 1993). For example, de Groot (1978) found that those at the highest level of expertise in chess chose the next move by evaluating the current situation in terms of principles derived from vast prior experience, rather than by calculating and evaluating the many move possibilities. Other work (Charness, 1981a, 1981b, 1991; Ericsson, 1996, 1997; Morrow, Leirer, Altieri, & Fitzsimmons, 1994; Walsh & Hershey, 1993) has similarly demonstrated that the expert characteristically uses deductive reasoning under conditions where the novice uses inductive reasoning. The expert is able to construct a framework within which to organize and effectively evaluate presented information, while the novice, with no expertise basis for constructing a framework, searches for patterns and does reasoning by trial-and-error evaluations. The expert apprehends large amounts of organized information, comprehends many relationships among elements of this information; infers possible continuations and extrapolations; and, as a result, is able to select the best from among many possibilities in deciding on the most likely outcome, consequence, or extension of relationships. The expert goes from the general (comprehension of relations, knowledge of principles) to the most likely specifics.

Expertise in problem solving also appears to involve a form of wide-span memory that is different from the forms of memory described (in current descriptions of intelligence) under the headings of *short-term memory*, *short-term apprehension and retrieval* (SAR), *instantaneous memory* (Sperling, 1960), and *working memory* (e.g., Baddeley, 1994). de Groot (1946, 1978) may have been the first to recognize a distinction between this expert memory and other forms of memory. He described how, with increasing expertise, subjects became better able to rapidly access alternative chess moves of increasingly higher quality, and then base their play on these complex patterns rather than engage in extensive search. Ericsson and Kintsch (1995) described such memory as a capacity that emerges as expertise develops. It becomes a defining feature of advanced levels of expertise (Ericsson & Delaney, 1996; Ericsson & Kintsch, 1995). It is a form of working memory, but it is functionally in-

dependent of what heretofore has been described as working memory. As noted earlier in this chapter, to distinguish it in language from this latter—which has been referred to as *short-term working memory* (STWM)—it is referred to as *expertise wide-span memory* (EWSM). It is a capacity for holding relatively large amounts of information (large relative to STWM) in immediate awareness for periods of several minutes. It functions as an aid to solving problems and behaving expertly. EWSM is different from STWM in respect to two major features: apprehension–retention limits and access in a sequence.

The apprehension–retention limits of STWM are small and of short duration. For example, the apprehension limits for the recency effect in serial position memory, which is often taken as an indicator of short-term memory, are only about three (plus or minus one), and this retention fades to zero in less than a few (estimated to be 10) seconds (Glanzer & Cunitz, 1966). The apprehension limits for the primacy effect also are only about three (plus or minus one), with duration less than a few seconds. In a near-classic article, Miller (1956) characterized the apprehension limits for forward span memory as the "magical number seven plus or minus two," and the duration of this memory (without rehearsal) is no more than 30 seconds. These kinds of limits have been demonstrated under conditions of competition for a limited resource, as in studies in which subjects are required to retain information while performing another task (Baddeley, 1993; Carpenter & Just, 1989; Stankov, 1988). The limits seen in the Sperling (1960) effect are larger than seven, but there is no consolidation of this memory and the span fades within milliseconds; it is regarded as indicator of apprehension alone, not a measure of short-term retention (memory).

For EWSM, the apprehension limits are substantially larger, and the retention limits are substantially longer, than any of the limits accepted as indicating STWM. Just how much larger and longer these limits are is not clear, but chess experts, for example, appear to be able to hold many more than seven elements of separate games within the span of immediate awareness for as long as several minutes (Ericsson & Kintsch, 1995; Gobet & Simon, 1996). In playing blindfold chess

(Ericsson & Staszewski, 1989; Holding, 1985; Koltanowski, 1985), the expert is literally never able to see the board; all the outcomes of sequences of plays must be kept within a span of immediate apprehension. The number of elements the expert retains in such representations is much more than seven, and this retention lasts over several minutes.

It has been argued that successive chunking in STWM is sufficient to account for feats of memory displayed by experts, and thus to obviate any need for a concept of EWSM (Chase & Simon, 1973; Gobet & Simon, 1996). Chase and Simon (1973) reasoned that high-level chess memory was mediated by a large number (10,000, they estimated) of acquired patterns regarded as chunks, which could be hierarchically organized. The analyses of Richman, Gobet, Staszewski, and Simon (1996) suggested that the number of such chunks would have to be in excess of 100,000, rather than 10,000. In any case, the mechanism suggested by Chase and Simon was direct retrieval of relevant moves cued by perceived patterns of chess positions that are stored in a form of STWM. They rejected a suggestion (Chase & Ericsson, 1982) that storage of generated patterns in long-term memory is possible within periods as brief as the 5-second presentations that were observed. Cooke, Atlas, Lane, and Berger (1993) and Gobet and Simon (1996), however, showed that this assumption is plausible. They found that highly skilled chess players could recall information from up to nine chess positions that had been presented one after the other as rapidly as one every 5 seconds without pauses. In the retrievals of blindfold chess, the number of chunks would appear to be larger than seven—and if chunks are maintained in a hierarchy or other such template, the representation would be changed with successive moves, and the number of sequences of such changes is larger than seven. Yet experts were able to use information of moves that were more than seven sequences removed from the point of decision.

Similarly, in studies of experts playing multiple games of chess presented on a computer screen, Saariluoma (1991) found that a chess master could simultaneously play six different games, each involving more than

seven relationships. The expert appeared to retain representations of many more than seven chess positions in a flexibly accessible form while moving from one game to another.

STWM is characterized by sequencing in retention, but such sequencing seems to be unimportant in EWSM. In STWM, maximum span is attained only if items are retained and retrieved in the temporal order of apprehension. If a task requires retrieval in a different order, the number of elements recalled is substantially reduced; memory span backward, for example, is only about three to four, compared with the seven of forward span. In descriptions of chess experts displaying EWSM, on the other hand, information is almost as readily accessed from the middle or end of a sequence as from the beginning (Charness & Bosman, 1990).

The Ericsson and Kintsch (1995) analyses thus make the case that while chunking helps to explain short-term memory that is somewhat larger than seven plus two, it is not fully adequate to account for the very large apprehension, long retention, and flexibility of access that experts display. In particular, if the different sequences experts access are regarded as chunks that must be maintained if the retrieval of experts is to be adequately described, the number of such chunks must be considerably larger than seven plus two, and they must be retained longer than a few seconds. Thus chunking cannot be the whole story (Ericsson & Kintsch, 1995; Gobet & Simon, 1996).

How might EWSM work? Our theory is that the development of expertise sensitizes the person to become more nearly aware of the large amount of information that is, for a very short period of time, available to all people (not just experts), but ordinarily is not accessed. Sperling's (1960) work indicates that for a split second, the human is aware of substantially more information than is indicated by estimates of the limits of STWM. Similarly, the studies of Biederman (e.g., 1995) demonstrate that we can recognize complex visual stimuli involving many more than seven elements and retain them for longer than 60 seconds. However, most of the information that comes into immediate awareness fades from awareness very quickly. It fades partly because new information enters awareness to take the place of previous information; it fades also because meaningful organizing systems are not immediately available to enable a perceiver to organize the incoming information. Biederman's findings demonstrate that information that is seen only briefly but is organized by the perceiver can be retained for long periods of time. Thus, if meaningful systems for organizing information are built up through expertise development (the systems of EWSM), and such systems are available in the immediate situation, then large amounts of briefly seen information might be organized in accordance with this system and retained for long periods of time for use in problem solving in an area of expertise. Such organized information (seen only briefly) would not be replaced by other incoming information. However, the briefly seen information would need to be that of a domain of expertise. The development of expertise would not, in general, improve memory; it would do so only in a limited domain.

Further Notes on the Development of Expertise

What we now know about expertise suggests that it is developed through intensive practice over extended periods of time and is maintained through continued efforts in regular, well-structured practice (Anderson, 1990; Ericsson, 1996; Ericsson & Charness, 1994; Ericsson, Krampe, & Tesch-Romer, 1993; Ericsson & Lehmann, 1996; Walsh & Hershey, 1993). What is described as *well-structured practice* is essential for effective development of expertise. Such practice is not simply repetition and is not measured simply by number of practice trials. The practice must be designed to identify and correct errors and to move one to ever-higher levels of performance. There should be goals and appropriate feedback. It was found that in developing expertise in chess, self-directed practice (using books and studying sequences of moves made by expert players) could be as effective as coach-directed practice (Charness, 1981a, 1981b, 1991; Ericsson, 1996).

Just how long it takes to reach the highest levels of expertise—one's own asymptote—is not known with precision for any domain. A "10-year rule" has been given as an approximation for domains characterized by complex problem solving, but this has been much debated (Anderson, 1990; Charness, Krampe, & Mayr, 1996; Ericsson & Charness, 1994; Ericsson, Krampe, & Tesch-Romer, 1993). The upshot of the debate is that the time it takes to become expert varies with domain, the amount and quality of practice and coaching, the developmental level at which dedication to becoming an expert begins, health, stamina, and a host of other variables. Ten years is a very rough estimation for some domains, such as chess and medical diagnosis (Ericsson, 1996).

Since it takes time (i.e., years) to reach high levels of expertise in complex problem solving, and expertise in such domains is developed (at least partially) through the period of adulthood, it follows that expertise abilities can improve in adulthood. Indeed, the research literature is consistent in showing that across different domains of expertise, people beginning at different ages in adulthood advance from low to asymptotic high levels of expertise (Ericsson, Krampe, & Heizmann, 1993). Advanced levels of expertise in certain games (e.g., chess, go) and in financial planning have been attained and maintained by older adults (Charness & Bosman, 1990; Charness et al., 1996; Ericsson & Charness, 1994; Kasai, 1986; Walsh & Hershey, 1993). Rabbitt (1993) found that among novices, crossword-solving ability was positively correlated with test scores indicating Gf ($r = .72$) and negatively correlated with age ($r = -.25$), just as Gf is so correlated; however, among experts crossword-solving ability was positively associated with age ($r = +.24$) and correlated near zero with Gf. The results of Bahrick (1984), Bahrick and Hall (1991), Conway, Cohen, and Stanhope (1991), Walsh and Hershey (1993), and Krampe and Ericsson (1996) indicate that continued practice is required to maintain a high level of expert performance: If the abilities of expertise are not used, they decline. To the extent that practice is continued, expertise is maintained over periods of years and decades.

It also appears from the extant (albeit sparse) evidence that high levels of EWSM can be maintained into advanced age. Baltes (1997) found that in domains of specialization, older adults could access information more rapidly than young adults. Charness (1981a, 1981b, 1991) found no age decrement in the depth of search for the next move and the quality of the resulting moves in chess.[6] Such findings suggest that there may be little or no decline with age for complex thinking abilities if these abilities are developed within a domain of expertise.

Also suggesting that expertise abilities indicative of intelligence can be developed and maintained in adulthood are results obtained by Krampe and Ericsson (1996) for speeded abilities. They obtained seven operationally independent measures of speed in a sample of classical pianists who ranged from amateurs to concert performers with international reputations, and who ranged in age from the mid-20s to the mid-60s. Regardless of age, experts performed better than amateurs on all music-related speeded tasks. Age-related decline was found at the highest level of expertise, but reliably for only one of the seven measures, and the decline was notably smaller than for persons at lower levels of expertise. The single best predictor of performance on all music-related tasks was the amount of practice participants had maintained during the previous 10 years.

In samples of practicing typists of different ages, Salthouse (1985) found that although abilities of finger-tapping speed, choice reaction time, and digit–symbol substitution that would seem to be closely related to typing ability declined systematically with age, typing ability as such did not: Older typists attained the same typing speed as younger typists. The older typists had longer eye spans, which enabled them to anticipate larger chunks of the material to be typed. Salthouse interpreted this as a compensatory mechanism. It can also be viewed as indicating a more advanced level of expertise, for, seemingly, it would relate to improving the skill of a typist of any age.

In a study of spatial visualization in architects of different ages and levels of expertise, Salthouse (1991) found that high-level experts consistently scored above low-level experts at every age. In the abilities of expertise, elderly high-level experts scored higher than youthful low-level experts. With practice to increase and maintain expertise, cognitive abilities (of expertise) increased with advancing age.

Expertise: Conclusions, Implications, and Extrapolations

Thus it seems that some kinds of expertise require, and indicate, high levels of the abilities that indicate human intelligence. Attaining such expertise involves developing deductive reasoning ability to solve very difficult problems. Also developed is EWSM, which enables one to remain aware of, and work with, large amounts of information in the area of expertise. This facilitates expertise deductive reasoning. Cognitive speed ability also develops in the domain of expertise as high levels of expertise are attained. Very possibly there are other abilities that develop under the press to acquire expertise. Research should be directed at identifying such abilities. These expertise abilities are different from the somewhat comparable abilities of fluid reasoning (Gf), working memory (SAR), and cognitive speed (Gs) that also characterize human intelligence.

It takes many years to develop a high level of expertise. Ten years is a rough estimate. Even more time is needed to develop the highest levels. Much of this development must occur in adulthood. High levels of the abilities of expertise are displayed primarily in adults (not younger people). Expertise abilities of older high-level experts exceed the comparable abilities of younger persons at lower levels of expertise.

Expertise abilities of intelligence are expected to increase (on average) in adulthood; that is, such abilities will increase at least in some people and during some parts of adulthood (perhaps mainly the early parts—the first 20 years, say). Burnout is common in activities that require intense dedication and work. After working intensely for years to develop expertise, one can reach a limit, begin to lose interest and focus, and become lax in maintaining and continuing to develop the abilities of one's expertise. Those abilities would then decline. People often switch fields after burning out in a particular field, and such switching might be accompanied by launching a program to develop expertise in the new field. This could occur at fairly advanced ages in adulthood. In this way, too, abilities of expertise could be expected to increase through much of adulthood.

Thus, our theory specifies that the deductive reasoning, EWSM, and cognitive speediness abilities associated with the development of expertise increase concomitantly with the decreases that have been found for Gf, STWM, and speediness defined outside a domain of expertise. It is possible that increase in expertise abilities necessarily results in decline in nonexpertise abilities, for the devotion of time, energy, and other resources to the development of expertise may of necessity take time, energy, and other resources away from maintenance of Gf, SAR, and Gs.

Such hypothesizing flows from sparse findings. The hypotheses may be correct, but perhaps for only a small number of people. The extant results have often come from studies of small samples. The adults in these cases may be exceptional. There have been no longitudinal follow-up studies to determine the extent to which people become exceptional and maintain that status. If such development occurs only in a few cases, there are good questions to ask about how the development might be fostered in most people. There is need for further research.

GENERAL SUMMARY

The present state of science thus indicates that human intelligence is a melange of many abilities that are interrelated in many ways. The abilities and their interrelationships are determined by many endogenous (genetic, physiological, neurological) and exogenous (experiential, nutritional, hygienic) influences. These influences operate over many minutes, months, and years of life; they may be more and less potent in some developmental periods than in others. There is very little we know, and much more we don't know, about these interrelationships and determinants.

It is unlikely that there is one central determinant running through the entire melange of abilities. If there is one such influence, the extant evidence suggests it must be weak, barely detectable among a chorus of other determinants. If g exists, it will be difficult to ferret it out from all the other influences that operate to produce intellectual abilities. Small influences can be hugely important, of course, but we have no inkling that is true for g (if, indeed, there is a g). Assertions that g has been discovered do nothing to help lo-

cate a possible g, or to indicate the importance of such an agent if it were to be found.

It is known that almost any task that can be made up to measure a cognitive ability correlates positively with tests of almost every other cognitive ability. Very few exceptions to this generalization have been found, but there are a couple. The first is found in samples of very young children—under 2–3 years of age. In such samples, measures involving motor skill and speediness have been found to be correlated near zero or perhaps even negatively with measures of awareness of concepts (i.e., the beginnings of vocabulary). The second exception is found in very homogeneous samples of young adults—all very nearly of the same age, same educational level, same ethnicity, same socioeconomic status, and so forth. Again, measures in which there is much emphasis on speediness correlate near zero, perhaps negatively, with tests that require solving difficult problems. With these two exceptions, cognitive ability tests are positively intercorrelated. This is referred to as a condition of *positive manifold*.

It is the evidence of positive manifold that is referred to in assertions that g has been discovered. But a positive manifold is not sufficient evidence of a single process. There are many ways for positive manifold to occur that do not involve one common factor (as described particularly well by Thomson, 1916, many decades ago).

Many variables that are not ability variables are positively correlated with ability variables (as well as among themselves). This does not indicate g. Variables scored in the "good" direction generally correlate positively with other things scored in the "good" direction (high ability correlates positively with ego strength, ambition, morale, family income, healthful habits, etc.), and variables scored in the "not good" direction generally correlate positively with other things scored in the "not good" direction (low ability correlates positively with neuroticism, other psychopathologies, inattentiveness, hyperactivity, boredom, lack of energy, delinquency, poverty, birth stress, etc.). Just as it is argued (e.g., by Jensen, 1998) that one can obtain a good measure of g by adding up scores on different ability tests that are positively intercorrelated, so one might argue that by taking into account the presence of a long list of the above-mentioned negative things and the absence of a long list of positive things, one can obtain a good measure of a *c* factor—*c* standing for *crud*.[7] The evidence for such a *c* factor is of the same form as the evidence said to exist for a *g* factor. The problems with the science of the *c* factor are the same as the problems with the science of the *g* factor. In both cases, many, many things can operate to produce the positive manifold of variable intercorrelations. In both cases, it is not a scientific simplification to claim (or imply) that one thing produces this positive manifold. In both cases, something like a bond theory of many causes (Thomson, 1916) is a more plausible model of the data than a one-common-factor model.

The extant evidence indicates that within the manifold of positive intercorrelations among cognitive abilities, there are pockets of substantially higher intercorrelations among some abilities, coupled with lower correlations of these abilities with other abilities. Such patterns of intercorrelations give rise to theories that separate sets of influences produce distinct common factors. Results from many studies now point to 80-some such distinct common factors operating at a primary level, and some eight or nine common factors operating at a second-order level.

Several indicators of primary-level influences interrelate to indicate a second-order factor that rather well represents Spearman's hypotheses that human intelligence is characterized by keenness of apprehension, ability to discern extant relationships, and ability to extrapolate to generate new, implied relationships. It seems that a capacity for attaining and maintaining focused attention is an integral part of this clutch of abilities. This capacity for concentration appears to enable speed in apprehending and scanning fundaments and possible relationships among fundaments in working toward solutions to complex problems. This capacity, coupled with abilities for apprehending the elements of problems, holding them in a span of awareness, identifying relationships amont the elements, and working out the implications of these relationships, define *fluid reasoning* (Gf).

Gf does not represent one and only one common-factor influence running through all abilities that indicate the nature of human intelligence. Certain other primary-level indicators interrelate to indicate a second-order factor of ready acquisition of information. It is manifested in acquisition of knowledge about the language, concepts, and information of the dominant culture. The abilities of the factor are the abilities the society seeks to pass from one generation to the next through various processes of acculturation, particularly those of formal education. This set of abilities is labeled *crystallized knowledge* and symbolized as Gc.[8]

Gc and Gf together do not represent two and only two common-factor influences running through all abilities that indicate the nature of human intelligence. There are also common-factor influences representing separate forms of memory. One of these, labeled *short-term working memory* (STWM) or *short-term apprehension and retrieval* (SAR), indicates span and capacity for holding information in awareness for very short periods of time (less than a minute) while, for example, working on a problem such as would be solved through the processes of Gf. A second form of memory indicates a facility for consolidating information in a manner that enables it to be stored and retrieved minutes, hours, and days later. This facility is labeled *tertiary storage and retrieval* (TSR). A third form of EWSM stems from extended intense practice in developing cognitive expertise.

Primary-level abilities also interrelate to indicate second-order factors representing cognitive functions associated with perceptual modalities. One such factor indicates functions that facilitate visualization; this is labeled *broad visualization* (Gv). Another set of relationships is for abilities of listening and hearing and comprehending intricacies of sounds; it is referred to as *auditory ability* (Ga). There are very possibly somewhat comparable cognitive functions spinning off from the other sensory modalities, but there has been virtually no study of such possibilities.

Speed of reacting, speed of deciding, speed of movement, speed of perceiving, various speeds in solving various different kinds of problems, speed in thinking, and other aspects of speed of responding and behaving are involved in very intricate ways in almost all the abilities that are regarded as indicating human intelligence. Five common factors involving different sets of indicators of speediness have been identified at what is approximately a second-order level among primary factors of speediness. These indicators of speediness do not indicate a general factor for speed of thinking, however. Nor do any of the speed factors represent a sine qua non of the other second-order systems. Indeed, as concerns Gf in particular, a capacity for behaving slowly (which seems to indicate focused concentration) largely accounts for any relationship between reasoning and speed of thinking; that is, an ability to concentrate seems to determine quick thinking in solving the difficult, abstract problems that characterize Gf. It may be true that capacity for focusing concentration largely accounts for the speediness of the speed factors and their relationships to other broad cognitive factors, but these hypotheses have not been examined. Good research is needed in this area.

The systems involved in retaining information in immediate awareness, concentration, and reasoning with novel problems decline, on average, in adulthood. Yet an important referent for the concept of intelligence is expertise: high-level ability to deal successfully with complex problems in which the solutions require advanced, deep understanding of a knowledge domain. Cognitive capability systems involved in retrieving information from the store of knowledge (TSR) and the store of knowledge itself (Gc) increase over much of the period of adulthood development. These increases point to the development of expertise, but the Gc and TSR measures tap only surface-like indictors of expertise abilities. They do no indicate the depth of knowledge, the ability to deal with many aspects of a problem, the reasoning, and the speed in considering possibilities that characterize high-level expertise performances. Gc and TSR do not measure the feats of reasoning and memory that characterize the most sublime expressions of adult intelligence. These capabilities have been described in studies of experts in games (e.g., chess and go), in medical diagnosis, and in financial planning. Factor-analytic studies have demonstrated that expert performances depend on abilities of deductive reasoning and EWSM, abilities that are quite independent of the Gf, SAR, and Gs abilities of intel-

ligence. Within a circumscribed domain of knowledge, EWSM provides an expert with much more information in the immediate situation than is available through the system for STWM. EWSM appears to sublimate to a form of deductive reasoning that utilizes a complex store of information to effectively anticipate, predict, evaluate, check, analyze, and monitor in problem solving within the knowledge domain. These abilities appear to characterize mature expressions of intelligence. Years of intensive, well-structured learning and regular practice are needed to develop and maintain these abilities. To the extent that such practice occurs through the years of adulthood, these abilities will increase; to this extent, important abilities of intelligence will not decline with advancing age.

NOTES

1. It is realized that what is considered first-order or second-order in a factor analysis depends on what is to be put into the analysis. If items are put into analysis, for example, the first-order factors are likely to be equivalent to the tests that are normally put into a first-order analysis, and the second-order factors among items correspond to the first-order factors among tests. Also, if tests are carefully chosen to represent one and only one first-order factor, the first-order factors will indicate the second-order factors among the usual factorings of tests. The order of a factor thus depends on the sampling of the elements to indicate that factor. It is with awareness of these possibilities that researchers have considered the sampling of elements and arrived at the classifications here referred to as *primary abilities* and *second-order* abilities.
2. This is the case, too, when nine second-order factors are considered.
3. That is, age is the primary marker for development, although by no means the only such marker (Nesselroade & Baltes, 1979).
4. The longitudinal findings generally suggest that declines set in somewhat earlier than is indicated by cross-sectional findings.
5. If the elements of the memory are not arranged in accordance with patterns that are part of expertise understanding—as when chess pieces are located in a quite arbitrary manner on a chessboard—the expert's memory is no better than the nonexpert's, and the memory span is approximately seven plus or minus two, as it is for other unrelated material.

6. Indeed, a large majority of the intercorrelations are positive.
7. Indeed, Herrnstein and Murray (1994) obtained such a composite, scored in the opposite direction, and called it "The Middle Class Values Index." The thought of calling it a *crud* factor is owed to Paul Meehl, who referred to it in this manner in a conversation with Horn many years ago.
8. The terms *crystallized* and *fluid* in the labels for Gc and Gf, respectively, were affixed by Cattell (1957) to represent his hypothesis that Gf is a necessary determinant of Gc—it "flows" into production of a Gc that then becomes fixed, rather in the way that polyps produce the calcareous skeletons that constitute a coral reef. The sparse evidence at hand suggests that something like this process may operate in the early years of development, but that as development proceeds, Gc may precede and do more to determine Gf than the reverse.

REFERENCES

Alexander, H. B. (1935). Intelligence, concrete and abstract. *British Journal of Psychology* (Monograph Suppl. No. 19).

Anderson, J. R. (1990). *Cognitive psychology and its implications* (3rd ed.). New York: W. H. Freeman.

Atkinson, R. C., & Shiffrin, R. M. (1968). Human memory: A proposed system and its control processes. In K. W. Spence & J. T. Spence (Eds.), *The psychology of learning and motivation* (Vol. 2, pp. 89–105). New York: Academic Press.

Baddeley, A. (1993). Working memory or working attention? In A. Baddeley & L. Weiskrantz (Eds.), *Attention: Selection, awareness, and control: A tribute to Donald Broadbent* (pp. 152–170). Oxford: Clarendon Press.

Baddeley, A. (1994). Memory. In A. M. Colman (Ed.), *Companion encyclopedia of psychology* (Vol. 1, pp. 281–301). London: Routledge.

Bahrick, H. P. (1984). Semantic memory content in permaslore: 50 years of memory for Spanish learned in school. *Journal of Experimental Psychology: General, 113,* 1–29.

Bahrick, H. P., & Hall, L. K. (1991). Lifetime maintenance of high school mathematics content. *Journal of Experimental Psychology: General, 120,* 20–33.

Baltes, P. B. (1997). On the incomplete architecture of human ontogeny: Selection, optimization, and compensation as foundation of developmental theory. *American Psychologist, 52,* 366–380.

Biederman, I. (1995). Visual object recognition. In S. F. Kosslyn & D. N. Osherson (Eds.), *An invitation to cognitive science: Vol. 2. Visual cognition* (2nd ed., pp. 121–165). Cambridge, MA: MIT Press.

Birren, J. E. (1974). Psychophysiology and speed of response. *American Psychologist, 29,* 808–815.

Bors, D. A., & Forrin, B. (1995). Age, speed of information processing, recall, and fluid intelligence. *Intelligence, 20,* 229–248.

Botwinick, J. (1978). *Aging and behavior: A comprehensive integration of research findings.* New York: Springer.

Botwinick, J., & Storandt, M. (1997). *Memory related functions and age.* Springfield, IL: Charles C. Thomas.

Bower, G. H. (1972). Mental imagery and associative learning. In L. W. Gregg (Ed.), *Cognition in learning and memory* (pp. 213–228). New York: Wiley.

Bower, G. H. (1975). Cognitive psychology: An introduction. In W. K. Estes (Ed.), *Handbook of learning and cognitive processes* (Vol. 1, pp. 3–27). New York: Erlbaum.

Broadbent, D. E. (1966). The well-ordered mind. *American Educational Research Journal, 3,* 281–295.

Brown, W., & Stephenson, W. (1933). A test of the theory of two factors. *British Journal of Psychology, 23,* 352–370.

Burt, C. (1909). Experimental tests of general intelligence. *British Journal of Psychology, 3,* 94–177.

Burt, C. (1949). Subdivided factors. *British Journal of Statistical Psychology, 2,* 41–63.

Carroll, J. B. (1993). *Human cognitive abilities: A survey of factor analytic studies.* New York: Cambridge University Press.

Carpenter, P. A., & Just, M. A. (1989). The role of working memory in language comprehension. In D. Clahr & K. Kotovski (Eds.), *Complex information processing: The impact of Herbert A. Simon* (pp. 31–68). Hillsdale, NJ: Erlbaum.

Cattell, R. B. (1941). Some theoretical issues in adult intelligence testing. *Psychological Bulletin, 38,* 592.

Cattell, R. B. (1957). *Personality and motivation structure and measurement.* Yonkers, NY: World.

Cattell, R. B. (1971). *Abilities: Their structure, growth and action.* Boston: Houghton-Mifflin.

Cattell, R. B. (1979). Are culture-fair intelligence tests possible and necessary? *Journal of Research and Development in Education, 12,* 1–13.

Cavanaugh, J. C. (1997). *Adult development and aging* (3rd ed.). New York: ITP.

Charness, N. (1981a). Search in chess: Age and skill differences. *Journal of Experimental Psychology: Human Perception and Performance, 7*(2), 467–476.

Charness, N. (1981b). Visual short-term memory and aging in chess players. *Journal of Gerontology, 36*(5), 615–619.

Charness, N. (1991). Expertise in chess: The balance between knowledge and search. In K. A. Ericsson & J. Smith (Eds.), *Toward a general theory of expertise: Prospects and limits* (pp. 30–62). Cambridge, UK: Cambridge University Press.

Charness, N., & Bosman, E. A. (1990). Expertise and aging: Life in the lab. In T. M. Hess (Ed.), *Aging and cognition: Knowledge organization and utilization* (pp. 343–386). New York: Elsevier.

Charness, N., Krampe, R, & Mayr, U. (1996). The role of practice and coaching in entrepreneurial skill domains: An international comparison of life-span chess skill acquisition. In K. A. Ericsson (Ed.), *The road to excellence* (pp. 51–80). Mahwah, NJ: Erlbaum.

Chase, W. G., & Ericsson, K. A. (1982). Skill and working memory. In G. H. Bower (Ed.), *The psychology of learning and motivation* (Vol. 16, pp. 1–58). New York: Academic Press.

Chase, W. G., & Simon, H. A. (1973). Perception in chess. *Cognitive Psychology, 4*, 55–81.

Cohen, J. (1959). The factorial structure of the WISC at ages 7.6, 10.6, and 13.6. *Journal of Consulting Psychology, 23*, 289–299.

Cohn, N. B., Dustman, R. E., & Bradford, D. C. (1984). Age-related decrements in Stroop color test performance. *Journal of Clinical Psychology, 40*, 1244–1250.

Conway, M. A., Cohen, G., & Stanhope, N. (1991). On the very long-term retention of knowledge acquired through formal education: Twelve years of cognitive psychology. *Journal of Experimental Psychology: General, 120*, 395–409.

Cooke, N. J., Atlas, R. S., Lane, D. M., & Berger, R. C. (1993). Role of high-level knowledge in memory for chess positions. *American Journal of Psychology, 106*, 321–351.

Craik, F. I. M. (1977). Age differences in human memory. In J. E. Birren & K. W. Schaie (Eds.), *Handbook of the psychology of aging* (pp. 55–110). New York: Van Nostrand Reinhold.

Craik, F. I. M., & Trehub, S. (Eds.). (1982). *Aging and cognitive processes.* New York: Plenum Press.

Cunningham, W. R., & Tomer, A. (1990). Intellectual abilities and age: Concepts, theories and analyses. In A. E. Lovelace (Ed.), *Aging and cognition: Mental processes, self awareness and interventions* (pp. 279–406). Amsterdam: Elsevier.

de Groot, A. D. (1946). *Het denken vun den schaker* [Thought and choice in chess]. Amsterdam: North-Holland.

de Groot, A. D. (1978). *Thought and choice in chess.* The Hague, Netherlands: Mouton.

Detterman, D. K. (Ed.). (1993). *Current topics in human intelligence* (Vol. 1). Norwood, NJ: Ablex.

El Kousey, A. A. H. (1935). The visual perception of space. *British Journal of Psychology* (Monograph Suppl. No. 20).

Ericsson, K. A. (1996). The acquisition of expert performance. In K. A. Ericsson (Ed.), *The road to excellence* (pp. 1–50). Mahwah, NJ: Erlbaum.

Ericsson, K. A. (1997). Deliberate practice and the acquisition of expert performance: An overview. In H. Jorgensen & A. C. Lehmann (Eds.), *Does practice make perfect?: Current theory and research on instrumental music practice* (pp. 9–51). Norges musikkhogskole: NMH-publikasjoner.

Ericsson, K. A., & Charness, N. (1994). Expert performance. *American Psychologist, 49*, 725–747.

Ericsson, K. A., & Delaney, P. F. (1998). Working memory and expert performance. In R. H. Logie & K. J. Gilhooly (Eds.), *Working memory and thinking: Current issues in thinking and reasoning* (pp. 93–114). Hove, UK: Psychology Press/Erlbaum.

Ericsson, K. A., & Kintsch, W. (1995). Long-term working memory. *Psychological Review, 105*, 211–245.

Ericsson, K. A., Krampe, R. T., & Heizmann, S. (1993). Can we create gifted people? In *CIBA Foundation Symposium: The origins and development of high ability* (pp. 22–249). Chichester, UK: Wiley.

Ericsson, K. A., Krampe, R. T., & Tesch-Romer, C. (1993). The role of deliberate practice in the acquisition of expert performance. *Psychological Review, 100*, 363–406.

Ericsson, K. A., & Lehmann, A. C. (1996). Expert and exceptional performance: Evidence of maximal adaptation to task constraints. *Annual Review of Psychology, 47*, 273–305.

Ericsson, K. A., & Staszewski, J. (1989). Skilled memory and expertise: Mechanisms of exceptional performance. In D. Klahr & K. Kotovsky (Eds.), *Complex information processing* (pp. 235–268). Hillsdale, NJ: Erlbaum.

Estes, W. K. (1974). Learning theory and intelligence. *American Psychologist, 29*, 740–749.

Eysenck, H. J. (1987). Speed of information processing, reaction time, and the theory of intelligence. In P. A. Vernon (Ed.), *Speed of information processing and intelligence* (pp. 21–68). Norwood, NJ: Ablex.

Flanagan, D. P., Genshaft, J. L., & Harrison, P. L. (Eds.). (1997). *Contemporary intellectual assessment: Theories, tests, and issues.* New York: Guilford Press.

Gathercole, S. E. (1994). The nature and uses of working memory. In P. Morris & M. Gruneberg (Eds.), *Theoretical aspects of memory* (pp. 50–78). London: Routledge.

Glanzer, M., & Cunitz, A. R. (1966). Two storage mechanisms in free recall. *Journal of Verbal Learning and Verbal Behavior, 5*, 351–360.

Gobet, F., & Simon, H. A. (1996). Templates in chess memory: A mechanism for recalling several boards. *Cognitive Psychology, 31*, 1–40.

Guilford, J. P. (1956). The structure of the intellect. *Psychological Bulletin, 53*, 276–293.

Guilford, J. P. (1964). Zero intercorrelations among tests of intellectual abilities. *Psychological Bulletin, 61*, 401–404.

Gustafsson, J. E. (1984). A unifying model for the structure of intellectual abilities. *Intelligence, 8*, 179–203.

Harwood, E., & Naylor, G. F. K. (1971). Changes in the constitution of the WAIS intelligence pattern with advancing age. *Australian Journal of Psychology, 23*, 297–303.

Hasher, L., & Zacks, R. T. (1988). Working memory, comprehension, and aging: A review and a new view. In G. H. Bower (Ed.), *The psychology of learning and motivation* (Vol. 22, pp. 193–225). San Diego, CA: Academic Press.

Herrnstein, R. J., & Murray, C. (1994). *The bell curve: Intelligence and class structure in American life*. New York: Free Press.

Hetzog, C. (1989). Influences of cognitive slowing on age differences. *Developmental Psychology, 25*, 636–651.

Holding, D. H. (1985). *The psychology of chess skill*. Hillsdale, NJ: Erlbaum.

Horn, J. L. (1965). *Fluid and crystallized intelligence: A factor analytic and developmental study of the structure among primary mental abilities*. Unpublished doctoral dissertation, University of Illinois.

Horn, J. L. (1968). Organization of abilities and the development of intelligence. *Psychological Review, 75*, 242–259.

Horn, J. L. (1989). Models for intelligence. In R. Linn (Ed.), *Intelligence: Measurement, theory and public policy* (pp. 29–73). Urbana: University of Illinois Press.

Horn, J. L. (1991). Measurement of intellectual capabilities: A review of theory. In K. S. McGrew, J. K. Werder, & R. W. Woodcock (Eds.), *Woodcock–Johnson technical manual* (pp. 197–246). Allen, TX: DLM.

Horn, J. L. (1994). The theory of fluid and crystallized intelligence. In R. J. Sternberg (Ed.), *The encyclopedia of intelligence* (pp. 443–451). New York: Macmillan.

Horn, J. L. (1998). A basis for research on age differences in cognitive capabilities. In J. J. McArdle & R. Woodcock (Eds.), *Human cognitive abilities in theory and practice* (pp. 57–91). Chicago: Riverside.

Horn, J. L. (2002). Selections of evidence, misleading assumptions, and oversimplifications: The political message of *The Bell Curve*. In J. Fish (Ed.), *Race and intelligence: Separating science from myth* (pp. 297–325). Mahwah, NJ: Erlbaum.

Horn, J. L., & Cattell, R. B. (1967). Age differences in fluid and crystallized intelligence. *Acta Psychologica, 26*, 107–129.

Horn, J. L., Donaldson, G., & Engstrom, R. (1981). Apprehension, memory and fluid intelligence decline in adulthood. *Research on Aging, 3*, 33–84.

Horn, J. L., & Hofer, S. M. (1992). Major abilities and development in the adult period. In R. J. Sternberg & C. A. Berg (Eds.), *Intellectual development* (pp. 44–99). New York: Cambridge University Press.

Horn, J. L., & Noll, J. (1994). A system for understanding cognitive capabilities. In D. K. Detterman (Ed.), *Current topics in intelligence* (pp. 151–203). Norwood, NJ: Ablex.

Horn, J. L., & Noll, J. (1997). Human cognitive capabilities: Gf-Gc theory. In D. P. Flanagan, J. L. Genshaft, & P. I. Harrison (Eds.), *Contemporary intellectual assessment* (pp. 53–91). New York: Guilford Press.

Hundal, P. S., & Horn, J. L. (1977). On the relationships between short-term learning and fluid and crystallized intelligence. *Applied Psychological Measurement, 1*, 11–21.

Jackson, M. A. (1960). The factor analysis of the Wechsler Scale. *British Journal of Statistical Psychology, 33*, 79–82.

Jensen, A. R. (1982). Reaction time and psychometric g. In H. J. Eysenck (Ed.), *A model for intelligence* (pp. 93–132). New York: Springer-Verlag.

Jensen, A. R. (1987). Psychometric g as a focus of concerted research effort. *Intelligence, 11*, 193–198.

Jensen, A. R. (1993). Why is reaction time correlated with psychometric g? *Current Directions in Psychological Science, 2*(2), 53–56.

Jensen, A. R. (1998). *The g factor: The science of mental ability*. London: Praeger.

Kasai, K. (1986). *Ido de atama ga yoku naru hon* [Becoming smart with GO]. Tokyo, Japan: Shikai.

Kaufman, A. S. (1990). *Assessing adolescent and adult intelligence*. Boston: Allyn & Bacon.

Kausler, D. H. (1990). *Experimental psychology, cognition, and human aging*. New York: Springer.

Koltanowski, G. (1985). *In the dark*. Coraopolis, PA: Chess Enterprises.

Krampe, R. T., & Ericsson, K. A. (1996). Maintaining excellence: Deliberate practice and elite performance in young and older pianists. *Journal of Experimental Psychology: General, 125*, 331–359.

Madden, D. J. (1983). Aging and distraction by highly familiar stimuli during visual search. *Developmental Psychology, 19*, 499–507.

Madden, D. J., & Nebes, R. D. (1980). Aging and the development of automaticity in visual search. *Developmental Psychology, 16*, 277–296.

Masanaga, H., & Horn, J. L. (2000). Characterizing mature human intelligence: expertise development. *Learning and Individual Differences, 12*, 5–33.

Masanaga, H., & Horn, J. L. (2001). Expertise and age-related changes in components of intelligence. *Psychology and Aging, 16*, 293–311.

McArdle, J. J., Hamagami, F., Meredith, W., & Bradway, K. P. (2001). Modeling the dynamic hypotheses of Gf-Gc theory using life-span data. *Learning and Individual Differences, 12*, 53–79.

McArdle, J. J., & Woodcock, R. (Eds.). (1998). *Human cognitive abilities in theory and practice*. Itasca, IL: Riverside.

McDowd, J. M., & Birren, J. E. (1990). Aging and attentional processes. In J. E. Birren & K. W. Schaie (Eds.), *Handbook of the psychology of aging* (3rd ed., pp. 222–233). New York: Academic Press.

McDowd, J. M., & Craik, F. I. M. (1988). Effects of aging and task difficulty on divided attention performance. *Journal of Experimental Psychology: Human Perception and Performance, 14*(20), 267–280.

McGrew, K. S. (1994). *Clinical interpretation of the Woodcock–Johnson Tests of Cognitive Ability—Revised*. Boston: Allyn & Bacon.

McGrew, K. S., & Flanagan, D. P. (1998). *The Intelligence Test Desk Reference (ITDR)*. Boston: Allyn & Bacon.

McGrew, K. S., Werder, J. K., & Woodcock, R. W. (1991). *WJ-R technical manual*. Chicago: Riverside.

Miller, G. A. (1956). The magical number seven, plus or minus two: some limits on our capacity for processing information. *Psychological Review, 63*, 81–97.

Morrow, D., Leirer, V., Altieri, P., & Fitzsimmons, C. (1994). When expertise reduces age differences in performance. *Psychology and Aging, 9*, 134–148.

Nesselroade, J. R., & Baltes, P. B. (Eds.). (1979). *Longitudinal research in the study of behavior and development*. New York: Academic Press.

Nettelbeck, T. (1994). Speediness. In R. J. Sternberg (Ed.), *Encyclopedia of human intelligence* (pp. 1014–1019). New York: Macmillan

Noll, J., & Horn, J. L. (1998). Age differences in processes of fluid and crystallized intelligence. In J. J. McArdle & R. W. Woodcock (Eds.), *Human cognitive abilities in theory and practice* (pp. 263–281). Chicago: Riverside.

Perfect, T. J., & Maylor, E. A. (Eds.). (2000). *Models of cognitive aging*. Oxford: Oxford University Press.

Plude, D. J., & Hoyer, W. J. (1985). Attention and performance: Identifying and localizing age deficits. In N. Charness (Ed.), *Aging and human performance* (pp. 47–99). New York: Wiley.

Rabbitt, P. (1965). An age-decrement in the ability to ignore irrelevant information. *Journal of Gerontology, 20*, 233–238.

Rabbitt, P. (1993). Crystal quest: A search for the basis of maintenance of practice skills into old age. In A. Baddeley & L. Weiskrantz (Eds.), *Attention: Selection, awareness, and control* (pp. 188–230). Oxford: Clarendon Press.

Rabbitt, P., & Abson, V. (1991). Do older people know how good they are? *British Journal of Psychology, 82*, 137–151.

Richman, H. B., Gobet, H., Staszewski, J. J., & Simon, H. A. (1996). Perceptual and memory processes in the acquisition of expert performance: The EPAM model. In K. A. Ericsson (Ed.), *The road to excellence* (pp. 167–188). Mahwah, NJ: Erlbaum.

Rimoldi, H. J. (1948). Study of some factors related to intelligence. *Psychometrika, 13*, 27–46.

Roediger, H. L., & Crowder, R. G. (1975). Spacing of lists in free recall. *Journal of Verbal Learning and Verbal Behavior, 14*, 590–602.

Saariluoma, P. (1991). Aspects of skilled imagery in blindfold chess. *Acta Psychologica, 77*, 65–89.

Salthouse, T. A. (1985). Speed of behavior and its implications for cognition. In J. E. Birren & K. W. Schaie (Eds.), *Handbook of the psychology of aging* (2nd ed., pp. 400–426). New York: Van Nostrand Reinhold.

Salthouse, T. A. (1987). The role of representations in age differences in analogical reasoning. *Psychology and Aging, 2*, 357–362.

Salthouse, T. A. (Ed.). (1991). *Theoretical perspectives on cognitive aging*. Hillsdale, NJ: Erlbaum.

Salthouse, T. A. (1992). Influence of processing speed on adult age differences in working memory. *Acta Psychologica, 79*, 155–170.

Salthouse, T. A. (1993). Speed mediation of adult age differences in cognition. *Developmental Psychology, 29*, 727–738.

Salthouse, T. A., Kausler, D. H., & Saults, J. S. (1990). Age, self-assessed health status, and cognition. *Journal of Gerontology, 45*, 156–160.

Salthouse, T. A., & Somberg, B. L. (1982). Isolating the age deficit in speeded performance. *Journal of Gerontology, 37*, 59–63.

Saunders, D. R. (1959). On the dimensionality of the WAIS battery for two groups of normal males. *Psychological Reports, 5*, 529–541.

Schaie, K. W. (1990). Perceptual speed in adulthood: Cross sectional and longitudinal studies. *Psychology and Aging, 4*(4), 443–453.

Schaie, K. W. (1996). *Intellectual development in adulthood: The Seattle longitudinal study*. Cambridge, UK: Cambridge University Press

Spearman, C. (1904). "General intelligence," objectively determined and measured. *American Journal of Psychology, 15*, 210–293.

Spearman, C. (1927). *The abilities of man: Their nature and measurement*. London: Macmillan.

Spearman, C. (1939). Thurstone's work re-worked. *Journal of Educational Psychology, 30*(1), 1–16.

Sperling, G. (1960). The information available in brief visual presentations. *Psychological Monographs, 74*, 498–450.

Stankov, L. (1988). Single tests, competing tasks, and their relationship to the broad factors of intelligence. *Personality and Individual Differences, 9*, 25–33.

Stankov, L., & Horn, J. L. (1980). Human abilities revealed through auditory tests. *Journal of Educational Psychology, 72*, 21–44.

Stephenson, W. (1931). Tetrad-differences for verbal sub-tests relative to non-verbal sub-tests. *Journal of Educational Psychology, 22*, 334–350.

Thomson, G. A. (1916). A hierarchy without a general factor. *British Journal of Psychology, 8*, 271–281.

Thurstone, L. L. (1938). *Primary mental abilities* (Psychometric Monographs, No. 1). Chicago: University of Chicago Press.

Thurstone. L. L. (1947). *Multiple factor analysis*. Chicago: University of Chicago Press.

Vernon, P. E. (1950). *The structure of human abilities*. London: Methuen.

Walsh, D. A. (1982). The development of visual information processes in adulthood and old age. In F. I. M. Craik & S. Trehub (Eds.), *Aging and cognitive processes* (pp. 99–125). New York: Plenum Press.

Walsh, D. A., & Hershey, D. A. (1993). Mental models and the maintenance of complex problem solving skills in old age. In J. Cerella, J. Rybash, W. Hoyer, & M. Commons (Eds.), *Adult information processing: Limits on loss* (pp. 553–584). San Diego, CA: Academic Press.

Waugh, N. C., & Norman, D. A. (1965). Primary memory. *Psychological Review, 72,* 89–104.

Wickens, C. D., Braune, R., & Stokes, A. (1987). Age differences in the speed and capacity of information processing I: A dual-task approach. *Psychology and Aging, 2,* 70–78.

Woodcock, R. W. (1995). Theoretical foundations of the WJ-R measures of cognitive ability. *Journal of Psychoeducational Assessment, 8,* 231–258.

Woodcock, R. W. (1996). *The Woodcock–Johnson Psycho-Educational Battery—Revised.* Itasca, IL: Riverside.

4

The Three-Stratum Theory of Cognitive Abilities

JOHN B. CARROLL

The three-stratum theory of cognitive abilities is an expansion and extension of previous theories. It specifies what kinds of individual differences in cognitive abilities exist and how those kinds of individual differences are related to one another. It provides a map of all cognitive abilities known or expected to exist and can be used as a guide to research and practice. It proposes that there are a fairly large number of distinct individual differences in cognitive ability, and that the relationships among them can be derived by classifying them into three different strata: stratum I, "narrow" abilities; stratum II, "broad" abilities; and stratum III, consisting of a single "general" ability.

ORIGIN OF THE THEORY

The theory was developed in the course of a major survey (Carroll, 1993a, 1994) of research over the past 60 or 70 years on the nature, identification, and structure of human cognitive abilities. That research involved the use of the mathematical technique known as *factor analysis*. Necessarily, the work also involved the analysis of correlations among scores on psychological tests and other kinds of assessments of individuals. This is because factor analysis concerns the structure of correlations among such variables—that is, the question of how many *factors* or *latent traits* are indicated by a set of correlations arranged in a matrix such that all the correlations among variables are shown systematically.

In my survey, I used factor analysis to examine more than 460 sets of data (hereafter, *datasets*) from the relevant literature. In most cases these datasets had been previously analyzed by the original investigators, but I felt it necessary to reanalyze them because I wanted to take advantage of important technical advances in factor-analytic methodology that were not used by the original investigators, usually because they were not yet available at the time of the original data analysis. I also considered it desirable to analyze the datasets in as consistent a way as possible to facilitate making valid general conclusions.

Before beginning my survey, I considered how best to select datasets, because it was going to be impossible to reanalyze all of what I estimated as more than 2,000 datasets available in the relevant literature published over the years 1930–1985 (approximately)

Since the publication of the first edition of this text, John B. Carroll has passed away. The present chapter is therefore a reprint of his chapter in the first edition.

in many countries—mainly English-speaking countries such as the United States, Canada, Great Britain, and Australia, but also other countries such as France, Germany, Japan, Spain, and even Russia. I established several criteria for selecting datasets: (1) Each dataset should contain a substantial number of variables reflecting performance on cognitive tasks typical of those used in intelligence and aptitude tests or in research in cognitive psychology; (2) the dataset should be based on a substantial number of individuals (preferably more than, say, 100) taken from a defined population of children, adolescents, or adults that had been tested in a consistent way; (3) the published form of the dataset should present the matrix of correlations among its variables, thus permitting reanalysis; and (4) sufficient information about the sample and the variables must have been available to permit at least tentative interpretation of the findings.

In the end, more than 480 datasets were selected, but a small number (about 15) turned out to contain mathematical inconsistencies that could not be resolved. Thus reanalysis of these datasets was not feasible. Many of the datasets were from research by prominent investigators of cognitive abilities such as Thurstone (1938), Thurstone and Thurstone (1941), Guilford (1967), Guilford and Hoepfner (1971), Cattell (1971), Horn (1965), and Vernon (1961); for this reason, the three-stratum theory has similarities to certain theories espoused by some of these investigators (e.g., Horn's fluid–crystallized theory) (see Horn & Noll, 1997, and Horn & Blankson, Chapter 3, this volume).

At this point it is necessary to introduce the concept of *stratum* and to describe certain features of the reanalyses performed in my survey. It was probably Thurstone (1947) who created a related concept—the *order* of a factor analysis. A *first-order* factor analysis is the application of factor-analytic techniques directly to a correlation matrix of the original variables in the dataset; it results in one or more *first-order factors*. A *second-order* factor analysis is the application of factor-analytic techniques to the matrix of correlations among the first-order factors (if there are two or more, and if the correlations are other than zero) of a dataset; it results in one or more *second-order factors*. A *third-order* factor analysis is the application of factor-analytic techniques to the matrix of correlations among the second-order factors (if there are two or more) of a dataset; usually it results in a single *third-order factor,* but it could result in more than one such factor. This process could be repeated at still higher orders, but it would rarely be necessary, because at each successive order the number of resulting factors becomes ever smaller. (A large number of original variables would be necessary, to permit analysis at the fourth order, for example.)

The concept of order (of a factor, or of a factor analysis) is therefore tied to operations in the application of factor analysis to a particular dataset. Usually, the variables in a dataset are scores on a variety of psychological tests; the factor analysis produces first-order factors that correspond to clusters of tests such that within each cluster, the tests are similar in the contents or psychological processes they involve. A dataset might, for example, yield three first-order factors—one being a "verbal" factor with loadings on vocabulary and reading comprehension tests, another being a "spatial" factor with loadings on formboard and paper-folding tests, and still another being a "memory span" factor with loadings on a series of memory span tests. If these factors are correlated, a second-order factor might be interpreted as a "general intelligence" factor.

Suppose, however, the variables in a dataset are individual test items (e.g., the individual items on a vocabulary test). A first-order factor analysis of the matrix of correlations among vocabulary items might produce one or more factors; if one factor were found, it might indeed be a "vocabulary" or "verbal" factor, but if two or more factors were found, the investigator might be prompted to identify these factors by their different contents (a factor of "literary vocabulary," a factor of "scientific vocabulary," etc.). A second-order factor analysis of the correlations among such factors would probably produce a "general vocabulary" factor, which might be similar to the first-order vocabulary or verbal factor produced in the analysis of a more typical battery of psychological tests. Thus a vocabulary factor might be a first-order factor in one case but a second-order factor in another case. Similarly, a "general" factor might be a second-order factor in one case but a third-order factor in another case.

As factor analysis is essentially a technique of classifying abilities, Cattell (1971) introduced the term *stratum* to help in characterizing factors, in an absolute sense, in terms of the narrowness or breadth of their content. In the conduct of my survey and in interpreting results, I called the first-order factors resulting from analysis of typical sets of psychological tests *factors at the first stratum*, or *stratum I factors*. (Almost all the datasets were composed of typical sets of psychological tests.) *Stratum II factors* were second-order factors from such datasets, and *stratum III factors* were third-order factors from such datasets. Frequently, however, datasets did not produce third-order factors; they produced only one second-order factor, which was often interpretable as a *general* factor similar to the general factor that occurred as a third-order factor in some other datasets. Thus the stratum of a factor is relative to the variety and diversity of the variables covered by it. Sometimes it is the same as the order of a factor, but in other cases it is not; its stratum is assigned in terms of its perceived breadth or narrowness. It is possible that some factors are so narrow or specific (in content) that their stratum is less than 1. This would be the case for highly specific kinds of vocabulary knowledge identified by factor analysis of the items of a vocabulary test, as mentioned previously. For convenience, however, the three-stratum theory omits mention of such narrow factors, of which there could be many.

The three-stratum theory thus postulates that most factors of interest can be classified as being at a certain stratum, and that the total array of cognitive ability factors contains factors at three strata—namely, first, second, and third. At the third or highest stratum is a general factor (often called *g*). The second stratum is composed of a relatively small number (perhaps about 10) of "broad" factors, including *fluid intelligence, crystallized intelligence, general memory and learning, broad visual perception, broad auditory perception, broad retrieval ability, broad cognitive speediness,* and *processing speed*. At the first stratum (or stratum I), there are numerous first-order factors, roughly grouped under the second-stratum factors as shown in Figure 4.1. Some are "level" factors in the sense that their scores indicate the level of mastery, along a difficulty scale, that the individual is able to demonstrate. Others are

"speed" factors in the sense that their scores indicate the speed with which the individual performs tasks or the individual's rate of learning in learning and memory tasks.

Rationale and Impetus for Generating the Theory

The theory was intended to constitute a provisional statement about the enumeration, identification, and structuring of the total range of cognitive abilities known or discovered thus far. In this way it was expected to replace, expand, or supplement previous theories of the structure of cognitive abilities, such as Thurstone's (1938) theory of primary mental abilities, Guilford's (1967) structure-of-intellect theory, Horn and Cattell's (1966) Gf-Gc theory, or Wechsler's (1974; see also Matarazzo, 1972) theory of verbal and performance components of intelligence.

OPERATIONALIZATION AND APPLICATION OF THE THEORY

Component Parts of the Theory

The theory consists of an enumeration of the cognitive abilities that have been found thus far, with statements concerning the nature and generality of these abilities, the types of tasks that require them, and the types of tests that can be used to measure them. In effect, it also consists of statements about the structure of the abilities in terms of the assignment of abilities to one of three strata of different degrees of generality. Second-order factors subsumed by the third-order general factor are related to each other by virtue of their loadings on the general factor; some of these are more related to the general factor than others. Similarly, first-order factors subsumed by a given second-order factor are related to each other by virtue of their loadings on that second-order factor.

All the abilities covered by the theory are assumed to be "cognitive" in the sense that cognitive processes are critical to the successful understanding and performance of tasks requiring these abilities, most particularly in the *processing of mental information*. In many cases, they go far beyond the kinds of intelligences measured in typical batteries of intelligence tests. The abilities are roughly classified as follows:

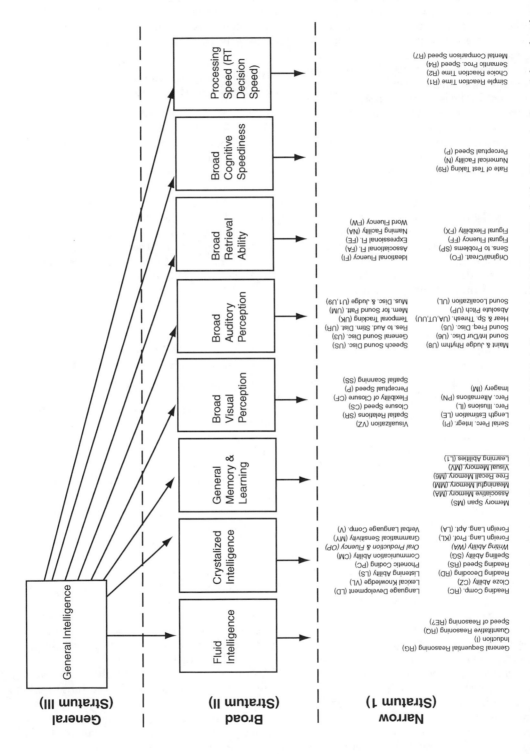

FIGURE 4.1. The three-stratum structure of cognitive abilities. From Carroll (1993a). Copyright © 1993 by Cambridge University Press. Adapted and reproduced by permission. *Note:* Stratum I factors are differentiated as "level" (plain type), "speed and level" (italics type), and "rate" (underlined) factors.

72

Abilities in the domain of language
Abilities in the domain of reasoning
Abilities in the domain of memory and learn-
ing
Abilities in the domain of visual perception
Abilities in the domain of auditory reception
Abilities in the domain of idea production
Abilities in the domain of cognitive speed
Abilities in the domain of knowledge and
achievement
Miscellaneous domains of ability (e.g., abili-
ties in the sensory domain, attention abil-
ities, cognitive styles, and administrative
abilities)

It must be stressed that this theory is only
provisional. Further research may suggest
that it should be revised, either in small or in
radical ways. It is becoming clear that present methods of measuring abilities may not
adequately cover all the abilities that exist or
that are important in practical life.

Operationalization of the Theory

Thus far, the three-stratum theory has not
been operationalized in any formal sense, in
terms of either actual batteries of tests or
other assessment procedures that are specifically designed to measure the abilities specified by the theory. A detailed description of
the theory as it pertains to the different domains of ability, including higher-stratum
abilities, can be found in relevant chapters of my book, *Human Cognitive Abilities*
(Carroll, 1993a). Most of these chapters describe representative tests or other procedures drawn from research studies or from
well-known batteries of tests whereby the
relevant factors of ability can be measured.
Other sources of information about tests for
measuring the abilities specified by the three-
stratum theory are handbooks by Jonassen
and Grabowski (1993) and Fleishman and
Reilly (1992).

**Applications of the Theoretical Model
for Practice and Research**

The three-stratum theory is intended chiefly
to provide guidance for further research
concerning cognitive abilities and their structure. For example, if new abilities are identified, the theory provides guidance as to
where such abilities should fit in the struc-

ture already established—whether they are
truly new or merely subvarieties of abilities
previously identified.

In research, also, the theory plays an
important role in presentation of factor-
analytic results. Matrices of factor loadings
show the loadings of tests (or other variables) on the different factors, at different
strata. Most often it is found that a given test
has significant loadings (say, greater than .3)
on more than one factor; for example, a test
might have such a loading on the general factor (at stratum III), a significant loading on
one or more of the stratum II factors, and a
significant loading on one or more of the
stratum I factors. In other cases, a test's significant loadings might occur only on a general factor and one of the stratum I factors.
In either case, the display of the test's loadings provides useful information about what
the test measures and the extent to which it
measures different factors. It is important to
realize that the scores of most tests reflect influences of more than one factor, usually factors at different strata.

The theory has similar uses in professional
practice. As was mentioned previously, it
provides what is essentially a "map" of all
known cognitive abilities. Such a map can be
used in interpreting scores on the many tests
used in individual assessment by clinical psychologists, school psychologists, industrial
psychologists, and others. Such scores can be
assessed in terms of the abilities they most
probably measure. The map also suggests
what abilities may need to be assessed in particular cases that require selection of appropriate tests (see Alfonso, Flanagan, &
Radwan, Chapter 9, this volume; Flanagan
& McGrew, 1997).

**EMPIRICAL SUPPORT
FOR THE THEORY**

The empirical support for this theory resides
in the reanalyses of the more than 460
datasets that were presented in Carroll
(1993a), where I offered arguments to justify
the procedures I used. The reanalyses themselves were presented in the form of detailed
hierarchical orthogonalized factor matrices
contained in a set of computer disks (Carroll,
1993b). Reviews of the book have been
highly favorable (Brand, 1993; Brody, 1994;

Burns, 1994; Eysenck, 1994; Nagoshi, 1994; Sternberg, 1994); thus it would seem that experts in the field have entered no serious objections to the results or the theory. It is possible, however, that more critical reviews will eventually appear, raising questions about certain features of the theory.

Relations with Other Theories

The three-stratum theory is an expansion and extension of most of the previous theories of cognitive abilities—in particular (in rough chronological order), those of Spearman (1927), Thurstone (1938), Vernon (1961), Horn and Cattell (1966; see Horn & Noll, 1997, and Horn & Blankson, Chapter 3, this volume), Hakstian and Cattell (1978), and Gustafsson (1989). Even in 1927, Spearman offered what was essentially a two-stratum theory; the latter authors presented further and more detailed evidence of the hierarchical structure of abilities.

The three-stratum theory differs more radically from the structure-of-intelligence theory offered by Guilford (1967) and Guilford and Hoepfner (1971). These investigators initially did not accept the notion of higher-order factors of intelligence; only in more recent papers did Guilford (1981, 1985) admit the possibility of higher-order factors, and some of Guilford's former colleagues have started to reanalyze his data in terms of higher-order factors (Bachelor, Michael, & Kim, 1994). The three-stratum theory has resemblances to the theory of *multiple intelligences* offered by Gardner (see Chen & Gardner, 1997 and Chapter 5, this volume). The various broad abilities show rough correspondences to Gardner's seven [now eight—Ed.] intelligences; however, Gardner seems not to accept the concept of an overarching general ability, nor does he accept the notion of a hierarchical structure of abilities. Apparently he regards his seven intelligences as being completely independent of each other, despite a plethora of evidence that this is not the case.

BEYOND TRADITIONAL THEORIES OF INTELLIGENCE

The three-stratum theory reflects advances in the behavioral sciences in a number of ways.

The Influence of Recent Advances in Psychometrics

In psychometrics, research over the past 50 years has increasingly emphasized that *intelligence,* or IQ, is not a single thing, but a complex, composite structure of a number of intelligences. A psychometric technique put forward by Schmid and Leiman (1957), the orthogonalization of hierarchical factor matrices, made it possible to formulate more exactly how this composite structure of intelligences could be conceptualized. The Schmid and Leiman technique has become popular only in recent years, but it has become one of the major bases of the three-stratum theory.

Other major bases of the three-stratum theory have been improvements in measurement theory and computational methods. A major advance in measurement theory has been the so-called item response theory (see mainly Lord & Novick, 1968), which presents a model of the relation of ability to test item performance and assists in the design of more valid and reliable ability tests. Although the conduct of a comprehensive factor-analytic study requires large logistic resources in assembling tests, test subjects, and test data, analysis of data has become increasingly easier with the advent of modern high-speed computers, particularly personal computers. The availability of personal computers enormously facilitated the reanalyses of large numbers of datasets in the Carroll studies (1993a, 1993b).

Influence of Recent Advances in Cognitive Psychology

The three-stratum theory reflects advances in cognitive psychology because these advances make it easier to interpret findings from factor analysis in terms of the properties of cognitive tasks (as represented in the psychological tests studied by factor analysis). Also, cognitive research has made it possible to focus attention on various cognitive tasks that were largely ignored in psychometrics (e.g., the sentence verification task and category-sorting tasks).

How the Three-Stratum Theory Departs from Traditional Paradigms

Above all, the three-stratum theory emphasizes the multifactorial nature of the domain of cognitive abilities and directs attention to many types of ability usually ignored in traditional paradigms. It implies that individual profiles of ability levels are much more complex than previously thought, but at the same time it offers a way of structuring such profiles, by classifying abilities in terms of strata. Thus a general factor is close to former conceptions of intelligence, whereas second-stratum factors summarize abilities in such domains as visual and spatial perception. Nevertheless, some first-stratum abilities are probably of importance in individual cases, such as the phonetic coding ability that is likely to describe differences between normal and dyslexic readers.

Future Directions in Research and Application

Much work remains to be done in the factor-analytic study of cognitive abilities. The map of abilities provided by the three-stratum theory undoubtedly has errors of commission and omission, with gaps to be filled in by further research, including the development of new types of testing and assessment and the factorial investigation of their relationships with each other and with better-established types of assessment.

The theory needs to be further validated by acquiring information about the importance and relevance of the various abilities it specifies. In this endeavor, cognitive psychology can help by investigating the basic information-processing aspects of such abilities. Developmental and educational psychology can assist by investigating the development, stability, and educability of abilities—not only those such as IQ, which has been studied extensively, but also the other types of abilities in different domains specified by the theory.

Moreover, the three-stratum theory has implications for studies in neuropsychology and human genetics. For example, the theory specifies, on the basis of factor-analytic studies, a certain structure for memory abilities. Does this structure have parallels in theories of brain function (Crick, 1994; Schacter & Tulving, 1994)? Similarly, the structure of abilities specified by the theory currently says little about the relative roles of genetic and environmental influences on these abilities; such influences can be investigated by considering them in relation to different

strata of abilities (Plomin & McClearn, 1993). Thus far, we have a considerable amount of information on the heritability of the third-stratum factor g, but relatively little on how much genes influence the development of lower-stratum abilities such as broad visual perception and perceptual speed.

The theory has major implications for practical assessment of individuals in clinical. educational, or industrial settings. It appears to prescribe that individuals should be assessed with regard to the *total range* of abilities the theory specifies. Any such prescription would of course create enormous problems; generally there would not be sufficient time to conduct assessments (by tests, ratings, interviews, personal observations, etc.) of all the abilities that exist. Even if there were, there is a lack of appropriate tests for many abilities. Research is needed to spell out how the assessor can select what abilities need to be tested in particular cases. The conventional wisdom is that abilities close to g are the most important to test or assess, but if this policy is followed too strictly, many abilities that are important in particular cases would probably be missed. Only the future will enable us to appreciate these possibilities adequately.

REFERENCES

Bachelor, P., Michael, W. B., & Kim, S. (1994). First-order and higher-order semantic and figural factors in structure-of-intellect divergent production measures. *Educational and Psychological Measurement, 54,* 608–619.

Brand, C. (1993, October 22). The importance of the g factor [Review of Carroll, 1993a]. *Times Higher Educational Supplement,* p. 22.

Brody, N. (1994). Cognitive abilities [Review of Carroll, 1993a]. *Psychological Science, 5,* 63, 65–68.

Burns, R. B. (1994). Surveying the cognitive terrain [Review of Carroll, 1993a]. *Educational Researcher, 23*(2), 35–37.

Carroll, J. B. (1993a). *Human cognitive abilities: A survey of factor-analytic studies.* New York: Cambridge University Press.

Carroll, J. B. (1993b). *Human cognitive abilities: A survey of factor-analytic studies.* Appendix B: Hierarchical factor matrix files. New York: Cambridge University Press.

Carroll, J. B. (1994). Cognitive abilities: Constructing a theory from data. In D. K. Detterman (Ed.), *Current topics in human intelligence: Vol. 4. Theories of intelligence* (pp. 43–63). Norwood, NJ: Ablex.

Cattell, R. B. (1971). *Abilities: Their structure, growth, and action.* Boston: Houghton Mifflin.

Chen, J.-Q., & Gardner, H. (1997). Alternative assessment from a multiple intelligences theoretical perspective. In D. P. Flanagan, J. L. Genshaft, & P. L. Harrison (Eds.), *Contemporary intellectual assessment: Theories, tests, and issues* (pp. 105–121). New York: Guilford Press.

Crick, F. (1994). *The astonishing hypothesis: The scientific search for the soul.* New York: Scribner's.

Eysenck, H. J. (1994). [Special review of Carroll, 1993a.] *Personality and Individual Differences, 16,* 199.

Flanagan, D. P., & McGrew, K. S. (1997). A cross-battery approach to assessing and interpreting cognitive abilities: Narrowing the gap between practice and cognitive science. In D. P. Flanagan, J. L. Genshaft, & P. L. Harrison (Eds.), *Contemporary intellectual assessment: Theories, tests, and issues* (pp. 314–325). New York: Guilford Press.

Fleishman, E. A., & Reilly, M. E. (1992). *Handbook of human abilities: Definitions, measurements, and job task requirements.* Palo Alto, CA: Consulting Psychologists Press.

Guilford, J. P. (1967). *The nature of human intelligence.* New York: McGraw-Hill.

Guilford, J. P. (1981). Higher-order structure-of-intellect abilities. *Multivariate Behavioral Research, 16,* 411–435.

Guilford, J. P. (1985). The structure-of-intellect model. In B. B. Wolman (Ed.), *Handbook of intelligence: Theories, measurements, and applications* (pp. 225–266). New York: Wiley.

Guilford, J. P., & Hoepfner, R. (1971). *The analysis of intelligence.* New York: McGraw-Hill.

Gustafsson, J. E. (1989). Broad and narrow abilities in research on learning and instruction. In R. Kanfer, P. L. Ackerman, & R. Cudeck (Eds.), *Abilities, motivation, and methodology: The Minnesota Symposium on Learning and Individual Differences* (pp. 203–237). Hillsdale, NJ: Erlbaum.

Hakstian, A. R., & Cattell, R. B. (1978). Higher-stratum ability structures on a basis of twenty primary abilities. *Journal of Educational Psychology, 70,* 657–669.

Horn, J. L. (1965). *Fluid and crystallized intelligence: A factor analytic study of the structure among primary mental abilities.* Unpublished doctoral dissertation, University of Illinois, Urbana/Champaign.

Horn, J. L., & Cattell, R. B. (1966). Refinement of the theory of fluid and crystallized general intelligences. *Journal of Educational Psychology, 57,* 253–270.

Horn, J. L., & Noll, J. (1997). Human cognitive capabilities: Gf-Gc theory. In D. P. Flanagan, J. L. Genshaft, & P. L. Harrison (Eds.), *Contemporary intellectual assessment: Theories, tests, and issues* (pp. 53–91). New York: Guilford Press.

Jonassen, D. H., & Grabowski, B. L. (Eds.). (1993). *Handbook of individual differences, learning, and instruction.* Hillsdale, NJ: Erlbaum.

Lord, F. M., & Novick, M. R. (1968). *Statistical theories of mental test scores.* Reading, MA: Addison-Wesley.

Matarazzo, J. D. (1972). *Wechsler's measurement and appraisal of adult intelligence* (5th ed.). Baltimore: Williams & Wilkins.

McGrew, K. S. (1997). Analysis of the major intelligence batteries according to a proposed comprehensive Gf-Gc framework. In D. P. Flanagan, J. L. Genshaft, & P. L. Harrison (Eds.), *Contemporary intellectual assessment: Theories, tests, and issues* (pp. 151–179). New York: Guilford Press.

Nagoshi, C. T. (1994). The factor-analytic guide to cognitive abilities [Review of Carroll, 1993a]. *Contemporary Psychology, 39,* 617–618.

Plomin, R., & McClearn, G. E. (Eds.). (1993). *Nature, nurture, and psychology.* Washington, DC: American Psychological Association.

Schacter, D. L., & Tulving, E. (Eds.). (1994). *Memory systems 1994.* Cambridge, MA: MIT Press.

Schmid, J., & Leiman, J. M. (1957). The development of hierarchical factor solutions. *Psychometrika, 22,* 53–61.

Spearman, C. (1927). *The abilities of man: Their nature and measurement.* New York: Macmillan.

Sternberg, R. J. (1994). 468 factor-analyzed data sets: What they tell us and don't tell us about human intelligence [Review of Carroll, 1993a]. *Psychological Science, 5,* 63–65.

Thurstone, L. L. (1938). *Primary mental abilities* (Psychometric Monographs, No. 1). Chicago: University of Chicago Press.

Thurstone, L. L. (1947). *Multiple factor analysis: A development and expansion of the vectors of mind.* Chicago: University of Chicago Press.

Thurstone, L. L., & Thurstone, T. G. (1941). *Factorial studies of intelligence* (Psychometric Monographs, No. 2). Chicago: University of Chicago Press.

Vernon, P. E. (1961). *The structure of human abilities* (2nd ed.). London: Methuen.

Wechsler, D. (1974). *Wechsler Intelligence Scale for Children—Revised.* New York: Psychological Corporation.

5

Assessment Based on Multiple-Intelligences Theory

JIE-QI CHEN
HOWARD GARDNER

How smart are you? "I'm pretty smart," you may be thinking. When we ask this question at talks or workshops, we hear responses like "That's not an easy question. If I compare myself to my colleagues, I'd have to say I'm about average," or "I'm not sure. I have a hard time with some job demands and sometimes have doubts about my competence."

Consider a second question: *How are you smart?* This question tends to elicit answers like "I'm an articulate speaker and I enjoy writing, but I have trouble with math, especially statistics," or "I'm good at designing charts and other graphics, but it's hard for me to express my ideas in words," or "I learn to play musical instruments easily, because I have a good sense of pitch and rhythm."

Although both questions concern human capability or competence, they reflect different models of intelligence. The underlying notion of the first question is that intelligence is a single overall property with one dimension, along which everyone can be arrayed. Moreover, this general mental ability can be measured reasonably well by a variety of standardized tests, especially by IQ tests designed specifically for this purpose (Eysenck, 1979; Jensen, 1993; Sattler, 2001; Snyderman & Rothman, 1988). In this view, IQ and scores on other standardized tests of

intelligence have predictive value for many educational, economic, and social outcomes (Herrnstein & Murray, 1994; Jensen, 1969, 1987).

In contrast, the second question reflects a stance that recognizes many discrete facets of cognition and acknowledges that people have different cognitive strengths. In this view, the array of intelligences cannot be assessed adequately with a brief sampling of short-answer psychological tasks in a decontextualized situation. Rather, they are more validly documented by the use of contextually rich instruments and an authentic assessment approach that sample a range of discrete cognitive capacities.

In this chapter, we describe the theoretical model that prompts the second question—the theory of *multiple intelligences* (MI; Gardner, 1993b, 1999)—and present it as the basis for an alternative approach to assessment. We begin by providing an overview of the theory, including the definition of an intelligence, criteria for identifying intelligences, and basic principles. We then chart the challenges posed to traditional conceptions of intelligence, particularly the psychometric view of intelligence and Piaget's theory of cognitive development. Moving from theory to practice, we identify general features of the MI approach to assessment, including descriptions of measures, materials, and contexts. We then introduce two instruments that incorporate features of the MI approach to assessment. We also report on empirical studies that support the validity of the MI-based approach to assessment with findings of differentiated, rather than general, profiles of individual cognitive abilities. We conclude the chapter with a discussion of the MI-based assessment approach in light of recent empirical work in the field and the advancement of MI theory itself.

AN OVERVIEW OF MI THEORY

MI theory grew from the efforts of Howard Gardner to reconceptualize the nature of intelligence. Introduced in his 1983 book, *Frames of Mind,* and refined in subsequent writings, the theory contends that human intelligence is neither a single complex entity nor a unified set of processes—hitherto the dominant view in the field of psychology. Instead, Gardner posits that there are several relatively autonomous intelligences, and that an individual's profile reflects a unique configuration of these intellectual capacities.

Definition of Intelligence

In his most recent formulation, *Intelligence Reframed* (1999), Gardner defines *intelligence* as "a biopsychological potential to process information that can be activated in a cultural setting to solve problems or create products that are of value in a culture" (p. 33). By considering intelligence a potential, Gardner asserts its emergent and responsive nature, thereby differentiating his theory from traditional ones, in which human intelligence is fixed and innate. Whether a potential will be activated depends in large part on the values of the culture in which an individual grows up and, relatedly, on the opportunities available in that culture. Gardner also acknowledges the role of personal decisions made by individuals, their families, and others in their lives. These activating forces result in the development and expression of a range of abilities, or intelligences, from culture to culture and also from individual to individual.

Gardner's definition of intelligence differs from other formulations in that it considers the creation of products, such as sculptures and computers, to be as important an expression of intelligence as abstract problem solving. Traditional theories do not recognize created artifacts as manifestations of intelligence and therefore are limited in both conceptualization and measurement.

Criteria for Identifying Intelligences

In the process of developing MI theory, Gardner considered the range of adult end states that are valued in diverse cultures around the world. To identify the abilities that support these end states, he examined empirical data from disciplines that had not been considered previously in defining human intelligence (Gardner, 1993b). The results of Gardner's extensive analyses consistently supported his emerging notion of specific and relatively independent sets of cognitive abilities. His examination of these datasets proceeded in light of eight criteria for identifying an intelligence. More specifically, to be defined as an *intelligence*, an ability is tested in terms of the following eight criteria (Gardner, 1993b):

- An intelligence should be isolable in cases of brain damage, and there should be evidence for its plausibility and autonomy in evolutionary history. These two criteria were derived from biology.
- Two criteria came from developmental psychology: An intelligence has to have a distinct developmental history with a definable set of expert end-state performances, and it must exist within special populations such as idiot savants and prodigies.
- Two criteria emerged from traditional psychology: An intelligence demonstrates relatively independent operation through the results of specific skill training, and also through low correlation to other intelligences in psychometric studies.
- Two criteria were derived from logical analysis: An intelligence must have its own identifiable core operation or set of operations, and must be susceptible to encoding in a symbol system (such as language, numbers, graphics, or musical notations).

Using these criteria to identify intelligences, Gardner grounded the development of MI theory in the analysis of empirical data. His account of intelligences is derived from his comprehensive and systematic review of empirical data from studies in biology, neuropsychology, developmental psychology, and cultural anthropology (Gardner, 1993b). The methodology Gardner used to develop MI theory is a drastic departure from the psychological testing approach typically used to develop assessments of intelligence. As Vygotsky (1978) argued, however, "Any fundamentally new approach to a scientific problem inevitably leads to new methods of investigation and analysis. The invention of new methods that are adequate to the new ways in which problems are posed requires far more than a simple modification of previously accepted methods" (p. 58).

Identified Intelligences

To date, Gardner has identified eight intelligences. We describe each, along with a mention of individuals who would presumably excel in a particular intelligence.

1. *Linguistic intelligence*, exemplified by writers and poets, describes the ability to perceive and generate spoken or written language.
2. *Logical–mathematical intelligence*, used by mathematicians, scientists, and computer programmers, involves the ability to appreciate and utilize numerical, abstract, and logical reasoning to solve problems.
3. *Musical intelligence*, seen in musical performers and composers, entails the ability to create, communicate, and understand meanings made out of sound.
4. *Spatial intelligence*, necessary for graphic designers and architects, refers to the ability to perceive, modify, transform, and create visual and/or spatial images.
5. *Bodily–kinesthetic* intelligence, exemplified by dancers and athletes, deals with the ability to use all or part of one's body to solve problems or fashion products.
6. *Naturalistic intelligence*, critical for archeologists and botanists, concerns the ability to distinguish among critical features of the natural environment.
7. *Interpersonal intelligence*, essential for leaders and teachers, describes the ability to recognize, appreciate, and contend with the feelings, beliefs, and intentions of other people.
8. *Intrapersonal intelligence* involves the ability to understand oneself—including emotions, desires, strengths, and vulnerabilities—and to use such information effectively in regulating one's own life. The self-description by a person strong in intrapersonal intelligence would closely resemble the description offered by those who know the person well.

Though the linguistic and logical–mathematical intelligences have been emphasized in psychometric testing and school settings, the eight intelligences in the MI framework have equal claims to priority and are seen as equally valid and important (Gardner, 1987a, 1987b, 1993b). Gardner does not claim either that this roster of intelligences is exhaustive or that the particular labels or delineations among the intelligences are definitive; rather, his aim is to establish support for a pluralistic view of intelligence. The identification of intelligences is based on empirical evidence and can be revised on the basis of new empirical findings (Gardner, 1994, 2003).

Characteristics of Intelligences

For Gardner (1993b, 2003), all people with typical functioning are capable of drawing on all of the intelligences. However, presumably for both hereditary and environmental reasons, each individual is distinguished by a particular *profile of intelligences*. An individual's profile features his or her particular combination of relatively stronger and weaker intelligences that are used to solve problems or to fashion products. These relative strengths and weaknesses are important sources of individual differences (Kornhaber, Krechevsky, & Gardner, 1990).

Intelligences are subject to encoding in varied symbol systems. Each intelligence can be expressed through one or more symbol systems, such as spoken or written language, numbers, music notation, picturing, or mapping. These varied symbol systems, each with particular problem-solving features and information-processing capacities, contribute to the relative independence of intelligences. It is also through symbol systems that intelligences are applied in specific domains or bodies of knowledge within a culture, such as mathematics, art, basketball, and medicine (Gardner, 1993b, 1999).

Although related, the concepts of *intelligence* and *domain* are readily distinguishable (Gardner, 1993b). The former refers to biological and psychological potentials within an individual, whereas the latter speaks of a body of knowledge valued and exercised within a culture. A particular intelligence may be deployed in many domains. For example, spatial forms of intelligence may operate in the domains of visual arts, navigation, and engineering. Similarly, performance in a domain may require the use of more than one intelligence. For example, the domain of musical performance involves bodily–kinesthetic and interpersonal as well as musical intelligences.

Intelligences cannot be viewed merely as a group of raw computational capacities. The world is wrapped in meanings. Over the long haul, intelligences can be implemented only to the extent that they partake of these meanings and enable the individual to develop into a functioning, symbol-using member of his or her community. An individual's intelligences, to a great extent, are shaped by cultural influences and refined by educational processes. It is through the process of education that "raw" intellectual competencies are developed and individuals are prepared to assume mature cultural roles. Rich educational experiences are essential for the development of each individual's particular configuration of interests and abilities (Gardner, 1991, 1993a, 1993b).

CHALLENGES TO TRADITIONAL CONCEPTIONS OF INTELLIGENCE

Challenges to the Psychometric View of Intelligence and Its Approach to Assessment

MI theory challenges the psychometric view of intelligence and its approach to assessment on several fronts. First, MI theory questions the conception of *intelligence* as a single entity that is general, stable, and representative of the entire range of cognitive behaviors (Gould, 1981; Herrnstein & Murray, 1994; Neisser et al., 1996; Plomin & Petrill, 1997; Sameroff, Seifer, Baldwin, & Baldwin, 1993; Snyderman & Rothman, 1987). In his extensive survey of literature on human intelligence, Gardner (1993b) noted that research on both typical and atypical populations has produced results that are inconsistent with the claims for general intelligence.

To be sure, we are aware that, based on correlations among psychological tests and subtests, numerous studies report finding a positive manifold, supporting the claim that an underlying factor contributes to performance on all or a majority of the measures of intellect. However, almost all of the measures used in these studies are paper-and-pencil tests, and most of the tests measure primarily logical–mathematical and linguistic intelligences or require that blend of intelligences for success on the psychometric instrument. Furthermore, the skills measured for each intelligences often represent a narrow range of that intelligence's applications. For example, linguistic intelligence is usually measured only through knowledge of vocabulary and reading comprehension. Other linguistic abilities, such as creative writing, persuasive argument, and reporting, are rarely included. Given that conventional psychological tests measure primarily two intelligences, sample a narrow range of knowledge and skills for each intelligence, and rely on the same means of measurement, it is not surprising that scores on these tests are correlated. MI theory predicts, however, that when a wide range of areas is assessed, individuals will display a differentiated profile of abilities, and correlations among diverse abilities will not be high (Gardner & Walters, 1993; Walters & Gardner, 1986).

In addition to the problems with measures used in traditional psychometric research, the measurement of so-called "general intelligence" is often used to array individuals in terms of how smart they are in a global sense. Such a notion gives rise to the idea of a cognitive elite; it encourages the inference that some people are at the top from the start, and that those who are not among the elite cause our social problems (Gardner, 1995; Gould, 1994). In schools today, the notion of general intelligence explicitly or implicitly contributes to the massive use of standardized achievement tests for accountability purposes. Based on mean scores on an achievement test, for example, some schools are rated as model exemplars whereas others are considered failures, and some children are promoted whereas others are labeled at risk at a very early age. Yet many of these tests measure only a narrow range of the intelligences and fail to offer appropriate opportunities for all children to demonstrate their intellectual strengths.

Arguing that intelligence tests focus primarily on linguistic and logical–mathematical forms of thinking, we recognize that some current intelligence tests do measure more than two cognitive abilities (Guilford, 1967; McGrew, 1997; Sternberg, 1985a, 1985b, 1996, 1997; See also various chapters in this volume). In his triarchic theory, for example, Sternberg identifies three basic kinds of information–processing components that underlie intelligent thought, referred to as *metacomponents, performance components,* and *knowledge acquisition components,* and various tests have been developed on the basis of the theory's tenets (Sternberg, 1985a, 1988, 1996, and Chapter 6, this volume). Carroll's work (Carroll, 1993 and Chapter 4, this volume) measures up to eight different intellectual components, including crystallized intelligence, visual ability, auditory intelligence, general memory and learning, retrieval, speed of processing, cognitive speediness, and fluid intelligence. Guilford (1967) claims the need to evaluate 120 components of intelligence. These intelligence tests, however, are based on "horizontal" theories of intelligence. That is, mental faculties measured in these tests putatively function similarly in all content areas and operate according to one general law. In contrast, MI theory is a "vertical" conceptualization of intelligence. According to MI theory, intelligences are sensitive to content areas. One should not assume a single "horizontal" capacity, such as memory, perception, or speed of processing, that necessarily cuts across domains. As such, individuals can be rapid or slow learners or can exhibit novel or stereotypical thinking in any one of the eight intelligences, without predictable consequences for any of the other intelligences (Gardner, 1993d).

With regard to how intelligence is measured, we acknowledge that the continuum of testing instruments ranges from those that are mass-produced, standardized, paper-and-pencil tests to those that feature interaction between test takers and test administrators and use a variety of materials, such as blocks, pictures, and geometric shapes. Despite this range, tests at all points on the continuum that are based on the psychometric view tend to be one-shot experiences and exclude capacities that cannot be readily measured through the use of such limited tasks as short-answer questions, block design, or picture arrangement. MI theory argues that the capacities excluded, such as artistic ability, athletic competence, and interpersonal skills, are also intelligences. For assessment to be accurate and complete, these intelligences must be measured in as direct and contextually appropriate a way as possible. This approach both expands the range of what is measured and permits assessment of the intelligences as an individual applies them in meaningful ways.

Challenges to Piaget's Theory of Cognitive Development and His Assessment Method

Piaget's account of cognitive development presents a theoretically distinct perspective. Departing from the psychometric view, Piaget emphasized the developmental nature of intelligence and the qualitatively, rather than quantitatively, different mind of the child. Piaget was also interested chiefly in the universal properties of the human intellect rather than individual differences (Piaget, 1954, 1977; Piaget & Inhelder, 1969). However, Piaget's theory is similar to the psychometric view in claiming that the mental structures that characterize developmental stages are best represented as a single entity or unified set of processes. In Piaget's theory, mental structures are general rather than specific and universal rather than cultural. In this limited respect, his theory views intelligence as a single entity.

The universal or general quality of mind in Piaget's theory is defined in terms of logical–mathematical thought about the physical aspects of the world, including the understanding of causality, time, and space. However, as argued above, logical–mathematical thinking is only one kind of human intelligence; it does not reflect the core operations of other forms of intelligence. In contrast to Piaget's belief, MI theory challenges the assumption that there are general structures that are applied to every domain. Rather, what exist in the mind of the child at a moment in time are specific skills in a variety of domains, each skill functioning at a certain level of mastery with respect to that domain (Chen, 1993; Feldman, 1994; Krechevsky & Gardner, 1990).

As for assessment, Piaget is famous for his creation and creative use of the clinical method. *Clinical method* refers to the way in which a researcher or an assessor interacts with a child by asking the child to complete tasks with concrete materials and answer specific questions about the reasoning involved (Piaget, 1929). Unlike psychometric testing, Piaget's clinical method emphasizes the interaction between adult and child. It also provides opportunities to explore the reasoning behind the child's task performance. We should note that, as in psychometric testing, Piagetian tasks are usually administered in a laboratory setting. Assessment materials and procedures, such as conservation tasks and follow-up questions, are decontextualized and may seem foreign to young children (Donaldson, 1988; Fischer & Bidell, 1992; Flavell, 1982; Flavell, Miller, & Miller, 2002). Because MI theory stresses the use of intelligences to solve problems or fashion products, MI-based assessment relies preferentially on meaningful tasks in contexts that are familiar to children.

With regard to the use of assessment information, Piaget assumes that cognitive development is essentially the result of the child's spontaneous tendencies to learn about the world, with the particular features of the environment playing a relatively minor role in the process (Piaget, 1954, 1977). In contrast, MI theory argues that for progressive and productive growth to occur in any intellectual domain, quite specific environmental conditions must be systematically presented and sustained over time. These environmental forces may be material, technological, social, or cultural in nature. The role of educators is not to wait passively for cognition to develop, but rather to orchestrate a variety of environmental conditions that will catalyze, facilitate, and enable developmental progress in diverse intellect domains (Feldman, 1994; Gardner, 1993c; Vygotsky, 1978).

ASSESSMENT FROM THE MI PERSPECTIVE

MI theory calls for a significant departure from traditional concepts of intelligence. Although this was not Gardner's initial intention, MI theory has also led to the development of alternative forms of assessment (Chen, Krechevsky, & Viens, 1998; Krechevsky, 1998). A risk to any innovation is the danger that it will be assimilated in terms of traditional forms and distorted in the process. And, in fact, there have been repeated requests for standardized paper-and-pencil MI tests, and several such instruments have been developed by test makers (Gardner, 1993d). To avoid inadvertently producing another psychometrically inspired tracking approach, in this section we describe the central features of an MI approach to assessment, including measures, instruments, materials, context, and purpose.

Measures: Valuing Intellectual Capacities in a Wide Range of Domains

As described earlier, MI theory maintains that human intelligence is pluralistic, that each intelligence is relatively autonomous, and that all of the intelligences are of potentially equal import. Assessment based on MI theory incorporates a range of measures designed to tap the different facets of each intellectual capacity.

In emphasizing the measurement of intellectual capacities in a wide range of domains, it is important to note that we do not deny the existence of some yet-to-be determined relationship among cognitive abilities; nor do we propose that standard psychometric measures be abolished overnight. Instead, we advocate the development of alternative methods of assessment, as well as the assessment of a broader range of skills and abilities. The MI approach to assessment recognizes both those students who excel in linguistic and logical pursuits and those students who have cognitive and personal strengths in other intelligences. By virtue of the wider range it measures, MI types of assessment identify more students who are "smart," albeit in different ways (Gardner, 1984, 1986, 1993a).

It has been documented that students who have trouble with some academic subjects, such as reading or math, are not necessarily inadequate in all areas (Chen, 1993; Comer, 1988; Levin, 1990; Slavin & Madden, 1989). The challenge is to provide comparable opportunities for these students to demonstrate their strengths and interests. When the students recognize that they are good at something, and when this accomplishment is acknowledged by teachers and classmates, the students are far more likely to experience success and feel valued. In some instances, the sense of success in one area may make students more likely to engage in areas where they feel less comfortable. When that occurs, the systematic use of multiple measures goes beyond its initial purpose of identifying diverse cognitive abilities and becomes a means of bridging student strengths in one area to other areas of learning (Chen, Krechevsky, & Viens, 1998).

Instruments: Using Media Appropriate to the Domain

Based on the contention that each intelligence exhibits particular problem-solving features and operational mechanisms, MI theory argues that *intelligence-fair* instruments are needed in order to assess the unique capacities of each intelligence. Such instruments engage the key abilities of particular intelligences, allowing one to look directly at the functioning of each intellectual capacity, rather than forcing the individual to reveal his or her intelligence through the customary lens of a linguistic or logical instrument.

For example, when an intelligence-fair instrument is used, bodily intelligence can be assessed by recording how a person learns and remembers a new dance or physical exercise. To consider a person's interpersonal intelligence, it is necessary to observe how he or she interacts with and influences others in different social situations. It is important to note that what is assessed is never an intelligence in pure form. Intelligences are always expressed in the context of specific tasks, domains, and disciplines. For example, there is no "pure" spatial intelligence; instead, there is spatial intelligence as expressed in a child's puzzle solution, route finding, block building, or basketball passing (Gardner, 1993b).

Materials: Engaging Children in Meaningful Activities and Learning

MI theory argues that the intelligences are manifested through a wide variety of artifacts and human efforts. For an assessment to be meaningful, the selection of assessment materials must be a careful and deliberate process. Although materials alone do not lead to meaningful assessment, *intelligence-sensitive* materials are more likely to invite questions, stimulate curiosity, facilitate discoveries, promote communications, and encourage the use of imagination and multiple symbol systems (Rinaldi, 2001).

Assessment based on MI theory is responsive to the fact that children have had different environmental and educational experiences. Considering that each intelligence is an expression of the interplay among biological, psychological, and environmental factors, children's prior experience with assessment materials directly affects their performance on tasks. For example, children who have little experience with blocks are less likely to do well in a block design task. Similarly, it would be unfair to assess a child's musical ability by asking him or her to play a xylophone if the child has never seen such a musical instrument. In recognition of the role that experience plays, the MI approach to assessment aims to use materials that are familiar to children. To the extent that children are not familiar with materials, they are given ample opportunities to explore materials prior to any formal assessment.

Materials used in many current intelligence tests, including pictures, geometric shapes, and manipulatives, are familiar to most children in industrial societies. Yet such materials provide little intrinsic attraction because they have little meaning to children's daily lives. For assessment to be meaningful for students and instructive for teachers, it should occur in the context of students' working on problems and projects that genuinely engage them, hold their interest, and motivate them to do well. Such assessments may not be as easy to design as a standardized multiple-choice test, but they are more likely to elicit a student's full repertoire of skills and to yield information that is useful for subsequent learning and instruction (Gardner, 1993a; Linn, 2000; Wiggins, 1998).

Context: Focusing on Ecological Validity and Relevance for Instruction

To assess intelligences, the first and foremost criterion for creating context is *ecological validity* (Gardner, 1993d); that is, the assessment environment must be natural, familiar, and ongoing. Learning is not a one-shot experience; accurate assessment is not, either. Instead, it is an ongoing process that should be fully integrated into the natural learning environment. When a child's ability is measured through a one-shot test or assessment, the child's profile of abilities is often incomplete and may be distorted. In contrast, when assessment is naturally embedded in the learning environment, it allows teachers to observe children's performances in various situations over time. Such observations make it possible to use multiple samples of a child's ability to document the dynamics and variation of the child's performances within and across domains, and so to portray the child's intellectual profile more accurately.

MI types of assessment blur the traditional distinction between assessment and instruction. A teacher uses the results of an MI-based assessment to plan instruction; as instruction proceeds, the teacher has new opportunities to assess a child's developing competence. In this process, assessment and instruction inform and enhance each other. Initially, methods for ongoing assessment will need to be introduced to students explicitly; over time, however, assessment will occur with increasing spontaneity and therefore will require little explicit recognition or labeling by either the student or the teacher (Gardner, 1993a).

Integrating authentic tasks and teacher observations over time, assessment based on MI theory does not typically function as a norm-referenced instrument. As clinically oriented scientists, we are wary of the establishment of a universal norm by which individuals' intelligences could be compared. Rather, intelligence in the MI framework is defined as a potential with a pluralist, responsive, and dynamic nature. MI-based assessment involves performance standards or criterion references that teachers or educators can use to guide and evaluate their observations. In contrast to norm-referenced tests, which feature decontextualized and impartial judgments of students' perfor-

mance, MI-based assessment is open to incorporating the clinical judgments of classroom teachers. In so doing, it places greater value on the experience and expertise of teachers who are knowledgeable about the context of the assessment and directly responsible for using the results (Darling-Hammond & Ancess, 1996; Darling-Hammond & Snyder, 1992; Linn, 2000; Meisels, Bickel, Nicholson, Xue, & Atkins-Burnett, 2001; Moss, 1994).

Purpose: Portraying Complete Intellectual Profiles to Support Learning and Teaching

Traditional tests—achievement, readiness, intelligence, and the like—are often used to rank-order and sort students based on a single quantitative score. Reference to single test scores leads to an almost exclusive focus on deficits when a score is relatively low. Consequently, psychologists often spend more time rank-ordering students than they do helping them. And educators often focus too much on remediating students' deficits, rather than on recognizing their strengths and extending these to other areas of learning. Seemingly objective scores on these standardized tests disguise the complex nature of human intelligence. In the process, the scores also limit children's range of learning potentials and narrow their opportunities for success in school.

Instead of ranking, labeling, and focusing on deficits, the purpose of MI types of assessment is to support each student on the basis of his or her complete intellectual profile—strengths, interests, and weaknesses. When it is deemed appropriate, students join the assessment process. They are informed of what can be expected in terms of assessment tasks. They help develop performance standards. They are also encouraged to learn to evaluate their own strengths and weaknesses. During an assessment, the assessor provides feedback to the student that is helpful immediately, such as suggestions about what to study or work on, and pointers on which work habits are productive and which are not. It is especially important that feedback include concrete suggestions and information about relative strengths the student can build upon, regardless of his or her rank within a comparable group of student

(Chen, Krechevsky, & Viens, 1998; Gardner, 1993a). The narrative profile can be further shared with parents and future teachers to strengthen the development of individualized educational plans.

Finally, it is important to note that the identification of intellectual strengths and weaknesses of individuals is not the endpoint of MI types of assessment. The purpose of portraying a complete intellectual profile is to help educators understand each child as completely as possible and then mobilize his or her intelligences to achieve specific educational goals. MI-based assessments promote achievement of these goals by assisting educators in selecting appropriate instructional strategies and pedagogical approaches, based on a comprehensive and in-depth understanding of each child.

MI-BASED ASSESSMENT TOOLS IN EARLY EDUCATION

Armed with findings about human cognition and its development, and in light of the perceived need for an alternative to formal testing, Gardner and his colleagues at Harvard University's Project Zero began more than a decade ago to design programs featuring new approaches to assessment (Gardner, 1993a; Krechevsky, 1998). Since then, there have been numerous efforts to develop MI-based assessments throughout the United States and across the world (Adams, 1993; Armstrong, 1994; Hsueh, 2003; Lazear, 1994; McNamee, Chen, Masur, McCray, & Melendez, 2003; Shearer, 1996; Stefanakis, 2003; Teels, 2000; Wu, 2003; Yoong, 2001). Below we describe two of these efforts: the Spectrum Assessment System and Bridging: Assessment for Teaching. Although both instruments are designed for use with young children, the principles and features of the instruments are applicable to the assessment of individuals across the age span.

Spectrum Assessment System

The Spectrum Assessment System was developed by the staff of Project Spectrum at the Harvard Graduate School of Education during the 1980s and 1990s. Project Spectrum, codirected by Gardner at Harvard and David Feldman at Tufts University, was a 10-year research project dedicated to the development of an innovative approach to assessment and curriculum for the preschool and early primary school years. Project Spectrum's work is based on the view that each child exhibits a distinctive profile of cognitive abilities or a spectrum of intelligences. These intelligences are not fixed; rather, they can be enhanced by educational opportunities, such as an environment rich with stimulating materials that support learning and self-expression. The name of the project reflects its mission to recognize diverse intellectual strengths in children.

The Spectrum Assessment System includes three components: the Preschool Assessment Activities, the Observational Guidelines, and the Spectrum Profile (hereafter referred to as Activities, Guidelines, and Profiles) (Chen, Isberg, & Krechevsky, 1998; Chen, Krechevsky, & Viens, 1998; Krechevsky, 1991, 1998). The Activities include 15 activities in seven domains of knowledge: language, mathematics, music, visual arts, social understanding, science, and movement (see Appendix 5.1). To facilitate the use of assessment findings, Spectrum researchers developed assessment activities in domains that are compatible with school curricula.

The assessments are embedded in meaningful, hands-on activities that share a number of distinctive features: (1) The activities give children inviting materials to manipulate, such as toy figures or a Play-Doh birthday cake; (2) they are intelligence-fair, using materials appropriate to particular domains rather than relying on language and math as assessment vehicles; and (3) they examine abilities relevant to achieving fulfilling adult roles. Although Spectrum assessment activities measure skills that are valued by adult society, these skills are used in contexts that are meaningful to children. For example, to assess social understanding, children are encouraged to manipulate figures in a scaled-down, three-dimensional replica of their classroom; to assess math skills, children are asked to keep track of passengers getting on and off a toy bus.

Some activities are structured tasks that can be administered in a one-on-one situation; others are more spontaneous and can take place in a group setting. Each activity measures specific abilities, often requires particular materials, and is accompanied by written instructions for task administration. These instructions include a score sheet that identifies and describes different levels of the key abilities assessed in the activity, making a child's performance on many activities quantifiable.

The Guidelines are observational checklists in eight different domains (see Appendix 5.2). In the Guidelines, the domain of science in the Preschool Assessment Activities is divided into natural science and mechanical science; this move permits the assessor to capture the uses of different key abilities. Each guideline describes a set of key abilities and core elements similar to those measured in the Preschool Assessment Activities. *Key abilities* are the abilities that children need to perform tasks successfully in each domain. In the case of music, key abilities include music perception, production, and composition. Spectrum researchers further identify a set of *core elements*, or specific cognitive skills that help children exercise and execute the designated key ability. For example, core elements for music production include the abilities to maintain accurate pitch, tempo, and rhythmic patterns; to exhibit expressiveness when singing or playing an instrument; and to recall and reproduce musical properties (Chen, Isberg, & Krechevsky, 1998). By directing observations in terms of domains, key abilities, and core elements, the guidelines provide teachers with a means of focusing, organizing, and recording their observations of individual children. The guidelines also help teachers to systematize information they may be collecting in a more intuitive way.

The Activities and Guidelines can be used independently. However, when used together, they provide a more complete and accurate picture of a child's abilities. Because both instruments use similar sets of domain-specific key abilities to gauge a child's performance, comparing and contrasting results from the two assessments become straightforward and meaningful. The Activities help describe the child's place in a developmental process at a particular point in time, whereas the Guidelines direct observation so that the child's progress can be tracked over time. The Activities focus on degrees or levels of a child's relative strengths and weaknesses, while the Guidelines look at the use of these identified abilities across settings. Finally, the Activities permit close examination of one child at a time, making it possible to document the child's performance in detail. In contrast, the Guidelines help teachers obtain a rough approximation of the ways in which children differ from one another in the given learning environment (Chen, 2004).

The third component of the *Spectrum Assessment System* is the Profile—a narrative report based on the information obtained from the two assessment processes described above (Krechevsky, 1998; Ramos-Ford & Gardner, 1991). Using nontechnical language, the report focuses on the range of cognitive abilities examined by the Spectrum assessment instruments. It describes each child's relative strengths and weaknesses in terms of that child's own capacities, and only occasionally in relation to peers. Strengths and weaknesses are described in terms of the child's performance in different content areas. For example, a child's unusual sensitivity to different kinds of music might be described in terms of facial expressions, movement, and attentiveness during and after listening to various music pieces. It is important to note that the child's profile is described not only in terms of capacities, but also in terms of the child's preferences and inclinations. The report stresses the importance of ongoing assessment. The profile is not a static image, but a dynamic composition that reflects a child's interests, capabilities, and experiences at a particular point in time. Changes in the child's profile are inevitable as his or her life experience changes. The conclusion of the Profile typically includes specific recommendations to parents and teachers about ways to support identified strengths and improve weak areas (Adams & Feldman, 1993; Krechevsky, 1998).

Bridging: Assessment for Teaching

Bridging: Assessment for Teaching (hereafter referred to as Bridging), developed by McNamee, Chen, and the staff of the Bridging project, is a diagnostic assessment tool based on teacher observations of children engaged in a group of activities (McNamee & Chen, 2004). Bridging is designed to help teachers portray the intellectual strengths and learning approaches of young children between the ages of 3 and 8. Its central component is a set of 19 activities representing diverse curricular areas, including language and literacy, mathematics, sciences, performing arts, and visual arts (see Figure 5.1).

Bridging shares certain features with the Spectrum assessment, including the identification of children's diverse cognitive strengths, the use of engaging activities, and a focus on guided observation and careful documentation. It goes beyond the Spectrum assessment by emphasizing the connection between specific cognitive abilities and school learning—focusing on the operation of cognitive abilities in curricular areas; attending to what children learn, as well as how they learn in relation to various social grouping situations; and linking the assessment results to classroom teaching practices (McNamee & Chen, 2004).

Bridging is organized in terms of school subject areas rather than intelligences, for several reasons: (1) School subject areas reflect intellectual abilities valued in most cultures; (2) curricular areas offer children points of entry for the pursuit of intellectual development; and (3) aligning assessment areas with the subject areas studied in schools facilitates teachers' incorporation of the Bridging activities into ongoing curriculum planning.

As an assessment instrument, each Bridging activity produces two outcomes. The first is a description of the child's performance level, reflecting his or her mastery of particular skills and understanding of specific concepts in a subject area. The scale used is a rubric, with scores ranging from 0 to 10 for each activity. The rubric is constructed on the basis of the developmental progression in the mastery of key concepts—content-specific concepts essential to the development of knowledge in a subject area. For example, in the area of mathematics, key concepts for preschool and primary grades include number sense, classifying/comparing, spatial relationships, part–whole relationships, and communication of mathematical understanding (Charlesworth & Lind, 1999). The focus on key concepts in the Bridging assessment process provides teachers with a point of entry and a structure for organizing their thinking when conducting the activities, reviewing the assessment results, and planning and implementing curricula.

Bridging does not provide age norms for use in interpreting assessment results. Instead, it asks teachers to identify expected performance levels for a given grade or age at a particular point in the school year, usually October and May. Teachers then assess children in their classroom in relation to this expected level of performance. This method

Language Arts and Literacy	1. Reading a book (child's choice) 2. Reading a book (teacher's choice) 3. Dictating a story 4. Acting out stories
Visual Arts	5. Experimenting crayon technique 6. Drawing a self-portrait 7. Making apttern block pictures
Mathematics	8. Creating pattern block pinwheels 9. Solving pattern block puzzles 10. Counting 11. Subtracting 12. Fair share 13. Estimating
Sciences	14. Exploring shadows and light 15. Assembling a nature display 16. Building a model car
Performing Arts	17. Moving to music 18. Playing an instrument 19. Singing a song

FIGURE 5.1. Areas and activities of bridging.

makes use of teachers' expertise and experience and gives them the opportunity to reflect on what they know (Darling-Hammond & Snyder, 1992; Eisner, 1977). A number of researchers have documented that such practice can help improve teachers' ability to observe students and to think critically about what they do (Bransford, Brown, & Cocking, 1999; Calfee & Hiebert, 1991; Meisels et al., 2001).

The second outcome of Bridging assessment is a description of a child's working approach when engaged in tasks. Whereas the first outcome focuses on the *content* of children's learning, the assessment of working approach provides information about the *process* of how individual children learn. A total of 14 working approach variables are observed across the 19 assessment activities. Half of the variables refer to evaluative qualities (e.g., planfulness, frustration tolerance); the other half portray descriptive qualities (e.g., playfulness, pace of work). Evaluative qualities describe working approaches that promote or hinder a child's performance. They are scored on a scale from 1 to 5, with higher scores indicating that a child' s working approach is more adaptive, goal-oriented, and organized, and thus more conducive to classroom learning. Descriptive qualities are noted but not scored. They indicate important individual differences, but are not qualities that can be judged on a scale in terms of lower and higher values (Masur, 2004).

Although *working approach* resembles *learning style*, in that both address the process dimension of learning, the two constructs differ in significant ways. For example, *learning styles* are usually defined as relatively stable traits within individuals across subject areas (Barbe & Milone, 1981; Dunn, 1988; Dunn, Dunn, & Price, 1996; Silver, Strong, & Perini, 1997), whereas *working approach* describes how a child interacts with materials and responds to the demands of a task in a specific subject area. Working approaches are not stable traits; rather, they are a profile of tendencies that may change over time and may vary depending on the nature of the activity the child is engaged in (Masur, 2004).

As the name indicates, Bridging begins with the assessment of children and leads to teaching based on knowledge gained from the assessment process. To facilitate the transition from assessment to teaching, Bridging includes a curriculum component with two elements: interpretation and application. The interpretation section translates performance scores into terms relevant to planning instruction. It also details children's behaviors, skills, or knowledge at given performance levels, to assist teachers with understanding the assessment results. The application section contains a variety of curricular ideas for working with children at their current level, while also guiding them toward further development in the subject area. These ideas and activities were developed with reference to best practices in the subject area or field. They are suggestive rather than prescriptive, because the most effective teaching comes from teachers who can draw on their in-depth understanding of children and subject areas as well as their expertise in the use of varied instructional strategies (McNamee & Chen, 2004).

Finally, it is important to point out that although Bridging is designed to portray diverse intellectual strengths and working approaches of young children, the unit of its analysis is the activity rather than the individual child—the primary focus of most existing assessment instruments. This shift is based on the conviction that intelligence is not a commodity located exclusively within the mind of an individual; rather, it is "in the air" among individuals when they interact with others or engage in activities (Leont'ev, 1981; McNamee, 2000; Vygotsky, 1978). By focusing on activity in the assessment process, we are able to study children in the context of classroom learning and to examine the social interactions that elicit, encourage, and mediate children's performance in school (McNamee & Chen, 2004). The attention to social dynamics distinguishes Bridging from many other MI-based approaches to assessment.

EMPIRICAL STUDIES OF CHILDREN'S DIVERSE COGNITIVE ABILITIES

Since the original publication of *Frames of Mind* in 1983, MI theory has attracted much attention in the fields of cognition and education. From its inception, MI theory has been based on a rigorous critical review of empirical work in disciplines ranging from neurobiology and developmental psychology to cultural anthropology (Gardner, 1993b). Gardner and his colleagues continue to monitor the considerable body of new data relevant to the claims of the theory. Some of the work is being done at Harvard's Project Zero (Adams, 1993; Chen, Krechevsky, & Viens, 1998; Gardner, 1993d; Kornhaber, 1999; Kornhaber & Krechevsky, 1995; Kornhaber, Veenema, & Fierros, 2003; Krechevsky, 1998; Winner, Rosenblatt, Windmueller, Davidson, & Gardner, 1986). Some is being done by researchers in the fields of cognition, education, and neuroscience, either explicitly investigating MI theory or conducting studies related to its positions (Diaz-Lefebvre, 2003; Rauscher, Shaw, & Ky, 1993; Rosnow, 1991; Rosnow, Skleder, Jaeger, & Rind, 1994; Rosnow, Skleder, & Rind, 1995; Silver et al., 1997; Wu, 2003). Below we describe four studies related to the validity of assessment based on MI theory. The first two studies used forms of the Spectrum Assessment System described earlier. The third and fourth studies used Bridging. Conducted with children of different age groups, different socioeconomic backgrounds, and varying risk factors, all four studies offer strong evidence that when a wide range of abilities is assessed, we are more likely to find differentiated profiles than a uniform level of general ability in young children. Furthermore, the identification of each child's areas of strength can be used to help them build skills in other areas of learning, thereby increasing the likelihood of their success in school.

Assessment and Study of Preschool Children's Cognitive Abilities

The primary purposes of the study by Adams (1993) were to examine the relationships among diverse cognitive abilities in preschool children and to describe the degree of variation in ability levels found within individual profiles. The sample in Adams's study consisted of 42 children (22 girls and 20 boys), 4 years of age. The children were predominantly white and from middle- to upper-income families. The assessment tasks, called the Spectrum Field Inventory, were adapted from the Spectrum Preschool Assessment Activities. A total of six tasks—dinosaur game, storytelling, art portfolio, assembly of functional objects, birthday task, and singing—were designed to measure mathematical, linguistic, artistic, mechanical, social, and musical abilities, respectively.

To examine possible relationships among the six tasks, Adams first generated a Pearson correlation matrix of all possible pairings of the task scores (see Table 5.1). As indicated in Table 5.1, 10 of the 15 correlations in the matrix were not significant. This finding runs counter to repeated reports of substantial positive correlations among IQ tests (Detterman & Daniel, 1989; Gould, 1981; Humphreys, 1982; Sattler, 2001).

To explore further the potential specificity

TABLE 5.1. Correlation Matrix of Group Scores on Six Spectrum Field Inventory Tasks

Tasks	Dinosaur (number sense)	Assembly (mechanical construction)	Singing (music production)	Art portfolio (visual arts)	Birthday party (social understanding)
Storytelling (language)	.44**	.15	−.14	.43*	.26
Dinosaur (number sense)		.41**	.21	.20	.25
Assembly (mechanical)			.06	.48**	.23
Singing (music production)				−.37	−.03
Art portfolio (visual arts)					.51**

Note. Data from Adams (1993).
*p < .05; **p < .01.

of intellectual abilities, Adams also analyzed each individual's levels of performance across tasks in relation to the group. Using the standard deviation as a criterion, Adams defined three levels of performance. *Strong*, *weak*, and *average* performances were defined as scores 1 standard deviation above the mean, 1 standard deviation below the mean, and between +1 and −1 standard deviations, respectively. Defining the three levels of performance in relation to the standard deviation provided a set of objective criteria for determining the degree of variability within an individual's set of scores.

Of the 42 children in Adams's study, 3 completed fewer than half of the six tasks and were eliminated from the analysis. In the remaining 39 profiles, only 4 children (10%) exhibited the same level of performance on all tasks. Of the remaining 35 children (90%) who performed at varying levels on the tasks, 16 (46%) earned scores that scattered over a range of 3–5 standard deviations, indicating that an individual's level of performance often varies when a diverse set of abilities is measured. In addition, each subject exhibited a pattern of performance on the Spectrum Field Inventory that was unique. On any single task, a number of individuals performed at the same level. However, when a range of areas was sampled, each individual's pattern of performance was highly likely to be distinct (Adams, 1993).

Study of Identifying At-Risk Children's Strengths

The study by Chen was designed to examine the impact of an MI-based intervention program on students at risk for school failure (Chen, 1993; Chen, Krechevsky, & Viens, 1998). Four first-grade classrooms with a total of 85 students participated in the study. All of the children resided in Somerville, Massachusetts, a low-socioeconomic-status residential area with some ethnic diversity. Of the 85 students, 15 were considered at risk for school failure, based on teacher evaluations of classroom behavior, measures of students' academic self-esteem and school adjustment, and scores on various achievement tests.

A central component in the intervention program was the introduction of "learning centers" in the classrooms. In the learning centers, children explored engaging activities in eight domains examined in the Spectrum Assessment System. Teachers in the four participating classrooms implemented learning center activities and integrated them into project-based curriculum units. The teachers and the project's researchers observed at-risk children while they engaged in learning center activities, and identified the children's strengths based on their demonstrated interest and competence. Interest was measured in terms of the frequency with which a child chose a particular domain-specific activity and the length of his or her involvement in that activity. Competence was evaluated with the Spectrum Observational Guidelines described earlier.

Using these methods, the teachers and researchers identified areas of strength for 13 of the 15 (87%) students with at-risk status. As seen in Table 5.2, these children's strengths spanned seven of the eight learning center areas. Also noteworthy, these children demonstrated more strengths in nonacademic areas than in academic ones—6, 3, and 3 identified strengths were in the areas of art, mechanics, and movement, respectively, versus 2 and 1 in the language and math areas. This result indicates that at-risk students, although they often perform poorly in traditional academic areas, are not necessarily low performers in all areas of learning. When a wide range of learning areas is made available for them to explore and to pursue, it is possible that children with at-risk status

TABLE 5.2. Identified Areas of Strength in At-Risk Children across Domains

Spectrum domain	Number of children with identified strength in domain[a]
Math	1
Social understanding	1
Science	2
Language	2
Mechanical	3
Movement	3
Visual arts	6

Note. Data from Chen (1993).
[a]Some children had more than one area of strength being identified.

will demonstrate competence and skills in a variety of areas.

Identifying and nurturing at-risk children's strengths could lead to further changes in their classroom behavior. This hypothesis was tested in Chen's (1993) study. Table 5.3 presents the findings based on observing children with at-risk status as they worked in areas of strength versus nonstrength areas, using the Child Behavioral Observation Scale (an instrument developed by Project Spectrum in 1990). A multivariate analysis of variance indicated a significant positive effect on all six measures when children worked in strength areas. The positive behaviors observed included increases in self-direction ($F = 3.98$, $p < .01$), self-confidence ($F = 3.96$, $p < .01$), positive classroom behavior ($F = 3.67$, $p < .01$), positive affect ($F = 3.96$, $p < .01$), self-monitoring ($F = 3.19$, $p < .01$), and active engagement ($F = 3.98$, $p < .01$). An analysis of individual participants indicated that all 15 students with at-risk status showed a statistically significant increase on at least one, and in some cases as many as five, of the aforementioned positive behaviors.

A plausible conclusion from this finding is that children with at-risk status tend to have positive experiences of being effective and productive when working in their areas of strength. This is significant, because it suggests the possibility of building on children's strengths. As children develop further competence in their areas of strength, they are more likely to experience feelings of satisfaction and self-worth. These feelings, in turn, may help children increase self-confidence

and self-esteem. Building on these changes holds promise as an alternative approach to boost at-risk children's academic achievement (Bolanos, 2003; Campbell, Campbell, & Dickinson, 1996; Chen, Krechevsky, & Viens, 1998; Hoerr, 2003; Kornhaber, 1999; Kornhaber & Krechevsky, 1997; Kornhaber et al., 2003).

As noted, many of the children who were at risk for school failure had strengths in areas other than language and math. Had the assessment been limited to these two areas, these children's strengths would have gone undetected and could not have served as a bridge for extending interest and involvement to other areas of the curriculum. Although assessment that samples only from linguistic and logical–mathematical intelligences may represent the extent of ability valued in a particular educational environment, it almost certainly does not reflect the true range of a child's intellectual potentials.

Studies of Young Children's Cognitive Profiles and Working Approach

Using Bridging, Chen, McNamee, and their project staff conducted two studies to investigate diverse cognitive profiles and developmental patterns in young children. In the first study, the Bridging staff administered all 19 Bridging assessment activities to a total of 92 children (47 prekindergarteners and 45 kindergarteners) in the city of Chicago. The participants represented a diverse population in terms of economic status (ranging from families on welfare to middle-class professional families) and ethnicity (more than 10 different languages were spoken in some classrooms). Child performance was scored according to specific rubric levels (0–10) designed for each Bridging activity.

Analysis of the data from the first study is still in progress. Two of the results from completed analyses are worth noting (McCray, Chen, & NcNamee, 2004). First, correlations between scores on activities did not indicate the operation of a general intelligence across activities. Specifically, only 4 out of 10 correlations in the partial correlation matrix of all possible scores from 19 activities in five Bridging assessment areas were significant, with correlation coefficients ranging from .27 to .44 (see Table 5.4). Second, individual profiles of performance on

TABLE 5.3. Mean Scores of At-Risk Students' Behavior when Working in Strength vs. Nonstrength Areas

Observed behavior	Areas of strength	Other areas
Self-direction	3.98**	2.25
Self-confidence	3.96**	2.33
Positive classroom behavior	3.67**	2.40
Positive affect	3.96**	2.58
Self-monitoring	3.19**	1.87
Activity engagement	4.26**	3.17

Note. Data from Chen (1993).
**$p < .01$.

TABLE 5.4. Partial Correlation Matrix of Group Scores on 19 Activities in Five Bridging Assessment Areas

Assessment activities and areas	Six mathematics activities	Three science activities	Three performing arts activities	Three visual arts activities
Four language arts and literacy activities	.27*	.22	.44**	.39**
Six mathematics activities		.13	−.03	.33**
Three science activities			−.13	.19
Three performing arts activities				−.06

*p < .05; ** p < .01.

the 19 activities were characterized by specificity rather than generality and uniformity. Each child's intellectual profile was analyzed in terms of two descriptive indicators: *range* and *variance*. Range referred to the distance between a subject's highest score and lowest score. (Scores on activities were converted to z scores for purposes of this analysis.) Variance indicated the average distance between a child's score on individual activities and the child's average score on all activities. Greater range and variance indicated that a child's level of performance varied as a function of activity. In terms of range, 88 out of 90 children in the study (98%) earned scores scattered over a range of 2–6 standard deviations. Of these 88 children, 31 (35%), 5 (5.6%), 1 (1%) and 1 (1%), had scores that ranged over 3, 4, 5, and 6 standard deviations respectively. With regard to variance, 49 out of 73 children (67%) scored above 0.6 (children with fewer than 14 activity scores were excluded from the variance analysis). Of these 49 children, 17 (23%), 16 (22%), 8 (11%), 5 (7%), and 3 (4%) children earned scores above 0.6, 0.7, 0.8, 0.9, and 1 variance, respectively. This study thus yielded a result similar to that reported by Adams (1993), but found even greater variability within individual profiles. Comparing the findings of the two studies suggests that the more diverse the population and the wider the range of areas assessed, the more likely it is that children will display profiles of specific ability. Diversity appears to be the rule rather than the exception in the expression of human intelligences (Gardner & Hatch, 1989).

The second study, by Masur (2004), was conducted in a Chicago public school serving a community of low-income African American families. Sixty-one children participated in the study, with an approximately equal number from each of three age groups: prekindergarten (average age 4 years, 6 months), kindergarten (average age 6.1 years), and second grade (average age 8.2 years). Children were assessed with 6 of the 19 Bridging activities: 4 related to the development of number concepts, 1 on geometry, and 1 on movement to music. Children participated in each activity twice: once with only the investigator and once in a small group. Children's efforts were scored in two ways: Bridging developmental rubrics (content measure) and a working approach scale (process dimension measure).

The primary purpose of Masur's study was to examine the process dimension of learning and its relationship to the content of learning. Findings of the study indicated that, first, there was a significant relationship between young children's level of task performance and the working approaches they used. Specifically, the evaluative working approach scores were significantly correlated with children's rubric scores at the .01 level, with correlation coefficients ranging from .31 to .72 for different working approach variables. Second, a child's working approach varied and was affected by many factors, including the content of the activity, years of schooling, and the child's areas of strength. In terms of the content of the activity, all seven evaluative working approach variables varied as a function of activity, and the differences in scores were significant at the .01 level. Based on the results of a regression analysis, activity accounted for 35% of the variance in working approaches, making it second only to years of schooling in terms of accounting for the observed variance (Masur, 2004)

Masur's findings are compelling both theoretically and practically. Theoretically, they provide evidence that children's information-processing and problem-solving capacities vary as functions of content area and the demands of the task. Practically, they suggest that teachers can improve student performance by helping them to develop more effective working approaches (Chen, Masar, & McCray, 2003; McNamee & Melendez, 2003).

DISCUSSION OF THE EMPIRICAL WORK AND IMPLICATIONS FOR MI-BASED ASSESSMENT

The studies described above provide empirical support for four critical points: (1) diversity and variation as the key to understanding human intelligence; (2) profile as a useful means to portray an individual's intellectual abilities; (3) working approach as a process dimension of a child's intellectual profile; and (4) activity as a viable unit for the analysis of an individual's intellectual abilities. These four points are discussed below in terms of their implications and applications to MI-based assessment.

Diversity and Variation as the Key to Understanding Human Intelligence

The findings reported above—that correlations among varied tasks were not consistently positive and high—differ from the well-known finding of substantial positive correlations among various tests of mental ability, often referred to as the *positive manifold* (Detterman & Daniel, 1989; Gardner, Kornhaber, & Wake, 1996). Although the positive manifold has served as a major source of evidence for psychometricians who claim that intelligence is a general ability, Gardner (1993b, 1993d) argues that it is, to a large extent, an artifact of test design. That is, positive manifold may reflect the measurement of restricted content using similar

techniques, rather than the structure of intelligence per se. Adding empirical weight to Gardner's argument, the results of the studies reported above indicate that when diverse cognitive abilities are measured directly, positive manifold is both reduced and attenuated.

In addition to the failure to find a positive manifold, the studies reported above *did* find that specificity and variability characterized the performance of the majority of subjects. The variability observed within subjects' sets of scores indicates that individuals often exhibited a range of competence, rather than a uniform level of ability, across domains. This finding held for children of different ages, different socioeconomic groups, and different degrees of risk for school failure. It suggests that when individuals are described in terms of either a single numerical score (e.g., IQ) or a global category (e.g., a Piagetian stage), meaningful variations within each individual's repertoire of abilities are concealed. By the same token, typical informal characterizations of intellectual abilities, such as "smart," "average," and "stupid," are also likely to be misleading and inaccurate. All children are likely to have strengths in some areas and weaknesses in others when a range of areas is considered.

Profile as a Useful Means to Portray an Individual's Intellectual Abilities

The means used to describe individuals shapes how differences among individuals are characterized. Because individuals' intellectual abilities are specific, so should be their descriptions. A profile specifying an individual's capabilities provides a comprehensive and detailed picture of the individual's cognitive strengths and weaknesses at a particular point in time. The use of profiles makes it impossible to describe differences among individuals in terms of a single linear relationship. Although it is still possible to rank-order individuals in each area assessed, individuals' positions will shift as rank orders are constructed for different content areas.

That constructing profiles differs from administering an IQ test or a set of Piagetian tasks is obvious. However, this approach also differs from those of pluralistic theorists such as Thurstone (1938), Guilford (1967), and Carroll (1993). MI-based assessment is not simply assessment of a wider range of abilities (e.g., memory, attention, symbol manipulation); it is assessment of a wider range of *domain-specific* abilities. Profiles based on such assessment describe individuals' intellectual abilities with respect to "vertical" rather than "horizontal" differences (Gardner, 1993b). The focus on measurement of various domain-specific abilities also makes it possible to study differentiated operational mechanisms and problem-solving capacities that underlie the expression of diverse intellectual abilities in individuals.

Working Approach as a Process Dimension of a Child's Intellectual Profile

The field of personality and cognition has long suggested that *style*—an individual's manner of approaching and accomplishing tasks—is an important dimension of cognitive activity (Dunn, 1988; Miller, 1991; Sternberg, 1989; Wolf & Gardner, 1978). Masur's (2004) work indicates that *working approach* is a significant contributing factor to children's interaction with content areas. As noted earlier, working approach is like style in that it describes the process of learning, but our construct is not a stable trait. Masur's finding of significant but low to moderate correlations between working approach and performance suggests that working approach may be an operative variable in children's content learning.

Masur's finding is thought-provoking, as it also suggests that working approach variables may be linked with characteristics of content areas. As shown in Masur's study, working approach variables varied by the content of the activity, and activity accounted for approximately one-third of the variance in all working approach variables together. This result implies that working approach is not a stable trait and may not be uniform in its operation across domains. Rather, it influences children's performance through its association with many other factors including particular content areas. Children's cognitive abilities are domain-specific; their working approaches appear to be also. That working approach is linked to content-specific performance could further differentiate the description of an individual's domain-specific competence and intellectual profile.

Activity as a Viable Unit for the Analysis of an Individual's Intellectual Abilities

The unit of analysis in Bridging is activity rather than the individual child. This is not just a methodological issue; it concerns the conception of intelligence as well. MI theory asserts that intelligence is distributed, in that human intelligence is so inextricably intertwined with people and objects that it is impossible to understand intellectual activities without also considering the use of tools and reliance on the contribution and efforts of other individuals (Gardner, 1993d). Children come to know the world through participation in activities where they interact with other human beings and materials. Activity mediates between a child's internal world of interests and proclivities on the one hand, and the external world of family, school, and community that requires children to learn the symbol systems and information important to the society or culture on the other (Project Zero & Reggio Children, 2001; Wertsch, 1981). Since activity interrelates internal and external factors, it reveals the "idiosyncratic individual" (Leont'ev, 1981, p. 47) as a complex creature influenced and shaped by biological, psychological, and social/cultural factors. Also, because activity involves a process "characterized by constant transformations" (Leont'ev, 1981, p. 65), it traces the individual change and growth that result from the interaction of internal and external factors. For these reasons, activity is a viable unit for studying children's intellectual abilities.

A shift in focus from the individual to activity does not ignore the individual. Rather, it places the individual in the context of physical and social interactions when his or her intellectual abilities are being examined (see Figure 5.2). As illustrated in Figure 5.2, development and learning in any activity system involve at least three interrelated and inseparable components—child, teacher/adult, and task. More specifically, the child brings his or her range of cognitive abilities and working approaches across domains to the activity; the task presents materials and goals that

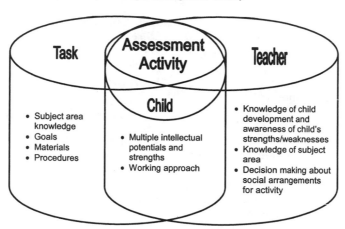

FIGURE 5.2. Activity as a unit of analysis.

embody knowledge and skills in subject areas; and the teacher makes decisions about patterns of interaction and support as he or she makes choices about grouping, instruction, and how to scaffold learning and development (McNamee & Chen, 2004).

In this conceptual framework, an individual cannot be taken outside of the activity to have his or her intellectual abilities observed and analyzed (Leont'ev, 1981; Rogoff, 1998). The processes of assessing should not, and cannot, be reduced to the individual actions of the child, the teacher, or the task. Similarly, the assessment results can be understood only by looking at the interactions of the child, teacher, and task. To exclude any of these elements from the equation is to miss opportunities for understanding the child in totality (Wertsch, 1981). Attending to activity in the assessment of diverse cognitive abilities makes it possible to (1) examine the context in which intellectual capacity is expressed through the interaction of the child, teacher, and task (Gutierrez & Rogoff, 2003); (2) determine the effects of various components on the child's performance; and (3) identify variables relevant to educational intervention. As such, MI-based assessment becomes a dynamic process aimed at building bridges between each child's current developmental status in subject areas and his or her future developmental course, as well as between the assessment of children and curriculum planning and implementation (McNamee & Chen, 2004; Gardner, 1998).

CONCLUSION

Many people criticize current educational practices, maintaining that a significant part of our educational malaise in the United States stems from the instruments used to assess student learning and the signals they send about what learning is valued (Baker, O'Neil, & Linn, 1993; Elmore, 2002; Gardner, 2000; Hargreaves & Earl, 2002; Horton & Bowman, 2002; Linn, Baker, & Betebenner, 2002; Meisels, 1992; Stiggins, 2002). These instruments often rely on a pencil-and-paper, short-answer format; sample only a small portion of intellectual abilities; and are administered only once or twice a year. Because this kind of instrument systematically ignores the wide range of abilities valued in our culture, it does little to help us recognize and nurture individuals' potentials. By constraining the curriculum and taking control of the learning process away from teachers and students, this kind of instrument actually discourages many students from discovering activities they enjoy and excel in (Chen, 2004; Gardner, 1993c; Hatch & Gardner, 1990).

Taking into account the psychological, biological, and cultural dimensions of cognition, MI theory presents a more comprehensive and scientifically compelling account of human intelligences than traditional intelligence theories do. The theory also provides an impetus for the development of new measures of the intelligences and the use of new, intelligence-fair forms of assessment. According to MI theory, the primary purpose of conducting an assessment should be to gather information for designing appropriate educational experiences and improving instruction.

To assess a child's distinctive intellectual abilities is not to create another means of labeling the child. Rather, the ultimate goal of an MI approach to assessment is to help create environments that foster the development of individual as well as group potential, promote deep understanding of disciplinary knowledge, and suggest alternative routes to the achievement of important educational goals. Clearly, this approach will require concerted efforts over a long period of time to develop appropriate instruments and to train individuals to administer and interpret them in a sensitive manner. We believe these efforts will help ensure that educators work not only to "leave no child behind," but also to inspire all children to achieve their highest potential.

APPENDIX 5.1. Project Spectrum Preschool Assessment Activities

Area	Measure	Activity
Movement	Creative movement	Biweekly movement curriculum
	Athletic movement	Obstacle course
Language	Invented narrative	Storyboard activity
	Descriptive narrative	Reporter activities
Mathematics	Counting/ strategy	Dinosaur game
	Calculating/ notation	Bus game
Social	Social analysis	Classroom model
	Social roles	Peer interaction checklist
Visual arts	Art production	Year-long collection of children's artwork
Music	Music production	Singing activities
	Music perception	Pitch matching games and song recognition
Science	Naturalist	Discovery area
	Logical inference	Treasure hunt game
	Hypothesis testing	Sink and float activity
	Mechanical construction	Assembly activity

APPENDIX 5.2. Project Spectrum Observational Guidelines

Visual Arts

Perception

- Is aware of visual elements in the environment and in artwork (e.g., color, lines, shapes, patterns, detail)
- Is sensitive to different artistic styles (e.g., can distinguish abstract art from realism, impressionism, etc.)

Production

Representation

- Is able to represent visual world accurately in two or three dimensions
- Is able to create recognizable symbols for common objects (e.g., people, vegetation, houses, animals) and coordinate elements spatially into unified whole
- Uses realistic proportions, detailed features, deliberate choice of color

Artistry

- Is able to use various elements of art (e.g., line, color, shape) to depict emotions, produce certain effects, and embellish drawings or three-dimensional work
- Conveys strong mood through literal representation (e.g., smiling sun, crying face) and abstract features (e.g., dark colors or drooping lines to express sadness); produces drawings or sculptures that appear "lively," "sad," or "powerful"
- Shows concern with decoration and embellishment
- Produces drawings that are colorful, balanced, and/or rhythmic

Exploration

- Is flexible and inventive in use of art materials (e.g., experiments with paint, chalk, clay)
- Uses lines and shapes to generate a wide variety of forms (e.g., open and closed, explosive and controlled) in two- or three-dimensional work
- Is able to execute a range of subjects or themes (e.g., people, animals, buildings, landscapes)

Mechanical Science

Visual–Spatial Abilities

- Is able to construct or reconstruct physical objects and simple machines in two or three dimensions
- Understands spatial relationships between parts of a mechanical object

Problem-Solving Approach with Mechanical Objects

- Uses and learns from trial-and-error approach
- Uses systematic approach in solving mechanical problems
- Compares and generalizes information

Understanding of Causal and Functional Relationships

- Infers relationships based on observation
- Understands relationship of parts to whole, the function of these parts, and how parts are put together

Fine Motor Skills

- Is adept at manipulating small parts or objects
- Exhibits good eye–hand coordination (e.g., hammers on head of nail rather than on fingers)

Movement

Body Control

- Shows an awareness of and ability to isolate and use different body parts
- Plans, sequences, and execute moves efficiently—movements do not seem random or disjointed
- Is able to replicate own movements and those of others

Sensitivity to Rhythm

- Moves in synchrony with stable or changing rhythms, particularly in music (e.g., child attempts to move with the rhythm, as opposed to being unaware of or disregarding rhythmic changes)
- Is able to set own rhythm and regulate it to achieve a desired effect

Expressivity

- Evokes moods and images through movement, using gestures and body postures; stimulus can be a verbal image, a prop, or music
- Is able to respond to mood or tonal quality of an instrument or music selection (e.g., uses light and fluid movements for lyrical music vs. strong and staccato movements for a march)

Generation of Movement Ideas

- Is able to invent interesting and novel movement ideas, verbally and/or physically, or offer extensions of ideas (e.g., suggesting that other children raise their arms to look like clouds floating in the sky)
- Responds immediately to ideas and images with original movements
- Choreographs a simple dance, perhaps teaching it to others

Responsiveness to Music

- Responds differently to different kinds of music
- Shows sensitivity to rhythm and expressiveness when responding to music
- Explores available space (vertical and horizontal) comfortably, using different levels, moving easily and fluidly around the space
- Anticipates others in a shared space
- Experiments with body in space (e.g., turning and spinning)

Music

Music Perception

- Is sensitive to dynamics (loud and soft)
- Is sensitive to tempo and rhythmic patterns
- Discriminates pitch
- Identifies musical and musicians' styles
- Identifies different instruments and sounds

Music Production

- Is able to maintain accurate pitch
- Is able to maintain accurate tempo and rhythmic patterns
- Exhibits expressiveness when singing or playing instrument
- Can recall and reproduce musical properties of songs and other compositions

Music Composition

- Creates simple compositions with some sense of beginning, middle, and end
- Creates simple notation system

Social Understanding

Understanding of Self

- Identifies own abilities, skills, interests, and areas of difficulty
- Reflects upon own feelings, experiences, and accomplishments
- Draws upon these reflections to understand and guide own behavior
- Shows insight into the factors that enable an individual to do well or have difficulty in an area

Understanding of Others

- Demonstrates knowledge of peers and their activities
- Attends closely to others
- Recognizes others' thoughts, feelings, and abilities
- Draws conclusions about others based on their activities

Assumption of Distinctive Social Roles

Leader

- Often initiates and organizes activities
- Organizes other children
- Assigns roles to others
- Explains how activity is carried out
- Oversees and directs activities

Facilitator

- Often shares ideas, information, and skills with other children
- Mediates conflict
- Invites other children to play
- Extends and elaborates other children's ideas
- Provides help when others need attention

Caregiver/Friend

- Comforts other children when they are upset
- Shows sensitivity to other children's feelings
- Shows understanding of friends' likes and dislikes

Mathematics

Numerical Reasoning

- Adept at calculations (e.g., can find shortcuts)
- Able to estimate
- Adept at quantifying objects and information (e.g., by record keeping, creating effective notation, graphing)
- Able to identify numerical relationships (e.g., probability, ratio)

Spatial Reasoning

- Finds spatial patterns
- Adept with puzzles
- Uses imagery to visualize and conceptualize a problem

Logical Problem Solving

- Focuses on relationships and overall structure of problem instead of isolated facts
- Makes logical inferences
- Generalizes rules

- Develops and uses strategies (e.g., when playing games)

Natural Science

Observational Skills

- Engages in close observation of materials to learn about their physical characteristics; uses one or more of the senses
- Often notices changes in the environment (e.g., new leaves on plants, insects on trees, subtle seasonal changes)
- Shows interest in recording observations through drawings, charts, sequence cards, or other methods

Identification of Similarities and Differences

- Likes to compare and contrast materials and/or events
- Classifies materials and often notices similarities and/or differences between specimens (e.g., compares and contrasts crabs and spiders)

Hypothesis Formation and Experimentation

- Makes predictions based on observations
- Asks "what if"-type questions and offers explanations for why things are the way they are
- Conducts simple experiments or generates ideas for experiments to test own or others' hypotheses (e.g., drops large and small rocks in water to see if one size sinks faster than the other; waters plant with paint instead of water)

Interest in/Knowledge of Nature Scientific Phenomena

- Exhibits extensive knowledge about various scientific topics; spontaneously offers information about these topics, or reports on own or others' experience with natural world
- Shows interest in natural phenomena, or related materials such as natural history books, over extended periods of time
- Regularly asks questions about things observed

Language

Invented Narrative/Storytelling

- Uses imagination and originality in storytelling
- Enjoys listening to or reading stories
- Exhibits interest in plot design and development, character elaboration and motivation, descriptions of settings, scenes or moods, use of dialogue, etc.
- Brings a sense of narrative to different tasks
- Shows performing ability or dramatic flair, in-

cluding a distinctive style, expressiveness, or an ability to play a variety of roles

Descriptive Language/Reporting

- Provides accurate and coherent accounts of events, feelings, and experiences (e.g., uses correct sequence and appropriate level of detail; distinguishes fact from fantasy)
- Provides accurate labels and descriptions for things
- Shows interest in explaining how things work, or describing a procedure
- Engages in logical argument or inquiry

Poetic Use of Language/Wordplay

- Enjoys and is adept at wordplay, such as puns, rhymes, metaphors
- Plays with word meanings and sounds
- Demonstrates interest in learning new words
- Uses words in a humorous fashion

ACKNOWLEDGMENT

We would like to express our sincere thanks to Margaret Adams for her insightful comments on and editorial changes to the chapter.

REFERENCES

Adams, M. (1993). *An empirical investigation of domain-specific theories of preschool children's cognitive abilities.* Unpublished doctoral dissertation, Tufts University.

Adams, M., & Feldman, D. H. (1993). Project Spectrum: A theory-based approach to early education. In R. Pasnak & M. L. Howe (Eds.), *Emerging themes in cognitive development: Vol. 2. Competencies* (pp. 53–76). New York: Springer-Verlag.

Armstrong, T. (1994). *Multiple intelligences in the classroom.* Alexandria, VA: Association for Supervision and Curriculum Development.

Baker, E. L., O'Neil, H. F., & Linn, R. L. (1993). Policy and validity prospects for performance-based assessment. *American Psychologist, 48,* 1210–1218.

Barbe, W. B., & Milone, M. N. (1981). What we know about modality strengths. *Educational Leadership, 38*(5), 378–380.

Bolanos, P. (2003, April). *Implementing MI in the key learning community.* Paper presented at the annual meeting of the American Educational Research Association, Chicago.

Bransford, J., Brown, A. L., & Cocking, R. R. (Eds.). (1999). *How people learn: Brain, mind, experience, and school.* Washington, DC: National Academy Press.

Calfee, R., & Hiebert, E. (1991). *Teacher assessment of achievement: Advances in program evaluation.* Greenwich, CT: JAI Press.

Campbell, L., Campbell, B., & Dickinson, D. (1996). *Teaching and learning through multiple intelligences.* Needham Heights, MA: Allyn & Bacon.

Carroll, J. B. (1993). *Human cognitive abilities: A survey of factor-analytic studies.* New York: Cambridge University Press.

Charlesworth, R., & Lind, K. K. (1999). *Math and science for young children* (5th ed.). Boston: Delmar.

Chen, J. Q. (1993, April). *Building on children's strengths: Project Spectrum intervention program for students at risk for school failure.* Paper presented at the biennial conference of the Society for Research in Child Development, New Orleans, LA.

Chen, J. Q. (2004). Project Spectrum approach to early education. In J. L. Roopnarine & J. E. Johnson (Eds.), *Approaches to early childhood education* (4th ed., pp. 251–279). Upper Saddle River, NJ: Merrill.

Chen, J. Q., Isberg, E., & Krechevsky, M. (Eds.). (1998). *Project Spectrum: Early learning activities.* New York: Teachers College Press.

Chen, J. Q., Krechevsky, M., & Viens, J. (1998). *Building on children's strengths: The experience of Project Spectrum.* New York: Teachers College Press.

Chen, J. Q., Masur, A., & McCray, J. (2003). *Assessing how children learn: Bridging assessment to teaching practice in early childhood classrooms.* Paper presented at the annual conference of the National Association for the Education of Young Children, Chicago.

Chen, J. Q., & McNamee, G. (2004). *Bridging: A diagnostic assessment for teaching and learning in early childhood classrooms.* Chicago: Erikson Institute.

Comer, J. P. (1988). Educating poor minority children. *Scientific American, 259*(5), 42–48.

Darling-Hammond, L., & Ancess, L. (1996). Authentic assessment and school development. In J. B. Baron & D. P. Wolf (Eds.), *Performance-based student assessment: Challenges and possibilities (95th yearbook of the National Society for the Study of Education)* (pp. 52–83). Chicago: University of Chicago Press.

Darling-Hammond, L., & Snyder, J. (1992). Reframing accountability: Creating learner-centered schools. In A. Lieberman (Ed.), *The changing contents of teaching (91st yearbook of the National Society for the Study of Education)* (pp. 11–36). Chicago: University of Chicago Press.

Detterman, D. K., & Daniel, M. H. (1989). Correlations of mental tests with each other and with cognitive variables are highest for low IQ groups. *Intelligence, 13,* 349–359.

Diaz-Lefebvre, R. (2003, April). *Multiple intelligences, learning for understanding and creative assessment: Some pieces to the puzzle of learning.* Paper presented at the annual meeting of the American Educational Research Association, Chicago.

Donaldson, M. (1988). *Children's minds.* London: Fontana.

Dunn, R. S. (1988). Teaching students through their perceptual strengths or preferences. *Journal of Reading, 31*(4), 304–309.

Dunn, R. S., Dunn, K. J., & Price, G. E. (1996). *Learning Style Inventory*. Lawrence, KS: Price Systems.

Eisner, E. W. (1977). On the uses of educational connoisseurship and criticism for evaluating classroom life. *Teachers College Record, 78*(3), 346–358.

Elmore, R. (2002). Testing trap: The single largest—and possibly most destructive—federal intrusion into America's public schools. *Harvard Magazine, 9–10,* 35–37, 97.

Eysenck, H. J. (1979). *The structure and measurement of intelligence*. Berlin: Springer-Verlag.

Feldman, D. H. (1994). *Beyond universals in cognitive development* (2nd ed.). Norwood, NJ: Ablex.

Fischer, K. W., & Bidell, T. R. (1992, Winter). Ever younger ages: Constructive use of nativist findings about early development. *SRCD Newsletter,* pp. 1–3.

Flavell, J. H. (1982). On cognitive development. *Child Development, 53,* 1–10.

Flavell, J. H., Miller, P. H., & Miller, S. A. (2002). *Cognitive development* (4th ed.). Upper Saddle River, NJ: Prentice-Hall.

Gardner, H. (1983). *Frames of mind: The theory of multiple intelligences*. New York: Basic Books.

Gardner, H. (1984). Assessing intelligence: A comment on "Testing intelligence without IQ test" by R. J. Sternberg. *Phi Delta Kappan, 65*(10), 699–700.

Gardner, H. (1986). The waning of intelligence tests. In R. Sternberg & D. Detterman (Eds.), *The acquisition of symbolic skills* (pp. 19–42). London: Plenum Press.

Gardner, H. (1987a). Beyond the IQ: Education and human development. *Harvard Educational Review, 57,* 187–193.

Gardner, H. (1987b). The theory of multiple intelligences. *Annals of Dyslexia, 37,* 19–35.

Gardner, H. (1991). *The unschooled mind: How children think and how schools should teach*. New York: Basic Books.

Gardner, H. (1993a). Assessment in context: The alternative to standardized testing. In H. Gardner, *Multiple intelligences: The theory in practice* (pp. 161–183). New York: Basic Books.

Gardner, H. (1993b). *Frames of mind: The theory of multiple intelligences* (10th-anniversary ed.). New York: Basic Books.

Gardner, H. (1993c). Intelligence in seven phases. In H. Gardner, *Multiple intelligences: The theory in practice* (pp. 213–230). New York: Basic Books.

Gardner, H. (1993d). *Multiple intelligences: The theory in practice*. New York: Basic Books.

Gardner, H. (1994). Multiple intelligences theory. In R. J. Sternberg (Ed.), *Encyclopedia of human intelligence* (pp. 740–742). New York: Macmillan.

Gardner, H. (1995, Winter). Cracking open the IQ box. *The American Prospect,* pp. 20, 71–80.

Gardner, H. (1998). The bridges of Spectrum. In J. Q. Chen, M. Krechevsky, & J. Viens, *Building on children's strengths: The experience of Project Spectrum* (pp. 138–145). New York: Teachers College Press.

Gardner, H. (1999). *Intelligence reframed: Multiple intelligences for the 21st century*. New York: Basic Books.

Gardner, H. (2000). *The disciplined mind: Beyond facts and standardized tests, the K–12 education that every child deserves*. New York: Penguin Books.

Gardner, H. (2003, April). *Multiple intelligences after twenty years*. Paper presented at the annual meeting of the American Educational Research Association, Chicago.

Gardner, H., & Hatch, T. (1989). Multiple intelligences go to school: Educational implications of the theory of multiple intelligences. *Educational Researcher, 18,* 4–10.

Gardner, H., Kornhaber, M. L., & Wake, W. K. (1996). *Intelligence: Multiple perspectives*. New York: Harcourt Brace College.

Gardner, H., & Walters, J. M. (1993). A rounded version. In H. Gardner, *Multiple intelligences: The theory in practice* (pp. 13–34). New York: Basic Books.

Gould, S. J. (1981). *The mismeasure of man*. New York: Norton.

Gould, S. J. (1994, November 28). Curveball. *The New Yorker,* pp. 139–149.

Guilford, J. P. (1967). *The nature of human intelligence*. New York: McGraw-Hill.

Gutierrez, K. D., & Rogoff, B. (2003). Cultural ways of learning: Individual Traits or repertoires of practice. *Educational Researcher, 32*(5), 19–25.

Hargreaves, A., & Earl, L. (2002). Perspectives on alternative assessment reform. *American Educational Research Journal, 39*(1), 69–95.

Hatch, T., & Gardner, H. (1990). If Binet had looked beyond the classroom: The assessment of multiple intelligences. *International Journal of Educational Research, 14*(5), 415–429.

Herrnstein, R. J., & Murray, C. (1994). *The bell curve: Intelligence and class structure in American Life*. New York: Free Press.

Hoerr, T. (2003, April). *How MI informs teaching at the New City School*. Paper presented at the annual meeting of the American Educational Research Association, Chicago.

Horton, C., & Bowman, B. T. (2002). *Child assessment at the preprimary level: Expert opinion and state trends* (Occasional Paper of Herr Research Center). Chicago: Erikson Institute.

Hsueh, W. C. (2003, April). *The development of a MI assessment for young children in Taiwan*. Paper presented at the annual meeting of the American Educational Research Association, Chicago.

Humphreys, L. G. (1982). The hierarchical factor model and general intelligence. In N. Hirschberg & L. G. Humphreys (Eds.), *Multivariate applications in the social sciences* (pp. 223–239). Hillsdale, NJ: Erlbaum.

Jensen, A. (1969). How much can we boost IQ and

scholastic achievement? *Harvard Educational Review, 39*(1), 1–123.

Jensen, A. (1987). Psychometric *g* as a focus of concerted research effort. *Intelligence, 11,* 193–198.

Jensen, A. (1993). Spearman's *g*: Links between psychometrics and biology. *Brain Mechanisms, 701,* 103–129.

Kornhaber, M. (1999). Multiple intelligences theory in practice. In J. Block, S. T. Everson, & T. R. Guskey (Eds.), *Comprehensive school reform: A program perspective* (pp. 179–191). Dubuque, IA: Kendall/Hunt.

Kornhaber, M., & Krechevsky, M. (1995). Expanding definition of learning and teaching: Notes from the MI underground. In P. W. Cookson, Jr. & B. Schneider (Eds.), *Creating school policy: Trends, dilemma, and prospects* (pp. 181–208). New York: Garland.

Kornhaber, M., Krechevsky, M., & Gardner, H. (1990). Engaging intelligence. *Educational Psychologist, 25*(3–4), 177–199.

Kornhaber, M., Veenema, S., & Fierros, E. (2003). *Multiple intelligences: Best ideas from research and practice.* Boston: Allyn & Bacon.

Krechevsky, M. (1991). Project Spectrum: An innovative assessment alternative. *Educational Leadership, 2,* 43–48.

Krechevsky, M. (1998). *Project Spectrum preschool assessment handbook.* New York: Teachers College Press.

Krechevsky, M., & Gardner, H. (1990). The emergence and nurturance of multiple intelligences: The Project Spectrum approach. In M. J. Howe (Ed.), *Encouraging the development of exceptional skills and talents* (pp. 222–245). Leicester, UK: British Psychological Society.

Lazear, D. (1994). *Seven pathways of learning: Teaching students and parents about multiple intelligences.* Tucson, AZ: Zephyr.

Leont'ev, A. N. (1981). The problem of activity in psychology. In J. W. Wertsch (Ed.), *The concept of activity in Soviet psychology* (pp. 37–71). Armonk, NY: Sharpe.

Levin, H. M. (1990). Accelerated schools: A new strategy for at risk students. *Policy Bulletin, 6,* 1–7.

Linn, R. (2000). Assessments and accountability. *Educational Researcher, 29*(2), 4–15.

Linn, R., Baker, E. L., & Betebenner, D. W. (2002). Accountability systems: implications of requirements of the No Child Left Behind Act of 2001. *Educational Researcher, 31*(6), 3–16.

Masur, A. (2004). *Working approach: A new look at the process of learning.* Unpublished doctoral dissertation, Erikson Institute, Chicago.

McCray, J., Chen, J. Q., & McNamee, G. (2004, April). *Identification and nurturance of diverse cognitive profiles in young children.* Paper presented at the annual conference of the American Educational Research Association, Seattle, WA.

McGrew, K. S. (1997). Analysis of major intelligence batteries according to a proposed comprehensive Gf-Gc framework. In D. P. Flanagan, J. L. Genshaft, & P. L. Harrison (Eds.), *Contemporary intellectual assessment: Theories, tests, and issues* (pp. 151–180). New York: Guilford Press.

McNamee, G. D. (2000). Child development research in early childhood classrooms. *Human Development, 43*(4–5), 246–251.

McNamee, G., & Chen, J. Q. (2004, August). *Assessing diverse cognitive abilities in young children's learning.* Paper presented at the 27th International Congress of the International Association for Cross-Cultural Psychology, Xi'an, China.

McNamee, G., & Melendez, L. (2003). *Assessing what children know and planning what to do next: Bridging assessment to teaching practice in early childhood classrooms.* Paper presented at the Annual Conference of the National Association for the Education of Young Children, Chicago.

Meisels, S. J. (1992). Doing harm by doing good: Iatrogenic effects of early childhood enrollment and promotion policies. *Early Childhood Research Quarterly, 7,* 155–174.

Meisels, S. J., Bickel, D. D., Nicholson, J., Xue, Y. G., & Atkins-Burnett, S. (2001). Trusting teachers' judgments: A validity study of a curriculum-embedded performance assessment in kindergarten to grade 3. *American Educational Research Journal, 38*(1), 73–95.

Miller, A. (1991). *Personality types: A modern synthesis.* Calgary, Alberta, Canada: University of Calgary Press.

Moss, P. (1994). Can there be validity without reliability? *Educational Researcher, 3,* 5–12.

Neisser, U., Boodoo, G., Bouchard, T. J., Boykin, A. W., Brody, N., Ceci, S., J., et al. (1996). Intelligence: Knowns and unknowns. *American Psychologist, 51,* 71–101.

Piaget, J. (1929). Introduction: Problems and methods. In J. Piaget, *The child's conception of the world* (pp. 1–32). New York: Harcourt, Brace.

Piaget, J. (1954). *The construction of reality in the child.* New York: Basic Books.

Piaget, J. (1977). The origins of intelligence in children. In H. Gruber & J. J. Vonche (Eds.), *The essential Piaget* (pp. 215–249). New York: Basic Books.

Piaget, J., & Inhelder, B. (1969). *The psychology of the child.* New York: Basic Books.

Plomin, R., & Petrill, S. A. (1997). Genetics and intelligences: What's new? *Intelligence, 24,* 53–77.

Project Zero & Reggio Children. (2001). *Making learning visible: Children as individual and group learners.* Reggio Emilia, Italy: Reggio Children.

Ramos-Ford, V., & Gardner, H. (1991). Giftedness from a multiple intelligences perspective. In N. Colangelo & G. A. Davis (Eds.), *Handbook of gifted education* (pp. 55–64). Boston: Allyn & Bacon.

Rauscher, F., Shaw, G. L., & Ky, K. N. (1993). Music and spatial task performance. *Nature, 365,* 611.

Rinaldi, C. (2001). Introduction. In Project Zero &

Reggio Children, *Making learning visible: Children as individual and group learners* (pp. 28–31). Reggio Emilia, Italy: Reggio Children.

Rogoff, B. (1998). Cognition as a collaborative process. In W. Damon (Series Ed.) & D. William, D, Kuhn, & R. S. Siegler (Vol. Eds.), *Handbook of child psychology: Vol. 2. Cognition, perception, and language* (5th ed., pp. 679–744). New York: Wiley.

Rosnow, R. L. (1991). Inside rumor: A personal journey. *American Psychologist, 46*(5), 484–496.

Rosnow, R. L., Skleder, A. A., Jaeger, M., & Rind, B. (1994). Intelligence and epistemics of interpersonal acumen: Testing some implications of Gardner's theory. *Intelligence, 19,* 93–116.

Rosnow, R. L., Skleder, A. A., & Rind, B. (1995). Reading other people: A hidden cognitive structure? *General Psychologist, 31,* 1–10.

Sameroff, A. J., Seifer, R., Baldwin, A., & Baldwin, C. (1993). Stability of intelligence from preschool to adolescence: The influence of social risk factors. *Child Development, 64,* 80–97.

Sattler, J. M. (2001). *Assessment of children: Cognitive applications* (4th ed.). San Diego, CA: Jerome M. Sattler.

Shearer, B. (1999). *Multiple intelligences developmental assessment scale.* Kent, OH: Multiple Intelligences Research and Consulting.

Silver, H., Strong, R., & Perini, M. (1997). Integrating learning styles and multiple intelligences. *Educational Leadership, 55*(1), 22–27.

Slavin, R. E., & Madden, N. A. (1989). What works for student at risk: A research synthesis. *Educational Leadership, 46*(5), 4–13.

Snyderman, M., & Rothman, S. (1987). Survey of expert opinion on intelligence and aptitude testing. *American Psychologist, 42,* 137–144.

Snyderman, M., & Rothman, S. (1988). *The IQ controversy, the media and public policy.* New Brunswick, NJ: Transaction.

Stefanakis, E. (2003, April). *Multiple intelligences and portfolios: A window into the learner's mind.* Paper presented at the annual meeting of the American Educational Research Association, Chicago.

Sternberg, R. J. (1985a). *Beyond IQ: A triarchic theory of human intelligence.* New York: Cambridge University Press.

Sternberg, R. J. (1985b). Cognitive approaches to intelligence. In B. B. Wolman (Ed.), *Handbook of intelligence: Theories, measurements, and applications* (pp. 59–118). New York: Wiley.

Sternberg, R. J. (1988). *The triarchic mind: A new theory of human intelligence.* New York: Viking.

Sternberg, R. J. (1989). Domain-generality versus domain-specificity: The life and impending death of a false dichotomy. *Merrill–Palmer Quarterly, 35*(1), 115–130.

Sternberg, R. J. (1996). *Successful intelligence: How practice and creative intelligence determine success in life.* New York: Simon & Schuster.

Sternberg, R. J. (1997). The triarchic theory of intelligence. In D. P. Flanagan, J. L. Genshaft, & P. L. Harrison (Eds.), *Contemporary intellectual assessment: Theories, tests, and issues* (pp. 92–104). New York: Guilford Press.

Stiggins, R. (2002). Assessment crisis: The absence of assessment for learning. *Phi Delta Kappan, 83*(10), 758–765.

Teels, S. (2000). *Rainbows of intelligence: Exploring how student learn.* Thousand Oaks, CA: Corwin Press.

Thurstone, L. L. (1938). *Primary mental abilities.* Chicago: University of Chicago Press.

Vygotsky, L. S. (1978). *Mind in society: The development of higher psychological processes* (M. Cole, V. John-Steiner, S. Scribner, & E. Souberman, Eds. & Trans.). Cambridge, MA: Harvard University Press.

Walters, J. M., & Gardner, H. (1986). The theory of multiple intelligences: Some issues and answers. In R. Sternberg & R. Wagner (Eds.), *Practical intelligences* (pp. 163–183). New York: Cambridge University Press.

Wertsch, J. W. (Ed.). (1981). *The concept of activity in Soviet psychology.* Armonk, NY: Sharpe.

Wiggins, G. (1998). *Educative assessment: Designing assessment to inform and improve student performance.* San Francisco: Jossey-Bass.

Winner, E., Rosenblatt, E., Windmueller, G., Davidson, L., & Gardner, H., (1986). Children's perceptions of "aesthetic" properties of the arts: Domain specific or pan-artistic? *British Journal of Developmental Psychology, 4,* 149–160.

Wolf, D., & Gardner, H. (1978). Style and sequence in early symbolic play. In M. Franklin & N. Smith (Eds.), *Early symbolization* (pp. 117–138). Hillsdale, NJ: Erlbaum.

Wu, W. T. (2003, April). *Multiple intelligences, educational reform, and successful careers.* Paper presented at the annual meeting of the American Educational Research Association, Chicago.

Yoong, S. (2001, November). *Multiple intelligences: A construct validation of the MIDAS Scale in Malaysia.* Paper presented at the International Conference on Measurement and Evaluation in Education, Penang, Malaysia.

6

The Triarchic Theory of Successful Intelligence

ROBERT J. STERNBERG

Some people seem to do what they do better than others, and so various cultures have created roughly comparable psychological constructs to try to explain, or at least to describe, this fact. The construct we have created we call *intelligence*. It is our way of saying that some people seem to adapt to the environments we both create and confront better than do others.

There have been numerous approaches to understanding the construct of intelligence, based on somewhat different metaphors for understanding the construct (Sternberg, 1990; see also essays in Sternberg, 2000). For example, some investigators seek to understand intelligence via what I have referred to as a geographic model, in which intelligence is conceived as a map of the mind. Such researchers have used psychometric tests to uncover the latent factors alleged to underlie intellectual functioning (see Carroll, Chapter 4, this volume). Other investigators have used a computational metaphor, viewing intelligence in much the way they view the symbolic processing of a computer (see Naglieri & Das, Chapter 7, this volume). Still others have followed an anthropological approach, viewing intelligence as a unique cultural creation. The approach I take in the triarchic theory proposed here can be viewed as a systems approach, in which many different aspects of intelligence are interrelated to each other in an attempt to understand how intelligence functions as a system.

The *triarchic theory of successful intelligence* (Sternberg, 1985a, 1988, 1997, 1999) explains in an integrative way the relationship between intelligence and (1) the internal world of the individual, or the mental mechanisms that underlie intelligent behavior; (2) experience, or the mediating role of the individual's passage through life between his or her internal and external worlds; and (3) the external world of the individual, or the use of these mental mechanisms in everyday life in order to attain an intelligent fit to the environment. The theory has three subtheories, one corresponding to each of the three relationships mentioned in the preceding sentence.

A crucial difference between this theory and many others is that the operationalizations (measurements) follow rather than precede the theory. Thus, rather than the theory's being derived from factor or other analyses of tests, the tests are chosen on the basis of the tenets of the theory. My colleagues and I have used many different kinds of tests (see Sternberg, 1985a, 1988, for reviews), such as analogies, syllogisms, verbal comprehension, prediction of future outcomes, and decoding of nonverbal cues. In every case, though, the choice of tasks has been dictated by the aspects of the theory that are being investigated, rather than the other way around.

DEFINITION OF SUCCESSFUL INTELLIGENCE

According to the proposed theory, *successful intelligence* is (1) the use of an integrated set of abilities needed to attain success in life, however an individual defines it, within his or her sociocultural context. People are successfully intelligent by virtue of (2) recognizing their strengths and making the most of them, at the same time that they recognize their weaknesses and find ways to correct or compensate for them. Successfully intelligent people (3) adapt to, shape, and select environments through (4) finding a balance in their use of analytical, creative, and practical abilities (Sternberg, 1997, 1999). Let us consider each element of the theory in turn.

The first element makes clear that there is no one definition of success that works for everyone. For some people, success is brilliance as lawyers; for others, it is originality as novelists; for others, it is caring for their children; for others, it is devoting their lives to God. For many people, it is some combination of things. Because people have different life goals, education needs to move away from single targeted measures of success, such as grade point average.

In considering the nature of intelligence, we need to consider the full range of definitions of success by which children can be intelligent. For example, in research we have done in rural Kenya (Sternberg et al., 2001), we have found that children who may score quite high on tests of an aspect of practical intelligence—knowledge of how to use natural herbal medicines to treat parasitic and other illnesses—may score quite poorly on tests of IQ and academic achievement. Indeed, we found an inverse relationship between the two skill sets, with correlations reaching the −.3 level. For these children, time spent in school takes away from time in which they learn the practical skills that they and their families view as needed for success in life. The same might be said, in the Western world, for many children who want to enter careers in athletics, theater, dance, art, music, carpentry, plumbing, entrepreneurship, and so forth. They may see time spent developing academic skills as time taken away from the time they need to develop practical skills relevant to meeting their goals in life.

The second element asserts that there are different paths to success, no matter what goal one chooses. Some people achieve success in large part through personal charm; others through brilliance of academic intellect; others through stunning originality; and yet others through working extremely hard. For most of us, there are at least a few things we do well, and our successful intelligence is dependent in large part upon making these things "work for us." At the same time, we need to acknowledge our weaknesses and find ways either to improve upon them or to compensate for them. For example, we may work hard to improve our skills in an area of weakness, or work as part of a team so that other people compensate for the kinds of things we do not do particularly well.

The third element asserts that success in life is achieved through some balance of adapting to existing environments, shaping those environments, and selecting new environments. Often, when we go into an environment—as do students and teachers in school—we try to modify ourselves to fit that environment. In other words, we adapt. But sometimes it is not enough to adapt: We are not content merely to change ourselves to fit the environment, but rather, also want to change the environment to fit us. In this case, we shape the environment in order to make it a better one for us and possibly for others as well. But there may come times when our attempts to adapt and to shape the environment lead us nowhere—when we simply cannot find a way to make the environment work for us. In these cases, we leave the old environment and select a new environment. Sometimes, the smart thing is to know when to get out.

Finally, we balance three kinds of abilities in order to achieve these ends: analytical abilities, creative abilities, and practical abilities. We need creative abilities to generate ideas, analytical abilities to determine whether they are good ideas, and practical abilities to implement the ideas and to convince others of the value of our ideas. Most people who are successfully intelligent are not equally endowed with these three abilities, but they find ways of making the three abilities work harmoniously together.

We have used five kinds of converging operations to test the theory of successful intelligence: cultural studies, factor-analytic studies, information-processing analyses, correlational analyses, and instructional studies (some of which are described below). This work is summarized elsewhere (e.g., Sternberg, 1985a, 1997, 2003). Examples of kinds of evidence in this work supporting the theory are the factorial separability of analytical, creative, and practical abilities; the substantial incremental validity of measures of practical intelligence over the validity of measures of academic (general) intelligence in predicting school and job performance; the usefulness of instruction based on the theory of successful intelligence, in comparison with other forms of instruction; and differences in the nature of what constitutes practical intelligence across cultures.

INTELLIGENCE AND THE INTERNAL WORLD OF THE INDIVIDUAL

Psychometricians, Piagetians, and information-processing psychologists have all recognized the importance of understanding the mental states or processes that underlie intelligent thought. In the triarchic theory, they seek this understanding by identifying and understanding three basic kinds of information-processing components, referred to as *metacomponents*, *performance components*, and *knowledge acquisition components*.

Metacomponents

Metacomponents are higher-order, executive processes used to plan what one is going to do, to monitor it while one is doing it, and evaluate it after it is done. These metacomponents include (1) recognizing the existence of a problem, (2) deciding on the nature of the problem confronting one, (3) selecting a set of lower-order processes to solve the problem, (4) selecting a strategy into which to combine these components, (5) selecting a mental representation on which the components and strategy can act, (6) allocating one's mental resources, (7) monitoring one's problem solving as it is happening, and (8) evaluating one's problem solving after it is done. Let us consider some examples of these higher-order processes.

Deciding on the nature of a problem plays a prominent role in intelligence. For example, the difficulty for young children as well as older adults in problem solving often lies not in actually solving a given problem, but in figuring out just what the problem is that needs to be solved (see, e.g., Flavell, 1977; Sternberg & Rifkin, 1979). A major feature distinguishing people with mental retardation from persons with typical functioning is the need of the former to be instructed explicitly and completely as to the nature of the particular task they are solving and how it should be performed (Butterfield, Wambold, & Belmont, 1973; Campione & Brown, 1979). The importance of figuring out the nature of the problem is not limited to persons with mental retardation. Resnick and Glaser (1976) have argued that intelligence is the ability to learn from incomplete instruction.

Selection of a strategy for combining lower-order components is also a critical aspect of intelligence. In early information-processing research on intelligence, including my own (e.g., Sternberg, 1977), the primary emphasis was simply on figuring out what study participants do when confronted with a problem. What components do participants use, and into what strategies do they combine these components?

Soon information-processing researchers began to ask why study participants use the strategies they choose. For example, Cooper (1982) reported that in solving spatial problems, and especially mental rotation problems, some study participants seem to use a holistic strategy of comparison, whereas others use an analytic strategy. She sought to figure out what leads study participants to the choice of one strategy over another. Siegler (1986) proposed a model of strategy selection in arithmetic computation problems that links strategy choice to both the rules and the mental associations participants have stored in long-term memory. MacLeod, Hunt, and Mathews (1978) found that study participants with high spatial abilities tend to use a spatial strategy in solving sentence–picture comparison problems, whereas study participants with high verbal abilities are more likely to use a linguistic strategy. In my own work, I have found that study participants tend to prefer strategies for analogical reasoning that place fewer demands on working memory (Sternberg & Ketron, 1982). In such strategies, study participants encode as few features as possible of complex stimuli, trying to disconfirm incorrect multiple-choice options on the basis of these few features, and then choosing the remaining answer as the correct one. Similarly, study participants choose different strategies in linear–syllogistic reasoning (spatial, linguistic, mixed spatial–linguistic), but in this task, they do not always capitalize on their ability patterns to choose the strategy most suitable to their respective levels of spatial and verbal abilities (Sternberg & Weil, 1980). In sum, the selection of a strategy seems to be at least as important for understanding intelligent task performance as the efficacy with which the chosen strategy is implemented.

Intimately tied up with the selection of a strategy is the selection of a mental representation for information. In the early literature on mental representations, the emphasis seemed to be on understanding how information is represented. For example, can individuals use imagery as a form of mental representation (Kosslyn & Koenig, 1995)? Investigators have realized that people are quite flexible in their representations of information. The most appropriate question to ask seems to be not how such information is represented but which representations are used in what circumstances. For example, I (Sternberg, 1977) found that analogy problems using animal names can draw on either spatial or clustering representations of the animal names. In the studies of strategy choice mentioned earlier, it was found that study participants can use either linguistic or spatial representations in solving sentence–picture comparisons (MacLeod et al., 1978) or linear syllogisms (Sternberg & Weil, 1980). We (Sternberg & Rifkin, 1979) found that the mental representation of certain kinds of analogies can be either more or less holistic, depending on the ages of the study participants. Younger children tend to be more holistic in their representations.

As important as any other metacomponent is the ability to allocate one's mental resources. Different investigators have studied resource allocation in different ways. Hunt and Lansman (1982), for example, have concentrated on the use of secondary tasks in assessing information processing and have proposed a model of attention allocation in the solution of problems that involve both a primary and a secondary task.

In my work, I have found that better problem solvers tend to spend relatively more time in global strategy planning (Sternberg, 1981). Similarly, in solving analogies, better analogical reasoners seemed to spend relatively more time encoding the terms of the problem than do poorer reasoners, but relatively less time in operating on these encodings (Sternberg, 1977; Sternberg & Rifkin, 1979). In reading as well, superior readers are better able than poorer readers to allocate their time across reading passages as a function of the difficulty of the passages to be read and the purpose for which the passages are being read (see Brown, Bransford, Ferrara, & Campione, 1983; Wagner & Sternberg, 1987).

Finally, monitoring one's solution process is a key aspect of intelligence (see also Brown, 1978). Consider, for example, the "missionaries and cannibals" problem, in which the study participants must "transport" a set of missionaries and cannibals across a river in a small boat without allowing the cannibals an opportunity to eat the missionaries—an event that can transpire only if the cannibals are allowed to outnumber the missionaries on either side of the river bank. The main kinds of errors that can be made are either to return to an earlier state in the problem space for solution (i.e., the problem solver goes back to where he or she was earlier in the solution process) or to make an impermissible move (i.e., the problem solver violates the rules, as in allowing the number of cannibals on one side to exceed the number of missionaries on that side) (Simon & Reed, 1976; see also Sternberg, 1982). Neither of these errors will result if a given subject closely monitors his or her solution processes. For young children, learning to count, a major source of errors in counting objects is to count a given object twice; again, such errors can result from failures in solution monitoring (Gelman & Gallistel, 1978). The effects of solution monitoring are not limited, of course, to any one kind of problem. One's ability to use the strategy of means–ends analysis (Newell & Simon, 1972)—that is, reduction of differences between where one is solving a problem and where one wishes to get in solving that problem—depends on one's ability to monitor just where one is in problem solution.

Performance Components

Performance components are lower-order processes that execute the instructions of the metacomponents. These lower-order components solve the problems according to the plans laid out by the metacomponents. Whereas the number of metacomponents used in the performance of various tasks is relatively limited, the number of performance components is probably quite large. Many of these performance components are relatively specific to narrow ranges of tasks (Sternberg, 1979, 1983, 1985a).

One of the most interesting classes of performance components is that found in inductive reasoning of the kind measured by tests such as matrices, analogies, series completions, and classifications. These components are important because of the importance of the tasks into which they enter: Induction problems of these kinds show the highest loading on the so-called *g*, or general intelligence factor (Carroll, Chapter 4, this volume; Horn & Blankson, Chapter 3, this volume; Jensen, 1980, 1998; Snow & Lohman, 1984; Sternberg & Gardner, 1982; see essays in Sternberg & Grigorenko, 2002). Thus identifying these performance components can give us some insight into the nature of the general factor. I am not arguing for any one factorial model of intelligence (i.e., one with a general factor) over others; to the contrary, I believe that most factor models are mutually compatible, differing only in the form of rotation that has been applied to a given factor space (Sternberg, 1977). The rotation one uses is a matter of theoretical or practical convenience, not of truth or falsity.

The main performance components of inductive reasoning are encoding, inference, mapping, application, comparison, justification, and response. They can be illustrated with reference to an analogy problem, such as "*Lawyer* is to *client* as *doctor* is to (a) *patient*, (b) *medicine*." In encoding, the subject retrieves from semantic memory semantic attributes that are potentially relevant for analogy solution. In inference, the subject discovers the relation between the first two terms of the analogy—here, *lawyer* and *client*. In mapping, the subject discovers the higher-order relation that links the first half of the analogy, headed by *lawyer*, to the second half of the analogy, headed by *doctor*. In applica-

tion, the subject carries over the relation inferred in the first half of the analogy to the second half of the analogy, generating a possible completion for the analogy. In comparison, the subject compares each of the answer options to the mentally generated completion, deciding which (if any) is correct. In justification, used optionally if none of the answer options matches the mentally generated solution, the subject decides which (if any) of the options is close enough to constitute an acceptable solution to the examiner. In response, the subject indicates an option, whether by means of pressing a button, making a mark on a piece of paper, or whatever.

Two fundamental issues have arisen regarding the nature of performance components as a fundamental construct in human intelligence. The first, mentioned briefly here, is whether their number simply keeps expanding indefinitely. Neisser (1982), for example, has suggested that it does. As a result, he views the construct as of little use. But this expansion results only if one considers seriously those components that are specific to small classes of problems or to single problems. If one limits one's attention to the more important, general components of performance, the problem simply does not arise—as shown, for example, in our (Sternberg & Gardner, 1982) analysis of inductive reasoning or in Pellegrino and Kail's (1982) analysis of spatial ability. The second issue is one of the level at which performance components should be studied. In so-called "cognitive correlates" research (Pellegrino & Glaser, 1979), theorists emphasize components at relatively low levels of information processing (Hunt, 1978, 1980; Jensen, 1982). In so-called "cognitive components" research (Pellegrino & Glaser, 1979), theorists emphasize components at relatively high levels of information processing (e.g., Mulholland, Pellegrino, & Glaser, 1980; Snow, 1980; Sternberg, 1977). Because of the interactive nature of human information processing, it would appear that there is no right or wrong level of analysis. Rather, all levels of information processing contribute to both task and subject variance in intelligent performance. The most expeditious level of analysis depends on the task and subject population: Lower-level performance components may be more important, for example, in studying more basic information-processing tasks, such as choice reaction time, or in studying higher-level tasks in children who have not yet automatized the lower-order processes that contribute to performance of these tasks.

Knowledge Acquisition Components

Knowledge acquisition components are used to learn how to do what the metacomponents and performance components eventually do. Three knowledge acquisition components appear to be central in intellectual functioning: (1) selective encoding, (2) selective combination, and (3) selective comparison.

Selective encoding involves sifting out relevant from irrelevant information. When new information is presented in natural contexts, relevant information for one's given purpose is embedded in the midst of large amounts of purpose-irrelevant information. A critical task for the learner is that of sifting the "wheat from the chaff," recognizing just what among all the pieces of information is relevant for one's purposes (see Schank, 1980).

Selective combination involves combining selectively encoded information in such a way as to form an integrated, plausible whole. Simply sifting out relevant from irrelevant information is not enough to generate a new knowledge structure. One must know how to combine the pieces of information into an internally connected whole (see Mayer & Greeno, 1972).

Selective comparison involves discovering a nonobvious relationship between new information and already acquired information. For example, analogies, metaphors, and models often help individuals solve problems. The solver suddenly realizes that new information is similar to old information in certain ways and then uses this information to form a mental representation based on the similarities. Teachers may discover how to relate new classroom material to information that students have already learned. Relating the new to the old can help students learn the material more quickly and understand it more deeply.

My emphasis on components of knowledge acquisition differs somewhat from the focus of some contemporary theorists in cognitive psychology, who emphasize what is already known and the structure of this knowledge (e.g., Chase & Simon, 1973; Chi, 1978; Keil, 1984). These various emphases are complementary. If one is interested in understanding, for example, differences in performance between experts and novices, clearly one would wish to look at the amount and structure of their respective knowledge bases. But if one wishes to understand how these differences come to be, merely looking at developed knowledge would not be enough. Rather, one would have to look as well at differences in the ways in which the knowledge bases were acquired. It is here that understanding of knowledge acquisition components will prove to be most relevant.

We have studied knowledge acquisition components in the domain of vocabulary acquisition (e.g., Sternberg, 1987; Sternberg & Powell, 1983). Difficulty in learning new words can be traced, at least in part, to the application of components of knowledge acquisition to context cues stored in long-term memory. Individuals with higher vocabularies tend to be those who are better able to apply the knowledge acquisition components to vocabulary-learning situations. Given the importance of vocabulary for overall intelligence, almost without respect to the theory or test one uses, utilization of knowledge acquisition components in vocabulary-learning situations would appear to be critically important for the development of intelligence. Effective use of knowledge acquisition components is trainable. I have found, for example, that just 45 minutes of training in the use of these components in vocabulary learning can significantly and fairly substantially improve the ability of adults to learn vocabulary from natural language contexts (Sternberg, 1987). This training involves teaching individuals how to learn meanings of words presented in context. The training consists of three elements. The first is teaching individuals to search out certain kinds of contextual cues, such as synonyms, antonyms, functions, and category memberships. The second is teaching mediating variables. For example, cues to the meaning of a word are more likely to be found close to the word than at a distance from it. The third is teaching process skills—encoding relevant cues, combining them, and relating them to knowledge one already has.

To summarize, then, the components of intelligence are important parts of the intelligence of the individual. The various kinds of components work together. Metacomponents activate performance and knowledge acquisition components. These latter kinds of components in turn provide feedback to the metacomponents. Although one can isolate various kinds of information-processing components from task performance using experimental means, in practice the components function together in highly interactive, and not easily isolable, ways. Thus diagnoses as well as instructional interventions need to consider all three types of components in interaction, rather than any one kind of component in isolation. But understanding the nature of the components of intelligence is not in itself sufficient to understand the nature of intelligence, because there is more to intelligence than a set of information-processing components. One could scarcely understand all of what it is that makes one person more intelligent than another by understanding the components of processing on, say, an intelligence test. The other aspects of the triarchic theory address some of the other aspects of intelligence that contribute to individual differences in observed performance, outside testing situations as well as within them.

INTELLIGENCE AND EXPERIENCE

Components of information processing are always applied to tasks and situations with which one has some level of prior experience (even if it is minimal experience). Hence these internal mechanisms are closely tied to one's experience. According to the experiential subtheory, the components are not equally good measures of intelligence at all levels of experience. Assessing intelligence requires one to consider not only components, but the level of experience at which they are applied.

Toward the end of the 20th century, a trend developed in cognitive science to study script-based behavior (e.g., Schank & Abelson, 1977), whether under the name of

script or under some other name, such as *schema* or *frame*. There is no longer any question that much of human behavior is scripted in some sense. However, from the standpoint of the present subtheory, such behavior is nonoptimal for understanding intelligence. Typically, one's actions when going to a restaurant, doctor's office, or movie theater do not provide good measures of intelligence, even though they do provide good measures of scripted behavior. What, then, is the relation between intelligence and experience?

According to the experiential subtheory, intelligence is best measured at those regions of the experiential continuum involving tasks or situations that are either relatively novel on the one hand, or in the process of becoming automatized on the other. As Raaheim (1974) pointed out, totally novel tasks and situations provide poor measures of intelligence: One would not want to administer, say, trigonometry problems to a first grader roughly 6 years old. But one might wish to administer problems that are just at the limits of the child's understanding, in order to test how far this understanding extends. Related is Vygotsky's (1978) concept of the *zone of proximal development*, in which one examines a child's ability to profit from instruction to facilitate his or her solutions of novel problems. To measure automatization skill, one might wish to present a series of problems—mathematical or otherwise—to see how long it takes for their solution to become automatic, and to see how automatized performance becomes. Thus both the slope and the asymptote (if any) of automatization are of interest.

Ability to Deal with Novelty

Several sources of evidence converge on the notion that the ability to deal with relative novelty is a good way of measuring intelligence. Consider three such sources of evidence. First, we have conducted several studies on the nature of insight, both in children and in adults (Davidson & Sternberg, 1984; Sternberg & Davidson, 1982). In the studies with children (Davidson & Sternberg, 1984), we separated three kinds of insights: insights of selective encoding, insights of selective combination, and insights of selective comparison. Use of these knowledge acquisition components is referred to as *insightful* when they are applied in the absence of existing scripts, plans, or frames. In other words, one must decide what information is relevant, how to put the information together, or how new information relates to old in the absence of any obvious cues on the basis of which to make these judgments. A problem is insightfully solved at the individual level when a given individual lacks such cues. A problem is insightfully solved at the societal level when no one else has these cues, either. In our studies, we found that children who are intellectually gifted are so in part by virtue of their insight abilities, which represent an important part of the ability to deal with novelty.

The critical finding was that providing insights to the children significantly benefited the nongifted, but not the gifted, children. (None of the children performed anywhere near ceiling level, so that the interaction was not due to ceiling effects.) In other words, the gifted children spontaneously had the insights and hence did not benefit from being given these insights. The nongifted children did not have the insights spontaneously and hence did benefit. Thus the gifted children were better able to deal with novelty spontaneously.

Another source of evidence for the proposed hypothesis relating coping with novelty to intelligence derives from the large literature on fluid intelligence, which is in part a kind of intelligence that involves dealing with novelty (see Cattell, 1971). Snow and Lohman (1984; see also Snow, Kyllonen, & Marshalek, 1984) multidimensionally scaled a variety of such tests and found the dimensional loading to follow a radex structure. In particular, tests with higher loadings on g, or general intelligence, fall closer to the center of the spatial diagram. The critical thing to note is that those tests that best measure the ability to deal with novelty fall closer to the center, and tests tend to be more removed from the center as their assessment of the ability to deal with novelty becomes more remote. In sum, evidence from the laboratories of others as well as mine supports the idea that the various components of intelligence that are involved in dealing with novelty, as measured in particular tasks and situations, provide particularly apt measures of intellectual ability.

Ability to Automatize
Information Processing

There are several converging lines of evidence in the literature to support the claim that automatization ability is a key aspect of intelligence. For example, I (Sternberg, 1977) found that the correlation between people–piece (schematic picture) analogy performance and measures of general intelligence increased with practice, as performance on these items became increasingly automatized. Skilled reading is heavily dependent on automatization of bottom-up functions (basic skills such as phonetic decoding), and the ability to read well is an essential part of crystallized ability—whether it is viewed from the standpoint of theories such as Cattell's (1971), Carroll's (1993), or Vernon's (1971), or from the standpoint of tests of crystallized ability, such as the verbal portion of the SAT. Poor comprehenders often are those who have not automatized the elementary, bottom-up processes of reading and hence do not have sufficient attentional resources to allocate to top-down comprehension processes. Ackerman (1987; Kanfer & Ackerman, 1989) has provided a three-stage model of automatization in which the first stage is related to intelligence, although the latter two appear not to be.

Theorists such as Jensen (1982) and Hunt (1978) have attributed the correlation between such tasks as choice reaction time and letter matching to the relation between speed of information processing and intelligence. Indeed, there is almost certainly some relation, although I believe it is much more complex than these theorists seem to allow for. But a plausible alternative hypothesis is that at least some of that correlation is due to the effects of automatization of processing: Because of the simplicity of these tasks, they probably become at least partially automatized fairly rapidly, and hence can measure both rate and asymptote of automatization of performance. In sum, then, although the evidence is far from complete, there is at least some support for the notion that rate and level of automatization are related to intellectual skill.

The ability to deal with novelty and the ability to automatize information processing are interrelated, as shown in the example of the automatization of reading described in this section. If one is well able to automatize, one has more resources left over for dealing with novelty. Similarly, if one is well able to deal with novelty, one has more resources left over for automatization. Thus performances at the various levels of the experiential continuum are related to one another.

These abilities should not be viewed in a vacuum with respect to the componential subtheory. The components of intelligence are applied to tasks and situations at various levels of experience. The ability to deal with novelty can be understood in part in terms of the metacomponents, performance components, and knowledge acquisition components involved in it. *Automatization* refers to the way these components are executed. Hence the two subtheories considered so far are closely intertwined. Now we need to consider the application of these subtheories to everyday tasks, in addition to laboratory ones.

INTELLIGENCE AND THE EXTERNAL WORLD OF THE INDIVIDUAL

According to the contextual subtheory, intelligent thought is directed toward one or more of three behavioral goals: *adaptation to an environment, shaping of an environment,* or *selection of an environment.* These three goals may be viewed as the functions toward which intelligence is directed. Intelligence is not aimless or random mental activity that happens to involve certain components of information processing at certain levels of experience. Rather, it is purposefully directed toward the pursuit of these three global goals, all of which have more specific and concrete instantiations in people's lives (Sternberg et al., 2000).

Adaptation

Most intelligent thought is directed toward the attempt to adapt to one's environment. The requirements for adaptation can differ radically from one environment to another—whether environments are defined in terms of families, jobs, subcultures, or cultures. Hence, although the components of intelligence required in these various contexts may be the same or quite similar, and although all of them may involve (at one time or another)

dealing with novelty and automatization of information processing, the concrete instantiations that these processes and levels of experience take may differ substantially across contexts. This fact has an important implication for our understanding of the nature of intelligence. According to the triarchic theory in general, and the contextual subtheory in particular, the processes, experiential facets, and functions of intelligence remain essentially the same across contexts, but the particular instantiations of these processes, facets, and functions can differ radically. Thus the content of intelligent thought and its manifestations in behavior will bear no necessary resemblance across contexts. As a result, although the mental elements that an intelligence test should measure do not differ across contexts, the vehicle for measurement may have to differ. A test that measures a set of processes, experiential facets, or intelligent functions in one context may not provide equally adequate measurement in another context. To the contrary, what is intelligent in one culture may be viewed as unintelligent in another.

Different contextual milieus may result in the development of different mental abilities. For example, Puluwat navigators must develop their large-scale spatial abilities for dealing with cognitive maps to a degree that far exceeds the adaptive requirements of contemporary Western societies (Gladwin, 1970). Similarly, Kearins (1981) found that Australian Aboriginal children probably develop their visual–spatial memories to a greater degree than do Australian children of European descent. The latter are more likely to apply verbal strategies to spatial memory tasks than are the Aboriginal children, who employ spatial strategies. This greater development is presumed to be due to the greater need the Aboriginal children have for using spatial skills in their everyday lives. In contrast, members of Western societies probably develop their abilities for thinking abstractly to a greater degree than do members of societies in which concepts are rarely dealt with outside their concrete manifestations in the objects of the everyday environment.

One of the most interesting differences among cultures and subcultures in the development of patterns of adaptation is in the matter of time allocation, a metacomponential function. In Western cultures in general, careful allocation of time to various activities is a prized commodity. Our lives are largely governed by careful scheduling at home, school, work, and so on. There are fixed hours for certain activities and fixed lengths of time within which these activities are expected to be completed. Indeed, the intelligence tests we use show our prizing of time allocation to the fullest. Almost all of them are timed in such a way as to make completion of the tests a nontrivial challenge. A slow or cautious worker is at a distinct disadvantage. Not all cultures and subcultures view time in the same way that we do. For example, among the Kipsigi, schedules are much more flexible; hence these individuals have difficulty understanding and dealing with Western notions of the time pressure under which people are expected to live (Super & Harkness, 1982). In Hispanic cultures, such as Venezuela, my own personal experience indicates that the press of time is taken with much less seriousness than it is in typical North American cultural settings. Even within the continental United States, though, there can be major differences in the importance of time allocation (Heath, 1983).

The point of these examples has been to illustrate how differences in environmental press and people's conception of what constitutes an intelligent response to it can influence just what counts as adaptive behavior. To understand intelligence, one must understand it not only in relation to its internal manifestations in terms of mental processes and its experiential manifestations in terms of facets of the experiential continuum, but also in terms of how thought is intelligently translated into action in a variety of different contextual settings. The differences in what is considered adaptive and intelligent can extend even to different occupations within a given cultural milieu. For example, I (Sternberg, 1985b) have found that individuals in different fields of endeavor (art, business, philosophy, physics) view intelligence in slightly different ways that reflect the demands of their respective fields.

Shaping

Shaping of the environment is often used as a backup strategy when adaptation fails. If one is unable to change oneself to fit the environment, one may attempt to change the environment to fit oneself. For example, repeated attempts to adjust to the demands of one's romantic partner may eventually lead to attempts to get the partner to adjust to oneself. But shaping is not always used in lieu of adaptation. In some cases, shaping may be used before adaptation is ever tried, as in the case of the individual who attempts to shape a romantic partner with little or no effort to shape him- or herself so as to suit the partner's wants or needs better.

In the laboratory, examples of shaping behavior can be seen in strategy selection situations where one essentially molds the task to fit one's preferred style of dealing with tasks. For example, in comparing sentence statements, individuals may select either a verbal or a spatial strategy, depending on their pattern of verbal and spatial ability (MacLeod et al., 1978). The task is "made over" in conformity to what they do best.

In some respects, shaping may be seen as the quintessence of intelligent thought and behavior. One essentially makes over the environment, rather than allowing the environment to make over oneself. Perhaps it is this skill that has enabled humankind to reach its current level of scientific, technological, and cultural advancement (for better or for worse). In science, the greatest scientists are those who set the paradigms (shaping), rather than those who merely follow them (adaptation). Similarly, the individuals who achieve greatest distinction in art and in literature are often those who create new modes and styles of expression, rather than merely following existing ones. It is not their use of shaping alone that distinguishes them intellectually, but rather a combination of their willingness to do it with their skill in doing it.

Selection

Selection involves renunciation of one environment in favor of another. In terms of the rough hierarchy established so far, selection is sometimes used when both adaptation and shaping fail. After attempting to both adapt to and shape a marriage, one may decide to deal with one's failure in these activities by "deselecting" the marriage and choosing the environment of the newly single. Failure to adjust to the demands of work environments, or to change the demands placed on one to make them a reasonable fit to one's interests, values, expectations, or abilities, may result in the decision to seek another job altogether. But selection is not always used as a last resort. Sometimes one attempts to shape an environment only after attempts to leave it have failed. Other times, one may decide almost instantly that an environment is simply wrong and feel that one need not or should not even try to fit into or to change it. For example, every now and then we get a new graduate student who realizes almost immediately that he or she came to graduate school for the wrong reasons, or who finds that graduate school is nothing at all like the continuation of undergraduate school he or she expected. In such cases, the intelligent thing to do may be to leave the environment as soon as possible, to pursue activities more in line with one's goals in life.

Environmental selection is not usually directly studied in the laboratory, although it may have relevance for certain experimental settings. Perhaps no research example of its relevance has been more salient than the experimental paradigm created by Milgram (1974), who, in a long series of studies, asked study participants to "shock" other study participants (who were actually confederates and who were not actually shocked). The finding of critical interest was how few study participants shaped the environment by refusing to continue with the experiment and walking out of it. Milgram has drawn an analogy to the situation in Nazi Germany, where obedience to authority created an environment whose horrors continue to amaze us to this day and always will. This example is a good one in showing how close matters of intelligence can come to matters of personality.

To conclude, adaptation, shaping, and selection are functions of intelligent thought as it operates in context. They may (although they need not) be employed hierarchically, with one path followed when another one fails. It is through adaptation, shaping, and selection that the components of intelligence, as employed at various levels of experience, become actualized in the real world. In this section, it has become clear that the modes of actualization can differ widely across individuals and groups, so that intelligence cannot be understood independently of the ways in which it is manifested.

INSTRUCTIONAL INTERVENTIONS BASED ON THE THEORY

The triarchic theory has been applied to instructional settings in various ways, with considerable success. The componential subtheory has been applied in teaching the learning of vocabulary from context to adult study participants (Sternberg, 1987), as mentioned earlier. Experimental study participants were taught components of decontextualization. There were three groups, corresponding to three types of instruction that were given based on the theory (see Sternberg, 1987, 1988). Control study participants either received no relevant material at all, or else received practical items but without theory-based instruction. Improvement occurred only when study participants were given the theory-based instruction, which involved teaching them how to use contextual cues, mediating variables such as matching parts of speech, and processes of decontextualization.

The experiential subtheory was the basis for the program (Davidson & Sternberg, 1984) that successfully taught insight skills (selective encoding, selective combination, and selective comparison) to children roughly 9–11 years of age. The program lasted 6 weeks and involved insight skills as applied to a variety of subject matter areas. An uninstructed control group received a pretest and a posttest, like the experimental group, but no instruction. We found that the experimental study participants improved significantly more than the controls, both when participants were previously identified as gifted and when they were not so identified. Moreover, we found durable results that lasted even 1 year after the training program, and we found transfer to types of insight problems not specifically used in the program.

The contextual subtheory served as the basis for a program called Practical Intelligence for Schools, developed in collaboration with a team of investigators from Harvard (Gardner, Krechevsky, Sternberg, & Okagaki, 1994; Sternberg, Okagaki, & Jackson, 1990). The goal of this program is to teach practical intellectual skills to children roughly 9–11 years of age in the areas of reading, writing, homework, and test taking. The program is completely infused into existing curricula. Over a period of years, we studied the program in a variety of school districts and obtained significant improvements for experimental versus uninstructed control study participants in a variety of criterion measures, including study skills measures and performance-based measures of performance in the areas taught by the program. The program has been shown to increase practical skills, such as those involved in doing homework, taking tests, or writing papers, as well as school achievement (Williams et al., 2002).

We have sought to test the theory of successful intelligence in the classroom. In a first set of studies, we explored the question of whether conventional education in school systematically discriminates against children with creative and practical strengths (Sternberg & Clinkenbeard, 1995; Sternberg, Ferrari, Clinkenbeard, & Grigorenko, 1996; Sternberg, Grigorenko, Ferrari, & Clinkenbeard, 1999). Motivating this work was the belief that the systems in most schools strongly tend to favor children with strengths in memory and analytical abilities. However, schools can be unbalanced in other directions as well.

One school we visited in Russia in 2000 placed a heavy emphasis upon the development of creative abilities—much more so than on the development of analytical and practical abilities. While on this trip, we were told of yet another school (catering to the children of Russian businessmen) that strongly emphasized practical abilities, and in which children who were not practically oriented were told that eventually, they would be working for their classmates who were practically oriented.

To validate the relevance of the theory of successful intelligence in classrooms, we have carried out a number of instructional studies. In one study, we used the Sternberg Triarchic Abilities Test (Sternberg, 1993). The test was administered to 326 children around the United States and in some other countries who were identified by their schools as gifted by any standard whatsoever (Sternberg et al., 1999). Children were se-

lected for a summer program in (college-level) psychology if they fell into one of five ability groupings: *high-analytical*, *high-creative*, *high-practical*, *high-balanced* (high in all three abilities), or *low-balanced* (low in all three abilities). Students who came to Yale were then assigned at random to four instructional groups, with the constraint that roughly equal numbers with each ability pattern be assigned to each group. Students in all four instructional groups used the same introductory psychology textbook (a preliminary version of Sternberg, 1995) and listened to the same psychology lectures. What differed among them was the type of afternoon discussion section to which they were assigned. They were assigned to an instructional condition that emphasized either memory, analytical, creative, or practical instruction. For example, in the memory condition, they might be asked to describe the main tenets of a major theory of depression. In the analytical condition, they might be asked to compare and contrast two theories of depression. In the creative condition, they might be asked to formulate their own theory of depression. In the practical condition, they might be asked how they could use what they had learned about depression to help a friend who was depressed.

Students in all four instructional conditions were evaluated in terms of their performance on homework, a midterm exam, a final exam, and an independent project. Each type of work was evaluated for memory, analytical, creative, and practical quality. Thus all students were evaluated in exactly the same way. Our results suggested the utility of the theory of successful intelligence. This utility showed itself in several ways.

First, we observed when the students arrived at Yale that the students in the high-creative and high-practical groups were much more diverse in terms of racial, ethnic, socioeconomic, and educational backgrounds than were the students in the high-analytical group, suggesting that correlations of measured intelligence with status variables such as these may be reduced by using a broader conception of intelligence. Thus the kinds of students identified as strong differed in terms of the populations from which they were drawn, in comparison with students identified as strong solely by analytical measures. More importantly, just by expanding the range of abilities measured, we discovered intellectual strengths that might not have been apparent through a conventional test.

Second, we found that all three ability tests—analytical, creative, and practical—significantly predicted course performance. When multiple-regression analysis was used, at least two of these ability measures contributed significantly to the prediction of each of the measures of achievement. In particular, for homework assignments, significant beta weights were obtained for analytical (.25) and creative (.16) ability measures; for the independent project, significant weights were obtained for the analytical (.14), creative (.22), and practical (.14) measures; for the exams, significant weights were obtained for the analytical (.24) and creative (.19) measures (Sternberg et al., 1999). Perhaps as a reflection of the difficulty of deemphasizing the analytical way of teaching, one of the significant predictors was always the analytical score. (However, in a replication of our study with low-income African American students from New York, Deborah Coates of the City University of New York found a different pattern of results. Her data indicated that the practical tests were better predictors of course performance than were the analytical measures, suggesting that which ability test predicts which criterion depends on population as well as mode of teaching.)

Third and most important, there was an aptitude–treatment interaction, whereby students who were placed in instructional conditions that better matched their pattern of abilities outperformed students who were mismatched. In particular, repeated-measures analysis revealed statistically significant effects of match for analytical and creative tasks as a whole. Three of five practical tasks also showed an effect. In other words, when students are taught in a way that fits how they think, they do better in school (see Cronbach & Snow, 1977, for a discussion of the difficulties in eliciting aptitude–treatment interactions). Children who have high levels of creative and practical abilities, but who are almost never taught or assessed in a way that matches their pattern of abilities, may be at a disadvantage in course after course, year after year.

A follow-up study (Sternberg, Torff, & Grigorenko, 1998) examined learning of so-cial studies and science by third graders and eighth graders. The 225 third graders were students in a very low-income neighborhood in Raleigh, North Carolina. The 142 eighth graders were largely middle- to upper-middle-class students studying in Baltimore, Maryland, and Fresno, California; these children were part of a summer program sponsored by the Johns Hopkins University for gifted students. In this study, students were assigned to one of three instructional conditions. Randomization was by classroom. In the first condition, they were taught the course that basically they would have learned had there been no intervention. The emphasis in the course was on memory. In a second condition, students were taught in a way that emphasized critical (analytical) thinking. In the third condition, they were taught in a way that emphasized analytical, creative, and practical thinking. All students' performance was assessed for memory learning (through multiple-choice assessments), as well as for analytical, creative, and practical learning (through performance assessments).

As expected, students in the successful-intelligence (analytical, creative, practical) condition outperformed the other students in terms of the performance assessments. For the third graders, respective means were highest for the triarchic (successful-intelligence) condition, second highest for the critical-thinking condition, and lowest for the memory condition for memory, analytical, and creative performance measures. For practical measures, the critical-thinking mean was insignificantly higher than the triarchic mean, but both were significantly higher than the memory mean. For the eighth graders, the results were similar. One could argue that this pattern of results merely reflected the way students were taught. Nevertheless, the result suggested that teaching for these kinds of thinking succeeded. More important, however, was the result that children in the successful-intelligence condition outperformed the other children even on the multiple-choice memory tests. In other words, to the extent that the goal is just to maximize children's memory for information, teaching for successful intelligence is still superior. It enables children to capitalize on their strengths and to correct or to compensate for their weaknesses, and it allows them to encode material in a variety of interesting ways.

We have now extended these results to reading curricula at the middle school and high school levels (Grigorenko, Jarvin, & Sternberg, 2002). In a study of 871 middle school students and 432 high school students, we taught reading either triarchically or through the regular curriculum. Classrooms were assigned randomly to treatments. At the middle school level, reading was taught explicitly. At the high school level, reading was infused into instruction in mathematics, physical sciences, social sciences, English, history, foreign languages, and the arts. In all settings, students who were taught triarchically substantially outperformed students who were taught in standard ways. Effects were statistically significant at the .001 level for memory–analytical, creative, and practical comparisons.

Thus the results of three sets of studies suggest that the theory of successful intelligence is valid as a whole. Moreover, the results suggest that the theory can make a difference not only in laboratory tests, but in school classrooms and even the everyday life of adults as well. At the same time, the studies have weaknesses that need to be remedied in future studies. The samples are relatively small and not fully representative of the entire U.S. population. Moreover, the studies have examined a limited number of alternative interventions. All interventions were of relatively short duration (up to a semester-long course). In addition, future studies should look at durability and transfer of training.

In sum, the triarchic theory serves as a useful basis for educational interventions and, in our own work, has shown itself to be a basis for interventions that improve students' performance relative to that of controls who do not receive the theory-based instruction.

BEYOND TRADITIONAL THEORIES OF INTELLIGENCE

The triarchic theory consists of three interrelated subtheories that attempt to account for the bases and manifestations of intelligent thought; as such, it represents an expanded view of intelligence that departs from traditional, general, and dichotomous theoretical perspectives. The componential subtheory relates intelligence to the internal world of the individual. The experiential subtheory relates intelligence to the experience of the individual with tasks and situations. The contextual subtheory relates intelligence to the external world of the individual. The elements of the three subtheories are interrelated: The components of intelligence are manifested at different levels of experience with tasks, and in situations of varying degrees of contextual relevance to a person's life. The components of intelligence are posited to be universal to intelligence; thus the components that contribute to intelligent performance in one culture do so in all other cultures as well. Moreover, the importance of dealing with novelty and the automatization of information processing to intelligence are posited to be universal. But the manifestations of these components in experience are posited to be relative to cultural contexts. What constitutes adaptive thought or behavior in one culture is not necessarily adaptive in another culture. Moreover, thoughts and actions that would shape behavior in appropriate ways in one context might not shape them in appropriate ways in another context. Finally, the environment one selects will depend largely on the available environments and on the fit of one's cognitive abilities, motivation, values, and affects to the available alternatives.

ACKNOWLEDGMENTS

Preparation of this chapter was supported by Grant No. REC-9979843 from the National Science Foundation and by government grants under the Javits Act Program (Grant Nos. R206R950001, R206R00001) as administered by the Institute of Educational Sciences (formerly the Office of Educational Research and Improvement), U.S. Department of Education. Grantees undertaking such projects are encouraged to express freely their professional judgment. This chapter therefore does not necessarily represent the positions or the policies of the U.S. government, and no official endorsement should be inferred.

REFERENCES

Ackerman, P. L. (1987). Individual differences in skill learning: An integration of psychometric and information processing perspectives. *Psychological Bulletin, 102,* 3–27.

Brown, A. L. (1978). Knowing when, where, and how to remember: A problem of metacognition. In R. Glaser (Ed.), *Advances in instructional psychology* (Vol. 1, pp. 77–165). Hillsdale, NJ: Erlbaum.

Brown, A. L., Bransford, J., Ferrara, R., & Campione, J. (1983). Learning, remembering, and understanding. In P. H. Mussen (Series Ed.) & J. Flavell & E. Markman (Vol. Eds.), *Handbook of child psychology: Vol. 3. Cognitive development* (4th ed., pp. 77–166). New York: Wiley.

Butterfield, E. C., Wambold, C., & Belmont, J. M. (1973). On the theory and practice of improving short-term memory. *American Journal of Mental Deficiency, 77*, 654–669.

Campione, J. C., & Brown, A. L. (1979). Toward a theory of intelligence: Contributions from research with retarded children. In R. J. Sternberg & D. K. Detterman (Eds.), *Human intelligence: Perspectives on its theory and measurement* (pp. 139–164). Norwood, NJ: Ablex.

Carroll, J. B. (1993). *Human cognitive abilities: A survey of factor-analytic studies.* New York: Cambridge University Press.

Cattell, R. B. (1971). *Abilities: Their structure, growth, and action.* Boston: Houghton Mifflin.

Chase, W. G., & Simon, H. A. (1973). The mind's eye in chess. In W. G. Chase (Ed.), *Visual information processing* (pp. 215–281). New York: Academic Press.

Chi, M. T. H. (1978). Knowledge structure and memory development. In R. S. Siegler (Ed.), *Children's thinking: What develops?* (pp. 73–96). Hillsdale, NJ: Erlbaum.

Cooper, L. A. (1982). Strategies for visual comparison and representation: Individual differences. In R. J. Sternberg (Ed.), *Advances in the psychology of human intelligence* (Vol. 1, pp. 77–124). Hillsdale, NJ: Erlbaum.

Cronbach, L. J., & Snow, R. E. (1977). *Aptitudes and instructional methods.* New York: Irvington.

Davidson, J. E., & Sternberg, R. J. (1984). The role of insight in intellectual giftedness. *Gifted Child Quarterly, 28*, 58–64.

Flavell, J. H. (1977). *Cognitive development.* Englewood Cliffs, NJ: Prentice-Hall.

Gardner, H., Krechevsky, M., Sternberg, R. J., & Okagaki, L. (1994). Intelligence in context: Enhancing students' practical intelligence for school. In K. McGilly (Ed.), *Classroom lessons: Integrating cognitive theory and classroom practice* (pp. 105–127). Cambridge, MA: Bradford Books.

Gelman, R., & Gallistel, C. R. (1978). *The child's understanding of number.* Cambridge, MA: Harvard University Press.

Gladwin, T. (1970). *East is a big bird.* Cambridge, MA: Harvard University Press.

Grigorenko, E. L., Jarvin, L., & Sternberg, R. J. (2002). School-based tests of the triarchic theory of intelligence: Three settings, three samples, three syllabi. *Contemporary Educational Psychology, 27*, 167–208.

Heath, S. B. (1983). *Ways with words: Language, life, and work in communities and classrooms.* New York: Cambridge University Press.

Hunt, E. B. (1978). Mechanics of verbal ability. *Psychological Review, 85*, 109–130.

Hunt, E. B. (1980). Intelligence as an information-processing concept. *British Journal of Psychology, 71*, 449–474.

Hunt, E. B., & Lansman, M. (1982). Individual differences in attention. In R. J. Sternberg (Ed.), *Advances in the psychology of human intelligence* (Vol. 1, pp. 207–254). Hillsdale, NJ: Erlbaum.

Jensen, A. R. (1980). *Bias in mental testing.* New York: Free Press.

Jensen, A. R. (1982). The chronometry of intelligence. In R. J. Sternberg (Ed.), *Advances in the psychology of human intelligence* (Vol. I, pp. 255–310). Hillsdale, NJ: Erlbaum.

Jensen, A. R. (1998). *The g factor.* Westport, CT: Praeger/Greenwood.

Kanfer, R., & Ackerman, P. L. (1989). Dynamics of skill acquisition: Building a bridge between intelligence and motivation. In R. J. Sternberg (Ed.), *Advances in the psychology of human intelligence* (Vol. 5, pp. 83–134). Hillsdale, NJ: Erlbaum.

Kearins, J. M. (1981). Visual spatial memory in Australian Aboriginal children of desert regions. *Cognitive Psychology, 13*, 434–460.

Keil, F. C. (1984). Transition mechanisms in cognitive development and the structure of knowledge. In R. J. Sternberg (Ed.), *Mechanisms of cognitive development* (pp. 81–99). San Francisco: Freeman.

Kosslyn, S. M., & Koenig, O. (1995). *Wet mind: The new cognitive neuroscience.* New York: Free Press.

MacLeod, C. M., Hunt, E. B., & Mathews, N. N. (1978). Individual differences in the verification of sentence–picture relationships. *Journal of Verbal Learning and Verbal Behavior, 17*, 493–507.

Mayer, R. E., & Greeno, J. G. (1972). Structural differences between learning outcomes produces by different instructional methods. *Journal of Educational Psychology, 63*, 165–173.

Milgram, S. (1974). *Obedience to authority.* New York: Harper & Row.

Mulholland, T. M., Pellegrino, J. W., & Glaser, R. (1980). Components of geometric analogy solution. *Cognitive Psychology, 12*, 252–284.

Neisser, U. (1982). *Memory observed.* New York: Freeman.

Newell, A., & Simon, H. A. (1972). *Human problem solving.* Englewood Cliffs, NJ: Prentice-Hall.

Pellegrino, J. W., & Glaser, R. (1979). Cognitive correlates and components in the analysis of individual differences. In R. J. Sternberg & D. K. Detterman (Eds.), *Human intelligence: Perspectives on its theory and measurement* (pp. 61–88). Norwood, NJ: Ablex.

Pellegrino, J. W., & Kail, R. (1982). Process analyses of spatial aptitude. In R. J. Sternberg (Ed.), *Advances in the psychology of human intelligence* (Vol. 1, pp. 311–365). Hillsdale, NJ: Erlbaum.

Raaheim, K. (1974). *Problem solving and intelligence.* Oslo: Universitetsforlaget.

Resnick, L. B., & Glaser, R. (1976). Problem solving and intelligence. In L. B. Resnick (Ed.), *The nature of intelligence* (pp. 205–230). Hillsdale, NJ: Erlbaum.

Schank, R. C. (1980). How much intelligence is there in artificial intelligence? *Intelligence, 4,* 1–14.

Schank, R. C., & Abelson, R. P. (1977). *Scripts, plans, goals, and understanding.* Hillsdale, NJ: Erlbaum.

Siegler, R. S. (1986). Unities across domains in children's strategy choices. In Perlmutter (Ed.), *The Minnesota Symposia on Child Psychology: Vol. 19. Perspectives on intellectual development* (pp. 1–48). Hillsdale, NJ: Erlbaum.

Simon, H. A., & Reed, S. K. (1976). Modeling strategy shifts in a problem solving task. *Cognitive Psychology, 8,* 86–97.

Snow, R. E. (1980). Aptitude processes. In R. E. Snow, P. A. Frederico, & W. E. Montague (Eds.), *Aptitude, learning, and instruction: Cognitive process analyses of aptitude* (Vol. 1, pp. 27–63). Hillsdale, NJ: Erlbaum.

Snow, R. E., Kyllonen, P. C., & Marshalek, B. (1984). The topography of ability and learning correlations. In R. J. Sternberg (Ed.), *Advances in the psychology of human intelligence* (Vol. 2, pp. 47–103). Hillsdale, NJ: Erlbaum.

Snow, R. E., & Lohman, D. F. (1984). Toward a theory of cognitive aptitude for learning from instruction. *Journal of Educational Psychology, 76,* 347–376.

Sternberg, R. J. (1977). *Intelligence, information processing, and analogical reasoning: The componential analysis of human abilities.* Hillsdale, NJ: Erlbaum.

Sternberg, R. J. (1979). The nature of mental abilities. *American Psychologist, 34,* 214–230.

Sternberg, R. J. (1981). Intelligence and nonentrenchment. *Journal of Educational Psychology, 73,* 1–16.

Sternberg, R. J. (1982). Reasoning, problem solving, and intelligence. In R. J. Sternberg (Ed.), *Handbook of human intelligence* (pp. 225–307). New York: Cambridge University Press.

Sternberg, R. J. (1983). Components of human intelligence. *Cognition, 15,* 1–48.

Sternberg, R. J. (1985a). *Beyond IQ: A triarchic theory of human intelligence.* New York: Cambridge University Press.

Sternberg, R. J. (1985b). Implicit theories of intelligence, creativity, and wisdom. *Journal of Personality and Social Psychology, 49,* 607–627.

Sternberg, R. J. (1987). Most vocabulary is learned from context. In M. G. McKeown & M. E. Curtis (Eds.), *The nature of vocabulary acquisition* (pp. 89–105). Hillsdale, NJ: Erlbaum.

Sternberg, R. J. (1988). *The triarchic mind: A new theory of human intelligence.* New York: Viking.

Sternberg, R. J. (1990). *Metaphors of mind.* New York: Cambridge University Press.

Sternberg, R. J. (1993). *Sternberg Triarchic Abilities Test.* Unpublished test.

Sternberg, R. J. (1995). *In search of the human mind.* Orlando, FL: Harcourt Brace.

Sternberg, R. J. (1997). *Successful intelligence.* New York: Plume.

Sternberg, R. J. (1999). The theory of successful intelligence. *Review of General Psychology, 3,* 292–316.

Sternberg, R. J. (Ed.). (2000). *Handbook of intelligence.* New York: Cambridge University Press.

Sternberg, R. J. (2003). Construct validity of the theory of successful intelligence. In R. J. Sternberg, J. Lautrey, & T. I. Lubart (Eds.), *Models of intelligence: International perspectives* (pp. 55–80). Washington, DC: American Psychological Association.

Sternberg, R. J., & Clinkenbeard, P. R. (1995). The triarchic model applied to identifying, teaching, and assessing gifted children. *Roeper Review, 17*(4), 255–260.

Sternberg, R. J., & Davidson, J. E. (1982, June). The mind of the puzzler. *Psychology Today,* pp. 37–44.

Sternberg, R. J., Ferrari, M., Clinkenbeard, P. R., & Grigorenko, E. L. (1996). Identification, instruction, and assessment of gifted children: A construct validation of a triarchic model. *Gifted Child Quarterly, 40,* 129–137.

Sternberg, R. J., Forsythe, G. B., Hedlund, J., Horvath, J., Snook, S, Williams, W. M., et al. (2000). *Practical intelligence in everyday life.* New York: Cambridge University Press.

Sternberg, R. J., & Gardner, M. K. (1982). A componential interpretation of the general factor in human intelligence. In H. J. Eysenck (Ed.), *A model for intelligence* (pp. 231–254). Berlin: Springer-Verlag.

Sternberg, R. J., & Grigorenko, E. L. (Eds.). (2002). *The general factor of intelligence: How general is it?* Mahwah, NJ: Erlbaum.

Sternberg, R. J., Grigorenko, E. L., Ferrari, M., & Clinkenbeard, P. (1999). A triarchic analysis of an aptitude-treatment interaction. *European Journal of Psychological Assessment, 15,* 1–11.

Sternberg, R. J., & Ketron, J. L. (1982). Selection and implementation of strategies in reasoning by analogy. *Journal of Educational Psychology, 74,* 399–413.

Sternberg, R. J., Nokes, K., Geissler, P. W., Prince, R., Okatcha, F., Bundy, D. A., et al. (2001). The relationship between academic and practical intelligence: A case study in Kenya. *Intelligence, 29,* 401–418.

Sternberg, R. J., Okagaki, L., & Jackson, A. (1990). Practical intelligence for success in school. *Educational Leadership, 48,* 35–39.

Sternberg, R. J., & Powell, J. S. (1983). Comprehending verbal comprehension. *American Psychologist, 38,* 878–893.

Sternberg, R. J., & Rifkin, B. (1979). The development of analogical reasoning processes. *Journal of Experimental Child Psychology, 27,* 195–232.

Sternberg, R. J., Torff, B., & Grigorenko, E. L. (1998). Teaching triarchically improves school achievement. *Journal of Educational Psychology, 90,* 374–384.

Sternberg, R. J., & Weil, E. M. (1980). An aptitude–strategy interaction in linear syllogistic reasoning. *Journal of Educational Psychology, 72,* 226–234.

Super, C. M., & Harkness, S. (1982). The infants' niche in rural Kenya and metropolitan America. In L. L. Adler (Ed.), *Cross-cultural research at issue* (pp. 47–55). New York: Academic Press.

Vernon, P. E. (1971). *The structure of human abilities.* London: Methuen.

Vygotsky, L. S. (1978). *Mind in society: The development of higher psychological processes* (M. Cole, V. John-Steiner, S. Scribner, & E. Souberman, Eds. & Trans.). Cambridge, MA: Harvard University Press.

Wagner, R. K., & Sternberg, R. J. (1987). Executive control in reading comprehension. In B. K. Britton & S. M. Glynn (Eds.), *Executive control processes in reading* (pp. 1–21). Hillsdale, NJ: Erlbaum.

Williams, W. M., Blythe, T., White, N., Li, J., Gardner, H., & Sternberg, R. J. (2002). Practical intelligence for school: Developing metacognitive sources of achievement in adolescence. *Developmental Review, 22,* 162–210.

7

Planning, Attention, Simultaneous, Successive (PASS) Theory

A Revision of the Concept of Intelligence

JACK A. NAGLIERI
J. P. DAS

ORIGINS OF THE THEORY

Authors of psychometric approaches to measurement of intelligence have become increasingly theory conscious, realizing the importance of explicitly stating the basis for derivation of the procedures. Without a theory, it is very difficult to evaluate the relevance and information value of the procedure.
—LIDZ (1991, p. 60)

The Planning, Attention, Simultaneous, and Successive (PASS; Naglieri & Das, 1997a) theory is rooted in the work of A. R. Luria (1966, 1973a, 1973b, 1980) on the functional aspects of brain structures. We used Luria's work as a blueprint for defining the important components of human intelligence (Das, Naglieri, & Kirby, 1994). Our efforts represent the first time that a specific researched neuropsychological theory was used to reconceptualize the concept of human intelligence.

Luria theorized that human cognitive functions can be conceptualized within a framework of three separate but related "functional units" that provide four basic psychological processes. The three brain systems are referred to as *functional units* because the neuropsychological mechanisms

work in separate but interrelated systems. Luria (1973b) stated that "each form of conscious activity is always a complex functional system and takes place through the combined working of all three brain units, each of which makes its own contribution" (p. 99). The four processes form a "working constellation" (Luria, 1966, p. 70) of cognitive activity. A child may therefore perform the same task with different contributions of the PASS processes, along with the application of the child's knowledge and skills.

Although effective functioning is accomplished through the integration of all processes as demanded by the particular task, not every process is equally involved in every task. For example, tasks like math calculation may be heavily weighted or dominated by a single process, while tasks such as reading decoding may be strongly related to another process. Effective functioning—for example, processing of visual information—also involve three hierarchical levels of the brain. Consistent with structural topography, these can be described in a simplified manner. First, there is the *projection area*, where the modality characteristic of the information is intact. Above the projection area is the *association area*, where information loses part of its modality tag. Above the association area is the *tertiary area* or *overlapping zone*, where information is amodal. This enables information to be integrated from various senses and processed at a higher level. Thus modality is most important at the level of initial reception, and less important at the level where information is integrated.

Description of the Three Functional Units

The function of the first unit provides regulation of cortical arousal and attention; the second codes information using simultaneous and successive processes; and the third provides for strategy development, strategy use, self-monitoring, and control of cognitive activities.

According to Luria, the first of these three functional units of the brain, the attention–arousal system, is located primarily in the brainstem, the diencephalon, and the medial regions of the cortex (Luria, 1973b). This unit provides the brain with the appropriate level of arousal or cortical tone, as well as directive and selective attention (Luria, 1973b). When a multidimensional stimulus array is presented to a person who is then required to pay attention to only one dimension, the inhibition of responding to other (often more salient) stimuli, and the allocation of attention to the central dimension, depend on the resources of the first functional unit. Luria stated that optimal conditions of arousal are needed before the more complex forms of attention, involving "selective recognition of a particular stimulus and inhibition of responses to irrelevant stimuli" (1973b, p. 271), can occur. Moreover, only when individuals are sufficiently aroused and their attention is adequately focused can they utilize processes in the second and third functional units.

The second functional unit is associated with the occipital, parietal, and temporal lobes posterior to the central sulcus of the brain. This unit is responsible for receiving, processing, and retaining information the person obtains from the external world. This unit involves simultaneous processing and successive processes. Simultaneous processing involves integrating stimuli into groups so that the interrelationships among the components are understood. For example, in

order to produce a diagram correctly when given the instruction "Draw a triangle above a square that is to the left of a circle under a cross," the relationships among the different shapes must be correctly comprehended. Whereas simultaneous processing involves working with stimuli that are interrelated, successive processing involves information that is linearly organized and integrated into a chain-like progression. For example, successive processing is involved in the decoding of unfamiliar words, production of syntactic aspects of language, and speech articulation. Following a sequence such as the order of operations in a math problem is another example of successive processing. In contrast, simultaneous processing involves integration of separate elements into groups.

The third functional unit is associated with the prefrontal areas of the frontal lobes of the brain (Luria, 1980). Luria stated that "the frontal lobes synthesize the information about the outside world . . . and are the means whereby the behavior of the organism is regulated in conformity with the effect produced by its actions" (1980, p. 263). This unit provides for the programming, regulation, and verification of behavior, and is responsible for behaviors such as asking questions, solving problems, and self-monitoring (Luria, 1973b). Other responsibilities of the third functional unit include the regulation of voluntary activity, conscious impulse control, and various linguistic skills such as spontaneous conversation. The third functional unit provides for the most complex aspects of human behavior, including personality and consciousness (Das, 1980).

Functional Units: Influences and Issues

Luria's organization of the brain into functional units accounts for cultural influences on higher cognition as well as biological factors. He stated that "perception and memorizing, gnosis and praxis, speech and thinking, writing, reading and arithmetic, cannot be regarded as isolated or even indivisible 'faculties' " (Luria, 1973b, p. 29). That is, we cannot, as phrenologists attempted to do, identify a "writing" spot in the brain; instead, we must consider the concept of units of the brain that provide a function. Luria (1973b) described the advantage of this approach:

It is accordingly our fundamental task not to "localize" higher human psychological processes in limited areas of the cortex, but to ascertain by careful analysis which groups of concertedly working zones of the brain are responsible for the performance of complex mental activity; when contributions made by each of these zones to the complex functional system; and how the relationship between these concertedly working parts of the brain in the performance of complex mental activity changes in the various stages of its development. (p. 34)

Activities such as reading and writing can be analyzed and linked as constellations of activities to specific working zones of the brain that support them (Luria, 1979, p. 141). Because the brain operates as an integrated functional system, however, even a small disturbance in an area can cause disorganization in the entire functional system (Das & Varnhagen, 1986).

Luria's concept of dynamic functional units provides the foundation for PASS processes. These basic psychological processes are firmly based on biological correlates, yet develop within a sociocultural milieu. In other words, they are influenced in part by the cultural experiences of the child. Luria (1979) noted that "the child learns to organize his memory and to bring it under voluntary control through the use of the mental tools of his culture" (p. 83). More recently, Kolb, Gibb, and Robinson (2003) have also noted that although "the brain was once seen as a rather static organ, it is now clear that the organization of brain circuitry is constantly changing as a function of experience" (p. 1). Similarly, Stuss and Benson (1990) recognize this interplay and especially the use of speech as a regulatory function when they state:

The adult regulates the child's behavior by command, inhibiting irrelevant responses. His child learns to speak, the spoken instruction shared between the child and adult are taken over by the child, who uses externally stated and often detailed instructions to guide his or her own behavior. By the age of 4 to 4½, a trend towards internal and contract speech (inner speech) gradually appears. The child begins to regulate and subordinate his behavior according to his speech. Speech, in addition to serving communication thought, becomes a major self-regulatory force, creating systems of

connections for organizing active behavior inhibiting actions irrelevant to the task at hand. (p. 34)

Luria stressed the role of the frontal lobes in language, organization, and direction of behavior and speech as a cultural tool that furthers the development of the frontal lobes and self-regulation. Cultural experiences thus actually help to accelerate the utilization of planning and self-regulation, as well as the other cognitive processes.

Luria (1979) also points out that abstraction and generalizations are themselves products of the cultural environment. Children learn, for example, to attend selectively to relevant objects through playful experiences and conversations with adults. Even simultaneous and successive processes are influenced by cultural experiences (e.g., learning songs, poems, rules of games, etc.). Naglieri (2003) has summarized the influence of social interaction on children's use of plans and strategies, and the resulting changes in performance on classroom tasks. This will be further discussed in a later section of this chapter, and by Naglieri in Chapter 20 of this volume.

The relationship between the third and first functional units is particularly strong. The first functional unit works in cooperation with, and is regulated by, higher systems of the cerebral cortex, which receive and process information from the external world and determine an individual's dynamic activity (Luria, 1973b). In other words, this unit has a reciprocal relationship with the cortex. It influences the tone of the cortex and is itself influenced by the regulatory effects of the cortex. This is possible through the ascending and descending systems of the reticular formation, which transmit impulses from lower parts of the brain to the cortex and vice versa (Luria, 1973b). For the PASS theory, this means that attention and planning are necessarily strongly related, because attention is often under the conscious control of planning. That is, our planning of behavior dictates the allocation of our limited attentional resources.

Three Functional Units and PASS Theory

Luria's concept of the three functional units used as the basis of the PASS theory is diagrammatically shown in Figure 7.1. Although rendering a complex functional system in two-dimensional space has its limitations, the diagram illustrates some of the important characteristics of the PASS theory. First, an important component of the theory is the role of a person's fund of information. Knowledge base is a part of each of the processes, because past experiences, learning, emotions, and motivations provide the background as well as the sources for the information to be processed. This information is received from external sources through their sense organs. When that sensory information is sent to the brain for analysis, central processes become active. However, internal cognitive information in the form of images, memory, and thoughts becomes part of the input as well. Thus the four processes operate within the context of an individual's

knowledge base and cannot operate outside the context of knowledge. "Cognitive processes rely on (and influence) the base of knowledge, which may be temporary (as in immediate memory) or more long term (that is, knowledge that is well learned)" (Naglieri & Das, 1997c, p. 145). Cognitive processing also influences knowledge acquisition, and learning can influence cognitive processing. Both are also influenced by membership in particular social and cultural milieus (Das & Abbott, 1995, p. 158). The importance of knowledge is therefore integral to the PASS theory. A person may read English very well and have good PASS processes, but may falter when required to read Japanese text—due to a deficient knowledge of Japanese, rather than a processing deficit.

Planning is a frontal lobe function. More specifically, it is associated with the pre-

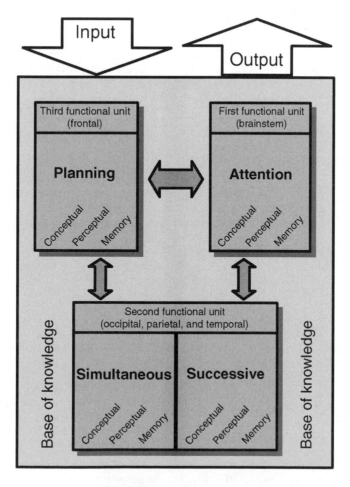

FIGURE 7.1. PASS theory.

frontal cortex and is one of the main abilities that distinguishes humans from other primates. The prefrontal cortex

> plays a central role in forming goals and objectives and then in devising plans of action required to attain these goals. It selects the cognitive skills required to implement the plans, coordinates these skills, and applies them in a correct order. Finally, the prefrontal cortex is responsible for evaluating our actions as success or failure relative to our intentions. (Goldberg, 2001, p. 24)

Planning therefore helps us select or develop the plans or strategies needed to complete tasks for which a solution is needed, and is critical to all activities where a child or adult has to determine how to solve a problem. It includes generation, evaluation, and execution of a plan, as well as self-monitoring and impulse control. Thus planning allows for the solution of problems; the control of attention, simultaneous, and successive processes; and selective utilization of knowledge and skills (Das, Kar, & Parrila, 1996).

Attention is a mental process that is closely related to the orienting response. The base of the brain allows the organism to direct focused selective attention toward a stimulus over time and to resist loss of attention to other stimuli. The longer attention is required, the more the activity is one that demands vigilance. Attention is controlled by intentions and goals, and involves knowledge and skills as well as the other PASS processes.

Simultaneous processing is essential for organization of information into groups or a coherent whole. The parietal, occipital, and temporal brain regions provide a critical "ability" to see patterns as interrelated elements. Because of the strong spatial characteristics of most simultaneous tasks, there is a strong visual–spatial dimension to activities that demand this type of processing. Simultaneous processing, however, is not limited to nonverbal content, as illustrated by the important role it plays in the grammatical components of language and comprehension of word relationships, prepositions, and inflections.

Successive processing is involved in the use of stimuli arranged in a specific serial order. Whenever information must be remembered or completed in a specific order, successive processing will be involved. Importantly, however, the information must not be able to be organized into a pattern (e.g., the number 9933811 organized into 99-33-8-11); instead, each element can only be related to those that precede it. Successive processing is usually involved with the serial organization of sounds and movements in order. It is therefore integral to, for example, working with sounds in sequence and early reading.

The PASS theory is an alternative to approaches to intelligence that have traditionally included verbal, nonverbal, and quantitative tests. Not only does this theory expand the view of what "abilities" should be measured, but it also puts emphasis on basic psychological processes and precludes the use of verbal achievement-like tests such as vocabulary. In addition, the PASS theory is an alternative to the anachronistic notion of a general intelligence. Instead, the functions of the brain are considered the building blocks of ability conceptualized within a cognitive processing framework. Although the theory may have its roots in neuropsychology, "its branches are spread over developmental and educational psychology" (Das & Varnhagen, 1986, p. 130). Thus the PASS theory of cognitive processing, with its links to developmental and neuropsychology, provides an advantage in explanatory power over the notion of general intelligence (Naglieri & Das, 2002).

OPERATIONALIZATION AND APPLICATION OF THE THEORY

The PASS theory is operationalized by the Cognitive Assessment System (CAS; Naglieri & Das, 1997a). This instrument is amply described in the CAS Interpretive Handbook (Naglieri & Das, 1997b) and by Naglieri in Chapter 20 of this book. We (Naglieri & Das, 1997a) generated tests to measure the PASS theory, following a systematic and empirically based test development program designed to obtain efficient measures of the processes that could be individually administered. The PASS theory was used as the foundation of the CAS, so the content of the test was determined by the theory and not influenced by previous views of ability. This is further elaborated in Chapter 20 of this book.

EMPIRICAL SUPPORT
FOR THE THEORY

Dillon (1986) suggested six criteria (validity, diagnosis, prescription, comparability, replicability/standardizability, and psychodiagnostic utility) for evaluation of a theory of cognitive processing. Naglieri (1989) evaluated the PASS model on these criteria, using the information available at that time; in this chapter, we use the same criteria to evaluate the current status of the PASS theory as operationalized by the CAS. This section includes summaries of research due to space limitations, but additional information is provided in Chapter 20 of this text and in other resources (Naglieri, 1999, 2003; Naglieri & Das, 1997b).

Validity

The fundamental validity of the PASS theory is rooted in the neuropsychological work of Luria (1966, 1973a, 1973b, 1980, 1982), who associated areas of the brain with basic psychological processes as described earlier in this chapter. Luria's research was based on an extensive combination of his and other researchers' understanding of brain functions, amply documented in his book *The Working Brain* (1973b). Using Luria's three functional units as a backdrop, Das and colleagues (Das, 1972; Das, Kirby, & Jarman, 1975, 1979; Das, Naglieri, & Kirby, 1994) initiated the task of finding ways to measure the PASS processes. These efforts included extensive analysis of the methods used by Luria, related procedures used within neuropsychology, experimental research in cognitive and educational psychology, and related areas. This work, subsequently summarized in several books (e.g., Das, Naglieri, & Kirby, 1994; Kirby, 1984; Kirby & Williams, 1991; Naglieri, 1999; Naglieri & Das, 1997b), demonstrated that the PASS processes associated with Luria's concept of the three functional units could be measured. This work also illustrated that the theoretical conceptualization of basic psychological processes had considerable potential for application.

Initial studies of the validity of the PASS theory included basic and essential elements for a test of children's cognitive competence, such as developmental changes. Researchers found that performance on early versions of tests of these processes showed evidence of developmental differences by age for children of elementary and middle school ages (Das, 1972; Das & Molloy, 1975; Garofalo, 1986; Jarman & Das, 1977; Kirby & Das, 1978; Kirby & Robinson, 1987; Naglieri & Das, 1988, 1997b) and for high school and college samples (Ashman, 1982; Das & Heemsbergen, 1983; Naglieri & Das, 1988).

We and our colleagues have also demonstrated that the constructs represented in the PASS theory are strongly related to achievement. A full discussion of those results is provided by Naglieri in Chapter 20 of this book. The results demonstrate that the PASS constructs are strongly related to achievement, and the evidence thus far suggests that the theory is more strongly related to achievement than are other measures of ability. Importantly, despite the fact that the measures of PASS processes do not include achievement-like subtests (e.g., vocabulary and arithmetic), the evidence demonstrates the utility of the PASS theory as operationalized by the CAS for predication of academic performance. Because one purpose of the CAS is to anticipate levels of academic performance on the basis of levels of cognitive functioning, these results provide critical support for the theory.

Diagnosis

There are two important aims of diagnosis: first, to determine whether variations in characteristics help distinguish one group of children from another; and second, to determine whether these data help with prescriptive decisions. Prescription is discussed in the next section; the question of diagnosis is addressed here. One way to examine the utility of PASS cognitive profiles is by analysis of the frequency of PASS cognitive weaknesses for children in regular and special educational settings. Naglieri (2000) has conducted such a study. A second way to examine diagnostic utility is by examination of specific populations (e.g., children with attention-deficit/hyperactivity disorder [ADHD] or learning disabilities). Both of these topics are summarized here; we begin with a discussion of PASS profiles in general, and then take a look at two particular groups of special children.

PASS Profiles

Glutting, McDermott, Konold, Snelbaker, and Watkins (1998) have suggested that research concerning profiles for specific children is typically confounded, because the "use of subtest profiles for both the initial formation of diagnostic groups and the subsequent search for profiles that might inherently define or distinguish those groups" (p. 601) results in methodological problems. They further suggested that researchers should "begin with unselected cohorts (i.e., representative samples, a proportion of which may be receiving special education), identify children with and without unusual subtest profiles, and subsequently compare their performance on external criteria" (p. 601). Naglieri (2000) followed this research methodology, using the PASS theory and his (Naglieri, 1999) concepts of *relative weakness* and *cognitive weakness*.

Naglieri (1999) described how to find disorders in one or more of the basic PASS processes as follows. A *relative weakness* is a significant weakness in relation to the child's mean PASS score determined using the ipsative methodology originally proposed by Davis (1956) and modified by Silverstein (1982, 1993). A problem with the approach is that a child may have a significant weakness that falls within the average range if the majority of scores are above average. In contrast, a *cognitive weakness* is found when a child has a significant intraindividual difference on the PASS scale scores of the CAS (according to the ipsative method), and the lowest score *also* falls below some cutoff designed to indicate what is typical or average. The difference between a relative weakness and a cognitive weakness, therefore, is that the determination of a cognitive weakness is based on dual criteria (a low score relative to the child's mean and a low score relative to the norm group). Naglieri further suggested that a cognitive weakness should be accompanied by an achievement test weakness comparable to the level of the PASS scale cognitive weakness. Children who have both a cognitive and an achievement test weakness should be considered candidates for special educational services if other appropriate conditions are also met (especially that the children's academic needs cannot be met in the regular educational environment).

Naglieri (2000) found that the relative-weakness method (the approach more commonly used in school psychology) identified children who earned average scores on the CAS as well as on achievement, and that approximately equal percentages of children from regular and special education classes had a relative weakness. Thus the concept of relative weakness did not identify children who achieved differently from children in regular education. By contrast, children with a cognitive weakness earned lower scores on achievement, and the more pronounced the cognitive weakness, the lower the achievement scores. Third, children with a PASS scale cognitive weakness were more likely to have been previously identified and placed in special education. Finally, the presence of a cognitive weakness was significantly related to achievement, whereas the presence of a relative weakness was not.

The findings for relative weakness partially support previous authors' arguments against the use of profile analysis for tests like the Wechsler (see Glutting et al., 1998, for a summary). The results for cognitive weakness support the PASS-theory-driven approach that includes the dual criteria of a significant profile with below-normal performance (Naglieri, 1999). The approach is also different from the subtest analysis approach, because the method uses the PASS theory-based-scales included in the CAS, rather than the traditional approach of analyzing a pattern of specific subtests. Finally, the approach is different because the focus is on cognitive, rather than relative, weaknesses (Naglieri, 1999).

Naglieri's (2000) findings support the view that PASS theory can be used to identify children with cognitive and related academic difficulties for the purpose of eligibility determination and, by extension, instructional planning. Naglieri (2003) and Naglieri and Pickering (2003) provide theoretical and practical guidelines about how a child's PASS-based cognitive weakness and accompanying academic weakness might meet criteria for special educational programming. If a child has a cognitive weakness on one of the four PASS constructs and comparable scores in reading and spelling, along with other appropriate data, the child may qualify for specific learning disability (SLD) services. The example presented in Figure 7.2 illustrates how this theory could be used to identify a child as having an SLD. The 1997 amendments to the Individuals with Disabilities Education Act define an SLD as "a disorder in one or more of the basic psychological processes [PASS processes are clearly consistent with this language] involved in understanding or in using language, spoken or written, that may manifest itself in an imperfect ability to listen, think, read, write, spell, or to do mathematical calculations" (p. 27). In the hypothetical case described here, there is a disorder in successive processing that is involved in the child's academic failure in reading and spelling. Assuming that the difficulty with successive processing has made attempts to teach the child ineffective, some type of special educational program may be appropriate.

The PASS theory provides a workable framework for determination of a disorder in basic psychological processes that can be integrated with academic performance and all other relevant information to help make a

diagnosis. Of course, the determination of an SLD or any other disorder is not made solely on the basis of PASS constructs, but these play an important role in the identification process. The connections between PASS and academic instruction (discussed elsewhere in this chapter and in Chapter 20) have also led researchers to begin an examination of the diagnostic potential of PASS profiles.

It is important to note that emphasis is placed at the PASS theoretical level rather than the specific subtest level. Subtests are simply varying ways of measuring each of the four processes, and by themselves have less reliability than the composite scale score that represents each of the PASS processes. It is also important to recognize that profile analysis of the PASS constructs should not be made in isolation or without vital information about a child's academic performance. The procedure described here illustrates that PASS profile analysis must include achievement variation, which allows differential di-

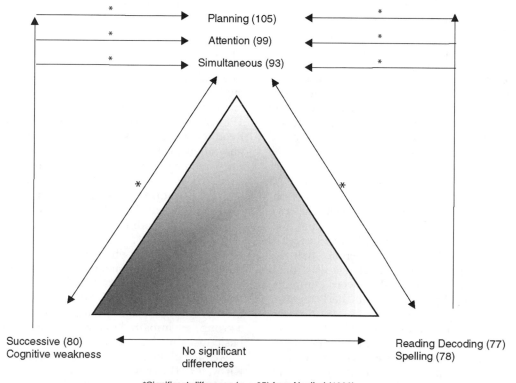

*Significant difference ($p < .05$) from Naglieri (1999).

FIGURE 7.2. Illustration of using the PASS theory (and scores on the CAS scales derived from this theory) to identify a child as having a basic psychological processing disorder model.

agnosis based upon a configuration of variables across tests rather than simply within one test. Thus a child with a written language disorder could have a cognitive weakness in planning, with similarly poor performance on tests that measure skills in writing a story (Johnson, Bardos, & Tayedi, 2003). In contrast, a child with an attention deficit may have a cognitive weakness in planning, along with behavioral disorganization, impulsivity, and general loss of regulation. Planning weaknesses may be seen in both children, but the larger context of their problems is different.

Children with ADHD

In contrast to an attention deficit, a planning deficit is hypothesized to be the distinguishing mark of ADHD within the constraints of PASS theory. A recent study by Naglieri, Goldstein, Iseman, and Schwebach (2003) is exemplary. The part of the study that is relevant here concerns the comparison between children with ADHD and the normative groups on two tests, the CAS and the Wechsler Intelligence Scale for Children—Third Edition (WISC-III). The purpose was to examine the assumption that the PASS theory and its derivative test, the CAS, may be particularly sensitive to the cognitive difficulties of children with ADHD, whereas a general intelligence test (the WISC-III) is inadequate for diagnosis of ADHD. Specifically, a low CAS Planning mean score was expected for the sample with ADHD. The results showed a large effect size for Planning between the children with ADHD and the standardization sample. However, in regard to the CAS Attention scale, a small effect size was observed. The differences between the two samples on the CAS Simultaneous and Successive scales were not significant. In regard to the WISC-III, the only difference that had a significant but small effect size was found when children with ADHD were compared to the normative samples on the Processing Speed Index.

Naglieri, Salter, and Edwards (2004) confirm the weakness of planning, but not attention, among children with ADHD in a recent report. Participants in the study were 48 children (38 males and 10 females) referred to an ADHD clinic. The contrast group consisted of 48 children (38 males and 10 females) in regular education. The results indicated that the children in regular education settings earned mean PASS scale scores on the CAS that were all above average, ranging from 98.6 to 103.6. In contrast, the experimental group earned mean scores close to the norm on the CAS Attention, Simultaneous, and Successive scales (ranging from 97.4 to 104.0), but a significantly lower mean score on the Planning scale (90.3).

The low mean Planning score for the children with ADHD in this study is consistent with the poor Planning performance reported in the previous study (Naglieri et al., 2003), as well as with previous research (Dehn, 2000; Paolitto, 1999) for children identified as having ADHD of the hyperactive–impulsive or combined types (Barkley, 1997). The consistency across these various studies suggests that some of these children have difficulty with planning rather than attentional processing as measured by the CAS. This finding is consistent with Barkley's (1997) view that ADHD is a failure of self-control (e.g., planning in the PASS theory) rather than a failure of attention. The PASS profiles of these groups have been different from those with reading failure and anxiety disorders (Naglieri et al., 2003).

Children with Reading Disability

The inability to engage in phonological coding has been suggested as the major cause of reading disability for children (Stanovich, 1988; Wagner, Torgesen, & Rashotte, 1994). Reading researchers generally agree that phonological skills play an important role in early reading. One of the most frequently cited articles in the field, by Torgesen, Wagner, and Rashotte (1994), argues that phonological skills are causally related to normal acquisition of reading skills. Support for this claim can also be found in the relationship between prereaders' phonological scores and their reading development 1–3 years later (e.g., Bradley & Bryant, 1985). A review by Share and Stanovich (1995) concluded that there is strong evidence that poor readers, as a group, are impaired in a very wide range of basic tasks in the phonological domain.

We have suggested (Das, Naglieri, & Kirby, 1994) that underlying a phonological skills deficit is a specific cognitive processing deficit that is involved in word-reading deficits. For example, successive processing can unite the various core correlates of word decoding; its binding strength increases if the word is a pseudoword, and further if it is to be read aloud, requiring pronunciation. The correlates are speech rate (fast repetition of three simple words), naming time (for naming simple short and familiar words arranged in rows, naming rows of single letters, or digits and color strips), and short-term memory for short lists of simple and short words. Of these tasks, speech rate correlates best with decoding pseudowords. Although the correlation with naming time is the next best one, it has, however, a slight edge over speech rate in decoding short familiar words (Das, Mishra, & Kirby, 1994). Thus in a discriminant-function analysis of normal readers versus children with dyslexia, it was shown that a test of strictly phonemic coding, such as phonemic separation, led to approximately 63% of correct classification, whereas two tests that involve articulation and very little phonemic coding (Speech Rate and Word Series, both Successive subtests in the CAS) contributed nearly 72% to correct classification. In other words, the discriminant-function analysis showed that the two subtests, Speech Rate and Word Series, were better at distinguishing normal readers from children with dyslexia than a direct test of phonemic segmentation was. Several studies on the relationship between PASS and reading disability have since supported the hypothesis that in predicting reading disability, distal processes (such as the PASS processes) are as important as proximal ones (such as phonological awareness and other tests of phonological coding) (Das, Parrila, & Papadopoulos, 2000).

Word reading and comprehension are two relatively separate skills. If some aspects of word-reading or decoding disability can be predicted by successive processing, disability in comprehension has been shown to be primarily related to deficits in simultaneous processing (Das, Kar, & Parrila, 1996; Das, Naglieri, & Kirby, 1994; Naglieri & Das, 1997c), as well as (to a relatively lesser extent) in successive processing and planning.

In concluding this section on the uses of PASS theory, we have presented some samples of empirical studies on all four processes that help in understanding the role of attention in attention deficits, planning in ADHD, and finally successive and simultaneous processing in reading disabilities. Moreover,

PASS theory has had several applications in areas of contemporary concern in education relating to diagnosis and placement, as Naglieri (1999) has discussed. Because of space limitations in this chapter, we cannot present them here. However, Chapter 20 of this book includes this discussion.

The research on PASS profiles has suggested that different homogeneous groups have distinctive weaknesses. Children with reading disabilities perform adequately on all PASS constructs except successive processing. This is consistent with Das's view (see Das, 2001; Das, Naglieri, & Kirby, 1994) that reading failure is the results of a deficit in sequencing of information (successive processing). Those with the combined type of ADHD perform poorly in planning (they lack cognitive control), but adequately on the remaining PASS constructs (Dehn, 2000; Naglieri et al., 2003; Paolitto, 1999). Children with the inattentive type of ADHD have adequate PASS scores except on attention (Naglieri & Pickering, 2003). Finally, Naglieri and colleagues (2003) found that children with anxiety disorders had a different PASS profile from those with ADHD. These findings suggest that the PASS theory and associated scores may have utility for differential diagnosis and, by extension, for instructional planning. Moreover, these findings provide some support for the diagnostic validity of the PASS theory.

Prescription

Dillon (1986) argued that the extent to which a theory of cognitive processing informs the user about interventions is an important dimension of validity. The PASS theory appears to have an advantage in this regard.

There are at least four main resources for applying the PASS theory to academic remediation and instruction, which we discuss briefly. The first is the PASS Remedial Program (PREP), developed by Das; the second is the Planning Facilitation Method, described by Naglieri; the third is Kirby and Williams's 1991 book *Learning Problems: A Cognitive Approach*; and the fourth is Naglieri and Pickering's (2003) book *Helping Children Learn: Intervention Handouts for Use in School and at Home*. The first two methods are based on empirical studies and discussed at length by Das

(2001), Das, Mishra, and Pool (1995), Das and colleagues (2000), and Naglieri (2003). The two books contain several reasonable approaches to academic interventions. The instructional methods use structured and directed instructions (PREP) as well as minimally structured instructions (Planning Facilitation). The books vary from very applied (Naglieri & Pickering, 2003) to more general (Kirby & Williams, 1991). In this chapter, the concepts behind the first two methods are more fully described in the sections that follow.

Description of the PREP

The PREP was developed as a cognitively based remedial program based on the PASS theory of cognitive functioning (Das, Naglieri, & Kirby, 1994). It aims at improving the processing strategies—specifically, simultaneous and successive processing—that underlie reading, while at the same time avoiding the direct teaching of word-reading skills such as phoneme segmentation or blending. PREP is also founded on the premise that the transfer of principles is best facilitated through inductive, rather than deductive, inference (see Das, 2001, for details). The program is accordingly structured so that tacitly acquired strategies are likely to be used in appropriate ways.

PREP was originally designed to be used with students in grades 2 and 3. Each of the 10 tasks involves both a global training component and a curriculum-related bridging component. The global components, which require the application of simultaneous or successive strategies, include structured non-reading tasks. These tasks also facilitate transfer by providing the opportunity for children to internalize strategies in their own way (Das et al., 1995). The bridging components involve the same cognitive demands as their matched global components—that is, simultaneous and successive processing. These cognitive processes have been closely linked to reading and spelling (Das, Naglieri, & Kirby, 1994).

Das and colleagues (1995) studied 51 grade 3 and grade 4 students with reading disabilities who exhibited delays of at least 12 months on either the Word Identification or Word Attack subtest of the Woodcock Reading Mastery Tests—Revised (WRMT-R). Participants were first divided into two groups: a PREP remediation group and a no-intervention control group. The PREP group received 15 sessions of training, involving groups of two students apiece, over a period of 2½ months. Children in the control group participated in regular classroom activities. After the intervention, both groups were tested again with the WRMT-R Word Identification and Word Attack subtests. The results indicated that although both groups gained during the intervention period, the PREP group gained significantly more on both Word Identification and Word Attack.

Carlson and Das (1997) report on two studies using a small-group version of the PREP for underachieving grade 4 students in Chapter 1 programs. In the first study, the experimental group received 15 hours of "add-on" training with PREP over an 8-week period. Both the PREP and control groups (22 and 15 students, respectively) continued to participate in the regular Chapter 1 program. The Word Attack and Word Identification subtests of the WRMT-R were administered at the beginning and the end of the study. The results showed significant improvement following training in PREP, as well as significant group × time interaction effects. The second study essentially replicated these results with a larger sample of grade 4 students. Since then, several other replication studies completed in the same school district have essentially reproduced the original results with children from grades 3, 4, 5, and 6, and with both bilingual (Spanish- and English-speaking) and monolingual (English-speaking only) children.

The effectiveness of a modified version of PREP (for an older group) was studied by Boden and Kirby (1995). A group of fifth- and sixth-grade students who were identified a year earlier as poor readers were randomly assigned to either a control or an experimental group. The control group received regular classroom instruction, and the experimental group received PREP in groups of four students for approximately 14 hours. As in previous studies, the results showed differences between the control and PREP groups on the WRMT-R Word Identification and Word Attack subtests after treatment. In relation to the previous year's reading scores, the PREP group performed significantly better than the control group.

Finally, the study by Parrila, Das, Kendrick, Papadopoulos, and Kirby (1999) was an extension of the above-described experiments, but with three important changes: (1) The control condition was a competing program given to a carefully matched group of children; (2) the participants were beginning readers in grade 1, and therefore younger than the grade 3 to grade 6 participants in the previous studies (8 of the 10 original PREP tasks were selected and modified for the grade 1 level); and (3) the training was shorter in duration than in most of the previous studies. The more stringent control condition was seen as an important test of the efficacy of PREP. The study attempted to demonstrate the efficacy of PREP by showing the advantage of PREP over the meaning-based reading program received by the control group.

Fifty-eight grade 1 children experiencing reading difficulties were divided into two matched remediation groups, one receiving the modified version of PREP and the other receiving the meaning-based program. Results showed a significant improvement of reading (WRMT-R Word Identification and Word Attack) for the PREP group, the gain in reading was greater than it was for the meaning-based training group. The relevance of the children's CAS profile was demonstrated as follows: Further results indicated that the high gainers in the PREP group were those with higher CAS Successive scores at the beginning of the program. In contrast, the high gainers in the meaning-based program were characterized by higher CAS Planning scores.

Taken together, the studies described here make a clear case for the effectiveness of PREP in remediating deficient reading skills during the elementary school years. These findings are further examined in Chapter 20 of this book.

Essentials of Planning Facilitation

The effectiveness of teaching children to be more strategic when completing in-class math calculation problems is well illustrated by research that has examined the relationship between strategy instruction and CAS Planning scores. Four studies have focused on planning and math calculation (Hald, 1999; Naglieri & Gottling, 1995, 1997; Naglieri & Johnson, 2000). The methods used by these researchers were based on similar research by Cormier, Carlson, and Das (1990) and Kar, Dash, Das, and Carlson (1992). The researchers utilized methods designed to stimulate children's use of planning, which in turn had positive effects on problem solving on nonacademic as well as academic tasks. The method was based on the assumption that planning processes should be facilitated rather than directly taught, so that the children would discover the value of strategy use without being specifically told to do so.

The Planning Facilitation Method has been applied with individuals (Naglieri & Gottling, 1995) and groups of children (Naglieri & Gottling, 1997; Naglieri & Johnson, 2000). Students completed mathematics worksheets that were developed according to the math curriculum in a series of baseline and intervention sessions over a 2-month period. During baseline and intervention phases, three-part sessions consisted of 10 minutes of math, followed by 10 minutes of discussion, followed by a further 10 minutes of math. During the baseline phase, discussion was irrelevant to the mathematics problems; in the intervention phase, however, a group discussion designed to encourage self-reflection was facilitated, so that the children would understand the need to plan and use efficient strategies.

The teachers provided questions or observations that facilitated discussion and encouraged the children to consider various ways to be more successful. Such questions included "How did you do the math?", "What could you do to get more correct?", or "What will you do next time?" The teachers made no direct statements such as "That is correct," or "Remember to use that same strategy." Teachers also did not provide feedback about the accuracy of previous math work completed, and they did not give mathematics instruction. The role of the teachers was to facilitate self-reflection and encourage the children to complete the worksheets in a planful manner. The positive effects of this intervention have been consistent across the research studies, as presented in Chapter 20 of this book.

Comparability

The extent to which cognitive processing constructs have relevance to some target task is an important criterion of validity for a theory, and one that is relevant to evaluation of the PASS theory. One example of the comparability of PASS and classroom performance can be found in the examination of the relationships between the attention portion of the theory and in-class behaviors of children.

Attention Tests and Teachers' Ratings of Attention

A good example of the comparability of PASS is the relationship between the constructs and classroom performance. Earlier in this chapter, we have discussed the relationship between PASS and academic achievement scores. In this section we look at one particular issue: the relationship between attention measures and ratings of attention in the classroom. This is an environment where a child must selectively attend to some stimuli and ignores others. The selectivity aspect relates to intentional discrimination between stimuli. Ignoring irrelevant stimuli implies that the child is resisting distraction. In terms of the PASS theory, this means that attention involves at least three essential dimensions, which are selection, shifting, and resistance to distraction. One way to examine the comparability of the PASS theory to classroom attention is therefore to look at the relationships between measures of attention and attending in the classroom.

Das, Snyder, and Mishra (1992) examined the relationship between teachers' rating of children's attentional behavior in the classroom and those children's performances on the CAS subtests of Expressive Attention and Receptive Attention. An additional test, Selective Auditory Attention, was included in this study; this test was taken from an earlier version of the CAS (Naglieri & Das, 1988). All three of these tasks had been shown to form a separate factor identified as Attention, which is independent of the three other PASS processes (Das et al., 1992).

Teachers' ratings of students' attention status in class were made with Das's Attention Checklist (ACL). This is a checklist containing 12 items that rate the degree to which attentional behavior is shown by a child. All the items on this checklist load on one factor that accounts for more than 70% of the variance, and the ACL has high reliability (alpha of .94; Das & Melnyk, 1989). In addition to the CAS and ACL, the children were given

the Conners 28-item rating scale. Das and colleagues (1992) found that the ACL and Conners Inattention/Passivity items were strongly correlated ($r = .86$), but that the correlation between the ACL and the Conners Hyperactivity scale was substantially lower ($r = .54$). This is logical, because the ACL is more a measure of inattention than of hyperactivity.

The correlations of ACL and the Attention subtest scores suggested that classroom behaviors and performance on measures of cognitive processing were related. The ACL correlated significantly ($p < .01$) with Expressive Attention ($r = .46$) and the Selective Auditory Attention false-detection score ($r = .37$). All other correlations with the ACL were not significant. The relationship between the ACL and children's performance on the CAS was further examined via factor analysis. Two factors were obtained: One had high loadings on the CAS Attention subtest scores (Receptive Attention and a smaller loading on Expressive Attention) and the omission score on the Selective Auditory Attention task, whereas the other factor had high loadings on the ACL, the commission errors on the Selective Auditory Attention task (which reflects distractibility), and the Expressive Attention task. Thus it was clear that the ACL, which measures teachers' ratings of attention in the classroom, was associated with performance on objective tasks that require resistance to distraction. Their common link is most probably failure of inhibition of attention to distractors. This was further supported in subsequent studies (Das, 2002). Therefore we suggest that attention as defined by the PASS theory is useful to explain why teachers' ratings of attention in the classroom correlated with performance on the two CAS tasks that require selectivity and resistance to distraction.

Replicability/Standardizability

The value of any theory of cognitive processing is ultimately related to the extent to which it can be uniformly applied across examiners and organized into a formal and standardized method to assure replication across practitioners. The availability of norms and interpretive guidelines provided the basis for accurate, consistent, and reliable interpretation of PASS scores as operationalized by the CAS (Naglieri & Das, 1997a). The CAS instrument is a reliable measure of PASS constructs normed on a large representative sample of children 5 through 17 years of age (see Naglieri, Chapter 20, this volume). In summary, we suggest that the CAS is acceptable as a reliable and valid assessment of the PASS processes, and that it can be used in a variety of settings for a number of different purposes, as shown in several books and the CAS interpretive handbook (Naglieri & Das, 1997b).

Psychodiagnostic Utility

Dillon's (1986) *psychodiagnostic utility* criterion deals with the ease with which a particular theory of cognitive processing can be used in practice. This criterion is linked to Messick's (1989) idea of *consequential validity* and emphasizes the transition from theory to practice, the extent to which the theory can be effectively applied. The best theory of intelligence, ability, or cognitive processing will ultimately have little impact on the lives of children unless the constructs (1) have been operationalized into a practical method that can be efficiently administered; (2) can be assessed in a reliable manner; and (3) yield scores that are interpretable within the context of some relevant comparison system. As we have mentioned here and in other publications, the PASS theory and the CAS appear to have sufficient applications for diagnosis and treatment. They have value in detecting the cognitive difficulties experienced by children in several diagnostic groups (children with dyslexia, ADHD/traumatic brain injury, and mental retardation [including Down syndrome]), as well as in constructing programs for cognitive enhancement (Das, 2002; Naglieri, 2003).

CONCLUDING REMARKS

The concept of general intelligence has enjoyed widespread use since it was originally described at the turn of the last century. Interestingly, Pintner (1923) noted over 80 years ago that although researchers were concerned with the measurement of separate faculties, processes, or abilities, they "borrowed from every-day life a vague term implying all-round ability and knowledge" and are still "attempting to define it more sharply and endow it with a stricter scientific connotation" (p. 53). Thus the concept of intelligence that has included the use of verbal, nonverbal, and quantitative tests to define and measure intelligence for about 100 years has been and remains just that—a concept in need of more clarity.

In some ways, PASS theory is an attempt to revive the intentions of early intelligence test developers by taking a multidimensional approach to the definition of ability. The most important difference between traditional IQ and PASS theory, therefore, lies in the use of cognitive processes rather than general ability. The multidimensional, rather than unidimensional, view of intelligence that the PASS theory provides is one of its distinguishing aspects (Das & Naglieri, 1992). It is a theory for which research has increasingly demonstrated utility (as summarized in this chapter and in Chapter 20), and practitioners have noted its consistency with the more modern demands placed on such tests. We suggest that PASS is a modern alternative to *g* and IQ, based on neuropsychology and cognitive psychology, and that it is well suited to meet the needs of psychologists practicing in the 21st century.

ACKNOWLEDGMENT

Preparation of this chapter was supported in part by Grant No. R215K010121 from the U.S. Department of Education.

REFERENCES

Ashman, A. F. (1982). Strategic behavior and linguistic functions of institutionalized moderately retarded persons. *International Journal of Rehabilitation Research, 5,* 203–214.

Barkley, R. A. (1997). *ADHD and the nature of self-control.* New York: Guilford Press.

Boden, C., & Kirby, J. R. (1995). Successive processing, phonological coding, and the remediation of reading. *Journal of Cognitive Education, 4,* 19–32.

Bradley, L., & Bryant, P. (1985). *Rhyme and reason in reading and spelling.* Ann Arbor MI: University of Michigan Press.

Carlson, J., & Das, J. P. (1997). A process approach to remediating word decoding deficiencies in Chapter 1 children. *Learning Disabilities Quarterly, 20,* 93–102.

Cormier, P., Carlson, J. S., & Das, J. P. (1990). Planning

ability and cognitive performance: The compensatory effects of a dynamic assessment approach. *Learning and Individual Differences, 2,* 437–449.

Das, J. P. (1972). Patterns of cognitive ability in non-retarded and retarded children. *American Journal of Mental Deficiency, 77,* 6–12.

Das, J. P. (1980). Planning: Theoretical considerations and empirical evidence. *Psychological Research* [W. Germany], *41,* 141–151.

Das, J. P. (1999). *PASS Reading Enhancement Program.* Deal, NJ: Sarka Educational Resources.

Das, J. P. (2001). *Reading difficulties and dyslexia.* Deal, NJ: Sarka Educational Resources.

Das, J. P. (2002). A better look at intelligence. *Current Directions in Psychology, 11,* 28–32.

Das, J. P., & Abbott, J. (1995). PASS: An alternative approach to intelligence. *Psychology and Developing Societies, 7*(2), 155–184.

Das, J. P., & Heemsbergen, D. (1983). Planning as a factor in the assessment of cognitive processes. *Journal of Psychoeducational Assessment, 1,* 1–16.

Das. J. P., Kar, B. C., & Parrila, R. K. (1996). *Cognitive planning: The psychological basis of intelligent behavior.* Thousand Oaks, CA: Sage.

Das, J. P., Kirby, J. R., & Jarman R. F. (1975). Simultaneous and Successive syntheses: An alternative model for cognitive abilities. *Psychological Bulletin, 82,* 87–103.

Das, J. P., Kirby, J. R., & Jarman, R. F. (1979). *Simultaneous and successive cognitive processes.* New York: Academic Press.

Das, J. P., & Melnyk, L. (1989). Attention checklist: A rating scale for mildly mentally handicapped adolescents. *Psychological Reports, 64,* 1267–1274.

Das, J. P., Mishra, R. K., & Kirby, J. R. (1994). Cognitive patterns of dyslexics: Comparison between groups with high and average nonverbal intelligence. *Journal of Learning Disabilities, 27,* 235–242.

Das, J. P., Mishra, R. K., & Pool, J. E. (1995). An experiment on cognitive remediation or word-reading difficulty. *Journal of Learning Disabilities, 28,* 66–79.

Das, J. P., & Molloy, G. N. (1975). Varieties of Simultaneous and Successive processing in children. *Journal of Educational Psychology, 67,* 213–220.

Das, J. P., & Naglieri, J. A. (1992). Assessment of attention, simultaneous–successive coding and planning. In H. C. Haywood & D. Tzuriel (Eds.), *Interactive Assessment* (pp. 207–232). New York: Springer-Verlag.

Das, J. P., Naglieri, J. A., & Kirby, J. R. (1994). *Assessment of cognitive processes.* Needham Heights: MA: Allyn & Bacon.

Das, J. P., Parrila, R. K., & Papadopoulos, T. C. (2000). Cognitive education and reading disability. In A. Kozulin & Y. Rand (Eds.), *Experience of mediated learning* (pp. 276–291). Amsterdam: Pergamon Press.

Das, J. P., Snyder, T. J., & Mishra, R. K. (1992). Assessment of attention: Teachers' rating scales and measures of selective attention. *Journal of Psychoeducational Assessment, 10,* 37–46.

Das, J. P., & Varnhagen, C. K. (1986). Neuropsychological functioning and cognitive processing. In J. E. Obzrut & G. W. Hynd (Eds.), *Child neuropsychology: Vol. 1. Theory and research* (pp. 117–140). New York: Academic Press.

Davis, F. B. (1959). Interpretation of differences among averages and individual test scores. *Journal of Educational Psychology, 50,* 162–170.

Dehn, M. J. (2000). *Cognitive Assessment System performance of ADHD children.* Paper presented at the annual convention of the National Association of School Psychologists, New Orleans, LA.

Dillon, R. F. (1986). Information processing and testing. *Educational Psychologist, 21,* 161–174.

Garofalo, J. (1986). Simultaneous synthesis, regulation and arithmetical performance. *Journal of Psychoeducational Assessment, 4,* 229–238.

Glutting, J. J., McDermott, P. A., Konold, T. R., Snelbaker, A. J., & Watkins, M. L. (1998). More ups and downs of subtest analysis: Criterion validity of the DAS with an unselected cohort. *School Psychology Review, 27,* 599–612.

Goldberg, E. (2001). *The executive brain: Frontal lobes and the civilized mind.* New York: Oxford University Press.

Hald, M. E. (1999). *A PASS cognitive processes intervention study in mathematics.* Unpublished doctoral dissertation, University of Northern Colorado.

Jarman, R. F., & Das, J. P. (1977). Simultaneous and successive synthesis and intelligence. *Intelligence, 1,* 151–169.

Johnson, J. A., Bardos, A. N., & Tayebi, K. A. (2003). Discriminant validity of the Cognitive Assessment System for students with written expression disabilities. *Journal of Psychoeducational Assessment, 21,* 180–195.

Kar, B. C., Dash, U. N., Das, J. P., & Carlson, J. S. (1992). Two experiments on the dynamic assessment of planning. *Learning and Individual Differences, 5,* 13–29.

Kirby, J. R. (1984). *Cognitive strategies and educational performance.* New York: Academic Press.

Kirby, J. R., & Das, J. P. (1978). Information processing and human abilities. *Journal of Educational Psychology, 70,* 58–66.

Kirby, J, R., & Robinson, G. L. (1987) Simultaneous and successive processing in reading disabled children. *Journal of Learning Disabilities, 20,* 243–252.

Kirby, J. R., & Williams, N. H. (1991). *Learning problems: A cognitive approach.* Toronto: Kagan & Woo.

Kolb, B., Gibb, R., & Robinson, T. E. (2003). Brain plasticity and behavior. *Current Directions in Psychological Science, 12,* 1–4.

Lidz, C. S. (1991). *Practitioner's guide to dynamic assessment.* New York: Guilford Press.

Luria, A. R. (1966). *Human brain and psychological processes.* New York: Harper & Row.

Luria, A. R. (1973a). The origin and cerebral organization of man's conscious action. In S. G. Sapir & A. C.

Nitzburg (Eds.), *Children with learning problems* (pp. 109–130). New York: Brunner/Mazel.

Luria, A. R. (1973b). *The working brain.* New York: Basic Books.

Luria, A. R. (1979). *The making of mind: A personal account of Soviet psychology.* Cambridge, MA: Harvard University Press.

Luria, A. R. (1980). *Higher cortical functions in man* (2nd ed.). New York: Basic Books.

Luria, A. R. (1982). *Language and cognition.* New York: Wiley.

Messick, S. (1989). Validity. In R. L. Linn (Ed.), *Educational measurement* (pp. 13–103). New York: American Council of Education/MacMillan.

Naglieri, J. A. (1989). A cognitive processing theory for the measurement of intelligence. *Educational Psychologist, 24,* 185–206.

Naglieri, J. A. (1999). *Essentials of CAS assessment.* New York: Wiley.

Naglieri, J. A. (2000). Can profile analysis of ability test scores work?: An illustration using the PASS theory and CAS with an unselected cohort. *School Psychology Quarterly, 15,* 419–433.

Naglieri, J. A. (2003). Current advances in assessment and intervention for children with learning disabilities. In T. E. Scruggs & M. A. Mastropieri (Eds.), *Advances in learning and behavioral disabilities: Vol. 16. Identification and assessment* (pp. 163–190). Greenwich, CT: JAI Press.

Naglieri, J. A., & Das, J. P. (1988). Planning–arousal–simultaneous–successive (PASS): A model for assessment. *Journal of School Psychology, 26,* 35–48.

Naglieri, J. A., & Das, J. P. (1997a). *Das–Naglieri: Cognitive Assessment System.* Itasca, IL: Riverside.

Naglieri, J. A., & Das, J. P. (1997b). *Das–Naglieri Cognitive Assessment System: Interpretive handbook.* Itasca, IL: Riverside.

Naglieri, J. A., & Das, J. P. (1997c). Intelligence revised. In R. Dillon (Ed.), *Handbook on testing* (pp. 136–163). Westport, CT: Greenwood Press.

Naglieri, J. A., & Das, J. P. (2002). Practical implications of general intelligence and PASS cognitive processes. In R. J. Sternberg & E. L. Grigorenko (Eds.), *The general factor of intelligence: How general is it?* (pp. 855–884). New York: Erlbaum.

Naglieri, J. A., Goldstein, S., Iseman, J. S., & Schwebach, A. (2003). Performance of children with attention deficit hyperactivity disorder and anxiety/depression on the WISC-III and Cognitive Assessment System (CAS). *Journal of Psychoeducational Assessment, 21,* 32–42.

Naglieri, J. A., & Gottling, S. H. (1995). A cognitive education approach to math instruction for the learning

disabled: An individual study. *Psychological Reports, 76,* 1343–1354.

Naglieri, J. A., & Gottling, S. H. (1997). Mathematics instruction and PASS cognitive processes: An intervention study. *Journal of Learning Disabilities, 30,* 513–520.

Naglieri, J. A., & Johnson, D. (2000). Effectiveness of a cognitive strategy intervention to improve math calculation based on the PASS theory. *Journal of Learning Disabilities, 33,* 591–597.

Naglieri, J. A., & Pickering, E. (2003). *Helping children learn: Instructional handouts for use in school and at home.* Baltimore: Brookes.

Naglieri, J. A., Salter, C. J., & Edwards, G. (2004). Assessment of children with ADHD and reading disabilities using the PASS theory and Cognitive Assessment System. *Journal of Psychoeducational Assessment, 22,* 93–105.

Paolitto, A. W. (1999). Clinical validation of the Cognitive Assessment System with children with ADHD. *ADHD Report, 7,* 1–5.

Parrila, R. K., Das, J. P., Kendrick, M., Papadopoulos, T., & Kirby, J. (1999). Efficacy of a cognitive reading remediation program for at-risk children in grade 1. *Developmental Disabilities Bulletin, 27,* 1–31.

Share, D. L., & Stanovich, K. E. (1995). Cognitive processes in early reading development: Accommodating individual differences into a model of acquisition. *Issues in Education, 1,* 1–57.

Silverstein, A. B. (1982). Pattern analysis as simultaneous statistical inference. *Journal of Consulting and Clinical Psychology, 50,* 234–240.

Silverstein, A. B. (1993). Type I, Type II, and other types of errors in pattern analysis. *Psychological Assessment, 5,* 72–74.

Stanovich, K. E. (1988). Explaining the differences between the dyslexic and the garden-variety poor reader: The phonological–core variable–difference model. *Journal of Learning Disabilities, 21,* 590–604, 612.

Stuss, D. T., & Benson, D. F. (1990). The frontal lobes and language. In E. Goldberg (Ed.), *Contemporary psychology and the legacy of Luria* (pp. 29–50). Hillsdale, NJ: Erlbaum.

Torgesen, J. K., Wagner, R. K., & Rashotte, C. A. (1994). Longitudinal studies of phonological processing and reading. *Journal of Learning Disabilities, 27,* 276–286.

Wagner, R. K., Torgesen, J. K., & Rashotte, C. A. (1994). Development of reading-related phonological processing abilities: New evidence of bi-directional causality from a latent variable longitudinal study. *Developmental Psychology, 30,* 73–87.

8

The Cattell–Horn–Carroll Theory of Cognitive Abilities

Past, Present, and Future

KEVIN S. McGREW

One of the most successful undertakings attributed to modern psychology is the measurement of mental abilities. Though rarely appreciated outside academe, the breakthrough in objectively gauging the nature and range of mental abilities is a pivotal development in the behavioral sciences. While this accomplishment has far-reaching implications for many areas of society, the full meaning of the test data has lacked a comprehensive theory that accounts for several major developments over the years. The track of data left by researchers remains diffuse without a clear signpost in the broad landscape of mental abilities.

—LAMB (1994, p. 386)

Since the beginning of our existence, humans have searched for order in their world. Today classification is thought of as essential to all scientific work (Dunn & Everitt, 1982). The reliable and valid classification of entities, and research regarding these entities and newly proposed entities, requires a "guide" or taxonomy (Bailey, 1994; Prentky, 1996). Although Lamb's (1994) lament about the lack of a clear signpost in the broad landscape of mental abilities had been true for decades, the crystallization of an empirically based psychometric taxonomy of human cognitive abilities finally occurred in the late 1980s to early 1990s.

In a chapter (McGrew, 1997) for the first edition of this volume, I predicted that progress in intelligence testing was being, and would continue to be energized, as a result of the articulation of this new consensus taxonomy of human cognitive abilities. The detailed description and articulation of the psychometric "table of human cognitive elements" in John "Jack" Carroll's (1993) *Hu-*

Portions of this chapter (inclusive of tables and figures) were previously published by the Institute for Applied Psychometrics,llc (*http://www.iapsych.com/chcpp/chcpp.html*). Copyright 2003 by the Institute for Applied Psychometrics,llc, Kevin S. McGrew. IAP grants permission to the publisher of this chapter to adapt this copyrighted material.

man Cognitive Abilities: A Survey of Factor-Analytic Studies, which concluded that the Cattell–Horn Gf-Gc theory was the most empirically grounded available psychometric theory of intelligence, resulted in my recommending that "all scholars, test developers, and users of intelligence tests need to become familiar with Carroll's treatise on the factors of human abilities" (McGrew, 1997, p. 151). I further suggested that practitioners heed Carroll's suggestion to "use his 'map' of known cognitive abilities to guide their selection and interpretation of tests in intelligence batteries" (p. 151). It was the purpose of that chapter to contribute, albeit in a small way, to the building of "a 'bridge' between the theoretical and empirical research on the factors of intelligence and the development and interpretation of psychoeducational assessment batteries" (p. 151).

This current chapter continues to focus on the construction of a theory-to-practice bridge, one grounded in the *Cattell–Horn–Carroll* (CHC) theory of cognitive abilities. The primary goals of this chapter are to (1) describe the evolution of contemporary CHC theory; (2) describe the broad and narrow CHC abilities; and (3) review structural evidence that supports the broad strokes of CHC theory.

THE EVOLUTION OF THE CHC THEORY OF COGNITIVE ABILITIES

Although various theories attempt to explain intelligent human behavior (Sternberg & Kaufman, 1998), "the most influential approach, and the one that has generated the most influential research, is based on psychometric testing" (Neisser et al., 1996, p. 95). The CHC theory of intelligence is the tent that houses the two most prominent psychometric theoretical models of human cognitive abilities (Daniel, 1997, 2000; Snow, 1998; Sternberg & Kaufman, 1998). CHC theory represents the integration of the Cattell–Horn Gf-Gc theory (Horn & Noll, 1977; see also Horn & Blankson, Chapter 3, this volume) and Carroll's three-stratum theory (Carroll, 1993, and Chapter 4, this volume). CHC is a psychometric theory, since it is primarily based on procedures assuming that "the structure of intelligence can be discovered by analyzing the interrelationship of scores on

mental ability tests. To develop these models, large numbers of people are given many types of mental problems. The statistical technique of factor analysis is then applied to the test scores to identify the 'factors' or latent sources of individual differences in intelligence" (Davidson & Downing, 2000, p. 37).

The psychometric study of cognitive abilities is more than the exploratory factor analysis (EFA) of a set of cognitive variables. Contemporary psychometric approaches differ from traditional psychometric approaches in three major ways: (1) There is greater use of confirmatory factor analysis (CFA) as opposed to EFA; (2) the structural analysis of items is now as important as the structural analysis of variables; and (3) item response theory models now play a pivotal role (Embretson & McCollam, 2000). Space limitations necessitate a focus only on the factor-analytic portions of the contemporary psychometric approach. It is also important to recognize that non-factor-analytic research, in the form of heritability, neurocognitive, developmental, and outcome prediction (occupational and educational) studies, provides additional sources of validity evidence for CHC theory (Horn, 1998; Horn & Noll, 1997).

Early Psychometric Heritage

Historical accounts of the evolution of the psychometric approach abound (e.g., see Brody, 2000; Carroll, 1993; Horn & Noll, 1997). Prior to 1930, the usual distinction made in cognitive abilities was between verbal and quantitative abilities (Corno et al., 2002). Key early historical developments that ultimately led to the emergence of CHC theory are listed in the first two sections of Table 8.1. The lack of a detailed treatment (in this chapter) of all the developments in Table 8.1 is a necessary constraint and in no way diminishes the importance of each contribution. In addition, the major steps that led to current CHC theory are illustrated in Figure 8.1. In the next section, CHC theory is described as it evolved through a series of major theory-to-practice bridging events that occurred during the past two decades. The goal is to establish an appropriate historical record of the events that transpired and the roles that different individuals played in this process.

TABLE 8.1. Significant Structural CHC Theoretical, Measurement, and Assessment Developments: A Continuum of Progress

Major CHC developments	Select comments
A. Early psychometric theory development	
1. Spearman's (1904, 1927) theory of *g* and *s* factors.	• Developed a "two-factor theory" (general intelligence factor, *g*, + specific factors, *s*) to account for correlations between measures of sensory discrimination (Galton tradition). *g* was hypothesized to represent a fixed amount of "mental energy." Spearman is generally credited with introducing the notion of factor analysis to the study of human abilities.
2. *The British tradition.* Using factor-analytic techniques that first extracted (from a matrix of correlations) the *g* factor, and then group factors of successively smaller breadth, primarily British researchers suggested full-fledged hierarchical structural models of intelligence (Burt, 1909, 1911, 1941, 1949a, 1949b; Vernon, 1950, 1961).	• According to Gustafsson (1988), Burt's model was to a great extent "logically constructed" and thus did not have major impact. In contrast, Horn stated that Burt's model was very influential (Horn & Noll, 1997). Vernon's (1950, 1961) model, which had a *g* factor at the apex of the hierarchy, and at the next level two major group factors (verbal–numerical–educational, or v:ed; spatial–practical–mechanical–physical, or k:m) received more widespread attention. The British models suggested that most of the variance of human intelligence was attributable to *g* and to very small group factors, and that the importance of the broader group factors was meager (Gustafsson, 1988).
3. *The American tradition.* Primary use of multiple-factor-analytic methods, with the rotation of factors according to the "simple-structure" criterion. This method did not readily identify a *g* factor. The correlations among oblique factors were typically factor-analyzed in turn to produce "second-order" factors (Cattell, 1941, 1957; Thurstone, 1938; Thurstone & Thurstone, 1941).	• Thurstone's theory posited seven to nine primary mental abilities (PMAs) that were *independent* of a higher-order *g* factor. Most modern hierarchical theories of intelligence have their roots in Thurstone's PMA theory (Horn & Noll, 1997). • The formal beginning of the Cattell–Horn Gf-Gc theory. *Fluid* (*Gf*) and *crystallized* (*Gc*) intelligence factors were extracted from second-order factor analysis of first-order (i.e., PMA) abilities.
4. System of "well-replicated common factors" (WERCOF abilities) established.	• Early summaries of the large body of PMA-based factor research suggested over 60 possible separate PMAs (Ekstrom, French, & Harman, 1979; French, 1951; French, Ekstrom, & Price, 1963; Guilford, 1967; Hakstian & Cattell, 1974; Horn, 1972).
B. Gf-Gc theory is extended	
1. Gv, Gsm, Glr, Gs added (Horn, 1965). Ga added; Gv, Gs, Glr refined (Horn, 1968).	• Postulation of additional broad *G* factors based on structural (factor-analytic), developmental, heritability, neurocognitive, and outcome criterion evidence research.
2. Evidence supports eight or nine broad abilities (Carroll & Horn, 1981).	• Despite a network of validity evidence supporting the broad strokes of Gf-Gc theory, by the early 1980s no individually administered clinical test battery reflected these findings. A gap between theory and applied measurement practice existed until 1989.
3. General hierarchical model of the structure of intelligence (HILI model) proposed by Gustafsson (1984, 1988).	• HILI model presented as general unifying framework for integrating British (Spearman, Burt, Vernon) and American (Thurston, Cattell, Horn) traditions of psychometric/theoretical research. Different models (e.g., Cattell–Horn, Vernon) could be viewed as "classes" of models within the general HILI framework. Gf was suggested to be identical to *g*.
4. Gq and English-language factors suggested (Horn, 1985–1991).	

(continued)

TABLE 8.1. *(continued)*

Major CHC developments	Select comments
C. First-generation Gf-Gc applied assessment and interpretation approaches	
1. Cattell–Horn Gf-Gc theory "discovered" by Woodcock. 2. Cattell Gf-Gc based WJ-R (Woodcock & Johnson, 1989) published.	• The "fortuitous" Horn–Carroll–Woodcock meeting. Horn and Cattell served as consultants to WJ-R revision team, resulting in first major Gf-Gc theory-to-practice "bridging" or cross-fertilization event, which had a major impact on the applied measurement of intelligence. Horn, Carroll, Woodcock, and McGrew independently factor-analyzed 1977 WJ as per CHC (Gf-Gc) theory and integrated results to form the WJ-R test specification design blueprint (1986–1987). The WJ-R represented the first individually administered battery designed as per Cattell–Horn Gf-Gc theory to measure nine broad abilities. Horn published an overview of Gf-Gc theory in a special appendix to the WJ-R technical manual (McGrew & Woodcock, 1991).
3. "Battery-free" Gf-Gc assessment concept is born. Gf-Gc-based confirmatory factor analysis (CFA) of multiple "cross-battery" data sets produces concept of cross-battery assessment and interpretation (Woodcock, 1990) and provides construct validity evidence for WJ-R and Gf-Gc theory.	• Individual tests from the major intelligence batteries (DAS, DTLA-3, K-ABC, SB-IV, WJ/WJ-R, WISC-R/WAIS/WAIS-R) were empirically classified at the *broad* Gf-Gc ability level. McGhee (1993) extended analyses to DAS and DTLA-3.
4. KAIT (Kaufman & Kaufman, 1993) Gf-Gc-based battery published.	• Provided composite scores for two broad abilities (Gf and Gc).
5. Informal "intelligent" Gf-Gc cross-battery approach to clinical test interpretation applied to the WJ-R Tests of Cognitive Abilities (McGrew, 1993).	• First presentation of an informal *clinical* approach to supplementing a test battery that was grounded in the available Gf-Gc cross-battery CFA studies.
D. Carroll's 1993 principia: *Human Cognitive Abilities*	
1. Carroll three-stratum (with *g*) model proposed.	• Presentation of the most comprehensive empirically based synthesis of the extant factor-analytic research on the structure of human cognitive abilities. A structure of intelligence was presented that included three hierarchical levels (strata) of abilities (narrow, broad, general), differing by breadth of generality. The resulting summary provided a working taxonomy of human cognitive abilities by which to guide research and intelligence testing practice.
2. Cattell–Horn (*g*-less) model supported as the most viable available psychometric model.	• Carroll and Cattell–Horn models differed primarily with regard to the existence of a *g* factor.
E. CHC investigations, integrations, and extensions	
1. English-language Grw factor defined (Woodcock, 1994).	• Confirmed Horn's previous identification of a language use factor.
2. Carroll three-stratum model validated across the lifespan with WJ-R norm data (Bickley, Keith, & Wolfe, 1995).	• In addition to supporting Carroll's three-stratum hierarchical model, results also supported Carroll's (1993) notion that "intermediate"-level abilities may exist between the three major strata of the model.

(continued)

TABLE 8.1. *(continued)*

Major CHC developments	Select comments
3. *Contemporary Intellectual Assessment* (CIA) book published (Flanagan, Genshaft, & Harrison, 1997).	• The first intellectual assessment book to include multiple chapters reflecting the bridging of Gf-Gc theory (e.g., Horn and Carroll chapters) and applied assessment and interpretation.
4. Horn and Carroll informally agree to Cattell–Horn–Carroll (CHC) umbrella theory terminology (1999).	

F. Second-generation CHC assessment and interpretation approaches emerge

1. All tests from major intelligence batteries logically classified at both the broad- and narrow-ability levels as per the first proposed synthesized Cattell–Horn and Carroll Gf-Gc model (McGrew, 1997).	• The lack of CFA cross-battery studies specifying both broad *and* narrow Gf-Gc factors led to expert-consensus content validity Gf-Gc narrow-ability test classifications.
2. Cross-battery assessment and interpretation approach formalized for the first time (Flanagan & McGrew, 1997).	• Cross-battery assessment approach introduced via the "three pillars of cross-battery assessment" (theory, construct relevant variance, construct representation) and a general operational framework.
3. Gf-Gc-based WJ-R and KAIT cross-battery CFA study completed (Flanagan & McGrew, 1998).	• Individual KAIT tests empirically classified at broad Gf-Gc level. The need to consider both the broad *and* narrow abilities in cross-battery CFA model specification and interpretation was presented.
4. *Intelligence Test Desk Reference (ITDR): Gf-Gc Cross-Battery Assessment* published (McGrew & Flanagan, 1998).	• First comprehensive description and formal operationalization of cross-battery assessment approach that can be applied to all major intelligence batteries and select special-purpose tests.
5. CHC-based WJ III published (Woodcock, McGrew, & Mather, 2001).	• WJ III is first individually administered battery designed/revised to ensure proper construct representation of nine broad CHC abilities via 2 + different narrow-ability test indicators for each broad ability domain. Horn and Cattell served as consultants to WJ III revision team.
6. Cross-battery approach refined (Flanagan, McGrew, & Ortiz, 2000; Flanagan & Ortiz, 2001) and extended to achievement test batteries (Flanagan, Ortiz, Alfonso, & Mascolo, 2002).	• First Wechsler CHC cross-battery approach presented. Additional special-purpose cognitive tests and tests from major individually administered achievement batteries classified as per CHC theory. The first operational model of learning disabilities based on CHC theory is presented.
7. CHC-based SB5 published (Roid, 2003).	• SB5 provides composite scores for five broad abilities (Gf, Gc, Gq, Gsm, Gv), via verbal and nonverbal test administration procedures. Horn, Cattell, and Woodcock served as consultants to revision team.

(continued)

TABLE 8.1. *(continued)*

Major CHC developments	Select comments
G. Post-Carroll (1993) CHC model evaluation and extensions (at broad [stratum II] level)	
1. Significant number of large- and small-sample studies employing large sets of ability indicators support the broad strokes (stratum II abilities) of CHC theory (McGrew & Evans, 2004).	• Broad abilities of Gf, Gc, Gv, Gsm, Glr, Gs, Gq, and Grw are validated as primary components of CHC model.
2. Empirical evidence suggest broad tactile (Gh) and kinesthetic (Gk) abilities (Pallier, Roberts, & Stankov, 2000; Stankov, 2000; Stankov, Seizova-Cajic, & Roberts, 2001).	• Results relevant to tactile–kinesthetic components of neuropsychological assessment. Domains need additional validity research.
3. Empirical evidence suggests broad olfactory (Go) domain (Danthiir, Roberts, Pallier, & Stankov, 2001).	• Possible broad olfactory (Go) ability is hypothesized, but currently lacks appropriate network of validity evidence. Additional research is needed.
4. Empirical evidence suggests that the cognitive speed portion of the CHC structural hierarchy may be more complex and differentiated than specified by Carroll or Cattell–Horn (Ackerman, Beier, & Boyle, 2002; O'Connor & Burns, 2003; Roberts & Stankov, 1999; Stankov, 2000). Evidence supports three broad speed ability domains (Gs, broad cognitive processing speed; Gt, broad decision speed; Gps, broad psychomotor speed).	• Perceptual speed (PS) ability has been identified as both a narrow and a broad ability (subsuming narrow pattern recognition, scanning, memory, and complex abilities) in different studies. • Decision time (DT) and movement time (MT) have been identified as both narrow and broad Gt abilities in different studies. • Research studies provide stronger support for the speed of reasoning (RE) ability, as well as the continued speculation that for every cognitive level ability, corresponding rate/fluency abilities exist. • Psychometric time ability, which appears similar to rate of test taking (R9) as defined by Carroll, is hypothesized as an intermediate ability between stratum II (broad) and stratum III (general, *g*). • The exact nature and ordering of empirically identified speed abilities in a cognitive speed hierarchy are not clear; additional research is needed.
5. Empirical evidence suggests broad domain-specific general knowledge (Gkn) ability distinct from Gc (Ackerman, Bowen, Beier, & Kanfer, 2001).	• Gkn ability is currently only identified at adult levels. • Development and emergence of Gkn may reflect the development of "wisdom" and "expertise."

Note. The listings in this table represent a continuum of conceptual progress, not necessarily a straight timeline. Key to abbreviations for test batteries: DAS, Differential Ability Scales; DTLA-3, Detroit Tests of Learning Aptitude—Third Edition; K-ABC, Kaufman Assessment Battery for Children; KAIT, Kaufman Adolescent and Adult Intelligence Test; SB-IV, Stanford–Binet Intelligence Scale: Fourth Edition; SB5, Stanford–Binet Intelligence Scales, Fifth Edition; WAIS(-R), Wechsler Adult Intelligence Scale(—Revised); WISC-R, Wechsler Intelligence Scale for Children—Revised; WJ(-R), Woodcock–Johnson Psycho-Educational Battery(—Revised); WJ III, Woodcock–Johnson III.

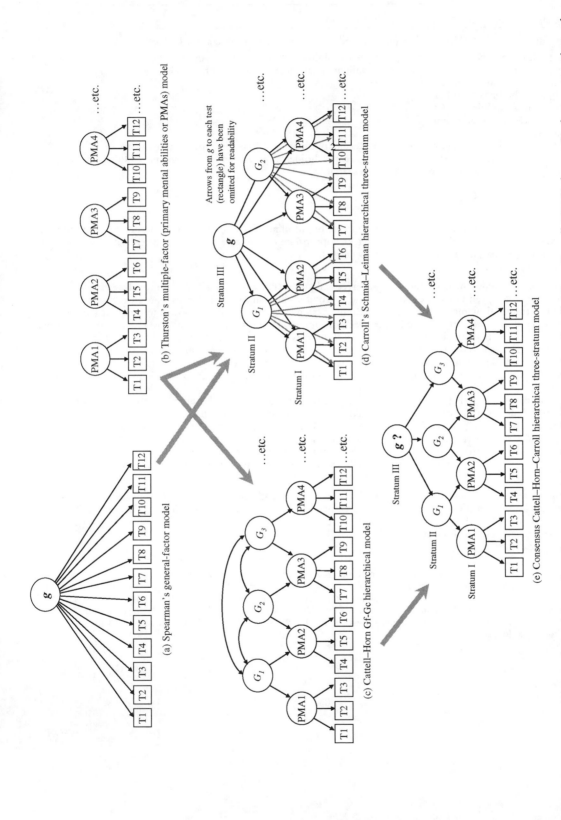

FIGURE 8.1. Major stages in the evolution of psychometric theories from Spearman's *g* to Cattell–Horn–Carroll (CHC) theory. Circles represent latent factors. Squares represent manifest measures (tests; T1, etc.). Double-headed arrows designate latent factor correlations. Single-headed path arrows designate factor loadings.

First-Generation Gf-Gc Applied Assessment and Interpretation Approaches

The integration of the Cattell–Horn Gf-Gc and Carroll three-stratum theories under the common CHC framework—and, more important, the subsequent impact of CHC theory on the applied field of intellectual test development and assessment—were due to a number of "bridging" events that occurred between 1985 and today. Only the major developments that resulted in the "cross-fertilization" of knowledge from the leading scholars in intelligence with that of applied test developers, or events that accelerated and/or changed the direction of the theory-to-practice fertilization, are highlighted below.

Cattell–Horn Gf-Gc Theory "Discovered"

By the middle to late 1980s, John Horn, a student of Raymond Cattell's, had concluded that the available research supported the presence of at least six to seven additional broad "G" abilities beyond Gf and Gc (see section B in Table 8.1). According to Horn and Noll (1997), the Cattell–Horn Gf-Gc theory evolved from a lengthy and systematic program of structural (factor-analytic) research by Cattell and Horn (Cattell & Horn, 1978; Hakstian & Cattell, 1978; Horn, 1968, 1976, 1988, 1991; Horn & Bramble, 1967; Horn & Cattell, 1966, 1967; Horn & Stankov, 1982; Rossman & Horn, 1972). The contribution of the Cattell–Horn Gf-Gc program of research to the development of psychometric theories of intelligence is impressive. During this same time period, Jan-Eric Gustafsson (1984, 1988) was similarly evaluating Gf-Gc models that included, in addition to a higher-order general intelligence (g) factor, a variety of Gf-Gc-flavored broad abilities. John Carroll was also publishing glimpses of his eventual three-stratum model of intelligence (Carroll, 1983, 1985; Carroll & Maxwell, 1979). Yet, at a time when the leading intelligence scholars were being drawn faster and faster toward the center of a psychometric vortex that would reveal a more or less common taxonomic structure of human cognitive abilities, the field of applied intelligence testing was largely ignorant of these develop-ments. The model of eight to nine broad Gf-Gc abilities had yet to hit the radar screen of practicing psychologists.

The seed that eventually blossomed and introduced CHC theory in the field of applied intelligence testing was planted in 1985, in the mind of one applied psychoeducational test developer of the times (viz., Richard Woodcock). The seed was planted during a presentation on Gf-Gc theory by John Horn at a 1985 conference honoring Lloyd Humphreys (see Schrank, Flanagan, Woodcock, & Mascolo, 2002). Hearing Horn's Gf-Gc presentation resulted in Woodcock's decision to consider the multiple-ability Gf-Gc theory as *the* model for a revision of the original Woodcock–Johnson Psycho-Educational Battery (WJ; Woodcock & Johnson, 1977; see sections C1–C2 in Table 8.1). The psychometric intelligence theory-to-practice bridge was now under construction.

Cattell–Horn Gf-Gc Theory Overview

By the late 1980s and early 1990s, scholars who routinely published in the rarified air of the journal Intelligence had generally recognized the Horn–Cattell Gf-Gc model as the best approximation of a taxonomic structure of human cognitive abilities. For example, Carroll (1993) stated, after his seminal review of the extant factor-analytic literature, that the Horn–Cattell Gf-Gc model "appears to offer the most well-founded and reasonable approach to an acceptable theory of the structure of cognitive abilities" (p. 62).

Gf-Gc theory received its original name because early versions (Cattell, 1943, 1963) of the theory only proposed two abilities: *fluid intelligence* (Gf) and *crystallized intelligence* (Gc). By 1991, Horn (1991) had already extended the Gf-Gc model of Cattell to the identification of 9–10 broad Gf-Gc abilities: *fluid intelligence* (Gf), *crystallized intelligence* (Gc), *short-term acquisition and retrieval* (SAR or Gsm), *visual intelligence* (Gv), *auditory intelligence* (Ga), *long-term storage and retrieval* (TSR or Glr), *cognitive processing speed* (Gs), *correct decision speed* (CDS), and *quantitative knowledge* (Gq).[1] The relative "newcomer" ability associated with the comprehension and expression of *reading and writing skills* (Grw) was added during this time period (Horn, 1988;

McGrew, Werder, & Woodcock, 1991; Woodcock, 1994; see section E1 in Table 8.1).

As illustrated in Figure 8.1, the Cattell–Horn Gf-Gc theory has its roots in Thurstone's (1938, 1947) theory of *primary mental abilities* (PMAs). In fact, according to Horn and Noll (1997), "to a considerable extent, modern hierarchical theories derive from this theory" (p. 62). At the time, Thurstone's PMA theory was at variance with the prevailing view that a higher-order *g* factor existed, and instead posited between seven and nine independent (orthogonal) PMAs: *induction* (I), *deduction* (D), *verbal comprehension* (V), *associative memory* (Ma), *spatial relations* (S), *perceptual speed* (P), *numerical facility* (N), and *word fluency* (Fw).[2] A large number of replication and extension studies confirmed Thurstone's PMAs and led to the eventual identification of over 60 abilities (Carroll, 1993; Horn & Noll, 1997; Jensen, 1998). Early pre-Carroll (1993) factor-analytic syntheses and summaries were published (Ekstrom, French, & Harman, 1979; French, 1951; French, Ekstrom, & Price, 1963; Guilford, 1967; Hakstian & Cattell, 1974; Horn, 1972) with the patterns of intercorrelations of the PMAs providing the rational for the specification of the higher-order broad *G* abilities in the Cattell–Horn Gf-Gc model (Horn & Noll, 1997; Horn & Masunaga, 2000). A thorough treatment of the contemporary Horn–Cattell Gf-Gc model can be found elsewhere in this volume (see Horn & Blankson, Chapter 3).

The "Fortuitous" Horn–Carroll–Woodcock Meeting

In the fall of 1985, I was engaged as a consultant and revision team member for the Woodcock–Johnson—Revised (WJ-R; Woodcock & Johnson, 1989). The first order of business was to attend a March 1986 "kickoff" revision meeting in Dallas, Texas. Woodcock invited a number of consultants, the two most noteworthy being John Horn and Carl Haywood. Revision team members were notified that it was important to hear Horn describe Gf-Gc theory, and also to determine whether "dynamic" testing concepts could be incorpo-

rated in the WJ-R.[3] At the last minute, the president of the publisher of the WJ (Developmental Learning Materials), Andy Bingham, made a fortuitous unilateral decision to invite (to the March 1986 WJ-R meeting) an educational psychologist he had worked with on the *American Heritage Word Frequency Book* (Carroll, Davies, & Richman, 1971). This educational psychologist, whom few members of the WJ-R revision team or the publisher's staff knew, was John B. Carroll.

The first portion of the meeting was largely devoted to a presentation of the broad strokes of Gf-Gc theory by Horn. With the exception of Carroll and Woodcock, most individuals present (myself included) were confused and struggling to grapple with the new language of "Gf this . . . Gc that . . . SAR . . . TSR . . . etc." During most of this time John Carroll sat quietly to my immediate left.

When asked for his input, Carroll pulled an old and battered square-cornered brown leather briefcase from his side, placed it on the table, and proceeded to remove a thick computer printout (of the old green and white barred tractor-feed variety associated with mainframe printers). Carroll proceeded to present the results of a just-completed Schmid–Leiman EFA of the correlation matrices from the 1977 WJ technical manual. A collective "Ah ha!" engulfed the room as Carroll's WJ factor interpretation provided a meaningful link between the theoretical terminology of Horn and the concrete world of WJ tests.

It is my personal opinion that this moment—a moment where the interests and wisdom of a leading applied test developer (Woodcock), the leading proponent of Cattell–Horn Gf-Gc theory (Horn), and one of the preeminent educational psychologists and scholars of the factor analysis of human abilities (Carroll) intersected (see section C in Table 8.1)—was the flash point that resulted in *all* subsequent theory-to-practice bridging events leading to today's CHC theory and related assessment developments. A fortuitous set of events had resulted in the psychometric stars' aligning themselves in perfect position to lead the way for every subsequent CHC assessment-related development.[4]

Publication of the Horn–Cattell Organized WJ-R Battery (1989)

With a Cattell–Horn Gf-Gc map in hand, I was directed to organize the available WJ factor- and cluster-analytic research studies (Kaufman & O'Neal, 1988; McGrew, 1986, 1987; McGue, Shinn, & Ysseldyke, 1979, 1982; Rosso & Phelps, 1988; Woodcock, 1978). Pivotal to this search for WJ Gf-Gc structure were factor analyses of the WJ correlation matrices by Carroll (personal communication, March 1986) and a WJ-based doctoral dissertation (Butler, 1987) directed by Horn. Woodcock and I, both freshly armed with rudimentary CFA skills and software, threw ourselves into reanalyses of the WJ correlation matrices. The result of this synthesis was the development of the WJ-R test development blueprint table (McGrew et al., 1991; Schrank et al., 2002), which identified existing WJ tests that were good measures of specific Gf-Gc abilities, as well as suggesting Gf-Gc "holes" that needed to be filled by creating new tests. The goal was for the WJ-R to have at least two or more cognitive tests measuring aspects of each of seven (Gf, Gc, Gv, Ga, Gsm, Glr, Gs) Cattell–Horn Gf-Gc broad abilities.

The publication of the WJ-R Tests of Cognitive Abilities (COG) represented the official "crossing over" of Gf-Gc theory from the domain of intelligence scholars and theoreticians to that of applied practitioners, particularly those conducting assessments in educational settings (see section C2 in Table 8.1). The WJ-R represented the first individually administered, nationally normed, clinical battery to close the gap between contemporary psychometric theory (i.e., Cattell–Horn Gf-Gc theory) and applied practice. According to Daniel (1997), the WJ-R was "the most thorough implementation of the multifactor model" (p. 1039) of intelligence. An important WJ-R component was the inclusion of a chapter by Horn (1991) in an appendix to the WJ-R technical manual (McGrew et al., 1991). Horn's chapter represented the first up-to-date comprehensive description of the Horn–Cattell Gf-Gc theory in a publication readily accessible to assessment practitioners. As a direct result of the publication of the WJ-R, "Gf-Gc as a second-language" emerged vigorously in ed-ucational and school psychology training programs, journal articles, books, and psychological reports, and it became a frequent topic on certain professional and assessment-related electronic listservs.

The Birth of "Battery-Free" Gf-Gc Assessment

In 1990, Woodcock published an article that, in a sense, provided a "battery-free" approach to Gf-Gc theoretical interpretation of all intelligence test batteries. In a seminal article summarizing his analysis of a series of joint CFA studies of the major intelligence batteries (i.e., the Kaufman Assessment Battery for Children [K-ABC], the Stanford–Binet Intelligence Scale: Fourth Edition [SB-IV], the Wechsler scales, the WJ, and the WJ-R; see section C3 in Table 8.1), Woodcock (1990), using empirical criteria, classified the individual tests of all the major batteries according to the Cattell–Horn Gf-Gc model.[5] For example, the WJ-R Visual–Auditory Learning test was classified by Woodcock as a strong measure of Glr, based on a median factor loading of .697 across 14 different analyses. Another example of a clear classification was the SB-IV Vocabulary test as a strong measure of Gc, based on a median factor loading of .810 across four analyses.

In the discussion of his results, Woodcock demonstrated how each individual test from each intelligence battery mapped onto the Cattell–Horn Gf-Gc taxonomy. The resulting tables demonstrated how each battery adequately measured certain Gf-Gc domains, but failed to measure, or measured poorly, other Gf-Gc domains.[6] More importantly, Woodcock (1990) suggested that in order to measure a greater breadth of Gf-Gc abilities, users of other instruments should use "cross-battery" methods to fill their respective Gf-Gc measurement voids. The concept of Gf-Gc *cross-battery assessment* was born, as well as a means to evaluate the cross-battery equivalence of scores from different batteries (Daniel, 1997).

In a sense, Woodcock had hatched the idea of Gf-Gc "battery-free" assessment, in which a common Gf-Gc assessment and interpretive taxonomy were deployed across intelligence batteries. Practitioners were no longer constrained to the interpretive structure provided by a specific intelligence battery.[7] Practitioners were given permission and a rationale to "think outside their test kits" in order to conduct more valid assessments. Based on Woodcock's (1990) findings, I (McGrew, 1993) subsequently described a Kaufman-like Gf-Gc supplemental testing approach for use with the WJ-R. Unwittingly, this was a clinical attempt to implement an informal cross-battery approach to assessment (see section C5 in Table 8.1). The development of the formal CHC cross-battery assessment approach was waiting in the wings, and blossomed during the next set of major CHC theory-to-practice bridging events.

Carroll's 1993 Principia: Human Cognitive Abilities

Carroll's 1993 book, *Human Cognitive Abilities: A Survey of Factor-Analytic Studies*, may represent in the field of applied psychometrics a work similar in stature to other so-called "principia" publications in other fields (e.g., Newton's three-volume *The Mathematical Principles of Natural Philosophy*, or *Principia* as it became known; Whitehead & Russell's *Principia Mathematica*; see section D in Table 8.1). Briefly, Carroll summarized a review and reanalysis of more than 460 different datasets that included nearly all the more important and classic factor-analytic studies of human cognitive abilities.

I am not alone in the elevation of Carroll's work to such a high stature. On the book cover, Richard Snow stated that "John Carroll has done a magnificent thing. He has reviewed and reanalyzed the world's literature on individual differences in cognitive abilities . . . no one else could have done it . . . it defines the taxonomy of cognitive differential psychology for many years to come." Burns (1994) was similarly impressed when he stated that Carroll's book "is simply the finest work of research and scholarship I have read and is destined to be *the classic study and reference work* on human abilities for decades to come" (p. 35; original emphasis). Horn (1998) described Carroll's (1993) work as a "tour de force summary and integration" that is the "definitive foundation for current theory" (p. 58); he also compared Carroll's summary to "Mendelyev's first presentation of a periodic table of elements in chemistry" (p. 58). Jensen (2004) stated that "on my first reading this tome, in 1993, I was reminded of the conductor Hans von Bülow's exclamation on first reading the full orchestral score of Wagner's *Die Meistersinger*, 'It's impossible, but there it is!' " (p. 4). Finally, according to Jensen,

> Carroll's magnum opus thus distills and synthesizes the results of a century of factor analyses of mental tests. It is virtually the grand finale of the era of psychometric *description and taxonomy* of human cognitive abilities. It is unlikely that his monumental feat will ever be attempted again by anyone, or that it could be much improved on. It will long be the key reference point and a solid foundation for the *explanatory* era of differential psychology that we now see burgeoning in genetics and the brain sciences. (p. 5; original emphasis)

The raw material reviewed and analyzed by Carroll was drawn from decades of tireless research by a diverse array of dedicated scholars (e.g., Spearman, Burt, Cattell, Gustaffson, Horn, Thurstone, Guilford, etc.). Carroll (1993) recognized that his theoretical model built on the research of others, particularly Cattell and Horn. According to Carroll, the Horn–Cattell Gf-Gc model "appears to offer the most well-founded and reasonable approach to an acceptable theory of the structure of cognitive abilities" (p. 62).

The beauty of Carroll's book was that for the first time ever, an empirically based taxonomy of human cognitive ability elements, based on the analysis (with a common method) of the extant literature since Spearman, was presented in a single, coherent, organized, systematic framework. Lubinski (2000) put a similar spin on the nature and importance of Carroll's principia when he stated that "Carroll's (1993) three-stratum theory is, in many respects, not new. Embryonic outlines are seen in earlier psychometric work (Burt, Cattell, Guttman, Humphreys, and Vernon, among others). But the empirical bases for Carroll's (1993) conclusions are unparalleled; readers should consult this source for a systematic detailing of more molecular abilities" (p. 412).

Carroll proposed a three-tier model of human cognitive abilities that differentiates abilities as a function of breadth. At the broadest level (stratum III) is a general intelligence factor, conceptually similar to Spearman's and Vernon's g. Next in breadth are eight broad abilities that represent "basic constitutional and long-standing characteristics of individuals that can govern or influence a great variety of behaviors in a given domain" (Carroll, 1993, p. 634). Stratum II includes the abilities of *fluid intelligence* (Gf), *crystallized intelligence* (Gc), *general memory and learning* (Gy), *broad visual perception* (Gv), *broad auditory perception* (Ga), *broad retrieval ability* (Gr), *broad cognitive speediness* (Gs), and *reaction time/decision speed* (Gt). Finally, stratum level I includes numerous narrow abilities that are subsumed by the stratum II abilities, which in turn are subsumed by the single stratum III g factor. Carroll's chapter in this volume (see Chapter 4) provides a more detailed summary of his model.

It is important to note that the typical schematic representation of Carroll's three-stratum model does not precisely mirror the operational structure generated by his EFA with the Schmid–Leiman orthogonalization procedure (EFA-SL). The typical depiction of Carroll's model looks much like the CHC theory model (Figure 8.1e). In reality, assuming a three-order (three-stratum) factor solution, Carroll's analyses looked more like Figure 8.1d, where the following elements are presented: (1) All tests' loading on the third-order g factor (arrows from g to T1–T12; omitted from figure); (2) salient loadings for tests on their respective first-order factor(s) (e.g., arrows from PMA1 to T1–T3); (3) salient loadings for tests on their respective second-order factor(s) (e.g., arrows from G_1 to T1–T6); (4) first-order factors' loading on their respective second-order factor(s) (e.g., arrows from G_1 to PMA1 and PMA2); and (5) second-order factors' loading on the third-order g factor (e.g., arrows from G_1 and G_2 to g).[8]

In a sense, Carroll provided the field of intelligence the much-needed "Rosetta stone" that would serve as a key for deciphering and organizing the enormous mass of human cognitive abilities structural literature that had accumulated since the days of Spearman. Carroll's work was also influential in creating the awareness among intelligence scholars, applied psychometricians, and assessment professionals, that understanding human cognitive abilities required

three-stratum vision. As a practical benefit, Carroll's work provided a common nomenclature for professional communication—a nomenclature that would go "far in helping us all better understand what we are measuring, facilitate better communication between and among professionals and scholars, and increase our ability to compare individual tests across and within intelligence batteries" (McGrew, 1997, p. 171).

The importance of the convergence on a provisional cognitive ability structural framework should not be minimized. Such a structure, grounded in a large body of convergent and discriminant validity research, is the first of at least a dozen conditions required for the building of an aptitude theory that can, in turn, produce a theory of aptitude–treatment interactions (Snow, 1998, p. 99).

CHC (Gf-Gc) Investigations, Integrations, and Extensions

The "CIA Book"

The collective influence of the Cattell–Horn Gf-Gc theory, Carroll's (1993) treatise, and the publication of the Cattell–Horn Gf-Gc-based WJ-R was reflected in the fact that nine chapters were either devoted to, or included significant treatment of, the Cattell–Horn Gf-Gc and/or Carroll three-stratum theories in Flanagan, Genshaft, and Harrison's (1997) edited volume *Contemporary Intellectual Assessment: Theories, Tests, and Issues* (often referred to as the "CIA book"). In turn, this publication was also a major theory-to-practice bridging event (see section E3 in Table 8.1), for three reasons.

First, the CIA book was the first one intended for university trainers and assessment practitioners that included chapters describing both the Cattell–Horn and Carroll models by the theorists themselves (Horn and Carroll). For those unfamiliar with the Horn Gf-Gc theory chapter in the WJ-R technical manual (McGrew et al., 1991), the CIA book provided a long-overdue introduction of the "state of the art" of contemporary psychometric theories of intelligence to the professional keepers of the tools of the intelligence-testing trade (e.g., school psychologists).

Second, Flanagan and I, while digesting

the implication of the need for three-stratum vision (as articulated by Carroll) and collaborating on a WJ-R–Kaufman Adolescent and Adult Intelligence Test (KAIT) cross-battery CFA study (see Flanagan & McGrew, 1998), realized that the prior Gf-Gc test classifications (Woodcock, 1990) described tests only at the broad-ability or stratum II level, and they needed to be "taken down to the next level"—to stratum I or the narrow-ability level.[9] In order to do so, a single taxonomy was needed. Neither the Cattell–Horn nor the Carroll model was picked over the other; instead, a "synthesized Carroll and Horn–Cattell Gf-Gc framework" (McGrew, 1997, p. 152) was developed, based on both Horn and Carroll's writings and a review of a previously unpublished EFA-SL of the WJ-R completed by Carroll (see section F1 in Table 8.1).

Finally, included in the CIA book was the first formal description of the assumptions, foundations, and operationalized set of principles for Gf-Gc cross-battery assessment (Flanagan & McGrew, 1997; see section F2 in Table 8.1). The cross-battery seed planted by Woodcock (1990) had given birth. The subsequent spreading of the assessment gospel as per Gf-Gc cross-battery (Flanagan & McGrew, 1997; Flanagan, McGrew, & Ortiz, 2000; Flanagan & Ortiz, 2001; Flanagan, Ortiz, Alfonso, & Mascolo, 2002; McGrew & Flanagan, 1998; see sections F4–F6 in Table 8.1) infused Gf–Gc theory into the minds of assessment practitioners and university training programs, regardless of their choice of favorite intelligence battery (e.g., the Cognitive Assessment System [CAS], the Differential Ability Scales [DAS], the K-ABC, the SB-IV, or the Wechsler Intelligence Scale for Children—Third Edition [WISC-III]). The formalization of Gf-Gc cross-battery assessment, primarily as the result of the work of Flanagan, was another significant theory-to-practice bridging event. Daniel (1997) described the cross-battery approach as "intriguing" and "creative work now being done to integrate and interpret all cognitive batteries within the framework of a single multifactor model" (p. 1043).

Gf-Gc cross-battery assessment did not discriminate among test kits on the basis of test name, heritage, publisher, type or color of carrying case, prominent authors (dead or alive), or presence or absence of manip-

ulatives or a performance scale. The cumulative impact of the introduction of Gf-Gc cross-battery assessment, following on the heels of the 1989 publication of the Gf-Gc organized WJ-R and Carroll's 1993 principia, established a Gf-Gc theory foothold in the field of applied intelligence testing. The intelligence theory-to-practice gap had narrowed fast. The CHC "tipping point" had been reached.[10]

CHC: The Rest of the Story

The first published record of the linking of Cattell–Horn–Carroll is in Flanagan and colleagues (2000), where it was stated that "a first effort to create a single Gf-Gc taxonomy for use in the evaluation and interpretation of intelligence batteries was the integrated Cattell–Horn–Carroll model (McGrew, 1997)" (p. 28).

The derivation of the name Cattell–Horn–Carroll (CHC) theory remains a mystery to many. To the best of my knowledge, the first formal published definition of CHC theory was presented in the WJ III technical manual (McGrew & Woodcock, 2001; see section F5 in Table 8.1):

> Cattell–Horn–Carroll theory of cognitive abilities. An amalgamation of two similar theories about the content and structure of human cognitive abilities (J. B. Carroll & J. L. Horn, personal communication, July 1999). The first of these two theories is Gf-Gc theory (Cattell, 1941; Horn, 1965) and the second is Carroll's (1993) three-stratum theory. CHC taxonomy is the most comprehensive and empirically supported framework available for understanding the structure of human cognitive abilities. (p. 9)

Despite the foothold Gf-Gc theory had achieved in the field of applied intelligence testing prior to 1999, the term "Gf-Gc" was often met with puzzled looks by recipients of psychological reports, sounded esoteric and nonmeaningful, and continued unintentionally to convey the inaccurate belief that the theory was a two-factor model (Gf and Gc), despite the fact that it had evolved to a model of eight or nine broad abilities. Having dealt with this communication problem since the publication of the WJ-R in 1989, Woodcock, together with the author of the Stanford–Binet Intelligence Scales, Fifth Edition (SB5; Roid, 2003) and staff members from Riverside Publishing, met with Horn and Carroll privately in Chapel Hill, North Carolina, to seek a common, more meaningful umbrella term that would recognize the strong structural similarities of their respective theoretical models, yet also recognize their differences. This sequence of conversations resulted in a verbal agreement that the phrase "Cattell–Horn–Carroll theory of cognitive abilities" made significant practical sense, and appropriately recognized the historical order of scholarly contribution of the three primary contributors (see section E4 in Table 8.1). That was it. The term *CHC theory* emerged from private personal communications in July 1999, and seeped into subsequent publications.[11]

CHC theory represents *both* the Cattell–Horn and Carroll models, in their respective splendor. Much like the phrase "information-processing theories or models," which provides an overarching theoretical umbrella for a spectrum of very similar (yet different) theoretical model variations (Lohman, 2001), CHC theory serves the same function for the "variations on a Gf-Gc theme" by Cattell–Horn and Carroll, respectively. Table 8.2 compares and contrasts the major similarities and differences between the Cattell–Horn Gf-Gc and Carroll three-stratum models. As described above, the CHC model (Figure 8.1e) used extensively in applied psychometrics and intelligence testing during the past decade is a consensus model. The specific organization and definitions of broad and narrow CHC abilities are summarized in Table 8.3.

In the next section, a review of the CHC-related structural factor-analytic research published during the past decade is presented.[12] The purpose of this review is to help the field iterate toward a more complete and better understanding of the structure of human cognitive abilities.

EMPIRICAL EVALUATIONS OF THE "COMPLETE" CHC MODEL

An acknowledged limitation of Carroll's (1993, p. 579) three-stratum model was the fact that his inferences regarding the relations between different factors at different levels (strata) emerged from data derived from a diverse array of studies and samples.

None of Carroll's datasets included the necessary breadth of variables to evaluate, in a single analysis, the general structure of his proposed three-stratum model. The sample sizes of most studies reviewed by Carroll were modest (median $n = 198$) and were limited in the breadth of variables analyzed (median number of variables = 19.6) (Roberts, Pallier, & Nelson-Goff, 1999). Some domains were weakly represented (e.g., Ga). According to Roberts and colleagues (1999), "no investigator has used [CFA] techniques to determine whether there is empirical support for the structure comprising the most salient aspects (i.e., Strata I and II) of Carroll's (1993) model" (p. 344).

This past decade has witnessed a number of EFA and/or CFA investigations that have included a wider range of CHC construct indicators. Collectively, these studies provide an opportunity to evaluate and validate the broad strokes of the CHC model (see Figure 8.1e and Table 8.3). Other studies, although not specifically designed to evaluate the CHC model, when viewed through a CHC lens provide additional support for major portions of the CHC model. The factor-analytic studies reviewed next were either (1) designed as per the CHC framework, (2) designed as per the Carroll and/or Cattell–Horn Gf-Gc models, and/or (3) were non-CHC studies that are now interpreted here through a post hoc CHC lens. Collectively, these studies provide empirical support for the broad strokes of contemporary CHC theory.

Large-Sample Studies

Studies with CHC-Designed Batteries

The most thorough evaluations of the structure of CHC theory are factor-analytic studies of variables from standardized test batteries administered to large, nationally representative samples. The most comprehensive evaluation of Carroll's three-stratum CHC model is the hierarchical cross-age (ages 6 through 90 years) multiple-group CFA of the WJ-R norm data by Bickley, Keith, and Wolfe (1995). Consistent with Carroll's (1993) conclusion that the structure of cognitive abilities is largely the same across ages, Bickley and colleagues found that the structure of cognitive abilities, as de-

TABLE 8.2. Comparison of Cattell–Horn and Carroll Theories of Human Cognitive Abilities

Cattell–Horn Gf-Gc theory	Carroll three-stratum theory	Salient similarities and differences
General intelligence (*g*)		
No	Yes	*g* (Carroll) vs. non-*g* (Cattell–Horn).
Broad abilities		
Fluid reasoning (Gf)	Fluid intelligence (Gf)	Similar.
Acculturation knowledge (Gc)	Crystallized intelligence (Gc)	Similar, with the exception that Carroll (1993 and Chapter 4, this volume) included reading and writing as narrow abilities under Gc. Horn (Horn & Noll, 1997; Horn & Masunaga, 2000) does not include reading and writing under Gc. Horn (1988) previously suggested a possible broad "language use" ability separate from Gc. Carroll (2003) subsequently noted a similar "language" factor in need of further research.
Short-term apprehension and retrieval abilities (SAR)	General memory and learning (Gy)	Carroll (1993) defined Gy as a broad ability that involves learning and memory abilities. Gy includes short-term memory span and other intermediate- to long-term memory abilities (e.g., associative, meaningful, and free-recall memory). Carroll indicated that "present evidence is not sufficient to permit a clear specification of the structure of learning and memory abilities" (p. 625). In contrast, Horn's *SAR* is more narrowly defined by short-term and working memory abilities (Horn & Noll, 1997; Horn & Masunaga, 2000). Horn includes intermediate and long-term associative and retrieval abilities under TSR/Glm.
Visual processing (Gv)	Broad visual perception (Gv)	Similar.
Auditory processing (Ga)	Broad auditory perception (Ga)	Similar.
Tertiary storage and retrieval (TSR/Glm)	Broad retrieval ability (Gr)	Carroll (1993) defined this domain primarily as the ready retrieval (fluency) and production of concepts or ideas from long-term memory (idea production). Horn also includes the same fluency of retrieval abilities, but adds a second category of abilities that involve the fluency of association in retrieval from storage over *intermediate* periods of time (minutes to hours). Carroll (1993 and Chapter 4, this volume) included these later abilities (e.g., associative memory) under Gy.
Processing speed (Gs)	Broad cognitive speediness (Gs)	Similar.
Correct decision speed (CDS)	Processing speed (RT decision speed) (Gt)	Horn's CDS (Horn & Mansunaga, 2000) appears to be defined as a more narrow ability (quickness in providing correct or incorrect answers to nontrivial tasks). Carroll's (1993) definition appears slightly broader (decision or reaction time as measured by reaction time paradigms).
Quantitative knowledge (Gq)		Horn (Horn & Noll, 1997; Horn & Masunaga, 2000) recognizes Gq as the understanding and application of math skills and concepts. Carroll (1993) reported separate narrow (stratum I) math achievement and knowledge abilities in a chapter on "Abilities in the Domain of Knowledge and Achievement." Carroll (2003) subsequently reported and acknowledged a Gq (Mathematics) factor.

Note. Complete, up-to-date definitions for each broad ability, plus narrow abilities under each broad ability, are presented in Table 8.3.

TABLE 8.3. Broad (Stratum II) and Narrow (Stratum I) CHC Ability Definitions

Fluid intelligence/reasoning (Gf): The use of deliberate and controlled mental operations to solve novel, "on-the-spot" problems (i.e., tasks that cannot be performed automatically). Mental operations often include drawing inferences, concept formation, classification, generating and testing hypotheses, identifying relations, comprehending implications, problem solving, extrapolating, and transforming information. Inductive reasoning (inference of a generalized conclusion from particular instances) and deductive reasoning (the deriving of a conclusion by reasoning; specifically, inference in which the conclusion about particulars follows necessarily from general or universal premises) are generally considered the hallmark indicators of Gf. Gf has been linked to *cognitive complexity*, which can be defined as a greater use of a wide and diverse array of elementary cognitive processes during performance.

General sequential (deductive) reasoning (RG): Ability to start with stated assertions (rules, premises, or conditions) and to engage in one or more steps leading to a solution to a problem. The processes are deductive as evidenced in the ability to reason and draw conclusions from given general conditions or premises to the specific. Often known as *hypothetico-deductive reasoning*.

Induction (I): Ability to discover the underlying characteristic (e.g., rule, concept, principle, process, trend, class membership) that underlies a specific problem or a set of observations, or to apply a previously learned rule to the problem. Reasoning from specific cases or observations to general rules or broad generalizations. Often requires the ability to combine separate pieces of information in the formation of inferences, rules, hypotheses, or conclusions.

Quantitative reasoning (RQ): Ability to inductively (I) and/or deductively (RG) reason with concepts involving mathematical relations and properties.

Piagetian reasoning (RP): Ability to demonstrate the acquisition and application (in the form of logical thinking) of cognitive concepts as defined by Piaget's developmental cognitive theory. These concepts include *seriation* (organizing material into an orderly series that facilitates understanding of relationships between events), *conservation* (awareness that physical quantities do not change in amount when altered in appearance), *classification* (ability to organize materials that possess similar characteristics into categories), etc.

Speed of reasoning (RE): Speed or fluency in performing reasoning tasks (e.g., quickness in generating as many possible rules, solutions, etc., to a problem) in a limited time. Also listed under Gs.

Crystallized intelligence/knowledge (Gc): "Can be thought of as the intelligence of the culture that is incorporated by individuals through a process of acculturation" (Horn, 1994, p. 443). Gc is typically described as a person's wealth (breadth and depth) of acquired knowledge of the language, information and concepts of specific a culture, and/or the application of this knowledge. Gc is primarily a store of verbal or language-based declarative (knowing "what") and procedural (knowing "how") knowledge, acquired through the "investment" of other abilities during formal and informal educational and general life experiences.

Language development (LD): General development or understanding and application of words, sentences, and paragraphs (not requiring reading) in spoken native-language skills to express or communicate a thought or feeling.

Lexical knowledge (VL): Extent of vocabulary (nouns, verbs, or adjectives) that can be understood in terms of correct word (semantic) meanings. Although evidence indicates that vocabulary knowledge is a separable component from LD, it is often difficult to disentangle these two highly correlated abilities in research studies.

Listening ability (LS): Ability to listen and understand the meaning of oral communications (spoken words, phrases, sentences, and paragraphs). The ability to receive and understand spoken information.

General (verbal) information (K0): Range of general stored knowledge (primarily verbal).

Information about culture (K2): Range of stored general cultural knowledge (e.g., music, art).

Communication ability (CM): Ability to speak in "real-life" situations (e.g., lecture, group participation) in a manner that transmits ideas, thoughts, or feelings to one or more individuals.

Oral production and fluency (OP): More specific or narrow oral communication skills than reflected by CM.

Grammatical sensitivity (MY): Knowledge or awareness of the distinctive features and structural principles of a native language that allows for the construction of words (morphology) and sentences (syntax). Not the skill in applying this knowledge.

Foreign-language proficiency (KL): Similar to LD, but for a foreign language.

Foreign-language aptitude (LA): Rate and ease of learning a new language.

(continued)

TABLE 8.3. *(continued)*

General (domain-specific) knowledge (**Gkn**): An individual's breadth and depth of acquired knowledge in specialized (demarcated) domains that typically do not represent the general universal experiences of individuals in a culture (Gc). Gkn reflects deep, specialized knowledge domains developed through intensive systematic practice and training (over an extended period of time), and the maintenance of the knowledge base through regular practice and motivated effort. The primary distinction between Gc and Gkn is the extent to which acquired knowledge is a function of the degree of cultural universality. Gc primarily reflects general knowledge accumulated via the experience of cultural universals.

Knowledge of English as a second language (KE): Degree of knowledge of English as a second language.

Knowledge of signing (KF): Knowledge of finger spelling and signing (e.g., American Sign Language) used in communication with persons with hearing impairments.

Skill in lip reading (LP): Competence in ability to understand communication from others by watching the movement of their mouths and expressions. Also known as *speech reading*.

Geography achievement (A5): Range of geography knowledge (e.g., capitals of countries).

General science information (K1): Range of stored scientific knowledge (e.g., biology, physics, engineering, mechanics, electronics).

Mechanical knowledge (MK): Knowledge about the function, terminology, and operation of ordinary tools, machines, and equipment. Since these factors were identified in research prior to the information/technology explosion, it is unknown whether this ability generalizes to the use of modern technology (e.g., faxes, computers, the Internet).

Knowledge of behavioral content (BC): Knowledge or sensitivity to nonverbal human communication/interaction systems (beyond understanding sounds and words; e.g., facial expressions and gestures) that communicate feelings, emotions, and intentions, most likely in a culturally patterned style.

Visual–spatial abilities (**Gv**): "The ability to generate, retain, retrieve, and transform well-structured visual images" (Lohman, 1994, p. 1000). The Gv domain represents a collection of different abilities emphasizing different processes involved in the generation, storage, retrieval, and transformation (e.g., mentally reversing or rotating shapes in space) of visual images. Gv abilities are measured by tasks (figural or geometric stimuli) that require the perception and transformation of visual shapes, forms, or images, and/or tasks that require maintaining spatial orientation with regard to objects that may change or move through space.

Visualization (Vz): The ability to apprehend a spatial form, object, or scene and match it with another spatial object, form, or scene with the requirement to rotate it (one or more times) in two or three dimensions. Requires the ability to mentally imagine, manipulate, or transform objects or visual patterns (without regard to speed of responding) and to "see" (predict) how they would appear under altered conditions (e.g., when parts are moved or rearranged). Differs from SR primarily by a deemphasis on fluency.

Spatial relations (SR): Ability to rapidly perceive and manipulate (mental rotation, transformations, reflection, etc.) visual patterns, or to maintain orientation with respect to objects in space. SR may require the identification of an object when viewed from different angles or positions.

Closure speed (CS): Ability to quickly identify a familiar meaningful visual object from incomplete (vague, partially obscured, disconnected) visual stimuli, without knowing in advance what the object is. The target object is assumed to be represented in the person's long-term memory store. The ability to "fill in" unseen or missing parts in a disparate perceptual field and form a single percept.

Flexibility of closure (CF): Ability to identify a visual figure or pattern embedded in a complex, distracting, or disguised visual pattern or array, when knowing in advance what the pattern is. Recognition of, yet the ability to ignore, distracting background stimuli is part of the ability.

Visual memory (MV): Ability to form and store a mental representation or image of a visual shape or configuration (typically during a brief study period), over at least a few seconds, and then to recognize or recall it later (during the test phase).

Spatial scanning (SS): Ability to quickly and accurately survey (visually explore) a wide or complicated spatial field or pattern and identify a particular configuration (path) through the visual field. Usually requires visually following the indicated route or path through the visual field.

Serial perceptual integration (PI): Ability to identify (and typically name) a pictorial or visual pattern when parts of the pattern are presented rapidly in serial order (e.g., portions of a line drawing of a dog are passed in sequence through a small "window").

Length estimation (LE): Ability to accurately estimate or compare visual lengths or distances without the aid of measurement instruments.

(continued)

TABLE 8.3. *(continued)*

Perceptual illusions (IL): The ability to resist being affected by the illusory perceptual aspects of geometric figures (i.e., not forming a mistaken perception in response to some characteristic of the stimuli). May best be thought of as a person's "response tendency" to resist perceptual illusions.

Perceptual alternations (PN): Consistency in the rate of alternating between different visual perceptions.

Imagery (IM): Ability to mentally depict (encode) and/or manipulate an object, idea, event or impression (that is not present) in the form of an abstract spatial form. Separate IM level and rate (fluency) factors have been suggested (see chapter text).

Auditory processing **(Ga):** Abilities that "depend on sound as input and on the functioning of our hearing apparatus" (Stankov, 1994, p. 157). A key characteristic of Ga abilities is the extent to which an individual can cognitively "control" (i.e., handle the competition between "signal" and "noise") the perception of auditory information (Gustafsson & Undheim, 1996), The Ga domain circumscribes a wide range of abilities involved in discriminating patterns in sounds and musical structure (often under background noise and/or distorting conditions), as well as the abilities to analyze, manipulate, comprehend, and synthesize sound elements, groups of sounds, or sound patterns. Although Ga abilities play an important role in the development of language abilities (Gc), Ga abilities do not require the comprehension of language (Gc).

Phonetic coding (PC): Ability to code, process, and be sensitive to nuances in phonemic information (speech sounds) in short-term memory. Includes the ability to identify, isolate, blend, or transform sounds of speech. Frequently referred to as *phonological* or *phonemic awareness.*

Speech sound discrimination (US): Ability to detect and discriminate differences in phonemes or speech sounds under conditions of little or no distraction or distortion.

Resistance to auditory stimulus distortion (UR): Ability to overcome the effects of distortion or distraction when listening to and understanding speech and language. It is often difficult to separate UR from US in research studies.

Memory for sound patterns (UM): Ability to retain (on a short-term basis) auditory events such as tones, tonal patterns, and voices.

General sound discrimination (U3): Ability to discriminate tones, tone patterns, or musical materials with regard to their fundamental attributes (pitch, intensity, duration, and rhythm).

Temporal tracking (UK): Ability to mentally track auditory temporal (sequential) events so as to be able to count, anticipate or rearrange them (e.g., reorder a set of musical tones). According to Stankov (2000), UK may represent the first recognition of the ability (Stankov & Horn, 1980) that is now interpreted as working memory (MW).

Musical discrimination and judgment (U1, U9): Ability to discriminate and judge tonal patterns in music with respect to melodic, harmonic, and expressive aspects (e.g., phrasing, tempo, harmonic complexity, intensity variations).

Maintaining and judging rhythm (U8): Ability to recognize and maintain a musical beat.

Sound intensity/duration discrimination (U6): Ability to discriminate sound intensities and to be sensitive to the temporal/rhythmic aspects of tonal patterns.

Sound frequency discrimination (U5): Ability to discriminate frequency attributes (pitch and timbre) of tones.

Hearing and speech threshold factors (UA, UT, UU): Ability to hear pitch and varying sound frequencies.

Absolute pitch (UP): Ability to perfectly identify the pitch of tones.

Sound localization (UL): Ability to localize heard sounds in space.

Short-term memory **(Gsm):** The ability to apprehend and maintain awareness of elements of information in the immediate situation (events that occurred in the last minute or so). A limited-capacity system that loses information quickly through the decay of memory traces, unless an individual activates other cognitive resources to maintain the information in immediate awareness.

Memory span (MS): Ability to attend to, register, and immediately recall (after only one presentation) temporally ordered elements and then reproduce the series of elements in correct order.

(continued)

TABLE 8.3. *(continued)*

Working memory (MW): Ability to temporarily store and perform a set of cognitive operations on information that requires divided attention and the management of the limited capacity resources of short-term memory. Is largely recognized to be the mind's "scratchpad" and consists of up to four subcomponents. The *phonological or articulatory loop* processes auditory–linguistic information, while the *visual–spatial sketchpad/scratchpad* is the temporary buffer for visually processed information. The *central executive mechanism* coordinates and manages the activities and processes in working memory. The component most recently added to the model is the episodic buffer. Recent research (see chapter text) suggests that MW is *not* of the same nature as the other 60+ narrow-factor-based, trait-like individual-difference constructs included in this table. MW is a theoretically developed construct (proposed to explain memory findings from experimental research) and not a label for an individual-difference-type factor. MW is retained in the current CHC taxonomy table as a reminder of the importance of this construct in understanding new learning and performance of complex cognitive tasks (see chapter text).

Long-term storage and retrieval **(Glr):** The ability to store and consolidate new information in long-term memory, and later fluently retrieve the stored information (e.g., concepts, ideas, items, names) through association. Memory consolidation and retrieval can be measured in terms of information stored for minutes, hours, weeks, or longer. Horn (Horn & Masunaga, 2000) differentiates two major types of Glr—fluency of retrieval of information over minutes or a few hours (*intermediate memory*), and fluency of association in retrieval from storage over days, months or years. Ekstrom et al. (1979) distinguished two additional characteristic processes of Glr: "(1) reproductive processes, which are concerned with retrieving stored facts, and (2) reconstructive processes, which involve the generation of material based on stored rules" (p. 24). Glr abilities have been prominent in creativity research, where they have been referred to as *idea production, ideational fluency,* or *associative fluency.*

Associative memory (MA): Ability to recall one part of a previously learned but unrelated pair of items (that may or may not be meaningfully linked) when the other part is presented (e.g., paired-associate learning).

Meaningful memory (MM): Ability to note, retain, and recall information (set of items or ideas) where there is a meaningful relation between the bits of information, the information comprises a meaningful story or connected discourse, or the information relates to existing contents of memory.

Free-recall memory (M6): Ability to recall (without associations) as many unrelated items as possible, in any order, after a large collection of items is presented (each item presented singly). Requires the ability to encode a "superspan collection of material" (Carroll, 1993, p. 277) that cannot be kept active in short-term or working memory.

Ideational fluency (FI): Ability to rapidly produce a series of ideas, words, or phrases related to a specific condition or object. Quantity, not quality or response originality, is emphasized. The ability to think of a large number of different responses when a given task requires the generation of numerous responses. Ability to call up ideas.

Associational fluency (FA): A highly specific ability to rapidly produce a series of words or phrases associated in meaning (semantically associated; or some other common semantic property) when given a word or concept with a restricted area of meaning. In contrast to FI, quality rather quantity of production is emphasized.

Expressional fluency (FE): Ability to rapidly think of and organize words or phrases into meaningful complex ideas under general or more specific cued conditions. Requires the production of connected discourse in contrast to the production of isolated words (e.g., FA, FW). Differs from FI in the requirement to rephrase given ideas rather than generating new ideas. The ability to produce different ways of saying much the same thing.

Naming facility (NA): Ability to rapidly produce accepted names for concepts or things when presented with the thing itself or a picture of it (or cued in some other appropriate way). The naming responses must be in an individual's long-term memory store (i.e., objects or things to be named have names that are very familiar to the individual). In contemporary reading research, this ability is called *rapid automatic naming* (RAN).

Word fluency (FW): Ability to rapidly produce isolated words that have specific phonemic, structural, or orthographic characteristics (independent of word meanings). Has been mentioned as possibly being related to the "tip-of-the-tongue" phenomenon (Carroll, 1993). One of the first fluency abilities identified (Ekstrom et al., 1979).

Figural fluency (FF): Ability to rapidly draw or sketch as many things (or elaborations) as possible when presented with a nonmeaningful visual stimulus (e.g., set of unique visual elements). Quantity is emphasized over quality or uniqueness.

Figural flexibility (FX): Ability to rapidly change set and try out a variety of approaches to solutions for figural problems that have several stated criteria. Fluency in successfully dealing with figural tasks that require a variety of approaches to a given problem.

(continued)

TABLE 8.3. *(continued)*

Sensitivity to problems (SP): Ability to rapidly think of a number of alternative solutions to practical problems (e.g., different uses of a given tool). More broadly may be considered imagining problems dealing with a function or change of function of objects and/or identifying methods to address the problems (Royce, 1973). Requires the recognition of the existence of a problem.

Originality/creativity (FO): Ability to rapidly produce unusual, original, clever, divergent, or uncommon responses (expressions, interpretations) to a given topic, situation, or task. The ability to invent unique solutions to problems or to develop innovative methods for situations where a standard operating procedure does not apply. Following a new and unique path to a solution. FO differs from FI in that FO focuses on the quality of creative responses, while FI focuses on an individual's ability to think of a large number of different responses.

Learning abilities (L1): General learning ability rate. Poorly defined by existing research.

Cognitive Processing Speed (Gs): The ability to automatically and fluently perform relatively easy or overlearned cognitive tasks, especially when high mental efficiency (i.e., attention and focused concentration) is required. The speed of executing relatively overlearned or automatized elementary cognitive processes.

Perceptual speed (P): Ability to rapidly and accurately search, compare (for visual similarities or differences) and identify visual elements presented side by side or separated in a visual field. Recent research (Ackerman, Beier, & Boyle, 2002; Ackerman & Cianciolo, 2000; Ackerman & Kanfer, 1993; see chapter text) suggests that P may be an *intermediate*-stratum ability (between narrow and broad) defined by four narrow subabilities:

1. *Pattern recognition (Ppr):* Ability to quickly recognize simple visual patterns.
2. *Scanning (Ps):* Ability to scan, compare, and look up visual stimuli.
3. *Memory (Pm):* Ability to perform visual-perceptual speed tasks that place significant demands on immediate short-term memory.
4. *Complex (Pc):* Ability to perform visual pattern recognition tasks that impose additional cognitive demands, such as spatial visualization, estimating and interpolating, and heightened memory span loads.

Rate of test taking (R9): Ability to rapidly perform tests that are relatively easy or overlearned (require very simple decisions). This ability is not associated with any particular type of test content or stimuli. May be similar to a higher-order *psychometric time* factor (Roberts & Stankov, 1999; Stankov, 2000). Recent research has suggested that R9 may better be classified as an *intermediate*-stratum ability (between narrow and broad) that subsumes almost all psychometric speeded measures (see chapter text).

Number facility (N): Ability to rapidly perform basic arithmetic (i.e., add, subtract, multiply, divide) and accurately manipulate numbers quickly. N does not involve understanding or organizing mathematical problems and is not a major component of mathematical/quantitative reasoning or higher mathematical skills.

Speed of reasoning (RE): Speed or fluency in performing reasoning tasks (e.g., quickness in generating as many possible rules, solutions, etc., to a problem) in a limited time. Also listed under Gf.

Reading speed (fluency) (RS): Ability to silently read and comprehend connected text (e.g., a series of short sentences, a passage) rapidly and automatically (with little conscious attention to the mechanics of reading). Also listed under Grw.

Writing speed (fluency) (WS): Ability to copy words or sentences correctly and repeatedly, or writing words, sentences, or paragraphs as quickly as possible. Also listed under Grw and Gps.

Decision/reaction time or speed (Gt): The ability to react and/or make decisions quickly in response to simple stimuli, typically measured by chronometric measures of reaction and inspection time. In psychometric methods, quickness in providing answers (correct or incorrect) to tasks of trivial difficulty (also known as *correct decision speed*, or CDS)—may relate to cognitive tempo.

Simple reaction time (R1): Reaction time (in milliseconds) to the onset of a single stimulus (visual or auditory) that is presented at a particular point of time. R1 is frequently divided into the phases of *decision time* (DT; the time to decide to make a response and the finger leaves a home button) and *movement time* (MT; the time to move finger from the home button to another button where the response is physically made and recorded).

Choice reaction time (R2): Reaction time (in milliseconds) to the onset of one of two or more alternative stimuli, depending on which alternative is signaled. Similar to R1, can be decomposed into DT and MT. A frequently used experimental method for measuring R2 is the Hick paradigm.

Semantic processing speed (R4): Reaction time (in milliseconds) when a decision requires some encoding and mental manipulation of the stimulus content.

Mental comparison speed (R7): Reaction time (in milliseconds) where stimuli must be compared for a particular characteristic or attribute.

(continued)

TABLE 8.3. *(continued)*

Inspection time (IT): The ability to quickly (in milliseconds) detect change or discriminate between alternatives in a very briefly displayed stimulus (e.g., two different-sized vertical lines joined horizontally across the top).

Psychomotor speed (**Gps**): The ability to rapidly and fluently perform body motor movements (movement of fingers, hands, legs, etc.), independently of cognitive control.

Speed of limb movement (R3): The ability to make rapid specific or discrete motor movements of the arms or legs (measured after the movement is initiated). Accuracy is not important.

Writing speed (fluency) (WS): Ability to copy words or sentences correctly and repeatedly, or writing words, sentences, or paragraphs as quickly as possible. Also listed under Grw and Gps.

Speed of articulation (PT): Ability to rapidly perform successive articulations with the speech musculature.

Movement time (MT): Recent research (see summaries by Deary, 2003; Nettelbeck, 2003; see chapter text) suggests that MT may be an intermediate-stratum ability (between narrow and broad strata) that represents the second phase of reaction time as measured by various elementary cognitive tasks. The time taken to physically move a body part (e.g., a finger) to make the required response is MT. MT may also measure the speed of finger, limb, or multilimb movements or vocal articulation (*diadochokinesis*; Greek for "successive movements") (Carroll, 1993; Stankov, 2000); it is also listed under Gt.

Quantitative knowledge (**Gq**): A person's wealth (breadth and depth) of acquired store of declarative and procedural quantitative knowledge. Gq is largely acquired through the "investment" of other abilities, primarily during formal educational experiences. It is important to recognize that RQ, which is the ability to reason inductively and deductively when solving quantitative problems, is not included under Gq, but rather is included in the Gf domain. Gq represents an individual's store of acquired mathematical knowledge, not reasoning with this knowledge.

Mathematical knowledge (KM): Range of general knowledge about mathematics. Not the performance of mathematical operations or the solving of math problems.

Mathematical achievement (A3): Measured (tested) mathematics achievement.

Reading/writing (**Grw**): A person's wealth (breadth and depth) of acquired store of declarative and procedural reading and writing skills and knowledge. *Grw* includes both basic skills (e.g., reading and spelling of single words) and the ability to read and write complex connected discourse (e.g., reading comprehension and the ability to write a story).

Reading decoding (RD): Ability to recognize and decode words or pseudowords in reading, using a number of subabilities (e.g., grapheme encoding, perceiving multiletter units and phonemic contrasts, etc.).

Reading comprehension (RC): Ability to attain meaning (comprehend and understand) connected discourse during reading.

Verbal (printed) language comprehension (V): General development, or the understanding of words, sentences, and paragraphs in native language, as measured by reading vocabulary and reading comprehension tests. Does not involve writing, listening to, or understanding spoken information.

Cloze ability (CZ): Ability to read and supply missing words (that have been systematically deleted) from prose passages. Correct answers can only be supplied if the person understands (comprehends) the meaning of the passage.

Spelling ability (SG): Ability to form words with the correct letters in accepted order (spelling).

Writing ability (WA): Ability to communicate information and ideas in written form so that others can understand (with clarity of thought, organization, and good sentence structure). Is a broad ability that involves a number of other writing subskills (knowledge of grammar, the meaning of words, and how to organize sentences or paragraphs).

English usage knowledge (EU): Knowledge of the "mechanics" (capitalization, punctuation, usage, and spelling) of written and spoken English-language discourse.

Reading speed (fluency) (RS): Ability to silently read and comprehend connected text (e.g., a series of short sentences, a passage) rapidly and automatically (with little conscious attention to the mechanics of reading). Also listed under Gs.

Writing speed (fluency) (WS): Ability to copy words or sentences correctly and repeatedly, or writing words, sentences, or paragraphs as quickly as possible. Also listed under Gs and Gps.

(continued)

TABLE 8.3. *(continued)*

Psychomotor abilities **(Gp):** The ability to perform body motor movements (movement of fingers, hands, legs, etc.) with precision, coordination, or strength.

Static strength (P3): The ability to exert muscular force to move (push, lift, pull) a relatively heavy or immobile object.

Multilimb coordination (P6): The ability to make quick specific or discrete motor movements of the arms or legs (measured after the movement is initiated). Accuracy is not relevant.

Finger dexterity (P2): The ability to make precisely coordinated movements of the fingers (with or without the manipulation of objects).

Manual dexterity (P1): Ability to make precisely coordinated movements of a hand, or a hand and the attached arm.

Arm–hand steadiness (P7): The ability to precisely and skillfully coordinate arm–hand positioning in space.

Control precision (P8): The ability to exert precise control over muscle movements, typically in response to environmental feedback (e.g., changes in speed or position of object being manipulated).

Aiming (AI): The ability to precisely and fluently execute a sequence of eye–hand coordination movements for positioning purposes.

Gross body equilibrium (P4): The ability to maintain the body in an upright position in space, or regain balance after balance has been disturbed.

Olfactory abilities **(Go):** Abilities that depend on sensory receptors of the main olfactory system (nasal chambers). The cognitive and perceptual aspects of this domain have not yet been widely investigated (see chapter text).

Olfactory memory (OM): Memory for odors (smells).

Olfactory sensitivity (OS): Sensitivity to different odors (smells).

Tactile abilities **(Gh):** Abilities that depend on sensory receptors of the tactile (touch) system for input and on the functioning of the tactile apparatus. The cognitive and perceptual aspects of this domain have not yet been widely investigated (see chapter text).

Tactile sensitivity (TS): The ability to detect and make fine discriminations of pressure on the surface of the skin.

Kinesthetic abilities **(Gk):** Abilities that depend on sensory receptors that detect bodily position, weight, or movement of the muscles, tendons, and joints. The cognitive and perceptual aspects of this domain have not yet been widely investigated.

Kinesthetic sensitivity (KS): The ability to detect, or be aware, of movements of the body or body parts, including the movement of upper body limbs (arms), and the ability to recognize a path the body previously explored without the aid of visual input (blindfolded).

Note. Many of the ability definitions in this table, or portions thereof, were originally published in McGrew (1997); these, in turn, were developed from a detailed reading of *Human Cognitive Abilities: A Survey of Factor-Analytic Studies* (Carroll, 1993). The two-letter narrow-ability (stratum I) factor codes (e.g., RG), as well as most of the broad-ability factor codes (e.g., Gf), are from Carroll (1993). The McGrew (1997) definitions have been revised and extended here, based on a review of a number of additional sources. Primary sources include Carroll (1993), Corsini (1999), Ekstrom et al. (1979), Fleishman and Quaintance (1984), and Sternberg (1994). An ongoing effort to refine the CHC definitions of abilities can be found in the form of the Cattell–Horn–Carroll (CHC) Definition Project (*http://www.iapsych.com/chcdef.htm*).

fined by eight broad abilities (Gf, Gv, Gs, Glr, Gc, Ga, Gsm, Gq) and a higher-order g ability, was invariant from childhood to late adulthood. The authors concluded that "this study provides compelling evidence that the three-stratum theory may form a parsimonious model of intelligence. The fact that it is also grounded in a strong foundation of vast, previous research also lends strong support for the acceptance of the model" (p. 323).

More recently, in the large, nationally representative WJ III standardization sample, we (McGrew & Woodcock, 2001) reported a CHC-based CFA of 50 test variables from ages 6 through late adulthood. Support was found for a model consisting of a higher-order g factor that subsumed the broad abilities of Gf, Gc, Gv, Ga, Gsm, Glr, Gs, Grw, and Gq. A comparison with four alternative models found the CHC model to be the most plausible representation of the structure in the data.

Subsequently, we (Taub & McGrew, 2004) used multiple-group CFAs to evaluate the factorial cross-age invariance of the WJ III COG from ages 6 through 90+. In addition to supporting the construct validity of a higher-order g and seven lower-order broad CHC factors (Gf, Gc, Gv, Ga, Gsm, Glr, Gs), our analyses supported the invariance of the WJ III COG measurement and CHC theoretical frameworks. These findings are consistent with those of Bickley and colleagues (1995) and provide additional support for the validity of the broad- and general-stratum abilities of CHC theory (from childhood through adulthood).

Of particular interest to the current chapter is the fact that in his last formal publication, Carroll (2003) applied his factor-analytic procedures and skills to an investigation of the structure of the 1989 WJ-R norm data. The purpose of Carroll's analyses was to compare the viability of three different views of the structure of human cognitive abilities. To paraphrase Carroll, these views can be characterized as follows:

1. *Standard multifactorial model*. This is the classic view of Spearman (Spearman, 1927, Spearman & Wynn Jones, 1950) and others (e.g., Carroll, 1993; Jensen, 1998; Thurstone & Thurstone, 1941) that a general (g) intelligence factor exists, as well as a variety of less general "broad" abilities.

2. *Limited structural analysis model*. This model also posits the presence of higher-order g ability, as well as lower-order broad abilities; however, it suggests that fluid intelligence (Gf) is highly correlated with, and may be identical with, g. This model is primarily associated with Gustafsson and others (Gustafsson, 1984, 1989, 2001; Gustafsson & Balke, 1993; Gustafsson & Undheim, 1996).

3. *Second-stratum multiplicity model*. This is a g-less model that also includes broad abilities, but suggests that the nonzero intercorrelations among lower-stratum factors do not support the existence of g. This is largely the view of Horn and Cattell (Cattell, 1971; Horn, 1998; Horn & Noll, 1997).

Carroll (2003) judged the WJ-R norm data to be a "sufficient" dataset for "drawing conclusions about the higher-stratum structure of cognitive abilities" (p. 8). Carroll submitted the 16- and 29-variable WJ-R correlation matrices (reported in McGrew et al., 1991) to the same EFA-SL procedures used in his 1993 survey. These EFA-based results, in turn, served as the starting point for a CFA intended to compare the three different structural model views of intelligence vis-à-vis the model comparison statistics provided by structural equation modeling (SEM) methods.[13]

Briefly, Carroll (2003) concluded that "researchers who are concerned with this structure in one way or another . . . can be assured that a general factor g exists, along with a series of second-order factors that measure broad special abilities" (p. 19). Carroll further stated that "doubt is cast on the view that emphasizes the importance of a Gf factor. . . . these data tend to discredit the limited structural analysis view and the second-stratum multiplicity view" (p. 17). Interestingly, in these analyses Carroll used the broad-ability nomenclature of CHC theory when reporting support for the broad abilities of Gf, Gc, Gv, Ga, Gsm, Glr, Gs, Gq, and language (composed of reading and writing tests; also known as Grw).

The most recent morphing of the long line of Stanford–Binet Intelligence Scales (the SB5; Roid, 2003) was guided extensively by the work of both Carroll and Horn (see Roid, 2003, pp. 7–11); consultation from authors of the CHC-designed WJ III (see

Roid, Woodcock, & McGrew, 1997; see also Roid, 2003, p. v); and a review of the CHC-organized cross-battery research literature of Flanagan, myself, and colleagues (see Roid, 2003, pp. 8–9). The result is a CHC-organized battery designed to measure five broad cognitive factors: Fluid Reasoning (Gf), Quantitative Reasoning (Gq), Crystallized Knowledge (Gc), Short-Term Memory (Gsm), and Visual Processing (Gv). Not measured are the broad abilities of Grw, Ga, Glr, and Gs. CFA reported in the SB5 manual indicates that the five-factor model (Gf, Gq, Gc, Gsm, Gv) was the most plausible model when compared to four alternative models (one-, two-, three-, and four-factor models).

Studies with Other Batteries

Recently, Roberts and colleagues (2000) examined the factor structure of the Armed Services Vocational Aptitude Battery (ASVAB) in terms of Gf-Gc theory and Carroll's (1993) three-stratum model. In two samples (n = 349, n = 6,751), adult subjects were administered both the ASVAB and marker tests from the Educational Testing Service Kit of Factor-Referenced Cognitive Tests (Ekstrom, French, Harman, & Derman, 1976). EFA and CFA supported a model that included the broad abilities of Gf, Gc, Gsm (SAR), Gv, Glr (TSR), and Gs.[14]

Although not using the language of CHC theory, Tulsky and Price's (2003) recent CFA of the Wechsler Adult Intelligence Scale—Third Edition (WAIS-III) and Wechsler Memory Scale—Third Edition (WMS-III) national standardization conorming sample also supports the CHC model. Of the six factors retained in their final cross-validated model, three factors can clearly be interpreted as broad CHC factors: Gs (Processing Speed), Gc (Verbal Comprehension), and Gv (Perceptual Organization). Tulsky and Price's Visual Memory factor could be classified as Gv (MV). The factor Tulsky and Price interpreted as Auditory Memory was defined by salient loadings from the WMS-III Logical Memory I and II, Verbal-Paired Associates I and II, and the Word List I and II tests—tests that have previously been classified according to CHC theory (see Flanagan et al., 2000) as measures of Glr (i.e., MM, MA, M6).[15] Finally, the factor defined by the WMS-III Spatial Span and WAIS-III

Digit Span, Letter–Number Sequencing, and Arithmetic tests was interpreted by Tulsky and Price as Working Memory (Gsm-MW). An alternative interpretation of the Working Memory factor could be Numerical Fluency (Gs-N), due to of the common use of numerals in all tasks (e.g., Digit Span, Letter–Number Sequencing, and Arithmetic all require the manipulation of numbers; Spatial Span performance might be aided via the subvocal counting of the shapes to be recalled).

Finally, Tirre and Field's (2002) systematic investigation of the structure of the Ball Aptitude Battery (BAB), when viewed through a CHC lens, provides additional support for the broad strokes of the CHC model. These investigators reported the results of three separate cross-battery CFAs (the BAB and the Comprehensive Ability Battery; the BAB and the ASVAB; and the BAB and the General Aptitude Test Battery) and their reanalysis of the Neuman, Bolin, and Briggs (2000) BAB study. Although Tirre and Field reported 15 different types of factors across all studies, only those factors replicated in at least two of the samples are discussed here. These included g (General Cognitive Ability), Gps (Perceptual Motor Speed), Gs-P (Clerical Speed), Gf (Reasoning), Gc (Verbal), and Gq (Numerical Ability). Two additional Glr-type factors emerged and were defined by slightly different combinations of tests in the different analyses. What Tirre and Field labeled Episodic Memory appears to be a Glr "level" factor defined primarily by the combination of Associative Memory (MA) and Meaningful Memory (MM) measures. In contrast, their Creativity factor was defined by Glr "rate" measures requiring rapid or fluent generation of ideas (FI—Ideational Fluency). Tirre and Field interpreted an additional factor as representing "Broad Retrieval Ability." However, in two of the three investigations where this factor emerged, the strongest factor loadings were for Gf tests (BAB Inductive Reasoning, BAB Analytical Reasoning).

Small-Sample Studies

A number of small-sample studies, many of which analyzed joint (cross-battery) datasets, provide additional support for the broad strokes of CHC theory.

In a study of 179 adults, Roberts, Pallier, and Stankov (1996) used EFA with a collection of 25 cognitive measures that have been used for decades in many intelligence research studies (i.e., not a single nationally normed battery). Six CHC factors were identified. The broad factors reported included Gf, Gc, Gsm (SAR), Gv, Ga, and Gs. With the exception of a seventh separate Induction (I) factor that was correlated with Gf, the six-factor structure is consistent with CHC theory. In a study that used some of the same measures, as well as measures of tactile and kinesthetic abilities, Roberts, Stankov, Pallier, and Dolph (1997) used a combination of EFA and CFA on a set of 35 variables administered to 195 college and adult subjects. In addition to the possibility of a broad tactile–kinesthetic ability (discussed later in this chapter), this study provided support for the CHC abilities of Gc, Gf, Gv, Gsm (SAR), and a blended Gs-Gt.

Li, Jordanova, and Lindenberger (1998) also included 3 measures of tactile abilities together with 14 research tests of cognitive abilities in a study designed to explore the relations between perceptual abilities and g in a sample of 179 adults. Embedded in the causal model, to operationally represent g, were five first-order factors consistent with the CHC model: Gs (Perceptual Speed), Gf (Reasoning), and Gc (Knowledge). Two additional factors, labeled Memory and Fluency, appear to represent the "level" (MA/MM) and "rate" (FI) components of Glr when viewed through a CHC lens.

Reed and McCallum (1995) presented the results of an EFA for 104 elementary school subjects who had been administered 18 tests from the Gf-Gc-designed WJ-R and 6 tests from the Universal Nonverbal Intelligence Test (UNIT; Bracken & McCallum, 1998). The original WJ-R and UNIT correlation matrix was subsequently submitted to a CHC-designed CFA (McGrew, 1997), and the results supported a model consisting of Gf, Gv, Gs (P), Glr (MA), Gc, Ga (PC), and Gsm (MS).[16] McGhee and Liberman (1994) also used EFA methods to investigate the dimensionality of 18 measures selected from a variety of psychoeducational batteries. In a small sample of 50 second-grade students, six distinct CHC cognitive factors were identified: Gv (MV), Gsm (MS), Gv (SR), Gc, Ga (PA), and Gq (KM).[17] In addition, two tests

requiring the drawing of designs represented a visual–motor factor that corresponds to abilities within Carroll's (1993) domain of broad psychomotor ability. Fifteen of the WJ-R tests were also subjected to an EFA together with 12 tests from the Detroit Tests of Learning Aptitude—Adult in a sample (n = 50) of elderly adults (Buckhalt, McGhee, & Ehrler, 2001). Buckhalt and colleagues (2001) reported evidence in support of eight CHC broad abilities (Glr, Gc, Gsm, Ga, Gq, Gf, Gv, and Gs).[18]

Cross-battery studies including tests from the KAIT (Kaufman & Kaufman, 1993) have also supported portions of the CHC model. In a sample of 255 normal adolescent and adult subjects, Kaufman, Ishikuma, and Kaufman (1994) completed an EFA of 11 tests from the WAIS-R, 8 tests from the KAIT, 2 tests from the Kaufman Functional Academic Skills Test (Kaufman & Kaufman, 1994a), and 3 tests from the Kaufman Short Neuropsychological Assessment Procedure (Kaufman & Kaufman, 1994b). Referring to their interpretation as a "Horn analysis," Kaufman and colleagues provided support for four CHC domains. Distinct Gc and Gf factors were identified. In addition, a Gsm (MS) factor was evident, which the authors labeled, in Horn's terminology, SAR. Kaufman and colleagues also presented what they termed a blended Gv-Gf factor. Inspection of the most salient tests on this blended factor (viz., WAIS-R Object Assembly, .84; Block Design, .75; Picture Completion, .61; Picture Arrangement, .61) suggests that broad Gv is a more defensible interpretation of the factor (see McGrew & Flanagan, 1998; Woodcock, 1990).

Two additional studies using the KAIT tests deserve comment. Although using a mixture of Cattell–Horn and Luria–Das terminology to interpret the factors, Kaufman's (1993) EFA of 8 KAIT and 13 K-ABC tests in a sample of 124 children ages 11–12 years supplied evidence for six CHC domains. Kaufman's KAIT and K-ABC factor results supported the validity of the Gc and Gf abilities. Kaufman's Achievement factor could be interpreted as a blend of Grw and Gq. Two different visual factors were identified and were labeled Simultaneous Processing and Broad Visualization by Kaufman. Post hoc CHC reinterpretations (see McGrew, 1997; McGrew & Flanagan, 1998) suggest that these two factors could be interpreted as broad Gv (salient loadings for K-ABC Photo Series, .80; Matrix Analogies, .61; Triangles, .61; Spatial Memory, .58; KAIT Memory for Block Designs, .32) and narrow Visual Memory (Gv-MV; KAIT Memory for Block Designs, .44, K-ABC Gestalt Closure, .42, K-ABC Hand Movements, .40) factors. Finally, the factor defined by K-ABC Number Recall and Word Order could be interpreted as Memory Span (Gsm-MS) rather than Sequential Processing.

We (Flanagan & McGrew, 1998) conducted a CHC-designed cross-battery CFA study of the KAIT tests together with select WJ-R and WISC-III tests in a nonwhite sample of 114 students in sixth, seventh, and eighth grades. Although a variety of specific hypotheses were tested at the stratum I (narrow-ability) level, support was found at the broad-factor level for the CHC abilities of Gf, Gc, Gv (MV and CS), Ga (PC), Gsm (MS), Glr (MA), Gs (P), and Grw. This study is notable in that it represented the first CHC-designed cross-battery study to attempt to evaluate, where possible in the model, all three strata of the CHC theory (see Table 8.1).

A number of recent studies have extended the CHC cross-battery research via the use of WJ III tests as CHC factor markers. In a sample of 155 elementary-school-age subjects who had been administered 18 WJ III tests and 12 tests from the Das–Naglieri CAS (Naglieri & Das, 1997), Keith, Kranzler, and Flanagan's (2001) CFA provided support for the CHC abilities of Gf, Gc, Gv, Ga (PC), Gsm, Glr (MA), and Gs. In what may be the most comprehensive CHC-organized cross-battery investigation to date we (McGrew et al., 2001) analyzed 53 different tests (26 from the WJ III, 6 from the KAIT, 11 from the WAIS-III, and 10 from the WMS-III) in a mixed university sample with and without learning disabilities (n = 200). CFAs provided support for the broad CHC abilities of Gf, Gc, Gv, Ga, Gsm, Glr, Grw, Gq, and Gs. Finally, in a more recent attempt to specify a three-stratum CHC cross-battery model, we (Phelps, McGrew, Knopik, & Ford, in press) analyzed the performance of 148 elementary-school-age students on 12 WISC-III tests and 29 WJ III tests. The best-fitting CFA model provided support for a CHC framework that included the broad abilities of Gf, Gc, Gv, Ga, Gsm, Glr, and Gs.

Empirical Evaluations: Summary and Conclusions

Collectively, the large- and small-sample structural validity studies published during the past decade support the broad strokes (i.e., the stratum II abilities) of contemporary CHC theory. The broad abilities of Gf, Gc, Gv, Ga, Gsm, Glr, Gs, Gq, and Grw have been validated in and across studies that have included a sufficient breadth of CHC indicators to draw valid conclusions. Although using the Cattell–Horn Gf-Gc theory as a guide, Stankov (2000) reached a similar conclusion (with the exception that he did not include Grw in his review).

It is likely that no single comprehensive study will ever include the necessary breadth of variables to allow for a definitive test of the complete structure of human cognitive abilities. Instead, increasingly better-designed and comprehensive studies, when viewed collectively through a CHC-organized theoretical lens, will provide for increasingly refined solutions that approximate the ideal. The research studies just reviewed, as well as contemporary reviews of recent factor-analytic research, will contribute to the ongoing search for increasingly satisfactory approximations of a psychometric model of the structure of human cognitive abilities. For example, a recent review (McGrew & Evans, 2004) of the factor-analytic research during the preceding decade (1993–2003) argues for a number of *internal* (i.e., elaboration on the nature of existing well-established broad CHC factors) and *external* (i.e., research that suggests new broad-ability domains or domains that have been only been partially investigated) extensions (Stankov, 2000). CHC model extensions have focused on the broad abilities of general knowledge (Gkn), tactile abilities (Gh), kinesthetic abilities (Gk), olfactory abilities (Go), and three separate broad speed abilities (Gs, general cognitive speed; Gt, decision/reaction time or speed; and Gps, psychomotor speed).[19]

BETWIXT, BEHIND, AND BEYOND g

g: Betwixt Horn and Carroll

The CHC model presented in Figure 8.1e reveals a quandary for users of CHC theory—namely, "to g [Carroll] or not to g [Horn]?"

To properly evaluate the relative merits of the *g* versus no-*g* positions would require extensive reading of the voluminous *g* literature. No fewer than three books or major papers (Brand, 1996; Jensen, 1998; Nyborg, 2003) have been devoted exclusively to the topic of *g* during the past decade. The existence and nature of *g* have been debated by the giants in the field of intelligence since the days of Spearman, with no universal resolution. The essence of the Cattell–Horn versus Carroll *g* conundrum is best summarized by Hunt (1999):

> Carroll notes that abilities in the second-order stratum (e.g., Gc and Gf) are positively correlated. This led Carroll to conclude that there is a third, highest-level stratum with a single ability in it: general intelligence. Here Carroll differs with the interpretations of Cattell and Horn. Cattell and Horn acknowledge the correlation, but regard it as a statistical regularity produced because it is hard to define a human action that depends on just one of the second-order abilities. Carroll sees the same correlation as due to the causal influence of general intelligence. It is not clear to me how this controversy could be resolved. (p. 2)

Even if no such "thing" as *g* exists, applied psychologists need to be cognizant of the reality of the positive manifold among the individual tests in intelligence batteries which is practically operationalized in the form of the global composite IQ score (Daniel, 2000).[20] Also, the positive manifold among cognitive measures often must be included in research designs to test and evaluate certain hypotheses. Researchers using the CHC model must make a decision whether *g* should be included in the application of the model in research. Brief summaries of the respective Horn and Carroll positions are presented below.

Horn on *g*

Horn (see, e.g., Horn & Masunaga, 2000) typically presents two lines of evidence against the "*g* as a unitary process" position. Structurally, Horn and Masunaga (2000) argue that "batteries of tests well selected to provide reliable measures of the various processes thought to be indicative of general intelligence do not fit the one common factor (i.e., Spearman *g*) model. This has been demonstrated time and time again" (p. 139). The statement also challenges Jensen's (1984, 1993) *g* argument in the form of the "indifference of the indicator" (see Horn, 1998). Horn (e.g., Horn & Noll, 1997; Horn & Masunaga, 2000) further argues that Carroll's (1993) research reveals no fewer than eight *different* general factors, with the general factor from one battery or dataset not necessarily being the same as the general factor in other batteries or datasets. More specifically, Horn and Noll (1997) argue: "The problem for theory of general intelligences is that the factors are not the same from one study to another. . . . The different general factors do not meet the requirements for the weakest form of invariance (Horn & McArdle, 1992) or satisfy the conditions of the Spearman model. The general factors represent different mixture measures, not one general intelligence" (p. 68). That is, the general factors fail to meet the *same factor requirement* (Horn, 1998, p. 77).

Second, in what is probably the more convincing portion of Horn's argument, research reveals that "the relationships that putative indicators of general intelligence have with variables of development, neurological functioning, education, achievement, and genetic structure are varied" (Horn & Masunaga, 2000, p. 139). That is, the broad CHC abilities demonstrate differential relations with (1) different outcome criteria (e.g., in the area of academic achievement, see Evans, Floyd, McGrew, & Leforgee, 2002; Floyd, Evans, & McGrew, 2003; McGrew, 1993; McGrew & Hessler, 1995, McGrew & Knopik, 1993); (2) developmental growth curves; (3) neurological functions; and (4) degree of heritability. "The many relationships defining the construct validities of the different broad factors do not indicate a single unitary principle" (Horn & Masunaga, 2000, p. 139). See Horn and Noll (1997) and Horn and Blankson (Chapter 3, this volume) for additional information.

Carroll on *g*

As presented earlier in this chapter, Carroll (2003), in his final publication, tested the *g* versus no-*g* versus "*g* is Gf" models in the WJ-R norm data. He concluded that "researchers who are concerned with this structure in one way or another...can be assured that a general factor *g* exists, along with a series of second-order factors that measure broad special abilities" (p. 19). He further stated that "doubt is cast on the view that emphasizes the importance of a Gf factor. . . . these data tend to discredit the limited structural analysis view and the second-stratum multiplicity view" (p. 17).

The primary basis for Carroll's belief in *g* stems not necessarily from the positive correlations among dissimilar tasks, but rather "from the three-stratum model that, for a well-designed dataset, yields factors at different strata, including a general factor" (Carroll, 1998, pp. 12–13). Carroll (1998) believed that for each factor in his three-stratum theory, there is a specific "state or substate" (e.g., "structured patterns of potentialities latent in neurons"; Carroll, 1998, p. 10) existing within an individual that accounts for the performance on tasks requiring a specific latent ability—"we can infer that *something* is there" (Carroll, 1998, p. 11; original emphasis). By extension, the emergence of a *g* factor in his EFA-SL work must reflect some form of specific state or substate within an individual.

Carroll (2003) further argued that the different *g* factors he reported (Carroll, 1993) do represent the same construct, given the underlying assumptions and procedures of the EFA-SL approach. In response to Horn's arguments, Carroll stated that Horn

conveniently forgets a fundamental principle on which factor analysis is based (a principle of which he is undoubtedly aware)—that the nature of a single factor discovered to account for a table of intercorrelations does not necessarily relate to special characteristics of the variables involved in the correlation matrix; it relates only to characteristics or underlying measurements (latent variables) that are common to those variables. I cannot regard Horn's comment as a sound basis for denying the existence of a factor *g*, yet he succeeded in persuading himself and many others to do exactly this for an extended period of years. (p. 19)

Finally, in a personal communication received just prior to his passing away, Carroll (personal communication, June 30, 2003) provided the following comments regarding the "proof" of *g*:

It is important to recognize that in my paper published in the Nyborg book occurs the first modern, real, scientific proof of *g*—in contrast to the many unacceptable "proofs" claimed by

Spearman, Burt, Pearson, and others. It used the features of a complete proof advanced by LISREL technologies. Jöreskog has discussed these features in his many writings . . . of particular interest are the proofs of the status of *g*, Gc, and Gf, as provided in the Nyborg chapter . . . in the sense *g*, Gc and Gf could be independently established, plus several other factors, (e.g. Gv, Ga). It was truly marvelous that enough data from these factors had accumulated to make their independence specifiable.

The "general factor" appears to pertain only to very general items of general knowledge—e.g., items of knowledge that are common to most people, present only as specified by parameters of "item difficulty." *g* thus appears not to pertain to the many items of knowledge incorporated in Gf or Gc. These items of knowledge are in some way special—classified under Gf or Gc (or some combination of these). It appears that a human being becomes a "member of society" only by acquiring aspects of special knowledge (either fluid or crystallized, or some combination of them).

Behind *g*: Working Memory?

Regardless of whether *g* can be proven to represent a specific essence of the human mind, those working in the field of applied intelligence testing need to be familiar with recent research suggesting that certain cognitive processes may lie *behind* the general factor. The integration of a century of psychometric research with contemporary information-processing theories has resulted in important strides in understanding human intelligence (Kyllonen, 1996). Although slightly different information-processing models have been hypothesized and researched, in general the four-source consensus model (Kyllonen, 1996) will suffice for this chapter. According to Kyllonen (1996), the four primary components or sources of this model are *procedural knowledge, declarative knowledge, processing speed* (Gs), and *working memory* (MW).[21]

One of the most intriguing findings from the marriage of psychometric and information-processing models, first reported by Kyllonen and Christal (1990), is that "individual differences in working memory capacity may be what are responsible for individual differences in general ability" (Kyllonen, 1996, p. 61). This hypothesis was proposed by Kyllonen (Kyllonen, 1996; Kyllonen & Christal, 1990), based on very high latent factor correlations (.80 to the mid-.90s) between measures of MW and Gf in a variety of adult samples. Attempts to understand the relation between MW and higher-order cognition "have occupied researchers for the past 20 years" (Kane, Bleckley, Conway, & Engle, 2001, p. 169). Since 1990, the concept of MW has played a central role in research attempting to explain individual differences in higher-level cognitive abilities, such as language comprehension (Gc; Engle, Cantor, & Carullo, 1992; Just & Carpenter, 1992), reading and mathematics (Grw and Gq; Hitch, Towse, & Hutton, 2001; Leather & Henry, 1994), reasoning or general intelligence (Gf and g; Ackerman, Beier, & Boyle, 2002; Conway, Cowan, Bunting, Themault, & Minkoff, 2002; Engle, Tuholski, Laughlin, & Conway, 1999; Fry & Hale, 1996, 2000; Kyllonen & Christal, 1990; Süß, Oberauer, Wittmann, Wilhelm, & Schulze, 2002), and long-term memory performance (Park et al., 1996; Süß et al., 2002).

The theoretical explanations for the consistently strong MW→Gf or g criterion relations differ primarily in terms of the different cognitive resources proposed to underlie MW performance (Lohman, 2000). More specifically, *multiple-resource* and *resource-sharing* models have been proposed (Bayliss, Jarrold, Gunn, & Baddeley, 2003). Some examples of resources hypothesized to influence MW performance are storage capacity, processing efficiency, the central executive, domain-specific processes, and controlled attention (Bayliss et al., 2003; Engle et al., 1999; Kane et al., 2001). Researchers have hypothesized that the reason why MW is strongly associated with complex cognition constructs (e.g., Gf) is that considerable information must be actively maintained in MW, especially when some active transformation of information is required. Even if the transformation "process" is effective, it must be performed within the limits of the working memory system. Therefore, although many different processes may be executed in the solution of a task, individual differences in the processes may primarily reflect individual differences, not working memory resources (Lohman, 2000, p. 325). A detailed treatment of the different theoretical explanations for working memory is beyond the scope of the current chapter and is not necessary in the current context. Figure 8.2 presents schematic summaries of four of the primary SEM investigations (published

during the past decade) that shed additional insights on the causal relations between MW and g or Gf.[22]

In the causal models portrayed in Figure 8.2, MW demonstrates a significant effect on all dependent variables (primarily Gf or g).[23] With the exception of the Süß and colleagues (2002) models (Figures 8.2d and 8.2e), the strength of the MW → Gf/g (.38 to .60) relations are lower than those reported by Kyllonen and Christal (1990). The weakest MW → Gf relationship (.38) was in the only sample of children and adolescents (Figure 8.2a). This finding may suggest a weaker relationship between the construct of MW and complex cognitive reasoning during childhood. In contrast, when the two different MW components (MW1 and MW2) are considered together in the two alternative Süß and colleagues models, MW collectively exerts a strong influence on g (MW1 = .65; MW2 = .40; Figure 8.2d) and Gf (MW1 = .70; MW2 = .24; Figure 8.2e).

It is important to note that in most studies that have explored the relation between MW and psychometric constructs, Gs is typically included as a direct precursor to MW (see Figures 8.2a and 8.2c). Collectively, the MW → criterion studies suggest that MW may be a significant causal factor working *behind the scenes* when complex cognitive performance is required (e.g., Gf or g). Missing from this literature are studies that include a broader and more complete array of CHC indicators and factors in larger and more carefully selected samples. This limitation is addressed below.

WJ III CHC MW → g Studies

For the purposes of this chapter, select tests from the CHC-designed WJ III COG battery were used to investigate the relations between measures of information-processing efficiency (viz., Gs, MS, and MW) and complex cognitive ability (operationalized in the form of g). In the causal model, g was operationally defined as a second-order latent factor composed of five well-identified latent CHC factors (Gf, Gc, Glr, Ga, and Gv; McGrew & Woodcock, 2001).[24] Consistent with the extant literature, Gs was specified to be a direct precursor to MW, although all models also tested for significant direct paths from Gs to g. In addition, given that MW subsumes the rote storage role of MS, a sepa-

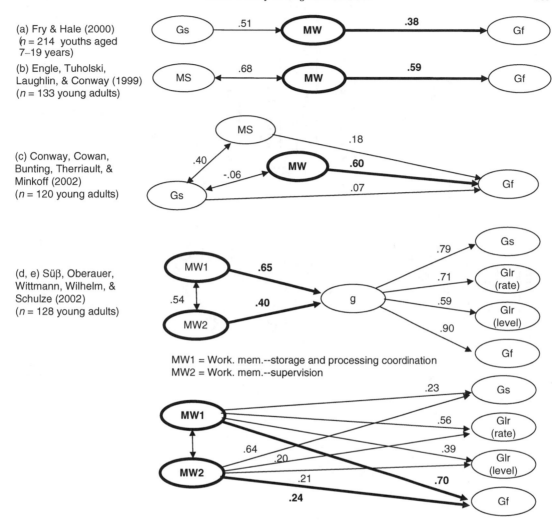

FIGURE 8.2. Working memory →complex cognitive abilities (viz., *g* and Gf) causal models reported from 1993–2003. Ovals represent latent factors. Single-headed arrows represent causal paths (effects). Double-headed arrows represent latent factor correlations. Manifest test indicators and residuals have been omitted for readability purposes. Factors have been renamed from original sources as per CHC theory.

rate MS factor with a direct effect on MW was specified. The inclusion of both MS and MW latent factors is consistent with the research models of Engle and colleagues (1999). The final model is represented in Figure 8.3.

For each of five age-differentiated nationally representative samples (each of which ranged in size from approximately 1,000 to 2,200 subjects; see McGrew & Woodcock, 2001), the same initial model was specified. In addition to the direct MW → *g* path, a direct Gs → *g* path was also tested in each sample (see Figure 8.3).[25] The results summarized in Figure 8.3 and Table 8.4 are im-

portant to note, as they allow for the investigation of the MW - *g* relationship in large, nationally representative samples. In addition, the latent factor constructs defined in these analyses are represented by the same indicators across all samples—a condition rarely achieved across independent research studies (e.g., see Figure 8.2). This later condition provides for configural invariance of the models across samples. The parameters presented in Figure 8.3 are for the 14- to 19-year-old sample. Table 8.4 presents the key parameters and model fit statistics for all samples.

The results presented in Figure 8.3 and Ta-

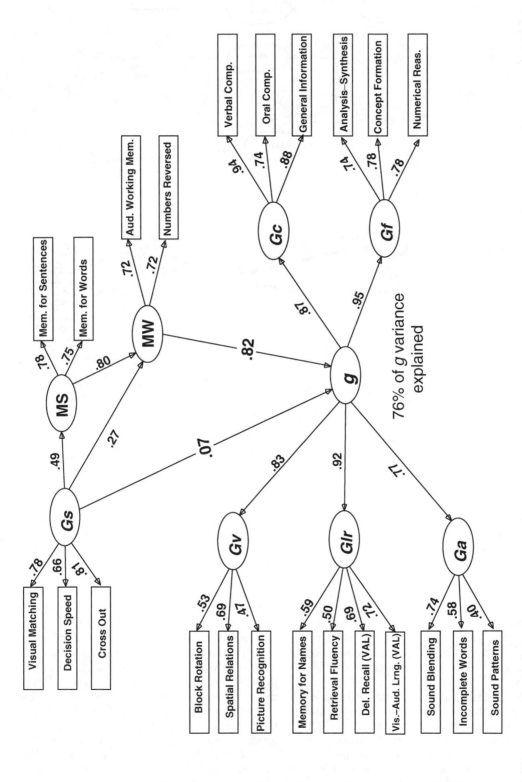

FIGURE 8.3. WJ III CHC information processing MW →g causal model (ages 14–19). Ovals represent latent factors. Rectangles represent manifest measures (tests). Single-headed arrows to tests from ovals designate factor loadings. Single-headed arrows between ovals represent causal paths (effects). Test and factor residuals have been omitted for readability purposes.

TABLE 8.4. Select Model Parameters and Fit Statistics for WJ III CHC MW →g Models (see Figure 8.3)

Age group (in years)	% g variance explained	Structural (causal) MW, MS, Gs, g paths						Select model fit statistics					
		MW to g path	Gs to g path	Gs to g total direct + indirect effects	Gs to MS path	MS to MW path	Gs to MW path	GFI[a]	AGFI[b]	CFI[c]	RMSEA[d]	RMSEA[e] (low)	RMSEA[e] (high)
6–8	86%	.93	—	.79	.44	.63	.46	.88	.84	.93	.078	.074	.081
9–13	80%	.90	—	.60	.40	.70	.39	.94	.92	.94	.054	.052	.056
14–19	76%	.82	.07	.61	.49	.80	.27	.93	.91	.94	.058	.055	.061
20–39	80%	.83	.09	.67	.50	.80	.30	.90	.87	.93	.068	.065	.071
40–90+	84%	.73	.22	.81	.61	.63	.43	.88	.84	.93	.078	.074	.081

[a]GFI, goodness-of fit index;

[b]AGFI, adjusted goodness-of fit index;

[c]CFI, normed comparative fit index;

[d]RMSEA, root-mean-square error of approximation;

[e]RMSEA low/high, 95% confidence band for lower and upper limits of RMSEA.

ble 8.4 are consistent with the previously summarized MW → *g* research literature. Across all five samples, the MW → *g* direct-effect path ranged from .73 to .93. Clearly, working memory (MW) potentially exerts a large causal effect on complex cognitive performance (i.e., *g*) when defined by the combined performance on five latent CHC factors (i.e., Gf, Gc, Glr, Ga, Gv). The trend for the MW → *g* path to decrease with increasing age (.93, .90, .82, .83, .73) may be of significant substantive interest to developmental psychologists and intelligence researchers studying the effect of aging within the CHC framework (e.g., see Horn & Masunaga, 2000; Park et al., 1996; Salthouse, 1996). Also of interest is the finding, consistent with prior research (Fry & Hale, 1996, 2000), that Gs did not demonstrate a direct effect on *g* in the childhood samples. However, starting in late adolescence (ages 14–19), Gs begins to demonstrate small yet significant direct effects on *g* (.07 and .09 from ages 14 to 39), and a much more substantial effect at middle age and beyond (.22). These developmental trends suggest the hypothesis that during an individual's formative years (ages 6–13), MW exerts a singular and large (.90 to .93) direct effect on complex cognitive task performance (i.e., *g*). In adolescence, MW appears to decrease slightly in direct influence on *g*, while Gs concurrently increases in importance, particularly during the latter half of most individuals' lives (40 years and above).

It is important to note that in all models, Gs exerts indirect effects on *g* via two routes (i.e., Gs → *MS* → *MW* → *g*; Gs → *MW* → *g*). The total effects (direct + indirect) of Gs on *g* have been calculated via standard path-model-tracing rules, and are summarized in Table 8.4. The range of total Gs → *g* effects is large (.60 to .81). Clearly, these analyses suggest that Gs and MW both exert large and significant influence on complex cognitive performance (i.e., *g*). Collectively, the total effects of Gs + MW (information-processing efficiency)[26] account for 76% to 86% of the CHC-defined *g* factor.

Behind *g*: Summary

The WJ III CHC MW → *g* analyses and research studies presented here continue to

suggest an intriguing relation between measures of cognitive efficiency (Gs and MW) and complex cognitive performance (viz., Gf and *g*). As articulated by Kyllonen (1996),

> the remarkable finding is the consistency with which the working memory capacity factor has proven to be the central factor in cognition abilities . . . working memory capacity is more highly related to performance on other cognitive tests, and is more highly related to learning, both short-term and long-term, than is any other cognitive factor. (pp. 72–73)

Leaping from these findings to the conclusion that MW is the basis of Spearman's *g* (Süß et al., 2002) or Gf (Kyllonen & Christal, 1990) is not the intent of this section of this chapter. Alternative claims for the basis of *g* (e.g., processing/reaction time) exist (see Nyborg, 2003). The important conclusion here is that appropriately designed CHC MW → *g* outcome studies can make important contributions to research focused on increasing our understanding of the nature and importance of working memory, as well as the specific cognitive resources that contribute to a variety of cognitive and academic performances. According to Süß and colleagues (2002),

> The strong relationship between working memory and intelligence paves the way for a better understanding of psychometric ability concepts through theories of cognition. Establishing this general association, however, is only the first step. Working memory itself is not a precisely defined construct. It is widely accepted that working-memory capacity is an important limited resource for complex cognition; however, which functions of working memory affect which part of the cognitive process in a given reasoning task is not well understood. . . . Now that the relationship between working memory and intelligence has been established on a molar level, further research with more fine-grained analyses need to be done. (pp. 285–286)

Beyond *g*: CHC Lower-Stratum Abilities Are Important

"The *g* factor (and highly *g*-loaded test scores, such as the IQ) shows a more far-reaching and universal practical validity than any other coherent psychological construct yet discovered" (Jensen, 1998, p. 270). The strength of g's prediction, together with past attempts to move "beyond g" (i.e., the addition of specific abilities to g in the prediction and explanation of educational and occupational outcomes), historically have not met with consistent success. In his American Psychological Association presidential address, McNemar (1964) concluded that "the worth of the multi-test batteries as differential predictors of achievement in school has not been demonstrated" (p. 875). Cronbach and Snow's (1977) review of the aptitude–treatment interaction research similarly demonstrated that beyond general level of intelligence (g), few, if any, meaningful specific ability–treatment interactions existed. Jensen (1984) also reinforced the preeminent status of g when he stated that "g accounts for all of the significantly predicted variance; other testable ability factors, independently of g, add practically nothing to the predictive validity" (p. 101).

In applied assessment settings, attempts to establish the importance of specific abilities above and beyond the full scale IQ (research largely based on the Wechsler batteries) score have typically meet with failure. As a result, assessment practitioners have been admonished to "just say no" to the practice of interpreting subtest scores in individual intelligence batteries (McDermott, Fantuzzo, & Glutting, 1990; McDermott & Glutting, 1997). The inability to move beyond g has provided little optimism for venturing beyond an individual's full scale IQ score in the applied practice of intelligence test interpretation. However, Daniel (2000) believes that these critics have probably "overstated" their case, given some of the techniques they have used in their research.[27]

Despite the "hail to the g" mantra, several giants in the field of intelligence have continued to question the "conventional wisdom" of complete deference to g. Carroll (1993) concluded that "there is no reason to cease efforts to search for special abilities that may be relevant for predicting learning" (p. 676). In a subsequent publication, Carroll (1998) stated: "It is my impression that there is much evidence, in various places, that special abilities (i.e., abilities measured by second- or first-stratum factors) contribute significantly to predictions" (p. 21). Snow (1998) struck a similar chord when he stated that

certainly it is often the case that many ability–learning correlations can be accounted for by an underlying general ability factor. Yet, there are clearly situations, such as spatial-mechanical, auditory, or language learning conditions, in which special abilities play a role aside from G. (p. 99)

In the school psychology literature, various authors (Flanagan, 2000; McGrew, Flanagan, Keith, & Vanderwood, 1997; Keith, 1999) have suggested that advances in theories of intelligence (viz., CHC theory), the development of CHC-theory-driven intelligence batteries (viz., WJ-R, WJ III), and the use of more contemporary research methods (e.g., SEM) argue for continued efforts to investigate the effects of g and specific abilities on general and specific achievements. A brief summary of CHC-based g + specific abilities $\rightarrow$ achievement research follows.

CHC g + Specific Abilities $\rightarrow$ Achievement SEM Studies

Using a Gf-Gc framework, Gustafsson and Balke (1993) reported that some specific cognitive abilities may be important in explaining school performance beyond the influence of g when (1) a Gf-Gc intelligence framework is used; (2) cognitive predictor and academic criterion measures are both operationalized in multidimensional hierarchical frameworks; and (3) cognitive abilities $\rightarrow$ achievement relations are investigated with research methods (viz., SEM) particularly suited to *understanding and explaining* (vs. simply *predicting*). The key advantage of the SEM method is that it allows for the simultaneous inclusion of casual paths (effects) from a latent g factor, plus specific paths for latent factors subsumed by the g factor, to a common dependent-variable factor (e.g., reading). This is not possible when multiple-regression methods are used.

Drawing on the research approach outlined by Gustafsson and Balke (1993), several CHC-designed studies completed during the past decade have identified significant CHC narrow or broad effects on academic achievement, above and beyond the effect of g. Using the Cattell–Horn Gf-Gc-based WJ-R norm data, we (McGrew et al., 1997;

Vanderwood, McGrew, Flanagan, & Keith, 2002) found, depending on the age level (five grade-differentiated samples from grades 1–12), that the CHC abilities of Ga, Gc, and Gs had significant cross-validated effects on reading achievement, above and beyond the large effect of *g*. In the grades 1–2 cross-validation sample (*n* = 232; McGrew et al., 1997), there was a strong direct effect of *g* on reading, which was accompanied by significant specific effects for Ga (.49) on word attack skills and Gc (.47) on reading comprehension. In math, specific effects beyond the high direct *g* effect were reported at moderate levels (generally .20 to .30 range) for Gs and Gf, while Gc demonstrated high specific effects (generally .31 to .50 range). Using the same WJ-R norm data, Keith (1999) employed the same *g* + specific abilities → achievement SEM methods in an investigation of general (*g*) and specific effects on reading and math as a function of ethnic group status. Keith's findings largely replicated the McGrew and colleagues (1997) results and suggested that CHC *g* + specific abilities → achievement relations are largely invariant across ethnic group status.

In a sample of 166 elementary-school-age students, Flanagan (2000) applied the same methodology used in the McGrew and colleagues (1997), Keith (1999), and Vanderwood and colleagues (2002) studies to a WISC-R + WJ-R "cross-battery" dataset. A strong (.71) direct effect for *g* on reading was found, together with significant specific effects for Ga (.28) on word attack and Gs (.15) and Gc (.42) on reading comprehension. More recently, I (McGrew, 2002) reported the results of similar modeling studies with the CHC-based WJ III. In three age-differentiated samples (ages 6–8, 9–13, 14–19), in addition to the ubiquitous large effect for *g* on reading decoding (.81 to .85), significant specific effects were reported for Gs (.10 to .35) and Ga (.42 to .47).

Beyond *g*: Summary

Collectively, the CHC-based *g* + specific abilities → achievement SEM studies reported during the last decade suggest that even when *g* (if it does exist) is included in causal modeling studies, certain specific lower-stratum CHC abilities display significant causal effects on reading and math achieve-

ment. Critics could argue that the trivial increases in model fit and the amount of additional achievement variance explained (vis-à-vis the introduction of specific lower-order CHC paths) is not statistically significant (which is the case), and thus that Occam's razor would argue for the simpler models that only include *g*.[28] Alternatively, knee-jerk acceptance of Occam's razor can inhibit scientifically meaningful discoveries. As best stated by Stankov, Boyle, and Cattell (1995) in the context of research on human intelligence, "while we acknowledge the principle of parsimony and endorse it whenever applicable, the evidence points to relative complexity rather than simplicity. Insistence on parsimony at all costs can lead to bad science" (1995, p. 16).

In sum, even when a Carroll *g* model of the structure of human cognitive abilities is adopted, research indicates that a number of lower-stratum CHC abilities make important contributions to understanding academic achievement, above and beyond *g*.[29] Reschly (1997) reached the same conclusion when he stated, in response to the McGrew and colleagues (1997) paper, that "the arguments were fairly convincing regarding the need to reconsider the specific versus general abilities conclusions. Clearly, some specific abilities appear to have potential for improving individual diagnoses. Note, however, that it is potential that has been demonstrated" (p. 238).

CONCLUSIONS AND CAVEATS

"These are exciting times for those involved in research, development, and the use of intelligence test batteries" (McGrew, 1997, p. 172). This 1997 statement still rings true today. Central to this excitement have been the recognition and adoption, within both the theoretical and applied fields of intelligence research and intelligence testing, of the CHC theory of human cognitive abilities (or some slight variation) as the definitive psychometric theory upon which to construct a working taxonomy of cognitive differential psychology. I echo Horn's (1998) and Jensen's (2004) comparisons to the first presentation of Mendelyev's periodic table of elements in chemistry and to Hans von Bülow's "there it is!" declaration upon reading the score of Wagner's *Die Meistersinger*: The order brought to the study, measurement, and assessment of human cognitive abilities by Carroll's (1993) synthesis—a synthesis built on the shoulders of a crowd of psychometric giants (Horn and Jensen included)—has finally provided both intelligence scholars and practitioners with the first empirically based consensus Rosetta stone from which to organize research and practice. This is truly a marvelous development.

Human intelligence is clearly multidimensional. The past decade has witnessed the accumulation of evidence that supports the broad strokes of the hierarchical multiability CHC theory of human cognitive abilities. This new evidence, often derived from studies that gathered data with a wide breadth of ability indicators in large, nationally representative samples, validates the inclusion of the broad (stratum II) abilities of Gf, Gc, Gq, Grw, Glr, Gsm, Gv, Ga, Gs, and Gt in the CHC taxonomy. In addition, past and recent research suggests (see McGrew & Evans, 2004, for a summary) the need to attend to, and possibly incorporate, the additional broad domains of general knowledge (Gkn), tactile abilities (Gh), kinesthetic abilities (Gk), olfactory abilities (Go), and three separate broad speed abilities (Gs, general cognitive speed; Gt, decision/reaction time or speed; and Gps, psychomotor speed) in future research, measurement, and assessment activities. It is also important to note that CHC theory is not based solely on factor-analytic evidence. Developmental, outcome criterion prediction, heritability, and neurocognitive studies add to the network of validity evidence in support of contemporary CHC theory (see Horn & Noll, 1997).

Consistent with Carroll's (1998) self-critique and recommendations for future research, it is important to recognize that the CHC framework is "an open-ended empirical theory to which future tests of as yet unmeasured or unknown abilities could possibly result in additional factors at one or more levels in Carroll's hierarchy" (Jensen, 2004, p. 5). The importance of avoiding a premature "hardening" of the CHC categories has been demonstrated this past decade vis-à-vis the structural research on the domain of cognitive mental speed, where research now suggests a domain characterized by a complex hierarchical structure with a possible g speed factor at the same stratum level as psychometric g (see McGrew & Evans, 2004). In this case, the CHC taxonomy has been used as the open-ended framework described by Jensen (2004) and as Carroll's (1994) intended "guide and reference for future researchers" (p. 22).

The revisions, additions, and extensions to the CHC taxonomy suggested in this chapter are based on a reasoned review and evaluation of research (again, primarily factor-analytic) spanning the last decade. It is hoped that the proposed CHC theory modifications proposed here enhance the "search for the Holy Grail" of human cognitive ability taxonomies, at least by providing a minor positive movement toward convergence on a more plausible model. However, the proposed CHC taxonomic enhancements summarized here and elsewhere (McGrew & Evans, 2004) require additional research and replication. Reanalysis of Carroll's 460+ datasets with contemporary procedures (viz., CFA), combined with both CFA and Carroll EFA-based exploratory procedures of post-Carroll (1993) datasets, will help elucidate the validity of current and future proposed revisions of the CHC taxonomy.[30]

Finally, although additional cautions and limitations could be enumerated,[31] the seductive powers of a neat and hierarchically organized structural diagram of cognitive abilities must be resisted. Any theory that is derived primarily from a "rectilinear system of factors is ... not of a form that well describes natural phenomena" (Horn & Noll, 1997, p. 84). By extension, assessment professionals must humbly recognize the inherent artificial nature of assessment tools built upon linear mathematical models. As stated by MacCallum (2003),

> it is abundantly clear that psychological researchers make extensive use of mathematical models across almost all domains of research. . . . It is safe to say that these models all have one thing in common: *They are all wrong.* Simply put, our models are implausible if taken as exact or literal representations of real world phenomena. They cannot capture the complexities of the real world which they purport to represent. At best, they can provide an approximation of the real world that has some substantive meaning and some utility. (pp. 114–115, original emphasis)

IMPLICATIONS AND FUTURE DIRECTIONS

One never notices what has been done; one can only see what remains to be done. . . .

—MARIE CURIE

Space does not allow a thorough discussion of all potential implications of contemporary CHC theory. As a result, only three major points are offered for consideration.

First, the structural research of the past decade demonstrates the dynamic and unfolding nature of the CHC taxonomy. Additional research is needed to better elucidate the structure of abilities in the broad domains of Gkn, Gk, Gh, and Go. In addition, Carroll's primary focus on identifying an overall structural hierarchy necessitated a deliberate ignoring of datasets with small numbers of variables within a single broad domain (Carroll, 1998). I believe that more focused "mining" within each broad (stratum II) domain is rich with possible new discoveries, and will be forthcoming soon. Studies with a molar focus on variables within a single broad domain can provide valuable insights into the structure and relations of the narrow abilities within that domain. With the foundational CHC structure serving as a working map, researchers can return to previously ignored or recently published datasets, armed with both EFA and CFA tools, to seek a better understanding of the narrow (stratum I) abilities. In turn, test developers and users of tests of intelligence need to continue to develop and embrace tools and procedures grounded in the best contemporary psychometric theory (viz., CHC theory; see recommendations by Flanagan et al., 2000; McGrew, 1997; McGrew & Flanagan, 1998).

Second, CHC theory needs to move beyond the mere description and cataloguing of human abilities to provide multilens explanatory models that will produce more prescriptive hypotheses (e.g., aptitude–treatment interactions). A particularly important area of research will be CHC-grounded investigations of the causal relations between basic information-processing abilities (e.g., processing speed and working memory—"behind *g*") and higher-order cognitive abilities (e.g., Gf, *g*, language, reading, etc.). The recent research in this area by a cadre of prominent researchers (Ackerman, Beier, & Boyle, 2002; Ardila, 2003; Baddeley, 2002; Bayliss et al., 2003; Cocchini, Logie, DellaSala, MacPherson, & Baddeley, 2002; Conway et al., 2002; Daneman & Merikle, 1996; Fry & Hale, 2000; Kyllonen, 1996; Lohman, 2001; Miyake, Friedman, Rettinger, Shah, & Hegarty, 2001; Oberauer, Süß, Wilhelm, & Wittmann, 2003; Paas, Renkl, & Sweller, 2003; Paas, Tuovinen, Tabbers, & VanGerven, 2003) has produced promising models for understanding the dynamic interplay of cognitive abilities during cognitive and academic performance.

In addition, a better understanding of human abilities is likely to require an equal emphasis on investigations of both the *content* and *processes* underlying performance on diverse cognitive tasks. In regard to content, the "faceted" hierarchical Berlin intelligence structure model (Beauducel, Brocke, & Liepmann, 2001; Süß et al., 2002) is a promising lens through which to view CHC theory. Older and lesser-used multivariate statistical procedures, such as multidimensional scaling (MDS), need to be pulled from psychometricians' closets to allow for the simultaneous examination of content (facets), processes, and processing complexity.[32] In addition, the promising "beyond *g*" (*g* + specific abilities) research should continue and be extended to additional domains of human performance. The evidence is convincing that a number of lower-stratum CHC abilities make important contributions to understanding academic and cognitive performance, above and beyond the effect of *g*.

Finally, it is time for the CHC taxonomy to go "back to the future" and revisit the original conceptualization of *aptitude,* as updated most recently by Richard Snow and colleagues (Corno et al., 2002). Contrary to many current erroneous assumptions, *aptitude* is not the same as *ability* or *intelligence*. According to Snow and colleagues, *aptitude* is more aligned with the concepts of *readiness, suitability, susceptibility,* and *proneness,* all of which suggest a "predisposition to respond in a way that fits, or does not fit, a particular situation or class of situations. The common thread is potentiality-a latent quality that enables the development or production, given specified conditions, of some more advanced performance" (Corno et al., 2002, p. 3).

Aptitudes represent the multivariate repertoire of a learner's degree of readiness (propensities) to learn and to perform well in general and domain-specific learning settings. As such, a person's aptitudes must include, along with cognitive and achievement abilities, *affective and conative characteristics*. Intelligence scholars and applied assessment personnel are urged to investigate the contemporary theoretical and empirical research that has married cognitive constructs (CHC and cognitive information processing) with affective and conative traits in the form of *aptitude trait complexes*. Snow and colleagues' aptitude model (Corno et al., 2002; Snow, Corno, & Jackson, 1996), and Ackerman and colleagues' model of intelligence as *process, personality, interests, and knowledge*, should be required reading for all involved in understanding and measuring human performance (Ackerman, 1996; Ackerman & Beier, 2003; Ackerman, Bowen, Beier, & Kanfer, 2001). The CHC taxonomy is the obvious cognitive cornerstone of a model of human aptitude.[33]

Yes. These are indeed exciting times in the ongoing quest to describe, understand, predict, explain, and measure human intelligence and performance.

ACKNOWLEDGMENTS

This chapter is dedicated to the memory of John "Jack" Carroll, "grandmaster of quantitative cognitive science" (Jensen, 2004, p. 1). I would like to thank Jeffrey Evans for his assistance in the literature review for this chapter.

NOTES

1. These broad abilities are defined in Table 8.3 in this chapter.
2. Different sources (Carroll, 1993; Horn & Noll, 1997; Jensen, 1998) list between seven and nine abilities, and also provide slightly different names for the Thurstone PMAs.
3. The 1977 WJ was, at the time, the only individually administered intelligence test battery to include miniature "learning" tasks. The possibility of revising these tests, or developing new tests, that reflected the dynamic assessment methods rooted in Vygotsky's (1978) *zone of proximal development* (Sternberg & Kaufman, 1998) resulted in the inclu-

sion of Carl Haywood, an recognized expert on the test–teach–test dynamic testing paradigm.

4. This was the first of a number of exhilarating meetings with Horn, Carroll, and primary WJ-R revision team members. These sessions also extended into the revision of the subsequent edition (WJ III). Horn and Carroll were generally in agreement regarding most aspects of the human cognitive ability taxonomy, with one exception—the existence of g. Suffice it to say, Horn (g does not exist) and Carroll (g exists) held strong and opposite views on the existence of g, and neither convinced the other during exchanges that often were quite "spirited." Their positions are described later in this chapter.
5. The reader is encouraged to read Woodcock's original 1990 article, to gain an appreciation for the significance of the work and why it has played such a significant role in the infusion of CHC theory into the practice of intelligence test development, assessment, and interpretation.
6. In fairness to these batteries, most were developed and published prior to the Cattell–Horn Gf-Gc model's morphing from a latent to a manifest model in the intelligence-testing literature. Hindsight is always 20-20.
7. The concept of applying a theoretical model not originally associated with a published battery to that battery was not a new idea (see Kaufman & Dopplet, 1976). Woodcock's unique contributions were extending this concept beyond application to the Wechsler scales to all available intelligence batteries; basing this "battery-free" interpretive philosophy on the most validated model of the structure of human cognitive abilities; and, most important, superimposing the Gf-Gc structure on batteries based on empirical evidence.
8. The interested reader should review Table 3.5 on pages 110–111 of Carroll (1993) for an example of a Carroll EFA-SL with three orders of factors. During his later years, Carroll recognized the advantages of CFA and encouraged others to use CFA methods to check his 1993 EFA-based results (Carroll, 1998). I had the fortunate opportunity to visit and work with Carroll in Fairbanks, Alaska, 4 weeks prior to his passing away. It was clear, as illustrated in his combined EFA + CFA WJ-R work (2003), that he had blended the two methodologies. His computer disks were full of unpublished EFA + CFA work that he had graciously completed for other researchers, or that represented his analysis of correlation matrices that had been included in manuscripts he had been asked to

review for a number of journals. His approach had clearly evolved to one of first obtaining results from his EFA-SL approach (as described in Chapter 3 of his 1993 book; see Figure 8.1d) and then using those results as the starting point for CFA refinement and model testing (as described in Carroll, 2003; see Figure 8.1e).

9. The complete process used to classify all tests from all major intelligence batteries at stratum I is first described in McGrew (1997).

10. A so-called "tipping point" is the "moment of critical mass, the threshold, the boiling point" (Gladwell, 2000, p. 12) where a movement that has been building over time, generally in small groups and networks, begins to influence a much wider audience.

11. Carroll recognized the CHC umbrella terminology in his last publication (2003), although he also was a bit puzzled over the details of the origin of "so-called CHC (Cattell–Horn–Carroll) theory of cognitive abilities" (p. 18). According to Carroll (2003), "even though I was to some extent involved in this change (as an occasional consultant to the authors and publisher), I am still not quite sure what caused or motivated it" (p. 18). In a personal conversation I had with Jack Carroll regarding this topic (at his daughter's home in Fairbanks, Alaska, on May 26, 2003), Carroll recognized the practical rational for the CHC umbrella term, but was planning to make it clear in the revision of his 1997 CIA chapter that although the CHC umbrella term might make practical sense, he felt strongly that human cognitive abilities consisted of at least three strata and that, in contrast to Horn's position, that g exists. He believed his last chapter publication (2003) provided convincing evidence for the existence of g. Carroll wanted to make it clear that the overarching CHC umbrella did not reflect his agreement with Horn on all aspects of the structure of human cognitive abilities. Chapter 4 of the present volume is a reprint of his chapter in the 1997 CIA book, and as such preserves his views.

12. Space constraints do not permit a review and summary of other forms of CHC empirical evidence (i.e., heritability, developmental, neurocognitive, outcome/criterion) published during the past decade.

13. See note 8.

14. Unless otherwise indicated, from this point on in this chapter, the factor names as reported by the original investigators are in parentheses. The factor names/CHC abbreviations preceding the names in parentheses reflect my own reinterpretation of the factors as per CHC theory.

15. In this particular paragraph, the factor codes in parentheses reflect my own interpretation and/or factor labeling.

16. The CHC classifications derived from this April 26, 1997 analysis are presented in McGrew and Flanagan (1998).

17. The factor interpretations presented here are based on my interpretation of the McGhee and Lieberman results. They used similar Gf-Gc terminology to provide slightly different, but very similar, factor interpretations.

18. The Buckhalt et al. (2001) Glr factor was defined primarily by measures of Glr, but also had a number of significant loadings from tests that measure Gv abilities. I have repeatedly seen the same type of factor in EFAs of the WJ-R and WJ III norm data.

19. See McGrew and Evans (2004) for a review of this literature and an explanation of the broad ability names and abbreviations reported here.

20. See Daniel (2000) for a discussion of the various issues involved in calculating practical composite IQ scores from intelligence batteries composed of different measures.

21. Another typical description of information-processing models makes distinctions between (1) memory systems—*short-term* and *long-term* memory; (2) types of knowledge—*declarative* and *procedural*; and (3) types of processing—*controlled* and *automatic* (Lohman, 2000).

22. For readability purposes, the manifest variables and certain other latent factors (age factors) were removed from all figures. In addition, based on a reading of the description of the variables used in each study, I changed the original latent factor names in accordance with CHC theory as described in this chapter. These interpretations do not necessarily reflect the interpretations of the authors of the original published studies.

23. Hambrick and Engle (2002) and Park and colleagues (1996) have reported similar causal models with memory performance as the dependent latent variable. In these studies, the MW direct causal paths were .30 and .44. In the Hambrick and Engle study, MW also had an indirect effect (.31) on memory performance that was mediated through a domain-specific knowledge (Gk) factor.

24. WJ III test indicators for the latent factors were selected based on the principles of (1) providing at least two qualitatively different narrow-ability indicators for each broad CHC factor; (2) using tests that were not factorially complex as determined from prior CFA studies (McGrew & Woodcock, 2001); and (3) using tests that were some of the best

WJ III CHC factor indicators (McGrew & Woodcock, 2001).

25. Given that the primary purpose of these analyses was to explore the relations between basic information-processing constructs (Gs and Gsm) and *g*, no effort was made to "tweak" the measurement models in each sample in search of slightly better-fitting models. The same configurially invariant measurement model was used across all five samples.

26. In the WJ III, the combination of Gs and MW (Gsm) is referred to, and is quantified as, Cognitive Efficiency (McGrew & Woodcock, 2001).

27. A nice summary of the issues involved in intelligence test profile analysis can be found in Daniel (2000).

28. For researchers, the essence of Occam's razor is that when two competing theories or models make the same level of prediction, the one that is simpler is better.

29. The *g* + specific abilities →achievement studies could be considered to represent the Carroll position on how cognitive abilities predict/explain academic achievement. The Horn position could similarly be operationally defined in research studies that use either SEM or multiple regression of the lower-order CHC variables on achievement (no *g* included in the models). The results of such Horn CHC → achievement models, completed in either the WJ-R or WJ III norm data, can be found in McGrew (1993), McGrew and Hessler (1995), McGrew and Knopik (1993), Evans and colleagues (2002), and Floyd and colleagues (2003). With the exception of Gv, all broad CHC abilities (Gf, Gc, Ga, Glr, Gsm, Gs) are reported to be significantly associated (at different levels that often vary within each ability domain by age) with reading, math, and writing achievement in the Horn CHC → achievement model.

30. See the Institute of Applied Psychometrics *Carroll Human Cognitive Abilities* (HCA) project for details on efforts to complete such analyses (*http://www.iapsych.com/chchca.htm*).

31. See Carroll (1994 and Chapter 4, this volume) and Horn and Noll (1997) for excellent self-criticisms of the CHC theory by the primary contemporary theory architects.

32. For example, in an unpublished MDS analysis of 50 different cognitive and achievement tests from the WJ III battery, I identified, in addition to the primary broad CHC abilities (e.g., Gv, Gf, Gc, etc.), three other dimensions (possibly reflecting intermediate-stratum abilities?) by which to organize and view the diverse array of CHC measures: (1) visual–spatial/figural vs. auditory linguistic;

(2) process dominant vs. product dominant; (3) automatic processes vs. controlled processes.

33. In the area of school learning, we (McGrew, Johnson, Cosio, & Evans, 2004) recently presented a research-synthesis-based comprehensive taxonomy (*essential student academic facilitators*) for organizing and understanding the conative and affective components of academic aptitude. The model includes the broad domains of *motivational orientation* (e.g., intrinsic motivation, academic goal orientation, etc.), *interests and attitudes* (e.g., academic interests, attitudes, values), *self-beliefs* (e.g., academic self-efficacy, self-concept, ability conception, etc.), *social/interpersonal abilities* (e.g., prosocial and problem behaviors, social goal setting, etc.), and *self-regulation* (e.g., planning, activation, monitoring, control and regulation, and reaction/reflection strategies).

REFERENCES

Ackerman, P. L. (1996). A theory of adult intellectual development: Process personality, interests, and knowledge. *Intelligence, 22*, 229–259.

Ackerman, P. L., & Beier, M. E. (2003). Intelligence, personality, and interests in the career choice process. *Journal of Career Assessment, 11*(2), 205–218.

Ackerman, P. L., Beier, M. E., & Boyle, M. O. (2002). Individual differences in working memory within a nomological network of cognitive and perceptual speed abilities. *Journal of Experimental Psychology: General, 131*(4), 567–589.

Ackerman, P. L., Bowen, K. R., Beier, M. E., & Kanfer, R. (2001). Determinants of individual differences and gender differences in knowledge. *Journal of Educational Psychology, 93*(4), 797–825.

Ackerman, P. L., & Cianciolo, A. T. (2000). Cognitive, perceptual-speed, and psychomotor determinants of individual differences during skill acquisition. *Journal of Experimental Psychology: Applied, 6*(4), 259–290.

Ackerman, P. L., & Kanfer, R. (1993). Integrating laboratory and field study for improving selection: Development of a battery for predicting air traffic controller success. *Journal of Applied Psychology, 78*(3), 413–432.

Ardila, A. (2003). Language representation and working memory with bilinguals. *Journal of Communication Disorders, 36*(3), 233–240.

Baddeley, A. D. (2002). Is working memory still working? *European Psychologist, 7*(2), 85–97.

Bailey, K. D. (1994). *Typologies and taxonomies: An introduction to classification techniques.* Thousand Oaks, CA: Sage.

Bayliss, D. M., Jarrold, C., Gunn, D. M., & Baddeley, A. D. (2003). The complexities of complex span: Explaining individual differences in working memory in children and adults. *Journal of Experimental Psychology: General, 132*(1), 71–92.

Beauducel, A., Brocke, B., & Liepmann, D. (2001). Perspectives on fluid and crystallized intelligence: Facets for verbal, numerical, and figural intelligence. *Personality and Individual Differences, 30*(6), 977–994.

Bickley, P. G., Keith, T. Z., & Wolfe, L. M. (1995). The three-stratum theory of cognitive abilities: Test of the structure of intelligence across the life span. *Intelligence, 20*(3), 309–328.

Bracken, B. A., & McCallum, R. S. (1998). *The Universal Nonverbal Intelligence Test.* Itasca, IL: Riverside.

Brand, C. R. (1996). Doing something about g. *Intelligence, 22*(3), 311–326.

Brody, N. (2000). History of theories and measurements of intelligence. In R. J. Sternberg (Ed.), *Handbook of intelligence* (pp. 16–33). New York: Cambridge University Press.

Buckhalt, J., McGhee, R., & Ehrler, D. (2001). An investigation of Gf-Gc theory in the older adult population: Joint factor analysis of the Woodcock–Johnson—Revised and the Detroit Test of Learning Aptitude—Adult. *Psychological Reports, 88*, 1161–1170.

Burns, R. B. (1994). Surveying the cognitive terrain. *Educational Researcher, 23*(2), 35–37.

Burt, C. (1909). Experimental tests of general intelligence. *British Journal of Psychology, 3*, 94–177.

Burt, C. (1911). Experimental tests of higher mental processes and their relation to general intelligence. *Journal of Experimental Pedagogy and Training, 1*, 93–112.

Burt, C. (1941). *Factors of the mind.* London: University of London Press.

Burt, C. (1949a). The structure of the mind: A review of the results of factor analysis. *British Journal of Psychology, 19*, 176–199.

Burt, C. (1949b). Subdivided factors. *British Journal of Statistical Psychology, 2*, 41–63.

Butler, K. J. (1987). *A factorial invariance study of intellectual abilities from late childhood to late adulthood.* Unpublished doctoral dissertation, University of Denver.

Carroll, J. B. (1983). Studying individual differences in cognitive abilities: Through and beyond factor analysis. In R. F. Dillon (Ed.), *Individual differences in cognition* (Vol. 1, pp. 1–33). New York: Academic Press.

Carroll, J. B. (1985). *Domains of cognitive ability.* Paper presented at the annual meeting of the American Association for the Advancement of Science, Los Angeles.

Carroll, J. B. (1993). *Human cognitive abilities: A survey of factor-analytic studies.* New York: Cambridge University Press.

Carroll, J. B. (1994). An alternative, Thurstonian view of intelligence. *Psychological Inquiry, 5*(3), 195–197.

Carroll, J. B. (1998). Human cognitive abilities: A critique. In J. J. McArdle & R. W. Woodcock (Eds.), *Human cognitive abilities in theory and practice* (pp. 5–24). Mahwah, NJ: Erlbaum.

Carroll, J. B. (2003). The higher-stratum structure of cognitive abilities: Current evidence supports g and about ten broad factors. In H. Nyborg (Ed.), *The scientific study of general intelligence: Tribute to Arthur R. Jensen* (pp. 5–22). Amsterdam: Pergamon Press.

Carroll, J. B., Davies, P., & Richman, B. (1971). *The American Heritage word frequency book.* Boston: Houghton Mifflin.

Carroll, J. B., & Horn, J. L. (1981). On the scientific basis of ability testing. *American Psychologist, 36*, 1012–1020.

Carroll, J. B., & Maxwell, S. E. (1979). Individual differences in cognitive abilities. *Annual Review of Psychology, 30*, 603–640.

Cattell, R. B. (1941). Some theoretical issues in adult intelligence testing. *Psychological Bulletin, 38*, 592.

Cattell, R. B. (1943). The measurement of adult intelligence. *Psychological Bulletin, 40*, 153–193.

Cattell, R. B. (1957). *Personality and motivation structure and measurement.* New York: World Book.

Cattell, R. B. (1963). Theory for fluid and crystallized intelligence: A critical experiment. *Journal of Educational Psychology, 54*, 1–22.

Cattell, R. B. (1971). *Abilities: Their structure, growth and action.* Boston: Houghton-Mifflin.

Cattell, R. B., & Horn, J. L. (1978). A check on the theory of fluid and crystallized intelligence with description of new subtest designs. *Journal of Educational Measurement, 15*, 139–164.

Cocchini, G., Logie, R. H., DellaSala, S., MacPherson, S. E., & Baddeley, A. D. (2002). Concurrent performance of two memory tasks: Evidence for domain-specific working memory systems. *Memory and Cognition, 30*(7), 1086–1095.

Conway, A. R. A., Cowan, N., Bunting, M. F., Therriault, D. J., & Minkoff, S. R. B. (2002). A latent variable analysis of working memory capacity, short-term memory capacity, processing speed, and general fluid intelligence. *Intelligence, 30*(2), 163–183.

Corno, L., Cronbach, L., Kupermintz, H., Lohman, D., Mandinach, E., Porteus, A., et al. (2002). *Remaking the concept of aptitude: Extending the legacy of Richard E. Snow.* Mahwah, NJ: Erlbaum.

Corsini, R. J. (1999). *The dictionary of psychology.* Philadelphia: Brunner/Mazel.

Cronbach, L. J., & Snow, R. E. (1977). *Aptitudes and instructional methods.* New York: Irvington.

Daneman, M., & Merikle, P. M. (1996). Working memory and language comprehension: A meta-analysis. *Psychonomic Bulletin and Review, 3*(4), 422–433.

Daniel, M. H. (1997). Intelligence testing: Status and trends. *American Psychologist, 52*(10), 1038–1045.

Daniel, M. H. (2000). Interpretation of intelligence test scores. In R. J. Sternberg (Ed.), *Handbook of intelligence* (pp. 477–491). New York: Cambridge University Press.

Danthiir, V., Roberts, R. D., Pallier, G., & Stankov, L. (2001). What the nose knows: Olfaction and cognitive abilities. *Intelligence, 29,* 337–361.

Davidson, J. E., & Downing, C. L. (2000). Contemporary models of intelligence. In R. J. Sternberg (Ed.), *Handbook of intelligence* (pp. 34–52). New York: Cambridge University Press.

Deary, I. (2003). Reaction time and psychometric intelligence: Jensen's contributions. In H. Nyborg (Ed.), *The scientific study of general intelligence: Tribute to Arthur R. Jensen* (pp. 53–76). San Diego, CA: Pergamon.

Dunn, G., & Everitt, B. S. (1982). *An introduction to mathematical taxonomy.* New York: Cambridge University Press.

Ekstrom, R. B., French, J. W., Harman, H. H., & Dermen, D. (1976). *Manual for kit of factor-referenced cognitive tests, 1976.* Princeton, NJ: Educational Testing Service.

Ekstrom, R. B., French, J. W., & Harman, H. H. (1979). Cognitive factors: Their identification and replication. *Multivariate Behavioral Research Monographs, 79*(2), 3–84.

Embretson, S. E., & McCollam, S. S. (2000). Psychometric approaches to understanding and measuring intelligence. In R. J. Sternberg (Ed.), *Handbook of intelligence* (pp. 423–444). New York: Cambridge University Press.

Engle, R. W., Cantor, J., & Carullo, J. J. (1992). Individual differences in working memory and comprehension: Test of four hypotheses. *Journal of Experimental Psychology, 18*(5), 972–992.

Engle, R. W., Tuhoski, S. W., Laughlin, J. E., & Conway, A. (1999). Working memory, short-term memory, and general fluid intelligence: A latent-variable approach. *Journal of Experimental Psychology: General, 128*(3), 309–331.

Evans, J. J., Floyd, R. G., McGrew, K. S., & Leforgee, M. H. (2002). The relations between measures of Cattell–Horn–Carroll (CHC) cognitive abilities and reading achievement during childhood and adolescence. *School Psychology Review, 31*(2), 246–262.

Flanagan, D. P. (2000). Wechsler-based CHC cross-battery assessment and reading achievement: Strengthening the validity of interpretations drawn from Wechsler test scores. *School Psychology Quarterly, 15*(3), 295–329.

Flanagan, D. P., Genshaft, J. L., & Harrison, P. L. (Eds.). (1997). *Contemporary intellectual assessment: Theories, tests, and issues.* New York: Guilford Press.

Flanagan, D. P., & McGrew, K. S. (1997). A cross-battery approach to assessing and interpreting cognitive abilities: Narrowing the gap between practice and science. In D. P. Flanagan, J. L. Genshaft, & P. L. Harrison (Eds.), *Contemporary intellectual assessment: Theories, tests, and issues* (pp. 314–325). New York: Guilford Press.

Flanagan, D. P., & McGrew, K. S. (1998). Interpreting intelligence tests from contemporary Gf-Gc theory:

Joint confirmatory factor analysis of the WJ-R and the KAIT in a non-white sample. *Journal of School Psychology, 36*(2), 151–182.

Flanagan, D. P., McGrew, K. S., & Ortiz, S. (2000). *The Wechsler Intelligence Scales and Gf-Gc Theory: A contemporary approach to interpretation.* Needham Heights, MA: Allyn & Bacon.

Flanagan, D. P., & Ortiz, S. (2001). *Essentials of cross-battery assessment.* New York: Wiley.

Flanagan, D. P., Ortiz, S. O., Alfonso, V. C., & Mascolo, J. T. (2002). *The achievement test desk reference (ATDR).* Boston: Allyn & Bacon.

Fleishman, E. A., & Quaintance, M. K. (1984). *Taxonomies of human performance.* Orlando, FL: Academic Press.

Floyd, R. G., Evans, J. J., & McGrew, K. S. (2003). Relations between measures of Cattell–Horn–Carroll (CHC) cognitive abilities and mathematics achievement across the school-age years. *Psychology in the Schools, 40*(2), 155–171.

French, J. W. (1951). *The description of aptitude and achievement tests in terms of rotated factors* (Psychometric Monographs, No. 5). Chicago: University of Chicago Press.

French, J. W., Ekstrom, R. B., & Price, L. R. (1963). *Manual and kit of reference tests for cognitive factors.* Princeton, NJ: Educational Testing Service.

Fry, A. F., & Hale, S. (1996). Processing speed, working memory, and fluid intelligence: Evidence for a developmental cascade. *Psychological Science, 7*(4), 237–241.

Fry, A. F., & Hale, S. (2000). Relationships among processing speed, working memory, and fluid intelligence in children. *Biological Psychology, 54*(1–3), 1–34.

Gladwell, M. (2000). *The tipping point: How little things can make a big difference.* Boston: Back Bay Books.

Guilford, J. P. (1967). *The nature of human intelligence.* New York: McGraw-Hill.

Gustafsson, J.-E. (1984). A unifying model for the structure of intellectual abilities. *Intelligence, 8,* 179–203.

Gustafsson, J.-E. (1988). Hierarchical models of individual differences in cognitive abilities. In R. J. Sternberg (Ed.), *Psychology of human intelligence* (Vol. 4, pp. 35–71). Hillsdale, NJ: Erlbaum.

Gustafsson, J.-E. (1989). Broad and narrow abilities in research on learning and instruction. In R. Kanfer, P. L. Ackerman, & R. Cudeck (Eds.), *Abilities, motivation, and methodology: The Minnesota Symposium on Learning and Individual Differences* (pp. 203–237). Hillsdale, NJ: Erlbaum.

Gustafsson, J.-E. (2001). On the hierarchical structure of ability and personality. In J. M. Collis & S. Messick (Eds.), *Intelligence and personality: Bridging the gap in theory and measurement* (pp. 25–42). Mahwah, NJ: Erlbaum.

Gustafsson, J.-E., & Balke, G. (1993). General and specific abilities as predictors of school achievement. *Multivariate Behavioral Research, 28*(4), 407–434.

Gustafsson, J.-E., & Undheim, J. O. (1996). Individual differences in cognitive functions. In D. C. Berliner & R. C. Calfer (Eds.), *Handbook of educational psychology* (pp. 186–242). New York: Macmillan.

Hakstian, A. R., & Cattell, R. B. (1974). The checking of primary ability structure on a basis of twenty primary abilities. *British Journal of Educational Psychology, 44,* 140–154.

Hakstian, A. R., & Cattell, R. B. (1978). Higher stratum ability structure on a basis of twenty primary abilities. *Journal of Educational Psychology, 70,* 657–659.

Hambrick, D. Z., & Engle, R. W. (2002). Effects of domain knowledge, working memory capacity, and age on cognitive performance: An investigation of the knowledge-is-power hypothesis. *Cognitive Psychology, 44*(4), 339–387.

Hitch, G. J., Towse, J. N., & Hutton, U. (2001). What limits children's working memory span? Theoretical accounts and applications for scholastic development. *Journal of Experimental Psychology: General, 130*(2), 184–198.

Horn, J. (1976). Human abilities: A review of research and theory in the early 1970's. *Annual Review of Psychology, 27,* 437–485.

Horn, J. (1998). A basis for research on age differences in cognitive abilities. In J. J. McArdle & R. W. Woodcock (Eds.), *Human cognitive abilities in theory and practice* (pp. 57–92). Mahwah, NJ: Erlbaum.

Horn, J. L. (1965). *Fluid and crystallized intelligence: A factor analytic study of the structure among primary mental abilities.* Unpublished doctoral dissertation, University of Illinois, Champaign.

Horn, J. L. (1968). Organization of abilities and the development of intelligence. *Psychological Review, 75,* 242–259.

Horn, J. L. (1972). State, trait and change dimensions of intelligence: A critical experiment. *British Journal of Educational Psychology, 42,* 159–185.

Horn, J. L. (1988). Thinking about human abilities. In J. R. Nesselroade (Ed.), *Handbook of multivariate psychology* (pp. 645–685). New York: Academic Press.

Horn, J. L. (1991). Measurement of intellectual capabilities: A review of theory. In K. S. McGrew, J. K. Werder, & R. W. Woodcock, *WJ-R technical manual* (pp. 197–232). Chicago: Riverside.

Horn, J. L. (1994). The theory of fluid and crystallized intelligence. In R. J. Sternberg (Ed.), *The encyclopedia of human intelligence* (pp. 443–451). New York: Macmillan.

Horn, J. L., & Bramble, W. J. (1967). Second-order ability structure revealed in rights and wrongs scores. *Journal of Educational Psychology, 58,* 115–122.

Horn, J. L., & Masunaga, H. (2000). New directions for research into aging and intelligence: The development of expertise. In T. J. Perfect & E. A. Maylor (Eds.), *Models of cognitive aging* (pp. 125–159). Oxford: Oxford University Press.

Horn, J. L., & Cattell, R. B. (1966). Refinement and test of the theory of fluid and crystallized intelligence. *Journal of Educational Psychology, 57,* 253–270.

Horn, J. L., & Cattell, R. B. (1967). Age differences in fluid and crystallized intelligence. *Acta Psychologica, 26,* 107–129.

Horn, J. L., & McArdle, J. J. (1992). A practical and theoretical guide to measurement invariance in aging research. *Experimental Aging Research, 18*(3–4), 117–144.

Horn, J. L., & Noll, J. (1997). Human cognitive capabilities: Gf-Gc theory. In D. P. Flanagan, J. L. Genshaft, & P. L. Harrison (Eds.), *Contemporary intellectual assessment: Theories, tests, and issues* (pp. 53–91). New York: Guilford Press.

Horn, J. L., & Stankov, L. (1982). Auditory and visual factors of intelligence. *Intelligence, 6*(2), 165–185.

Hunt, E. (1999). Intelligence and human resources: Past, present, and future. In P. L. Ackerman, P. Kyllonen, & R. Roberts (Eds.), *Learning and individual differences: Process, trait, and content determinants* (pp. 3–30). Washington, DC: American Psychological Association.

Jensen, A. R. (1984). Test validity: g versus the specificity doctrine. *Journal of Social and Biological Structures, 7,* 93–118.

Jensen, A. R. (1993). Spearman's hypothesis tested with chronometric information-processing tasks. *Intelligence, 17*(1), 47–77.

Jensen, A. R. (1998). *The g factor: The science of mental ability.* Westport, CT: Praeger.

Jensen, A. R. (2004). Obituary—John Bissell Carroll. *Intelligence, 32*(1), 1–5.

Just, M. A., & Carpenter, P. A. (1992). A capacity theory of comprehension: Individual differences in working memory. *Psychological Review, 99*(1), 122–149.

Kane, M. J., Bleckley, M. K., Conway, A. R. A., & Engle, R. W. (2001). A controlled-attention view of working-memory capacity. *Journal of Experimental Psychology: General, 130*(2), 169–183.

Kaufman, A. S., & Dopplet, J. E. (1976). Analysis of WISC-R standardization data in terms of the stratification variables. *Child Development, 47,* 165–171.

Kaufman, A. S., Ishikuma, T., & Kaufman, N. L. (1994). A Horn analysis of the factors measured by the WAIS-R, Kaufman Adolescent and Adult Intelligence Test (KAIT), and two new brief cognitive measures for normal adolescents and adults. *Assessment, 1,* 353–366.

Kaufman, A. S., & Kaufman, N. L. (1993). *Kaufman Adolescent and Adult Intelligence Test manual.* Circle Pines, MN: American Guidance Services.

Kaufman, A. S., & Kaufman, N. L. (1994a). *Manual for Kaufman Functional Academic Skills Test (K-FAST).* Circle Pines, MN: American Guidance Service.

Kaufman, A. S., & Kaufman, N. L. (1994b). *Manual for Kaufman Short Neuropsychological Assessment Procedure (K-SNAP).* Circle Pines, MN: American Guidance Service.

Kaufman, A. S., & O'Neal, M. (1988). Factor structure of the Woodcock–Johnson cognitive subtests from preschool to adulthood. *Journal of Psychoeducational Assessment, 6,* 35–48.

Keith, T. Z. (1999). Effects of general and specific abilities on student achievement: Similarities and differences across ethnic groups. *School Psychology Quarterly, 14*(3), 239–262.

Keith, T. Z., Kranzler, J. H., & Flanagan, D. P. (2001). What does the Cognitive Assessment System (CAS) measure?: Joint confirmatory factor analysis of the CAS and the Woodcock–Johnson Tests of Cognitive Ability (3rd edition). *School Psychology Review, 30*(1), 89–119.

Kyllonen, P. C. (1996). Is working memory capacity Spearman's *g*? In I. Dennis & P. Tapsfield (Eds.), *Human abilities: Their nature and measurement* (pp. 49–76). Mahwah, NJ: Erlbaum.

Kyllonen, P. C., & Christal, R. E. (1990). Reasoning ability is (little more than) working-memory capacity?! *Intelligence, 14*, 389–433.!

Lamb, K. (1994). Genetics and Spearman's "g" factor. *Mankind Quarterly, 34*(4), 379–391.

Leather, C. V., & Henry, L. A. (1994). Working memory span and phonological awareness tasks as predictors of early reading ability. *Journal of Experimental Child Psychology, 58*, 88–111.

Li, S., Jordanova, M., & Lindenberger, U. (1998). From good senses to good sense: A link between tactile information processing and intelligence. *Intelligence, 26*(2), 99–122.

Lohman, D. F. (1994). Spatially gifted, verbally inconvenienced. In N. Colangelo, S. G. Assouline, & D. L. Ambroson (Eds.), *Talent development: Vol. 2. Proceedings from the 1993 Henry B. and Jocelyn Wallace National Research Symposium on Talent Development* (pp. 251–264). Dayton, OH: Ohio Psychology Press.

Lohman, D. F. (2000). Complex information processing and intelligence. In R. J. Sternberg (Ed.), *Handbook of intelligence* (pp. 285–340). New York: Cambridge University Press.

Lohman, D. F. (2001). Issues in the definition and measurement of abilities. In J. M. Collis & S. Messick (Eds.), *Intelligence and personality: Bridging the gap in theory and measurement* (pp. 79–98). Mahwah, NJ: Erlbaum.

Lubinski, D. (2000). Scientific and social significance of assessing individual differences: "Sinking shafts at a few critical points." *Annual Review of Psychology, 51*, 405–444.

MacCallum, R. C. (2003). Working with imperfect models. *Multivariate Behavioral Research, 38*(1), 113–139.

McDermott, P. A., Fantuzzo, J. W., & Glutting, J. J. (1990). Just say no to subtest analysis: A critique on Wechsler theory and practice. *Journal of Psychoeducational Assessment, 8*, 290–302.

McDermott, P. A., & Glutting, J. J. (1997). Informing stylistic learning behavior, disposition, and achievement through ability subtests—or, more illusions of meaning? *School Psychology Review, 26*, 163–175.

McGhee, R., & Lieberman, L. (1994). Gf-Gc theory of human cognition: Differentiation of short-term auditory and visual memory factors. *Psychology in the Schools, 31*, 297–304.

McGrew, K. S. (1986). A review of the differential predictive validity of the Woodcock–Johnson Scholastic Aptitude clusters. *Journal of Psychoeducational Assessment, 4*, 307–317.

McGrew, K. S. (1987). Exploratory factor analysis of the Woodcock–Johnson Tests of Cognitive Ability. *Journal of Psychoeducational Assessment, 5*, 200–216.

McGrew, K. S. (1993). The relationship between the WJ-R Gf-Gc cognitive clusters and reading achievement across the lifespan. *Journal of Psychoeducational Assessment, Monograph Series: WJ-R Monograph*, 39–53.

McGrew, K. S. (1997). Analysis of the major intelligence batteries according to a proposed comprehensive Gf-Gc framework. In D. P. Flanagan, J. L. Genshaft, & P. L. Harrison (Eds.), *Contemporary intellectual assessment: Theories, tests, and issues* (pp. 151–179). New York: Guilford Press.

McGrew, K. S. (2002). *Advanced interpretation of the Woodcock–Johnson III*. Workshop presented at the annual convention of the National Association of School Psychologists, Chicago.

McGrew, K. S., & Evans, J. (2004). *Carroll Human Cognitive Abilities Project: Research Report No. 2. Internal and external factorial extensions to the Cattell–Horn–Carroll (CHC) theory of cognitive abilities: A review of factor analytic research since Carroll's seminal 1993 treatise*. St. Cloud, MN: Institute for Applied Psychometrics.

McGrew, K. S., & Flanagan, D. P. (1998). *The intelligence test desk reference (ITDR): Gf-Gc cross battery assessment*. Boston: Allyn & Bacon.

McGrew, K. S., Flanagan, D. P., Keith, T. Z., & Vanderwood, M. (1997). Beyond *g*: The impact of Gf-Gc specific cognitive abilities research on the future use and interpretation of intelligence tests in the schools. *School Psychology Review, 26*(2), 189–210.

McGrew, K. S., Gregg, N., Hoy, C., Stennett, R., Davis, M., Knight, D., et al. (2001). *Cattell–Horn–Carroll confirmatory factor analysis of the WJ III, WAIS-III, WMS-III and KAIT in a university sample*. Manuscript in preparation.

McGrew, K. S., & Hessler, G. L. (1995). The relationship between the WJ-R Gf-Gc cognitive clusters and mathematics achievement across the life-span. *Journal of Psychoeducational Assessment, 13*, 21–38.

McGrew, K. S., Johnson, D. R., Cosio, A., & Evans, J. (2004). *Increasing the chance of no child being left behind: Beyond cognitive and achievement abilities*. Minneapolis: University of Minnesota, Institute on Community Integration.

McGrew, K. S., & Knopik, S. N. (1993). The relationship between the WJ-R Gf-Gc cognitive clusters and writing achievement across the life-span. *School Psychology Review, 22*, 687–695.

McGrew, K. S., Werder, J. K., & Woodcock, R. W. (1991). *WJ-R technical manual*. Chicago: Riverside.

McGrew, K. S., & Woodcock, R. W. (2001). *Woodcock–Johnson III technical manual*. Itasca, IL: Riverside.

McGue, M., Shinn, M., & Ysseldyke, J. (1979). *Validity of the Woodcock–Johnson Psycho-Educational Battery with learning disabled students* (Research Report No. 15). Minneapolis: University of Minnesota, Institute of Research on Learning Disabilities.

McGue, M., Shinn, M., & Ysseldyke, J. (1982). Use of the cluster scores on the Woodcock–Johnson Psycho-Educational Battery with learning disabled students. *Learning Disability Quarterly, 5*, 274–287.

McNemar, Q. (1964). Lost: Our intelligence? Why? *American Psychologist, 19*, 871–872.

Miyake, A., Friedman, N. P., Rettinger, D. A., Shah, P., & Hegarty, P. (2001). How are visuospatial working memory, executive functioning, and spatial abilities related?: A latent-variable analysis. *Journal of Experimental Psychology: General, 130*(4), 621–640.

Naglieri, J., & Das, J. P. (1997). *Das–Naglieri Cognitive Assessment System (CAS)*. Itasca, IL: Riverside.

Neisser, U., Boodoo, G., Bouchard, T. J. Jr., Boykin, A. W., Brody, N., Ceci, S. J., et al. (1996). Intelligence: Knowns and unknowns. *American Psychologist, 51*(2), 77–101.

Nettelbeck, T. (2003). Inspection time and *g*. In H. Nyborg (Ed.), *The scientific study of general intelligence: Tribute to Arthur R. Jensen* (pp. 77–92). San Diego, CA: Pergamon.

Neuman, G. A., Bolin, A. U., & Briggs, T. E. (2000). Identifying general factors of intelligence: A confirmatory factor analysis of the Ball Aptitude Battery. *Educational and Psychological Measurement, 60*(5), 697–712.

Nyborg, H. (Ed.). (2003). *The scientific study of general intelligence: Tribute to Arthur R. Jensen*. Amsterdam: Pergamon Press.

Oberauer, K., Suß, H.-M., Wilhelm, O., & Wittman, W. W. (2003). The multiple faces of working memory: Storage, processing, supervision, and coordination. *Intelligence, 31*(2), 167–193.

O'Connor, T. A., & Burns, N. R. (2003). Inspection time and general speed of processing. *Personality and Individual Differences, 35*(3), 713–724.

Paas, F., Renkl, A., & Sweller, J. (2003). Cognitive load theory and instructional design: Recent developments. *Educational Psychologist, 38*(1), 1–4.

Paas, F., Tuovinen, J. E., Tabbers, H., & VanGerven, P. W. M. (2003). Cognitive load measurement as a means to advance cognitive load theory. *Educational Psychologist, 38*(1), 63–71.

Pallier, G., Roberts, R. D., & Stankov, L. (2000). Biological versus psychometric intelligence: Halstead's (1947) distinction revisited. *Archives of Clinical Neuropsychology, 15*(3), 205–226.

Park, D. C., Lautenschlager, G., Smith, A. D., Earles, J. L., Frieske, D., Zwahr, M., & Gaines, C. L. (1996). Mediators of long-term memory performance across the life span. *Psychology and Aging, 11*(4), 621–637.

Phelps, L., McGrew, K., Knopik, S., & Ford, L. (in press). The general (*g*), broad and narrow CHC stratum characteristics of the WJ III and WISC-III tests: A confirmatory cross-battery investigation. *School Psychology Quarterly*.

Prentky, R. A. (1996). Teaching machines. In R. J. Corsini & A. J. Auerbach (Eds.), *Concise encyclopedia of psychology* (2nd ed., Vol. 3, p. 509). New York: Wiley.

Reed, M. T., & McCallum, R. S. (1995). Construct validity of the Universal Nonverbal Intelligence Test (UNIT). *Psychology in the Schools, 32*, 277–290.

Reschly, D. (1997). Utility of individual ability measures and public policy choices for the 21st century. *School Psychology Review, 26*, 234–241.

Roberts, R. D., Nelson-Goff, G., Anjoul, F., Kyllonen, P. C., Pallier, G., & Stankov, L. (2000). The Armed Services Vocational Aptitude Battery (ASVAB): Little more than acculturated learning (Gc)!? *Learning and Individual Differences, 12*(1), 81–103.

Roberts, R. D., Pallier, G., & Nelson-Goff, G. (1999). Sensory processes within the structure of human cognitive abilities. In P. L. Ackerman, P. C. Kyllonen, & R. D. Roberts (Eds.), *Learning and individual differences* (Vol. 15, pp. 339–368). Washington, DC: American Psychological Association.

Roberts, R. D., Pallier, G., & Stankov, L. (1996). The basic information processing (BIP) unit, mental speed and human cognitive abilities: Should the BIP R.I.P.? *Intelligence, 23*, 133–155.

Roberts, R. D., & Stankov, L. (1999). Individual differences in speed of mental processing and human cognitive abilities: Toward a taxonomic model. *Learning and Individual Differences, 11*(1), 1–120.

Roberts, R. D., Stankov, L., Pallier, G., & Dolph, B. (1997). Charting the cognitive sphere: Tactile–kinesthetic performance within the structure of intelligence. *Intelligence, 25*, 111–148.

Roid, G. H. (2003). *Stanford–Binet Intelligence Scales, Fifth Edition*. Itasca, IL: Riverside.

Roid, G. H., Woodcock, R. W., & McGrew, K. S. (1997). *Factor analysis of the Stanford–Binet L and M Forms*. Unpublished manuscript, Riverside Publishing, Itasca, IL.

Rossman, B. B., & Horn, J. L. (1972). Cognitive, motivational and temperamental indicants of creativity and intelligence. *Journal of Educational Measurement, 9*, 265–286.

Rosso, M., & Phelps, L. (1988). Factor analysis of the Woodcock–Johnson with conduct disordered adolescents. *Psychology in the Schools, 25*, 105–110.

Royce, J. R. (1973). The conceptual framework for a multi-factor theory of individuality. In J. R. Royce (Ed.), *Multivariate analysis and psychological theory* (pp. 305–407). New York: Academic Press.

Salthouse, T. A. (1996). The processing-speed theory of adult age differences in cognition. *Psychological Review, 103*(3), 403–428.

Schrank, F. A., Flanagan, D. P., Woodcock, R. W., & Mascolo, J. T. (2002). *Essentials of WJ III cognitive abilities assessment*. New York: Wiley.

Snow, R. E. (1998). Abilities and aptitudes and achievements in learning situations. In J. J. McArdle & R. W. Woodcock (Eds.), *Human cognitive abilities in theory and practice* (pp. 93–112). Mahwah, NJ: Erlbaum.

Snow, R. E., Corno, L., & Jackson, D. (1996). Individual differences in affective and conative functions. In D. C. Berliner & R. C. Calfee (Eds.), *Handbook of educational psychology* (pp. 243–310). New York: Simon & Schuster Macmillan.

Spearman, C. E. (1904). "General Intelligence," objectively determined and measured. *American Journal of Psychiatry, 15,* 201–293.

Spearman, C. E. (1927). *The abilities of man: Their nature and measurement.* London: Macmillan.

Spearman, C. E., & Wynn Jones, L. (1950). *Human ability: A continuation of "The abilities of man."* London: Macmillan.

Stankov, L. (1994). The complexity effect phenomenon is an epiphenomenon of age-related fluid intelligence decline. *Personality and Individual Differences, 16*(2), 265–288.

Stankov, L. (2000). Structural extensions of a hierarchical view on human cognitive abilities. *Learning and Individual Differences, 12*(1), 35–51.

Stankov, L., Boyle, G. J., & Cattell, R. B. (1995). Models and paradigms in personality and intelligence research. In D. H. Saklofske & M. Zeidner (Eds.), *International handbook of personality and intelligence* (pp. 15–44). New York: Plenum Press.

Stankov, L., & Horn, J. L. (1980). Human abilities revealed through auditory tests. *Journal of Educational Psychology, 72,* 21–44.

Stankov, L., Seizova-Cajic, T., & Roberts, R. D. (2001). Tactile and kinesthetic perceptual processes within the taxonomy of human cognition and abilities. *Intelligence, 29*(1), 1–29.

Sternberg, R. J. (1994). *The encyclopedia of human intelligence.* New York: Macmillan.

Sternberg, R. J., & Kaufman, J. C. (1998). Human abilities. *Annual Review of Psychology, 49,* 1134–1139.

Suß, H.-M., Oberauer, K., Wittmann, W. W., Wilhelm, O., & Schulze, R. (2002). Working-memory capacity explains reasoning ability—and a little bit more. *Intelligence, 30*(3), 261–288.

Taub, G. E., & McGrew, K. S. (2004). A confirmatory factor analysis of Cattell–Horn–Carroll theory and cross-age invariance of the Woodcock–Johnson tests of cognitive abilities III. *School Psychology Quarterly, 19*(1), 72–87.

Thurstone, L. L. (1938). The perceptual factor. *Psychometrika, 3,* 1–17.

Thurstone, L. L. (1947). *Multiple factor analysis.* Chicago: University of Chicago Press.

Thurstone, L. L., & Thurstone, T. G. (1941). *Factorial studies of intelligence* (Psychometric Monographs, No. 2). Chicago: University of Chicago Press.

Tirre, W. C., & Field, K. A. (2002). Structural models of abilities measured by the Ball Aptitude Battery. *Educational and Psychological Measurement, 62*(5), 830–856.

Tulsky, D. S., & Price, L. R. (2003). The joint WAIS-III and WMS-III factor structure: Development and cross-validation of a six-factor model of cognitive functioning. *Psychological Assessment, 15*(2), 149–162.

Vanderwood, M. L., McGrew, K. S., Flanagan, D. P., & Keith, T. Z. (2002). The contribution of general and specific cognitive abilities to reading achievement. *Learning and Individual Differences, 13,* 159–188.

Vernon, P. E. (1950). *The structure of human abilities.* New York: Wiley.

Vernon, P. E. (1961). *The structure of human abilities* (2nd ed.). London: Methuen.

Vygotsky, L. S. (1978). Mind in society: The development of higher psychological processes. (M. Cole, V. John-Stiner, S. Scribner, & E. Souberman, Eds. & Trans.) Cambridge, MA: Harvard University Press.

Woodcock, R. W. (1978). *Development and standardization of the Woodcock–Johnson Psycho-Educational Battery.* Hingham, MA: Teaching Resources.

Woodcock, R. W. (1990). Theoretical foundations of the WJ-R measures of cognitive ability. *Journal of Psychoeducational Assessment, 8,* 231–258.

Woodcock, R. W. (1994). Measures of fluid and crystallized intelligence. In R. J. Sternberg (Ed.), *The encyclopedia of human intelligence* (pp. 452–456). New York: Macmillan.

Woodcock, R. W., & Johnson, M. B. (1977). *Woodcock–Johnson Psycho-Educational Battery.* Hingham, MA: Teaching Resources.

Woodcock, R. W., & Johnson, M. B. (1989). *Woodcock–Johnson Psycho-Educational Battery—Revised.* Chicago: Riverside.

Woodcock, R. W., McGrew, K. S., & Mather, N. (2001). *Woodcock–Johnson III.* Itasca, IL: Riverside.

III

Contemporary and Emerging Interpretive Approaches

Part III, "Contemporary and Emerging Interpretive Approaches," a section not found in the first edition of the text, includes chapters about applications of the latest theoretical models and contemporary psychometric research in the use and interpretation of intelligence tests. In Chapter 9, "The Impact of the Cattell–Horn–Carroll Theory on Test Development and Interpretation of Cognitive and Academic Abilities," Vincent C. Alfonso, Dawn P. Flanagan, and Suzan Radwan offer empirically guided recommendations regarding how psychologists can augment any major intelligence test battery to ensure that a greater breadth of cognitive abilities is measured and interpreted according to the integrated Cattell–Horn–Carroll model. Randy G. Floyd's Chapter 10, "Information-Processing Approaches to Interpretation of Contemporary Intellectual Assessment Instruments," provides a comprehensive description of the major information-processing theories of cognition and their use in interpreting test results. Chapter 11, "Advances in Cognitive Assessment of Culturally and Linguistically Diverse Individuals: A Nondiscriminatory Interpretive Approach," by Samuel O. Ortiz and Salvador Hector Ochoa, provides an application of recent theory and psychometric research in promoting valid assessment of individuals from diverse backgrounds.

In Chapter 12, "Issues in Subtest Profile Analysis," Marley W. Watkins, Joseph J. Glutting, and Eric A. Youngstrom examine the drawbacks and methodological weaknesses of traditional approaches to determining whether a profile of scores on a given intelligence test battery is unique, and therefore propose alternative methods of subtest/profile analysis. Part III concludes with Chapter 13 by Nancy Mather and Barbara J. Wendling, "Linking Cognitive Assessment Results to Academic Interventions for Students with Learning Disabilities." The largest group of children identified with disabilities in school settings consists of youngsters with learning disabilities, and Mather and Wendling's chapter has great relevance in assessment and planning effective interventions for these children.

9

The Impact of the Cattell–Horn–Carroll Theory on Test Development and Interpretation of Cognitive and Academic Abilities

VINCENT C. ALFONSO
DAWN P. FLANAGAN
SUZAN RADWAN

In recent years, the *Cattell–Horn–Carroll* (CHC) theory has had a significant impact on the measurement of cognitive abilities and the interpretation of intelligence test performance. The purpose of this chapter is to summarize the most salient ways in which CHC theory has influenced the field of intellectual assessment. The chapter begins with a brief summary of the evolution of CHC theory. Next, the specific ways in which current CHC theory and research have influenced test development are presented. Finally, the CHC cross-battery approach is described as one mechanism through which practitioners in the field of psychoeducational assessment have embraced CHC theory, particularly as it applies to test interpretation.

BRIEF HISTORY OF THE CHC THEORY

The CHC theory is the most comprehensive and empirically supported psychometric theory of the structure of cognitive and academic abilities to date. It represents the in-

tegrated works of Raymond Cattell, John Horn, and John Carroll (Flanagan, McGrew, & Ortiz, 2000; McGrew, Chapter 8, this volume; Neisser et al., 1996). Because it has an impressive body of empirical support in the research literature (e.g., developmental, neurocognitive, outcome criterion), it is used extensively as the foundation for selecting, organizing, and interpreting tests of intelligence and cognitive abilities (e.g., Flanagan et al., 2000; Flanagan & Ortiz, 2001; McGrew & Flanagan, 1998). Most recently, it has been used for classifying achievement tests to (1) facilitate interpretation of academic abilities, and (2) provide a foundation for organizing assessments for individuals suspected of having a learning disability (Flanagan, Ortiz, Alfonso, & Mascolo, 2002). In addition, CHC theory is the foundation on which many new and recently revised intelligence batteries have been based (see Kaufman, Kaufman, Kaufman-Singer, & Kaufman, Chapter 16, this volume; Roid & Pomplun, Chapter 15, this volume; Schrank, Chapter 17, this volume). Because the evolution of CHC theory is described in depth by

McGrew (Chapter 8, this volume) and Horn and Blankson (Chapter 3, this volume), only a brief overview is presented here.

Original Gf-Gc Theory: First Precursor to CHC Theory

The original Gf-Gc theory was a dichotomous conceptualization of human cognitive ability put forth by Raymond Cattell in the early 1940s. Cattell based his theory on the factor-analytic work of Thurstone conducted in the 1930s. Cattell believed that *fluid intelligence* (Gf) included inductive and deductive reasoning abilities that were influenced by biological and neurological factors, as well as incidental learning through interaction with the environment. He postulated further that *crystallized intelligence* (Gc) consisted primarily of acquired knowledge abilities that reflected, to a large extent, the influences of acculturation (Cattell, 1957, 1971).

In 1965, John Horn expanded the dichotomous Gf-Gc model to include four additional abilities, including *visual perception or processing* (Gv), *short-term memory* (*short-term acquisition and retrieval—SAR or Gsm*), *long-term storage and retrieval* (*tertiary storage and retrieval—TSR or Glr*), and *speed of processing* (Gs). Later he added *auditory processing ability* (Ga) to the theoretical model and refined the definitions of Gv, Gs, and Glr (Horn, 1968; Horn & Stankov, 1982).

In the early 1990s, Horn added a factor representing an individual's quickness in reacting (*reaction time*) and making decisions (*decision speed*). The abbreviation for this factor is Gt (Horn, 1991). Finally, factors for *quantitative ability* (Gq) and *broad reading/ writing ability* (Gw) were added to the model, based on the research of Horn (e.g., 1991) and Woodcock (1994), respectively. Based largely on the results of Horn's thinking and research, Gf-Gc theory expanded into an eight-factor model that became known as the Cattell–Horn Gf-Gc theory (Horn, 1991; see also Horn & Blankson, Chapter 3, this volume).

Carroll's Three-Stratum Theory: Second Precursor to CHC Theory

In his seminal review of the world's literature on human cognitive abilities, Carroll (1993) proposed that the structure of cognitive abilities could be understood best via three strata that differ in breadth and generality. The broadest and most general level of ability is represented by stratum III. According to Carroll, stratum III represents a general factor consistent with Spearman's (1927) concept of *g* and subsumes both broad (stratum II) and narrow (stratum I) abilities. The various broad (stratum II) abilities, are denoted with an uppercase G followed by a lowercase letter (e.g., Gf and Gc). The eight broad abilities included in Carroll's theory subsume a large number of narrow (stratum I) abilities (Carroll, 1993; see also Carroll, Chapter 4, this volume).[1]

The Cattell–Horn and Carroll Theories: Similarities and Differences

Figure 9.1 includes the Cattell–Horn Gf-Gc theory and Carroll's three-stratum theory (without the narrow abilities). These theories are presented together in order to highlight the most salient similarities and differences between them. Each theory posits that there are multiple broad (stratum II) abilities, and for the most part, the names and abbreviations associated with these abilities are similar or identical. Briefly, there are four major structural differences between the Carroll and Cattell–Horn theories. First, Carroll's theory includes a general ability factor (stratum III); the Cattell–Horn theory does not. Second, the Cattell–Horn theory includes quantitative knowledge and quantitative reasoning as a separate broad ability (i.e., Gq), whereas Carroll's theory includes quantitative reasoning as a narrow ability subsumed by Gf. This difference is depicted in Figure 9.1 by the arrow that leads from Gq in the Cattell–Horn theory to Gf in Carroll's theory. Third, the Cattell–Horn theory includes a broad reading/writing (Grw) factor; Carroll's theory includes reading and writing as narrow abilities subsumed by Gc. This difference is depicted in Figure 9.1 by the arrow that leads from Grw in the Cattell–Horn theory to Gc in Carroll's theory. Fourth, Carroll's theory includes short-term memory with other memory abilities, such as associative memory, meaningful memory, and free-recall memory, under Gy in Figure 9.1; the Cattell–Horn theory separates short-term memory (Gsm) from associative mem-

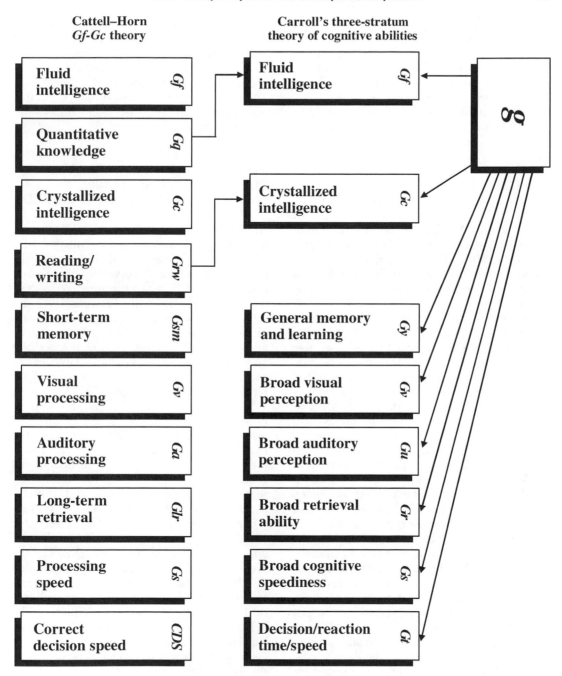

FIGURE 9.1. Comparison of Cattell–Horn Gf-Gc and Carroll three-stratum theories. Narrow abilities are omitted from this figure. From Flanagan, Ortiz, Alfonso, and Mascolo (2002). Published by Allyn and Bacon, Boston, MA. Copyright © 2002 by Pearson Education. Reprinted by permission.

ory, meaningful memory, and free-recall memory, because the latter abilities are purported to measure long-term retrieval (Glr in Figure 9.1). Notwithstanding these differences, Carroll (1993) concluded that the Cattell–Horn Gf-Gc theory represents the most reasonable approach to the structure of cognitive abilities currently available.

Current CHC Theory

In the late 1990s, McGrew (1997) attempted to resolve differences between the Cattell–Horn and Carroll models on the basis of his research. McGrew proposed an "integrated" Gf-Gc theory in Flanagan and colleagues (2000). This integrated theory became known as the Cattell–Horn–Carroll (CHC) theory of cognitive abilities shortly thereafter (see McGrew, Chapter 8, this volume, for details). CHC theory is depicted in Figure 9.2. This figure shows that CHC theory currently consists of 10 broad cognitive abilities and more than 70 narrow abilities.

The CHC theory presented in Figure 9.2 omits a g or general ability factor, primarily because the utility of the theory (as it is employed in assessment-related disciplines) is in clarifying individual cognitive and academic strengths and weaknesses, which are understood best through the operationalization of broad (stratum II) and narrow (stratum I) abilities (Flanagan & Ortiz, 2001). Others, however, believe that g is the most important ability to assess because it predicts the lion's share of the variance in multiple outcomes, both academic and occupational (e.g., Glutting, Watkins, & Youngstrom, 2003). Notwithstanding one's position on the importance of g in understanding various outcomes (particularly academic), there is considerable evidence that both broad and narrow CHC cognitive abilities explain a significant portion of variance in specific academic abilities, over and above the variance accounted for by g (e.g., McGrew, Flanagan, Keith, & Vanderwood, 1997; Vanderwood, McGrew, Flanagan, & Keith, 2002).

The various revisions of and refinements to the theory of fluid and crystallized intelligence over the past several decades, along with its mounting network of validity evidence, only began to influence intelligence test development recently—in the middle to late 1980s. Today, however, nearly every intelligence test developer acknowledges the importance of CHC theory in defining and interpreting cognitive ability constructs, and most have used this theory to guide directly the development of their intelligence tests. The increased importance given to CHC theory in intelligence test development is summarized next.

INTELLIGENCE TESTS PUBLISHED PRIOR TO 1998: WHAT ABILITIES WERE MEASURED?

Although there was substantial evidence of at least eight or nine broad cognitive Gf-Gc abilities by the late 1980s, the tests of the time did not reflect this diversity in measurement. Table 9.1 shows the intelligence batteries that were published between 1981 and 1997. The information presented in this table was derived from a series of joint factor analyses conducted by Woodcock (1990) and others (Carroll, 1993; Flanagan & McGrew, 1997; Horn, 1991; Keith, 1997; Keith, Kranzler, & Flanagan, 2001; McGrew, 1997; Phelps, McGrew, Knopik, & Ford, in press). As Table 9.1 shows, the majority of tests published prior to 1998 measured only two or three broad cognitive abilities well (i.e., included two or more measures of the broad ability). For example, this table shows that the Wechsler Preschool and Primary Scale of Intelligence—Revised (WPPSI-R), the Kaufman Assessment Battery for Children (K-ABC), the Kaufman Adolescent and Adult Intelligence Test (KAIT), the Wechsler Adult Intelligence Scale—Revised (WAIS-R), and the Cognitive Assessment System (CAS) batteries only measured two or three broad CHC abilities adequately. The WPPSI-R primarily measured Gv and Gc. The K-ABC primarily measured Gv and Gsm, and to a much lesser extent Gf, while the KAIT primarily measured Gc and Glr, and to a much lesser extent Gf and Gv. The CAS measured Gs, Gsm, and Gv. Finally, while the Differential Ability Scales (DAS), the Stanford–Binet Intelligence Scale: Fourth Edition (SB-IV), and the Wechsler Intelligence Scale for Children—Third Edition (WISC-III) did not provide sufficient coverage of abilities to narrow the gap between contemporary theory and practice, their comprehensive measurement of approxi-

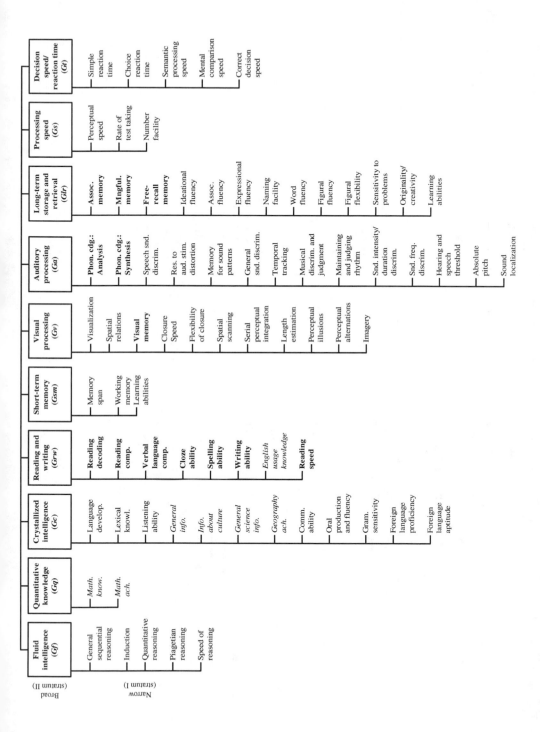

FIGURE 9.2. The Cattell–Horn–Carroll (CHC) theory of cognitive abilities. *Italic type* indicates abilities that were not included in Carroll's three-stratum theory, but were included by Carroll in the domains of knowledge and achievement. **Boldface type** indicates abilities that are placed under different CHC broad abilities than in Carroll's theory. These changes are based on the Cattell–Horn theory and/or recent research (see Flanagan et al., 2000; Flanagan & Ortiz, 2001; McGrew, 1997; McGrew & Flanagan, 1998). From Flanagan, Ortiz, Alfonso, and Mascolo (2002). Published by Allyn and Bacon, Boston, MA. Copyright © 2002 by Pearson Education. Reprinted by permission.

TABLE 9.1. Representation of Broad CHC Abilities on Nine Intelligence Batteries Published Prior to 1998

Battery	Gf	Gc	Gv	Gsm	Glr	Ga	Gs
WISC-III	—	Vocabulary Information Similarities Comprehension	Block Design Object Assembly Picture Arrangement Picture Completion Mazes	Digit Span	—	—	Symbol Search Coding
WAIS-R	—	Vocabulary Information Similarities Comprehension	Block Design Object Assembly Picture Completion Picture Arrangement	Digit Span	—	—	Digit–Symbol
WPPSI-R	—	Vocabulary Information Similarities Comprehension	Block Design Object Assembly Picture Completion Mazes Geometric Design	Sentences	—	—	Animal Pegs
KAIT	Mystery Codes Logical Steps	Definitions Famous Faces Auditory Comprehension Double Meanings	Memory for Block Designs	—	Rebus Learning Rebus Delayed Recall Auditory Delayed Recall	—	—
K-ABC	Matrix Analogies	—	Triangles Face Recognition Gestalt Closure Magic Window Hand Movements Spatial Memory Photo Series	Number Recall Word Order	—	—	—
CAS	—	—	Figure Memory Verbal Spatial Relations	Word Series Sentence Repetition	—	—	Matching Numbers Receptive Attention Planned Codes

190

	DAS	WJ-R	SB-IV
Number Detection Planned Connections Expressive Attention	Speed of Information Processing	Visual Matching Cross Out	—
	—	Incomplete Words Sound Blending Sound Patterns	—
	Recall of Objects	Memory for Names Visual–Auditory Learning Delayed Recall: Memory for Names Delayed Recall: Visual–Auditory Learning	—
Sentence Questions	Recall of Digits	Memory for Words Memory for Sentences Numbers Reversed	Memory for Sentences Memory for Digits
Nonverbal Matrices	Pattern Construction Block Building Copying Matching Letter-Like Forms Recall of Designs Recognition of Pictures	Spatial Relations Picture Recognition Visual Closure	Pattern Analysis Bead Memory Copying Memory for Objects Paper Folding and Cutting
	Similarities Verbal Comprehension Word Definitions Naming Vocabulary	Oral Vocabulary Picture Vocabulary Listening Comprehension Verbal Analogies	Verbal Relations Comprehension Absurdities Vocabulary
	Matrices Picture Similarities Sequential and Quantitative Reasoning	Concept Formation Analysis–Synthesis	Matrices Equation Building Number Series

Note. CHC classifications are based on the extant literature and primary sources such as Woodcock (1990), Horn (1991), Carroll (1993), McGrew (1997), and McGrew and Flanagan (1998). WISC-III, Wechsler Intelligence Scale for Children—Third Edition (Wechsler, 1991); WAIS-R, Wechsler Adult Intelligence Scale—Revised (Wechsler, 1981); WPPSI-R, Wechsler Preschool and Primary Scale of Intelligence—Revised (Wechsler, 1989); KAIT, Kaufman Adolescent and Adult Intelligence Test (Kaufman & Kaufman, 1993); K-ABC, Kaufman Assessment Battery for Children (Kaufman & Kaufman, 1983); CAS, Cognitive Assessment System (Das & Naglieri, 1997); DAS, Differential Ability Scales (Elliott, 1990); WJ-R, Woodcock–Johnson Psycho-Educational Battery—Revised (Woodcock & Johnson, 1989); SB-IV, Stanford–Binet Intelligence Scale: Fourth Edition (Thorndike, Hagen, & Sattler, 1986).

mately four CHC abilities, as depicted in Table 9.1, was nonetheless an improvement over the above-mentioned batteries. Table 9.1 shows that only the Woodcock–Johnson Psycho-Educational Battery—Revised (WJ-R) included measures of all broad cognitive abilities listed in the table. Nevertheless, most of the broad abilities were not measured adequately by the WJ-R (McGrew & Flanagan, 1998).

In general, Table 9.1 shows that Gf, Gsm, Glr, Ga, and Gs were not measured well by the majority of intelligence tests published prior to 1998. Therefore, it is clear that most test authors did not use the theory of fluid and crystallized intelligence and its corresponding research base to guide the development of their intelligence tests. As such, a substantial theory–practice gap existed; that is, theories of the structure of cognitive abilities were far in advance of the instruments used to operationalize them. In fact, prior to the mid-1980s, theory seldom played a role in intelligence test development. The numerous dashes in Table 9.1 exemplify the theory–practice gap that existed in the field of intellectual assessment at that time.

A METHOD DESIGNED TO NARROW THE THEORY–PRACTICE GAP: THE CHC CROSS-BATTERY APPROACH

As a result of his findings, Woodcock (1990) suggested that it might be necessary to "cross" batteries to measure a broader range of cognitive abilities. As such, the findings presented in Table 9.1 provided the impetus for the development of the cross-battery approach (McGrew & Flanagan, 1998). This approach to assessment (currently known as the *CHC cross-battery approach*, and referred to hereafter as the CB approach) is a time-efficient method of assessment and interpretation that is grounded in CHC theory and research. The CB approach provides a set of principles and procedures that allows practitioners to measure a wider range of abilities than that represented by most single intelligence or achievement batteries, in a theoretically and psychometrically defensible manner. In effect, the CB approach was developed to systematically replace the dashes in Table 9.1 with tests from another battery.

As such, this approach guides practitioners in the selection of tests, both core and supplemental, that together provide measurement of abilities that is considered sufficient in both breadth and depth for the purpose of addressing referral concerns. Furthermore, the CB approach details a hypothesis generation model of test interpretation that is grounded in current research. The section that follows briefly summarizes the three pillars or foundational sources of information that underlie the CB approach (Flanagan & Ortiz, 2001).

The Three Pillars of the CB Approach

The first pillar of the CB approach is CHC theory. This theory was selected to guide assessment and interpretation because it is based on a more thorough network of validity evidence than other contemporary multidimensional ability models of intelligence (see McGrew & Flanagan, 1998; Messick, 1992; Sternberg & Kaufman, 1998). According to Daniel (1997), the strength of this model is that it was arrived at "by synthesizing hundreds of factor analyses conducted over decades by independent researchers using many different collections of tests. Never before has a psychometric ability model been so firmly grounded in data" (pp. 1042–1043). Because the broad and narrow abilities that constitute CHC theory have been defined elsewhere in this book (see Horn & Blankson, Chapter 3, this volume; McGrew, Chapter 8, this volume), these definitions will not be reiterated here.

The second pillar of the CB approach consists of the CHC broad (stratum II) classifications of cognitive and academic ability tests. Specifically, based on the results of a series of cross-battery confirmatory factor analysis studies of the major intelligence batteries and task analyses of many test experts, Flanagan and colleagues classified all the subtests of the major cognitive and achievement batteries according to the particular CHC broad abilities they measured. To date, over 500 CHC broad-ability classifications have been made, based on the results of these studies. These classifications of cognitive and academic ability tests assist practitioners in identifying measures that assess various aspects of the broad abilities (such as Gf, Gc,

Gq, and Grw) represented in CHC theory. Classification of tests at the broad-ability level is necessary to improve upon the validity of cognitive assessment and interpretation. Specifically, broad-ability classifications ensure that the CHC constructs underlying assessments are minimally affected by *construct-irrelevant variance* (Messick, 1989, 1995). In other words, knowing what tests measure what abilities enables clinicians to organize tests into *construct-relevant* clusters—clusters containing only measures that are *relevant to* the construct or ability of interest.

The third pillar of the CB approach consists of the CHC narrow (stratum I) classifications of cognitive and academic ability tests. These classifications were originally reported in McGrew (1997). Subsequently, Caltabiano and Flanagan (2004) have provided content validity evidence for the narrow-ability classifications underlying the major intelligence and achievement batteries. Use of narrow-ability classifications were necessary to ensure that the CHC constructs underlying assessments are well represented. That is, the narrow-ability classifications of tests assist practitioners in combining qualitatively different indicators (or tests) of a given broad ability into clusters, so that appropriate inferences can be made from test performance. Taken together, the three pillars underlying the CB approach provide the necessary foundation for organizing assessments of cognitive and academic abilities that are theoretically driven, comprehensive, and valid.

IMPACT OF CHC THEORY AND CB CLASSIFICATIONS ON TEST DEVELOPMENT

In the past decade, Gf-Gc theory, and more recently CHC theory, have had a significant impact on the revision of old intelligence batteries and development of new ones. For example, a wider range of broad and narrow abilities is represented in current intelligence batteries than that which was represented in previous editions of these tests. Table 9.2 provides several salient examples of the impact that CHC theory and the resulting CB classifications have had on intelligence test

development over the past two decades. This table lists the major intelligence tests in the order in which they were revised, beginning with those tests with the greatest number of years between revisions (i.e., the K-ABC and its second edition, the KABC-II) and ending with newly developed tests and tests that at this writing have yet to be revised (e.g., the Wide Range Intelligence Test [WRIT] and DAS, respectively). As is obvious from a review of Table 9.2, CHC theory and CB classifications have had a significant impact on recent test development.

Of the seven intelligence batteries (including both comprehensive and brief measures) that were published since 2000, the test authors of three clearly used CHC theory and CB classifications as a blueprint for test development (i.e., the WJ III, SB5, and KABC-II), and the test authors of two were obviously influenced by CHC theory (i.e., the Reynolds Intellectual Assessment Scales [RIAS] and WRIT). Only the authors of the most recent Wechsler scales (i.e., the WPPSI-III, WISC-IV, and WAIS-III) have not stated explicitly that CHC theory was used as a guide for revision. Nevertheless, these authors acknowledge the research of Cattell, Horn, and Carroll in their most recent manuals (Wechsler, 2002, 2003). Presently, as Table 9.2 shows, nearly all intelligence batteries that are used with some regularity subscribe either explicitly or implicitly to CHC theory.

The obvious adherence to CHC theory may be seen also in Table 9.3. This table is identical to Table 9.1, except that it also includes the subtests from the most recent revisions of the tests from Table 9.2. A review of Table 9.3, which includes all intelligence batteries that have been published after 1998, shows that many of the gaps in measurement of broad cognitive abilities have been filled. Specifically, the majority of tests published after 1998 now measure four or five broad cognitive abilities adequately, as compared to two or three. For example, Table 9.3 shows that the WISC-IV, WAIS-III, WPPSI-III, KABC-II, and SB5 all measure four or five broad CHC abilities. The WISC-IV measures Gf, Gc, Gv, Gsm, and Gs, while the KABC-II measures Gf, Gc, Gv, Gsm, and Glr. The WAIS-III measures Gc, Gv, Gsm, and Gs adequately, and to a lesser extent Gf, while the WPPSI-III measures Gc, Gv/Gf, and Gs

TABLE 9.2. Impact of the CHC Theory on Intelligence Test Development

Test (year of publication) CHC impact	Revision (year of publication) CHC impact
K-ABC (1983) No obvious impact.	**KABC-II (2004)** Provides a second global score that includes crystallized ability. Includes several new subtests measuring reasoning. Interpretation of test performance may be based on CHC theory or Luria's theory. Provides assessment of five CHC broad abilities. (See Kaufman et al., Chapter 14, this volume.)
SB-IV (1986) Used a three-level hierarchical model of the structure of cognitive abilities to guide construction of the test. The top level included the general reasoning factor or g; the middle level included three broad factors called Crystallized Abilities, Fluid-Analytic Abilities, and Short-Term Memory; the third level included more specific factors, including Verbal Reasoning, Quantitative Reasoning, and Abstract/Visual Reasoning.	**SB5 (2003)** CHC theory has been used to guide test development. Increases the number of broad factors from four to five. Includes a Working Memory factor, based on research indicating its importance for academic success. (See Roid & Pomplum, Chapter 15, this volume.)
WAIS-R (1981) No obvious impact.	**WAIS-III (1997)** Enhances the measurement of fluid reasoning by adding the Matrix Reasoning subtest. Includes four Index scores that measure specific abilities more purely than the traditional IQs provided in the various Wechsler scales. Includes a Working Memory Index, based on recent research indicating its importance for academic success.
WPPSI-R (1989) No obvious impact.	**WPPSI-III (2002)** Incorporates measures of Processing Speed that yield a Processing Speed Quotient, based on recent research indicating the importance of processing speed for early academic success. Enhances the measurement of fluid reasoning by adding the Matrix Reasoning and Picture Concepts subtests.
WJ-R (1989) Modern Gf-Gc theory was used as the cognitive model for test development. Included two measures of each of eight broad abilities.	**WJ III (2001)** CHC theory has been used as a "blueprint" for test development. Includes two or three qualitatively different narrow abilities for each broad ability. The combined Cognitive and Achievement batteries of the WJ III include 9 of the 10 broad abilities subsumed in CHC theory.
WISC-III (1991) No obvious impact.	**WISC-IV (2003)** Eliminates Verbal and Performance IQs, adhering more closely to CHC theory. Replaces the Freedom from Distractibility Index with the Working Memory Index, a purer measure of working memory. Replaces the Perceptual Organization Index with the Perceptual Reasoning Index. Enhances the measurement of fluid reasoning by adding the Matrix Reasoning and Picture Concepts subtests. Enhances the measurement of processing speed with the addition of the Cancellation subtest.

(continued)

TABLE 9.2. (*continued*)

Test (year of publication) CHC impact	Revision (year of publication) CHC impact
RIAS (2003) Includes indicators of fluid and crystallized abilities.	
WRIT (2002) Has been developed to be consistent with current theories of intelligence. Evaluates multiple abilities. Provides Crystallized and Fluid IQs based on Cattell–Horn theory.	
CAS (1997) No obvious impact.	
KAIT (1993) Includes subtests organized according to the work of Horn and Cattell. Provides Fluid and Crystallized IQs.	
DAS (1990) No obvious impact.	

Note. K-ABC, Kaufman Assessment Battery for Children (Kaufman & Kaufman, 1983); KABC-II, Kaufman Assessment Battery for Children—Second Edition (Kaufman & Kaufman, 2004); SB-IV, Stanford–Binet Intelligence Scale: Fourth Edition (Thorndike et al., 1986); SB5, Stanford–Binet Intelligence Scales, Fifth Edition (Roid, 2003); WAIS-R, Wechsler Adult Intelligence Scale—Revised (Wechsler, 1981); WAIS-III, Wechsler Adult Intelligence Scale—Third Edition (Wechsler, 1997); WPPSI-R, Wechsler Preschool and Primary Scale of Intelligence—Revised (Wechsler, 1989); WPPSI-III, Wechsler Preschool and Primary Scale of Intelligence—Third Edition (Wechsler, 2002); WJ-R, Woodcock–Johnson Psycho-Educational Battery—Revised (Woodcock & Johnson, 1989); WJ III, Woodcock–Johnson III Tests of Cognitive Abilities (Woodcock, McGrew, & Mather, 2001); WISC-III, Wechsler Intelligence Scale for Children—Third Edition (Wechsler, 1991); WISC-IV, Wechsler Intelligence Scale for Children—Fourth Edition (Wechsler, 2003); RIAS, Reynolds Intellectual Assessment Scales (Reynolds & Kamphaus, 2003); WRIT, Wide Range Intelligence Test (Glutting, Adams, & Sheslow, 2002); CAS, Cognitive Assessment System (Das & Naglieri, 1997); KAIT, Kaufman Adolescent and Adult Intelligence Test (Kaufman & Kaufman, 1993); DAS, Differential Ability Scales (Elliott, 1990).

adequately. Finally, the SB5 measures four CHC broad abilities (i.e., Gf, Gc, Gv, Gsm).

Table 9.3 shows that the WJ III continues to include measures of all the major broad cognitive abilities and now measures these abilities well, particularly when it is used in conjunction with the Diagnostic Supplement (DS; Woodcock, McGrew, Mather, & Schrank, 2003). Moreover, a comparison of Tables 9.1 and 9.3 indicates that two broad abilities not measured by many intelligence batteries prior to 1998 are now measured by the majority of intelligence batteries available today—that is, Gf and Gsm. These broad abilities may be better represented on revised and new intelligence batteries because of the accumulating research evidence regarding their importance in overall aca-

demic success (Flanagan et al., 2002). Finally, Table 9.3 reveals that intelligence batteries continue to fall short in their measurement of three CHC broad abilities—specifically, Glr, Ga, and Gs. Thus, although there is greater coverage of CHC broad abilities now than there was only a few years ago, the need for the CB approach to assessment remains.

In sum, the CHC theory and the cognitive ability classifications of the CB approach have had a major impact on intelligence test development in recent years. The creators of some tests used CHC theory and CB classifications as a blueprint, while the developers of others adhered more loosely to the theory. It seems clear that the new generation of intelligence batteries has been influenced substantially by

TABLE 9.3. Representation of Broad CHC Abilities on Eight Intelligence Batteries Published after 1998

Battery	Gf	Gc	Gv	Gsm	Glr	Ga	Gs
WISC-IV	Matrix Reasoning Picture Concepts Arithmetic	Vocabulary Information Similarities Comprehension Word Reasoning	Block Design Picture Completion	Digit Span Letter–Number Sequencing	—	—	Symbol Search Coding Cancellation
WAIS-III[a]	Matrix Reasoning	Vocabulary Information Similarities Comprehension	Block Design Object Assembly Picture Arrangement Picture Completion	Digit Span Letter–Number Sequencing	—	—	Symbol Search Digit-Symbol Coding
WPPSI-III	Matrix Reasoning Picture Concepts	Vocabulary Information Similarities Comprehension Receptive Vocabulary Picture Naming Word Reasoning	Block Design Object Assembly Picture Completion	—	—	—	Coding Symbol Search
KABC-II	Pattern Reasoning Story Completion	Expressive Vocabulary Verbal Knowledge Riddles	Triangles Gestalt Closure Rover Block Counting Conceptual Thinking Face Recognition	Number Recall Word Order Hand Movements	Atlantis Rebus Atlantis Delayed Rebus Delayed	—	—
WJ III/DS	Concept Formation Analysis–Synthesis	Verbal Comprehension General	Spatial Relations Picture Recognition	Memory for Words Numbers Reversed	Visual–Auditory Learning Retrieval Fluency	Sound Blending Auditory Attention Incomplete Words	Visual Matching Decision Speed Pair Cancellation

	Number Series / Number Matrices	Information / Bilingual Verbal Comprehension	Planning / Visual Closure / Block Rotation	Auditory Working Memory / Memory for Sentences	Visual–Auditory Learning Delayed / Rapid Picture Naming / Memory for Names / Memory for Names Delayed	Sound Pattern–Voice / Sound Pattern–Music	Cross Out
SB5	Nonverbal Fluid Reasoning / Verbal Fluid Reasoning / Nonverbal Quantitative Reasoning / Verbal Quantitative Reasoning	Nonverbal Knowledge / Verbal Knowledge	Nonverbal Visual–Spatial Processing / Verbal Visual–Spatial Processing	Nonverbal Working Memory / Verbal Working Memory	—	—	—
RIAS	Odd-Item Out	Guess What / Verbal Reasoning	What's Missing	Verbal Memory / Nonverbal Memory	—	—	—
WRIT	Matrices	Verbal Analogies / Vocabulary	Diamonds	—	—	—	—

Note. CHC classifications are based on the extant literature and primary sources such as Woodcock (1990), Horn (1991), Carroll (1993), McGrew (1997), McGrew and Flanagan (1998), Caltabiano and Flanagan (2004), and Keith, Fine, Taub, Reynolds, and Kranzler (2004). WISC-IV, Wechsler Intelligence Scale for Children—Fourth Edition (Wechsler, 2003); WAIS-III, Wechsler Adult Intelligence Scale—Third Edition (Wechsler, 1997); WPPSI-III, Wechsler Preschool and Primary Scale of Intelligence—Third Edition (Wechsler, 2002); KABC-II, Kaufman Assessment Battery for Children—Second Edition (Kaufman & Kaufman, 2004); WJ III, Woodcock–Johnson III Tests of Cognitive Abilities (Woodcock, McGrew, & Mather, 2001); WJ III/DS, Diagnostic Supplement to the Woodcock–Johnson III Tests of Cognitive Abilities (Woodcock, McGrew, & Mather, 2003); SB5, Stanford–Binet Intelligence Scales, Fifth Edition (Roid, 2003); RIAS, Reynolds Intellectual Assessment Scales (Reynolds & Kamphaus, 2003); WRIT, Wide Range Intelligence Test (Glutting et al., 2002).

[a]Although the WAIS-III was published in 1997, it is included in this table because its predecessor, the Wechsler Adult Intelligence Scale—Revised, was included in Table 9.1, and because we wished to present all revised Wechsler scales in one table.

CHC theory and its expansive research base. In addition, the CHC ability classifications of the CB approach have influenced test development and continue to play a role in narrowing the theory–practice gap.

IMPACT OF CHC THEORY AND THE CB APPROACH ON TEST INTERPRETATION

We believe that perhaps the greatest contribution that CHC theory and the CHC CB approach have made to psychoeducational assessment involves interpretation of ability test performance. In this section, we explain how and why we believe this to be true, through a brief discussion of the following topics: (1) limitations of using one cognitive or achievement battery to answer most referrals of suspected learning disability; (2) psychometrically defensible means of evaluating data across batteries; (3) systematic approach to organizing assessments, generating/testing hypotheses, and making interpretations; (4) application to an operational definition of learning disability; and (5) application of CB interpretive methods to current intelligence batteries.

Limitations of Single Test Batteries

As a result of the theoretical and empirical work of John Carroll, John Horn, Richard Woodcock, Kevin McGrew, Dawn Flanagan, Tim Keith, and numerous others, it became clear that no single intelligence battery adequately measured all the broad abilities delineated in CHC theory. That is, almost no intelligence battery, particularly the Wechsler scales, contained a sufficient number of tests to measure the breadth of broad CHC abilities. Many of the broad abilities not measured by the Wechsler scales or by some other batteries, such as Gf, Ga, and Glr, have demonstrated a significant relationship to academic achievement. Therefore, perhaps the greatest limitation of a single intelligence battery is related to the assessment of children referred for suspected learning disabilities. Most single intelligence batteries do not measure all of the abilities considered important for understanding learning difficulties (see Flanagan et al., 2002). The CB approach

provides a systematic means of supplementing single intelligence batteries to ensure that the abilities considered most important vis-à-vis the referral are well represented in the assessment.

Psychometrically Defensible Means of Evaluating Data across Batteries

The CB approach provides a psychometrically defensible means of evaluating data within and across intelligence and achievement batteries. Following are some of the most salient ways in which the developers of the CB approach have made CHC-based assessment and interpretation across batteries defensible.

First, the CB approach provides professionals with a common, empirically based set of terms—in other words, a standard nomenclature that may be used to significantly reduce or eliminate miscommunication and misinterpretation within and across disciplines. This standard nomenclature also ensures that users of the CB approach will be less likely to make errors when combining cognitive or achievement tests (McGrew & Flanagan, 1998).

Second, the classification system of the CB approach is based on the results of theory-driven joint factor analyses and expert consensus studies. According to Kaufman (cited in Flanagan et al., 2000), the CB approach has current research at its foundation. It is based on sound theory and sound assessment principles.

Third, the use of the CB approach guards against two ubiquitous sources of invalidity in assessment—construct-irrelevant variance and construct underrepresentation (Messick, 1995). As stated earlier, the former source of invalidity is reduced or eliminated through the construction of broad-ability clusters, using the broad-ability classifications of the CB approach. The latter source of invalidity is reduced or eliminated through the construction of clusters that include tests measuring qualitatively different aspects of the broad ability following narrow-ability classifications. These procedures have been incorporated into the test use and interpretation procedures of two major intelligence batteries (the WISC-IV and KABC-II; Flanagan & Kaufman, 2004; Kaufman, Lichtenberger,

Fletcher-Janzen, & Kaufman, in press). For a point–counterpoint discussion of the psychometric characteristics of the CB approach, see Watkins, Glutting, and Youngstrom (2002), Watkins, Youngstrom, and Glutting (2002), and Ortiz and Flanagan (2002a, 2002b).

Systematic Approach to Organizing Assessments, Generating/Testing Hypotheses, and Making Interpretations

The CB approach provides practitioners with the means to organize assessments, generate and test hypotheses regarding an individual's functioning, and draw reliable and valid conclusions from cross-battery data in a systematic manner. The CB approach to assessment, decision making, and interpretation "provides an advancement over traditional practice in terms of both measurement and meaning" (Flanagan & Ortiz, 2001, p. 84). Practitioners who are familiar with the CB approach know that it is based on hypothesis-driven assessment and interpretation, which include a priori and a posteriori assumptions as well as recursive assessment activities. Through the use of this method, practitioners are likely to become more confident in their approach to data collection and interpretation, as well as their ability to make placement and other educationally relevant decisions.

Application to an Operational Definition of Learning Disability

In 2002, Flanagan and colleagues extended the CB approach to include academic ability tests, for several reasons. First, the measurement and interpretation of academic abilities are rarely grounded in theory. Second, CHC theory includes academic ability constructs in its structure (e.g., Gq and Grw). Third, information derived from intelligence and achievement batteries is seldom integrated and interpreted systematically. Through the inclusion of CHC classifications of academic achievement tests, the CB approach could be readily applied to the process of evaluating individuals with learning difficulties.

Flanagan and colleagues (2002) integrated CB interpretation guidelines, current CHC theory and research (including findings regarding the relations between cognitive and academic abilities), and recent research and developments in the field of learning disabilities, to conceptualize an operational definition of learning disabilities. This definition includes several levels of assessment and evaluation, each containing specific criteria that must be met before advancing to subsequent levels. Flanagan and colleagues suggest following this operational definition after an individual has not responded positively to appropriately designed and monitored interventions. It is only when criteria at all levels of the operational definition have been met that an individual may be diagnosed with a learning disability. Individuals who meet all criteria are characterized as having a below-average aptitude–achievement consistency (i.e., related cognitive and academic deficits) within an otherwise normal ability profile (i.e., intact abilities). Furthermore, the deficits are judged to be intrinsic to the individual, as opposed to being caused primarily by exclusionary factors (e.g., cultural differences, language differences, emotional disturbance, etc.). For a comprehensive description of this operational definition, see Mascolo and Flanagan (Chapter 24, this volume).

Application of CB Interpretive Methods to Current Intelligence Batteries

Kaufman and Kaufman, the authors of the KABC-II—the newest intelligence test in the field—have incorporated CB methods into their comprehensive interpretive approach (Kaufman & Kaufman, 2004; Kaufman et al., in press). For example, they place greater emphasis on normative (as opposed to ipsative) strengths and weaknesses; they have eliminated individual subtest analysis, focusing only on scale- or cluster-level interpretation; and they recommend interpreting only those abilities that are unitary (i.e., abilities defined by nonsignificant variations among the test scores that represent them). Similarly, CB interpretive procedures have been applied to the WISC-IV (Flanagan & Kaufman, 2004). In short, the leader of *intelligent* test interpretation, Alan S. Kaufman, has integrated his methods with the CB methods in an effort to advance the science of interpreting cognitive abilities.

CONCLUSIONS
AND FUTURE DIRECTIONS

CHC theory and the CB approach have influenced intelligence test development and interpretation. The new millennium has brought with it a new generation of intelligence tests. For the first time in the history of intelligence test development, theory has played a prominent role. The latest editions of the WJ, SB, and K-ABC are firmly grounded in CHC theory. The latest edition of the WISC represents the most significant revision of any Wechsler scale to date. Although not overtly based on any specific theory, the WISC-IV is more closely aligned with theory than previous editions and may be interpreted from the perspective of CHC theory (Flanagan & Kaufman, 2004). The CB approach may be used to operationalize CHC theory more fully by supplementing any single intelligence battery with relevant tests from other batteries. It seems clear that our current instrumentation and interpretive methods will serve to improve upon the practice of intellectual assessment.

The future of intelligence test development and interpretation will undoubtedly be influenced by CHC theory and research for many years to come. The findings of current research have already suggested the need to revise and refine the theory (Horn & Blankson, Chapter 3, this volume; McGrew, Chapter 8, this volume). Findings in the learning disabilities literature, as they relate to the abilities and processes most closely associated with academic skills, suggest that there is a need to represent *narrow* abilities more comprehensively on intelligence and achievement batteries.

Future research will probably continue to examine the importance of specific cognitive abilities in the explanation of academic outcomes, above and beyond the variance explained by *g*. Also, it is hoped that future research in the field of learning disabilities will be guided by CHC theory, and that the search for aptitude–achievement interactions will be revisited using CHC constructs as opposed to Wechsler's traditional clinical composites (i.e., Verbal and Performance IQs). In general, the infusion of CHC theory in related fields, such as learning disabilities, education, and neuropsychology, seems necessary to elucidate the utility of cognitive ability assessment in the design of educational treatment plans and interventions for individuals with learning difficulties.

NOTE

1. John Carroll's contribution to the first edition of this volume has been reprinted for this edition.

REFERENCES

Caltabiano, L., & Flanagan, D. P. (2004). *Content validity of new and recently revised intelligence tests: Implications for interpretation*. Manuscript in preparation.

Carroll, J. B. (1993). *Human cognitive abilities: A survey of factor-analytic studies*. Cambridge, England: Cambridge University Press.

Cattell, R. B. (1957). *Personality and motivation structure and measurement*. Yonkers, NY: World Book.

Cattell, R. B. (1971). *Abilities: Their structure, growth, and action*. Boston: Houghton Mifflin.

Daniel, M. H. (1997). Intelligence testing: Status and trends. *American Psychologist, 52*, 1038–1045.

Das, J. P., & Naglieri, J. A. (1997). *Das–Naglieri Cognitive Assessment System*. Itasca, IL: Riverside.

Elliott, C. D. (1990). *Differential Ability Scales*. San Antonio, TX: Psychological Corp.

Flanagan, D. P., & Kaufman, A. S. (2004). *Essentials of WISC-IV assessment*. New York: Wiley.

Flanagan, D. P., & McGrew, K. S. (1997). A cross-battery approach to assessing and interpreting cognitive abilities: Narrowing the gap between practice and cognitive science. In D. P. Flanagan, J. L. Genshaft, & P. L. Harrison (Eds.), *Contemporary intellectual assessment: Theories, tests, and issues* (pp. 314–325). New York: Guilford Press.

Flanagan, D. P., McGrew, K. S., & Ortiz, S. O. (2000). *The Wechsler intelligence scales and Gf-Gc theory: A contemporary approach to interpretation*. Needham Heights, MA: Allyn & Bacon.

Flanagan, D. P., & Ortiz, S. O. (2001). *Essentials of cross-battery assessment*. New York: Wiley.

Flanagan, D. P., Ortiz, S. O., Alfonso, V. C., & Mascolo, J. T. (2002). *The achievement test desk reference (ADTR): Comprehensive assessment and learning disabilities*. Boston: Allyn & Bacon.

Glutting, J. J., Adams, W., & Sheslow, D. (2002). *Wide Range Intelligence Test*. Wilmington, DE: Wide Range.

Glutting, J. J., Watkins, M. M., & Youngstrom, E. A. (2003). Multifactored and cross-battery ability assessments: Are they worth the effort? In C. R. Reynolds & R. W. Kamphaus (Eds.), *Handbook of psychological and educational assessment of chil-*

dren: Intelligence, aptitude, and achievement (2nd ed., pp. 343–377). New York: Guilford Press.

Horn, J. L. (1965). *Fluid and crystallized intelligence: A factor analytic and developmental study of the structure among primary mental abilities.* Unpublished doctoral dissertation, University of Illinois, Champaign.

Horn, J. L. (1968). Organization of abilities and the development of intelligence. *Psychological Review, 75,* 242–259.

Horn, J. L. (1991). Measurement of intellectual capabilities: A review of theory. In K. S. McGrew, J. K. Werder, & R. W. Woodcock, *WJ-R technical manual* (pp. 197–232). Chicago: Riverside.

Horn, J. L., & Stankov, L. (1982). Auditory and visual factors of intelligence. *Intelligence, 6,* 165–185.

Kaufman, A. S., & Kaufman, N. L. (1983). *Kaufman Assessment Battery for Children.* Circle Pines, MN: American Guidance Service.

Kaufman, A. S., & Kaufman, N. L. (1993). *Kaufman Adolescent and Adult Intelligence Test.* Circle Pines, MN: American Guidance Service.

Kaufman, A. S., & Kaufman, N. L. (2004). *Kaufman Assessment Battery for Children—Second Edition.* Circle Pines, MN: American Guidance Service.

Kaufman, A. S., Lichtenberger, E. O., Fletcher-Janzen, E., & Kaufman, N. L. (in press). *Essentials of KABC-II assessment.* New York: Wiley.

Keith, T. Z. (1997). Using confirmatory factor analysis to aid in understanding the constructs measured by intelligence tests. In D. P. Flanagan, J. L. Genshaft, & P. L. Harrison (Eds.), *Contemporary intellectual assessment: Theories, tests, and issues* (pp. 373–402). New York: Guilford Press.

Keith, T. Z., Fine, J. G., Taub, G. E., Reynolds, M. R., & Kranzler, J. H. (2004). *Hierarchical, multi-sample, confirmatory factor analysis of the Wechsler Intelligence Scale for Children—Fourth Edition: What does it measure?* Manuscript submitted for publication.

Keith, T. Z., Kranzler, J. H., & Flanagan, D. P. (2001). Independent confirmatory factor analysis of the Cognitive Assessment System (CAS): What does the CAS measure? *School Psychology Review, 28,* 117–144.

McGrew, K. S. (1997). Analysis of the major intelligence batteries according to a proposed comprehensive Gf-Gc framework. In D. P. Flanagan, J. L. Genshaft, & P. L. Harrison (Eds.), *Contemporary intellectual assessment: Theories, tests, and issues* (pp. 151–180). New York: Guilford Press.

McGrew, K. S., & Flanagan, D. P. (1998). *The intelligence test desk reference (ITDR): Gf-Gc cross-battery assessment.* Boston: Allyn & Bacon.

McGrew, K. S., Flanagan, D. P., Keith, T. Z., & Vanderwood, M. (1997). Beyond *g*: The impact of Gf-Gc specific cognitive abilities research on the future use and interpretation of intelligence tests in the schools. *School Psychology Review, 26,* 177–189.

Messick, S. (1989). Validity. In R. Linn (Ed.), *Educational measurement* (3rd ed., pp. 13–103). Washington, DC: American Council on Education.

Messick, S. (1995). Validity of psychological assessment: Validation of inferences from persons' responses and performances as scientific inquiry into score meaning. In A. E. Kazdin (Ed.), *Methodological issues and strategies in clinical research* (2nd ed., pp. 241–261). Washington, DC: American Psychological Association.

Neisser, U., Boodoo, G., Bouchard, T. J., Boykin, A. W., Brody, N., Ceci, S. J., et al. (1996). Intelligence: Knowns and unknowns. *American Psychologist, 51,* 77–101.

Ortiz, S. O., & Flanagan, D. P. (2002a, May). Cross-battery assessment revisited: Some cautions concerning "some cautions" (Part I). *Communique, 30*(7), 32–34.

Ortiz, S. O., & Flanagan, D. P. (2002b, June). Some cautions concerning "Some cautions concerning cross-battery assessment" (Part II). *Communique, 30*(8), 36–38.

Phelps, L., McGrew, K. S., Knopik, S. N., & Ford, L. (in press). The general (*g*) broad and narrow CHC stratum characteristics of the WJ III and WISC-III tests: A confirmatory cross-battery investigation. *School Psychology Quarterly.*

Reynolds, C. R.-, & Kamphaus, R. W. (2003). *Reynolds Intellectual Assessment Scales.* Lutz, FL: Psychological Assessment Resources.

Roid, G. H. (2003). *Stanford–Binet Intelligence Scales, Fifth Edition.* Itasca, IL: Riverside.

Spearman, C. E. (1927). *The abilities of man.* London: Macmillan.

Sternberg, R. J., & Kaufman, J. C. (1998). Human abilities. *Annual Review of Psychology, 49,* 479–502.

Thorndike, R. L., Hagen, E. P., & Sattler, J. M. (1986). *Stanford–Binet Intelligence Scale: Fourth Edition.* Chicago: Riverside.

Vanderwood, M. L, McGrew K. S., Flanagan, D. P., & Keith, T. Z. (2001). The contribution of general and specific cognitive abilities to reading achievement. *Learning and Individual Differences, 13,* 159–188.

Watkins, M. W., Glutting, J. J., & Youngstrom, E. A. (2002, October). Cross-battery assessment: Still concerned. *Communique, 31*(2), 42–44.

Watkins, M. W., Youngstrom, E. A., & Glutting, J. J. (2002, February). Some cautions concerning cross-battery assessment. *Communique, 30*(5), 16–20.

Wechsler, D. (1981). *Wechsler Adult Intelligence Scale—Revised.* San Antonio, TX: Psychological Corporation.

Wechsler, D. (1989). *Wechsler Preschool and Primary Scale of Intelligence—Revised.* San Antonio, TX: Psychological Corporation.

Wechsler, D. (1991). *Wechsler Intelligence Scale for Children—Revised.* San Antonio, TX: Psychological Corporation.

Wechsler, D. (1997). *Wechsler Adult Intelligence Scale—Third Edition.* San Antonio, TX: Psychological Corporation.

Wechsler, D. (2002). *Wechsler Preschool and Primary Scale of Intelligence—Third Edition.* San Antonio, TX: Psychological Corporation.

Wechsler, D. (2003). *Wechsler Intelligence Scale for Children—Fourth Edition.* San Antonio, TX: Psychological Corporation.

Woodcock, R. W. (1990). Theoretical foundations of the WJ-R measures of cognitive ability. *Journal of Psychoeducational Assessment, 8,* 231–258.

Woodcock, R. W. (1994). Measures of fluid and crystallized intelligence. In R. J. Sternberg (Ed.), *Encyclopedia of human intelligence* (pp. 452–456). New York: Macmillan.

Woodcock, R. W., & Johnson, M. B. (1989). *Woodcock–Johnson Psycho-Educational Battery—Revised.* Chicago: Riverside.

Woodcock, R. W., McGrew, K. S., & Mather N. (2001). *Woodcock–Johnson III Tests of Cognitive Abilities.* Itasca, IL: Riverside.

Woodcock, R. W., McGrew, K. S., Mather, N., & Schrank, F. A. (2003). *Diagnostic Supplement to the Woodcock–Johnson III Tests of Cognitive Abilities.* Itasca, IL: Riverside.

10

Information-Processing Approaches to Interpretation of Contemporary Intellectual Assessment Instruments

RANDY G. FLOYD

Despite considerable work in the 1970s and 1980s in applying cognitive psychology to individual differences and psychometric studies, this line of investigation is still in its early stages. Only a few of the more important types of abilities have been studied in detail, and at this writing many questions remain to be resolved.

—CARROLL (1993, p. 71)

Humans have long examined the internal workings of the mind—from Aristotle, to Descartes, to Wundt, to Binet, and to the modern cognitive scientists (Ashcraft, 1998; Bechtel & Graham, 1998; Sobel, 2001). For example, Wundt used the method of introspection to study sensations and perceptual experiences. Now cognitive scientists use intricate computer simulations to examine the rules that guide cognition and human behavior. In general, contemporary intellectual assessment instruments, as methods to study the human mind, rely upon measurement of individual differences in broadly defined cognitive abilities drawn from factor-analytic research. The study of individual differences in cognitive abilities, called the *psychometric approach* or the *differential paradigm*, has been useful because measures

of these abilities predict a number of socially important outcomes, such as academic attainments, occupational and social status, job performance, and income, to name a few (Godttfredson, 1997, 2002; Horn & Noll, 1997; Jensen, 1998; Neisser et al., 1996). Although a concentration on individual differences in the display of the broadly defined cognitive abilities may be useful for predictive purposes with large groups of people, such a concentration may be limiting in several ways to those interpreting assessment results for individuals. For one thing, a focus on ranking individuals based on summaries of item-level performance (i.e., subtest or composite scores) does little to explain why an individual has performed at a level above or below others in the comparison group. Furthermore, a focus on breadth of factors and scores representing them largely obscures an understanding of the particulars of cognitive performance, such as strategy use and the activation of specific mental operations.

Consistent with calls for greater integration between subfields within psychology (e.g., Anastasi, 1967; Cronbach, 1957; Glasser, 1981; McNemar, 1964; Sternberg, 1981), the thesis of this chapter is that (1) more attention should be paid to the research of cognitive psychologists and cognitive scientists when test developers are designing intellectual assessment instruments and interpretive frameworks for them; and (2) efforts should be made to identify and measure the micro-level cognitive processes that underlie cognitive abilities and that lead to individual differences. To that end, this chapter reviews and evaluates recent applications of cognitive systems to the interpretation of ability tests.

THE PSYCHOMETRIC APPROACH

The psychometric approach has a long history in psychology. This approach to studying cognitive abilities is based upon findings that scores stemming from the administration of cognitive tasks to groups of people reveal substantial individual differences. *Individual differences* may be defined as "derivations or variations along a variable or dimension that occur among members of any particular group" (Corsini, 1999, p. 481), or as "all the ways in which people differ from one another, especially psychological differences" (Colman, 2001, p. 389). Because of these individual differences, latent relations between scores can be identified via covariance structural analyses, such as factor analysis. The interpretation of most contemporary intellectual assessment instruments relies heavily upon identification of these latent relations surfacing from patterns of individual differences (e.g., Kamphaus, 2001; Kaufman & Lichtenberger, 2002; McGrew & Flanagan, 1998; Sattler, 2001; see Alfonso, Flanagan, & Radwan, Chapter 9, this volume). The descriptions of these relations may vary from very general labels, such as the *g* factor, to more specific labels, such as *reading decoding*.

Based on the structure provided by factor analysis and accompanying factor labels, an individual's *ability* can be inferred from comparison of individual performance to that of some larger group (viz., a norm group). Typically, an ability is defined as a "developed skill, competence, or power to do something, especially . . . existing capacity to perform some function, whether physical, mental, or a combination of the two, without further education or training" (Colman, 2001, p. 1). According to Carroll (1993), it is defined by "some kind of performance, or potential for performance" (p. 4). Thus, at its most basic level, an ability may be viewed as a discrete behavior that is either performed or not (e.g., saying the word "No" or writing the letter *X*). However, during intellectual assessments, an ability is more often viewed as a collection of related behaviors on which individuals vary in terms of efficiency and accuracy of performance. Thus these relative differences in performance define ability.

INFORMATION-PROCESSING APPROACHES

In the 1970s and 1980s, there was a surge of interest by cognitive psychologists in *information processing* as an alternative technology for understanding the measurement of human cognitive competencies. According to Sternberg (1981), "information processing" is generally defined as the sequence of mental operations and their products involved in performing a cognitive task" (p. 1182). Consistent with this definition, information-processing models of cognitive functioning emerged in which a computer system was used as the analogy (Hunt, Frost, & Lunneborg, 1973; Neisser, 1967; Newell & Simon, 1972). These models provided a description of the stages through which information is transformed from sensations to mental representations, analyzed within the cognitive system and expressed via some response. These stages of information processing were often represented in *box-and-arrow models* (Logan, 2000). Each stage typically represented an elementary information process (Newell & Simon, 1972). *Information processes* are defined as hypothetical constructs used by cognitive theorists to describe how persons apprehend, discriminate, select, and attend to certain aspects of the vast welter of stimuli that impinge on the sensorium to form internal representations that can be mentally manipulated, transformed, related to previous internal representations, stored in memory . . . and later retrieved from storage to govern the person's decision and behavior in a particular situation. (Jensen, 1998, pp. 205–206)

Thus, an elementary information process can be considered the fundamental mental event in which information is operated on to produce a response (Carroll, 1993; Posner & McLeod, 1982). For example, these processes may include the *encoding* of external information into the cognitive system, *comparison* of the new information to information stored in memory, selection of a response (e.g., either "same" or "different"), and execution of that response (saying either "same" or "different") (see Logan, 2000). Models of complex information processing dwarf simple models such as this one.

Models such as the modal model of memory, the working memory model, and the ACT-R theory represent some of the most advanced descriptions of the human information-processing system and its elementary information processes.

Modal Model of Memory

More than 35 years ago, Atkinson and Shiffrin (1968) presented a *modal model of memory* (see Figure 10.1). In many ways, it is the "granddaddy" of the comprehensive information-processing models. Since its initial presentation, this model has stimulated a large body of research that has led to support for its postulations as well as to modifications (Estes, 1999; Healy & McNamara, 1996; Raaijmakers, 1993; Shiffrin, 1999). The model specifies both structural features and control processes. The structural features represent the hardware and built-in programs of the cognitive system; they include the *sensory register*, multiple *short-term stores*, and the *long-term store*. The

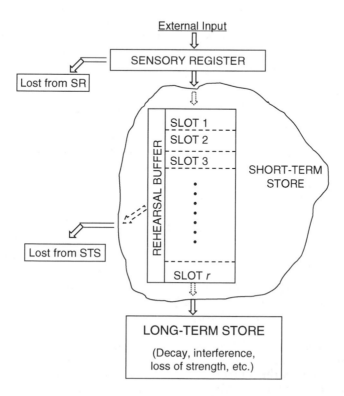

FIGURE 10.1. The modal model of memory. From Atkinson and Shiffrin (1968), page 113. Copyright 1968 by Academic Press. Reprinted by permission from Elsevier.

sensory register represents the temporary holding space for all stimuli from the environment detected by the sense organs (e.g., sounds, images). Unless it is attended to, this information is lost in milliseconds. If it is attended to, it is copied into one of the short-term stores associated with the sensory register. Atkinson and Shiffrin referred to some of these stores as *auditory–verbal–linguistic memory,* the *visual short-term store,* and the *haptic* (touch-related) *short-term store.* Because oral communication is ubiquitous and the objects of our attention are frequently labeled or coded verbally, the auditory–verbal–linguistic memory is perhaps the most vital to adaptive information processing. The limited-capacity stores are temporary holding areas for information in one's immediate awareness—*active* information. Such information, stored in a finite number of slots in the stores, is lost within approximately 30 seconds if it is not rehearsed or reactivated in some way. With use of storage strategies, information in the short-term stores is copied into the long-term store. The long-term store is considered a relatively permanent storage area—a warehouse of memories and acquired knowledge. The information in the long-term store may appear to be lost for a number of reasons: decay of the information, interference due to subsequent experiences, or weakening of the bonds between related units of information.

Control processes in the modal model of memory describe acquired programs that drive the operation of the structural system. Examples of control processes include rehearsal of information in the short-term store, verbal coding of stimuli, and memory storage and retrieval strategies. According to this model, the individual coordinates control processes to accomplish cognitive goals.

Working Memory Model

Baddeley's *working memory model* (Baddeley, 1986, 1994, 1996, 2001; Baddeley & Hitch, 1994) is a modification and extension of the modal model of memory (Atkinson & Shiffrin, 1968). Baddeley and colleagues developed the working memory model to increase the understanding of the functional or "working" operations carried out in the short-term stores. As such, working memory facilitates the manipulation and storage of information in the larger memory system, which includes sensory stores and a long-term store. According to Baddeley, working memory is composed of three subcomponents: the *central executive* and two slave systems, the *phonological loop* and the *visuo-spatial sketchpad* (see Figure 10.2). These slave systems largely represent two of the short-term stores identified by Atkinson and Shiffrin.

After receiving information via the auditory sensory store, the phonological loop holds and manipulates phonological (speech-based) stimuli. The phonological loop consists of two components: the *phonological short-term store* and the *articulatory rehearsal process.* The phonological short-term store retains speech-based information for a brief time according to its phonological structure. Baddeley (1986) suggested that this information gains obligatory access to the phonological store and becomes an auditory memory trace. Consistent with the auditory–verbal–linguistic memory store of Atkinson and Shiffrin (1968), the phonological store retains the structure of the information for 2–3 seconds before the corresponding memory trace fades. The articulatory rehearsal process functions to maintain or refresh the fading information in the phonological store through subvocal articulation.

The visuo-spatial sketchpad functions to hold and to manipulate visual and spatial information. Baddeley (1986) proposed that visual information and spatial information are operated on by separate elements of this system. Visual information is thought to rely on sensory coding and spatial information on motoric processes (Wilson & Emmorey, 1997). The visuo-spatial sketchpad has a structure similar to that of the phonological loop, in which one area holds visual and spatial information, and another element facilitates rehearsal of such information.

The central executive is described as an attentional control system that coordinates information processes performed in working memory. It represents, in effect, a *homunculus*—a little person who manipulates the workings of the cognitive system (Baddeley, 1996). The central executive performs two functions: processing and storage capabilities, and control activities (Gathercole, 1994). The processing and storage capabilities of the central executive include mainte-

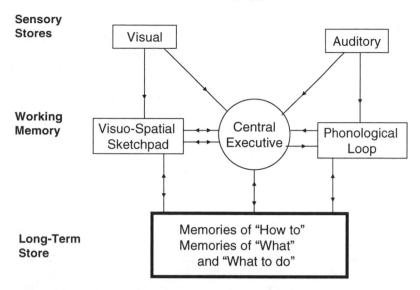

Sensory Stores Visual | Auditory

Working Memory Visuo-Spatial Sketchpad ↔ Central Executive ↔ Phonological Loop

Long-Term Store Memories of "How to" Memories of "What" and "What to do"

FIGURE 10.2. The working memory model. From Torgesen (1996), page 158. Copyright 1996 by Paul H. Brookes Publishing Co. Adapted by permission.

nance rehearsal, the analysis of information, and the storage and retrieval of memories held in the long-term store. The control activities include the management of attention and behavior and the regulation of information in the memory system.

Anderson's ACT-R

Whereas the modal memory and working memory models are models of memory, *adaptive control of thought—rational theory* (ACT-R, pronounced "act R") is more ambitious in its breadth and explanatory power (Anderson, 1983; Anderson & Lebiere, 1998). This evolving architecture[1] forms the basis for computer modeling of the higher-level cognitive processes leading to complex human behavior (Anderson, 1976, 1983, 1990, 1993; Anderson & Lebiere, 1998). For example, ACT-R has simulated behavior on several tasks like those seen on intellectual assessment instruments, such as mathematical problem solving, spatial reasoning, sentence memory, and nonverbal reasoning (Anderson et al., 2004).

The foundation of ACT-R is formed from units of procedural knowledge and units of declarative knowledge that are entered into its system. Procedural knowledge can be conceptualized as knowing *how* to perform a

behavior, and in ACT-R it comprises a repository of productions, which are if–then rules or strategies used to achieve goals. Declarative knowledge can be conceptualized as knowing *what* and *what to do*, and in ACT-R it comprises memories and other explicit knowledge called *chunks*. As evident in the representation of ACT-R in Figure 10.3, visual information from the environment enters the cognitive system through activation of the visual module. *Modules* represent programs or storehouses of knowledge used by the cognitive system. Following the model, information is then placed in a visual buffer. *Buffers* in ACT-R are similar to the sensory register and short-term stores of Atkinson and Shiffrin (1968) and the slave systems of Baddeley (1986). (Figure 10.3 emphasizes visual information processing and not phonological processing.) Once in the buffer, information may be acted upon by any number of productions from the central processing system, such as matching and selection. These productions are extracted from the procedural knowledge module and its associated buffer, and if needed, information from the declarative knowledge module may be extracted to assist in understanding the new information and reacting to it in an adaptive manner. When the central processing system prepares a response, the execution production may be activated in the manual (or motor) buffer, and the manual module can make a response.

Trends across Models

Across the three models, five trends are apparent. First, the physical nature of the information to be processed by the cognitive system affects how that information enters the cognitive system and to what structures it is routed. For example, both the working memory model and the ACT-R model specify an input channel for visual information and another for auditory information. Similarly, all three models include structures devoted to visual information and to auditory or phonological information. Second, all three of these models specify areas where active manipulation and integration of information takes place: short-term stores, the phonological loop and the visual-spatial sketchpad, and buffers. Third, all of the models describe repositories of knowledge in which new information may be stored and from which previously saved information may be extracted. Fourth, two of the models describe

an output or response mechanism. Finally, all three models describe processes as tools (or applications) serving specific functions in the cognitive system. Across the models, processes included activities such as articulatory rehearsal, verbal coding, memory storage and retrieval, attention maintenance, pattern matching, and response preparation.

NEED FOR INTEGRATION

It is logical that a focus on the structures and the molecular mental operations included in the modal model, the working memory model, and ACT-R may ultimately be more useful than a focus on the more global and relative abilities when engaged in intellectual assessment of individuals. I believe that there are at least four reasons for greater integration of information-processing models into interpretation of intellectual assessment instruments: (1) increasing interdisciplinary research and partnerships with cognitive psychology, cognitive science, and other fields drawing on information-processing models; (2) improving methods to generate validity

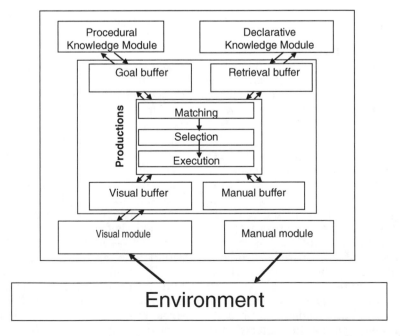

FIGURE 10.3. The adaptive control of thought-rational (ACT-R) architecture. From Anderson et al. (2004). Copyright 2004 by the American Psychological Association. Adapted by permission.

evidence for intellectual assessment instruments by looking at response processes; (3) aiding in the diagnosis and treatment of learning disabilities and other cognitive disabilities; and (4) explaining the reasons for individual differences in cognitive abilities with greater specificity.

Increasing Interdisciplinary Research and Partnerships

The information-processing metaphor is not only relevant to cognitive psychology and cognitive science, but it is also influential in educational psychology (Mayer, 1996) and developmental psychology (Klahr & Wallace, 1976; Thompson, 2000). For example, authors have applied information-processing models to the education of children (e.g., Borkowski, Carr, Rellinger, & Pressley, 1990). However, interpretive approaches linking assessment data to instructional interventions derived from these models appear to be minimal or nonexistent. Those involved in test interpretation would be wise to draw upon resources from these fields and to participate in more interdisciplinary research.

Item Development and Validity Evidence

A better understanding of the human information-processing system as well as the use of a common nomenclature to describe the global and more specific cognitive abilities would be useful during the development of items for assessment instruments (Irvine & Kyllonen, 2002; see also McGrew, Chapter 8, and Alfonso et al., Chapter 9, this volume, for a description of the CHC taxonomy of cognitive abilities). In fact, such evidence may be used to support the validity of an instrument in measuring a cognitive process or ability. For example, the *Standards for Educational and Psychological Testing* volume (American Educational Research Association, American Psychological Association, & National Council on Measurement in Education, 1999) states the following:

> Theoretical and empirical analyses of the response processes of test takers can provide evidence concerning the fit between the construct and the detailed nature of performance or response actually engaged in by examinees....

> Evidence based on response processes generally comes from analyses of individual responses. Questioning test takers about their performance strategies or responses to particular items can yield evidence that enriches the definition of the construct. (p. 12)

Identification of Learning Disabilities and Other Cognitive Deficits

There are frequent references to cognitive processes in the learning disability literature, and information-processing approaches have been deemed important to their understanding (e.g., Swanson, 1991, 1996). In addition, federal statutes describing and mandating the provision of services to those with learning disabilities refer to elementary information processes. For example, the 1997 amendments to the Individuals with Disabilities Education Act (IDEA, 1997) define a specific learning disability as "a disorder in one or more of the *basic psychological processes* [emphasis added] involved in understanding or in using language, spoken or written, that may manifest itself in an imperfect ability to listen, think, speak, read, write, spell, or to do mathematical calculations" (Sec. 602). Based on this definition, several U.S. states require that children demonstrate significant IQ–achievement discrepancies along with documented "processing deficits."

In light of recent discussions regarding proposed changes In the IDEA (1997) with regard to the learning disability category, the use of terms related to cognitive processing remain. For example, a position statement from the American Academy of School Psychology Ad Hoc Committee on Comprehensive Evaluation for Learning Disabilities (2004) stated that

> The core procedure of a comprehensive evaluation ofLD is an objective, norm-referenced assessment of the presence and severity of any strengths and weakness among the cognitive processes related to learning in the achievement area. These cognitive processes include (but are not limited to): knowledge, storage and retrieval, phonological awareness, reasoning, working memory, executive functioning, and processing speed. (p. 1)

A clearer understanding of the nature and measurement of these processes would be useful—if for no other reason than to guide the assessment of learning disabilities believed to stem from errors in information processes.

Cognitive Interventions and Education

Because elementary information processes are at a lower level of generality than latent factors and come closer to representing specific behaviors of interest, identification of these processes may benefit cognitive interventions and education. Sternberg (1981) optimistically asserted that "information processing analyses of mental abilities may enable us to diagnose and eventually remediate deficiencies in intellectual function at the level of process, strategies, and representations of information" (p. 1186). However, because cognitive interventions and education methods have focused on improving domain-general abilities (approximating factors, such as inductive and deductive reasoning), their results have been rather dismal (Corrigan & Yudofsky, 1996; Loarer, 2003). A more narrow focus on elementary information processes may be useful. For example, Loarer's (2003) *second-generation cognitive education methods* focus on these processes directly in the context in which they will be used.

Integration with Factor-Analytic Research

It is likely that many of the identified elementary information processes fit well into a hierarchical model of cognitive abilities specifying differing levels of generality. Although cognitive abilities are not processes, abilities likely stem from a combination of processes. As the intelligence-testing field moves toward a standard nomenclature for describing cognitive abilities at varying levels of generality (see McGrew, Chapter 8, this volume), elementary information processes will probably provide a clear link to narrow (stratum I) cognitive abilities (Carroll, 1988, 1993, 1998, and Chapter 4, this volume; Deary, 2001; Sternberg, 1977). With commonalities in use of stimulus materials, presumed cognitive processes, and kinds of outcomes and products, *some* narrow (stratum I) abilities may provide at least approximations of identification of cognitive processes (Carroll, 1976, 1988). In this vein, Sternberg (1977)

presented a schematic using Thurstone's (1938) *primary mental abilities* to indicate the importance of tasks and components below the level of general, broad-ability, and narrow-ability factors. I have adapted this schematic to incorporate a more contemporary factor-analytic model, the Cattell–Horn–Carroll (CHC) theory (see Figure 10.4). (Central tenets of the CHC theory are described in this volume by Horn & Blankson, Chapter 3; Carroll, Chapter 4; McGrew, Chapter 8; and Schrank, Chapter 17.)

APPLICATIONS OF INFORMATION-PROCESSING MODELS TO TEST INTERPRETATION

This section of the chapter reviews some of the approaches that have been used to increase understanding of the results of intellectual assessment instruments via integration of information-processing models. There are four general ways in which this integration has occurred: (1) identifying components representing information processes based on task analysis of test items by experts; (2) overlaying factor-analytic models of intelligence onto information-processing models; (3) creating test batteries designed to operationalize some information processes; and (4) modifying existing batteries to ferret out information processes. Examples of each of these approaches are described below.

Task-Analytic Approaches

Carroll's Coding Scheme for Cognitive Tasks

Carroll (1976) was one of the first scholars to call for an integration of the factor-analytic research and information-processing models. He stated, "What still seems needed is a general methodology and theory for interpreting psychometric tests as cognitive tasks, and for characterizing (but not necessarily classifying) factor-analytic factors . . . according to a model of cognitive processes" (p. 30). After completing a comprehensive review of the research examining elementary information processes, Carroll amended an information-processing model proposed by Hunt (1971) and, from it, developed a coding scheme for cognitive tasks (see Table 10.1). Carroll specified six general

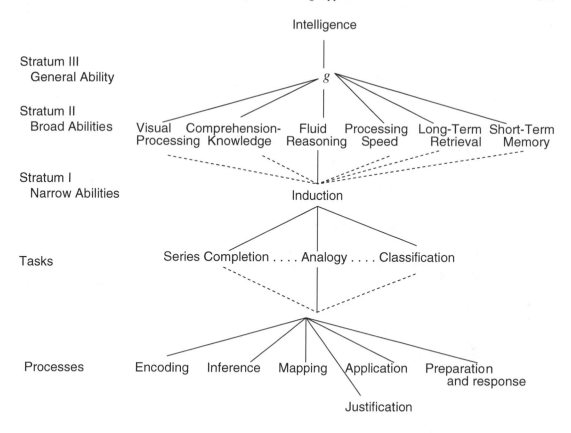

FIGURE 10.4. Possible relations between the three-stratum model described in the Cattell–Horn–Carroll theory, cognitive tasks, and processes underlying them. From Sternberg (1977), page 318. Copyright 1977 by Lawrence Erlbaum Associates. Adapted by permission.

elements in his coding scheme. As presented in Table 10.1, the first element describes some characteristics of the stimuli presented at the outset of a task, such as the number and nature of the stimuli used in an item. The second element focuses on the types of overt responses that must be made to respond to an item and the manner in which they are judged for accuracy. The third element focuses on the temporal parameters of steps in the task. For example, a time delay between presentation of the item and recall of its content would be coded. The fourth element focuses on the elementary information processes likely employed when performing the task. The fifth element includes speed-related influences or conditions on task performance. The final element focuses on the primary memory stores involved during task completion and their content. Memory stores included short-term memory stores,

long-term memory stores, and intermediate-term memory stores (i.e., working memory involving memory storage and retrieval). Content of the stores may range from simple stimuli, such as one-dimensional lines, to information focusing on word meaning.

Carroll (1976) used this scheme to deconstruct the steps involved in completing items from 48 tests found in the group-administered Kit of Reference Tests for Cognitive Factors (French, Ekstrom, & Price, 1963). He chose tests as "pure" measures of 24 factors and randomly selected two tests of each factor for coding. In order to delineate the probable "causes" of individual differences on these tests, Carroll presented a portion of the results organized according to the factors measured by the tests. These results included the descriptions of the primary memory store involved, the cognitive operations implied in task directions, and strate-

TABLE 10.1. Carroll's Provisional Coding Scheme for Cognitive Tasks

I. Types of stimuli presented at outset of task
  A. Number of stimulus classes
    a. One stimulus class (a word, picture, etc.)
    b. Two stimulus classes (as in many types of multiple-choice items, paired-associates learning, etc.)
  B. Description of the stimulus class(es)
    a. Complete
    b. Degraded (with visual or auditory "noise")
  C. Interpretability
    a. Unambiguous (immediately interpretable)
    b. Ambiguous (coded several ways)
    c. Anomalous (not immediately codable)
II. Overt responses to be made at end of task
  A. Number and type
    a. Select response from presented alternatives
    b. Produce one correct answer from operations to be performed
    c. Produce as many responses as possible (all different)
    d. Produce a specified number of responses (all different)
  B. Response mode
    a. Indicate choice of alternative (in some conventional way)
    b. Produce a single symbol (letter, numerical quantity)
    c. Write word
    d. Write phrase or sentence
    e. Write paragraph or more
    f. Make spoken response
    g. Make line or simple drawing
  C. Criterion for response acceptability
    a. Identity
    b. Similarity (or nonsimilarity) with respect to one or more features
    c. Semantic opposition
    d. Containment
    e. Correct result of serial operation
    f. Instance (subordinate of stimulus class)
    g. Superordinate
    h. Correct answer to verbal question ("fill in wh-")
    i. Comparative judgment
    j. Arbitrary association established in task
    k. Semantic and/or grammatical acceptability ("makes sense")
    l. Connectedness of lines or paths
III. Task structure
  A. Unitary (each item is completed on a single occasion)
  B. A temporal structure, such that stimuli are presented on one occasion and responses are made on another occasion (as in memory and learning tasks)
IV. Operations and strategies
  A. Number of operations and strategies for the task
  B. Type or description
    a. Identify, recognize, and interpret stimulus
    b. Educe identities or similarities between two or more stimuli
    c. Retrieve name, description, or instance from memory
    d. Store item in memory
    e. Retrieve associations, or general information, from memory
    f. Retrieve or construct hypotheses
    g. Examine different portions of memory
    h. Perform serial operations with data from memory
    i. Record intermediate result
    j. Use visual inspection strategy (examine different parts of visual stimulus)
    k. Reinterpret possibly ambiguous item
    l. Image, imagine, or otherwise form abstract representation of a stimulus
    m. Mentally rotate spatial configuration
    n. Comprehend and analyze language stimulus
    o. Judge stimulus with respect to specified characteristic

(continued)

TABLE 10.1. *(continued)*

      p. Ignore irrelevant stimuli
      q. Use a special mnemonic aid (specify)
      r. Rehearse associations
      s. Develop a specific search strategy (visual)
      t. Chunk or group stimuli or data from memory
  C. Is the operation specified in the task instructions?
      a. Yes, explicitly
      b. Implied but not explicitly stated
      c. Not specified or implied in instructions
  D. How dependent is acceptable performance on this operation or strategy?
      a. Crucially dependent
      b. Helpful, but not crucial
      c. Of dubious effect (may be positive or negative)
      d. Probably a hindrance, counterproductive
V. Temporal aspects of the operation strategy
  A. Duration (range of average duration)
      a. Irrelevant or inapplicable
      b. Very short (e.g., <200 msec)
      c. Middle range (e.g., <1 sec)
      d. Long (e.g., 1–5 sec)
      e. Longer (e.g., >5 sec)
  B. Individual differences in duration (or probability of strategy)
      a. Probably inconsequential
      b. Possibly relevant
      c. Probably wide individual differences (in likely test population)
  C. Criterion for termination of operation
      a. Irrelevant
      b. Upon arrival at recognizably correct solution (self-terminating)
      c. Not self-terminating in sense of (b) (i.e., the solution may be a guess, or subject may be satisfied with what is actually an incorrect solution)
VI. Memory storage involved
  A. Term
      a. Memory store involved
      b. Sensory buffer
      c. Short-term memory (a matter of seconds)
      d. Intermediate-term memory (a matter of minutes)
      e. Long-term or permanent memory (programs/production system housed there)—contents:
          i. Visual-representational (images or other abstract representations derived from visual perceptions
         ii. Auditory-representational (analogous to visual-representational, but in the auditory mode)
        iii. Lexicosemantic information (abstract representation of words, and their semantic and grammatical features and rules in English)
        iv. Quantitative information (abstract representation of numbers, number operations, and algorithms for dealing with quantitative information)
         v. Abstract concepts and "general logic" information (representations of various concepts, principles, and rules having to do with implication, inference, causality, sequencing, attributes, patterning, etc.)
        vi. Experiential information (related to an individual's general store of information about the self and the environment, and past experiences)
  B. Contents
      a. Nonspecific
      b. Visual in nature (general, nonspecific)
          i. Points, positions of points
         ii. Lines (one-dimensional)
        iii. Lines and curves (two-dimensional)
        iv. Geometric patterns and shapes
         v. Pictorial (objects, etc.)
            1. Subcategory (e.g., tools)
        vi. Real two-dimensional items
       vii. Maps, charts, grids
     viii. Representation of three-dimensional geometric shapes

(continued)

TABLE 10.1. *(continued)*

> 1. Pictures of three-dimensional geometric objects or situations
> 2. Faces
> ix. Real objects in three dimensions
> c. Auditory
> d. Graphemic, general
>> i. Letters
>> ii. Words (apart from their semantic information)
>> iii. Alphabetic order information
> e. Linguistic, general (of native language)
>> i. Lexical
>> ii. Syntactic
>> iii. Grammatical rules and features, general
>> iv. Semantic (meanings of words, syntactic features, etc.)
>> v. Nonverbal semantics (e.g., meanings of pictorial symbols)
> f. Numerical, mathematical, general
>> i. Digit symbols with meaning
>> ii. Elementary number operations and symbols
>> iii. Algorithms for dealing with quantitative relations
> g. Logic, general
>> i. Various abstract patterns (alternation, sequence, etc.)
>> ii. Attributes in which stimuli could vary
> h. Movements, kinesthetic "concepts"
> i. "Real-world" experiences, situation, facts, information
>> i. Subcategories (e.g., mechanical and electrical information)
> j. Arbitrary, new codings and associations established in the task situation
> C. Relevance of individual differences in the store
>> a. Most subjects will have required store
>> b. Doubtful that most subjects will have required store
>> c. Wide individual differences in this memory store are likely

Note. From Carroll (1976). Copyright 1976 by Lawrence Erlbaum Associates. Adapted by permission.

gies that may contribute to performance. In the coding scheme, Carroll distinguished between *operations*, which are "control processes that are explicitly specified, or implied, in the task instructions and fore-exercises that must be performed if the task is to be completed successfully" and *strategies*, which are considered "control processes that are not specified by task instructions, but may or may not be used (discovered) by a particular subject" (p. 42).

Table 10.2 presents results for four factors frequently measured by contemporary intellectual assessments. For example, the factor *lexical knowledge* is measured on tasks like Vocabulary from the *Wechsler Intelligence Scale for Children—Fourth Edition* (WISC-IV; Wechsler, 2003) and *Wechsler Adult Intelligence Scale—Third Edition* (WAIS-III; Wechsler, 1997). According to Carroll's (1976) coding, items on tests measuring this factor tap lexico-semantic information stored in the long-term store, and the operation performed is retrieval of the meanings of

the words presented. The factor *memory span* is measured by tasks such as Digits Forward from Digit Span. Items measuring memory span require that the information be held in the short-term memory stores, and individual differences are thought to stem at least partially from the speed in which information to be held is encoded, refreshed, and retrieved from the stores; the nature of that information (e.g., numbers, letters, words); and the capacity of the memory stores. Individuals may engage in strategies such as grouping information and vocal or subvocal rehearsal. *Perceptual speed* is measured by tasks like Coding and Symbol Search. These tasks require that the information be held in the short-term memory stores (whether coded as visual images or coded verbally as words). The primary operation would include searching for items, and individual differences would stem primarily from speed in doing so. *Induction* is measured by tasks such as Matrix Reasoning. Despite tasks measuring this factor typically being considered measures of novel reasoning, according to Carroll, such tasks tap abstract or logical information stored in the long-term store—perhaps procedural knowledge. The primary operation used is the search for information to form hypotheses for solving items, and individual differences stem primarily from the depth and breadth of this information stored in memory and the speed in which the information is retrieved and hypotheses tested. A strategy may include using a systematic–deductive manner of testing hypotheses.

Carroll's (1976) coding scheme provides a useful and well-developed method for understanding the information-processing characteristics underlying performance on subtest items. Of particular importance are his descriptions of the processes implied in task directions (i.e., operations) and his specification of the primary memory store involved in item-level performance. Despite this potential, I could not find another article, chapter,

or test that has utilized Carroll's coding scheme to classify items from intellectual assessment instruments. It is notable that, in reflecting on his work, Carroll (1987) wrote the following in a chapter published more than 10 years after developing this coding scheme: "As I now peruse the list of cognitive operations, strategies, and memory scores that I postulated in 1974, I cannot see that subsequent empirical work would cause me to modify my list in any substantial way, except possibly to make small revisions and add detail" (p. 240). Although the multifaceted nature of cognitive tasks renders it impossible to construct a classification system for elementary information processes that is invariant across persons (Jensen, 1998; Lohman, 1994, 2000), interpretation of these tasks will likely be enhanced by the use of Carroll's coding scheme—especially if more recent conceptualizations from cognitive psychology and cognitive science, such

TABLE 10.2. Results for Select Latent Factors from Carroll's Coding of Cognitive Tasks

| Factor | Principal type of memory involved | Cognitive processes/operations | | | |
		Addressing sensory buffers (attentional processes)	Addressing intermediate-term memory or long-term memory	Manipulations in executive and short-term memory	Strategies
Lexical knowledge	Long-term memory (lexico-semantic)		Retrieve word meanings (content)		
Memory span	Short-term memory (nonspecific)			Store in short-term memory (time, content) Retrieve from short-term memory (time, content)	Chunk or group stimulus items
Perceptual speed	Short-term memory (visual)	Visual search for specified items (time)		Comparison of visual stimuli	
Induction	Long-term memory (abstract logical)		Search hypotheses (content, time)		Serial operations to construct new hypotheses (probability that strategy would be used, time)

Note. Carroll's (1976) factor label for *lexical knowledge* was originally *verbal comprehension*. Based on Carroll (1987), "comparison of visual stimuli" was added to the *perceptual speed* entry. From Carroll (1976). Copyright 1976 by Lawrence Erlbaum Associates. Adapted by permission.

as *productions* (i.e., rules guiding operations or strategy use), are incorporated.

Sternberg's Componential Approach

Whereas Carroll (1976) began with the psychometric approach to understanding cognitive performance and used information-processing research to enrich the understanding of individual differences and associated latent abilities, Sternberg (1977) sought to replace the focus on individual differences and latent abilities with elementary information processes. His landmark 1977 book, *Intelligence, Information Processing, and Analogical Reasoning*, introduced *componential analysis*, a technique designed to "identify the component mental operations underlying a series of related information-processing tasks and to discover the organization of these component operations in terms of their relationships both to each other and to higher-order constellations of mental abilities" (p. 65). Sternberg equated components with elementary information processes described by cognitive psychologists. Componential analysis required the identification of the sequence and combination of components involved in cognitive performance and the construction of models to be tested. To demonstrate the utility of componential analysis, Sternberg offered a systematic task analysis of performance on items measuring analogical reasoning ability. Such items require examinees to complete analogies by inferring a rule or rules from information provided. Analogies may be represented by the equation "*A* is to *B* as *C* is to *D*," with *D* being the unknown answer. Sternberg's analyses of the cognitive components necessary to complete such analogies were expressed in flowcharts, including the one shown in Figure 10.5. These intensive task analyses described the elementary information processes supporting performance on such items.

As evident in both Figures 10.4 and 10.5, the components of analogical reasoning were labeled *encoding, inferring, mapping, justification*, and *preparing–responding*. Encoding refers to the process of identifying the attributes and other characteristics of each part of the analogy. Inference refers to the process of determining the relations between the first two elements in the analogy. Mapping refers to the process of determining the relations

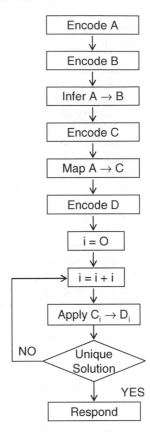

FIGURE 10.5. Flowchart describing the information processes involved in *induction* (i.e., analogical reasoning). From Sternberg (1977), page 139. Copyright 1977 by Lawrence Erlbaum Associates. Reprinted by permission.

between the first and third elements in the analogy. Application refers to the generation of rules to identify the missing element. Justification, considered an optional process, represents testing of hypotheses based on the prevailing rule from the application phase. Preparing–responding refers to the behaviors occurring before and after the elementary information processes that are involved directly in providing the missing element.

Although Sternberg's componential analysis appeared promising, a number of criticisms weakened the initial enthusiasm for this approach. For example, the identification of components seemed somewhat arbitrary and dependent on the researcher conducting the analysis, and the sheer number of possible components that could be identified for any given task mounted (Glass, Holyoak,

& Santa, 1979; Newell, 1990). In addition, the components, seen as distinct divisions of performance on a given task, were shown to be highly intercorrelated—probably indicating a higher-order cognitive ability that could be represented by a factor. As a result, according to Deary (2002), "the components have remained clever slices of test scores rather than validated mechanisms of mind" (p. 156). Vestiges of these components remain in Sternberg's triarchic theory (see Sternberg, Chapter 6, this volume), but Sternberg now describes three levels of components: *metacomponents* (control processes), *performance components* (lower-order processes used in execution of strategies for task performance), and *knowledge acquisition components* (learning new information and storing it in memory). In addition, these components serve as only one piece of intelligence behavior, along with experience and context.

Kaufman's Shared-Abilities Approach

Perhaps the most integrative interpretive framework for evaluating scores yielded by intellectual assessment instrument is that of Kaufman and Lichtenberger (Kaufman, 1994; Kaufman & Lichtenberger, 1999, 2000, 2002). This framework, incorporated in their *shared-abilities analysis*, has been most consistently applied to the subtests from the Wechsler intelligence scales (e.g., Wechsler, 1991, 1997). It integrates existing factor-analytic evidence and conceptions of intelligence and personality into a rudimentary information-processing model to promote the classification of cognitive tasks according to the abilities they measure.

Kaufman and Lichtenberger draw upon an information-processing model that is a synthesis of (1) Silver's (1993) model explaining deficiencies and deficits displayed by children with learning disabilities, and (2) Osgood's (1957) conception of channels of communication. Following an information-processing perspective, Silver's model includes *input, integration, storage,* and *output* stages. Input refers to the manner in which information enters the cognitive system (i.e., auditory–verbal or visual–motor channels). Integration refers to the mental operations facilitating the interpretation and processing of information that has entered

the cognitive system. Such operations include sequencing encoded information, inferring meaning from the encoded information, and integrating new information with the old. Storage represents the depositing of information in either the short-term store or the long-term store. Finally, output refers to the manner in which a response is expressed—typically through language or motor activity.

Paralleling Silver's model, Osgood's (1957) psycholinguistic approach refers to *channels of communication* and describes information processing in terms of *reception, association,* and *expression*. Osgood's conception of channels of communication refers to the pathways in when types of meaningful information travel. These channels include auditory–verbal or visual–motor pathways. The information-processing component reception mirrors Silver's input stage and refers to the perception and encoding of external information that is seen or heard. Association mirrors Silver's integration stage and refers to the mental manipulations used to relate new the information to existing knowledge or to transform the new information. Finally, expression mirrors Silver's output stage and refers to the manifestation of a response (viz., a vocal or motor response) stemming from information processing.

Based on their synthesis of these two models, Kaufman and Lichtenberger (2000, 2002) assert than any cognitive task can be classified according to four (or, most recently, five) criteria.[2] The first is specification of the channel of communication: auditory–verbal or visual–motor. The second is input/reception. The third is integration/association. The fourth is storage/memory. The fifth is output/expression. As part of the classification of each cognitive task, the level of emphasis on a criterion can be identified, and ties between performance on one task and another can be made according to their shared abilities. For example, the WISC-IV (Wechsler, 2003) and WAIS-III (Wechsler, 1997) Comprehension subtest, which requires the examinee to answer detailed questions about cultural phenomena, would follow the auditory–verbal channel, require adequate input/reception to understand the question, draw upon a complex interplay between integration/association and storage/memory processes to reason using prior knowledge, and probably lead to output/expression via verbalization. In contrast, the WISC-IV and WAIS-III Picture Completion subtest, which requires the identification of missing stimuli in pictures, would follow the visual–motor channel, require adequate reception to encode stimuli in the pictures, draw upon integration/association to compare the stimulus pictures to existing images of objects and settings, require little storage of information via storage/memory processes, and lead to output/expression via verbalization or motoric response (i.e., pointing).

In order to develop hypotheses regarding cognitive performance, Kaufman and Lichtenberger (Kaufman, 1994; Kaufman & Lichtenberger, 1999, 2000, 2002) have integrated the information-processing framework with existing factor-analytic evidence and conceptions of intelligence. Table 10.3 presents the specific abilities or components listed under each information-processing category. Note that much of the terminology is derived from Guilford (1967), Horn (1989), and Bannatyne (1974).

Although the shared-abilities analysis and its simple information-processing model may sensitize those interpreting intellectual assessment tasks (1) to the construct-irrelevant influences related to input (e.g., visual acuity problems) and output (e.g., motor deficits) and (2) to the fine-grained processes affecting performance, they have a number of limitations. First, the approach stems primarily from theoretically and logically derived analysis of subtests by its authors, and I have found no reviews or critical evaluations of

TABLE 10.3. Kaufman and Lichtenberger's Integrative Shared Abilities Organized by Information-Processing Categories

Input

Attention/concentration
Auditory–vocal channel
Complex verbal directions
Distinguishing essential from nonessential detail
Encode information for processing
Simple verbal directions
Understanding long questions
Understanding words
Visual–motor channel
Visual perception of abstract material
Visual perception of complete meaningful stimuli
Visual perception of meaningful stimuli

Integration/association and storage/memory

Achievement
Acquired knowledge
Cognition
Common sense
Concept formation
Convergent production
Crystallized intelligence
Culture-loaded knowledge
Evaluation
Facility with numbers
Figural cognition
Figural evaluation
Fluid intelligence
Fund of information
General ability
Handling abstract verbal concepts
Holistic (right-brain) processing

Integration/association and storage/memory
(continued)

Integrating brain function
Learning ability
Long-term memory
Memory
Nonverbal reasoning
Planning ability
Reasoning
Reproduction of models
Semantic cognition
Semantic content
Sequential
Short-term memory (auditory or visual)
Simultaneous processing
Social comprehension
Spatial
Spatial visualization
Symbolic content
Synthesis
Trial-and-error learning
Verbal concept formation
Verbal conceptualization
Verbal reasoning
Visual memory
Visual processing
Visual sequencing

Output

Much verbal expression
Simple vocal expression
Visual organization
Visual–motor coordination

Note. From Kaufman and Lichtenberger (2002). Published by Allyn and Bacon, Boston, MA. Copyright 2002 by Pearson Education. Adapted by permission.

the information-processing aspect of this interpretive approach. Although such creative work is necessary to guide the initial development of interpretive frameworks, there is little or no evidence supporting its use—in terms of diagnostic or eligibility accuracy or intervention development. Second, its model of information processing is somewhat dated and rather simplistic. It relies upon a few statements about processing deficits in children with learning disabilities, as well as a dated model of linguistics, rather than more recent research from cognitive psychologists and cognitive scientists. As a result, it fails to include an array of information-processing steps (e.g., memory retrieval) and necessary model components (e.g., long-term store, control processes) like those outlined above. It also tends to focus on general categories of information processing rather than specific processes. Finally, the integration of factor-analytic research in the model to represent the elementary information processes seems too vague and loosely integrated to be useful.

Factor-Analytic Overlay Models

In a series of articles, chapters, and other publications during the past decade, Woodcock and colleagues have developed an information-processing model that outlines the organization of and interactions among latent abilities (as specified in the CHC theory) and external and internal influences on cognitive performance (Dean, Decker, Woodcock, & Schrank, 2003; Dean & Woodcock, 1999; Mather & Woodcock, 2001; Woodcock, 1993, 1997, 1998). The most recent version of Woodcock's model is presented in Figure 10.6. Consistent with classic information-processing models and architectures, the horizontal dimension of the model represents the *input–processing–output loop*. It begins with physical stimuli being registered by the senses. If attended to, this information is encoded into immediate awareness, which is represented by the CHC broad cognitive ability *short-term memory* (Gsm) in the model. It represents the short-term store in the Atkinson and Shiffrin model and the phonological loop in the Baddeley model. Information then may be acted upon and expressed via motor or oral output, or entered again into the processing loop. Thick lines in the model re-

flect the "freeway" of cognitive processing—relatively automatic, high-speed paths. The vertical dimension of the model represents complexity of information processing, ranging from reflexes at the automatic level to complex mental operations such as reasoning at the highest levels.

Woodcock includes 10 relatively distinct, but somewhat general, abilities from CHC theory in the information-processing model. As noted above, immediate awareness is represented by short-term memory (Gsm). The *processing speed* (Gs) ability is conceptualized as a valve controlling the speed of information flow. Both of these abilities are grouped under the label *cognitive efficiency*. Woodcock and colleagues also include five abilities in the model that are considered *thinking abilities*. These abilities require application of programs devoted to sensory perception, storage and retrieval of information in the long-term store, and novel problem solving. These abilities include *tactile and kinesthetic thinking* (Gtk), *visual–spatial thinking* (Gv), *auditory processing* (Ga), *long-term retrieval* (Glr), and *fluid reasoning* (Gf). The model also includes *stores of acquired knowledge*, which represents the information stored in the largely permanent long-term store. Consistent with ACT-R (Anderson & Lebiere, 1998), Woodcock refers to the stores of acquired knowledge as storehouses of declarative and procedural knowledge. Although these stores could contain enumerable specific content areas, Woodcock focuses on three general abilities: *reading and writing* (Grw), *quantitative knowledge* (Gq), and *comprehension-knowledge* (Gc). However, it is likely that the thinking abilities, which are differentiated from the stores of acquired knowledge, are the result of related procedural memory modules and the action rules contained in them (i.e., productions).

In addition to these measurable components operationalized by existing assessment instruments (viz., the Woodcock–Johnson III; Woodcock, McGrew, & Mather, 2001a), Woodcock and colleagues also include an *executive control* component in the model, which is consistent with Baddeley's central executive. Executive control governs the choice and sequence of cognitive processes. For example, it can activate Woodcock's metaknowledge filter to search the stores

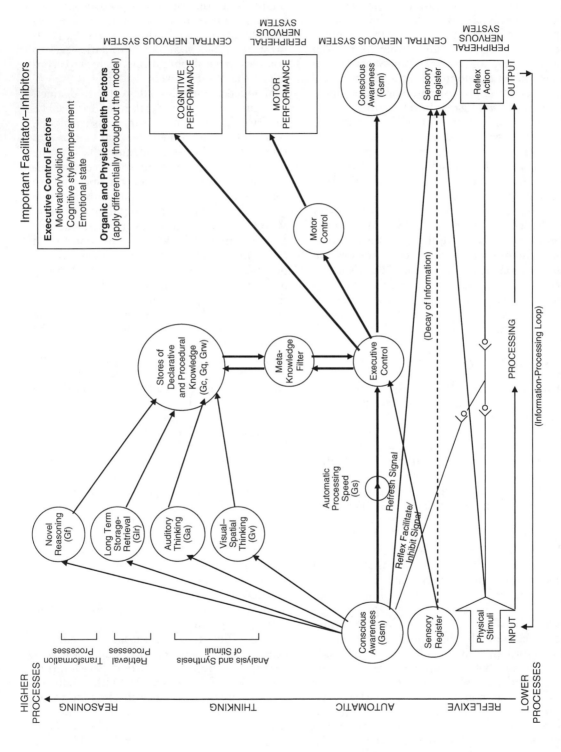

FIGURE 10.6. Dean and Woodcock's information-processing model. From Dean and Woodcock (1999), page 15. Copyright 1999 by Riverside Publishing. Reprinted by permission.

of acquired knowledge (i.e., the long-term store) for existing strategies or knowledge to be used during completion of a cognitive task. Finally, Woodcock maintains attention to situational and contextual influences on cognitive performance by the inclusion of *facilitators–inhibitors* in the model. Examples include distractions during testing and noncognitive person variables (e.g., sensory acuity deficits, fatigue, motivation, and behavioral styles).

Woodcock and colleagues' information-processing model serves as the basis for the Gf-Gc Diagnostic Worksheet (Woodcock, 1993, 1998), the WJ III Diagnostic Worksheet (Mather & Woodcock, 2001; Schrank & Woodcock, 2002), and the Dean–Woodcock Neuropsychological Assessment System neuropsychology model. The latest incarnation of this model and worksheet focuses on the interactions among cognitive ability scores from the Woodcock–Johnson III Tests of Cognitive Abilities (Woodcock, McGrew, & Mather, 2001c); achievement scores from the Woodcock–Johnson III Tests of Achievement (Woodcock, McGrew, & Mather, 2001b); sensory–motor scores from the Dean–Woodcock Sensory–Motor Battery (Dean & Woodcock, 2003b); and facilitators–inhibitors from the Dean–Woodcock Structured Interview (Dean & Woodcock, 2003c) and the Dean–Woodcock Emotional Status Exam (Dean & Woodcock, 2003a).

Although Woodcock and colleagues' information-processing model contains almost all of the same components as recent information-processing models from cognitive psychology and cognitive science. It is a very plausible organization of the interactions among the broad cognitive ability factors specified in CHC theory, it is clear that the cognitive ability factors came first, and that the factors were fitted to the information-processing model without great attention to their generality and to the processes required during completion of their constituent tests and test items. As a result, there are several problems with the organization of the model. As noted above, it is unclear how Woodcock's thinking abilities differ from procedural knowledge and related productions held in his stores of acquired knowledge. Review of prominent information-processing models also indi-

cates that a short-term store for visual information (in Baddeley's model, the visuo-spatial sketchpad) is probably necessary in comprehensive information-processing models, but it is absent in Woodcock and colleagues' model. A component representing this structure and related processes could be represented along with short-term memory to represent the holding areas for active information.

The operationalization of the factors in the information-processing model also seems problematic. More specifically, the inclusion of broad cognitive abilities, rather than more specific narrow abilities, leads to uncertainty in the use of the model for test interpretation. For example, consistent with covariance structural analyses, Picture Recognition from the Woodcock–Johnson III Tests of Cognitive Abilities (Woodcock et al., 2001c) is typically grouped with another test as a measure of visual–spatial thinking in the thinking ability section of the model. Picture Recognition requires examinees to hold images in mind and soon afterward identify them in an array of images. In the nomenclature of CHC theory, it measures visual memory or more generally visual short-term memory span. As a result, it should probably be placed in an area to represent the visuo-spatial sketchpad, as described above. In addition, abilities related to language processing are grouped under the same general factor, comprehension–knowledge, as are measures of cultural knowledge. Just because tests measuring similar processes covary to the degree that they measure as a single factor does not mean that they should be grouped together in a fine-grained information-processing analysis. Without attention to these more specific influences on item- and task-level performance, melding of measures of factors and information-processing models accomplishes little.

Test Batteries Developed to Assess Information Processes

The task-analytic models presented above that examine elementary information processes generally start with existing assessment instruments and evaluate them via information-processing frameworks. Similarly, the factor-analytic overlay models draw first upon existing classifications of tests according to empirically derived schemes and then integrate them with information-processing models. In contrast, several cognitive ability test batteries have been based on theory and knowledge regarding information processing, with less emphasis on structural evidence provided by factor analysis (see Keith, Kranzler, & Flanagan, 2001; Sternberg, 1984). Two test batteries whose developers have drawn on this top-down approach are discussed in this section.[3]

Das and Naglieri's Model

As described by Naglieri and Das (Chapter 7, this volume), their model of cognitive functioning specifies several interrelated cognitive operations—*planning, attention, simultaneous,* and *successive* (PASS) processes—that represent elementary information processes. Planning processes refer to the actions of executive control involved in governing the information-processing system, such as searching the long-term store for existing strategies and problem solving. This process mirrors the productions outlined in ACT-R (Anderson & Lebiere, 1998) and other production systems (Schunn & Klahr, 1998). Attention processes refer to the modulation of arousal and maintenance of mental focus across time. Simultaneous processing refers to perceiving, encoding, transforming, or otherwise utilizing bits of information occurring concurrently or as a group, whereas successive processing refers to the same processes involving bits of information presented in serial order (one after another).

Although the PASS model began as a relatively confined description of types of information processing (Das, Kirby, & Jarman, 1979), it later expanded to a theory of intelligence (Das, Naglieri, & Kirby, 1994; Naglieri & Das, 1997). However, it still maintains characteristics of an information-processing model by specifying input, processing, and output stages and knowledge stores (e.g., Das et al., 1994). For example, Naglieri and colleagues (e.g., Das et al., 1994; Naglieri & Das, 1997) provide a schematic outlining the interactions among the PASS processes within an information-processing model (see Figure 10.8). This schematic specifies sensory input mechanisms that process information in either a simultaneous or a successive manner. It also specifies a base of knowledge in the long-term store that can be stored or extracted and used via the PASS processes. As evident in Figure 10.7, all PASS processes may be preformed at the memory, conceptual, and perceptual levels. For example, simultaneous processes may be expressed at the memory level by drawing an image from memory. Finally, output mechanisms can be expressed in either a simultaneous or a successive manner. For instance, writing sentences typically requires successive motor output to group letters and words in the correct order on the written page.

Although at least one attempt was made to interpret existing intelligence tests from the perspective of PASS theory (Naglieri & Das, 1990), the PASS processes are best operationalized in the commercially published Cognitive Assessment System (CAS; Naglieri & Das, 1997; see Naglieri, Chapter 20, this volume). The CAS was designed to assess the PASS processes in children ages 5 through 17. Scores from its 12 subtests contribute to four scales representing each of the PASS processes. This battery stems from a long line of research and test development, and the body of research providing evidence to support this model is substantial (Das et al., 1994). For example, a search of the PsychInfo database using the terms "PASS theory" and "Cognitive Assessment System" revealed 49 published journal articles focusing on the content of the theory or research producing validity evidence for the CAS. However, the exhaustiveness of the PASS model is uncertain, and the relations between its components and those of more prominent information-processing models are unclear to me.

Kyllonen's Model

In order to measure a range of cognitive abilities during research studies examining personnel selection and training and the effects of stressors on cognition, Kyllonen and colleagues (Chaiken, Kyllonen, & Tirre, 2000; Kyllonen, 1995, 2002) developed the Cognitive Ability Measurement (CAM) battery. The battery includes almost 60 individual tests, and all are administered using a computer-based user interface. Tests were developed to operationalize the major elements and processes represented in early versions of the ACT architecture (ACT*; Anderson, 1983) via measurement of seven cognitive abilities. These abilities include

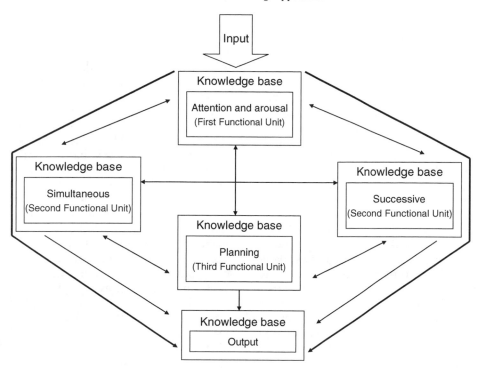

FIGURE 10.7. The planning, attention, simultaneous, and successive (PASS) process model. From Naglieri and Das (1990), page 315. Copyright 1990 by the Psychoeducational Corporation. Reprinted by permission.

working memory capacity, rate of learning of declarative knowledge (fact acquisition), rate of learning of procedural knowledge (skill acquisition), consolidated declarative knowledge, consolidated procedural knowledge, mental processing speed, and time estimation.

The CAM battery is structured according to a detailed taxonomy that highlights aspects of the tests that may influence performance on them (and accompanying scores). They include test paradigms, domains of knowledge, input modality, and response format (Kyllonen, 1995). To ensure broad construct representation in measurement of the elements and operations of the ACT architecture and to avoid "method variance" stemming primarily from similar test paradigms, the CAM battery draws from varying test paradigms to assess an ability. For example, in order to assess the rate of learning of declarative knowledge, test paradigms requiring free-recall learning, paired-associates learning, and implicit learning are employed. In order to avoid the measurement of abilities tied closely to the content acted upon by

the information processes, tests that vary in terms of the domain of knowledge (i.e., verbal, quantitative, and spatial) but measure the same ability and draw from the same test paradigm are included. Following the example regarding assessing rate of learning of declarative knowledge, the tests using the free-recall learning paradigm require working with representations of words or sentences, numbers, or visual–spatial stimuli. Similarly, tests may vary systematically according to the nature in which the test items are presented (e.g., in a visual or auditory input modality). Finally, tests are selected to vary systematically in their response formats. For example, response formats include pressing a key, touching a computer screen, manipulating a mouse, and vocalizing an answer. The authors of the CAM battery sought to develop at least one test that measures each of the seven cognitive abilities and that falls into each cell of this four-dimension taxonomy. As a result, the number of possible tests designed to measure *each* ability through different methods are many. This number would logically equal the (a) the number of test paradigms multiplied by (b) the number of domains of knowledge multiplied by (c) the number of input modalities multiplied by (d) the number of response formats.

The CAM battery has a well-supported architecture from which it was developed. It also is innovative because it was designed to tap into general levels of abilities by balancing out test-related influences. Unlike no other assessment battery, it allows for distinctions to be made between influences due to test demands, test content, input modality, and response format and those influences associated with a specific type of ability—perhaps a process. However, the CAM battery has been used primarily for research purposes and is not commercially available. Its multitude of individual tests (and an administration time of 5 to 12 hours; Kyllonen, 1995, 2002) would probably be too unwieldy for most psychologists and other professionals involved in psychoeducational assessments. Furthermore, it is unclear how a user would use the litany of scores stemming from such a battery. A starting point may be to identify relative strengths and weaknesses within tests measuring the same abilities or to identify relative strengths and weaknesses between tests measuring different abilities using the same parameters.

Test Batteries Modified to Assess Information Processes

Recently, existing intellectual assessment instruments have been modified to isolate some of the processes that may be interfering with performance or leading to weaknesses in abilities. Both the Wechsler Adult Intelligence Scale—Revised as a Neuropsychological Instrument (WAIS-R NI; Kaplan, Fein, Morris, & Delis, 1991) and the Wechsler Intelligence Scale for Children—Third Edition as a Process Instrument (WISC-III PI; Kaplan, Fein, Kramer, Delis, & Morris, 1999) are innovative test batteries designed to isolate information processes.[4] For example, the authors of the WISC-III PI state that this battery offers a "finer analysis of problem-solving behaviors and the parsing of component factors contributing to performance [that can] provide the examiner a deeper understanding of the child's level of information processing as well as a basis for generating tailored, individual interven-

tions" (Kaplan et al., 1999, p. 2). As evident by their titles, the test batteries draw upon the subtests from the Wechsler intelligence scales, but the task paradigms of the subtests are modified slightly to isolate some of the information processes.

The more recent and more well-developed of the two batteries is the WISC-III PI (Kaplan et al., 1999). The authors recommend that users of this battery, rather than interpreting the norm-based scores of examinees, should base interpretations on the type of task errors, behaviors during task completion, and comparisons between differing task paradigms. Following this recommendation, the WISC-III PI subtests are designed to remove requirements that may contribute construct-irrelevant influences on performance. There are adaptations to stimulus input, to the steps in replying, and to the nature of the cognitive task itself. Table 10.4 lists some of these adaptations. The battery also offers eight additional scoring criteria and provides the option of add-on administration procedures. Observations of performance during subtests may yield the frequency of these behaviors: requests for item repetition, pointing responses, and (on the Block Design subtest), use of extra blocks and breaks in the final configurations. In addition, there are several simple checklists of behaviors during the test administration that promote the recording of language skills, sensory response or motor stereotypies, social skills, cooperativeness, attention/concentration, and confidence. There is little doubt that the WAIS-R NI (Kaplan et al., 1991) and the WISC-III PI (Kaplan et al., 1999) are innovative and potentially useful models for test developers hoping to construct tests that isolate elementary information processes as much as possible. In addition, practitioners examining these batteries can be sensitized to the micro-level influences on performance.

CONCLUSIONS AND RECOMMENDATIONS FOR INTERPRETATION

Can the modern versions of the box-and-arrow models and a focus on elementary information processes aid the development of assessment instruments and facilitate more accurate interpretations of their scores? I

TABLE 10.4. Descriptions of the WISC-III Subtests and Their Modifications in the WISC-III PI

WISC-III subtest	Typical task requirements	Modifications to subtest or subtest scoring
Information	Children are required to answer orally presented questions about people, places, and things from U.S. culture.	Division of items by content categories: number facts, calendar facts, geography, science, and history. Provision of response options in multiple-choice format.
Vocabulary	Children are required to define orally presented words.	Words in items presented in images. Provision of response options in multiple-choice format.
Block Design	Children are required to construct geometric patterns from a model or visual image, using cubes, during a timed administration.	Provision of overlay on stimulus design that distinguishes individual blocks. Motor-free administration option.
Digit Span	Children are required to repeat orally presented digits in sequence or in reversed sequence.	Visual presentation of items. Letters presented rather than digits. Analysis of types of errors.
Arithmetic	Children are required to solve orally presented arithmetic problems without the use of paper and pencil.	Written response option.
Picture Completion	Children are required to identify important parts missing from pictures.	Division of items by pattern/symmetry items and knowledge-based items.
Picture Arrangement	Children are required to arrange a set of pictures into a logical story during a timed administration.	Ordering words on cards to make a sentence, rather than pictures to make a logical story.

believe so. In fact, it seems particularly important to have knowledge of the steps examinees *may* follow to successfully complete items from some intellectual assessment instruments and most all instruments measuring reading, writing, and mathematics. Regardless of the words used to describe these steps—*elementary information processes, propositions, chunks, components, operations,* or *processing stages*—greater understanding of them is likely to benefit individuals who seek comprehensive psychoeducational assessments for learning difficulties. The information I have reviewed so far has revealed that some progress has been made toward greater understanding. However, I am not convinced that interpretive strategies that are based on the information-processing models reviewed here have progressed to the point to which one can place confidence in judgments about the identification and measurement of information processes. Consis-

tent with Carroll's statement quoted at the beginning of this chapter, much work remains to be done for us to understand how best to measure these micro-level aspects of human information processing.

Processes as Hypothetical Constructs

How should psychologists and other professionals involved in psychoeducational assessments view cognitive processes and their measurement? We should view them as hypothetical constructs, which is consistent with Jensen's definition of information processes at the beginning of the chapter. Hypothetical constructs are things unseen. In the case of cognitive processes, they occur inside the "black box" of the mind (see Shaw, 2004). Although we can infer the existence of processes from an individual's responses on tasks and we can program computers to simulate them, representing and measuring an individual's elementary information processes in an accurate way using orally presented, paper-and-pencil, or typical computer-based tasks is probably beyond our grasp. Perhaps we should recognize that identifying an individual's errors in information processing will always be one based on reasoning and inference. This realization is demonstrated well by the interpretive framework of the WISC-III PI (Kaplan et al., 1999).

Processes as Steps

We should use the terms *process* or *processing* in the most informed way possible: to refer to the many unseen steps in completing a task and not to the sum or outcome of those steps. Shaw (2004) lamented that these terms are too often used superfluously. He stated, "*Language processing* means language. *Reading processing* means reading. *Information processing* means thinking. *Memory processing* means memory. The word [processing] adds nothing" (p. 34, original emphasis). Perhaps replacing "process" with "step" and "processing" with "steps" will ground us in the true meaning of the terms.

Norm-Referenced Scores as Abilities, Not Processes

We should probably avoid the interpretation of most norm-referenced scores from intellectual assessment instruments as indicating an elementary information process. Most of these scores are probably best seen as measures of cognitive abilities. These measures of cognitive abilities represent individual differences in the complete series of cognitive processes used when completing items, which are then aggregated into a subtest score, a composite score, or both. Because of this aggregation, ability scores should not be viewed as pure measures of distinct cognitive processes. This recommendation is reinforced by Carroll (1976), who stated,

> Nearly all cognitive tasks are complex, in the sense that they involve different kinds of memories and control processes. . . . It may be impossible, in principle, to identify "pure" factors of individual differences—probably not, at any rate, through the application of typical group-administered tests [and typical individually administered tests]. . . . The often-noted observation that all psychometric tests in the cognitive domain tend to be more or less positively correlated probably reflects the multifaceted nature of the tasks sampled in these tests. (p. 52)

During most complex tasks like those from contemporary intellectual assessment instruments, an examinee's performance is far too multifaceted to deconstruct it into distinct steps and accurately measure each of them.

There is little doubt that measures of cognitive abilities are affected by processes. For example, evidence abounds that tasks requiring attention to individual sounds measure a factor like broad auditory perception (see Carroll, 1993). However, we do not know if this factor emerges because of a common set of information processes used during task completion, because of similar task stimuli and related task paradigms, or because of some combination of these or other influences (cf. Kyllonen, 1995, 2002). Careful review of the different tasks measuring auditory processing indicates that many require somewhat different operations and strategies and draw on different types of knowledge for task completion. However, the task stimuli are the most similar among tasks measuring this factor. Perhaps the common processes at the input stage of information processing form a common bond between these tasks. On the other hand, the body of evidence examining tasks designed to measure processes, such as those measuring sequential and simultaneous processes, should be examined to determine if the small collection of processes they purportedly measure are in fact common across tasks varying in task stimuli, task paradigms, and task response formats. Based on recent research that has called into question the distinctions between the types of processes described in PASS theory and cognitive abilities described in CHC theory (e.g., Kaufman & Kaufman, 2004a; Keith et al., 2001), it is probable that these measures of processes also measure abilities.

A number of tests from commercially published intellectual assessment instruments may isolate groups of relatively unique information processes. These are relatively simple tasks (a) focusing on processes associated closely with sensory information held in short-term stores and (b) requiring few steps to complete items. One instance is the Picture Recognition test from the WJ III (Woodcock et al., 2001c; see also Schrank, Chapter 17, this volume). Each item requires examinees to study images of groups of people, animals, foods, plants, or objects for 5 seconds and then identify the images within a larger array after their removal. When considering possible processes, the examinee must sense and encode the images into the short-term store, retain that information for a brief period of time, match the mental representation of those images to those seen in the array, and respond by pointing or naming letters of the pictures in the array. (A facilitative strategy would include coding the images to be remembered according to some verbal label in order to draw upon the phonological store in addition to the visual store.) It seems logical that this test measures individual differences in the capacity of the short-term store most closely associated with visual information, like Baddeley's (1986) visual–spatial sketchpad. I suppose that all scores associated with such tasks that tap into small groups of processes would have relatively low g loadings because they involve fewer steps and components of the information processing system. For example, as reported in Floyd, Shaver, and McGrew (2003), the WJ III Picture Recognition test has a g loading of only .38 (g loadings below .50 are considered poor; see Kaufman, 1994). Some of the least complex cognitive tasks, such as those measuring reaction time, often also demonstrate very low g loadings (Carroll, 1993; Jensen, 1998). Although some test users may believe that measuring a distinct group of related information processes is very useful, it is probable that, when used in practice, the resulting scores will not possess the much-heralded predictive power of more complex measures. As a result, evidence of the clinical utility of these measures of distinct groups of processes is needed.

Processes at Item Level

If the interpretation of most norm-referenced scores largely precludes a focus on cognitive processes, what are the alternatives? As noted above, the best alternative may be to infer processes based on the item-level performance of individuals. For example, it makes sense to examine items in terms of in-fluences associated with *input* into the cognitive system and *output* via responses. At least these steps associated with information processing are observable to some extent. Labeling of these steps is modeled well by the interpretive approach of Kaufman and colleagues (Kaufman, 1994; Kaufman & Lichtenberger, 1999, 2000, 2002). Of particular importance are the stimuli used for test items and the manner in which they are conveyed to the examinee. For example, a person whose occupation requires frequent exposure and manipulation of numbers—such as an accountant—may perform better on short-term memory tasks when numbers are the task stimuli than when they are letters. Use of tasks requiring the same type of cognitive performance using different types of task stimuli may be helpful to examine hypotheses about the reasons for an individual's low levels of performance (see Kaplan et al. 1999; Kyllonen, 1995, 2002). However, the effects of practice across such alternate tasks may confound accurate measurement.

Attention to the manner in which participants must respond (i.e., output) should also be considered because abilities may be expressed better through one type of response versus another. The distinction between declarative and procedural memory, verbal and performance abilities, and verbal and nonverbal abilities are all consistent with this focus on output (see, e.g., Kaufman & Lichtenberger, 2002; Roid, 2003). At minimum, attention to the initial and the final steps taken when completing items will likely be very beneficial in identifying influences that interfere with the measurement of the intended constructs (see McGrew & Flanagan, 1998).

Here are two caveats. First, when I referred above to processes as the steps examinees *may* follow to complete an item or task, I italicized the word "may" because there is sufficient evidence to expect (1) variability within tasks across items for individuals and (2) variability in processes across individuals with different levels of abilities (see Lohman, 2000). Some processes may be very simple and lead to little variability across items or across individuals—like subtraction with borrowing—but most cognitive tasks are complex (Corno et al., 2002). This complexity probably leads to increased variability within and across individuals, which means that we should not abandon the focus on the individual during interpretation and that we should not trust that everyone follows the same processes during task completion.

Second, it is unclear to me how an individual's performance of most processes and the differences in the functioning of the structures in the cognitive system can ever be consistently and accurately inferred for complex cognitive tasks—even at the item level. In the case of memory stores and related operations, it may be possible to isolate the capacity to retain information in the short-term store for a brief period of time before producing a response (i.e., short-term memory). However, once information reaches a "deeper level" in the information processing system (such as the long-term store) or that information is transformed in some way, there is little way to distinguish between different content and operations of the varying memory structures. For example, during tasks in which previously retained information must be recalled, the breadth and depth of information stored in the long-term store would be targeted. However, other processes, such as retention or rehearsal of the item in the short-term store, information search and retrieval operations, and construction of the response before output, must all be employed. All of these processes are thought to be controlled by a central executive, which some scores purport to measure. Perhaps tasks can be distinguished on a relative scale in terms of involving more of one kind of process than others (see Kaufman & Kaufman, 2004a).

Processes of Achievement Tasks

Perhaps interpretive approaches supporting contemporary assessment techniques should focus *first* on the information processes associated with completion of academic and vocationally relevant tasks, such as reading and mathematics. There are two practical reasons for this conclusion. First, it appears that the standard set of steps to complete reading, mathematics, and writing tasks are relatively easy to identify and relatively uniform across persons. As noted above, the range of processes needed to correctly complete items from most tasks measuring these domains is much narrower than the range of processes needed for most tasks measuring cognitive abilities. Most achievement tests that focus on basic or functional levels of performance target procedural knowledge associated with the domain of interest and limit the number of operations or strategies to be used. The task stimuli also are generally uniform within the domain of interest (e.g., with reading, words or sentences), and responses modalities are similar across related tasks. For example, responses to mathematics calculation items often require written responses. The common processes required for tasks within each of these achievement domains make them viable targets for interpretative approaches based on information processing.

Second, task analysis of assessment techniques measuring achievement domains would probably help assessors engaged in psychoeducational assessment to reach a key goal: to provide parents, teachers, children, and other clients tangible strategies for improving performance during reading, mathematics, and writing. Rather than focusing on why a child constructs block designs slowly or inaccurately, and generalizing those findings to an achievement task, shouldn't we be first concerned about actual performance during that achievement task and the processes that lead to successful performance on it? Shouldn't assessment tasks focus on what an examinee does when reading, the process of speaking a foreign language in conversation, or the processes supporting acquisition of new vocabulary words? For example, a child's slow performance on a test of visual processing or a test of processing speed does not necessarily mean that the child will perform slowly on other tasks requiring encoding and responding to visual stimuli, such a reading or mathematics. For example, problems with visual–spatial orientation (relative to peers) identified during a test of visual processing may not affect performance on a test of mathematics calculations that requires such visual–spatial orientation, such as when adding down columns. However, if a child consistently makes errors in mathematics calculations when adding down columns but appears to have mastered the recall of addition facts, that child may be seen as having a problem with visual–spatial orientation during mathematics calculation tasks. Because this second conclusion is grounded in processes of the achievement task, it will probably lead to tangible benefits for the child being assessed through more effective interventions focusing on performance during mathematics. I believe that an analysis of processes stemming from performance on achievement tasks, like this example, best reflects the guidelines for identification of learning disabilities that call for identification of the *deficits or disorders in processes* contributing to the imperfect ability to listen, speak, read, write, spell, or to complete math problems (IDEA, 1997).

Many experienced professionals involved in testing already successfully engage in inferring processes by conducting careful analysis of examinees' errors at the item level during achievement tasks. To aid these and other professionals, more practical, authentic assessment tasks and interpretive frameworks could be developed to isolate processes during such tasks. Much has already been done in this vein by Berninger (2001) and by those using curriculum-based evaluation procedures like those described by Howell and Nolet (2000). Similarly, some prominent achievement test batteries, such as the second edition of the *Kaufman Test of Educational Achievement* (KTEA; Kaufman & Kaufman, 2004b), provide detailed error analysis techniques to aid in identification of processes not used or used errantly by test takers during reading decoding and spelling.

Processes from Research

I would be remiss if I did not recommend additional research and study in this area. First, I suspect that careful study of the body of research conducted using ACT-R (Anderson et al., 2004; Anderson & Lebiere, 1998) and other production systems will reveal insights that can be applied to the measurement of elementary information processes (see Carpenter, Just, & Shell, 1990). (A careful examination of this research and technology was beyond the scope of this chapter.) Second, there should be continued effort to refine their definitions and measurement of cognitive abilities and the most specific processes that underlie them (Das et al., 1994; McGrew, 1997). Because a consensus nomenclature of cognitive abilities is forming (see McGrew, Chapter 8, this volume), the connections between latent abilities mea-

sured by assessment instruments and the more specific processes that may be required to complete them may become more apparent. Third, I believe that Carroll's (1976) coding scheme may provide the richest method to evaluate items from existing individual assessment instruments. Test developers could utilize this method to provide a robust account of the processes required to complete items on their instruments and to allow for identification of possible construct-irrelevant influences on performance. However, more research may be needed to support the use of the coding scheme. For example, it is unknown whether independent researchers using this scheme would reliably code the same tasks in an identical manner, as Carroll acknowledged. It is probable that the recent surge of interest in *cognitive task analysis* when designing computer systems and other technology will produce techniques for improving Carroll's coding scheme (see Schraagen, Chipman, & Shalin, 2000). Finally, more research using interviews with examinees completing assessment instrument items, think-aloud protocols, and conceptual analyses should be conducted to facilitate a better understanding of information processes (Ericsson & Simon, 1993; Newstead, Bradon, Handley, Evans, & Dennis, 2002).

NOTES

1. Earlier incarnations of ACT-R include ACT-E (Anderson, 1976) and ACT* (Anderson, 1983). The most recent version of ACT-R is 5.0.

2. In earlier descriptions, the integration/association and storage/memory classifications were merged, due to difficulty differentiating these processes.

3. The second edition of the Kaufman Assessment Battery for Children (KABC-II; Kaufman & Kaufman, 2004a), which was designed to measure simultaneous and sequential processes, was not described in this chapter because it was not published when the penultimate daft of this chapter was written (see Kaufman et al., Chapter 16, this volume).

4. Like the KABC-II (Kaufman & Kaufman, 2004a), the WISC-IV as a Processing Instrument (Kaplan et al., 2004) was not described in this chapter because it was not published when the penultimate draft of this chapter was written. However, based on a review of mar-

keting material, the organization and adaptations to the subtests appear to be similar to those seen with the WISC-III PI.

ACKNOWLEDGMENT

Special thanks to James O. Rust who provided constructive feedback about an early draft of this chapter.

REFERENCES

American Academy of School Psychology Ad Hoc Committee on Comprehensive Evaluation for Learning Disabilities (2004). *Statement on comprehensive evaluation for learning disabilities*. Retrieved September 2, 2004, from http://espse.ed.psu.edu/spsy/aasp/AASPstateLD.pdf

American Educational Research Association, American Psychological Association, & National Council on Measurement in Education. (1999). *Standards for educational and psychological testing*. Washington, DC: American Educational Research Association.

Anastasi, A. (1967). Psychology, psychologists, and psychological testing. *American Psychologist, 22*, 297–306.

Anderson, J. R. (1976). *Language, memory and thought*. Hillsdale, NJ: Erlbaum.

Anderson, J. R. (1983). *The architecture of cognition*. Cambridge, MA: Harvard University Press.

Anderson, J. R. (1990). *The adaptive character of thought*. Hillsdale, NJ: Erlbaum.

Anderson, J. R., Bothell, D., Byrne, M. D., Douglas, S., Lebiere, C., & Qin, Y. (2004). An integrated theory of the mind. *Psychological Review, 111*, 1036–1060.

Anderson, J., & Lebiere, C. (1998). *The atomic components of thought*. Mahwah, NJ: Erlbaum.

Ashcraft, M. H. (1998). *Fundamentals of cognition*. New York: Longman.

Atkinson, R. C., & Shiffrin, R. M. (1968). Human memory: A proposed system and its control processes. In K. W. Spence & J. T. Spence (Eds.), *The psychology of learning and motivation* (pp. 89–195). New York: Academic Press.

Baddeley, A. (1986). *Working memory*. New York: Oxford University Press.

Baddeley, A. (1994). Working memory: The interface between memory and cognition. In D. L. Schacter & E. Tulving (Eds.), *Memory systems 1994* (pp. 351–367). Cambridge, MA: MIT Press.

Baddeley, A. (1996). Exploring the central executive. *Quarterly Journal of Experimental Psychology, 49A*, 5–28.

Baddeley, A. (2001). Is working memory still working? *American Psychologist, 56*, 851–864.

Baddeley, A. D., & Hitch, G. J. (1994). Development in the concept of working memory. *Neuropsychology, 8*, 485–493.

Bannatyne, A. (1974). Diagnosis: A note on recategorization of the WISC scaled scores. *Journal of Learning Disabilities, 7*, 272–274.

Bechtel, W., & Graham, G. (Eds.). (1998). *A companion to cognitive science*. Malden, MA: Blackwell.

Berninger, V. (2001). *Process Assessment of the Learner (PAL) Test Battery for Reading and Writing*. San Antonio, TX: Psychological Corporation.

Borkowski, J. G., Carr, M., Rellinger, E. A., & Pressley, M. (1990). Self-regulated strategy use: Interdependence of metacognition, attributions, and self-esteem. In B. F. Jones (Ed.), *Dimensions of thinking: Review of research* (pp. 53–92). Hillsdale, NJ: Erlbaum.

Carpenter, P. A., Just, M. A., & Shell, P. (1990). What one intelligence test measures: A theoretical account of the processing in the Raven Progressive Matrices Test. *Psychological Review, 97*, 404–431.

Carroll, J. B. (1976). Psychometric tests as cognitive tasks: A new structure of intellect. In L. B. Resnick (Ed.), *The nature of intelligence* (pp. 27–56). Hillsdale, NJ: Erlbaum.

Carroll, J. B. (1987). Psychometric approaches to cognitive abilities and processes. In S. H. Irvine & S. E. Newstead (Eds.), *Intelligence and cognition: Contemporary frames of reference* (pp. 217–251). Boston: Martinus Nijhoff.

Carroll, J. B. (1988). Cognitive abilities, factors, and processes. *Intelligence, 12*, 101–109.

Carroll, J. B. (1993). *Human cognitive abilities: A survey of factor analytic studies*. New York: Cambridge University Press.

Carroll, J. B. (1998). Human cognitive abilities: A critique. In J. J. McCardle & R. W. Woodcock (Eds.), *Human cognitive abilities in theory and practice* (pp. 5–24). Mahwah, NJ: Erlbaum.

Chaiken, S. R., Kyllonen, P. C., & Tirre, W. (2000). Organization and components of psychomotor ability. *Cognitive Psychology, 40*, 198–226.

Colman, A. M. (2001). *A dictionary of psychology*. New York: Oxford University Press.

Corno, L., Cronbach, L. J., Kupermintz, H., Lohman, D. F., Mandinach, E. B., Porteus, A. W., & Talbert, J. E. (2002). *Remaking the concept of aptitude: Extending the legacy of Richard E. Snow*. Mahwah, NJ: Erlbaum.

Corrigan, P. W., & Yudofsky, S. C. (Eds.). (1996). *Cognitive rehabilitation for neuropsychiatric disorders*. Washington, DC: American Psychiatric Press.

Corsini, R. J. (1999). *The dictionary of psychology*. Philadelphia: Brunner/Mazel.

Cronbach, L. J. (1957). The two disciplines of scientific psychology. *American Psychologist, 12*, 671–684.

Das, J. P., Kirby, J. R., & Jarman, R. F. (1979). *Simultaneous and successive cognitive processes*. New York: Academic Press.

Das, J. P., Naglieri, J. A., & Kirby, J. R. (1994). *Assessment of cognitive processes: The PASS theory of intelligence*. Needham Heights, MA: Allyn & Bacon.

Dean, R. S., Decker, S. L., Woodcock, R. W., &

Schrank, F. A. (2003). A cognitive neuropsychology assessment system. In F. A. Schrank & D. P. Flanagan (Eds.), *WJ III clinical use and interpretation* (pp. 345–376). New York: Academic Press.

Dean, R. S., & Woodcock, R. W. (1999). *The WJ–R and Bateria–R in neuropsychological assessment* (Research Report No. 3). Itasca, IL: Riverside.

Dean, R. S., & Woodcock, R. W. (2003a). *Dean–Woodcock Emotional Status Exam*. Itasca, IL: Riverside.

Dean, R. S., & Woodcock, R. W. (2003b). *Dean–Woodcock Sensory–Motor Battery*. Itasca, IL: Riverside.

Dean, R. S., & Woodcock, R. W. (2003c). *Dean–Woodcock Structured Interview.* Itasca, IL: Riverside.

Deary, I. J. (2001). Human intelligence differences: Toward a combined experimental-differential approach. *Trends in Cognitive Science, 4,* 164–170.

Deary, I. J. (2002). g and cognitive elements of information processing: An agnostic view. In R. J. Sternberg & E. L. Grigorenko (Eds.), *The general factor of intelligence: How general is it?* (pp. 151–181). Mahwah, NJ: Erlbaum.

Ericsson, K. A., & Simon, H. A. (1993). *Protocol analysis: Verbal reports as data* (rev. ed.). Cambridge, MA: MIT Press.

Estes, W. K. (1999). Models of human memory: A 30–year retrospective. In C. Izawa (Ed.), *On human memory: Evolution, progress, and reflections on the 30th anniversary of the Atkinson–Shiffrin model* (pp. 59–86). Mahwah, NJ: Erlbaum.

Floyd, R. G., Shaver, R. B., & McGrew, K. S. (2003). Interpretation of the Woodcock–Johnson III Tests of Cognitive Abilities: Acting on evidence. In F. A. Schrank & D. P. Flanagan (Eds.), *WJ III clinical use and interpretation* (pp. 1–46, 403–408). New York: Academic Press.

French, J. W., Ekstrom, R. B., & Price, L. A. (1963). *Kit of Reference Tests for Cognitive Factors*. Princeton, NJ: Education Testing Service.

Gathercole, S. E. (1994). Neuropsychology and working memory: A review. *Neuropsychology, 8,* 494–505.

Glass, A. L., Holyoak, K. J., & Santa, J. L. (1979). *Cognition*. Reading, MA: Addison-Wesley.

Glasser, R. (1981). The future of testing: A research agenda for cognitive psychology and psychometrics. *American Psychologist, 36,* 923–936.

Godttfredson, L. S. (1997). Why g matters: The complexity of everyday life. *Intelligence, 24,* 79–132.

Godttfredson, L. S. (2002). g: Highly general and highly practical. In R. J. Sternberg & E. L. Grigorenko (Eds.), *The general factor of intelligence: How general is it?* (pp. 331–380). Mahwah, NJ: Erlbaum.

Guilford, J. P. (1967). *The nature of human intelligence*. New York: McGraw-Hill.

Healy, A. F., & McNamara, D. S. (1996). Verbal learning and memory: Does the modal model still work? *Annual Review of Psychology, 47,* 143–172.

Horn, J. L. (1989). Cognitive diversity: A framework for learning. In P. L. Ackerman, R. J. Sternberg, & R. Glaser (Eds.), *Learning and individual differences* (pp. 61–116). New York: Freeman.

Horn, J. L., & Noll, J. (1997). Human cognitive capabilities: Gf-Gc theory. In D. P. Flanagan, J. L. Genshaft, & P. L. Harrison (Eds.), *Contemporary intellectual assessment: Theories, tests, and issues* (pp. 53–93). New York: Guilford Press.

Howell, K. W., & Nolet, V. (2000). *Curriculum-based evaluation: Teaching and decision making* (3rd ed.). Scarborough, ON, Canada: Wadsworth.

Hunt, E. (1971). What kind of computer is man? *Cognitive Psychology, 2,* 57–98.

Hunt, E., Frost, N., & Lunneborg, C. (1973). Individual differences in cognition: A new approach to intelligence. In G. H. Bower (Ed.), *The psychology of learning and motivation: Advances in research and theory* (pp. 87–122). New York: Academic Press.

Individuals with Disabilities Education Act Amendments of 1997, Pub. L. No. 105–17, 20 U.S.C. 33, §§ 1400 *et seq.* (1997)

Irvine, S., & Kyllonen, P. C. (2002). *Generating items for cognitive tests: Theory and practice*. Hillsdale, NJ: Erlbaum.

Jensen, A. R. (1998). *The g factor: The science of mental ability*. Westport, CT: Preager.

Kamphaus, R. W. (2001). *Clinical assessment of child and adolescent intelligence* (2nd ed.). Boston: Allyn & Bacon.

Kaplan, E., Delis, D., Fein, D., Maerlender, A., Morris, R., & Kramer, J. (2004). *WISC-IV Integrated*. San Antonio, TX: Harcourt Assessment.

Kaplan, E., Fein, D., Kramer, J., Delis, D., & Morris, R. (1999). *WISC-III as a Process Instrument*. San Antonio, TX: Psychological Corporation.

Kaplan, E., Fein, D., Morris, R., & Delis, D. (1999). *WAIS-R as a Neuropsychological Instrument*. San Antonio, TX: Psychological Corporation.

Kaufman, A. S. (1994). *Intelligent testing with the WISC-III*. New York: Wiley.

Kaufman, A. S., & Kaufman, N. L. (2004a). *Kaufman Assessment Battery for Children, Second Edition manual*. Circle Pines, MN: American Guidance Service.

Kaufman, A. S., & Kaufman, N. L. (2004b). *Kaufman Test of Educational Achievement, Second Edition manual*. Circle Pines, MN: American Guidance Service.

Kaufman, A. S., & Lichtenberger, E. O. (1999). *Essentials of WAIS-III assessment*. New York: Wiley.

Kaufman, A. S., & Lichtenberger, E. O. (2000). *Essentials of WISC-III and WPPSI-R assessment*. New York: Wiley.

Kaufman, A. S., & Lichtenberger, E. O. (2002). *Assessing adolescent and adult intelligence* (2nd ed.). Boston: Allyn & Bacon.

Keith, T. Z., Kranzler, J. H., & Flanagan, D. P. (2001). What does the Cognitive Assessment System (CAS) measure? Joint confirmatory factor analysis of the

CAS and the Woodcock–Johnson Tests of Cognitive Ability (3rd ed.). *School Psychology Review, 30,* 89–119.

Klahr, D., & Wallace, J. G. (1976). *Cognitive development: An information-processing view.* Hillsdale, NJ: Erlbaum.

Kyllonen, P. C. (1995). CAM: A theoretical framework for cognitive abilities measurement. In D. Detterman (Ed.), *Current topics in human intelligence: Vol. 4. Theories of intelligence* (pp. 307–359). Norwood, NJ: Ablex.

Kyllonen, P. C. (2002). Item generation for repeated testing of human performance. In S. Irvine & P. C. Kyllonen (Eds.), *Generating items for cognitive tests: Theory and practice* (pp. 251–275). Hillsdale, NJ: Erlbaum.

Loarer, E. (2003). Cognitive training for individuals with deficits. In R. J. Sternberg, J. Lautrey, & T. I. Lubart (Eds.), *Models of intelligence: International perspectives* (pp. 243–260). Washington, DC: American Psychological Association.

Logan, G. (2000). Information-processing theories. In A. E. Kazdin (Ed.), *Encyclopedia of psychology* (pp. 294–297). Washington, DC: American Psychological Association.

Lohman, D. F. (1994). Component scores as residual variation (or why the intercept correlates best). *Intelligence, 19,* 1–11.

Lohman, D. F. (2000). Complex information processing and intelligence. In R. J. Sternberg (Ed.), *Handbook of intelligence* (pp. 285–340). Cambridge, UK: Cambridge University Press.

Mather, N., & Woodcock, R. W. (2001). *Examiner's manual. Woodcock–Johnson III Tests of Cognitive Abilities.* Itasca, IL: Riverside.

Mayer, R. E. (1996). Learners as information processors: Legacies and limitations of educational psychology's second metaphor. *Educational Psychologist, 31*(3/4), 151–161.

McGrew, K. S. (1997). Analysis of the major intelligence batteries according to a proposed comprehensive Gf-Gc framework. In D. P. Flanagan, J. L. Genshaft, & P. L. Harrison (Eds.), *Contemporary intellectual assessment: Theories, tests, and issues* (pp. 131–150). New York: Guilford Press.

McGrew, K. S., & Flanagan, D. P. (1998). *The intelligence test desk reference (ITDR): Gf-Gc cross-battery assessment.* Boston: Allyn & Bacon.

McNemar, Q. (1964). Lost: Our intelligences. *American Psychologist, 19,* 871–882.

Naglieri, J. A., & Das, J. P. (1990). Planning, attention, simultaneous, and successive (PASS) cognitive processes as a model for intelligence. *Journal of Psychoeducational Assessment, 8,* 303–337.

Naglieri, J. A., & Das, J. P. (1997). *Das–Naglieri Cognitive Assessment System.* Itasca, IL: Riverside.

Neisser, U. (1967). *Cognitive psychology.* Englewood Cliffs, NJ: Prentice-Hall.

Neisser, U., Boodoo, G., Bouchard, T. J., Boykin, A. W., Brody, N., Ceci, S. J., et al. (1996). Intelligence: Knowns and unknowns. *American Psychologist, 51,* 77–101.

Newell, A. (1990). *Unified theories of cognition.* Cambridge, UK: Cambridge University Press.

Newell, A., & Simon, H. A. (1972). *Human problem solving.* Englewood Cliffs, NJ: Prentice-Hall.

Newstead, S., Bradon, P., Handley, S., Evans, J., & Dennis, I. (2002). Using the psychology of reasoning to predict the difficulty of analytical reasoning problems. In S. Irvine & P. C. Kyllonen (Eds.), *Generating items for cognitive tests: Theory and practice* (pp. 35–51). Hillsdale, NJ: Erlbaum.

Osgood, C. E. (1957). A behavioristic analysis of perception and language as cognitive phenomena. In J. S. Bruner, E. Brunswick, E. Festinger, K. F. Muenzinger, C. E. Osgood, & D. Rapaport (Eds.), *Contemporary approaches to cognition* (pp. 75–118). Cambridge, MA: Harvard University Press.

Posner, M. I., & McLeod, P. (1982). Information processing models-in search of elementary operations. *Annual Review of Psychology, 22,* 477–514.

Raaijmakers, J. G. W. (1993). The story of the two-store model of memory: Past criticisms, current status, and future directions. In D. E. Meyer & S. Kornblum (Eds.), *Attention and performance XIV: Synergies in experimental psychology, artificial intelligence, and cognitive neuroscience* (pp. 467–487). Cambridge, MA: MIT Press.

Roid, G. H. (2003). *Stanford–Binet Intelligence Scale, Fifth Edition.* Itasca, IL: Riverside.

Sattler, J. M. (2001). *Assessment of children: Cognitive applications* (4th. ed.). San Diego, CA: Author.

Schraagen, J. M., Chipman, S. F., & Shalin, V. L. (Eds.). (2000). *Cognitive task analysis.* Mahwah, NJ: Erlbaum.

Schrank, F. A., & Woodcock, R. W. (2002). *Report Writer for the WJ III Compuscore and Profiles Program* [Computer software]. Itasca, IL: Riverside.

Shaw, S. R. (2004). Disordered processing. *NASP Communiqué, 32*(5), 33–34.

Shiffrin, R. M. (1999). 30 years of memory. In C. Izawa (Ed.), *On human memory: Evolution, progress, and reflections on the 30th anniversary of the Atkinson-Shiffrin model* (pp. 17–33). Mahwah, NJ: Erlbaum.

Schunn, C. D., & Klahr, D. (1998). Production systems. In W. Bechtel & G. Graham (Eds.), *A companion to cognitive science* (pp. 542–551). Malden, MA: Blackwell.

Silver, L. B. (1993). Introduction and overview to the clinical concepts of learning disabilities. *Child and Adolescent Psychiatric Clinics of North America, 2,* 181–192.

Sobel, C. P. (2001). *The cognitive sciences: An interdisciplinary approach.* Mountain View, CA: Mayfield.

Sternberg, R. (1977). *Intelligence, information processing, and analogical reasoning.* Hillsdale, NJ: Erlbaum.

Sternberg, R. (1981). *Testing and cognitive psychology. American Psychologist, 36,* 1181–1189.

Sternberg, R. (1984). The Kaufman Assessment Battery

for Children: An information-processing analysis and critique. *Journal of Special Education, 18*, 269–279.

Swanson, H. L. (1991). Learning disabilities, distinctive encoding, and hemispheric resources: An information-processing perspective. In J. E. Obrzut & G. W. Hynd (Eds.), *Neuropsychological foundations of learning disabilities: A handbook of issues, methods, and practice* (pp. 241–285). San Diego, CA: Academic Press.

Swanson, H. L. (1996). Information processing: An introduction. In K. D. Reid, W. P. Hresko, & H. L. Swanson (Eds.), *Cognitive approaches to learning disabilities* (3rd ed., pp. 251–285). Austin, TX: Pro-Ed.

Thompson, R. M. (2000). *Comparing theories of child development* (5th ed.). Belmont, CA: Wadsworth.

Thurstone, L. L. (1938). *Primary mental abilities* (Psychometric Monographs, No. 1). Chicago: University of Chicago Press.

Torgesen, J. K. (1996). A model of memory from an information processing perspective: The special case of phonological memory. In G. R. Lyon & N. A. Krasnegor (Eds.), *Attention, memory, and executive function* (pp. 157–184). Baltimore: Brookes.

Wechsler, D. (1991). *Wechsler Intelligence Scale for Children—Third Edition*. San Antonio, TX: Psychological Corporation.

Wechsler, D. (1997). *Wechsler Adult Intelligence Scale—Third Edition*. San Antonio, TX: Psychological Corporation.

Wechsler, D. (2003). *Wechsler Intelligence Scale for Children—Fourth Edition*. San Antonio, TX: Psychological Corporation.

Wilson, M., & Emmorey, K. (1997). A visuo-spatial "phonological loop" in working memory: Evidence from American Sign Language. *Memory and Cognition, 25*, 313–320.

Woodcock, R. W. (1993). An information processing view of the Gf-Gc theory. *Journal of Psychoeducational Assessment Monograph Series: Woodcock–Johnson Psycho-Educational Assessment Battery—Revised*, pp. 80–102. Cordova, TN: Psychoeducational Corporation.

Woodcock, R. W. (1997). The Woodcock–Johnson Tests of Cognitive Ability—Revised. In D. P. Flanagan, J. L. Genshaft, & P. L. Harrison (Eds.), *Contemporary intellectual assessment: Theories, tests, and issues* (pp. 230–246). New York: Guilford Press.

Woodcock, R. W. (1998). Extending Gf-Gc theory into practice. In J. J. McArdle & R. W. Woodcock (Eds.), *Human cognitive abilities in theory and practice* (pp. 137–156). Mahwah, NJ: Erlbaum.

Woodcock, R. W., McGrew, K. S., & Mather, N. (2001a). *Woodcock–Johnson III*. Itasca, IL: Riverside.

Woodcock, R. W., McGrew, K. S., & Mather, N. (2001b). *Woodcock–Johnson III Tests of Achievement*. Itasca, IL: Riverside.

Woodcock, R. W., McGrew, K. S., & Mather, N. (2001c). *Woodcock–Johnson III Tests of Cognitive Abilities*. Itasca, IL: Riverside.

11

Advances in Cognitive Assessment of Culturally and Linguistically Diverse Individuals

A Nondiscriminatory Interpretive Approach

SAMUEL O. ORTIZ
SALVADOR HECTOR OCHOA

Practitioners who engage in the assessment of culturally and linguistically diverse individuals often recognize that the process involves an array of complex issues, many of which may not have been adequately covered during graduate training. Even when such issues are included as a regular component of psychological coursework and curricula, there is often limited opportunity for direct supervision in the actual process of assessment with diverse individuals. As a result, practitioners who recognize the problems facing them in such types of evaluation may still not have any idea regarding what procedural alterations or methodological changes should be included in evaluation practices. The search for any information and guidance on nondiscriminatory assessment practices often proves rather futile because the literature tends to be long on describing what the issues are but short on what to do about them. For example, the American Psychological Association (APA) has published "Guidelines for Providers of Psychological Services to Ethnic, Linguistic, and Culturally Diverse Populations" (APA,

1993), which emphasizes the need for psychologists to acknowledge the influences of language and culture on behavior, and to consider those factors when working with diverse groups. The guidelines also include admonitions regarding appraisal of the validity of the methods and procedures used for assessment and interpretation. What should be done when the validity is deemed questionable or precisely what should have been done to reduce bias and maintain validity in the first place are unfortunately absent from this and other guidelines.

In the absence of clear methodological frameworks for reducing the potential biasing aspects of evaluation with culturally and linguistically diverse learners, practitioners have resorted to a variety of methods drawn primarily from clinical lore and based only loosely on theoretical or empirical foundations. For example, the most obvious issue to be addressed when working with linguistically different individuals is the language or communication barrier that results from the difference between the language spoken by the examiner and examinee. In contrast, issues related to cultural differences, those between the examinee and the individuals on whom the test was normed, tends to receive little if any attention (Ortiz & Flanagan, 1998). The subtle, but more powerful effect of culture on test performance is thus overshadowed by attempts to deal with the more obvious issue of language—so much so that practitioners are often satisfied if this single issue is addressed (e.g., either by use of an interpreter or referring the individual for evaluation by a professional who speaks the individual's language). The focus on language issues is neither resolved in such a simple manner nor a guarantee of automatic bias reduction. Consider that:

> mere possession of the capacity to communicate in an individual's native language does not ensure appropriate, non-discriminatory assessment of that individual. Simple translation and/or interpretation of standardized testing batteries or test items does not represent current best practices in the field. Traditional assessment practices and their inherent biases can be easily replicated in any number of languages. (Flanagan, McGrew, & Ortiz, 2000, p. 291)

When guidelines are offered in the literature regarding specific practices and procedures, such as appropriate instrument selection, alterations and modifications to administration, or interpretive procedures, and so forth, they tend to be rather piecemeal and do not address the broader issues regarding a comprehensive approach to nondiscriminatory evaluation (Gonzalez, Brusca-Vega, & Yawkey, 1997; GoPaul-McNicol & Thomas-Presswood, 1998; Hamayan & Damico, 1991). Fair and equitable assessment of individuals from diverse backgrounds is not accomplished via any single methodological shortcut, regardless of how promising it may be. In the end, practitioners are often left with little instruction in how best to integrate appropriate procedures and methods into a broader, nondiscriminatory assessment paradigm (Ysseldyke, 1979).

Given the lack of applied information available to practitioners, it should be no surprise that the issues involved in bilingual, cross-cultural, nondiscriminatory assessment are too often distilled to finding simple answers to complex questions. For example, practitioners routinely resort to asking what is the "best" tool to use in evaluation of diverse individuals. But even such straightforward questions rarely lead to equally straightforward responses and the solutions sought by practitioners are likely to remain rather complicated. This does not mean, however, that the ability to understand and apply nondiscriminatory procedures requires an inordinate amount of professional effort or training. To the contrary, it is the purpose and intention of this chapter to present two recent developments related to the assessment of culturally and linguistically diverse individuals that can provide substantial benefits to assessment practice. Indeed, the procedures to be described in this chapter have been chosen as examples of emerging and innovative approaches that place practical yet sophisticated nondiscriminatory methods firmly within the reach of any professional evaluator.

Practitioners are cautioned not to assume that comprehensive nondiscriminatory assessment of diverse individuals can be accomplished solely through the use of these methods. As noted previously, fair and equitable assessment of diverse individuals rests first and foremost on the application and use of a systematic, broad framework wherein methods specifically designed to reduce bias are incorporated (see Ortiz, 2002). Nevertheless, when applied judiciously, the techniques that will be discussed can aid practitioners significantly in two important aspects of the assessment process: determining the modality for testing and reduction of bias in interpretation.

THE MULTIDIMENSIONAL ASSESSMENT MODEL FOR BILINGUAL INDIVIDUALS

Because evaluation should be tailored to the specific referral question and purpose of assessment, practitioners are required to make a wide range of decisions regarding how to develop and implement the most appropriate practices and procedures. The decision regarding what approach to take in any evaluation is critical with respect to the fundamental issue of validity. The degree to which meaningful interpretations can be drawn from test results is tied directly to the confidence the evaluator has in the validity of the results. Therefore, selecting the approach that is most likely to produce fairer and more equitable estimates of an individual's true abilities and knowledge is not a factor that can be taken lightly. For example, one aspect of this decision-making process involves determination of the mode(s) and language(s) of assessment. The most common recommendation regarding the evaluation of linguistically different individuals tends to be a nonverbal approach. Despite such persistent but misguided clinical prescriptions favoring the use of this modality, there are a wide variety of factors to be considered before a nonverbal approach could be judged as the most appropriate or most valid.

The Multidimensional Assessment Model for Bilingual Individuals (MAMBI; Ochoa & Ortiz, in press) was created specifically to assist practitioners in determining what is likely the best approach to take in the evaluation of diverse school-aged children that will lead to the most valid results. Although the general principles are applicable to adults as well, the MAMBI is geared more toward decisions regarding evaluations to be conducted on children where the interactions between education and cognitive and language development serve to greatly complicate the process. Consider that in the case of school-aged children, there are at least three important variables to evaluate in determining the appropriate modality: (1) current degree of language proficiency in both English and the native language; (2) current and previous type(s) of educational program(s); and (3) current grade level. This information directly influences the choice regarding assessment modality, which itself involves consideration of four different approaches, including: (1) reduced culture/language testing; (2) testing in the native language; (3) testing in English; and (4) bilingual testing. Making the process more complicated is the fact that these approaches are not mutually exclusive and may be used in combination with each other as may be appropriate.

Management of all of these variables is clearly a difficult task even for experienced professionals. In response, Ochoa and Ortiz (in press) developed the MAMBI, which is illustrated in Figure 11.1 and represents the first systematic integration of the major variables central to making determinations regarding assessment modality with diverse individuals.

As depicted in Figure 11.1, the MAMBI provides an integration of three of the primary variables involved in the decision-making process and represented as language profile, instructional programming/history, and current grade level. An explanation of the variables, including the reason for inclusion and the relevance to decisions regarding modality of assessment, follows.

Language Profile

Language is a developmental process that has four commonly accepted and predictable stages: (1) preproduction, (2) early production, (3) speech-emergence, and (4) intermediate fluency. These stages are meant only to provide distinctions in the acquisition of different language skills and abilities and should be viewed as ordered periods along a broader continuum of development. In general, individuals begin to learn their native language from birth and, in the absence of any communicative disorder, progress through these identifiable stages and acquire greater and greater levels of proficiency and fluency in the language. The process of language acquisition moves through the four stages rather rapidly, in as little as 3 to 5 years. By the time individuals are ready to begin formal schooling, around the age of 5, they have developed proficiency that falls somewhere between the latter part of the speech emergence stage to the beginning part of the intermediate fluency stage, perhaps best described as "beginning fluency," and preserves the continuous nature of development.

Difficulties in the assessment of linguistically diverse individuals arise as a consequence of two important conditions: (1) the presence of a second language acquisition process [i.e., L2, usually English] occurring at the same time as the native language acquisition process [i.e., L1]; and (2) differences in the developmental trajectory between L1 and L2 resulting from different starting points. The former condition, the fact that an individual is bilingual or speaks more than one language, is readily recognized by evaluators who understand the impact it may have on communication efforts during testing. But the latter often escapes notice or is only poorly understood. For many immigrants in the United States, the L2 process often begins at a point

FIGURE 11.1. The Ochoa and Ortiz Multidimensional Assessment Model for Bilingual Individuals (MAMBI).

Instructional program/history	Currently in a bilingual education program, in lieu of or in addition to receiving ESL services								Previously in bilingual education program, now receiving English-only or ESL services								All instruction has been in an English-only program with or without ESL services							
Current grade	K–4				5–7				K–4				5–7				K–4				5–7			
Assessment mode	NV	L1	L2	BL	NV	L1	L2	BL	NV	L1	L2	BL	NV	L1	L2	BL	NV	L1	L2	BL	NV	L1	L2	BL
Language profile 1 L1 minimal/L2 minimal	⊘	✓		✓	⊘	✓	✓	✓	⊘	✓		✓	⊘	✓	✓	✓	⊘	✓	✓*	✓	⊘	✓	✓	✓
Language profile 2 L1 emergent/L2 minimal	⊘	✓		✓	⊘	✓	✓	✓	⊘	✓		✓	⊘	✓	✓	✓	⊘	✓	✓*	✓	■	■	■	■
Language profile 3 L1 fluent/L2 minimal		⊘				⊘	✓			⊘				⊘	✓		■	■	■	■	■	■	■	■
Language profile 4 L1 minimal/L2 emergent	⊘	✓		✓	⊘	✓	✓	✓	⊘	✓	✓	✓	⊘	✓	✓	✓	⊘	✓	✓#	✓	⊘	✓	✓	✓
Language profile 5 L1 emergent/L2 emergent	⊘	✓	✓	✓	⊘	✓	✓	✓	⊘	✓	✓	✓	⊘	✓	✓	✓	⊘	✓	✓#	✓	⊘	✓	✓	✓
Language profile 6 L1 fluent/L2 emergent		⊘	✓			⊘	✓	✓		⊘	✓			⊘	✓	✓	■	■	■	■	■	■	■	■
Language profile 7 L1 minimal/L2 fluent	■	■	■	■		⊘			■	■	■	■		⊘			■	■	■	■	■	■	■	■
Language profile 8 L1 emergent/L2 fluent	■	■	■	■			⊘		■	■	■	■		⊘			■	■	■	■	■	■	■	■
Language profile 9 L1 fluent/L2 fluent	■	■	■	■		⊘			■	■	■	■		⊘			■	■	■	■	■	■	■	■

CALP level 1–2 = minimal proficiency; CALP level 3 = emergent proficiency; CALP level 4–5 = fluent level of proficiency.

NV = Assessment conducted primarily in a nonverbal manner with English-language-reduced/acculturation-reduced measures.

L1 = Assessment conducted in the first language learned by the individual (i.e., native or primary language).

L2 = Assessment conducted in the second language learned by the individual, which in most cases refers to English.

BL = Assessment conducted relatively equally in both languages learned by the individual (i.e., the native language and English).

■ = Combinations of language development and instruction that are improbable or due to other factors (e.g., Saturday school, foreign-born adoptees, delayed school entry).

⊘ = Recommended mode of assessment that should take priority over other modes and that is most likely to be the most accurate estimate of the student's true abilities.

✓ = Secondary or optional mode of assessment that may provide additional valuable information, but that is likely to result in an underestimate of the student's abilities.

✓* = This mode of assessment is not recommended for students in K–2, but may be informative in 3–4; however, results are likely to be an underestimate of true ability.

✓# = This mode of assessment is not recommended for students in K–1, but may be informative in 2–4; however, results are likely to be an underestimate of true ability.

FIGURE 11.1. The Ochoa and Ortiz Multidimensional Assessment Model for Bilingual Individuals (MAMBI). Adapted from Ochoa and Ortiz (in press). Copyright by The Guilford Press. Adapted by permission.

other than birth—that is, some period of time after the L1 process has already been in place. The acquisition of L2 is generally initiated by the public school system where the learning of English is mandatory. Because language development, particularly more advanced levels of proficiency, are directly influenced by schooling, it is important to consider the differing levels of proficiency in L1 and L2 an individual possesses in order to make appropriate decisions regarding modality of assessment.

The MAMBI operationalizes in terms of "language profile" and is determined by the combination of the levels of proficiency an individual possesses in both L1 and L2. Proficiency levels follow the concepts developed by Cummins (1984) known as basic interpersonal communication skills (BICS) and cognitive academic language proficiency (CALP). In the MAMBI, the concept of BICS is not utilized, as Cummins has described it as mostly a social or conversational level of proficiency. Rather, it is the concept of CALP that forms the basis of proficiency to denote the language profiles in the MAMBI because CALP development is directly dependent upon formal schooling and represents the type of advanced language abilities that are required for school success (Cummins, 1984).

According to Ochoa and Ortiz (in press), a CALP level of 1–2 is considered *minimal* proficiency; a CALP level of 3 is operationally defined as an *emergent* level of proficiency; and a CALP level of 4–5 is operationally defined as a *fluent* level of proficiency. These categories are meant only to provide some distinction in language ability, but it should be recognized that in fact there are no direct measures of actual CALP available because the concept itself has not been developed enough by Cummins to permit clear operationalization of it as a construct. The level of CALP is determined primarily by considering multiple sources of data, which may include results from tests that provide estimates of CALP (e.g., Woodcock–Muñoz Language Survey; Woodock & Muñoz-Sandoval, 1996), as well as other informal measures of language functioning and proficiency. Ochoa and Ortiz caution that no single score or procedure should be used as the sole criterion for determining level of CALP

and that the purpose of making the distinctions is to provide clear differentiation between individuals who are at distinctly different stages of language development.

Detailed discussion of the differences between the various language profiles is beyond the scope of this chapter. For example, language profiles 7 and 8 are blacked out in Figure 11.1 because they represent extremely unusual or illogical developmental patterns that are unlikely to exist. The reader is referred to Ochoa and Ortiz (in press) for more information regarding specific descriptions of each profile and their relation to other factors in the model that are also important in assessment. For the present purpose, practitioners need only recognize that there are many combinations of language proficiency that can result even in individuals who speak only two languages and that the developmental stages for each language have relevance in making decisions regarding how best to approach an assessment and what type of testing may be most appropriate for a given case.

Current Grade Level

Another important variable to consider in making informed decisions regarding an assessment approach is the current grade level of the individual, particularly for school-aged children. Obviously, this is one of the more simple data to collect as grade level is a relatively unambiguous issue. In the MAMBI, Ochoa and Ortiz (in press) provide only two categories for evaluating and considering grade level: kindergarten through fourth grade (K–4) and fifth through seventh grade (5–7).

As noted previously, formal schooling affects the nature and course of language development. The development of CALP is predicated upon formal schooling and, according to Cummins (1984), takes about 5 to 7 years to develop. With respect to the language profile proficiency levels described in the prior section, a fluent CALP level would thus not be expected until about fifth grade at the earliest. Hence, the division of schooling between the fourth and fifth grades in the MAMBI. Such a division appears to have substantial face validity in the sense that school curricula generally tend to shift in terms of instruction at about this point. That is, the early part of the school curriculum is occupied primarily with instruction in the basic skills—learning to read, write, and do math. Such instruction often forms the bulk of the first 4 years of education. By the fourth grade or so, it is generally expected that most students have developed grade-expected skill levels so that the curriculum now begins to shift away from direct skill instruction toward more conceptual development. This shift is often described by educators as moving from "learning to read" to "reading to learn." That research indicates CALP begins to appear at this point is probably no mere coincidence but rather a testament to the observations and experiences of educators related to the interaction between cognitive and linguistic development.

The two categories developed by Ochoa and Ortiz (in press) are thus intended to distinguish individuals who have not yet had sufficient education and would not be expected to have developed fluent CALP levels from those individuals who have had time and who, under appropriate circumstances, should have developed fluent levels of CALP. The importance of this information in determining the modality of assessment is relatively clear in that individuals with more limited (minimal or emergent) CALP levels would benefit more from nonverbal approaches, whereas those with higher (fluent) levels of CALP would not necessarily need or require a nonverbal approach. Likewise, individuals with relatively similar levels of language proficiency might be best evaluated through a bilingual approach, one that takes both languages into account simultaneously, irrespective of the particular level of proficiency. In all cases, however, knowledge of grade level sets the standard for what to expect in terms of development. In the evaluation of culturally and linguistically diverse individuals, it is when expected development is not met that evaluators need to probe the conditions that may have impeded it. Apart from actual or true disability, perhaps the most important factor affecting an individual's cognitive and linguistic development (and as a consequence their academic performance) is related to instructional programming and history.

Instructional Programming/History

The third variable depicted in Figure 11.1 refers to the nature and type of instructional programming a pupil has received. Individuals who enter the U.S. public school system and who are not native English speakers can expect to receive a variety of different instructional services related to English language acquisition, including total immersion (English only), English as a second language (ESL), transitional bilingual education (early-exit), maintenance bilingual education (late-exit), and two-way bilingual education (dual-language or dual-immersion). Each of these types of programming directly affects cognitive and linguistic development and carry with them predictable academic consequences and outcomes (Thomas & Collier, 1997). It is the degree and manner in which each type of programming affects development that merits the attention of practitioners and bears upon decisions regarding assessment modality.

One of the more consistent findings in the education of language minority children is that high-level instruction in the core subject areas (particularly language arts) given in the native language for at least 4 to 5 years, and accompanied by instruction that specifically fosters the development of English, ultimately leads to the same rates of academic achievement as their monolingual English-speaking peers (August & Hakuta, 1997; Ramirez, Wolfson, Talmadge, & Merino, 1986; Thomas & Collier, 1997). It has been postulated that the reason for their success rests on the development of CALP in the native language, which allows for transfer of cognitive and linguistic abilities into the second language (Cummins, 1984). In other words, normal cognitive and linguistic development is not altered or inhibited by such pedagogical methods as they are in the case of English immersion, ESL, and early-exit bilingual programs.

Given the importance of educational programming with respect to development, Ochoa and Ortiz (in press) describe three categories relating to educational circumstances and history. The first category includes pupils who are currently in a well-implemented bilingual education program, in lieu of or in addition to receiving any

ESL services. Because both maturation and proper programming are essential to CALP development, current grade level becomes relevant given that children in grades K–4 would not yet be expected to have reached fluent levels, whereas those in grades 5–7 and above would. The second category for educational programming and history that may describe the experience of English-language learners concerns those individuals who were previously in a bilingual program but are now receiving English-only instruction or ESL services. Individuals in this educational circumstance were likely in transitional-type bilingual education programs where native language instruction was terminated no later than third grade—unfortunately, just before the development of fluent levels of CALP. The third category described by Ochoa and Ortiz is perhaps the most frequent experience encountered by English learners and is the case where all instruction has been in English only, with or without ESL services. The interruption of the native language process and introduction of English as a second language process upon school entrance generally means that such students will not have been afforded the opportunity to develop fluent levels of CALP in either L1 or L2, greatly compromising academic success.

In making the decision regarding modality of assessment, practitioners need to consider other important factors. For example, individuals who began learning English before the age of 10 will often display no perceptible accent and will have pronunciation that is indistinguishable from that of native English speakers. The lack of an accent is not an indicator of proficiency but only a marker regarding when learning of the language began. In addition, English learners who are not given the benefit of a maintenance type of bilingual program will display the effects of *language loss* or *language deterioration* (also known as *subtractive bilingualism*). Another important consideration involves age at school entrance. Many English learners enter the U.S. public school system beyond the age of 5 and the nature and extent of any education they may have received in their native country will affect cognitive and linguistic development and affect decisions regarding assessment modalities. And last,

differences in L1 and L2 proficiency are often described in terms of "dominance" and used to guide assessment modality—that is, assessment is conducted in the dominant language. Such an approach tends to neglect the fact that bilingual individuals do not cease to be bilingual simply because they have become dominant in English. Bilingual individuals simply cannot be equated to or treated as monolinguals regardless of their English proficiency or fluency (Bialystok, 1991; Grosjean, 1989).

Selection of Assessment Modality

In the MAMBI, Ochoa and Ortiz (in press) attempt to integrate the three variables discussed previously and have formulated recommendations regarding various approaches to the assessment process. The importance regarding careful consideration and deliberate selection of the most appropriate assessment modality is conducted for the purposes of obtaining the most valid test results. To this end, they defined the four basic approaches in evaluation, including: (1) nonverbal assessment [NV]; (2) assessment primarily in the native language [L1]; (3) assessment primarily in English [L2]; and (4) true bilingual assessment [BL].

Nonverbal assessment is defined by Ochoa and Ortiz (in press) as an approach to evaluation that is conducted primarily in a nonverbal or "language-reduced" manner using tests that are either designed specifically to be free of oral language requirements or that incorporate reductions in the need or demand for English language proficiency. Such tests are often purported to be culture fair or culture reduced, but such claims are usually overstated (Flanagan & Ortiz, 2001; Ortiz, 2001, 2002). In many cases, this approach is perhaps most valid and best suited for individuals with very low levels (minimal or emergent) of proficiency in either L1 or L2, assuming no other factors may exist to make the approach inappropriate. This would include individuals characterized by language profiles 1, 2, 4, and 5. In contrast, use of a nonverbal approach with those English learners who have reached fluent levels of CALP in L1 or L2 may not provide optimal results. These individuals will have language profiles 3, 6, or 9 and the rationale is that by virtue of having developed CALP, the attenuating influence of the linguistic demands of any given tests is reduced and becomes less of, but certainly not a negligible, concern in testing.

The second assessment modality described by Ortiz and Ochoa (in press) in the MAMBI is assessment that is conducted primarily in the native language or L1 testing. Use of this approach seeks to measure an individual's abilities in their native language in cases where it is felt that measurement in English would be largely invalid or where it may provide additional information beyond any English-language testing that may be administered. However, this modality presents problems for practitioners who are not bilingual and who lack the capability to administer native language tests, albeit they may employ translators/interpreters to assist in the process. Ochoa and Ortiz recommend that native-language testing will be most valid for individuals who have language profiles 3, 6, or 9 (i.e., where L1 is at the fluent level). Because such individuals have developed a high degree of proficiency in their native language, it would be imprudent to ignore that development, which forms a considerable part of their entire linguistic repertoire.

The third assessment modality described by Ochoa and Ortiz (in press) involves assessment in English (L2). The approach is straightforward and involves the administration of psychological tests in English. Unfortunately, the many potential problems and impediments to normal language development that occur as a function of educational programming and the fact that English is generally the individual's second, not native, language makes this approach to assessment largely unsuitable as the preferred or recommended modality in the evaluation of linguistically diverse populations. In the MAMBI, English-language testing is not recommended as the approach most likely to lead to valid results for any language profile except 9. Only individuals who have reached high levels of proficiency in English (L2 fluent) can be considered viable candidates for assessment in English that would be considered reasonably fair estimates of true functioning. Practitioners are cautioned, however, not to overestimate the validity of results obtained from the use of tests administered in English, even when the individual may be fluent in English. Standardized, norm-referenced tests tend to have norms that are not entirely appropriate for use with English-language learners or even those who have become English-dominant and may continue to provide underestimates of actual ability. Nonetheless, testing in English is an acceptable option for those individuals who have reached age-appropriate levels of language development in English.

The last modality incorporated by Ochoa and Ortiz (in press) into the MAMBI is described as bilingual assessment. Bilingual assessment is often misunderstood and is not the same as assessment of bilinguals. Whereas assessment of bilinguals involves the administration of tests in English only to bilingual individuals by monolingual English-speaking evaluators, bilingual assessment involves the use of bilingual methods and procedures by bilingual evaluators (Ortiz, 2002). At present there are no actual "bilingual" tests and the task of standardizing bilingual interaction, which involves spontaneous code-switching as desired or needed, appears exceedingly difficult if not impossible to accomplish. Given this limitation, Ochoa and Ortiz suggest that bilingual assessment is the recommended testing modality primarily for individuals with language profile 9 (L1 fluent/L2 fluent) and as a secondary option for those with language profiles 1, 2, and 5, where both languages are at low and relatively similar levels of development. Individuals with these profiles have yet to develop CALP in their native language or English. Depending on their educational experiences, the total verbal repertoire of individuals with language profile 1, 2, or 5 may be shared across L1 and L2. Thus, the most valid form of assessment in such cases will be those where a true bilingual approach is utilized and that allows individuals to express themselves in whatever language may be necessary at any given moment or for any particular purpose.

In sum, the MAMBI clearly represents a sophisticated integration of several important and relevant variables that affect decisions regarding how best to approach assessment with bilingual individuals in order to gather the most reliable and valid data possible. Other issues in assessment, particularly those related to interpretation of results, cannot be obviated solely by this method. Beyond this, significant limitations in current instruments and procedures exist and will affect practitioners' ability to generate completely fair and equitable estimates of performance. Therefore, practitioners should not assume that, after following the guidelines offered by Ochoa and Ortiz (in press), unbiased or nondiscriminatory results are inevitable. The authors of the MAMBI assert that their recommendations regarding selection of the most appropriate assessment modality are meant only to assist in reducing, not entirely eliminating, the potential discriminatory aspects of assessing bilingual individuals. Moreover, cautions regarding the degree of validity that may be expected from test results are incorporated into the MAMBI and practitioners should be aware of the limitations of any assessment modality, irrespective of how appropriate it may be.

THE CULTURE–LANGUAGE TEST CLASSIFICATIONS AND CULTURE–LANGUAGE INTERPRETIVE MATRIX

It was noted that the MAMBI was designed to address fundamental concerns with data validity as a function of assessment modality. Once it has been determined what approach is likely to be the most fair and equitable method, practitioners must still wrestle with problems that relate to interpreting data in as nondiscriminatory a manner as possible. This issue also boils down to one of validity in that confidence in the meaning and conclusions drawn from test results rests upon the degree to which the evaluator is certain that what has been measured is actual ability and not some other construct (e.g., level of acculturation or English-language proficiency). Until practitioners can assess the degree to which cultural and linguistic factors have or have not systematically influenced obtained test results, validity cannot be established and any inferences that may be drawn subsequently remain of questionable validity.

To address issues related to validity and less discriminatory assessment of results, practitioners can look to the development of the Culture–Language Test Classifications (C-LTC; Flanagan et al., 2000; McGrew & Flanagan, 1998) and its companion Culture–

Language Interpretive Matrix (C-LIM; Flanagan & Ortiz, 2001; Ortiz, 2001, 2004; Ortiz & Flanagan, 1998). The C-LTC was initially developed as an extension of the CHC theoretical classifications presented as the basis of the CHC Cross-Battery assessment and interpretive approach (Flanagan et al., 2000; McGrew & Flanagan, 1998). The C-LIM evolved shortly afterward as a further refinement of the C-LTC designed specifically to aid in interpretation by allowing practitioners to evaluate the degree to which cultural and linguistic influences may have affected test results (Flanagan & Ortiz, 2001; Ortiz, 2001, 2004). Although the C-LTC and the C-LIM were initially linked to the CHC Cross-Battery approach, the authors assert that it can be used independently and its utility does not depend on the use or application of any particular assessment procedure. Whereas the MAMBI sought to guide the selection of an appropriate test modality, the C-LTC and C-LIM are designed to guide interpretation once it has been determined that standardized tests will be used.

In an appeal for less discriminatory practices, Figueroa (1990a, 1990b) suggested that application of defensible theoretical frameworks in the assessment of culturally and linguistically diverse individuals was an important avenue to explore. In addition, he admonished practitioners to pay particular attention to the cultural and linguistic dimensions of tests that were often ignored or misunderstood in evaluation. In response to such issues, Ortiz and Flanagan (1998), Flanagan and Ortiz (2001), and Flanagan and colleagues (2000) developed the C-LTC, essentially a classification system for cognitive ability tests based on two critical test dimensions: degree of cultural loading and degree of linguistic demand. These two dimensions were deliberately selected because they have been identified as factors that have a significant and powerful relationship to test performance for individuals who are culturally and linguistically diverse that can render results invalid (Figueroa, 1990a, 1990b; Sandoval, Frisby, Geisinger, Scheuneman, & Grenier, 1998; Valdés & Figueroa, 1994). The classifications of the standardized, norm-referenced tests included in the C-LTC represented a departure from the more common classifications related to the theoretical construct to be measured. Instead, the C-

LTC categorized tests on the basis of the degree to which each was culturally loaded and the extent of its inherent linguistic demands. In effect, a rather new and unique frame of reference from which to view test performance was created. An example of the C-LTC for various subtests of the Wechsler Intelligence Scale for Children—IV (WISC-IV; Wechsler, 2004) is presented in Figure 11.2.

As is evident in Figure 11.2, the C-LTC is organized as a matrix with degree of cultural loading as the variable along the vertical axis and degree of linguistic demand along the horizontal axis. Each variable is subdivided into three levels (low, moderate, and high) that are intended to further distinguish the classifications. The final result is a 3×3 matrix with nine distinct cells, some of which contain tests that share a particular combination of cultural loading and linguistic demand. Again, it is important to note that the classifications are not based on cognitive ability constructs, that is, two tests within the same cell are not there because they measure the same thing (e.g., visual processing), but rather because they have similar levels of cultural loading and linguistic demand.

Cultural Loading Classifications

According to Flanagan and Ortiz (2001), degree of cultural loading represents the degree to which a given subtest requires specific knowledge of or experience with mainstream U.S. culture. The subtests depicted in Figure 11.2 were classified in terms of several culturally related characteristics, including whether there was an emphasis on a particular thought or conceptual process, the actual content or materials involved in the task, and the nature of an expected response. Attention was also given to aspects of the communicative relationship between examinee and examiner (i.e., culturally specific elements apart from actual oral language, such as affirmative head nods, pointing, etc.) (see McCallum & Bracken, 1997). These characteristics were chosen in accordance with the findings of various researchers (e.g., Jensen, 1974; Valdés & Figueroa, 1994) who have noted that more process-oriented tests, and those containing more novel stimuli and communicative requirements, tend to yield less discriminatory estimates of functioning or ability.

Degree of linguistic demand

	Low	Moderate	High
Low	**MATRIX REASONING** (*Gv*-SR, Vz) Cancellation (*Gs*-P, R9)	**BLOCK DESIGN** (*Gv*-SR, Vz) **SYMBOL SEARCH** (*Gs*-P, R9) **DIGIT SPAN** (*Gsm*-MS, MW) **CODING** (*Gs*-R9)	**LETTER–NUMBER SEQUENCING** (*Gsm*-MW)
Moderate		**ARITHMETIC** (*Gq*-A3) Picture Concepts (*Gc*-K0, *Gf*-I)*	
High	Picture Completion (*Gc*-K0, *Gv*-CF)*		**INFORMATION** (*Gc*-K0) **SIMILARITIES** (*Gc*-LD, VL) **VOCABULARY** (*Gc*-VL, LD) **COMPREHENSION** (*Gc*-K0, LS) Word Reasoning (*Gc*-VL, *Gf*-I)*

Degree of cultural loading (vertical axis label)

FIGURE 11.2. Cultural loading and linguistic demand classifications of the WISC-IV subtests. Tests marked with an asterisk demonstrate mixed loadings on the two separate factors indicated. From Ortiz (2004). Copyright 2004 by John Wiley & Sons. Adapted by permission.

Linguistic Demand Classifications

Flanagan and Ortiz (2001) define degree of linguistic demand as the amount of linguistic facility required by a given test based on three factors: (1) verbal versus nonverbal language requirements on the part of the examiner (in administration of the test); (2) receptive language requirements on the part of the examinee; and (3) expressive language requirements on the part of the examinee. Similar to the cultural loading classifications, the subtests in Figure 11.2 are organized according to a three-level category system (i.e., high, moderate, and low). Degree of linguistic demand was selected as another important variable known to affect test performance for linguistically diverse individuals. The literature is clear that lack of English language proficiency is a highly attenuating factor in test performance and represents an important dimension of tests that must be evaluated accordingly (Cummins, 1984; Figueroa, 1990a; Hakuta, 1986; Jensen, 1974, 1976, 1980; Sandoval et al., 1998; Valdés & Figueroa, 1994),

Application of the information provided about the WISC-IV subtests in Figure 11.2 rests on the premise that selection of a set of tests known to assess a particular construct, combined with consideration of the relevant cultural and linguistic dimensions of such tests, provides more reliable, valid, and interpretable assessment data than the data ordinarily obtained via traditional methods. As noted previously, individuals who are less acculturated to mainstream U.S. culture, and/or who have lower English proficiency, tend to perform lower than their monolingual English-speaking peers raised in mainstream U.S. culture from birth (Figueroa, 1990a, 1990b; Hamayan & Damico, 1991; Jensen, 1974; Mercer, 1979; Valdés & Figueroa, 1994). Consequently, scores for diverse individuals are expected to be better approximations of true ability for tests that are lower in cultural loading and linguistic demand, and poorer estimates of true ability for tests that are higher in cultural loading and linguistic demand. By examining factors relevant to the background of diverse individuals (e.g., level of English and other language proficiency, language of instruction, educational and familial history, degree of acculturation, etc.), practitioners can select tests that

are more suitable and less discriminatory. Although there will be individual considerations, given individual variations in experience and proficiency, *in general tests with lower cultural loadings and lower linguistic demands should be selected over tests that are classified higher.* For example, administration of the Picture Concepts subtest is expected, according to the literature, to be a fairer estimate of ability (in this case, Gc) than would administration of the Information subtest (which also measures Gc), because Picture Concepts is lower in terms of both cultural loading and linguistic demand. In the case of Information, acculturation and language proficiency play a larger role; therefore, the obtained results are likely to be less accurate estimates of true ability.

The C-LTC represents an important tool for practitioners because it outlines in systematic fashion two variables that have detrimental effects on the test performance of culturally and linguistically diverse individuals. Originally, the classifications were meant only to guide test selection in a manner similar to, but much less sophisticated than, what is provided by the MAMBI. By selecting tests that were less culturally loaded and less linguistically demanding, Ortiz and Flanagan (1998) believed that practitioners could construct batteries that would measure cognitive constructs in a manner that was more fair and equitable. However, it became apparent that some abilities, particularly those related to language skills and verbal ability, simply could not be measured through culturally or linguistically reduced tests. The development of the C-LIM (Flanagan & Ortiz, 2001) addressed this issue, not by seeking out new tests but by providing a way to assess the degree to which cultural or linguistic factors may or may not have affected test results.

The CHC Culture–Language Matrix

The classification of tests according to shared levels of cultural loading and linguistic demand helped to identify tests that might result in more equitable estimates of true ability when used with culturally and linguistically diverse individuals. But this was not the only benefit from the manner in which the tests were classified. In accordance with decades of research on the test performance of bilinguals, Flanagan and Ortiz (2001) realized that the arrangement of the classifications meant that results of tests contained in the upper left cell (low cultural loading/low linguistic demand) would be fairer and hence higher on average than results of tests classified in the lower right cell (high cultural loading/high linguistic demand). Data from numerous studies supported not only the classifications themselves but also the nature of expected patterns of performance for diverse individuals (Brigham, 1923, 1930; Cummins, 1984; Figueroa, 1990a; Gould, 1996; Jensen, 1974, 1976, 1980; Sanchez, 1932, 1934; Valdés & Figueroa, 1994; Yerkes, 1921). This pattern is illustrated in Figure 11.3.

Although placed in an orthogonal arrangement, the two factors in Figure 11.3 are actually correlated to some degree. Nevertheless, the arrows in the illustration depict the three possible ways in which the test results of diverse individuals may be attenuated. First, test performance may decrease solely as a function of the increasing cultural loading of tests. Similarly, test performance may decrease solely as a function of the increasing linguistic demands of tests. And finally, test performance may decrease as a function of the combination of both cultural loading and linguistic demand. This information, coupled with knowledge regarding an individual's cultural and linguistic experience, makes it possible to accomplish defensible interpretation through analysis of the patterns formed by test data.

The value of understanding this declining pattern of performance lies in its predictability, not only for diverse groups, but also for diverse individuals. To the degree that the pattern of scores obtained by an individual from a diverse background matches the expected decline in performance portrayed by the arrows moving from left to right, from top to bottom, or from the upper left to the lower right, examiners can infer whether what has been measured is actual ability or level of English-language proficiency, level of acculturation, both, or even something else. In other words, if scores are available for tests within any of the cells, an average may be taken and that cell average would be expected typically to decline in magnitude from left to right and top to bottom. Thus, in cases where such a typical and expected pattern of scores is evident in the cells across the matrix, it can be said that the primary effect on test performance was not due to actual abil-

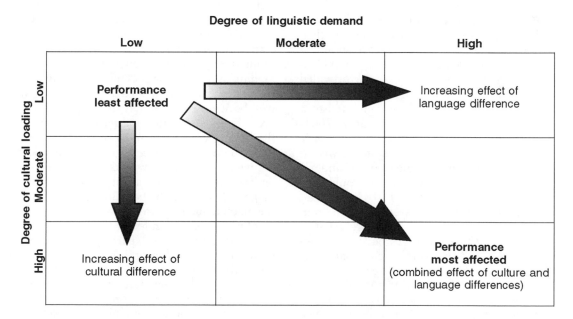

FIGURE 11.3. Pattern of expected test performance for culturally and linguistically diverse individuals. From Flanagan and Ortiz (2001). Copyright 2001 by John Wiley & Sons. Adapted by permission.

ity but rather level of acculturation, limited English language proficiency, or both acting as systematic influences on performance. Conversely, when a typical pattern for diverse individuals is *not* found—that is, the scores do not follow or match the expected direction of decline—then it can be concluded that some other factor (e.g., a disability) apart from cultural or linguistic differences has influenced the results. Failure to identify a clear pattern of decline implies that cultural or linguistic factors cannot be viewed as the primary or only factors affecting the results, albeit they may be contributing to some part of the pattern. Flanagan and Ortiz (2001) have developed a simple worksheet designed to facilitate evaluation of test results obtained from evaluations of diverse individuals. Practitioners need only make a few minor calculations in order to use the worksheet, which is presented in Figure 11.4.

To begin the process of evaluating the relative influence of culture and language on test performance, practitioners should first insert the names of any tests that may have been used during the course of evaluation into the appropriate cells according to degree of cultural loading and linguistic demand. The appropriate cells are determined by the classifications contained in the C-LTC. Additional spaces are provided in each cell in the event that several tests need to be entered together. The next step is to write the corresponding standard score obtained for each individual subtest in each cell in the space provided next to the test name. In some cases, standard scores may need to be converted to a common metric. Flanagan and Ortiz (2001) recommend using the deviation IQ metric (mean = 100; *SD* = 15). For example, Wechsler scaled scores have a mean of 10 and *SD* of 3. Thus, a scaled score of 12 would convert to a deviation IQ of 110. Tables that provide a simple conversion between standard scores are readily available to assist in this process. Once all scores have been converted, the third step is to calculate an overall mean or average score for each cell. The score obtained for any subtest in which it is the only test within the cell is used as the average for that cell. For cells in which there are no tests, no average is calculated. Flanagan and Ortiz caution strongly that the "cell average" is simply an arithmetic short-

hand that represents aggregate performance on a group of tests that have been classified together on the basis of cultural and linguistic characteristics. The scores do not have any relation to any type of construct or ability and should not be viewed as indications of any real or latent variable. Such derived scores represent nothing more than an individual's average performance on tests that share similar levels of cultural loading and linguistic demand, and there is no inherent meaning or implied construct for the cell average, and it should not be interpreted in any other manner or ascribed any other meaning.

After all cell averages are calculated, practitioners should examine the matrix to determine whether or not the results follow the expected pattern of decline, as illustrated in Figure 11.3. According to Flanagan and Ortiz (2001), if the overall pattern of test scores obtained for a given individual approximates any of the three patterns expected for diverse individuals (decline in performance due to cultural loading, linguistic demand, or both), it may be reasonably interpreted that the results reflect the systematic attenuating effect on performance of cultural or linguistic differences, or both. Scores in cells that decrease from the top to the bottom of the matrix would indicate a direct effect of cultural loading (lack of acculturation). Likewise, scores in cells that decrease from left to right in the matrix would indicate a direct effect of linguistic demand (limited English proficiency). Were cultural loading and linguistic demand largely uncorrelated, such independent effects might well be seen. Because they are related, however, the most common pattern to emerge in the testing of diverse individuals would be one where scores in cells at the upper left corner of the matrix would be highest and decrease in magnitude in the cells that move diagonally toward the bottom right corner of the matrix. Such a pattern would indicate the combined effect of cultural loading and linguistic demand on test performance. In the opinion of the evaluator, if any of these patterns are evident in the data, considerable support would be generated for the hypothesis that the individual's scores are more a reflection of cultural or linguistic differences, or both, than they are valid estimates of actual ability or knowledge. In other words, the emergence of typical and expected pat-

Name of examinee: _____ Date: _____

Degree of linguistic demand

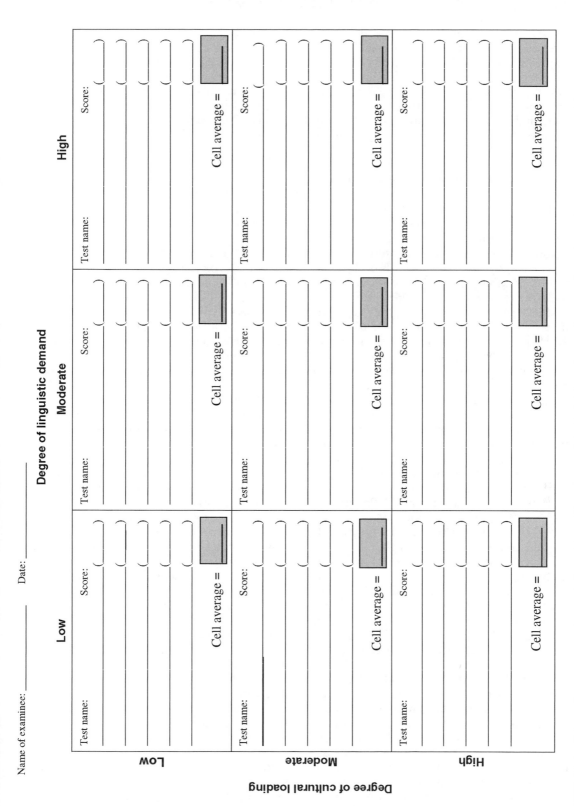

	Low	Moderate	High
Low	Test name: ____ Score: ____ ... Cell average = ____	Test name: ____ Score: ____ ... Cell average = ____	Test name: ____ Score: ____ ... Cell average = ____
Moderate	Test name: ____ Score: ____ ... Cell average = ____	Test name: ____ Score: ____ ... Cell average = ____	Test name: ____ Score: ____ ... Cell average = ____
High	Test name: ____ Score: ____ ... Cell average = ____	Test name: ____ Score: ____ ... Cell average = ____	Test name: ____ Score: ____ ... Cell average = ____

Degree of cultural loading

FIGURE 11.4. Culture–language matrix worksheet. From Flanagan and Ortiz (2001). Copyright 2001 by John Wiley & Sons. Adapted by permission.

247

terns of performance cast serious doubt on the validity of obtained results and practitioners should refrain from attempting to interpret the findings. However, if examination of the obtained test data reveals patterns that are not consistent with those expected or predicted for diverse individuals (i.e., any pattern that deviates from a clear, declining pattern similar to the declining ones previously described), it is reasonable to assume that other factors, including the possibility of a disability, is responsible for the dispersion of results. Flanagan and Ortiz (2001) state, however, that failure to identify a typical declining pattern of performance does not automatically imply that measured performance is wholly valid. Diagnosis of dysfunction or disability should be bolstered by a wide range of data and multiple sources of evidence that converge to support the practitioner's professional opinion. Ortiz (2001, 2004) has further stated that proper evaluation of results using the C-LIM requires solid information regarding the degree to which an individual differs from the mainstream (i.e., the individual's level of acculturation) and the individual's level of English language proficiency. Although the literature reveals that on average expected performance tends to drop by about one full standard deviation (15 points) in cells with the highest degree of cultural loading and linguistic demand (Cummins, 1984; Figueroa, 1990a; Jensen, 1974, 1976, 1980; Valdés & Figueroa, 1994), individuals who are more fully acculturated and who possess higher levels of English proficiency will score correspondingly higher. In a similar vein, individuals who are not acculturated and who speak very little English (such as recent immigrants) will score correspondingly lower. Thus, this information is crucial in establishing reasonable expectations of test performance decrements.

Much like the MAMBI, the C-LTC and C-LIM should not be relied upon as the only guide for decisions related to test selection or interpretation. Rather, the information contained in the classifications and the interpretive matrix is intended to supplement assessment and evaluation practices applied within the context of a comprehensive, systematic framework for nondiscriminatory assessment. When used in conjunction with other relevant assessment information (e.g., direct observations, review of records, interviews, language proficiency testing, socioeconomic status, developmental data, family history, etc.), these classifications may lead to a significant decrease in bias related to the use of standardized tests.

SUMMARY

The two approaches described in this chapter, the MAMBI and the C-LTC/C-LIM, were selected not only because they represent innovative approaches in the assessment of culturally and linguistically diverse individuals but also because they are methods that can be utilized and adopted by virtually any practitioner. That is, they do not require that examiners have linguistic competency beyond English, although it is recommended that practitioners have reasonable command of the knowledge bases and multicultural competencies required for such endeavors. Taken together, the MAMBI and the C-LTC/C-LIM offer practitioners highly sophisticated tools that can be readily applied in the evaluation of individuals from diverse backgrounds. These methods integrate the pertinent and most crucial variables involved in the evaluation of culturally and linguistically diverse populations in a way that is accessible to practitioners without requiring extensive training or experience. Moreover, because these procedures do not require any new or additional assessment competencies, all practitioners now have the means to deal with some of the more difficult tasks facing them—notably, addressing the fundamental issue of validity in evaluation.

Development of the two methods described in this chapter was driven largely by the issue of validity. In both cases, the guidance offered to practitioners rests on the premise that selection and use of a set of tests that share a similar modality as well as similar cultural and linguistic dimensions provides more reliable, valid, and interpretable assessment data than the data ordinarily obtained via traditional methods. Individuals who are less acculturated to the U.S. mainstream and who have less English proficiency as compared to their same-age peers are known to perform more poorly in comparison to their monolingual English-speaking peers as a function of the degree of difference between them (Figueroa, 1990a, 1990b; Hamayan & Damico, 1991; Jensen, 1974; Mercer, 1979; Valdés & Figueroa, 1994). By examining factors relevant to the background of diverse individuals (e.g., level of English and other language proficiency, language of instruction, educational and familial history, degree of acculturation, etc.), practitioners can use these methods to select an approach to assessment that is less discriminatory and leads to fairer and more equitable estimates of true performance and to evaluate the relative influence of cultural and linguistic factors on test performance.

Whenever standardized, norm-referenced tests are used in the course of evaluating the cognitive abilities of culturally and linguistically diverse individuals, the possibility always exists that what was actually measured in the evaluation was level of acculturation and English language proficiency than actual ability. Although they do not represent a complete solution to the many problems and obstacles facing practitioners seeking to evaluate the intellectual functioning of individuals from diverse backgrounds, application of the MAMBI and the C-LTC/C-LIM provide powerful new tools for reducing many of the most difficult aspects of nondiscriminatory assessment. If used in conjunction with other sources of information and data, these methods are believed to be extremely practical approaches that can assist practitioners in making defensible and educated decisions regarding equitable assessment with culturally and linguistically diverse individuals.

REFERENCES

American Psychological Association (APA). (1993). Guidelines for providers of psychological services to ethnic, linguistic, and culturally diverse populations. *American Psychologist, 48*(1), 45–48.

August, D., & Hakuta, K. (Eds.). (1997). *Improving schooling for language-minority children: A research agenda.* Washington, DC: National Academy Press.

Bialystok, E. (1991). *Language processing in bilingual children.* New York: Cambridge University Press.

Brigham, C. C. (1923). *A study of American intelligence.* Princeton, NJ: Princeton University Press.

Brigham, C. C. (1930). Intelligence tests of immigrant groups. *Psychological Review, 37,* 158–165.

Cummins, J. C. (1984). *Bilingual and special education: Issues in assessment and pedagogy.* Austin, TX: Pro-Ed.

Figueroa, R. A. (1990a). Assessment of linguistic minority group children. In C. R. Reynolds & R. W. Kamphaus (Eds.), *Handbook of psychological and educational assessment of children: Intelligence and achievement* (pp. 671–696). New York: Guilford Press.

Figueroa, R. A. (1990b). Best practices in the assessment of bilingual children. In A. Thomas & J. Grimes (Eds.), *Best practices in school psychology II* (pp. 93–106). Washington, DC: National Association of School Psychologists.

Flanagan, D. P., & Ortiz, S. O. (2001). *Essentials of cross-battery assessment.* New York: Wiley.

Flanagan, D. P., McGrew, K. S., & Ortiz, S. O. (2000). *The Wechsler intelligence scales and Gf-Gc theory: A contemporary approach to interpretation.* Boston: Allyn & Bacon.

Gonzalez, V., Brusca-Vega, R., & Yawkey, T. (1997). *Assessment and instruction of culturally and linguistically diverse students with or at risk of learning problems: From research to practice.* Needham Heights, MA: Allyn & Bacon.

Gopaul-McNicol, S., & Thomas-Presswood, T. (1998). *Working with linguistically and culturally different children: Innovative clinical and educational approaches.* Needham Heights, MA: Allyn & Bacon.

Gould, S. J. (1996). *The mismeasure of man.* New York: Norton.

Grosjean, F. (1989). Neurolinguists beware!: The bilingual is not two monolinguals in one person. *Brain and Language, 36,* 3–15.

Hakuta, K. (1986). *Mirror of language: The debate on bilingualism.* New York: Basic Books.

Hamayan, E. V., & Damico, J. S. (1991). *Limiting bias in the assessment of bilingual students.* Austin, TX: Pro-Ed.

Jensen, A. R. (1974). How biased are culture-loaded tests? *Genetic Psychology Monographs, 90,* 185–244.

Jensen, A. R. (1976). Construct validity and test bias. *Phi Delta Kappan, 58,* 340–346.

Jensen, A. R. (1980). *Bias in mental testing.* New York: Free Press.

McCallum, R. S., & Bracken, B. A. (1997). The Universal Nonverbal Intelligence Test. In D. P. Flanagan, J. L. Genshaft, & P. L. Harrison (Eds.), *Contemporary intellectual assessment: Theories, tests, and issues* (pp. 268–280). New York: Guilford Press.

McGrew, K. S., & Flanagan, D. P. (1998). *The intelligence test desk reference (ITDR): Gf-Gc cross-battery assessment.* Boston: Allyn & Bacon.

Mercer, J. R. (1979). *System of Multicultural Pluralistic Assessment: Technical manual.* New York: Psychological Corporation.

Ochoa, S. H., & Ortiz, S. O. (in press). Cognitive assessment of culturally and linguistically diverse individuals. In R. Rhodes, S. H. Ochoa, & S. O. Ortiz (Eds.), *Assessment of culturally and linguistically diverse students*. New York: Guilford Press.

Ortiz, S. O. (2001). Assessment of cognitive abilities in Hispanic children. *Seminars in Speech and Language,* 22(1), 17–37.

Ortiz, S. O. (2002). Best practices in nondiscriminatory assessment. In A. Thomas & J. Grimes (Eds.), *Best practices in school psychology IV* (pp. 1321–1336). Washington, DC: National Association of School Psychologists.

Ortiz, S. O. (2004). Use of the WISC-IV with culturally and linguistically diverse populations. In D. P. Flanagan & A. S. Kaufman (Eds.), *Essentials of WISC-IV assessment* (pp. 245–254). New York: Wiley.

Ortiz, S. O., & Flanagan, D. P. (1998). Gf-Gc cross-battery interpretation and selective cross-battery assessment: Referral concerns and the needs of culturally and linguistically diverse populations. In K. S. McGrew & D. P. Flanagan (Eds.), *The intelligence test desk reference (ITDR): Gf-Gc cross-battery assessment* (pp. 401–444). Boston: Allyn & Bacon.

Ortiz, S. O., & Flanagan, D. P. (2002). Best practices in working with culturally and linguistically diverse children and families. In A. Thomas & J. Grimes (Eds.), *Best practices in school psychology IV* (pp. 1351–1372). Washington, DC: National Association of School Psychologists.

Ramirez, J. D., Wolfson, R., Talmadge, G. K., & Merino, B. (1986). *First year report: Longitudinal study of immersion programs for language minority chil-dren* (Submitted to U.S. Department of Education, Washington, DC). Mountain View, CA: SRA Associates.

Sanchez, G. I. (1932, March). Scores of Spanish-speaking children on repeated tests. *Pediatric Seminar and Journal of Genetic Psychology,* pp. 223–231.

Sanchez, G. I. (1934). Bilingualism and mental measures: A word of caution. *Journal of Applied Psychology, 18,* 756–772.

Sandoval, J., Frisby, C. L., Geisinger, K. F., Scheuneman, J. D., & Grenier, J. R. (Eds.). (1998). *Test interpretation and diversity: Achieving equity in assessment.* Washington, DC: American Psychological Association.

Thomas, W., & Collier, V. (1997). *Language minority student achievement and program effectiveness.* Washington DC: National Clearinghouse for Bilingual Education.

Valdés, G., & Figueroa, R. A. (1994). *Bilingualism and testing: A special case of bias.* Norwood, NJ: Ablex.

Wechsler, D. (2004). *Wechsler Intelligence Scale for Children—Fourth Edition (WISC-IV).* San Antonio, TX: Harcourt Assessment.

Woodcock, R. W., & Muñoz-Sandoval, A. F. (1996). *Batería Woodcock–Muñoz: Pruebas de Habilidad Cognitiva—Revisada.* Itasca, IL: Riverside.

Yerkes, R. M. (1921). Psychological examining in the United States Army. *Memoirs of the National Academy of Sciences, 15,* 1–890.

Ysseldyke, J. E. (1979). Issues in psychoeducational assessment. In G. D. Phye & D. Reschly (Eds.), *School psychology: Perspectives and issues* (pp. 87–116). New York: Academic Press.

12

Issues in Subtest Profile Analysis

MARLEY W. WATKINS
JOSEPH J. GLUTTING
ERIC A. YOUNGSTROM

More than 250 million standardized tests are administered to public school students each year in the United States (Salvia & Ysseldyke, 1998). Although much school-based testing is accomplished in groups, a substantial number of standardized tests are also employed in individual evaluations. For example, millions of children served in special education programs have participated in individual psychoeducational evaluations (U.S. Department of Education, 2001). Individual evaluations to determine special education eligibility often include a standardized measure of intellectual functioning. Of the available individual intelligence tests, the Wechsler scales are the most frequently used (Kaufman & Lichtenberger, 2000). Among school-age children, the Wechsler Intelligence Scale for Children (WISC; Wechsler, 1949), Wechsler Intelligence Scale for Children—Revised (WISC-R; Wechsler, 1974), and Wechsler Intelligence Scale for Children—Third Edition (WISC-III; Wechsler, 1991) have been the most popular (Kamphaus, Petoskey, & Rowe, 2000; Oakland & Hu, 1992) for decades.

Typically, interpretation of individual intelligence tests is based on a hierarchical, top-down model that first considers the global IQ scores. Next, to extract more information from the test, distinct patterns or profiles of subtest scores are analyzed.

Finally, individual subtests are considered in isolation. This practice of interpreting the pattern of subtest scores attained by children on individual measures of intelligence is known as *subtest profile analysis*. Based on these principles, elaborate subtest interpretation systems (Kaufman, 1994; Sattler, 2001) have achieved wide popularity in school psychology training and practice (Alfonso, Oakland, LaRocca, & Spanakos, 2000; Groth-Marnat, 1997; Kaufman, 1994; Pfeiffer, Reddy, Kletzel, Schmelzer, & Boyer, 2000). For example, approximately 74% of school psychology training programs place moderate to great emphasis on the use of subtest scores in their individual cognitive assessment courses (Alfonso et al., 2000). Among a sample of school psychologists, Pfeiffer and colleagues (2000) found that almost 70% reported profile analysis to be a useful feature of the WISC-III, and 29% reported that they derived specific value from individual WISC-III subtests.

PURPOSES

Profile analysis has typically been applied for two major purposes: (1) diagnostically discriminating average and exceptional children, and (2) identifying specific cognitive strengths and weaknesses. Wechsler (1958) himself may have encouraged the process of diagnostically interpreting children's subtest profiles when he advanced the hypothesis that childhood schizophrenia could be identified by high scores on the Picture Completion and Object Assembly subtests and low scores on the Picture Arrangement and Digit Symbol subtests. Eventually, more than 75 patterns of subtest variation were identified for the Wechsler series alone (McDermott, Fantuzzo, & Glutting, 1990). Currently, many different subtest profiles are purportedly diagnostic of learning and emotional problems (e.g., Kaufman, 1994).

To identify cognitive strengths and weaknesses, specific patterns of subtest scores are presumed to substantially invalidate global intelligence indices (Groth-Marnat, 1997), so that subtest patterns, rather than IQ composites, become the focus of interpretation. Subtests that are significantly higher or lower than a child's own average are considered relative strengths or weaknesses, respectively. Next, hypotheses concerning the underlying causes of significant subtest variations are identified by locating abilities thought to be shared by two or more subtests. Extensive lists of the abilities presumed to underlie each subtest are provided by Kaufman (1994), Sattler (2001), and Kaufman and Lichtenberger (2000). Finally, these hypotheses are used to generate educational and psychological interventions and remedial suggestions (Zeidner, 2001).

BRIEF HISTORICAL REVIEW OF PROFILE ANALYSIS RESEARCH

Scatter

Attempts to analyze IQ subtest variations date back to the inception of standardized intelligence testing (Zachary, 1990). For example, Binet suggested that the passes and failures of psychotic or alcoholic examinees would exhibit more *scatter* across age levels on his scale than would other examinees (see Matarazzo, 1985). Early researchers hypothesized that subtest scatter would predict scholastic potential or membership in exceptional groups (Harris & Shakow, 1937). Uneven subtest scores were assumed to be signs of pathology or of greater potential than indicated by averaged IQ composites. Hundreds of studies were conducted to test these

hypotheses. Based on their analysis of decades of IQ subtest scatter research, Kramer, Henning-Stout, Ullman, and Schellenberg (1987) found no evidence that subtest scatter uniquely identified any diagnostic group, and they opined that "we regard scatter analysis as inefficient and inappropriate" (p. 45). A narrative review of 70 years of research on subtest scatter also arrived at pessimistic conclusions concerning its diagnostic accuracy (Zimmerman & Woo-Sam, 1985). Although isolated studies found abnormal scatter within clinical groups, differences tended to disappear when adequate comparison samples were used. Zimmerman and Woo-Sam (1985) observed that "extensive scatter proved to be both typical and 'normal,' and thus of limited use as a diagnostic feature" (p. 878).

Similar negative results were reported in a longitudinal study of the WISC-R. Moffitt and Silva (1987) concluded that perinatal, neurological, and health problems did not cause extreme Verbal IQ–Performance IQ (VIQ-PIQ) discrepancies, and found that neither behavior problems nor motor problems were significantly related to VIQ-PIQ scores. Furthermore, VIQ-PIQ score discrepancies were unreliable across time. That is, the majority of children with extreme VIQ-PIQ score discrepancies did not maintain such a large difference when tested with the WISC-R 2 years later. Thus "VIQ-PIQ discrepancies are of doubtful diagnostic value" (Moffitt & Silva, 1987, p. 773).

The quantitative combination of results from 94 studies (N = 9,372) also demonstrated that subtest scatter and scatter between VIQ and PIQ failed to uniquely identify children with learning disabilities (LDs) (Kavale & Forness, 1984). For example, the average VIQ-PIQ difference for children with LDs was only 3.5 points—a difference found in 79% of the normal population. In sum, subtest scatter was determined to be of "little value in LD diagnosis" (Kavale & Forness, 1984, p. 139).

Subtest Profiles

Given the popularity of the Wechsler scales, Wechsler subtest profiles have been the source of much research. For example, the validity of using WISC and WISC-R subtests for diagnosing LDs was the focus of a meta-analysis by Kavale and Forness (1984). This quantitative summary of 94 studies revealed that "the differential diagnosis of LD using the WISC, although intuitively appealing, appears to be unwarranted" because "regardless of the manner in which WISC subtests were grouped and regrouped, no recategorization, profile, pattern, or factor cluster emerged as a 'clinically' significant indicator of LD" (Kavale & Forness, 1984, p. 150).

Taking another approach, Mueller, Dennis, and Short (1986) statistically clustered the WISC-R subtest data of 119 samples of nonexceptional and exceptional children (N = 13,746) to determine whether profiles would emerge that were diagnostically characteristic of various disabilities. Results indicated that WISC-R subtest profiles were typically marked by general intellectual level but could not reliably distinguish among diagnostic groups. Like Kavale and Forness (1984), Mueller and colleagues concluded that Wechsler subtest profiles were not helpful in differentiating among children with emotional and learning impairments, and they recommended that IQ tests be used only to estimate global intellectual functioning.

The poor diagnostic accuracy of subtest profiles has generalized across tests and cultures. For example, Rispens and colleagues (1997) analyzed the ability of subtest profiles from the Dutch version of the WISC-R to distinguish among 511 children with conduct disorder, mood disorder, anxiety disorder, attention deficit disorder, and other psychiatric disorders. Rispens and colleagues found that subtest patterns did not significantly differ across the various groups and concluded that "WISC profiles . . . cannot contribute to differential diagnosis" (p. 1593).

Subtest profiles have also been found to be unexceptional markers when empirically generated subtest profiles serve as a normative standard against which subtest profiles obtained from clinical groups are compared. If subtest profiles are markers of disability, then unique profiles should be found in the sample with disabilities. On the other hand, if subtest profiles are not distinctive of disability, profiles from the sample without disabilities should replicate for the sample with disabilities. To test this hypothesis, Watkins and Kush (1994) applied normative WISC-R subtest profiles (McDermott,

Glutting, Jones, Watkins, & Kush, 1989) to 1,222 students with LDs, emotional handicaps, and mental retardation. They found that 96% of the children with disabilities displayed subtest profiles that were similar to those of the WISC-R standardization sample. No statistical or logical patterns could be detected in the subtest scores of the 4% of students with disabilities who exhibited profiles dissimilar to those of the standardization sample.

Another normative comparison applied the Wechsler Adult Intelligence Scale—Revised (WAIS-R) standardization sample core profiles to 161 adults with brain damage and found that 82% exhibited typical or normal subtest profiles (Ryan & Bohac, 1994). Patients with unique profiles did not differ on the basis of age, education, or organic etiology, so the atypical profiles did not contribute any diagnostic information. The WAIS-R core profiles were also applied to 194 college students with LDs (Maller & McDermott, 1997). Almost 94% of these students were found to have normatively typical subtest profiles. Unique profiles were disparate and not indicative of subtypes of LDs.

Historical Review: Summary

Subtest scatter had been determined to be clinically ineffectual as early as 1937 (Harris & Shakow, 1937). Cautions concerning the accuracy of subtest profiles were frequent (McNemar, 1964; Simensen & Sutherland, 1974). By 1983, Frank was able to say that "in spite of the fact that the Wechsler looked like it would be ideal for a comparative study of the intellectual/cognitive behavior of various psychopathological types, 40 years of research has failed to support that idea" (p. 79). A cumulative body of research evidence has shown that neither subtest scatter nor subtest profiles demonstrate acceptable accuracy in discriminating among diagnostic groups.

METHODOLOGICAL, STATISTICAL, AND PSYCHOMETRIC PROBLEMS WITH SUBTEST PROFILE ANALYSIS

Fundamental methodological, statistical, and psychometric problems cause subtest analysis results to be more illusory than real and to represent more of a shared professional myth (Faust, 1990) than clinically astute detective work (Kaufman, 1994). Although a large number of problems have been identified (Glutting, Watkins, & Youngstrom, 2003; Watkins, 2003), this chapter concentrates on four major issues: *reliability*, *ipsative measurement*, *group mean differences*, and *inverse probabilities*.

Reliability

The weak reliability of subtest scores has been repeatedly demonstrated. For example, none of the WISC-III subtests reached the internal-consistency reliability criterion of ≥ .90 recommended by Salvia and Ysseldyke (1998) for making decisions about individuals. Similar results were found on the Wechsler Adult Intelligence Scale—Third Edition (WAIS-III; Wechsler, 1997), where the median internal consistency of the subtests was .85, and the Wechsler Intelligence Scale for Children—Fourth Edition (WISC-IV; Wechsler, 2003), where the median internal consistency of the subtests was .86.

The stability of subtest scores across time has also been inadequate for individual decisions. After administering the Dutch version of the WISC-R to a group of children three times at 6-month intervals, Neyens and Aldenkamp (1996) concluded that, "subtest scores show only fair to good, or even poor stability, which suggests that changes in subtest scores, as stated by many researchers, should not [be taken] into account when evaluating the cognitive development of children of normal intelligence" (p. 168). More recently, Smith, Smith, Bramlett, and Hicks (1999) tested a small sample of rural school children with the WISC-III and again 3 years later. The median stability coefficient for the subtests was .59, compared to .83 for the composite IQ scores. Using a large national sample of students twice tested for special education eligibility (N = 667), Canivez and Watkins (1998) found a median subtest stability coefficient of .68 and a median stability coefficient of .87 for the IQ composites. Even short-term stability coefficients have been inadequate for individual decisions. For example, the median short-term stability of the Stanford–Binet Intelligence Scales, Fifth Edition (Roid, 2003) subtests was .825, in contrast to .90 for the Full Scale IQ (FSIQ)

score, and the median WISC-IV short-term stability coefficient was .78 for subtests, compared to .89 for the FSIQ.

However, these published reliability coefficients are overestimates of the typical reliability of subtest scores, for at least two reasons. First, they were calculated by test companies or researchers who paid close attention to standardization procedures and double-checked scoring accuracy (Feldt & Brennan, 1993; Thorndike, 1997). In clinical practice, administration, clerical, and scoring errors are ubiquitous (Belk, LoBello, Ray, & Zachar, 2002). Second, internal-consistency and stability reliability coefficients do not take into account all types of measurement error. For example, Schmidt, Le, and Ilies (2003) found that the reliability of a measure of general mental ability was overestimated by about 7% when transient measurement error was ignored.

Even worse, subtest profile analysis involves the comparison of multiple difference scores. The reliability of the difference between two scores is lower than the reliability of either score alone (Feldt & Brennan, 1993). The increased error generated by the use of difference scores makes even the best subtest-to-subtest comparison unstable (e.g., the reliability of the WISC-III Block Design and Vocabulary subtests is .87, but the reliability of their difference is .76).

Ipsative Measurement

Many subtest interpretative systems move away from *normative* measurement and instead rely on *ipsative* measurement principles (Cattell, 1944). That is, subtest scores are subtracted from mean composite scores for an individual. Thereby, the scores are transformed into person-relative metrics and away from their original population-relative metric (McDermott et al., 1990). Ipsative measurement is concerned with how a child's subtest scores relate to his or her personalized, average performance, and discounts the influence of global intelligence (Jensen, 2002). For example, two hypothetical students' normative (population-relative) and ipsative (person-relative) scores are displayed in Table 12.1. These two students have identical ipsative scores, but their normative scores are very different.

TABLE 12.1. Normative (Population-Relative) and Ipsative (Person-Relative) Scores for Two Hypothetical Examinees

Subtest	Student A		Student B	
	Norm. score	Ipsative score	Norm. score	Ipsative score
A	3	−4	10	−4
B	7	0	14	0
C	11	+4	18	+4
Mean	7	0	14	0

The ipsative perspective holds intuitive appeal, because it seems to isolate and amplify aspects of cognitive ability. Nevertheless, transformation of the score metric from normative to ipsative is psychometrically problematic. For example, McDermott and colleagues (1990) demonstrated that the ipsatization of WISC-R scores produced a loss of almost 60% of that test's reliable variance. McDermott and Glutting (1997) replicated those results with the Differential Ability Scales (DAS; Elliott, 1990) and WISC-III. They found that, on average, ipsative scores lost two-thirds to three-fourths of the reliable information provided by normative scores.

This information loss has been concretely demonstrated by analyzing the stability of ipsative subtest profiles. The temporal stability of subtest profiles among 303 randomly selected children tested twice as part of WISC-R validation studies, and among 189 children twice tested for special education eligibility, was computed (McDermott, Fantuzzo, Glutting, Watkins, & Baggaley, 1992). Classificatory stability of relative cognitive strengths and weaknesses identified by subtest elevations and depressions was near chance levels for both groups of children. Livingston, Jennings, Reynolds, and Gray (2003) also found that the stability of WISC-R subtest profiles across a 3-year test–retest interval was too low for clinical use.

Similar temporal instability of subtest patterns was found for 579 students who were twice tested for special education eligibility with the WISC-III across a 2.8-year interval (Watkins & Canivez, 2004). Based on 66 subtest composites, subtest-based strengths and weaknesses replicated across test–retest occasions at chance levels (median kappa =

.02). Because subtest-based cognitive strengths and weaknesses are unreliable, recommendations based on them will also be unreliable.

Both practical and theoretical analyses suggest that the mathematical properties of ipsative methods are profoundly different from those of familiar normative methods (Hicks, 1970; McDermott et al., 1990, 1992). Thus ipsative subtest scores cannot be interpreted as if they possessed the psychometric properties of normative scores. Based on this evidence, Jensen (2002) concluded that "the ipsative use of test batteries like the Wechsler scales, the Kaufman scales, and the Stanford–Binet IV is nearly worthless" (p. 11).

Group Mean Differences

Identification of IQ subtest profiles has generally been based upon statistically significant group differences. That is, a group of children with a particular disorder is identified, and their mean subtest score is compared to the mean subtest score of a group of children without the disorder. Statistically significant subtest score differences between the two groups are subsequently interpreted as evidence that the profile is diagnostically accurate for individuals. However, differences in group mean scores may not support individual interpretation. Nor does statistical significance of group differences equate to individual discrimination. As noted by Elwood (1993), "significance alone does *not* reflect the size of the group differences nor does it imply the test can discriminate subjects with sufficient accuracy for clinical use" (p. 409; original emphasis).

This situation illustrates reliance on classical validity methods instead of the more appropriate clinical utility approach (Wiggins, 1988). Average group subtest score differences indicate that *groups* can be discriminated. This classical validity approach cannot be uncritically extended to conclude that mean group differences are distinctive enough to differentiate among *individuals*. Figures 12.1 and 12.2 illustrate this dilemma. They display hypothetical score distributions of children from nondisabled and disabled populations. Group mean differences are clearly discernible in both, but the overlap between distributions in Figure 12.2 makes it difficult to determine group mem-

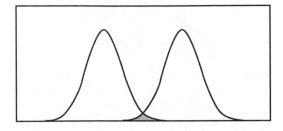

FIGURE 12.1. Hypothetical test score distributions from nondisabled (left) and disabled (right) populations that overlap (shaded region) only at the extremes.

bership accurately for those individuals in the shaded region. Although real score distributions are more similar to Figure 12.2, many researchers and clinicians act as if Figure 12.1 describes the relative score distributions.

There are four possible outcomes when one is using test scores to diagnose a disability: *true positive*, *true negative*, *false positive*, and *false negative*. Two outcomes are correct (true positive and true negative), and two are incorrect (false positive and false negative). True positives are children with disabilities who are correctly identified as such by the test. False positives are children identified by the test as having a disability who do not actually have one. In contrast, false negatives are children with disabilities who are not identified by the test as having disabilities. A test with a low false-negative rate has high sensitivity, and a test with a low false-positive rate has high specificity.

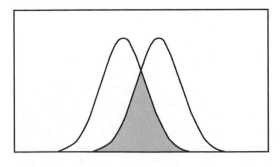

FIGURE 12.2. Hypothetical test score distributions from nondisabled (left) and disabled (right) populations that show considerable overlap (shaded region).

The relative proportion of correct and incorrect diagnostic decisions depends on the cut score used. For example, a cut score at the mean of the normal distribution in Figure 12.2 produces both a high true-positive and a high false-positive rate. That is, it correctly identifies those who are disabled, but it makes many mistakes for those who are not disabled. In contrast, a cut score at the mean of the disabled distribution makes few false-positive errors but many false-negative errors. Figure 12.2 graphically displays the tradeoffs between sensitivity and specificity that are always encountered when test scores are used to differentiate groups (Zarin & Earls, 1993).

Beyond cut scores, the accuracy of diagnostic decisions is dependent on the base rate or prevalence of the particular disability in the population being assessed. Very rare disabilities are difficult for a test to identify accurately (Meehl & Rosen, 1955). This issue is relevant for psychological practice and research, because many disabilities are by definition unusual or rare.

Although sensitivity and specificity are both desirable attributes of a diagnostic test, they are dependent on the cut score and prevalence rate. Thus neither provides a unique measure of diagnostic accuracy (McFall & Treat, 1999). In contrast, by systematically using all possible cut scores of a diagnostic test and graphing true-positive against false-positive decision rates, one can determine the full range of that test's diagnostic utility. Designated the *receiver operating characteristic* (ROC), this procedure was originally applied more than 50 years ago to determine how well an electronics receiver was able to distinguish signal from noise (Dawson-Saunders & Trapp, 1990). Because they are not confounded by cut scores or prevalence rates, ROC methods were subsequently widely adopted in the physical (Swets, 1988), medical (Dawson-Saunders & Trapp, 1990), and psychological (Swets, 1996) sciences. More recently, ROC methods were strongly endorsed for evaluating the accuracy of psychological assessments (McFall & Treat, 1999; Swets, Dawes, & Monahan, 2000).

As illustrated in Figure 12.3, the main diagonal of a ROC curve represents chance diagnostic accuracy. The more accurate the

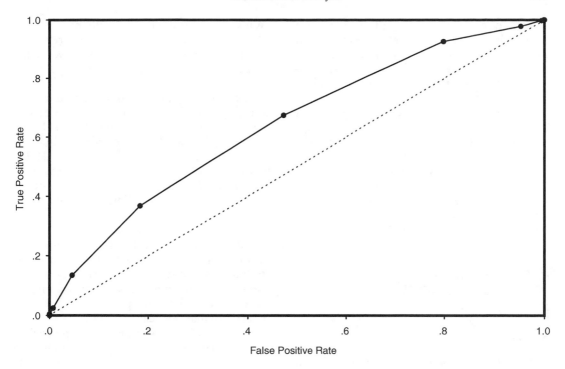

FIGURE 12.3. ROC curve for the WISC-III LDI for 445 students with LDs and 2,200 students without disabilities (AUC = .64). Data from Watkins, Kush, and Schaefer (2002); see this article for a full report of this study.

test, the further the ROC curve will deviate toward the upper left of the graph. This can be quantified by calculating the *area under the curve* (AUC), which provides an overall accuracy index of the test (Henderson, 1993). AUC values can range from .5 to 1.0. An AUC value of .5 signifies that the test has chance discrimination. In contrast, an AUC value of 1.0 denotes perfect discrimination. AUC values of .5 to .7 indicate low test accuracy, .7 to .9 indicate moderate test accuracy, and .9 to 1.0 indicate high test accuracy (Swets, 1988). More practically, the AUC can be interpreted in terms of two students: one drawn at random from the nondisabled population, and one randomly selected from the disabled population. The AUC is the probability that the test will correctly identify the student from the disabled population.

Clinical utility statistics (e.g., sensitivity, specificity, ROC) must be considered when one is evaluating the accuracy of test scores used to differentiate individuals. Group sep-aration is necessary, but not sufficient, for accurate decisions about individuals.

Inverse Probabilities

Another fatal flaw in much subtest profile research is the use of inverse probabilities. Although related to the group–individual problem, it is particularly pernicious in clinical practice. Specifically, it is generally not understood that the probability of a particular score on a diagnostic test, given membership in a diagnostic group, is different from the probability of membership in a diagnostic group, given a particular score on a diagnostic test (McFall & Treat, 1999). For example, the probability of being a chronic smoker, given a diagnosis of lung cancer, is about .99, but the probability of having lung cancer, given chronic smoking, is only around .10 (Gambrill, 1990). That is, 99% of patients with lung cancer are chronic smokers, but only 10% of smokers develop lung cancer.

This quandary can be illustrated with a hypothetical subtest analysis example. A small group of children with LDs are located, and their WISC subtest scores are analyzed. It is found that many of these children exhibit a profile marked by relatively depressed scores on four specific subtests. Thus the probability of this subtest profile is high, given that a child has an LD. However, clinical use of subtest profiles is predicated on a different probability—namely, determining the probability that a referred child has an LD, given the subtest profile. Inverse probabilities systematically overestimate prospective accuracy (Dawes, 1993).

RECENT PROFILE ANALYSIS RESEARCH

Diagnosis

Scatter

Tables of subtest scatter have been included in the WISC-III, WAIS-III, and WISC-IV manuals. Accompanying these tables is the comment that subtest scatter has "frequently been considered diagnostically significant" (Wechsler, 2003, p. 46). Thus clinical interest in subtest scatter has remained high.

It is often asserted that the presence of marked subtest variability reduces the predictive validity of the IQs (Kaufman, 1994). When this hypothesis was tested with the WAIS-III, it was found to be incorrect for predicting memory indices (Ryan, Kreiner, & Burton, 2002). However, Fiorello, Hale, McGrath, Ryan, and Quinn (2002) applied regression commonality analysis to WISC-III factor scores used to predict achievement. They concluded that a general intelligence factor (g) did not exist for about 80% of their sample, and they suggested that factor variability justified profile analysis. The scientific status of g is too complex to explicate for this chapter, but the results of Fiorello and colleagues run counter to massive amounts of existing research (Jensen, 1998). When multiple regression is applied, there is no universally accepted definition of predictor importance (Azen & Budescu, 2003) and there is no consensus on which method is best employed to explain the relative importance of multiple correlated predictors

(Whittaker, Fouladi, & Williams, 2002). More critically, Pedhazur (1997) reported that communality analysis is not "a valid approach for ascertaining relative importance of variables" (p. 275).

To test the predictive validity and diagnostic utility of WISC-III subtest scatter, two samples of students were analyzed: the 1,118 students in the WISC-III/Wechsler Individual Achievement Test (WIAT; Wechsler, 1992) linking sample, and the 1,302 students with LDs from 46 states from Smith and Watkins (2004). For predictive validity, the FSIQ of the WISC-III/WIAT sample was entered as a predictor in multiple regression, followed by the absolute amount of subtest scatter among the 10 mandatory subtests. The FSIQ was substantially predictive of WIAT reading achievement ($R = .70$), but the addition of subtest scatter did not improve prediction ($R = .70$). In terms of diagnostic utility, subtest scatter of the WISC-III/WIAT sample was compared to the subtest scatter of the sample with LDs. Figure 12.4 shows that the discrimination was at chance levels (AUC = .51).

The value of WISC-III subtest scatter as a diagnostic indicator was also analyzed by Daley and Nagle (1996) among 308 children with LDs. They found that "subtest scatter and Verbal–Performance discrepancies do not appear to hold any special utility in the diagnosis of learning disabilities" (p. 331). These negative results were replicated in several other studies (Dumont & Willis, 1995; Greenway & Milne, 1999; Iverson, Turner, & Green, 1999). More definitive research was conducted by Watkins (1999), using the WISC-III standardization sample as a normative comparison group. Subtest variability as quantified by range and variance exhibited no diagnostic utility in distinguishing 684 children with LDs from the 2,200 children of the WISC-III standardization sample. Likewise, the number of subtests deviating from examinees' VIQ, PIQ, and FSIQ by ±3 points exhibited no diagnostic utility in distinguishing the children of the WISC-III standardization sample from 684 children with LDs (Watkins & Worrell, 2000). Based upon these results, Watkins and Worrell concluded that "using subtest variability as an indicator of learning disabilities would constitute a case of acting in opposition to scientific evidence" (2000, p. 308).

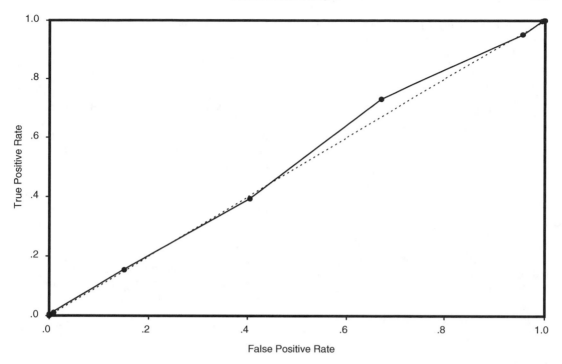

FIGURE 12.4. ROC analysis of 10-subtest scatter between 1,118 students in the WIAT norm sample and 1,302 students with LDs (AUC = .51).

Subtest Profiles

ACID Profile

The ACID subtest profile is probably the most venerable. Based on the Arithmetic, Coding, Information, and Digit Span subtests, it has been applied to the WISC, WISC-R, and WISC-III. Most recently, Prifitera and Dersh (1993) compared percentages of children with WISC-III ACID profiles from samples with LDs and attention-deficit/hyperactivity disorder (ADHD) to percentages showing the ACID profile in the WISC-III standardization sample. Their findings uncovered a greater incidence of ACID profiles in clinical samples, with approximately 5% of the children with LDs and 12% of those with ADHD showing the ACID profile, while such a configuration occurred in only 1% of the cases from the WISC-III standardization sample. Based upon these data, Prifitera and Dersh (1993) concluded that ACID profiles "are useful for diagnostic purposes" because "the presence of a pattern or poses"

patterns would suggest strongly that the disorder is present" (pp. 50–51).

Ward, Ward, Hatt, Young, and Mollner (1995) investigated the prevalence of the WISC-III ACID profile among children with LDs (N = 382) and found a prevalence rate of 4.7% (vs. the expected rate of 1%). Obtaining similar ACID results from a sample of children with LDs (N = 165), Daley and Nagle (1996) suggested practitioners "investigate the possibility of a learning disability" (p. 330) when confronted by an ACID profile.

The studies described above relied on the group mean difference approach to incorrectly infer diagnostic utility. Watkins, Kush, and Glutting (1997a) evaluated the diagnostic utility of the WISC-III ACID profile among children with LDs. As in previous research, ACID profiles were more prevalent among children with LDs (N = 612) than among nondisabled children (N = 2,158). However, when ACID profiles were used to classify students into disabled and nondisabled groups, they operated with considerable error. At best, only 51% of the children identified by a positive ACID profile were previously diagnosed as having LDs. These data indicated that a randomly selected child with an LD had a more severe ACID profile than a randomly selected child without an LD about 60% of the time (AUC = .60). Although marginally better than chance, the degree of accuracy was quite low (cf. classificatory criteria presented by Swets, 1988).

SCAD Profile

Whereas the ACID profile has a long history, the SCAD profile (based on the Symbol Search, Coding, Arithmetic, and Digit Span subtests) seems to have been first studied by Prifitera and Dersh in 1993. Kaufman (1994) opined that Arithmetic, Coding, and Digit Span have "been quite effective at identifying exceptional groups from normal ones, and . . . are like a land mine that explodes on a diversity of abnormal populations but leaves most normal samples unscathed" (p. 213). Kaufman concluded that the SCAD profile is "an important piece of evidence for diagnosing a possible abnormality" (p. 221); it "won't identify the type of exceptionality, but [the profile is] likely to be valuable for making a presence–absence decision and helping to pinpoint specific areas of deficiency" (p. 214).

Prifitera and Dersh (1993) found the SCAD profile to be more common within a sample of children with LDs (n = 99) and another sample of children with ADHD (n = 65) than within the WISC-III standardization sample. Using this imbalance of prevalence rates as guidance, Prifitera and Dersh suggested that the subtest configuration would be "useful in the diagnosis of LD and ADHD" (p. 53).

These claims were tested by Watkins, Kush, and Glutting (1997b) with children who were enrolled in learning and emotional disability programs (N = 365). When these children were compared to the WISC-III standardization sample via diagnostic utility statistics, an AUC of .59 was generated. Thus, contrary to Kaufman's (1994) assertion, SCAD subtest scores were not found to be important evidence for diagnosing exceptionalities.

Learning Disability Index

The Learning Disability Index (LDI; Lawson & Inglis, 1984) is of particular interest, because it was hypothesized to relate to specific neuropsychological deficits of students with LDs. Lawson and Inglis (1984) conjectured that WISC-R subtests are sensitive to the presence of LDs in direct proportion to their verbal saturation, which is in turn related to left-hemisphere dysfunction. This theoretical link between test and brain functioning is important, because contemporary definitions of LDs specify an endogenous etiology related to "central nervous system dysfunction" (Hammill, 1990, p. 82).

Comparisons of groups of students with and without LDs found significantly higher mean LDI scores among students with LDs than among students in regular education (Bellemare, Inglis, & Lawson, 1986; Clampit & Silver, 1990). Statistically significant LDI differences between groups were subsequently interpreted as evidence that the LDI is diagnostically effective. For example, Kaufman (1990) concluded that the LDI taps a sequential–simultaneous processing dimension and is "quite valuable for distinguishing learning-disabled children from normal children" (p. 354).

However, mean differences between groups are insufficient for individual diagnostic decisions. Consequently, more appropriate diagnostic utility statistics were applied to the WISC-III LDI scores of 2,053 students previously diagnosed with LDs and 2,200 students without LDs. Subsamples of students with specific reading (n = 445) and math (n = 168) disabilities permitted more refined assessment of the efficacy of the LDI. ROC analyses revealed that the LDI resulted in a correct diagnostic decision only 55–64% of the time (Watkins, Kush, & Schaefer, 2002). See Figure 12.3 for an illustrative ROC curve for students with specific reading disabilities (n = 445) compared to the 2,200 students in the normative sample. These results demonstrated that the LDI is an invalid diagnostic indicator of LDs.

Diagnosis: Summary

When properly analyzed, data have consistently failed to find subtest scatter or subtest profiles to be diagnostically accurate. Based on their review of IQ subtest scatter research, Kline, Snyder, Guilmette, and Castellanos (1992) suggested that psychologists "have pursued scatter analysis . . . with little success. It is time to move on" (p. 11). That suggestion was reiterated by McGrew and Knopik (1996), who remarked that "considering the years of study attributed to the concept of scatter and the lack of an empirical foundation, it is recommended that future research efforts be directed elsewhere" (p. 362). Clearly, there is no scientific support for the use of subtest scatter to inform diagnosis or prediction.

Likewise, results have been consistent in indicating that subtest profiles offer little diagnostic advantage. Limited space prohibits reviews of research regarding other subtest profiles, but diagnostic utility results have been unfailingly negative (Glutting, McDermott, Watkins, Kush, & Konold, 1997; Glutting, McGrath, Kamphaus, & McDermott, 1992; Gussin & Javorsky, 1995; Lowman, Schwanz, & Kamphaus, 1996; Oh, Glutting, & McDermott, 1999; Piedmont, Sokolove, & Fleming, 1989; Smith & Watkins, 2004; Teeter & Korducki, 1998; Watkins, 1996). Sattler (2001) also concluded that subtest profiles "cannot be used for classification purposes or to arrive at a diagnostic label" (p. 299). Similar cautions regarding the use of subtests for diagnostic decisions have been offered by Kaufman and Lichtenberger (2000) and Kamphaus (2001). Unmistakably, abundant scientific evidence and expert consensus recommend against the use of subtest profiles for the diagnosis of childhood learning and behavior disorders.

Specific Cognitive Strengths and Weaknesses

Although there is general agreement that IQ subtest-based diagnosis should be avoided, the use of subtest profiles to identify specific cognitive strengths and weaknesses is frequently recommended. As articulated by Kaufman and Lichtenberger (1998), the examiner "must generate hypotheses about an individual's assets and deficits" (p. 192). Next, the examiner must "confirm or deny these hypotheses by exploring multiple sources of evidence" (p. 192). Finally, "well-validated hypotheses must then be translated into meaningful, practical recommendations" (p. 192) concerning interventions, instructional strategies, and remediation activities (Groth-Marnat, 1997).

Subtest interpretation systems provide hundreds of hypotheses to consider when IQ subtest patterns are obtained (Kaufman, 1994; Sattler, 2001). The enormous number of hypotheses makes it impossible to review the entire scientific literature. However, subtest profiles are often assumed to be related to a wide variety of learning and behavioral variables (Kaufman, 1994; Sattler, 2001).

Academic Achievement

One way to test the utility and validity of subtest scores is to decompose profiles into their elemental components. The unique, incremental predictive validity of each component can then be analyzed separately to determine what aspect or aspects, if any, of the subtest profile are related to academic performance. To this end, Cronbach and Gleser (1953) cautioned that subtest profiles contain only three types of information: *elevation*, *scatter*, and *shape*. Elevation information is represented by a person's aggregate performance (i.e., mean normative score) across subtests. Profile scatter is defined by how widely scores in a profile diverge from its mean. Scatter is typically operationalized by the standard deviation of the subtest scores in a profile. Finally, shape information reflects where "ups and downs" occur in a profile. Even if two profiles have the same elevation and scatter, their high and low points may be different.

Watkins and Glutting (2000) tested the incremental validity of WISC-III subtest profile level, scatter, and shape in forecasting academic performance. WISC-III subtest profiles were decomposed into their three fundamental elements and sequentially regressed onto reading and mathematics achievement scores for nonexceptional (n = 1,118) and exceptional (n = 538) children. Profile elevation was statistically and practically significant for both nonexceptional (R = .72 to .75) and exceptional (R = .36 to .61) children. Profile scatter did not aid in the prediction of achievement. Profile shape accounted for an additional 5–8% of the variance in achievement measures: One pattern of relatively high verbal scores positively predicted both reading and mathematics achievement, and a pattern of relatively low scores on the WISC-III Arithmetic subtest was negatively related to mathematics. Beyond these two somewhat intuitive patterns, profile shape information had inconsequential incremental validity for both nonexceptional and exceptional children. In other words, it was the averaged, norm-referenced information (i.e., elevation) contained in subtest profiles that best predicted achievement. This information is essentially redundant to that conveyed by global intelligence scores.

Similar results have been obtained by other researchers with a variety of intelligence tests (e.g., the WISC-R, Stanford–Binet, Woodcock–Johnson, etc.) (Glutting, Youngstrom, Ward, Ward, & Hale, 1997; Hale & Raymond, 1981; Hale & Saxe, 1983; Kahana, Youngstrom, & Glutting, 2002; Kline et al., 1992; McDermott & Glutting, 1997; McGrew & Knopik, 1996; Ree & Carretta, 1997; Youngstrom, Kogos, & Glutting, 1999). Interestingly, research has consistently demonstrated that general mental ability also accounts for the vast majority of the predictable variance in job learning among adults (Ree & Carretta, 2002; Schmidt, 2002). Given these results, Kline and colleagues (1992) concluded that "the most useful information from IQ-type tests is the overall elevation of the child's profile. Profile shape information adds relatively little unique information, and therefore examiners should not overinterpret particular patterns of scores" (p. 431). Thorndike (1986) similarly concluded that 80–90% of the predictable variance in scholastic performance is accounted for by general ability, with only 10–20% accounted for by all other scores in IQ tests. From these findings, it has been concluded that subtest scatter and shape offer minimal assistance for generating hypotheses about children's academic performance.

Learning Behaviors

Teacher ratings of child learning behaviors, as operationalized by the Learning Behaviors Scale (LBS; McDermott, Green, Francis, &

Stott, 1996), reflect four relatively independent subareas: competence motivation, attitude toward learning, attention/persistence, and strategy/flexibility. The DAS and LBS were conormed with a nationally representative sample of 1,250 children. When DAS and LBS scores were compared, DAS global ability accounted for 8.2% of learning behavior, and DAS subtests only increased the explained variance by 1.7%.

Test Session Behaviors

It is widely assumed that astute test session observation and clinical insight allow psychologists to draw valid inferences regarding an examinee's propensities and behaviors outside the testing situation (Sparrow & Davis, 2000). That is, a quiet child during testing is assumed to be retiring in other situations, an active child is inferred to be energetic in the classroom, and so on. However, a synthesis of research on test session behaviors found that the average correlation between test session behaviors and conduct in other environments was only .18 (Glutting, Youngstrom, Oakland, & Watkins, 1996).

Among the normative sample of the Guide to the Assessment of Test Session Behavior (Glutting & Oakland, 1993), a standardized test session observation scale, there was little differential variability across WISC-III subtests (Oakland, Broom, & Glutting, 2000). In fact, global ability accounted for 9.2% of test session behaviors, and the addition of WISC-III subtests only explained another 3.2% (McDermott & Glutting, 1997).

Behavioral Adjustment

Subtest profiles are commonly assumed to reflect dispositions that allow inferences about school behavior and adjustment. To test this assumption, a nationally representative sample of 1,200 children was administered the DAS, and their teachers independently provided standardized ratings of school and classroom behaviors on the Adjustment Scales for Children and Adolescents (ASCA; McDermott, Marston, & Stott, 1993). The ASCA provides measures of six core syndromes: attention-deficit hyperactivity, solitary aggressive (provocative), solitary aggressive (impulsive), oppositional defiant, diffident, and avoidant. Following the method of Kaufman (1994), the 5% of children with the most unusual DAS subtest profiles were identified and then matched on the basis of age, race, gender, parent education levels, and overall IQs to an equal number of comparison group children without unusual subtest profiles. There were no significant differences between these two groups on the six ASCA behavioral scales. Nor were there significant differences on academic tests. Thus academic and behavioral problems were not related to unusual DAS subtest profiles (Glutting, McDermott, Konold, Snelbaker, & Watkins, 1998).

This negative result was replicated by an analysis of the relationships between IQs from the WISC-III and classroom behaviors measured by the ASCA (Glutting et al., 1996). Four of the 56 correlations between the WISC-III and ASCA reached statistical significance at $p < .05$, but this ratio barely exceeded the expected chance rate of three significant correlations. The average coefficient was also low (average $r = -.04$, with a 95% confidence interval of $-.20$ to $+.13$) and indicated that as much as 99% of the score variation was unique to each instrument. These meager results were not surprising: "11 previous investigations showed an average relationship of $-.19$ between children's scores on individually administered IQ tests and their home and school behavior" (Glutting et al., 1996, p. 103).

Specific Strengths
and Weaknesses: Summary

Most hypotheses generated from subtest variation "are either untested by science or unsupported by scientific findings" (Kamphaus, 1998, p. 46). The evidence that exists regarding relationships between subtest profiles and socially important academic and behavioral outcomes is, at best, weak: Subtest profile information contributes 2–8% variance beyond general ability to the prediction of achievement, and 2–3% to the prediction of learning behaviors and test session behaviors. Hypothesized relationships between subtest profiles and measures of psychosocial behavior have persistently failed to achieve statistical or clinical signifi-

cance. Thus "neither subtest patterns nor profiles of IQ have been systematically found to be related to personality variables" (Zeidner & Matthews, 2000, p. 585). After reviewing the research on subtest analysis, Hale and Green (1995) concluded that "knowledge of a child's subtest profile does not appreciably help the clinician in predicting either academic achievement levels or behavioral difficulties" (p. 98). Thus hypotheses derived from subtest analysis "are based on the clinician's acumen and not on any sound research base" (Kamphaus, 2001, p. 598).

GENERAL CONCLUSIONS

Many researchers have found the popularity of IQ subtest profile analysis to greatly outstrip its meager scientific support (Braden, 1997; Bray, Kehle, & Hintze, 1998; Gresham & Witt, 1997; Kamphaus, 2001; Reynolds & Kamphaus, 2003; Watkins, 2000, 2003). Although subtest profile analysis has not demonstrated adequate reliability, diagnostic utility, or treatment validity, it continues to be endorsed by assessment specialists and applied widely in training and practice.

Apparently, subtest profile interpretation flourishes due to its intuitive appeal (Bracken, McCallum, & Crain, 1993) and clinical tradition (Shaw, Swerdlik, & Laurent, 1993). Subtest-based interpretation systems are often justified by prescientific arguments without consideration for the professional obligations of psychologists (American Educational Research Association, American Psychological Association, & National Council on Measurement in Education, 1999), the limitations of clinical judgment (Garb, 2003), or the demands of scientific reasoning (Gibbs, 2003). Scientific psychological practice cannot be sustained by clinical conjectures, personal anecdotes, and unverifiable beliefs that have consistently failed empirical validation. Given the paucity of empirical support, subtest profile analysis can best be described as reliance on clinical delusions, illusions, myths, or folklore. Consequently, psychologists should eschew interpretation of cognitive subtest profiles.

REFERENCES

Alfonso, V. C., Oakland, T. D., LaRocca, R., & Spanakos, A. (2000). The course on individual cognitive assessment. *School Psychology Review, 29,* 52–64.

American Educational Research Association, American Psychological Association, & National Council on Measurement in Education. (1999). *Standards for educational and psychological testing.* Washington, DC: American Educational Research Association.

Azen, R., & Budescu, D. V. (2003). The dominance analysis approach for comparing predictors in multiple regression. *Psychological Methods, 8,* 129–148.

Belk, M. S., LoBello, S. G., Ray, G. E., & Zachar, P. (2002). WISC-III administration, clerical, and scoring errors made by student examiners. *Journal of Psychoeducational Assessment, 20,* 290–300.

Bellemare, F. G., Inglis, J., & Lawson, J. S. (1986). Learning disability indices derived from a principal components analysis of the WISC-R: A study of learning disabled and normal boys. *Canadian Journal of Behavioral Science, 18,* 86–91.

Bracken, B. A., McCallum, R. S., & Crain, R. M. (1993). WISC-III subtest composite reliabilities and specificities: Interpretive aids. *Journal of Psychoeducational Assessment Monograph Series, Advances in Psychological Assessment: Wechsler Intelligence Scale for Children—Third Edition,* pp. 22–34.

Braden, J. P. (1997). The practical impact of intellectual assessment issues. *School Psychology Review, 26,* 242–248.

Bray, M. A., Kehle, T. J., & Hintze, J. M. (1998). Profile analysis with the Wechsler scales: Why does it persist? *School Psychology International, 19,* 209–220.

Canivez, G. L., & Watkins, M. W. (1998). Long-term stability of the Wechsler Intelligence Scale for Children—Third Edition. *Psychological Assessment, 10,* 285–291.

Cattell, R. B. (1944). Psychological measurement: Normative, ipsative, interactive. *Psychological Review, 51,* 292–303.

Clampit, M. K., & Silver, S. J. (1990). Demographic characteristics and mean profiles of learning disability index subsets of the standardization sample of the Wechsler Intelligence Scale for Children—Revised. *Journal of Learning Disabilities, 23,* 263–264.

Cronbach, L. J., & Gleser, G. C. (1953). Assessing similarity between profiles. *Psychological Bulletin, 50,* 456–473.

Daley, C. E., & Nagle, R. J. (1996). Relevance of WISC-III indicators for assessment of learning disabilities. *Journal of Psychoeducational Assessment, 14,* 320–333.

Dawes, R. M. (1993). Prediction of the future versus an understanding of the past: A basic asymmetry. *American Journal of Psychology, 106,* 1–24.

Dawson-Saunders, B., & Trapp, R. G. (1990). *Basic and clinical biostatistics.* Norwalk, CT: Appleton & Lange.

Dumont, R., & Willis, J. O. (1995). Intrasubtest scatter on the WISC-III for various clinical samples vs. the standardization sample: An examination of WISC folklore. *Journal of Psychoeducational Assessment, 13,* 271–285.

Elliott, C. D. (1990). *Differential Ability Scales: Introductory and technical handbook.* San Antonio, TX: Psychological Corporation.

Elwood, R. W. (1993). Psychological tests and clinical discriminations: Beginning to address the base rate problem. *Clinical Psychology Review, 13,* 409–419.

Faust, D. (1990). Data integration in legal evaluations: Can clinicians deliver on their premises? *Behavioral Sciences and the Law, 7,* 469–483.

Feldt, L. S., & Brennan, R. L. (1993). Reliability. In R. L. Linn (Ed.), *Educational measurement* (3rd ed., pp. 105–146). Phoenix, AZ: Oryx Press.

Fiorello, C. A., Hale, J. B., McGrath, M., Ryan, K., & Quinn, S. (2002). IQ interpretation for children with flat and variable test profiles. *Learning and Individual Differences, 13,* 115–125.

Frank, G. (1983). *The Wechsler enterprise: An assessment of the development, structure, and use of the Wechsler tests of intelligence.* New York: Pergamon Press.

Gambrill, E. (1990). *Critical thinking in clinical practice: Improving the accuracy of judgments and decisions about clients.* San Francisco: Jossey-Bass.

Garb, H. N. (2003). Clinical judgment and mechanical prediction. In I. B. Weiner (Series Ed.) & J. R. Graham & J. A. Naglieri (Vol. Eds.), *Handbook of psychology: Vol. 10. Assessment psychology* (pp. 27–42). New York: Wiley.

Gibbs, L. E. (2003). *Evidence-based practice for the helping professions: A practical guide with integrated multimedia.* Pacific Grove, CA: Brooks/Cole.

Glutting, J. J., McDermott, P. A., Konold, T. R., Snelbaker, A. J., & Watkins, M. W. (1998). More ups and downs of subtest analysis: Criterion validity of the DAS with an unselected cohort. *School Psychology Review, 27,* 599–612.

Glutting, J. J., McDermott, P. A., Watkins, M. W., Kush, J. C., & Konold, T. R. (1997). The base rate problem and its consequences for interpreting children's ability profiles. *School Psychology Review, 26,* 176–188.

Glutting, J. J., McGrath, E. A., Kamphaus, R. W., & McDermott, P. A. (1992). Taxonomy and validity of subtest profiles on the Kaufman Assessment Battery for Children. *Journal of Special Education, 26,* 85–115.

Glutting, J. J., & Oakland, T. (1993). *Guide to the assessment of test-session behavior.* San Antonio, TX: Psychological Corporation.

Glutting, J. J., Watkins, M. W., & Youngstrom, E. A. (2003). Multifactored and cross-battery ability assessments: Are they worth the effort? In C. R. Reynolds & R. W. Kamphaus (Eds.), *Handbook of psychological and educational assessment of children: Intelligence, aptitude, and achievement* (2nd ed., pp. 343–374). New York: Guilford Press.

Glutting, J. J., Youngstrom, E. A., Oakland, T., & Watkins, M. W. (1996). Situational specificity and generality of test behaviors for samples of normal and referred children. *School Psychology Review, 25*, 94–107.

Glutting, J. J., Youngstrom, E. A., Ward, T., Ward, S., & Hale, R. L. (1997). Incremental efficacy of WISC-III factor scores in predicting achievement: What do they tell us? *Psychological Assessment, 9*, 295–301.

Greenway, P., & Milne, L. (1999). Relationship between psychopathology, learning disabilities, or both and WISC-III subtest scatter in adolescents. *Psychology in the Schools, 36*, 103–108.

Gresham, F. M., & Witt, J. C. (1997). Utility of intelligence tests for treatment planning, classification, and placement decisions: Recent empirical findings and future directions. *School Psychology Quarterly, 12*, 249–267.

Groth-Marnat, G. (1997). *Handbook of psychological assessment* (3rd ed.). New York: Wiley.

Gussin, B., & Javorsky, J. (1995). The utility of the WISC-III Freedom from Distractibility in the diagnosis of youth with attention deficit hyperactivity disorder in a psychiatric sample. *Diagnostique, 21*, 29–40.

Hale, R. L., & Green, E. A. (1995). Intellectual evaluation. In L. A. Heiden & M. Hersen (Eds.), *Introduction to clinical psychology* (pp. 79–100). New York: Plenum Press.

Hale, R. L., & Raymond, M. R. (1981). Wechsler Intelligence Scale for Children—Revised patterns of strengths and weaknesses as predictors of the intelligence achievement relationship. *Diagnostique, 7*, 35–42.

Hale, R. L., & Saxe, J. E. (1983). Profile analysis of the Wechsler Intelligence Scale for Children—Revised. *Journal of Psychoeducational Assessment, 1*, 155–162.

Hammill, D. D. (1990). On defining learning disabilities: An emerging consensus. *Journal of Learning Disabilities, 23*, 74–84.

Harris, A. J., & Shakow, D. (1937). The clinical significance of numerical measures of scatter on the Stanford–Binet. *Psychological Bulletin, 34*, 134–150.

Henderson, A. R. (1993). Assessing test accuracy and its clinical consequences: A primer for receiver operating characteristic curve analysis. *Annals of Clinical Biochemistry, 30*, 521–539.

Hicks, L. E. (1970). Some properties of ipsative, normative, and forced-choice normative measures. *Psychological Bulletin, 74*, 167–184.

Iverson, G. L., Turner, R. A., & Green, P. (1999). Predictive validity of WAIS-R VIQ–PIQ splits in persons with major depression. *Journal of Clinical Psychology, 55*, 519–524.

Jensen, A. R. (1998). *The g factor: The science of mental ability*. Westport, CT: Praeger.

Jensen, A. R. (2002). SASP interviews: Arthur R. Jensen. *SASP News, 2*(4), 8–19.

Kahana, S. Y., Youngstrom, E. A., & Glutting, J. J. (2002). Factor and subtest discrepancies on the Differential Ability Scales: Examining prevalence and validity in predicting academic achievement. *Assessment, 9*, 82–93.

Kamphaus, R. W. (1998). Intelligence test interpretation: Acting in the absence of evidence. In A. Prifitera & D. H. Saklofske (Eds.), *WISC-III clinical use and interpretation: Scientist-practitioner perspectives* (pp. 39–57). San Diego, CA: Academic Press.

Kamphaus, R. W. (2001). *Clinical assessment of child and adolescent intelligence* (2nd ed.). Boston: Allyn & Bacon.

Kamphaus, R. W., Petoskey, M. D., & Rowe, E. W. (2000). Current trends in psychological testing of children. *Professional Psychology: Research and Practice, 31*, 155–164.

Kaufman, A. S. (1990). *Assessing adolescent and adult intelligence*. Boston: Allyn & Bacon.

Kaufman, A. S. (1994). *Intelligent testing with the WISC-III*. New York: Wiley.

Kaufman, A. S., & Lichtenberger, E. O. (1998). Intellectual assessment. In A. S. Bellack & M. Hersen (Eds.), *Comprehensive clinical psychology: Vol. 4. Assessment* (pp. 187–238). New York: Elsevier.

Kaufman, A. S., & Lichtenberger, E. O. (2000). *Essentials of WISC-III and WPPSI-R assessment*. New York: Wiley.

Kavale, K. A., & Forness, S. R. (1984). A meta-analysis of the validity of Wechsler scale profiles and recategorizations: Patterns or parodies? *Learning Disability Quarterly, 7*, 136–156.

Kline, R. B., Snyder, J., Guilmette, S., & Castellanos, M. (1992). Relative usefulness of elevation, variability, and shape information from WISC-R, K-ABC, and Fourth Edition Stanford–Binet profiles in predicting achievement. *Psychological Assessment, 4*, 426–432.

Kramer, J. J., Henning-Stout, M., Ullman, D. P., & Schellenberg, R. P. (1987). The viability of scatter analysis on the WISC-R and the SBIS: Examining a vestige. *Journal of Psychoeducational Assessment, 5*, 37–47.

Lawson, J. S., & Inglis, J. (1984). The psychometric assessment of children with learning disabilities: An index derived from a principal components analysis of the WISC-R. *Journal of Learning Disabilities, 17*, 517–522.

Livingston, R. B., Jennings, E., Reynolds, C. R., & Gray, R. M. (2003). Multivariate analyses of the profile stability of intelligence tests: High for IQs, low to very low for subtest analyses. *Archives of Clinical Neuropsychology, 18*, 487–507.

Lowman, M. G., Schwanz, K. A., & Kamphaus, R. W. (1996). WISC-III third factor: Critical measurement issues. *Canadian Journal of School Psychology, 12*, 15–22.

Maller, S. J., & McDermott, P. A. (1997). WAIS-R profile analysis for college students with learning disabilities. *School Psychology Review, 26*, 575–585.

Matarazzo, J. D. (1985). Psychological assessment of intelligence. In H. I. Kaplan & B. J. Sadock (Eds.),

Comprehensive textbook of psychiatry (Vol. 1, 4th ed., pp. 502–513). Baltimore: Williams & Wilkins.

McDermott, P. A., Fantuzzo, J. W., & Glutting, J. J. (1990). Just say no to subtest analysis: A critique on Wechsler theory and practice. *Journal of Psychoeducational Assessment, 8,* 290–302.

McDermott, P. A., Fantuzzo, J. W., Glutting, J. J., Watkins, M. W., & Baggaley, R. A. (1992). Illusion of meaning in the ipsative assessment of children's ability. *Journal of Special Education, 25,* 504–526.

McDermott, P. A., & Glutting, J. J. (1997). Informing stylistic learning behavior, disposition, and achievement through ability subtests—or, more illusions of meaning? *School Psychology Review, 26,* 163–175.

McDermott, P. A., Glutting, J. J., Jones, J. N., Watkins, M. W., & Kush, J. (1989). Core profile types in the WISC-R national sample: Structure, membership, and applications. *Psychological Assessment, 1,* 292–299.

McDermott, P. A., Green, L. F., Francis, J. M., & Stott, D. H. (1996). *Learning Behaviors Scale.* Philadelphia: Edumetric & Clinical Science.

McDermott, P. A., Marston, N. C., & Stott, D. H. (1993). *Adjustment Scales for Children and Adolescents.* Philadelphia: Edumetric & Clinical Science.

McFall, R. M., & Treat, T. A. (1999). Quantifying the information value of clinical assessments with signal detection theory. *Annual Review of Psychology, 50,* 215–241.

McGrew, K. S., & Knopik, S. N. (1996). The relationship between intra-cognitive scatter on the Woodcock–Johnson Psycho-Educational Battery—Revised and school achievement. *Journal of School Psychology, 34,* 351–364.

McNemar, Q. (1964). Lost: Our intelligence? Why? *American Psychologist, 19,* 871–882.

Meehl, P. E., & Rosen, A. (1955). Antecedent probability and the efficiency of psychometric signs, patterns, or cutting scores. *Psychological Bulletin, 52,* 194–216.

Moffitt, T. E., & Silva, P. A. (1987). WISC-R Verbal and Performance IQ discrepancy in an unselected cohort: Clinical significance and longitudinal stability. *Journal of Consulting and Clinical Psychology, 55,* 768–774.

Mueller, H. H., Dennis, S. S., & Short, R. H. (1986). A meta-exploration of WISC-R factor score profiles as a function of diagnosis and intellectual level. *Canadian Journal of School Psychology, 2,* 21–43.

Neyens, L. G. J., & Aldenkamp, A. P. (1996). Stability of cognitive measures in children of average ability. *Child Neuropsychology, 2,* 161–170.

Oakland, T., Broom, J., & Glutting, J. (2000). Use of freedom from distractibility and processing speed to assess children's test-taking behaviors. *Journal of School Psychology, 38,* 469–475.

Oakland, T., & Hu, S. (1992). The top 10 tests used with children and youth worldwide. *Bulletin of the International Test Commission, 19,* 99–120.

Oh, H.-J., Glutting, J. J., & McDermott, P. A. (1999). An epidemological-cohort study of DAS processing speed factor: How well does it identify concurrent achievement and behavior problems? *Journal of Psychoeducational Assessment, 17,* 362–375.

Pedhazur, E. J. (1997). *Multiple regression in behavioral research: Explanation and prediction* (3rd ed.). Fort Worth, TX: Harcourt Brace.

Pfeiffer, S. I., Reddy, L. A., Kletzel, J. E., Schmelzer, E. R., & Boyer, L. M. (2000). The practitioner's view of IQ testing and profile analysis. *School Psychology Quarterly, 15,* 376–385.

Piedmont, R. L., Sokolove, R. L., & Fleming, M. Z. (1989). An examination of some diagnostic strategies involving the Wechsler intelligence scales. *Psychological Assessment, 1,* 181–185.

Prifitera, A., & Dersh, J. (1993). Base rates of WISC-III diagnostic subtest patterns among normal, learning-disabled, and ADHD samples. *Journal of Psychoeducational Assessment, WISC-III Monograph,* pp. 43–55.

Ree, M. J., & Carretta, T. R. (1997). What makes an aptitude test valid? In R. F. Dillon (Ed.), *Handbook on testing* (pp. 65–81). Westport, CT: Greenwood Press.

Ree, M. J., & Carretta, T. R. (2002). g2K. *Human Performance, 15,* 3–23.

Reynolds, C. R., & Kamphaus, R. W. (2003). *Reynolds Intellectual Assessment Scales and the Reynolds Intellectual Screening Test professional manual.* Lutz, FL: Psychological Assessment Resources.

Rispens, J., Swaab, H., van den Oord, E. J. C. G., Cohen-Kettenis, P., van Engeland, H., & van Yperen, T. (1997). WISC profiles in child psychiatric diagnosis: Sense or nonsense? *Journal of the American Academy of Child and Adolescent Psychiatry, 36,* 1587–1594.

Roid, G. H. (2003). *Stanford–Binet Intelligence Scales, Fifth Edition: Technical manual.* Itasca, IL: Riverside.

Ryan, J. J., & Bohac, D. L. (1994). Neurodiagnostic implications of unique profiles of the Wechsler Adult Intelligence Scale—Revised. *Psychological Assessment, 6,* 360–363.

Ryan, J. J., Kreiner, D. S., & Burton, D. B. (2002). Does high scatter affect the predictive validity of WAIS-III IQs? *Applied Neuropsychology, 9,* 173–178.

Salvia, J., & Ysseldyke, J. E. (1998). *Assessment* (7th ed.). Boston: Houghton Mifflin.

Sattler, J. M. (2001). *Assessment of children: Cognitive applications* (4th ed.). San Diego, CA: Jerome M. Sattler.

Schmidt, F. L. (2002). The role of general cognitive ability and job performance: Why there cannot be a debate. *Human Performance, 15,* 187–210.

Schmidt, F. L., Le, H., & Ilies, R. (2003). Beyond alpha: An empirical examination of the effects of different sources of measurement error on reliability estimates for measures of individual differences constructs. *Psychological Methods, 8,* 206–224.

Shaw, S. R., Swerdlik, M. E., & Laurent, J. (1993). Review of the WISC-III. In B. Bracken & R. S. McCallum (Eds.), *Advances in psychoeducational assessment* (pp. 151–160). Brandon, VT: Clinical Psychology.

Simensen, R. J., & Sutherland, J. (1974). Psychological assessment of brain damage: The Wechsler scales. *Academic Therapy, 10,* 69–81.

Smith, C. B., & Watkins, M. W. (2004). Diagnostic utility of the Bannatyne WISC-III pattern. *Learning Disabilities Research and Practice, 19,* 49–56.

Smith, T., Smith, B. L., Bramlett, R. K., & Hicks, N. (1999, April). *WISC-III stability over a three year period.* Paper presented at the annual meeting of the National Association of School Psychologists, Las Vegas, NV.

Sparrow, S. S., & Davis, S. M. (2000). Recent advances in the assessment of intelligence and cognition. *Journal of Child Psychology and Psychiatry, 41,* 117–131.

Swets, J. A. (1988). Measuring the accuracy of diagnostic systems. *Science, 240,* 1285–1293.

Swets, J. A. (1996). *Signal detection theory and RIC analysis in psychology and diagnosis: Collected papers.* Mahwah, NJ: Erlbaum.

Swets, J. A., Dawes, R. M., & Monahan, J. (2000). Psychological science can improve diagnostic decisions. *Psychological Science in the Public Interest, 1,* 1–26.

Teeter, P. A., & Korducki, R. (1998). Assessment of emotionally disturbed children with the WISC-III. In A. Prifitera & D. H. Saklofske (Eds.), *WISC-III clinical use and interpretation: Scientist-practitioner perspectives* (pp. 119–138). San Diego, CA: Academic Press.

Thorndike, R. L. (1986). The role of general ability in prediction. *Journal of Vocational Behavior, 29,* 332–339.

Thorndike, R. M. (1997). *Measurement and evaluation in psychology and education* (6th ed.). Upper Saddle River, NJ: Merrill.

U.S. Department of Education. (2001). *Twenty-first annual report to Congress on the implementation of the Individuals with Disabilities Education Act.* Jessup, MD: Author.

Ward, S. B., Ward, T. J., Hatt, C. V., Young, D. L., & Mollner, N. R. (1995). The incidence and utility of the ACID, ACIDS, and SCAD profiles in a referred population. *Psychology in the Schools, 32,* 267–276.

Watkins, M. W. (1996). Diagnostic utility of the WISC-III developmental index as a predictor of learning disabilities. *Journal of Learning Disabilities, 29,* 305–312.

Watkins, M. W. (1999). Diagnostic utility of WISC-III subtest variability among students with learning disabilities. *Canadian Journal of School Psychology, 15,* 11–20.

Watkins, M. W. (2000). Cognitive profile analysis: A shared professional myth. *School Psychology Quarterly, 15,* 465–479.

Watkins, M. W. (2003). IQ subtest analysis: Clinical acumen or clinical illusion? *Scientific Review of Mental Health Practice, 2,* 118–141.

Watkins, M. W., & Canivez, G. L. (2004). Temporal stability of WISC-III subtest composite: Strengths and weaknesses. *Psychological Assessment, 16,* 133–138.

Watkins, M. W., & Glutting, J. J. (2000). Incremental validity of WISC-III profile elevation, scatter, and shape information for predicting reading and math achievement. *Psychological Assessment, 12,* 402–408.

Watkins, M. W., & Kush, J. C. (1994). Wechsler subtest analysis: The right way, the wrong way, or no way? *School Psychology Review, 23,* 640–651.

Watkins, M. W., Kush, J. C., & Glutting, J. J. (1997a). Discriminant and predictive validity of the WISC-III ACID profile among children with learning disabilities. *Psychology in the Schools, 34,* 309–319.

Watkins, M. W., Kush, J. C., & Glutting, J. J. (1997b). Prevalence and diagnostic utility of the WISC-III SCAD profile among children with disabilities. *School Psychology Quarterly, 12,* 235–248.

Watkins, M. W., Kush, J. C., & Schaefer, B. A. (2002). Diagnostic utility of the Learning Disability Index. *Journal of Learning Disabilities, 35,* 98–103.

Watkins, M. W., & Worrell, F. C. (2000). Diagnostic utility of the number of WISC-III subtests deviating from mean performance among students with learning disabilities. *Psychology in the Schools, 37,* 303–309.

Wechsler, D. (1949). *Wechsler Intelligence Scale for Children.* New York: Psychological Corporation.

Wechsler, D. (1958). *The measurement and appraisal of adult intelligence* (4th ed.). Baltimore: Williams & Wilkins.

Wechsler, D. (1974). *Wechsler Intelligence Scale for Children—Revised.* New York: Psychological Corporation.

Wechsler, D. (1991). *Wechsler Intelligence Scale for Children—Third Edition.* San Antonio, TX: Psychological Corporation.

Wechsler, D. (1992). *Wechsler Individual Achievement Test.* San Antonio, TX: Psychological Corporation.

Wechsler, D. (1997). *Wechsler Adult Intelligence Scale—Third Edition.* San Antonio, TX: Psychological Corporation.

Wechsler, D. (2003). *Wechsler Intelligence Scale for Children—Fourth Edition: Technical and interpretive manual.* San Antonio, TX: Psychological Corporation.

Whittaker, T. A., Fouladi, R. T., & Williams, N. J. (2002). Determining predictor importance in multiple regression under varied correlational and distributional conditions. *Journal of Modern Applied Statistical Methods, 1,* 354–366.

Wiggins, J. S. (1988). *Personality and prediction: Principles of personality assessment.* Malabar, FL: Krieger.

Youngstrom, E. A., Kogos, J. L., & Glutting, J. J. (1999). Incremental efficacy of Differential Ability Scales factor scores in predicting individual achievement criteria. *School Psychology Quarterly, 14,* 26–39.

Zachary, R. A. (1990). Wechsler's intelligence scales: Theoretical and practical considerations. *Journal of Psychoeducational Assessment, 8,* 276–289.

Zarin, D. A., & Earls, F. (1993). Diagnostic decision making in psychiatry. *American Journal of Psychiatry, 150,* 197–206.

Zeidner, M. (2001). Invited foreword and introduction. In J. J. W. Andrews, D. H. Saklofske, & H. L. Janzen (Eds.), *Handbook of psychoeducational assessment: Ability, achievement, and behavior in children.* San Diego, CA: Academic Press.

Zeidner, M., & Matthews, G. (2000). Intelligence and personality. In R. J. Sternberg (Ed.), *Handbook of intelligence* (pp. 581–610). New York: Cambridge University Press.

Zimmerman, I. L., & Woo-Sam, J. M. (1985). Clinical applications. In B. B. Wolman (Ed.), *Handbook of intelligence: Theories, measurements, and applications* (pp. 873–898). New York: Wiley.

13

Linking Cognitive Assessment Results to Academic Interventions for Students with Learning Disabilities

NANCY MATHER
BARBARA J. WENDLING

In a recent conversation in the teachers' lounge, Mr. Calloway, the special education teacher, suggested to Ms. Sammons, the third-grade teacher, that Steve, a child struggling with reading, should be given an intelligence test. Mr. Calloway noted that the results would help them gain a better understanding of Steve's abilities and provide insights into why he was having so much difficulty with reading. Ms. Sammons replied, "Why bother? I'd just get back a bunch of numbers and still not know how to help Steve learn to read." Conceivably, Ms. Sammons's candid response would be representative of the opinion of many general education teachers if they were questioned about the usefulness and value of intelligence testing. Her comment also illustrates the present-day disassociation between assessment results and prescriptive interventions. Although these types of tests are usually part of an evaluation for learning disabilities, do they actually help with the selection of effective academic interventions?

The use and validity of intelligence and cognitive ability tests for prescribing treatments have been widely debated (e.g., Good, Vollmer, Creek, Katz, & Chowdhri, 1993; Messick, 1989; Reschly & Ysseldyke, 2002).

Unfortunately, in the field of learning disabilities (LD), the driving force for many public school assessments has been the determination of eligibility for services, rather than the careful design of individualized intervention programs. Clearly, the goal of most assessments should be to create an educational plan designed to produce improved outcomes for the individual (Heller, Holtzman, & Messick, 1982; Reschly, 1992).

Most clinicians would agree that the results obtained from tests that measure cognitive abilities lead to inferences regarding cognition, behavior, and academic functioning. Most would also concur that additional supportive qualitative and quantitative data are needed for the results to be accurately interpreted and fully understood. Results from any single test, regardless of content, provide only a narrow, static view of a person. In contrast, results from comprehensive assessments provide a multidimensional view of the person, where abilities, achievements, temperament, motivations, experiences, and behaviors are all considered as factors that contribute to academic performance and influence the selection of appropriate interventions.

Thus the selection of accommodations and instructional interventions is based upon in-

terviews and observations of actual performance within settings, as well as the results
from both cognitive and academic testing.
Results from cognitive tests can, however,
help an evaluator develop an initial hypothesis that leads to the selection of other appropriate assessments and culminates in the selection of appropriate accommodations and
strategies. They can also help an evaluator
create a stronger rationale for why a person
needs and is legally entitled to specific accommodations. For example, low scores on
timed measures may suggest to an evaluator
that the individual will need extended time
on tests or require more time when reading
assignments and may benefit from an instructional strategy that is designed to promote reading fluency and rate. Before drawing these conclusions, however, the evaluator
will need additional data, including reports
from classroom teachers, as well as measures
of reading rate. When viewed together, the
low scores on timed tests, the teacher reports
of slow reading, and the scores indicating a
compromised reading rate may all support
the conclusion that additional time is an
appropriate accommodation. The findings
may also indicate that the person will benefit from an intervention designed to improve reading fluency and rate—such as the
repeated-readings procedure, a strategy designed for individuals who read slowly despite adequate word recognition (Meyer &
Felton, 1999; Samuels, 1979). When viewed
as one piece of the diagnostic puzzle and
integrated with other data, results from tests
of intelligence and cognitive ability can help
evaluators draw meaningful insights to help
design specific intervention plans for students with LD.

In this chapter, we do not focus on a
specific test instrument, but rather on the
common cognitive constructs and abilities
that are measured by these instruments,
how these constructs relate to LD, and possible implications for intervention. The relationships between certain cognitive abilities and academic performance are well
established (e.g., vocabulary and reading
comprehension), whereas others are not
(e.g., processing speed and word identification). Furthermore, some cognitive constructs are commonly measured on many
intelligence tests (e.g., vocabulary and
memory), whereas others currently are not

(e.g., phonological awareness and rapid automatized naming).

GENERAL ISSUES

Before discussing how performance on specific cognitive abilities can provide insight
into the selection of interventions, four general issues related to the use of cognitive assessments with students with LD are discussed: (1) the need for and provision of
differentiated instruction, (2) the limitations
of global IQ scores, (3) the overreliance on
ability–achievement discrepancies for eligibility, and (4) the use of profile analysis.

Need for and Provision of Differentiated Instruction

Historically, the field of LD has been based
on the belief that individualized educational
planning makes a difference because children
differ in their abilities and therefore should
be taught and treated differently (Kavale &
Forness, 1998; Whitener, 1989). A child who
has difficulty memorizing information requires a different type of instruction from
that needed by one who memorizes facts easily. A child who works slowly needs more
time than one who works rapidly. A child
who struggles to pay attention requires more
novelty and structure than one who attends
easily. In some cases, these marked differences in learning and behavior are neurologically based (Semrud-Clikeman et al.,
2000; Shaywitz, 1998, 2003; Shaywitz et al.,
2003).

Although 99% of teachers believe that students process and learn information differently, and that instruction is more effective if
the materials and methods are matched to
students' unique learning styles (Reschly,
1992), differentiated instruction does not always occur. Unfortunately, even after a comprehensive assessment has been completed
and an appropriate plan developed, many
students with LD receive the same treatment
goals and teaching strategies as their normally achieving peers (Reynolds & Lakin,
1987). To explore the implementation of differentiated instruction, Schumm, Moody,
and Vaughn (2000) interviewed third-grade
teachers who served students with LD in inclusive classrooms. Overall, the teachers re-

ported using whole-class instruction that included the same materials for all students, regardless of performance levels. All students were expected to read grade-level materials, even if they could not pronounce the words. Furthermore, students with LD did not receive instruction directed at improving their word analysis skills. One teacher voiced strong opposition to providing instruction in word analysis, stating, "By the time they come to third grade they really should have those skills" (quoted in Schumm et al., 2000, p. 483). With undifferentiated instruction and minimal direct instruction in reading, the students with LD made little academic improvement, and their attitudes toward reading declined as well.

The use of undifferentiated instruction does not, of course, negate the value of cognitive ability tests for educational planning, but it does suggest that teachers may not perceive the value of carefully constructed individualized plans or even attempt to implement them. The resulting perception may then be to discredit the value and need for cognitive ability testing or standardized testing in general, because the findings do not influence educational programming. Clearly, for students with LD, differential, remedial instruction that addresses the source of the problem will be more effective than global approaches that do not (Aaron, 1997).

Limitations of Global Scores

One major problem with the use of intelligence tests for the diagnosis of LD has been an overreliance on global scores that do not convey useful information for educational planning. A full-scale IQ score simply represents the individual's relative standing compared to the selected norm group, based on his or her performance at a specific point in time on a specific set of tasks designed to measure the test authors' conceptualization of intelligence. Stanovich (1999) has aptly defined intelligence as "the statistical amalgamation of a panoply of different cognitive processes" (p. 352). Throughout the 20th century, the limited utility of global ability scores for describing the performance of individuals with LD has been recognized (Kavale & Forness, 1995; Orton, 1925; Reid, Hresko, & Swanson, 1996). As early

as 1938, Stern reflected upon the limited value of global IQ scores:

> To be sure there has been and there still is exaggerated faith in the power of numbers. For example, "an intelligence quotient" may be of provisional value as a first crude approximation when the mental level of an individual is sought; but whoever imagines that in determining this quantity he has summed up "the" intelligence of an individual once and for all, so that he may dispense with the more intensive qualitative study, leaves off where psychology should begin. (p. 60)

Unfortunately, in the field of LD, systems of educational classification have been based upon special claims that IQ scores measure intellectual potential—a belief that is neither conceptually nor psychometrically justifiable (Stanovich, 1999).

Tests also vary in the abilities that are assessed, and the types of tasks administered then influence the obtained score. If the tasks primarily measure the student's strengths, then a higher score is obtained but if they measure the student's weaknesses, a lower score is obtained. Because intelligence tests often measure certain aspects of the disability or the weak cognitive processes, Orton (1925) cautioned that for individuals with reading problems, full-scale scores provide an entirely erroneous estimate of the person's intellectual capabilities. Similarly, Fletcher and colleagues (1998) have observed: "To the extent that the child who reads poorly has a significant language disorder, scores on a language-based IQ test will underestimate the child's aptitude for learning in other areas" (p. 200). Composite scores mask the contribution made by reading-related cognitive abilities, so that the correlations and comparisons between these measures must be interpreted with caution (Vellutino, 2001).

The important factor to consider is what abilities are being measured by a certain test and to what aspects of academic performance these abilities are most related. Students with LD often obtain lower scores than normally achieving peers on measures of phonological awareness, rate, memory, and perceptual speed (Gregg, Davis, Coleman, Wisenbaker, & Hoy, 2004; Shessel & Reiff, 1999). They will therefore receive lower scores on intelligence tests that place a greater emphasis on these abilities, and higher scores on tests that place more emphasis on acquired knowledge and reasoning. Specific abilities also influence performance in different academic areas, making some abilities better predictors of certain tasks than others. For example, because they do not require vocabulary or higher-level reasoning, lower-level tasks, such as measures of perceptual speed, are not particularly good predictors of reading comprehension. In contrast, measures of vocabulary and acquired knowledge are good predictors of reading comprehension, but may underpredict or overpredict how well a person will do in math computation. The major considerations are that content differences among various intelligence and cognitive ability tests result in full-scale score differences, and within these subsets of measures, some are better predictors or more closely related to certain types of academic performance than others.

Overreliance on Ability–Achievement Discrepancies

Although intelligence tests are routinely administered to children as one component of a comprehensive evaluation, this practice in many public school settings has been driven more by policy than by diagnostic value. The difficulty in developing a qualitative definition of an LD, combined with the need to make funding decisions, prompted school districts to use statistical methods to identify students with LD (Silver & Hagin, 2002). For several decades, a common use of a full-scale IQ score has been to predict achievement. Results from an IQ test (usually a global score) were compared directly to the standard scores from achievement tests to determine a discrepancy. Based upon an arbitrary cutting point (e.g., 16 or 22 points), a significant discrepancy was deemed necessary to be eligible for services. The most psychometrically sound procedures employed a correction for the effects of statistical regression.

Much has been written about the limitations of using an IQ–achievement discrepancy for the identification of LD (e.g., Berninger, 2001; Fletcher et al., 2001; Lyon, 1995; Mather & Healey, 1990; Vellutino, 2001), as well as the need to abandon this type of discrepancy (Flowers, Meyer, Lovato, Wood, & Felton, 2000; Fuchs, Mock, Morgan, & Young, 2003). To complicate matters further, state and school district guidelines have varied in regard to the specific method used to define a discrepancy, as well as the magnitude of the discrepancy needed to qualify for services. Therefore, a child may be identified as having an LD in one district, but then may be denied services in another, depending on the state and local criteria or on the personal philosophy of an independent evaluator who assesses the child (Berninger, 1996). In discussing the discrepancy procedure, Simpson and Buckhalt (1990) have stated:

> Although the formula method may have some appeal because it requires less clinical competence and judgement, the fact remains that reducing an important diagnostic decision to a mathematical equation gives a false sense of objectivity to a contrived procedure that is still essentially subjective. (p. 274)

Recent discussions surrounding the reauthorization of the Individuals with Disabilities Education Act (IDEA, 1997; U.S. Department of Education, 2000) as well as the report from the President's Commission on Excellence in Special Education (2002), downplay the need for intelligence testing and advocate a shift away from an IQ–achievement discrepancy as the sole criterion for LD service eligibility. If intelligence tests are not needed as part of the eligibility process, it is likely that their use in public schools will decline. In fact, if a noncategorical approach to service delivery is adopted, as some have recommended, the need for intelligence testing would be reduced or eliminated altogether (Tilly, Grimes, & Reschly, 1993). Under this new framework, emphasis would be placed on prereferral interventions, and attention would focus on more frequent data collection designed to reveal the effectiveness of educational interventions. LD would be redefined as inadequate response to intervention. Unfortunately, as the consensus grows that the IQ–achievement discrepancy should be abandoned, a valid and validated replacement does not exist (Fuchs et al., 2003).

Even within a response-to-treatment model, Fuchs and colleagues (2003) recommend the use of cognitive assessments for students who do not respond to treatments, because without their use the LD construct will disappear altogether and lead to a bin of so-called "high-incidence disabilities." In response to the recently revised IDEA guidelines, Hale, Naglieri, Kaufman, and Hale (2004) reiterate that a child with LD has a disorder in one or more of the basic psychological processes. To align the definition of LD with evaluation procedures, they suggest that the following clarification be added to the law: "In determining whether a child has a specific learning disability, a local educational agency should include reliable and valid norm-referenced measures of basic psychological processes" (p. 13). For the results of these tests to be useful, however, the focus needs to be on obtaining information that is relevant to behavioral and academic functioning, rather than simply·providing an estimate of global ability or calculating an IQ–achievement discrepancy. Even though a student may be deemed ineligible for certain services, all evaluations need to address the referral concerns and propose solutions. As Cruickshank (1977) stated, "Diagnosis must take second place to instruction, and must be a tool of instruction, not an end in itself" (p. 194). The purpose of testing cognitive abilities is to determine the person's unique strengths and weaknesses. In the case of LD, the identified underlying cognitive weaknesses are often directly linked to the specific difficulties in various aspects of school achievement.

Use of Profile Analysis

The documentation of strengths and weaknesses is often accomplished through profile analysis and consideration of the underlying processes involved in reading, writing, and math. Although identifying an individual's strengths and weaknesses can contribute to educational planning, this practice has been discouraged because of legitimate psychometric concerns. Glutting, McDermott, and Konold (1997; see also Watkins, Glutting, & Youngstrom, Chapter 12, this volume) have described the various problems with interpreting individual differences through profile analysis, reminding psychologists to "just say no." Although danger does exist in profile analysis when the differences among

abilities are minimal and insignificant, significant intraindividual discrepancies among abilities are precisely how intelligence tests can contribute to LD determination and educational planning. As long as interpretation is performed within the context of all data, this type of analysis is supported by the following statement from the *Standards for Educational and Psychological Testing* (American Educational Research Association, American Psychological Association, & National Council on Measurement in Education, 1999):

> Because each test in a battery examines a different function, ability, skill, or combination thereof, the test taker's performance can be understood best when scores are not combined or aggregated, but rather when each score is interpreted within the context of all other scores and assessment data. For example, low scores on timed tests alert the examiner to slowed responding as a problem that may not be apparent if scores on different kinds of tests are combined. (p. 123)

A growing body of research supports the usefulness of factor or specific ability scores in identifying the cognitive processing problems that specifically inhibit school learning (e.g., Evans, Floyd, McGrew, & Leforgee, 2002; Flanagan, Ortiz, Alfonso, & Mascolo, 2002; Gregg et al., 2004; Hale, Fiorello, Kavanagh, Hoeppner, & Gaitherer, 2001; McGrew, Flanagan, Keith, & Vanderwood, 1997). As examples, Berninger and Abbott (1994) described oral language and orthographic skills as the best predictors of reading. Adams (1990) found that a child's level of phonemic awareness in kindergarten was the best predictor of reading success in elementary school. Others have described the relationship between slow rapid automatized naming (RAN; see later discussion) and poor reading skills (e.g., Denckla & Rudel, 1974; Torgesen, 1997; Wolf, Bowers, & Biddle, 2000).

Researchers continue to document the relationships among specific cognitive, linguistic, and academic abilities, identifying prerequisite skills and delineating early indicators of risk. The evolution of theory- and research-based tests measuring multiple abilities has also given professionals the opportunity to gain a better understanding of an individual's unique characteristics. Hannon and Daneman (2001) have described the increasing focus on theory:

> With the advent and dominance of the information-processing approach to cognition, the emphasis has switched from measurement to theory. The goal is no longer simply to quantify individual differences in intellectual tasks, but also to explain the individual differences in terms of the architecture and processes of the human information-processing system. (p. 103)

Assessments should then focus on understanding a person's information-processing capabilities, including the factors that can facilitate performance. As Gardner (1999; see also Chen & Gardner, Chapter 5, this volume) has suggested, "We shouldn't ask how smart you are, but rather how are you smart?" Understanding the "constraints" (e.g., limited instruction, specific cognitive or linguistic weaknesses, limited cultural experiences, poor motivation) that affect performance, as well as the multidimensional impact of these constraints (Berninger, 1996), is also important. Because the various constraints affect different aspects of academic functioning, they can help inform the type and extent of accommodations and instruction needed. Interpretation of intraindividual differences and a determination of how these differences affect performance is then the cornerstone for linking the results of cognitive ability tests to meaningful instructional plans.

One basic concept underlying identification of LD is that the difficulty does not extend too far into other domains. In other words, the problem is relatively specific, circumscribed, or domain-specific (Stanovich, 1999). The academic problem is best described as a reading disability, math disability, or spelling disability that is presumably caused by weaknesses in specific cognitive or linguistic processes. The first part of an evaluation is then to determine an initial domain-specific classification (Stanovich, 1999); the next part is to identify the deficient cognitive processes that underlie the disorder (Robinson, Menchetti, & Torgesen, 2002). LD is caused by inherent weaknesses in underlying cognitive processes (Robinson et al., 2002). The assessment process can then be viewed as an ability-oriented evalua-

tion designed to help formulate the problem and then determine specific interventions (Fletcher, Taylor, Levin, & Satz, 1995).

COGNITIVE ABILITIES AND ACADEMIC INTERVENTIONS

Within the last 50 years, numerous researchers have explored the proximal causes of academic failure and have attempted to determine exactly which factors have predictive value. Interest in the predictive value of cognitive and linguistic factors is fueled by a desire to identify young children who are most at risk for failure, particularly in the area of reading. Ideally, a predictor or subset of predictors will accurately differentiate between the children who will struggle with certain academic subjects and those who will not, so that intervention efforts can begin early (Bishop, 2003).

Several cognitive and linguistic factors have been linked to the academic difficulties experienced by children with LD. Even though we discuss these cognitive abilities separately, Horn (1991) has admonished that attempting to measure cognitive abilities in isolation "is like slicing smoke" (p. 198). Cognitive and academic abilities are interrelated, and various combinations of abilities are employed as a person completes specific tasks.

Consider the various skills required to take notes while listening to a lecture. The note taker must have attention, knowledge of the topic, vocabulary, memory to hold on to important points, and writing skill. A student may struggle with note taking for any or all of these reasons. In addition, the prediction of performance for students with LD may be improved when several factors are considered (Gregg et al., 2004). For example, when combined, measures of working memory and language comprehension appear to provide the best prediction of reading comprehension ability (Daneman & Carpenter, 1980).

In some circumstances, performance is influenced by something other than what a test was designed to measure. Stern (1938) noted: "It should never, of course, be supposed possible to test a definite, narrowly circumscribed separate capacity of thought with any one of these tests. Other abilities are always involved" (p. 315). He continued:

> Yet this is in no sense to be construed as a defect in the tests. On the contrary, they provide a favorable opportunity for observing the process of thinking in all its complexity. One must not be content to calculate the score for each performance. A completed test, which according to the system of scoring is thrown out as erroneous or deficient in performance, may very frequently result from the fact that *other* kinds of thinking than those expected have intervened, but which may have significance in terms of the subject's particular intellectual approach. (p. 316; original emphasis)

Thus Stern emphasized that intelligence tests are valuable beyond the mere production of scores, because careful observation during performance and analysis of the psychological processes that led to the test answer can deepen an evaluator's insight into the structure and functioning of cognitive abilities. Accordingly, we reemphasize the value of forming, exploring, confirming, or rejecting diagnostic hypotheses that are based upon test scores, as well as careful, systematic observations of behavior.

Vocabulary, Acquired Knowledge, and Language Comprehension

Unless they are designed primarily to measure nonverbal abilities, most intelligence batteries contain measures of vocabulary, acquired knowledge, and language comprehension. Often described as *crystallized intelligence, verbal or oral language abilities,* or *stores of acquired knowledge,* these abilities are highly correlated with achievement and are good predictors of academic success (Anastasi, 1988; Johnson, 1993). Because most of the measures of crystallized intelligence rely on language, crystallized intelligence can be equated with verbal intelligence (Carroll, 1993; Hunt, 2000) and has often been used as a key indicator of giftedness (Benbow & Lubinski, 1996). These subtests typically measure aspects of cultural knowledge, rather than specialized knowledge specific to a domain. Lawyers, physicians, and astronomers all possess a lot of knowledge, but about different things (Hunt, 2000). If the measures included specialized knowledge, no defensible way of ordering people in

terms of the knowledge they possess would exist.

Verbal abilities and knowledge have a strong and consistent relationship with reading (Evans et al., 2002), mathematics (Floyd, Evans, & McGrew, 2003), and writing (McGrew & Knopik, 1993) across the lifespan. The most fully substantiated relationship is with reading comprehension and written expression. Both reading comprehension and written expression depend upon background knowledge to understand and create messages, familiarity with sentence structures, verbal reasoning abilities, and a broad and deep vocabulary (McCardle, Scarborough, & Catts, 2001). Words and the concepts they represent are thus the building blocks of literacy (Bell & Perfetti, 1994; Cunningham, Stanovich, & Wilson, 1990; Perfetti, Marron, & Foltz, 1996).

Unlike other cognitive abilities, crystallized intelligence has been described as a maintained ability rather than a vulnerable ability, because it continues to develop until midlife and does not decline with age as significantly as other abilities (Horn, 1991). On growth curves, the rate of growth for crystallized intelligence is much greater than other abilities, and it shows a less rapid rate of decline (McGrew & Woodcock, 2001).

Reasons for Differences in Performance

Some people will have weaknesses on these tests because of language impairments, whereas others will have weaknesses because of limited experiences with language and a lack of educational experiences and opportunities (Carlisle & Rice, 2002). In addition, tests of general knowledge, vocabulary, and language comprehension most often reflect the culture and language of the norm group. Therefore, individuals from diverse cultural and/or linguistic backgrounds or from low socioeconomic levels often obtain lower scores on measures of acquired knowledge.

A person's vocabulary is influenced by three main factors: (1) familiarity with words, (2) the depth of conceptual understanding of those words, and (3) the ability to retrieve words as needed (Gould, 2001). A student may understand the meaning of a word, but have difficulty using the word correctly when speaking. These word-finding or word-retrieving difficulties may also negatively influence performance on the verbal subtests found on many intelligence measures. If a person obtains a low score on a vocabulary measure, the evaluator must determine whether that low score is a result of limited verbal knowledge, limited cultural experiences, or difficulty in retrieving verbal labels (a problem more closely linked to associative memory).

Implications

In discussing the reasons for reading comprehension failure, Perfetti and colleagues (1996) distinguish between the processes involved in comprehension (e.g., working memory and comprehension monitoring) and knowledge—which includes word meanings or vocabulary, as well as *domain knowledge* (i.e., the concepts specific to a domain, such as physics, biology, or history). Clearly, knowledge is an important component underlying reading comprehension that contributes to individual differences in reading (Hannon & Daneman, 2001). A person's level of acquired knowledge, including domain knowledge obtained through life experiences, school, or work, is highly predictive of academic performance. Breadth and depth of knowledge and a robust oral vocabulary suggest that the person will excel on tasks involving language-learning abilities, whereas limited knowledge and a poor vocabulary suggest that the person will struggle. Since many academic tasks require linguistic competence, individuals with low verbal abilities are likely to encounter academic difficulties in most areas and will need increased opportunities and experiences to improve linguistic abilities, including vocabulary and world knowledge. In general, people who have difficulty understanding or using spoken language will have difficulty with the aspects of reading, writing, and mathematics that depend upon language-specific processes, such as reading comprehension and math problem solving.

Gough and Tunmer (1986) proposed a simple equation for determining an estimate of reading comprehension: decoding × spoken language comprehension = reading comprehension. Although this equation would result in an accurate prediction for most people, it would not for individuals with specific reading disabilities, because their verbal abil-

ities are typically more advanced than their decoding skills. Essentially, what distinguishes individuals with reading disabilities from other poor readers is that their listening comprehension ability is higher than their ability to decode words (Rack, Snowling, & Olson, 1992). Thus measures of verbal abilities, including listening comprehension, can be used to provide the best estimate of how much a poor reader could get from written text if his or her deficient decoding skills were resolved (Stanovich, 1999).

Beyond third grade, individuals with good verbal ability and good reading skills acquire knowledge and new vocabulary primarily through reading. In contrast, individuals with good verbal ability but poor reading skills are much more likely to learn new vocabulary through oral discussions (Carlisle & Rice, 2002). Unfortunately, since reading rather than listening is used to acquire more complex syntax and abstract vocabulary, poor readers will tend to fall behind good readers on verbal tasks as they progress through school. Since many intelligence tests include vocabulary measures, a poor reader's relative standing on the verbal scores tends to decline, compared to that of normally achieving peers. As a result, poor language contributes to a lower IQ score, as well as to poor reading (Fletcher et al., 1998; Strang, 1964).

The relationship between intelligence measures and reading ability is reciprocal, in that reading experience influences intelligence test scores, and cognitive and academic tests assess many of the same underlying abilities (e.g., vocabulary, general information) (Aaron, 1997). Older students with reading difficulties may have depressed performance on measures of oral language because of limited experiences with text. Strang (1964) summarized this problem:

> Intelligence tests are not a sure measure of innate ability to learn. They measure "developed ability," not innate or potential intelligence. Previous achievement affects the test results. The poor reader is penalized on the verbal parts of the test. The fact that his store of information is limited by the small amount of reading he has done also works against him. (p. 212)

Thus for students with reading disabilities, lack of exposure to print contributes to reduced knowledge and vocabulary, and these deficiencies in language-based abilities are likely to increase over time (Vellutino, Scanlon, & Lyon, 2000). This phenomenon, nicknamed the "Matthew effect" from the Biblical reference that the rich get richer and the poor get poorer (Stanovich, 1986; Walberg & Tsai, 1983), alters the course of development in education-related cognitive skills (Stanovich, 1993). In other words, poor reading contributes to lowered verbal ability and knowledge. Furthermore, measures of verbal ability and listening comprehension may underestimate potential for achievement among students with attentional or language-processing problems, as well as among students for whom English is a second language (Berninger & Abbott, 1994; Fletcher et al., 1998).

Interventions

An individual with limited knowledge or vocabulary is likely to experience difficulty learning new knowledge or vocabulary unless the knowledge can be associated with prior knowledge (Beck, Perfetti, & McKeown, 1982). Individuals with limited verbal abilities benefit from structured instruction in vocabulary and knowledge and preteaching of relevant vocabulary. Ideally, an individual's home and school environments are language-rich, with many opportunities and experiences to reinforce learning. A variety of strategies can be used to help individuals understand the nature of related words and concepts (Joyce, Weil, & Showers, 1992). One important way language develops is through social interactions with more knowledgeable language users (Vygotsky, 1962). As teachers and students work together to attain educational goals, they can model the process of learning by talking about these processes as they perform tasks. Thus modeling and thinking aloud are useful for promoting language development.

Phonological Processing

Phonological awareness, another component of oral language, is important to an understanding of reading disabilities. *Phonological awareness* refers to the ability to attend to various aspects of the sound structure of speech, whereas *phonemic awareness* refers to the understanding that speech can be divided or sequenced into a series of discrete sounds. The importance of phonological processing to reading and spelling achievement has been extensively documented (e.g., Ehri, 1998; Morris et al., 1998; Snow, Burns, & Griffin, 1998; Torgesen, 1998; Wagner, Torgesen, Laughon, Simmons, & Rashotte, 1993). In addition, phonological awareness has a reciprocal relationship with the development of reading and spelling; learning to read and spell helps develop phonological processing. Rack and colleagues (1992) have hypothesized that phonological awareness underlies the establishment of the graphemic memory store that is required for written language.

Because phonological awareness abilities are prerequisites for success in reading and spelling competence, they should be assessed, especially in cases where the referral questions are related to poor word identification or spelling skill.

Reasons for Differences in Performance

Cultural and linguistic differences have an impact on the development of phonological awareness. Individuals who have had limited exposure to the sounds of language, have limited oral language, have not been read to during the preschool years, or come from a low socioeconomic environment may have difficulty discriminating and manipulating speech sounds.

Implications

A weakness in phonological processing is a common factor among individuals with early reading problems (Fletcher & Foorman, 1994; Share & Stanovich, 1995; Siegel & Ryan, 1988; Stanovich & Siegel, 1994). Phonological processes are critical for the development of reading and spelling skills (Adams, 1990; Goswami & Bryant, 1990; Gough, 1996). Results from longitudinal studies suggest that 75% of children who struggle with reading in third grade will still be poor readers at the end of high school, primarily because of problems in phonological awareness (Francis, Shaywitz, Stuebing, Shaywitz, & Fletcher, 1996; Lyon, 1998). Individuals with poor phonological abilities typically make less progress in basic word-reading skills than normally achieving peers. Even spelling problems in young adults often reflect specific problems in the phonological aspects of language (Moats, 2001).

Recent findings have documented the neuroanatomical differences between the brains of poor readers and those of normally achieving readers (Shaywitz, 2003). The evolution of functional magnetic resonance imaging or fMRI technology has made it possible to discover exactly which parts of the brain are engaged during phonological tasks. Good readers engage both the front and back of the brain as they perform phonological processing tasks, whereas poor readers appear to use only the front of the brain. In addition, some children who show phonologically based reading difficulties also exhibit difficulties in retrieval of math facts (Ashcraft, 1987, 1992; Light & DeFries, 1995).

Interventions

Regardless of etiology, poor phonological awareness indicates a need for intervention (Lyon, 1996; Shaywitz, Escobar, Shaywitz, Fletcher, & Makuch, 1992). Identification of children with poor phonological awareness can often occur by kindergarten (Wise & Snyder, 2001). Once children have been identified, direct and explicit instruction involving the relationships among phonemes and graphemes is most effective (National Reading Panel, 2000) and results in improved word reading (Jenkins & O'Conner, 2001). Without this direct instruction in phonemic awareness and sound–symbol associations, individuals with phonologically based reading problems will not attain adequate reading levels (Frost & Emery, 1995).

The National Reading Panel (2000) has identified phonemic awareness as one of the five key components to effective reading instruction. The most important phonological ability for reading is *blending* (the ability to push together sounds), whereas the most important ability for spelling is *segmentation* (the ability to break apart the speech sounds in a word). Explicit, sequenced, multisensory instruction at the appropriate level, delivered by highly trained teachers to groups of six or fewer, appears most effective for increasing phonological awareness (Wise & Snyder, 2001).

Short-Term Memory and Working Memory

Two types of memory are discussed briefly in this section: *short-term memory* or *memory span*, and *working memory*. Currently, the relationship between short-term memory and working memory has been described in three different ways: (1) the two as similar constructs; (2) working memory as a subset of short-term memory; and (3) short-term memory as a subset of working memory (Engle, Tuholski, Laughlin, & Conway, 1999). For purposes of this discussion, we address these constructs as being related, but distinct.

Short-term memory is a limited-capacity system that requires apprehending and holding information in immediate awareness. Most adults can hold seven pieces of information (plus or minus two) at one time. Short-term memory can be thought of as the "use it or lose it" memory. When new information requires a person's short-term memory, the previous information held is either stored or discarded. Common short-term memory tasks include sentence repetition tasks and repeating digits or words in serial order. Research has documented the importance of memory span to achievement (Flanagan et al., 2002), and to the development of verbal abilities (Engle et al., 1999). Memory span also appears to be significantly related to basic writing skills, particularly spelling (Berninger, 1996; Lehto, 1996).

Working memory has been described as a brain-based function in which plans can be retained temporarily as they are being formed, transformed, or executed (Miller, Galanter, & Pribram, 1960). Similarly, Baddeley (1990) has described working memory as a system for temporarily storing and manipulating information while executing complex cognitive tasks that involve learning, reasoning, and comprehension. Jensen (1998) has described it as the "mind's scratchpad." Thus working memory is engaged when information in short-term memory must be maintained, while other information is being manipulated or transformed in some manner. An example of a common working memory task is listening to numbers in a forward sequence and then restating them in reverse order. Working memory shows a strong connection to fluid intelligence and reasoning ability (Kyllonen & Christal, 1990), whereas short-term memory does not (Engle et al., 1999).

Strong connections exist between working memory and many areas of academic performance (Baddeley, 1986). As examples, significant correlations have been found between working memory and reading comprehension (Coltheart, 1987; Just & Carpenter, 1992; Perfetti & Goldman, 1976), language comprehension (King & Just, 1991), vocabulary acquisition (Daneman & Green, 1986; Gathercole & Baddeley, 1993), spelling (Ormrod & Cochran, 1988), math computation (Ashcraft & Kirk, 2001; Wilson & Swanson, 2001), and math problem solving (Logie, Gilhooly, & Wynn, 1994). Children who have both reading and math disabilities often have difficulty on tasks involving working memory (Evans et al., 2002; Floyd et al., 2003; Reid et al., 1996; Siegel & Ryan, 1988; Wilson & Swanson, 2001), as do children who only have difficulties in math. Both verbal working memory tasks and visual–spatial working memory tasks appear to be important predictors of math ability (Wilson & Swanson, 2001)

Reasons for Differences in Performance

The capacity of working memory will vary, based upon how efficiently an individual performs the specific processes demanded by the task (Daneman & Green, 1986). Some memory span and working memory tasks involve language processing, whereas others involve the processing and retention of digits. Thus reading comprehension is more highly related to verbal measures than to measures of mathematical span (Daneman & Tardif, 1987).

In addition to significant problems with memory, difficulties in several other areas can cause performance on memory tasks to appear impaired. For example, a processing problem such as central auditory processing disorder may negatively affect performance on auditory memory tasks. Depending on the demands of the memory task (e.g., sentence repetition), language proficiency can be a factor. Knowledge of syntax and vocabulary helps facilitate performance on sentence repetition tasks, placing individuals with different linguistic backgrounds at a distinct disadvantage. Because the stimulus is presented briefly and only once on most memory tasks, performance can be affected by attention or anxiety. Results from recent studies suggest that individuals with high math anxiety demonstrate smaller working memory spans when performing math-related tasks (Ashcraft & Kirk, 2001).

Implications

Above-average performance on memory tasks can indicate good attention. If information can be dealt with quickly, then the limited capacity system of short-term memory will not be overloaded, and more attention can be directed to higher-level tasks. Good working memory facilitates proficiency in higher-level abilities, such as reading comprehension, math problem solving, and written expression.

In contrast, individuals with limited memory abilities may (1) appear inattentive; (2) have difficulty following directions or recalling sequences (e.g., months of the year); (3) have trouble memorizing factual information; (4) have difficulty following a lecture or a class discussion; (5) have trouble taking notes; or (6) struggle to comprehend what has been stated or read. For reading comprehension to occur, an individual must decode the words to obtain meaning. If decoding is labored, then fluency is reduced, and greater demands are placed on working memory, diminishing comprehension.

In math, weaknesses in memory span and working memory may contribute to difficulties in retrieving basic facts or solving algorithms. Individuals with math disabilities appear to have difficulty holding information in their minds while completing other processes (Geary, 1996). They may understand the rules, but forget the numerical information or have trouble following the steps of an algorithm in order. They know fewer facts and forget them more quickly than other children. Other characteristics of individuals with math disabilities suggest difficulties in the storage and retrieval process. Difficulties in learning basic number facts do not necessarily mean that a person has poor memory. Limited knowledge can also result from insufficient exposure, poor instruction, or attentional weaknesses, rather than specific math disabilities (Robinson et al., 2002).

Interventions

To accommodate individuals with memory difficulties, oral directions need to be short—or, better yet, written down. In addition, oral instructions can be supported with visual cues, such as demonstrations, pictures, or graphic representations. Accommodations for memory difficulties often involve reducing the amount of information that must be memorized. For example, a teacher can provide a student with a fact chart or calculator, rather than requiring that all math facts be memorized.

Practice, review, and specific instruction in memory strategies can also improve performance. The more routines are practiced, the more automatic the tasks become (Buchel, Coull, & Friston, 1999). This automaticity is especially important for activities that require rapid, efficient responses, such as pronouncing words or responding quickly to math facts.

Many of the methods and strategies that focus on basic math skills have common elements. Teachers are encouraged to review prerequisite information and previously learned skills, provide practice distributed over time, and introduce new skills carefully and systematically. Validated instructional techniques to improve math performance include (1) providing immediate feedback through demonstration and modeling of the correct computational procedure, (2) setting goals, (3) using peers and computers, (4) providing practice to promote fluency with facts, (5) using "talk-alouds" while solving problems, (6) teaching specific strategies for computation and problem solving, and (7) using a concrete-to-abstract teaching sequence (Mastropieri, Scruggs, & Shiah, 1991).

In the concrete-to-abstract teaching sequence, the concrete level involves the use of objects or manipulative devices; the semiconcrete level involves representations such as tallies; and the abstract level involves actual numbers. Direct and systematic instruction through this sequence can help students transform their concrete understandings into the abstract level of numbers. Students may also benefit from the use of mnemonic strategies as aids to remembering the steps in math operations.

Some students will require specific accommodations such as the use of books on tape, permission to tape-record lectures, and the provision of study guides and lecture notes. In addition, individuals who struggle on tasks involving memory need to understand how their difficulties with memory affect their learning, so that they can request specific accommodations when needed.

Long-Term Retrieval and Rapid Automatized Naming

Long-term retrieval is another type of memory process that involves associative memory or the process of storing and retrieving information. Problems with this process can affect how effectively new information is stored, as well as how efficiently it is retrieved. Long-term retrieval is not to be confused with the actual information being stored or recalled which is considered to be crystallized or verbal intelligence. Word-finding difficulties (discussed briefly earlier in connection with verbal abilities) are in some cases problems with the retrieval process.

Associative memory, a narrow ability of long-term retrieval, appears to be an important ability at the early stages of reading (Evans et al., 2002) and math development (Floyd et al., 2003). Acquisition of basic reading or math skills requires the individual to associate pairs of information, such as phonemes (speech sounds) with graphemes (letters), and to store this information for later use. The acquisition of alphabetic knowledge (grapheme–phoneme correspondence) can be described as a visual–verbal paired-associate learning task (Hulme, 1981; Manis, Seidenberg, Stallings, et al., 1999). Results from one recent study indicated that paired-associate learning accounted for unique variance in reading, even when the powerful influence of phonological awareness was controlled for (Windfuhr & Snowling, 2001). These findings suggest that difficulties in recalling associations may impose an independent constraint on learning to read.

Both letter sound knowledge and letter name knowledge have also been identified as strong predictors of reading attainment (Adams, 1990; Muter, Hulme, Snowling, & Taylor, 1997). These aspects of literacy development require the ability to form associations between visual and verbal representations, store those associations, and retrieve them later as needed. In addition, several studies have reported that individuals with dyslexia have difficulties associating verbal labels with visual stimuli (Holmes & Castles, 2001; Vellutino, 1995).

The same basic memory problem that results in common features of reading disabilities, such as difficulties retaining letter–sound correspondences and retrieving words from memory, may also contribute to the fact retrieval problems of many children with math disabilities. Conceivably, a weakness in the long-term storage and retrieval process is a core difficulty that helps explain the high prevalence of comorbidity of reading and math disabilities (Robinson et al., 2002).

Naming facility, another narrow ability of long-term retrieval, has also been identified as a key predictor of early reading achievement (Scarborough, 1998). Carroll (1993) classifies naming facility as a narrow ability of long-term retrieval that is sometimes referred to as *speed of lexical access*, or the efficiency with which individuals retrieve and pronounce letters or words.

One type of naming facility has been referred to as *rapid automatized naming* (RAN) (Denckla & Rudel, 1974). On these types of tasks, a person is typically shown an array of (6–8 in a row, with a total of 30–50) objects, colors, letters, or digits that repeat a pattern, and is asked to name the stimuli as quickly as possible. Unlike other long-term retrieval tasks, these measures are timed, and the person is asked to name the symbols as quickly as possible. Although RAN has been the focus of extensive research in recent years, use of this type of assessment began with the original work of Geschwind (1965) and Denckla and Rudel (1974). Since this time, many studies have demonstrated a connection between slow naming speed and subsequent poor reading skill (e.g., Perfetti, 1994; Wagner et al., 1993; Wolf & Bowers, 1999). Both phonemic awareness and RAN appear to account for independent variance in later reading scores and to relate to distinct aspects of reading development (Manis, Seidenberg, & Doi, 1999).

To attempt to refine explanations of reading failure, Wolf and Bowers (1999) have proposed a theory referred to as the *double-deficit hypothesis*. According to this theory, three major subtypes of poor readers exist: (1) ones with phonological deficits, (2) ones with naming speed deficits, and (3) ones with a combination of the two. Wolf and Bowers have hypothesized that the RAN tasks tap the nonphonological skills related to reading, such as the processes involved in the serial scanning of print. Presumably, children who are slow to name symbols are slower to form orthographic representations of words (Bowers, Sunseth, & Golden, 1999)—abilities related to the visual aspects of reading. If common letter patterns are not recognized easily and quickly, orthographic pattern knowledge, and subsequently reading rate, will be slow to develop (Bowers & Wolf, 1993).

Some evidence also suggests that RAN differentially predicts reading, based upon level of reading skill. For example, Meyer, Wood, Hart, and Felton (1998) found that RAN tasks had predictive power only for poor readers. Manis, Seidenberg, and Doi (1999) summarized what existing research suggests about RAN: (1) RAN appears to be independent of phonology and to contribute independent variance to word identification and comprehension; (2) the independent contribution appears larger with younger children and individuals with reading disabilities; (3) RAN does not relate to the ability to read phonically regular nonsense words; (4) RAN appears to be more closely related to tasks involving orthography than to tasks involving phonology; (5) RAN is related to both the accuracy and speed of reading words, but the relationship is stronger with speeded measures; and (6) the relationship of RAN to reading skills past the early period of acquisition has not been resolved.

Reasons for Differences in Performance

As with other measures of memory, tasks measuring long-term retrieval may be affected by attention or anxiety. Individuals with math disabilities have difficulty learning basic facts and then, once facts are stored, have difficulty accessing them (Geary, 1996). This difficulty appears to be similar to the word retrieval difficulties common in individuals with reading disabilities. Another problem noted in the retrieval process is the inability to inhibit the recall of related but unnecessary information when one is trying to retrieve a specific answer. For example, an individual not only may recall 9 as the answer to 4 + 5, but may also recall 6, the number following the 4-5 sequence, or 20, the product of 4 × 5. Thinking of these extraneous facts slows down the process of getting to the correct answer and increases the chance for error.

Word retrieval difficulties can also impede the effortless retrieval of numbers, letters, and words. German (2001) has described three types of word-finding errors as "slip of the tongue" (recalling the wrong word), "tip of the tongue" (unable to recall the word), and "twist of the tongue" (mispronouncing the target word). An individual manifesting word-finding difficulties is not necessarily lacking "knowledge," but may be unable to retrieve and express that knowledge on demand. Higbee (1993) has distinguished between *available* and *accessible* information. Available information is known and stored. Accessible information is available information that is retrievable. When known information cannot be recalled, a word-finding difficulty is present.

As with word retrieval difficulties, differences in performance on RAN tasks can also be attributed to a variety of cognitive and linguistic processes. Wolf, Bowers, and Biddle (2000) describe serial naming speed as similar to reading because it involves a "combination of rapid, serial processing, and integration of attention, perceptual, conceptual, lexical, and motoric subprocesses" (p. 393). A person may have slow naming speed because of any one, or several of, the multiple processes underlying these tasks. Morris and colleagues (1998) have described this specific subtype of reading disability as a "rate deficit." Students with this deficit were impaired on tasks requiring rapid serial naming, but not on measures of phonological awareness. Conceivably, rapid sequential processing is common to naming speed, processing speed, and reading tasks, and slow naming speed reflects a global deficit in the rapid execution of a variety of cognitive processes (Kail, Hall, & Caskey, 1999). What-

ever RAN measures, it may be partially subsumed under the rubric of processing speed (Denckla & Cutting, 1999).

Implications

High performance on associative storage and retrieval tasks suggests that an individual will be successful in learning new information and recalling stored information. Such individuals may learn associations quickly and recall stored facts with ease. Long-term retrieval helps an individual retrieve and demonstrate knowledge. Low performance on this ability suggests that the individual will experience difficulty storing new information and recalling previously learned information. These individuals may have difficulty acquiring phoneme–grapheme knowledge, memorizing math facts, and completing fill-in-the-blank tests that require the precise recall of specific information.

Presently, more is known about RAN than about other associative memory abilities. The best predictive measures of early reading achievement appear to be a combination of letter identification, phonological awareness, and RAN (Adams, 1990; Bishop, 2003). In addition, children with weaknesses in both RAN and phonemic awareness appear to be the most resistant to reading intervention (Wolf & Bowers, 1999). In a recent study, Vaughn, Linan-Thompson, and Hickman (2003) found that low RAN scores were the single best predictor of treatment resistors among second-grade students. Children with only naming speed deficits (no weaknesses in phonological awareness) are characterized by problems in word identification, fluency, and comprehension (Wolf, Bowers, & Biddle, 2000). Although future research is likely to confirm the exact processes involved in RAN tasks, students with naming deficits appear to have a poorer prognosis for reading success than do other subgroups (Korhonen, 1991). Denckla (1979) described these students as a "hard-to-learn" group.

Although the double-deficit theory attempts to explain two cognitive correlates of reading failure, poor phonological awareness and slow naming speed are not the only tasks that differentiate poor readers from good readers. For example, Ackerman, Holloway, Youngdahl, and Dykman (2001) found that in addition to these factors, poor readers were lower than normally achieving peers on orthographic tasks, attention ratings, arithmetic achievement, and all Wechsler Intelligence Scale for Children—Third Edition factors except the Perceptual Organization Index. Wolf (1999) has also acknowledged the importance of using multidimensional models for explaining reading difficulties:

> ... this new conceptualization of reading disabilities was ironically, named too quickly. To be sure, double deficit captures the phenomenon of study—that is, the importance of understanding the separate and combined effects of two core deficits—but it fails miserably in redirecting our simultaneous attention as a field to the entire profile of strengths and limitations manifest in children with reading disabilities. Only when we develop truly multi-dimensional models of deficits and strengths will our diagnostic and remedial efforts be best matched to individual children. (p. 23)

Interventions

Individuals with difficulties in associative memory and retrieval will require repeated opportunities and more practice to learn new information. Carroll (1989) suggested: "The degree of learning or achievement is a function of the ratio of the time actually spent on learning to the time needed to learn" (p. 26). Students who have trouble retaining associations require more time to learn. The strategies that may be most useful include limiting the amount of information presented at one time, and using multisensory and meaning-based instructional approaches that help a person make connections and retain new learning. Examples of approaches include verbal rehearsal, active learning, use of manipulatives, and real-life projects. Smith and Rivera (1998) found that demonstration plus a permanent model was an effective strategy for helping children master computational mathematics, especially learning math skills and organizing and remembering the sequence of multistep algorithms. In addition, techniques that activate the emotional center of the brain by using humor, dramatizations, or movement can enhance learning (Leamnson, 2000). The most effective strategies help a learner form associations between new and learned information by activating prior knowledge, so that the learning of new information occurs in the context of what the learner already knows (Marzano, 1992).

Another helpful method to facilitate recall is instruction in the use of mnemonic strategies. For example, the *keyword* method involves associating new words to visual images to help students recall word meanings and learn new vocabulary (Mastropieri, 1988). Three steps are used: *recoding, relating*, and *retrieving*. For recoding, students change the new vocabulary word into a known word, the keyword, which has a similar sound and is easily pictured. For relating, students associate the keyword with the definition of the new vocabulary word through a mental image or a sentence. For retrieving, students think of the keyword, remember the association, and then retrieve the definition.

Specific programs that address the challenges imposed by slow rapid naming times are also under development. For example, Wolf, Miller, and Donnelly (2000) describe the RAVE-O program, which emphasizes fluency through rapid recognition of the most frequent orthographic multiletter patterns in the language.

Visual–Spatial Thinking

Many intelligence tests include visual–spatial tasks because they are inherently less verbal in nature. Carroll (1993) described broad *visual–spatial ability* as including the narrow abilities of *spatial relations, visualization, visual memory, closure speed, spatial scanning*, and a number of others that are not typically included on intelligence tests. Thus a wide range of these abilities exists, and they emphasize the processes of image generation, storage, retrieval, and transformation (Lohman, 1994).

Results from current research do not indicate a strong relationship between visual–spatial abilities and academic performance (Ackerman et al., 2001; Flanagan et al., 2002; McGrew & Flanagan, 1998). This is not to say that such abilities are unimportant to academic success. Clearly, spelling involves a visual component of retrieving a mental image of the word to spell, but the visual–spatial tasks on intelligence measures have little relationship with spelling competence (Liberman, Rubin, Duques, & Carlisle, 1985; Sweeney & Rourke, 1985; Vellutino, 1979). This lack of correlation is probably found because the types of visual–spatial tasks traditionally included on intelligence tests, such as manipulating patterns, assembling objects, or noting visual details in pictures, differ from the types of visual–orthographic processing abilities that are required for efficient reading and spelling. Visual–spatial abilities are often three-dimensional in nature, and should therefore not be confused with the orthographic processing abilities that include the visual representations of the writing system (Berninger, 1990).

Visual–spatial thinking abilities do appear, however, to be somewhat related to math performance. Children with math disabilities appear to have difficulties in visual memory and visual–spatial working memory (Fletcher, 1985; McLean & Hitch, 1999). Rourke and Finlayson (1978) found that students with math disabilities scored lower on measures of visual-perceptual and visual–spatial ability than students who had comorbid math and reading disabilities. Still others have suggested that visual–spatial abilities are related to performance on higher-level mathematics, but not to basic math skills (Flanagan et al., 2002).

Reasons for Differences in Performance

Several factors can influence performance on visual–spatial tasks. One consideration is identifying the many narrow abilities that are typically measured by such tasks. For example, an individual may have strengths in visual memory of objects, but weaknesses in spatial relations. Other factors, such as speed (on timed visual–spatial tasks), attention, motivation, and working memory, can influence performance. Problems in visual–motor coordination can also affect performance on timed visual–spatial tasks that involve the use of manipulatives, such as moving and assembling blocks or puzzle pieces.

Implications

Strengths or weaknesses in visual–spatial ability as measured by current intelligence tests do not appear to lead to specific recommendations for instruction. For example, it

would be erroneous to conclude that a student with high scores on visual–spatial tasks would benefit from a sight word approach to teaching reading, or that a student with low scores would benefit from a phonics approach to reading instruction. Many individuals, including those in clinical groups, demonstrate average scores on visual–spatial tasks with simultaneous low achievement. For example, Dean and Woodcock (1999) found that visual processing was one of the highest scores in two clinical groups: individuals with learning disorders and those with language disorders. Furthermore, visual processing scores do not differentiate between college students with and without LD (McGrew & Woodcock, 2001). In many children with reading disabilities, visual–spatial skills are better developed than other abilities (Fletcher et al., 1995). These findings provide further evidence that visual processing abilities remain relatively intact in clinical groups, and therefore are not good predictors of academic performance.

Although much of the emphasis in the field of learning disabilities has been placed on students who struggle with the acquisition and use of spoken and written language, a smaller subset of students evidence symptoms characteristic of what have been referred to as *nonverbal learning disabilities* (NVLD). Two major characteristics of NVLD are poor spatial organization and inattention to visual details—abilities related to visual–spatial thinking. In addition, many students with NVLD are poorly organized and appear unfocused. Although they may be described as inattentive and distractible, these observed behaviors result from a reduced capacity for self-directed behavior, rather than from poor attention (Fletcher et al., 1995). A student with NVLD often has strengths in word decoding, spelling, and rote memory, but encounters extreme difficulty with reading comprehension, computational arithmetic, and mathematical problem solving (Rourke, 1995). The student may also have social difficulties, find reasoning difficult, and struggle to acquire new skills, particularly motor skills. Difficulties in dealing with novel and complex materials are especially evident. Since a large proportion of the communication in an average conversation is nonverbal in nature, a student with NVLD may also miss information about what is being communicated, and then may be unsure of how to respond (Rothenberg, 1998). Because a student with NVLD has early strengths in the development of general declarative knowledge and vocabulary, identification of problems tends to occur in later grades. As the student moves through school, tasks that require higher-level spatial–analytic abilities, such as writing themes and problem solving, become increasingly difficult. Thus, when considered in an educational setting, measures of visual–spatial thinking may be most useful for documenting strengths and identifying students with NVLD.

Interventions

For individuals with strengths in visual–spatial abilities, teachers may enhance the student's performance by instruction with pictures, diagrams, or graphic organizers. Color coding may also be useful to illustrate steps or highlight important information. Individuals with strengths in visual–spatial thinking often excel in tasks such as visualizing and drawing three-dimensional objects. Furthermore, teaching specific learning strategies, such as the use of imagery, graphic organizers, and puzzles, may significantly improve less skilled individuals' performances on visual–spatial tasks. Another strategy, verbal labeling, uses language to describe visual forms as they are manipulated and represented spatially (Kibel, 1992).

In general, students with NVLD benefit when interventions are highly concrete and as verbal as possible. Prior to the introduction of new information or skills, students need to feel in control of the environment. The most effective methods are highly structured and provide external guidance. Expectations may need to be simplified, broken down, or modified. A student with NVLD benefits from consistency and predictability, so relatively static learning environments are often best. Because verbal abilities are typically unimpaired, teaching the student how to use self-talk to reinforce routines or procedures can help with the completion of simple as well as more complex tasks. Rourke (1995) recommends using a "part-to-whole" verbal teaching approach by presenting information in a logical sequence, one step at a time, so that the student can pay attention to details. The guiding principles for treating

children with NVLD are that interventions should be verbal, highly concrete, and systematic, and should reinforce organization and structure (Fletcher et al., 1995).

Processing Speed

One commonly identified characteristic of intelligent behavior is mental quickness (Nettelbeck, 1994). *Processing speed* is the ability to perform simple cognitive tasks quickly and fluently over a sustained period of time. McGrew and Flanagan (1998) define processing speed as the ability to perform cognitive tasks automatically, especially when under pressure to maintain focused attention and concentration; they state that "attentive speediness" encapsulates the essence of processing speed. From an information-processing perspective, speediness and automaticity of processing underlie efficient performance (Kail, 1991; Lohman, 1989). Processing information quickly frees up limited resources so that higher-level thinking can occur.

Perceptual speed is a narrow ability of processing speed; Carroll (1993) describes it as the ability to search for and compare visual symbols. This ability is strongly related to reading achievement throughout the elementary school years (McGrew et al., 1997), math achievement throughout the elementary school years and into adulthood (McGrew & Hessler, 1995), and writing achievement (McGrew & Knopik, 1993; Williams, Zolten, Rickert, Spence, & Ashcraft, 1993). Thus the ability to process symbols rapidly is strongly related to academic performance, particularly in the elementary school years. In a study investigating the differences between normally achieving readers and those with reading disabilities, the rate of visual processing was slower for students with reading disabilities (Kruk & Willows, 2001).

Reasons for Differences in Performance

When an evaluator is considering a person's performance on processing speed tasks, several additional factors need to be considered. Performance on these tasks can be affected by motivation and attention. Personality style can also affect performance on speeded tasks, as can cultural differences. Some cultures do not value speeded performance as an important behavioral attribute. In general, individuals who are reflective will work more slowly, carefully reviewing their options before responding. Some gifted individuals exhibit a relative weakness on speeded tasks, because they reflect and check answers before making a decision. In contrast, individuals who are impulsive may work quickly and carelessly.

Implications

High performance on processing speed tasks indicates that a person is able to process information quickly, freeing up resources for higher-level thinking. Low performance on processing speed tasks suggests that the person may process visual symbols slowly or be inattentive. A distinction exists between *automatic* and *conceptual* processing (Schneider & Shiffrin, 1977). The automatic processes require little attentional resources, whereas the conceptual processes are controlled and require the application of knowledge and strategies. Processing speed appears to be most closely related to the lower-order academic tasks that become increasingly automatic with repeated practice, such as reading words quickly, knowing multiplication facts, or spelling words with accuracy. Although processing speed weaknesses appear to be related to reading disabilities, the relationship is not fully understood at this time. Two consistent findings have emerged, however, from the research on individuals with LD: (1) Individuals both with and without LD exhibit a range of responses on a variety of speeded tasks, and the intercorrelations between different speeded tasks often differ for both groups; and (2) individuals with LD typically obtain lower scores than normally achieving individuals on a variety of speeded tasks (Ofiesh, Mather, & Russell, in press).

Thus the issue of extended time has particular relevance for students with reading disabilities. In considering the provision of time accommodations on exams, Kelman and Lester (1997) advise educational authorities to consider whether or not speed is a genuine academic virtue in the particular context. If not, the test should be untimed. In the very few cases where speed is judged to be necessary, no one should be provided accommodations.

Interventions

Individuals with slow processing speed will often require specific accommodations, particularly when measures of reading rate and academic fluency are compromised as well. These individuals may need extended time, as well as shortened directions and assignments. They may also benefit from instructional interventions designed to increase reading rate and fluency.

To date, one study has explored the relationship between extended test time and processing speed (Ofiesh, 2000). Results indicated that the Visual Matching and Cross Out tests of the Woodcock–Johnson Psycho-Educational Battery—Revised Tests of Cognitive Ability (Woodcock & Johnson, 1989) were fair indicators of the need for extended time, and that the Digit Symbol test of the Wechsler Adult Intelligence Scale—Revised (Wechsler, 1981) was not. Additional research regarding the relationship between specific speeded tests and the need for extended test time could help evaluators justify recommendations and provide a rationale for the need for the accommodation of extended time (Ofiesh et al., in press).

Fluid Reasoning

Fluid reasoning involves the ability to solve novel problems using inductive or deductive reasoning. A number of intelligence tests include fluid reasoning tasks, such as matrices, sequences, or analogies.

Some individuals with LD tend to have great difficulties in abstracting principles from experiences (Geary, 1993; Swanson, 1987). Parmar, Cawley, and Frazita (1996) found that the performance of individuals with math disabilities declined differentially when irrelevant information was included in the word problems. Some students with reading and math disabilities appear to struggle with making generalizations (Ackerman & Dykman, 1995). These inferential reasoning difficulties then interfere with an individual's ability to "classify an event as belonging to a category" (Bruner, 1971, p. 93), and thereby affect success at mathematical problem solving. Unfortunately, little is known about the breadth, depth, and course of the developmental and generalization capabilities of children (Pressley & Woloshyn, 1995), but a growing body of research indicates that poor inferential reasoning is one cause of reading comprehension problems (Wise & Snyder, 2001).

Reasons for Differences in Performance

Performance on fluid reasoning tasks may vary for a number of reasons. One reason is the use of effective strategies. Results from one study indicated that high achievers are more attentive and use more effective strategies (e.g., talking through a task) that help them learn and practice the task at hand, whereas low achievers use less effective strategies for task completion (e.g., guessing, carelessness, attending to inappropriate contextual clues) (Anderson, Brubaker, Alleman-Brooks, & Duffy, 1985).

Another reason for differences in performance is mental flexibility. Individuals who have mental flexibility are able to anticipate what is expected on a task and change the approach when needed, resulting in more successful outcomes (Kronick, 1988). In contrast, individuals with rigid cognitive styles may be unable to use their knowledge except when the context closely resembles the original learning situation (Westman, 1996). Performance can also vary, depending upon the type of reasoning task. Some tasks require reasoning with language (e.g., analogies), whereas others require nonverbal problem solving (e.g., matrices).

Implications

Individuals with high performance on fluid reasoning tasks are likely to succeed in higher-level thinking tasks, such as those involved in math reasoning or reading comprehension. They will typically display mental flexibility when approaching problem-solving tasks, shifting strategies to accomplish their goalls. Individuals with low performance on fluid reasoning tasks are more likely to experience difficulty with higher-level thinking tasks. They may display rigidity when attempting new things and continue to apply a strategy that does not work.

Interventions

Extending and refining knowledge requires examining it in a deeper, more analytical way by doing such things as comparing, classifying, inducing, deducing, analyzing errors, constructing support, abstracting, and analyzing perspectives (Marzano, 1992). These types of thinking skills require that the brain uses multiple and complex systems of retrieval and integration (Lowery, 1998). Experiential learning appears to activate the area of the brain responsible for higher-order thinking (Sousa, 1998). Therefore, instruction that combines physical activities with problem-solving tasks can help connect the motor cortex with the frontal lobes, where thinking occurs, and can thus increase memory and learning (Kandel & Squire, 2000). Learning can be demonstrated in multiple ways, such as dramatizations, experiments, visual displays, music, or inventions.

Providing opportunities for individuals to develop their metacognitive skills and higher-order thinking skills is important; such opportunities may include engaging in reflective discussions about the lessons or using thought journals. Teaching students to use self-questioning techniques, identify main ideas and themes, classify and categorize objects, attend to organizational cues, and implement strategies can lead to significant gains in inferential skills. Strategy instruction—that is, teaching individuals how to learn—has also proven to be effective in improving the performance and achievement of students with LD (e.g., Deshler, Ellis, & Lenz, 1996; Pressley & Woloshyn, 1995). This type of instruction appears to be more effective for higher-order, conceptual tasks than for lower-order tasks (Deshler et al., 1996).

CONCLUSION

If the same instructional approaches are used with all students, regardless of individual differences, the available resources should not be consumed by evaluating intellectual and cognitive abilities. In discussing the assessment of intellectual functioning, Wasserman (2003) indicates that one of applied psychology's biggest failures of the 20th century is that intellectual assessments have not been systematically linked to effective interventions. He notes, however, that reasons exist for guarded optimism, because some of the newer remedial programs use principles derived from cognitive instruction. First, however, changes are needed in fundamental assessment paradigms. Wasserman states: "Challenges to conventional thinking in intelligence assessment have laid the groundwork for a paradigm shift, and . . . new tests delivering additional applied value to the practitioner have the greatest likelihood of success in the future" (2003, p. 438). These tests should help evaluators identify the impaired cognitive abilities that contribute to learning problems, assess how the test scores fit with those of diagnostic groups who have similar patterns of learning problems, and prescribe interventions that have been demonstrated to be effective with children who have similar test score profiles.

A child with LD has a psychological processing disorder (Hale et al., 2004). This disorder then affects and inhibits some aspect of academic performance. Fortunately, research continues to document and increase our understandings of the relationships among various cognitive abilities and achievement. When used by skilled clinicians, results from intelligence tests can contribute to diagnostic hypotheses that then are reaffirmed or rejected, depending upon additional observations and information. To reiterate Stern's (1938) advice, the determination of appropriate conclusions requires intensive, qualitative study. Modern tests of intelligence and cognitive abilities, as well as modern views of cognitive processing, can help us identify and plan interventions for students with LD if we (1) look beyond global scores to specific cognitive abilities that have established relationships to achievement; (2) identify and address problems at an early age; and (3) implement effective, differentiated instruction. If we follow these principles, these evaluations can provide important information that helps us understand the nature and severity of the learning disability. Based upon our diagnostic conclusions, we can then select the interventions that will be the most effective.

REFERENCES

Aaron, P. G. (1997). The impending demise of the discrepancy formula. *Review of Educational Research, 67,* 461–502.

Ackerman, P. T., & Dykman, R. A. (1995). Reading-disabled students with and without comorbid arithmetic disability. *Developmental Neuropsychology, 11,* 351–371.

Ackerman, P. T., Holloway, C. A., Youngdahl, P. L., & Dykman, R. A. (2001). The double-deficit theory of reading disability does not fit all. *Learning Disabilities Research and Practice, 16,* 152–160.

Adams, M. J. (1990). *Beginning to read: Thinking and learning about print.* Cambridge, MA: MIT Press.

American Educational Research Association, American Psychological Association, & National Council on Measurement in Education. (1999). *Standards for educational and psychological testing.* Washington, DC: American Educational Research Association.

Anastasi, A. (1988). *Psychological testing* (6th ed.). New York: Macmillan.

Anderson, L. M., Brubaker, N. L., Alleman-Brooks, J., & Duffy, G. S. (1985). A qualitative study of seatwork in first-grade classrooms. *Elementary School Journal, 86,* 123–140.

Ashcraft, M. H. (1987). Children's knowledge of simple arithmetic: A developmental model and simulation. In J. Bisanz, C. J. Brainerd, & R. Kail (Eds.), *Formal methods in developmental psychology: Progress in cognitive developmental research* (pp. 302–338). New York: Springer-Verlag.

Ashcraft, M. H. (1992). Cognitive arithmetic: A review of data and theory. *Cognition, 44,* 75–106.

Ashcraft, M. H., & Kirk, E. P. (2001). The relationships among working memory, math anxiety, and performance. *Journal of Experimental Psychology: General, 130,* 224–237.

Baddeley, A. D. (1986). *Working memory.* New York: Oxford University Press.

Baddeley, A. D. (1990). *Human memory: Theory and practice.* Boston: Allyn & Bacon.

Beck, I. L., Perfetti, C. A., & McKeown, M. G. (1982). The effects of long-term vocabulary instruction on lexical access and reading comprehension. *Journal of Educational Psychology, 74,* 506–521.

Bell, L. C., & Perfetti, C. A. (1994). Reading skill: Some adult comparisons. *Journal of Educational Psychology, 86,* 244–255.

Benbow, C. P., & Lubinski, D. (Eds.). (1996). *Intellectual talent: Psychometric and social issues.* Baltimore: Johns Hopkins University Press.

Berninger, V. W. (1990). Multiple orthographic codes: Key to alternative instructional methodologies for developing orthographic phonological connections underlying word identification. *School Psychology Review, 19,* 518–533.

Berninger, V. W. (1996). *Reading and writing acquisi-*

tion: *A developmental neuropsychological perspective*. Boulder, CO: Westview Press.

Berninger, V. W. (2001). Understanding the "lexia" in dyslexia: A multidisciplinary team approach to learning disabilities. *Annals of Dyslexia, 51,* 23–48.

Berninger, V. W., & Abbott, R. D. (1994). Redefining learning disabilities: Moving beyond aptitude–achievement discrepancies to failure to respond to validated treatment protocols. In G. R. Lyon (Ed.), *Frames of reference for the assessment of learning disabilities: New views on measurement issues* (pp. 163–183). Baltimore: Brookes.

Bishop, A. G. (2003). Prediction of first-grade reading achievement: A comparison of fall and winter kindergarten screenings. *Learning Disability Quarterly, 26,* 189–200.

Bowers, P. G., Sunseth, K., & Golden, J. (1999). The route between rapid naming and reading progress. *Scientific Studies of Reading, 3,* 31–53.

Bowers, P. G., & Wolf, M. (1993). Theoretical links between naming speed, precise timing mechanisms, and orthographic skill in dyslexia. *Reading and Writing: An Interdisciplinary Journal, 5,* 69–85.

Bruner, J. S. (1971). *The relevance of education.* New York: Norton.

Buchel, C., Coull, J. T., & Friston, K. J. (1999). The predictive value of changes in effective connectivity for human learning. *Science, 283,* 1538–1541.

Carlisle, J. F., & Rice, M. S. (2002). *Improving reading comprehension: Research-based principles and practices.* Baltimore: York Press.

Carroll, J. B. (1989). Factor analysis since Spearman: Where do we stand? What do we know? In R. Kanfer, P. L. Ackerman, & R. Cudeck (Eds.), *Abilities, motivation, and methodology* (pp. 43–67). Hillsdale, NJ: Erlbaum.

Carroll, J. B. (1993). *Human cognitive abilities: A survey of factor-analytic studies.* New York: Cambridge University Press.

Coltheart, M. (Ed.). (1987). *Attention and performance XII: The psychology of reading.* Hove, UK: Erlbaum.

Cruickshank, W. M. (1977). Least-restrictive placement: Administrative wishful thinking. *Journal of Learning Disabilities, 10,* 193–194.

Cunningham, A. E., Stanovich, K. E., & Wilson, M. R. (1990). Cognitive variation in adult college students differing in reading ability. In T. H. Carr & B. A. Levy (Eds.), *Reading and its development: Component skills approaches* (pp. 129–159). San Diego, CA: Academic Press.

Daneman, M., & Carpenter, P. A. (1980). Individual differences in working memory and reading. *Journal of Verbal Learning and Verbal Behavior, 19,* 450–466.

Daneman, M., & Green, I. (1986). Individual differences in comprehending and producing words in context. *Journal of Memory and Language, 25,* 1–18.

Daneman, M., & Tardif, T. (1987). Working memory and reading skill re-examined. In M. Coltheart (Ed.), *Attention and performance XII: The psychology of reading* (pp. 491–508). Hove, UK: Erlbaum.

Dean, R. S., & Woodcock, R. W. (1999). *The WJ-R and Bateria-R in neuropsychological assessment* (Research Report No. 3). Itasca, IL: Riverside.

Denckla, M. B. (1979). Childhood learning disabilities. In K. M. Heilman & E. Valenstein (Eds.), *Clinical neuropsychology* (pp. 535–573). New York: Oxford University Press.

Denckla, M. B., & Cutting, L. E. (1999). History and significance of rapid automatized naming. *Annals of Dyslexia, 49,* 29–42.

Denckla, M. B., & Rudel, R. (1974). Rapid automatized naming of pictured objects, colors, letters and numbers by normal children. *Cortex, 10,* 186–202.

Deshler, D. D., Ellis, E. S., & Lenz, B. K. (1996). *Teaching adolescents with learning disabilities: Strategies and methods* (2nd ed). Denver, CO: Love.

Ehri, L. C. (1998). Grapheme–phoneme knowledge is essential for learning to read words in English. In J. L. Metsala & L. C. Ehri (Eds.), *Word recognition in beginning literacy* (pp. 3–40). Mahwah, NJ: Erlbaum.

Engle, R. W., Tuholski, S. W., Laughlin, J. E., & Conway, A. R. A. (1999). Working memory, short-term memory, and general fluid intelligence: A latent-variable approach. *Journal of Experimental Psychology: General, 128,* 309–331.

Evans, J. J., Floyd, R. G., McGrew, K. S., & Leforgee, M. H. (2002). The relations between measures of Cattell–Horn–Carroll (CHC) cognitive abilities and reading achievement during childhood and adolescence, *School Psychology Review, 31,* 246–262.

Flanagan, D. P., Ortiz, S. O., Alfonso, V. C., & Mascolo, J. T. (2002). *The achievement test desk reference (ATDR): Comprehensive assessment of learning disabilities.* Boston: Allyn & Bacon.

Fletcher, J. M. (1985). Memory for verbal and nonverbal stimuli in learning disabilities subgroups: Analysis by selective reminding. *Journal of Experimental Child Psychology, 40,* 244–259.

Fletcher, J. M., & Foorman, B. R. (1994). Issues in the definition and measurement of learning disabilities: The need for early intervention. In G. R. Lyon (Ed.), *Frames of reference for the assessment of learning disabilities: New views on measurement issues* (pp. 185–200). Baltimore: Brookes.

Fletcher, J. M., Francis, D. J., Shaywitz, S. E., Lyon, G. R., Foorman, B. R., Stuebing, K. K., et al. (1998). Intelligent testing and the discrepancy model for children with learning disabilities. *Learning Disabilities Research & Practice, 13,* 186–203.

Fletcher, J. M., Lyon, G. R., Barnes, M., Stuebing, K. K., Francis, D. J., Olson, R. K., et al. (2001, August). *Classification of learning disabilities: An evidence-based evaluation.* Paper presented at the U.S. Department of Education LD Summit, Washington, DC.

Fletcher, J. M., Taylor, H. G., Levin, H. S., & Satz, P. (1995). Neuropsychological and intellectual assessment of children. In H. Kaplan & B. Sadock (Eds.), *Comprehensive textbook of psychiatry* (pp. 581–601). Baltimore: Williams & Wilkins.

Floyd, R. G., Evans, J. J., & McGrew, K. S. (2003). Relations between measures of Cattell–Horn–Carroll (CHC) cognitive abilities and mathematics achievement across the school-age years. *Psychology in the Schools, 60,* 155–171.

Flowers, L., Meyer, M., Lovato, J., Wood, F., & Felton, R. (2000). Does third grade discrepancy status predict the course of reading development? *Annals of Dyslexia, 50,* 49–71.

Francis, D. J., Shaywitz, S. E., Stuebing, K. K., Shaywitz, B. A., & Fletcher, J. M. (1996). Developmental lag versus deficit models of reading disability: A longitudinal, individual growth curves study. *Journal of Educational Psychology, 88,* 3–17

Frost, J. A., & Emery, M. J. (1995, August). *Academic interventions for children with dyslexia who have phonological core deficits.* Reston, VA: Council for Exceptional Children. (ERIC Digest No. 539)

Fuchs, D., Mock, D., Morgan, P. L., & Young, C. L. (2003). Responsiveness to intervention: Definitions, evidence, and implications for the learning disabilities construct. *Learning Disabilities Research & Practice, 18,* 157–171.

Gardner, H. (1999). *Reframing intelligence.* New York: Basic Books.

Gathercole, S. E., & Baddeley, A. D. (1993). Phonological working memory: A critical building block for reading development and vocabulary acquisition. *European Journal of Psychology, 8,* 259–272.

Geary, D. C. (1993). Mathematical disabilities: Cognitive, neuropsychological, and genetic components. *Psychological Bulletin, 114,* 345–362.

Geary, D. C. (1996). *Children's mathematical development: Research and practical application.* Washington, DC: American Psychological Association.

German, D. J. (2001). *It's on the tip of my tongue.* Chicago: Word Finding Materials.

Geschwind, N. (1965). Disconnection syndrome in animals and man (Parts I, II). *Brain, 88,* 237–294, 585–644.

Glutting, J. J., McDermott, P. A., & Konold, T. R. (1997). Ontology, structure, and diagnostic benefits of a normative subtest taxonomy from the WISC-III standardization sample. In D. P. Flanagan, J. L. Genshaft, & P. L Harrison (Eds.), *Contemporary intellectual assessment: Theories, tests, and issues* (pp. 349–372). New York: Guilford Press.

Good, R. H., Vollmer, M., Creek, R. J., Katz, L., & Chowdhri, S. (1993). Treatment utility of the Kaufman Assessment Battery for Children: Effects of matching instruction and student processing strength. *School Psychology Review, 22,* 8–26.

Goswami, U., & Bryant, P. (1990). *Phonological skills and learning to read.* Hove, UK: Erlbaum.

Gough, P. B. (1996). How children learn to read and why they fail. *Annals of Dyslexia, 46,* 3–20.

Gough, P. B., & Tunmer, W. E. (1986). Decoding, reading, and reading disability. *Remedial and Special Education, 7,* 6–10.

Gould, B. W. (2001). Curricular strategies for written expression. In A. M. Bain, L. L. Bailet, & L. C. Moats (Eds.), *Written language disorders: Theory into practice* (2nd ed., pp.185–220), Austin, TX: PRO-ED.

Gregg, N., Davis, M., Coleman, C., Wisenbaker, J., & Hoy, C. (2004). *Implications for accommodation decisions at the postsecondary level.* Unpublished manuscript, University of Georgia.

Hale, J. B., Fiorello, C. A., Kavanagh, J. A., Hoeppner, J. B., & Gaitherer, R. A. (2001). WISC-III predictors of academic achievement for children with learning disabilities: Are global and factor scores comparable? *School Psychology Quarterly, 16*(1), 31–35.

Hale, J. B., Naglieri, J. A., Kaufman, A. S., & Kavale, K. A. (2004). Specific learning disability classifications in the new Individuals with Disabilities Education Act: The danger of good ideas. *The School Psychologist, 58*(1), 6–29.

Hannon, B., & Daneman, M. (2001). A new tool for measuring and understanding individual differences in the component processes of reading comprehension. *Journal of Educational Psychology, 93*(1), 103–128.

Heller, K., Holtzman, W., & Messick, S. (Eds.). (1982). *Placing children in special education: A strategy for equity.* Washington, DC: National Academy Press.

Higbee, K. L. (1993). *Your memory, how it works and how you improve it.* New York: Paragon House.

Holmes, V. M., & Castles, A. E. (2001). Unexpectedly poor spelling in university students. *Scientific Studies of Reading, 5,* 319–350.

Horn, J. L. (1991). Measurement of intellectual capabilities: A review of theory. In K. S. McGrew, J. K. Werder, & R. W. Woodcock, *WJ-R technical manual* (pp. 197–232). Itasca, IL: Riverside.

Hulme, C. (1981). *Reading retardation and multisensory teaching.* London: Routledge & Kegan Paul.

Hunt, E. (2000). Let's hear it for crystallized intelligence. *Learning and Individual Differences, 12,* 123–129.

Individuals with Disabilities Education Act Amendments of 1997, Pub. L. No. 105–17, 20 U.S.C. 33, §1400 et seq. (1997).

Jenkins, J., & O'Connor, R. E. (2001, August). *Early identification and intervention for young children.* Paper presented at the U.S. Department of Education LD Summit, Washington, DC.

Jensen, A. R. (1998). *The g factor: The science of mental ability.* Westport, CT: Praeger.

Johnson, D. J. (1993). Relationship between oral and written language. *School Psychology Review, 22,* 595–609.

Joyce, B., Weil, M., & Showers, B. (1992). *Models of teaching* (4th ed.). Needham Heights, MA: Allyn & Bacon.

Just, M. A., & Carpenter, P. A. (1992). A capacity theory of comprehension: Individual differences in working memory. *Psychological Review, 99,* 122–149.

Kail, R. (1991). Developmental change in speed of processing during childhood and adolescence. *Psychological Bulletin, 109,* 490–501.

Kail, R., Hall, L. K., & Caskey, B. J. (1999). Processing speed, exposure to print, and naming speed. *Applied Psycholinguistics, 20,* 303–314.

Kandel, E. R., & Squire, L. R. (2000). Neuroscience: Breaking down scientific barriers to the study of brain and mind. *Science, 290,* 1113–1120.

Kavale, K. A., & Forness, S. R. (1995). *The nature of learning disabilities: Critical elements of diagnosis and classification.* Hillsdale, NJ: Erlbaum.

Kavale, K. A., & Forness, S. R. (1998). The politics of learning disabilities. *Learning Disability Quarterly, 21,* 245–273.

Kelman, M., & Lester, G. (1997). *Jumping the queue: An inquiry into the legal treatment of students with learning disabilities.* Cambridge, MA: Harvard University Press.

Kibel, M. (1992). Linking language to action. In T. R. Miles & E. Miles (Eds.), *Dyslexia and mathematics* (pp. 42–57). London: Routledge.

King, J., & Just, M. A. (1991). Individual differences in syntactic processing: The role of working memory. *Journal of Memory and Language, 30,* 580–602.

Korhonen, T. T. (1991). Neuropsychological stability and prognosis of subgroups of children with learning disabilities. *Journal of Learning Disabilities, 24,* 48–57.

Kronick, D. (1988). *New approaches to learning disabilities: Cognitive, metacognitive, and holistic.* Philadelphia: Grune & Stratton.

Kruk, R. S., & Willows, D. M. (2001). Backward pattern masking of familiar and unfamiliar materials in disabled and normal readers. *Cognitive Neuropsychology, 18*(1), 19–37.

Kyllonen, P. C., & Christal, R. E. (1990). Reasoning ability is (little more than) working memory capacity?! *Intelligence, 14,* 389–433.

Leamnson, R. (2000). Learning as biological brain change. *Change, 32*(6), 34–40.

Lehto, J. (1996). Working memory capacity and summarizing skills in ninth graders. *Scandinavian Journal of Psychology, 37*(1), 84–92.

Liberman, I. Y., Rubin, H., Duques, S., & Carlisle, J. (1985). Linguistic abilities and spelling proficiency in kindergartners and adult poor spellers. In D. B. Gray & J. F. Kavanaugh (Eds.), *Biobehavioral measures of dyslexia* (pp. 163–176). Parkton, MD: York Press.

Light, J. G., & DeFries, J. C. (1995). Comorbidity of reading and mathematics disabilities; Genetic and environmental etiologies. *Journal of Learning Disabilities, 28,* 96–106.

Logie, R. H., Gilhooly, K. J., & Wynn, C. (1994).

Counting on working memory in arithmetic problem solving. *Memory and Cognition, 21,* 11–22.

Lohman, D. F. (1989). Human intelligence: An introduction to advances in theory and research. *Review of Educational Research, 59,* 333–373.

Lohman, D. F. (1994). Spatial ability. In R. J. Sternberg (Ed.), *Encyclopedia of human intelligence* (pp. 1000–1007). New York: Macmillan.

Lowery, L. (1998). How new science curriculums reflect brain research. *Educational Leadership, 56*(3), 26–30.

Lyon, G. R. (1995). Toward a definition of dyslexia. *Annals of Dyslexia, 45,* 3–27.

Lyon, G. R. (1996). State of research. In S. Cramer & W. Ellis (Eds.), *Learning disabilities: Lifelong issues* (pp. 3–61). Baltimore: Brookes.

Lyon, G. R. (1998). Why reading is not natural. *Educational Leadership, 3,* 14–18.

Manis, F. R., Seidenberg, M. S., & Doi, L. M. (1999). See Dick RAN: Rapid naming and the longitudinal prediction of reading subskills in first and second graders. *Scientific Studies of Reading, 3,* 129–157.

Manis, F. R., Seidenberg, M. S., Stallings, L., Joanisse, M., Bailey, C., Freedman, L., et al. (1999). Development of dyslexic subgroups: A one-year follow up. *Annals of Dyslexia, 49,* 105–134.

Marzano, R. J. (1992). *A different kind of classroom: Teaching with dimensions of learning.* Alexandria, VA: Association for Supervision and Curriculum Development.

Mastropieri, M. A. (1988). Using the keyboard (*sic*) method. *Teaching Exceptional Children, 20*(2), 4–8.

Mastropieri, M. A., Scruggs, T. E., & Shiah, S. (1991). Mathematics instruction for learning disabled students: A review of the research. *Learning Disabilities Research & Practice, 6,* 89–98.

Mather, N., & Healey, W. C. (1990). Deposing aptitude–achievement discrepancy as the imperial criterion for learning disabilities. *Learning Disabilities: A Multidisciplinary Journal, 1*(2), 40–48.

McCardle, P., Scarborough, H. S., & Catts, H. W. (2001). Predicting, explaining, and preventing children's reading difficulties. *Learning Disabilities Research and Practice, 16,* 230–239.

McGrew, K. S., & Flanagan, D. P. (1998). *The intelligence test desk reference (ITDR): Gf-Gc cross-battery assessment.* Needham Heights, MA: Allyn & Bacon.

McGrew, K. S., Flanagan, D. P., Keith, T. Z., & Vanderwood, M. (1997). Beyond g: The impact of Gf-Gc specific cognitive abilities research on the future use and interpretation of intelligence tests in the schools. *School Psychology Review, 26,* 177–189.

McGrew, K. S., & Hessler, G. L. (1995). The relationship between the WJ-R Gf-Gc cognitive clusters and mathematics achievement across the life-span. *Journal of Psychoeducational Assessment, 13,* 21–38.

McGrew, K. S., & Knopik, S. N. (1993). The relationship between the WJ-R Gf-Gc cognitive clusters and writing achievement across the life span. *School Psychology Review, 22*, 687–695.

McGrew, K. S., & Woodcock, R. W. (2001). *Woodcock–Johnson III Technical manual*. Itasca, IL: Riverside.

McLean, J. F., & Hitch, G. J. (1999). Working memory impairments in children with specific arithmetic learning difficulties. *Journal of Experimental Child Psychology, 74*, 240–260.

Messick, S. (1989). Validity. In R. Linn (Ed.), *Educational measurement* (3rd ed., pp. 104–131). Washington, DC: American Council on Education.

Meyer, M. S., & Felton, R. H. (1999). Repeated reading to enhance fluency: Old approaches and new directions. *Annals of Dyslexia, 49*, 283–306.

Meyer, M. S., Wood, F. B., Hart, L. A., & Felton, R. H. (1998). Selective predictive value of rapid automatized naming in poor readers. *Journal of Learning Disabilities, 31*, 106–117.

Miller, G., Galanter, E., & Pribram, K. (1960). *Plans and the structure of behavior*. New York: Holt.

Moats, L. C. (2001). Spelling disability in adolescents and adults. In A. M. Bain, L. L. Bailet, & L. C. Moats (Eds.), *Written language disorders: Theory into practice* (2nd ed., pp. 43–75). Austin, TX: Pro-Ed.

Morris, R. D., Stuebing, K. K., Fletcher, J. M., Shaywitz, S. E., Lyon, G. R., Shankweiler, D. P., et al. (1998). Subtypes of reading disability: Variability around a phonological core. *Journal of Educational Psychology, 90*, 347–373.

Muter, V., Hulme, C., Snowling, M., & Taylor, S. (1997). Segmentation, not rhyming predicts early progress in learning to read. *Journal of Experimental Child Psychology, 65*, 370–398.

National Reading Panel. (2000). *Report of the National Reading Panel: Teaching children to read: An evidence-based assessment of the scientific research literature on reading and its implications for reading instruction*. Washington, DC: National Institute of Child Health and Human Development.

Nettelbeck, T. (1994). Speediness. In R. J. Sternberg (Ed.), *Encyclopedia of human intelligence* (pp. 1014–1019). New York: Macmillan.

Ofiesh, N. S. (2000). Using processing speed tests to predict the benefit of extended test time for university students with learning disabilities. *Journal of Postsecondary Education and Disability, 14*, 39–56.

Ofiesh, N., Mather, N., & Russell, A. (in press). Using speeded cognitive, reading, and academic measures to determine the need for extended test time among university students with learning disabilities. *Journal of Psychoeducational Assessment*.

Ormrod, J. E., & Cochran, K. F. (1988). Relationship of verbal ability and working memory to spelling achievement and learning to spell. *Reading Research and Instruction, 28*, 33–43.

Orton, S. T. (1925). Word-blindness in school children. *Archives of Neurology and Psychiatry, 14*, 581–615.

Parmar, R. S., Cawley, J. R., & Frazita, R. R. (1996). Word problem-solving by students with and without math disabilities. *Exceptional Children, 62*, 415–429.

Perfetti, C. A. (1994). Reading. In R. J. Sternberg (Ed.), *Encyclopedia of human intelligence* (pp. 923–930). New York: Macmillan.

Perfetti, C. A., & Goldman, S. R. (1976). Discourse memory and reading comprehension skill. *Journal of Verbal Learning and Verbal Behavior, 14*, 33–42.

Perfetti, C. A., Marron, M. A., & Foltz, P. W. (1996). Sources of comprehension failure: Theoretical perspectives and case studies. In C. Cornoldi & J. Oakhill (Eds.), *Reading comprehension difficulties: Processes and intervention* (pp. 137–165). Mahwah, NJ: Erlbaum.

President's Commission on Excellence in Special Education. (2002). *A new era: Revitalizing special education for children and their families*. Retrieved from http://www.ed.gov/inits/commissionsboards/whspecialeducation/reports.html

Pressley, M., & Woloshyn, V. (Eds.). (1995). *Cognitive strategy instruction that really improves children's academic performance*. Cambridge, MA: Brookline Books.

Rack, J. P., Snowling, M., & Olson, R. (1992). The nonword reading deficit in developmental dyslexia: A review. *Reading Research Quarterly, 27*, 28–53.

Reid, D. K., Hresko, W. P., & Swanson, H. L. (1996). *Cognitive approaches to learning disabilities*. Austin, TX: PRO-ED.

Reschly, D. J. (1992). Mental retardation: Conceptual foundations, definitional criteria, and diagnostic operations. In S. R. Hooper, G. W. Hynd, & R. E. Mattison (Eds.), *Developmental disorders: Diagnostic criteria and clinical assessment* (pp. 23–67). Hillsdale, NJ: Erlbaum.

Reschly, D. J., & Ysseldyke, J. E. (2002). School psychology paradigm shift. In A. Thomas & J. Grimes (Eds.), *Best practices in school psychology IV* (pp. 17–31). Washington, DC: National Association of School Psychologists.

Reynolds, M. C., & Lakin, K. C. (1987). Noncategorical special education for mildly handicapped students. A system for the future. In M. C. Wang, M. C. Reynolds, & H. J. Walberg (Eds.), *The handbook of special education: Research and practice* (Vol. 1, pp. 331–356). Oxford: Pergamon Press.

Robinson, C. S., Menchetti, B. M., & Torgesen, J. K. (2002). Toward a two-factor theory of one type of mathematics disabilities. *Learning Disabilities Research and Practice, 17*, 81–90.

Rothenberg, S. (1998). Nonverbal learning disabilities and social functioning: How can we help? *Journal of the Learning Disabilities Association of Massachusetts, 8*(4), 10.

Rourke, B. P. (1995). *Syndrome of nonverbal learning disabilities: Neurodevelopmental manifestations*. New York: Guilford Press.

Rourke, B. P., & Finlayson, M. A. L. (1978). Neuropsychological significance of variations in patterns of academic performance: Verbal and visual–spatial abilities. *Journal of Abnormal Child Psychology, 6,* 121–133.

Samuels, S. J. (1979). The method of repeated readings. *Reading Teacher, 32,* 403–408.

Scarborough, H. S. (1998). Predicting the future achievement of second graders with reading disabilities: Contributions of phonemic awareness, verbal memory, rapid naming, and IQ. *Annals of Dyslexia, 48,* 115–136.

Schneider, W., & Shiffrin, R. M. (1977). Controlled and automatic human information processing: Detection, search, and attention. *Psychological Review, 84,* 1–66.

Schumm, J. S., Moody, S. W., & Vaughn, S. (2000). Grouping for reading instruction: Does one size fit all? *Journal of Learning Disabilities, 33,* 477–488.

Semrud-Clikeman, M., Steingard, R. J., Filipeck, P., Biederman, J., Bekken, K., & Renshaw, P. F. (2000). Using MRI to examine brain–behavior relationships in males with attention deficit disorder with hyperactivity. *Journal of the American Academy of Child and Adolescent Psychiatry, 39,* 477–484.

Share, D. L., & Stanovich, K. E. (1995). Cognitive processes in early reading development: Accommodating individual differences into a model of acquisition. *Issues in Education: Contributions from Educational Psychology, 1,* 1–57.

Shaywitz, S. E. (1998). Dyslexia. *New England Journal of Medicine, 338,* 307–312.

Shaywitz, S. E. (2003). *Overcoming dyslexia: A new and complete science-based program for overcoming reading problems at any level.* New York: Knopf.

Shaywitz, S. E., Escobar, M. D., Shaywitz, B. A., Fletcher, J. M., & Makuch, R. (1992). Evidence that dyslexia may represent the lower tail of a normal distribution of reading ability. *New England Journal of Medicine, 326,* 145–150.

Shaywitz, S. E., Shaywitz, B. A., Fulbright, R. K., Skudlarski, P., Mencl, W. E., Constable, R. T., et al. (2003). Neural systems for compensation and persistence: Young adult outcome of childhood reading disability. *Biological Psychiatry, 54,* 25–33.

Shessel, I., & Reiff, H. B. (1999). Experiences of adults with learning disabilities: Positive and negative impacts and outcomes. *Learning Disability Quarterly, 22,* 305–316.

Siegel, L. S., & Ryan, E. B. (1988). Development of grammatical sensitivity, phonological, and short-term memory in normally achieving and learning disabled children. *Developmental Psychology, 24,* 28–37.

Silver, A. A., & Hagin, R. A. (2002). *Disorders of learning in childhood* (2nd ed.). New York: Wiley.

Simpson, R. G., & Buckhalt, J. A. (1990). A non-formula discrepancy model to identify learning disabilities. *School Psychology International, 11,* 273–279.

Smith, D. D., & Rivera, D. P. (1998). Mathematics. In B. Wong (Ed.), *Learning about learning disabilities* (2nd ed., pp. 346–374). San Diego, CA: Academic Press.

Snow, C., Burns, S., & Griffin, P. (1998). *Preventing reading difficulties in young children.* Washington, DC: National Academy Press.

Sousa, D. (1998). Brain research can help principals reform secondary schools. *NASSP Bulletin, 82*(598), 21–28.

Stanovich, K. E. (1986). Matthew effects in reading: Some consequences of individual differences in the acquisition of literacy. *Reading Research Quarterly, 21,* 360–407.

Stanovich, K. E. (1993). The construct validity of discrepancy definitions of reading disability. In G. R. Lyon, D. B. Gray, J. F. Kavanagh, & N. A. Krasnegor (Eds.), *Better understanding learning disabilities: New views from research and their implications for education and public policies* (pp. 273–307). Baltimore: Brookes.

Stanovich, K. E. (1999). The sociopsychometrics of learning disabilities. *Journal of Learning Disabilities, 32,* 350–361.

Stanovich, K. E., & Siegel, L. S. (1994). Phenotypic performance profile of children with reading disabilities: A regression-based test of the phonological–core variable–difference model. *Journal of Educational Psychology, 86,* 24–53.

Strang, R. (1964). *Diagnostic teaching of reading.* New York: McGraw-Hill.

Stern, W. (1938). *General psychology from the personalistic standpoint.* New York: Macmillan.

Swanson, H. L. (1987). Information-processing theory and learning disabilities: An overview. *Journal of Learning Disabilities, 20,* 3–7.

Sweeney, J. E., & Rourke, B. P. (1985). Spelling disability subtypes. In B. P. Rourke (Ed.), *Neuropsychology of learning disabilities: Essentials of subtype analysis* (pp. 133–144). New York: Guilford Press.

Tilly, W. D., Grimes, J. P., & Reschly, D. J. (1993). Special education system reform: The Iowa story. *Communique, 22,* 1–4.

Torgesen, J. K. (1997). The prevention and remediation of reading disabilities: Evaluating what we know from research. *Journal of Academic Language Therapy, 1,* 11–47.

Torgesen, J. K. (1998). Catch them before they fall: Identification and assessment to prevent failure in young children. *American Educator, 22,* 32–39.

U.S. Department of Education. (2000). *Twenty-second annual report to Congress on the implementation of the Individuals with Disabilities Education Act.* Washington, DC: Author.

Vaughn, S., Linan-Thompson, S., & Hickman, P. (2003). Response to instruction as a means of identifying students with reading/learning disabilities. *Exceptional Children, 69,* 391–409.

Vellutino, F. R. (1979). *Dyslexia: Theory and research.* Cambridge, MA: MIT Press.

Vellutino, F. R. (1995). Semantic and phonological coding in poor and normal readers. *Journal of Exceptional Child Psychology, 59,* 76–123.

Vellutino, F. R. (2001). Further analysis of the relationship between reading achievement and intelligence: A response to Naglieri. *Journal of Learning Disabilities, 34*, 306–310.

Vellutino, F. R., Scanlon, D. M., & Lyon, G. R. (2000). Differentiating between difficult-to-remediate and readily remediated poor readers: More evidence against the IQ–achievement discrepancy definition of reading disability. *Journal of Learning Disabilities, 33*, 223–238.

Vygotsky, L. S. (1962). *Thought and language.* Cambridge, MA: MIT Press.

Wagner, R. K., Torgesen, J. K., Laughon, P., Simmons, K., & Rashotte, C. A. (1993). The development of young readers' phonological processing abilities. *Journal of Educational Psychology, 85*, 83–103.

Walberg, H. J., & Tsai, S. (1983). Matthew effects in education. *American Educational Research Journal, 20*, 359–373.

Wasserman, J. D. (2003). Assessment of intellectual functioning. In J. R. Graham & J. A. Naglieri (Eds.), *Handbook of psychology* (pp. 417–442). New York: Wiley.

Wechsler, D. (1981). *Wechsler Adult Intelligence Scale—Revised.* New York: Psychological Corporation.

Westman, J. C. (1996). Concepts of dyslexia. In L. R. Putnam (Ed.), *How to become a better reading teacher: Strategies for assessment and intervention* (pp. 65–73). Englewood Cliffs, NJ: Merrill.

Whitener, E. M. (1989). A meta-analytic review of the effect on learning of the interaction between prior achievement and instructional support. *Review of Educational Research, 59*, 65–86.

Williams, J., Zolten, A. J., Rickert, V. I., Spence, G. T.,

& Ashcraft, E. W. (1993). Use of nonverbal tests to screen for writing dysfluency in school-age children. *Perceptual and Motor Skills, 76*, 803–809.

Wilson, K. M., & Swanson, H. L. (2001). Are mathematics disabilities due to a domain-general or a domain-specific working memory deficit? *Journal of Learning Disabilities, 34*, 237–248.

Windfuhr, K. L., & Snowling, M. J. (2001). The relationship between paired associate learning and phonological skills in normally developing readers. *Journal of Experimental Child Psychology, 80*, 160–173.

Wise, B. W., & Snyder, L. (2001, August). *Judgments in identifying and teaching children with language-based reading difficulties.* Paper presented at the U.S. Department of Education LD Summit, Washington, DC.

Wolf, M. (1999). What time may tell: Towards a new conceptualization of developmental dyslexia. *Annals of Dyslexia, 49*, 3–27.

Wolf, M., & Bowers, P. G. (1999). The double-deficit hypothesis for the developmental dyslexias. *Journal of Educational Psychology, 91*, 415–438.

Wolf, M., Bowers, P. G., & Biddle, K. (2000). Naming speed processes, timing, and reading: A conceptual review. *Journal of Learning Disabilities, 33*, 387–407.

Wolf, M., Miller, L., & Donnelly, K. (2000). Retrieval, automaticity, vocabulary, elaboration, orthography (RAVE-O): A comprehensive, fluency-based reading intervention program. *Journal of Learning Disabilities, 33*, 375–386.

Woodcock, R. W., & Johnson, M. B. (1989). *Woodcock–Johnson Psychoeducational Battery—Revised.* Itasca, IL: Riverside.

IV

New and Revised
Intelligence Batteries

Part IV of this textbook focuses on recently developed or revised individual, standardized, norm-referenced intelligence tests. The methods of assessment used with the Binet and Wechsler scales dominated the 1900s. However, developers of new tests and recent revisions of tests for assessing intelligence have attempted to move beyond the tradition established by the early Binet and Wechsler scales and to incorporate strong theoretical and research foundations into intellectual assessment. The chapters in Part IV describe major intelligence tests, most of which were published or revised in the late 1990s and early 2000s, and the latest research about these tests. Most of the assessment instruments included here were revised or initially developed since the first edition of this textbook was published in 1997. Part IV chapters summarize information about instruments such as the most recent revisions of the Wechsler, Stanford–Binet, Kaufman, and Woodcock–Johnson scales and the new Reynolds Intellectual Assessment Scales. The chapters in Part IV were written by the authors or developers of the new tests, who provide information about the tests' psychometric and research foundations and their applications in the comprehensive assessment of abilities.

Chapter 14, "The Wechsler Scales," by Jianjun Zhu and Larry Weiss, includes information about the latest revisions of these scales: the Wechsler Intelligence Scale for Children—Fourth Edition, Wechsler Preschool and Primary Scale of Intelligence—Third Edition, and Wechsler Adult Intelligence Scale—Third Edition. In Chapter 15, Gale H. Roid and Mark Pomplun present "The Stanford-Binet Intelligence Scales, Fifth Edition." James C. Kaufman, Alan S. Kaufman, Jennie Kaufman-Singer, and Nadeen L. Kaufman are authors of Chapter 16, "The Kaufman Assessment Battery for Children—Second Edition and the Kaufman Adolescent and Adult Intelligence Test."

"The Woodcock–Johnson III Tests of Cognitive Ability" are described in Chapter 17 by Fredrick A. Schrank. Chapter 18, "The Differential Ability Scales," was authored by Colin D. Elliott. (The chapter primarily describes the existing DAS, published in 1990, although a second edition of the instrument is currently in preparation.) Chapter 19, "The Universal Nonverbal Intelligence Test: A Multidimensional Measure of Intelligence," was authored by R. Steve McCallum and Bruce A. Bracken. The UNIT uses a model of intelligence that includes two tiers (memory and reasoning) and two organizational strategies (symbolic and nonsymbolic) of intelligence. Chapter 20, "The Cognitive Assessment System," by Jack A. Naglieri, describes an instrument based on the planning, attention, simultaneous, and successive (PASS) theory presented in Chapter 7. The newest intelligence tests presented in the textbook are described in Chapter 21, "Introduction to the Reynolds Intellectual Assessment Scales and the Reynolds Intellectual Screening Test," written by Cecil R. Reynolds and Randy W. Kamphaus.

In general, the authors of Chapters 14 through 21 provide descriptions of their assessment instruments and discuss the instruments' theoretical and research underpinnings, organization and format, and psychometric characteristics. The authors also provide recommendations for interpreting the abilities measured by their instruments. Finally, the chapters provide summaries of the specific ways in which these intelligence tests differ from traditional approaches, descriptions of how the tests reflect advances in intellectual assessment, and brief case studies.

14

The Wechsler Scales

JIANJUN ZHU
LARRY WEISS

The Wechsler intelligence scales are a family of individually administered instruments for assessing the intellectual functioning of children and adults. Since the original publication of the Wechsler–Bellevue Intelligence Scale in 1939, the Wechsler scales have had a tremendous influence on the field of psychological assessment. They are the most frequently used intelligence tests and have made significant contribution to clinical and school psychology practice (Harrison, Kaufman, Hickman, & Kaufman, 1988; Kaufman & Lichtenberger, 1999; Sattler & Ryan, 2001; Wasserman & Maccubbin, 2002; Watkins, Campbell, Nieberding, & Hallmark, 1995). The Wechsler intelligence scales are also the most researched instruments. An immense volume of literature related to their clinical utility and psychometric properties has been accumulated since the original publication of each instrument (Kamphaus, 1993; Kaufman, 1994; Psychological Corporation, 1997, 2002; Wechsler, 2002, 2003).

Although Wechsler borrowed many ideas from existing measures (see Zachary, 1990), his scales represent significant innovations in the history of intelligence testing. Based on his considerable clinical expertise, Wechsler united the finest aspects of others' work to create a family of intelligence scales that are comprehensive, clinically useful, ecologically valid, and theoretically sound. Table 14.1 provides a history of cognitive assessment instruments authored and published under the Wechsler name.

THEORY AND STRUCTURE OF THE WECHSLER SCALES

Although there is overwhelming evidence of research supporting their clinical utility, the Wechsler scales have been criticized for the lack of a strong theoretical basis (Beres, Kaufman, & Perlman, 2000; Kaufman & Lichtenberger, 1999). Such critiques have led at least one commentator to believe that "it is a matter of luck that many of the Wechsler subtests are neurologically relevant" (McFie, 1975, p. 14). It is very hard to believe, however, that Wechsler could develop a family of intelligence scales that are so clinically useful without a deep understanding of the nature of intelligence and the guidance of certain explicit or implicit theories of intelligence (Zhu, Weiss, Prifitera, & Coalson, 2003). A careful review of Wechsler's publications and test manuals (e.g., Wechsler, 1939, 1950, 1974, 1975, 1981, 1997a, 2002, 2003) suggests that the development of each edition of the Wechsler scales was clearly based on the contemporary theory of the time.

While Wechsler was more of a clinician and test developer than a theorist, he was deeply influenced by two key theorists of in-

TABLE 14.1. History of the Wechsler Scales

—	WISC-IV (2003)	—	—
WAIS-III (1997a)	WISC-III (1991)	WPPSI-III (2002)	WMS-III (1997c)
WAIS-R (1981)	WISC-R (1974)	WPPSI-R (1989)	WMS-R (1987)
WAIS (1955)	WISC (1949)	WPPSI (1967)	WMS (1945)
Wechsler–Bellevue—Form I (1939)	Wechsler–Bellevue—Form II (1946)	—	—

Note. WAIS, Wechsler Adult Intelligence Scale; WISC, Wechsler Intelligence Scale for Children; WPPSI, Wechsler Preschool and Primary Scale ofIntelligence; WMS, Wechsler Memory Scale. -R means —Revised, -III means —Third Edition, and -IV means —Fourth Edition.

telligence at the time, Charles E. Spearman and Edward L. Thorndike. Wechsler was obviously influenced by Spearman's *g* or general intelligence theory (Kaufman & Lichtenberger, 1999; Psychological Corporation, 1997; Tulsky, Zhu, & Prifitera, 2000). He believed that intelligence is not equal to intellectual abilities; as he saw it, the construct of intelligence is a *global* entity aggregated of specific abilities that are qualitatively different (Wechsler, 1939, 1950, 1974, 1975, 1981). Wechsler (1981) wrote:

> Intelligence is multifaceted as well as multidetermined. What it always calls for is not a particular ability but an overall competency or global capacity, which in one way or another enables a sentient individual to comprehend the world and to deal effectively with its challenges. (p. 8)

Furthermore, also clearly influenced by Thorndike, Wechsler conceived of intelligence as comprising elements or abilities that are qualitatively different. Therefore, he believed that intelligence could best be measured by a wide array of tests. Wechsler (1974) wrote: "Intelligence can manifest itself in many forms, and an intelligence scale, to be effective as well as fair, must utilize as many different languages (tests) as possible" (p. 5). Wechsler was innovative in his incorporation of scores for Verbal and Performance scales, in addition to an overall composite score. However, the early versions of the Wechsler scales grouped subtests into Verbal and Performance scales mainly because of clinical and practical considerations. Such a split did not imply that these were the only abilities involved in the tests. It was only one of several ways in which the tests could be grouped (Wechsler, 1958).

Several decades of factor-analytic studies of intelligence measures have accumulated significant evidence supporting the theoretical foundation of the Wechsler scales. For instance, after analyzing the factor structure of more than 450 datasets, Carroll (1993) demonstrated that a general intelligence factor was present through those datasets. On the other hand, Cohen (1952a, 1952b, 1957a, 1957b, 1959), Horn (1991, 1994), and Carroll (1993) also provided strong evidence indicating that intelligence is composed of specific narrow abilities that appear to cluster into higher-order ability domains.

Although Wechsler did not develop his intelligence scales according to modern intelligence theory, the theory he used to guide test development, either explicitly or implicitly (Zachary, 1990), has many similarities to modern theories of intelligence assessment. For instance, using both Wechsler Adult Intelligence Scale—Third Edition (WAIS-III) and Wechsler Memory Scale—Third Edition (WMS-III) normative data and a structural equating modeling approach, Tulsky and Price (2003) demonstrated that these two Wechsler scales assess six domains of cognitive functioning: Verbal Comprehension, Perceptual Organization (or Perceptual Reasoning), Processing Speed, Working Memory, Auditory Memory, and Visual Memory. These cognitive domains are very consistent with those specified by contemporary theories and measures of intelligence (Carroll, 1993 and Chapter 4, this volume; Horn, 1991).

Although the modern Wechsler intelligence scales continue the excellence of their predecessors, their theoretical foundation has been strengthened to reflect the changes and advances in contemporary intelligence theories. It is important to note that the latest versions of the Wechsler intelligence scales have not been developed according to any single doctrine of intelligence theory. Like their predecessors, while focusing on the clinical and ecological validity of the tests, the modern Wechsler intelligence scales bridge the ideas of several different intelligence theories. At each revision of the Wechsler intelligence scales, not only have the normative data been updated; the test blueprint has also been carefully redesigned to reflect advances in theoretical and practical foundations of cognitive and neuropsychological assessment. Therefore, if the original Wechsler scales were based on implicit theory, the modern Wechsler scales are clearly driven by ongoing clinical research and theoretical development.

For instance, because several theories of cognitive functioning emphasize the importance of fluid reasoning (Carpenter & Just, 1989; Carpenter, Just, & Shell, 1990; Carroll, 1993 and Chapter 4, this volume; Cattell, 1943, 1963; Cattell & Horn, 1978; Daneman & Carpenter, 1980; de Jonge & de Jonge, 1996; Sternberg, 1995), the Wechsler scales have incorporated new subtests, such as Matrix Reasoning, Picture Concepts, and Word Reasoning, to enhance the measurement of fluid reasoning. Recent literature has also suggested that working memory is a key component of learning (Fry & Hale, 1996; Kyllonen, 1987; Kyllonen & Christal, 1989, 1990; Perlow, Jattuso, & Moore, 1997; Swanson, 1999; Woltz, 1988). Cognitive psychologists have come to believe that working memory is the most important predictor of individual differences in learning ability and fluid reasoning. It is responsible for differences among learners on a wide variety of learning tasks. The greater an individual's working memory capabilities are, the greater his or her attention and learning capabilities are. Inspired by this literature, the developers of the WAIS-III and Wechsler Intelligence Scale for Children—Fourth Edition (WISC-IV) have redesigned the Arithmetic subtest, provided separate norms for Digit Span Forward and Backward, and developed a Letter–Number Sequencing subtest to enhance the measure of working memory domain. In addition, contemporary research has shown that the processing speed is an important domain of cognitive func-

tioning (Carroll, 1993 and Chapter 4, this volume; Deary & Stough, 1996; Horn & Noll, 1997). It is sensitive to such neurological conditions as epilepsy, attention-deficit/hyperactivity disorder (ADHD), and traumatic brain injury (Donders, 1997). Processing speed may be especially important to assess in children because of its relationship to neurological development, other cognitive abilities, and learning. Improvements in children's performance on measures of processing speed are mirrored by age-related changes in the number of transient connections to the central nervous system and increases in myelinization (Berthier, DeBlois, Poirier, Novak, & Clifton, 2000; Cepeda, Kramer, & Gonzalez de Sather, 2001; Kail, 2000; Kail & Salthouse, 1994). Clinical research in developmental cognitive neuropsychology suggests a dynamic interplay among working memory, processing speed, and reasoning (Carpenter et al., 1990; Fry & Hale, 1996; Kail & Salthouse, 1994; Schatz, Kramer, Albin, & Matthay, 2000). For example, more rapid processing of information may reduce demands on working memory and facilitate reasoning. Therefore, all of the latest Wechsler scales include subtests designed to measure the processing speed domain. The recent advances in contemporary intelligence theories have inspired all these changes.

The developers of the most recent Wechsler scales have also made significant efforts to remove confounding variables so that the scales tap relatively pure cognitive domains. These efforts include providing factor index scores, reducing the weights of time bonus, providing separate norms for Digit Span Forward and Backward and for Block Design with and without bonus, dropping or redesigning subtests that have split loadings, and so forth. Meanwhile, the Wechsler research team has also remained fully aware that the ecological validity and clinical utility of the test cannot be sacrificed. A century of cognitive research has proven that human cognitive functions form a dynamically unified entity. They are interrelated and interact with each other in the context of ecological environment. They "appear to behave differently when alone from what they do when operating in concert" (Wechsler, 1975, p. 138). Therefore, it is almost impossible and meaningless to measure a pure cognitive function.

Overemphasizing the need to assess pure cognitive functions may increase the risk of losing the ecological validity and the clinical utility of a test. Measuring psychometrically pure factors of discrete domains may be useful diagnostically, but it does not necessarily result in information that is clinically rich or practically useful in real-world applications (Zachary, 1990). This may be why some so-called "theory-based" intelligence tests have had a hard time establishing their clinical utility.

In addition, assessment results of the Wechsler intelligence scales are very consistent with those from the modern "theory-based" intelligence scales. This is supported by the fact that many subtests utilized by the latter scales obviously measure constructs similar to those tapped by the subtests of the Wechsler scales. In addition, the correlations between the Full Scale IQ (FSIQ) of Wechsler scales and the Differential Ability Scales (DAS) General Cognitive Ability (GCA) score or the Kaufman Adolescent and Adult Intelligence Test (KAIT) Composite Intelligence score are quite high, ranging from .81 to .91 (Elliott, 1990; Kaufman & Kaufman, 1993).

DESCRIPTION OF SUBTESTS AND COMPOSITES

The WISC-IV has a total of 15 subtests, including 10 core subtests and 5 supplemental subtests. The WAIS-III is composed of 14 subtests, including 11 core subtests and 3 supplemental or optional subtests. The Wechsler Preschool and Primary Scale of Intelligence—Third Edition (WPPSI-III) consists of 14 subtests, including 7 core subtests and 7 supplemental or optional subtests.

Table 14.2 lists the subtests of the three instruments, and the IQ and Index scales to which each subtest contributes. The subtests noted with a check mark are core subtests that contribute to IQ or factor Index scores. The subtests noted with a check mark enclosed in parentheses are supplemental and can substitute for core subtests that contribute to the same scale. Those subtests noted with an asterisk are optional subtests. For instance, the Receptive Vocabulary subtest of the WPPSI-III is a core subtest for ages 2 years, 6 months to 3 years, 11 months (2:6– 3:11) and an optional subtest for ages 4:0– 7:3. That is why it is noted with both a check mark and an asterisk.

Subtest Descriptions and Rationales

Vocabulary

The Vocabulary subtest consists of two types of items: picture naming and word definition. For picture items, the examinee names pictures that are displayed in the stimulus book. For verbal items, the examinee gives definitions for words that the examiner reads aloud. When verbal items are presented, children ages 9–16 and adults are also shown the words in the Stimulus Book. An example of a Vocabulary item is "What does *conceive* mean?" Vocabulary is designed to measure an individual's acquired knowledge and verbal concept formation. It also measures an individual's crystallized intelligence, fund of knowledge, verbal conceptualization, verbal reasoning, learning ability, long-term memory, and degree of language development. Other abilities that may be used during this task include auditory perception and comprehension, verbal conceptualization, abstract thinking, and verbal expression (Bannatyne, 1974; Cooper, 1995; Kaufman, 1994; Kaufman & Lichtenberg, 1999; Politano & Finch, 1996; Ryan & Smith, 2003; Sattler & Saklofske, 2001). Factor analysis indicates that the Wechsler Vocabulary subtest loads on the Verbal Comprehension factor. It is a good measure of *g* and has an ample amount of specificity (Kaufman & Lichtenberg, 1999; Sattler & Saklofske, 2001).

Similarities

The examinee is presented with two words that represent common concepts and is asked to describe how they are alike. An example of a Similarities item is "In what way are fishes and birds alike?" To make this test more age-appropriate, the WPPSI-III uses a slightly different testing format. The child is read an incomplete sentence containing two concepts that share a common characteristic and is asked to complete the sentence by providing a response that reflects the shared characteristic. An example of a Similarities sentence completion item is "Finish what I

TABLE 14.2. Subtests and Related Composite Scores of the Wechsler Scales

WISC-IV (2003)	Contribution to IQ and factor Index scales				
	VCI	PRI	WMI	PSI	FSIQ
Vocabulary	√				√
Similarities	√				√
Comprehension	√				√
Information	(√)				(√)
Word Reasoning	(√)				(√)
Letter–Number Sequencing			√		√
Digit Span			√		√
Arithmetic			(√)		(√)
Block Design		√			√
Matrix Reasoning		√			√
Picture Concepts		√			√
Picture Completion		(√)			(√)
Coding				√	√
Symbol Search				√	√
Cancellation				(√)	(√)

WAIS-III (1997)	Contribution to IQ and factor Index scales						
	VIQ	PIQ	FSIQ	VCI	POI	WMI	PSI
Vocabulary	√		√	√			
Similarities	√		√	√			
Information	√		√	√			
Comprehension	√		√	√			
Arithmetic	√		√			√	
Digit Span	√		√			√	
Letter–Number Sequencing						√	
Block Design		√	√		√		
Matrix Reasoning		√	√		√		
Picture Completion		√	√		√		
Picture Arrangement		√	√		(√)		
Digit Symbol–Coding		√	√				√
Symbol Search		(√)	(√)				√
Object Assembly (Optional)		*	*				

WPPSI-III (2002)	Contribution to IQ and factor Index scales				
	VIQ	PIQ	PSI	FSIQ	GLC
Vocabulary	√			√	
Information	√			√	
Word Reasoning	√			√	
Similarities	(√)			(√)	
Comprehension	(√)			(√)	
Block Design		√		√	
Matrix Reasoning		√		√	
Picture Concepts		√		√	
Picture Completion		(√)		(√)	
Object Assembly		(√)		(√)	
Coding			√	√	
Symbol Search			√	(√)	
Receptive Vocabulary	√*			√*	*
Picture Naming	*			*	*

Note. VCI, Verbal Comprehension Index; PRI, Perceptual Reasoning Index; WMI, Working Memory Index; PSI, Processing Speed Index; FSIQ, Full Scale IQ; VIQ, Verbal IQ; PIQ, Performance IQ; POI, Perceptual Organization Index. GLC is an optional index score designed to provide a quick measure of children's general language abilities. The two subtests that contribute to GLC are Picture Naming and Receptive Vocabulary. See text for an explanation of check marks and asterisks.

say: Fishes and birds are both _____ ."
The Similarities subtest is designed to measure verbal reasoning, concept formation, and verbal problem solving. It also involves auditory comprehension, memory, distinction between nonessential and essential features, and verbal expression (Bannatyne, 1974; Cooper, 1995; Glasser & Zimmerman, 1967; Kaufman, 1994; Kaufman & Lichtenberg, 1999; Politano & Finch, 1996; Ryan & Smith, 2003; Sattler & Saklofske, 2001). This subtest loads on the Verbal Comprehension factor and is a good measure of g. It also has an adequate to ample amount of specificity across different Wechsler scales (Kaufman & Lichtenberg, 1999; Sattler & Saklofske, 2001).

Comprehension

The Comprehension subtest requires the examinee to answer questions based on his or her understanding of general principles and social situations (e.g., "What is the advantage of keeping money in a bank?"). The subtest is designed to measure verbal reasoning and conceptualization, verbal comprehension and expression, the ability to evaluate and use past experience, verbal problem solving, and the ability to demonstrate practical information. The task also involves knowledge of conventional standards of behavior, social judgment and maturity, social orientation, and common sense (Bannatyne, 1974; Groth-Marnat, 1997; Kaufman, 1994; Kaufman & Lichtenberg, 1999; Politano & Finch, 1996; Ryan & Smith, 2003; Sattler & Saklofske, 2001). Comprehension loads on the Verbal Comprehension factor and is a good measure of g. Its specificity is adequate to ample.

Information

The examinee answers questions that address a broad range of general knowledge topics (e.g., "Name the country that launched the first man-made satellite"). It is designed to measure an individual's ability to acquire, retain, and retrieve general factual knowledge. It involves crystallized intelligence, long-term memory, and the ability to retain and retrieve information from school and the environment. Other skills that may

be used are auditory perception and comprehension, as well as verbal expressive ability (Cooper, 1995; Groth-Marnat, 1997; Horn, 1985; Kaufman, 1994; Kaufman & Lichtenberg, 1999; Politano & Finch, 1996; Ryan & Smith, 2003; Sattler & Saklofske, 2001). This subtest loads on the Verbal Comprehension factor. It is a good measure of g and has an adequate to ample amount of specificity (Kaufman & Lichtenberg, 1999; Sattler & Saklofske, 2001).

Word Reasoning

The examinee is asked to identify the common concept being described in a series of clues. A new subtest for the WPPSI-III and WISC-IV, Word Reasoning is related to tasks measuring verbal reasoning, such as the Word Context subtest of the Delis–Kaplan Executive Function System (Delis, Kaplan, & Kramer, 2001), the Riddles subtest of the Kaufman Assessment Battery for Children, and cloze tasks (i.e., tasks requiring the child to complete missing portions of a sentence). An example of a Word Reasoning item is "It is used for transportation, and it goes on water. What is it?" These tasks have been shown to measure verbal comprehension, analogical and general reasoning ability, verbal abstraction, domain knowledge, the ability to integrate and synthesize different types of information, and the ability to generate alternative concepts (Ackerman, Beier, & Bowen, 2000; Alexander & Kulikowich, 1991; Delis et al., 2001; DeSanti, 1989; McKenna & Layton, 1990; Newstead, Thompson, & Handley, 2002; Ridgeway, 1995). The subtest is a good measure of g and has an ample amount of specificity.

Block Design

The Block Design subtest requires the examinee to view a constructed model or a picture in the Stimulus Book, and to use one-color or two-color blocks to recreate the design within a specified time limit. Figure 14.1 presents an example of a Block Design item. This subtest is designed to measure the ability to analyze and synthesize abstract visual stimuli. It also involves nonverbal concept formation, visual perception and organization, visual–spatial problem solving, visual non-

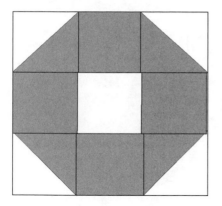

FIGURE 14.1. An example of a Block Design item.

verbal reasoning, simultaneous processing, visual–motor coordination, learning, and the ability to separate figure and ground in visual stimuli (Cooper, 1995; Groth-Marnat, 1997; Kaufman, 1994; Kaufman & Lichtenberg, 1999; Politano & Finch, 1996; Ryan & Smith, 2003; Sattler & Saklofske, 2001). Cooper (1995) suggests that it involves visual observation and matching abilities for younger children, as well as the ability to integrate visual and motor processes. Factor analysis suggests that Block Design subtest loads on the Perceptual Organization/Perceptual Reasoning factor. It is a fairly good measure of *g* and has an adequate to ample amount of specificity (Kaufman & Lichtenberg, 1999; Sattler & Saklofske, 2001).

Picture Concepts

For each Picture Concepts item, the examinee is presented with two or three rows of pictures and chooses one picture from each row to form a group with a common characteristic. This is a new core subtest for the WPPSI-III and WISC-IV. Figure 14.2 presents an example of a Picture Concepts item. Although verbal mediation may be involved, Picture Concepts is considered the nonverbal counterpart of Similarities (Wechsler, 2002, 2003). It is designed to measure abstract, categorical reasoning ability. Items are sequenced to reflect increasing demands on abstract reasoning ability (Deak & Maratsos, 1998; Flavell, 1985; Shulman, Yirmiya, & Greenbaum, 1995). Factor analysis demonstrates that this subtest loads on the Perceptual Organization/Perceptual Responding factor. It also has fairly good *g* loading and an ample amount of specificity.

Matrix Reasoning

For each Matrix Reasoning item, the examinee looks at an incomplete matrix and selects the missing portion from five response options. It is a new core subtest for the Wechsler scales. Figure 14.3 presents an example of a Matrix Reasoning item. This subtest is designed to enhance the measurement of fluid intelligence, nonverbal

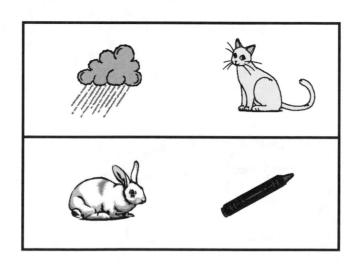

FIGURE 14.2. An example of a Picture Concepts item.

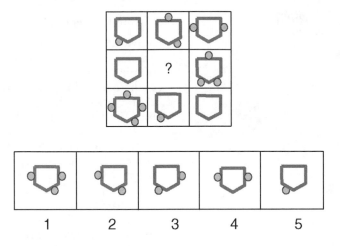

FIGURE 14.3. An example of a Matrix Reasoning item.

reasoning, analogical reasoning, nonverbal problem solving, and spatial visualization (Kaufman & Lichtenberg, 1999; Ryan & Smith, 2003; Sattler & Ryan, 2001). This subtest loads on the Perceptual Organization/Perceptual Reasoning factor. It is a good measure of *g* and has an ample amount of specificity (Kaufman & Lichtenberg, 1999; Sattler & Ryan, 2001).

Picture Completion

The Picture Completion task requires the examinee to view a picture and then point to or name the important part missing within a specified time limit. Figure 14.4 shows an example of a Picture Completion item. This subtest is designed to measure visual perception and organization, concentration, visual discrimination, visual recognition of essential details of objects, reasoning, and long-term memory (Cooper, 1995; Kaufman,

1994; Kaufman & Lichtenberg, 1999; Politano & Finch, 1996; Ryan & Smith, 2003; Sattler & Saklofske, 2001). The subtest loads on the Perceptual Organization/Perceptual Reasoning factor. It is a fair measure of *g* and has an adequate to ample amount of specificity (Kaufman & Lichtenberg, 1999; Sattler & Saklofske, 2001).

Digit Span

The Digit Span subtest is composed of two parts: Digit Span Forward and Digit Span Backward. Digit Span Forward requires the examinee to repeat numbers in the same order as those read aloud by the examiner, and Digit Span Backward requires the examinee to repeat the numbers in the reverse order of that presented by the examiner. Each item of Digit Span Forward and Digit Span Backward is composed of two trials with the same

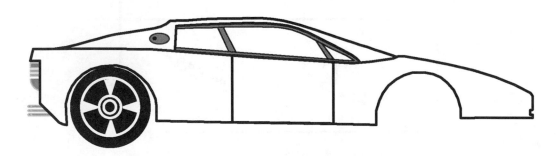

FIGURE 14.4. An example of a Picture Completion item.

span. This subtest measures auditory short-term memory, sequencing skills, attention, and concentration (Groth-Marnat, 1997; Kaufman, 1994; Kaufman & Lichtenberg, 1999; Ryan & Smith, 2003; Sattler & Saklofske, 2001). The Digit Span Forward task involves rote learning and memory, attention, encoding, and auditory processing. The Digit Span Backward task involves working memory, transformation of information, mental manipulation, and visual–spatial imaging (Groth-Marnat, 1997; Hale, Hoeppner, & Fiorello, 2002; Kaufman, 1994; Reynolds, 1997; Sattler & Saklofske, 2001). The shift from the Digit Span Forward task to the Digit Span Backward task requires cognitive flexibility and mental alertness. Digit Span loads on the Working Memory factor. It is a fair measure of *g* and has an ample amount of specificity (Kaufman & Lichtenberg, 1999; Sattler & Saklofske, 2001).

Letter–Number Sequencing

The examinee is read a sequence of numbers and letters, and recalls the numbers in ascending order and the letters in alphabetical order. Letter–Number Sequencing is a new subtest for the WAIS-III and WISC-IV. This subtest is based in part on the work of Gold, Carpenter, Randolph, Goldberg, and Weinberger (1997), who developed a similar task for individuals with schizophrenia. The task involves sequencing, mental manipulation, attention, mental flexibility, auditory working memory, visual–spatial imaging, and processing speed (Crowe, 2000; Kaufman & Lichtenberg, 1999; Ryan & Smith, 2003; Sattler & Ryan, 2001; Wechsler, 1997b, 2003). Factor analysis reveals that this subtest loads on the Working Memory factor. It is a fair measure of *g* and has an ample amount of specificity (Kaufman & Lichtenberg, 1999).

Arithmetic

The examinee mentally solves a series of orally presented arithmetic problems within a specified time limit. Items were developed to increase the working memory demands while simultaneously making the mathematical knowledge required to complete the subtest task more age-appropriate. To ensure

that the test loads on the Working Memory factor, the difficulty of the mathematical calculation was set very low, so that most examinees can solve the problems correctly if they are presented the problem visually with numbers directly. Performing the Arithmetic task involves auditory verbal comprehension, mental manipulation, concentration, attention, working memory, long-term memory, and numerical reasoning ability. It may also involve sequencing, fluid reasoning, and logical reasoning (Groth-Marnat, 1997; Kaufman, 1994; Kaufman & Lichtenberg, 1999; Politano & Finch, 1996; Ryan & Smith, 2003; Sattler & Saklofske, 2001; Sternberg, 1993). The subtest loads mainly on the Working Memory factor. It often shows a secondary loading on the Verbal Comprehension factor, due to heavy involvement of auditory verbal comprehension. It is a good measure of *g* and has an adequate to ample amount of specificity (Kaufman & Lichtenberg, 1999; Sattler & Saklofske, 2001).

Coding

The examinee copies symbols that are paired with simple geometric shapes or numbers. Using a key, the examinee draws each symbol in its corresponding shape or box within a specified time limit. Figure 14.5 presents an example of a Coding task. In addition to visual–motor processing speed, the subtest measures short-term memory, learning ability, visual perception, visual–motor coordination, visual scanning ability, cognitive flexibility, attention, and motivation (Cooper, 1995; Groth-Marnat, 1997; Kaufman, 1994; Sattler & Saklofske, 2001). It may also involve visual and sequential processing (Kaufman, 1994; Kaufman & Lichtenberg, 1999; Politano & Finch, 1996; Ryan & Smith, 2003; Sattler & Saklofske, 2001). Factor analysis indicates that the Coding subtest loads on the Processing Speed factor. It is a fair measure of *g* and an ample amount of specificity (Kaufman & Lichtenberg, 1999)

Symbol Search

The examinee scans a search group and indicates whether the target symbol(s) matches any of the symbols in the search group with-

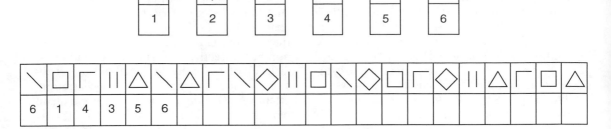

FIGURE 14.5. An example of a Coding Task.

in a specified time limit. Figure 14.6 presents an example of a Symbol Search task. In addition to visual–motor processing speed, the subtest also involves short-term visual memory, visual–motor coordination, cognitive flexibility, visual discrimination, and concentration. It may also tap auditory comprehension, perceptual organization, and planning and learning ability (Kaufman, 1994; Kaufman & Lichtenberg, 1999; Politano & Finch, 1996; Ryan & Smith, 2003; Sattler & Saklofske, 2001). This subtest loads on the Processing Speed factor. It is a fair measure of *g* and has an adequate to ample amount specificity for most age ranges covered by the Wechsler scales. However, it does not have adequate specificity for ages 16–29 and 55–89 (Kaufman & Lichtenberg, 1999; Sattler & Ryan, 2001).

Object Assembly

For all items, the examinee fits the pieces of a puzzle together to form a meaningful whole within specified time limits. It is designed to assess perceptual organization, integration and synthesis of part–whole relationships, and use of sensory–motor feedback. It also involves spatial ability, fluid ability, visual–motor reasoning, trial-and-error learning, visual–motor coordination, cognitive flexibility, persistence, motor coordination, and dexterity (Cooper, 1995; Politano & Finch, 1996; Ryan & Smith, 2003; Sattler & Saklofske, 2001; Wechsler, 1991). Kaufman (1994) also suggest that simultaneous processing, nonverbal reasoning, speed of mental processing, and anticipation of relationships are involved. Scores on this subtest may be influenced by a child's experience with puzzles, visual-perceptual problems, or response to time pressures (Kaufman, 1994; Kaufman & Lichtenberg, 1999). The results of factor analysis suggest that Object Assembly loads on the Perceptual Organization/Perceptual Reasoning factor. It is a fair measure of *g* for most age groups. However, it has an adequate to ample amount of specificity for WPPSI-III age ranges (Kaufman & Lichtenberg, 1999; Sattler & Saklofske, 2001).

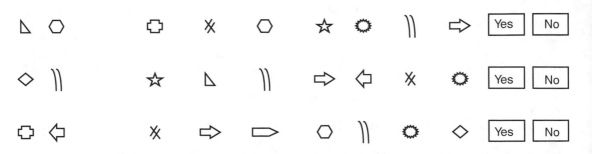

FIGURE 14.6. An example of a Symbol Search Task.

Picture Arrangement

The examinee is presented with a set of picture cards that tell a story in a specified order and asked to rearrange the cards into a logical sequence within the specified time limit. Performing the Picture Arrangement task involves nonverbal reasoning, problem solving, planning ability, visual organization, visual sequencing, social reasoning, integrated brain functioning, acquired knowledge, and verbal mediation (Kaufman, 1994; Kaufman & Lichtenberg, 1999; Politano & Finch, 1996; Ryan & Smith, 2003; Sattler & Saklofske, 2001). Factor-analytic work reveals that Picture Arrangement has split loadings on both the Perceptual Organization/Perceptual Reasoning and Verbal Comprehension factors. Its g loading is from .60 to .62.

Cancellation

Cancellation is a new supplemental subtest for the WISC-IV. The examinee scans both a random and a structured arrangement of pictures and marks target pictures within a specified time limit. It is similar to previously developed cancellation tasks, designed to measure processing speed, visual selective attention, vigilance, and visual neglect (Bate, Mathias, & Crawford, 2001; Gauthier, Dehaut, & Joanette, 1989; Geldmacher, 1996; Halligan, Marshall, & Wade, 1989; Wojciulik, Husain, Clarke, & Driver, 2001). Cancellation loads on the Processing Speed factor. Although it is not a measure of g, it has an ample amount of specificity.

Receptive Vocabulary

Receptive Vocabulary is a new subtest developed for the WPPSI-III. It is a core verbal subtest for ages 2:6–3:11 and an optional verbal subtest for ages 4:0–7:3. For each item, the child looks at a group of four pictures and points to the one the examiner names aloud. This subtest taps concept formation, auditory and visual discrimination, auditory processing, auditory memory, integration of visual perception and auditory input, and receptive language ability (Brownell, 2000a; Robinson & Saxon, 1999; Semel, Wigg, & Secord, 1995; Wechsler,

2002). This subtest loads on the Verbal Comprehension factor. It is a good measure of g and has an adequate amount of specificity.

Picture Naming

Picture Naming is a new supplemental Verbal subtest for WPPSI-III. For each item, the child names a picture that is displayed in the stimulus book. This subtest taps concept formation, expressive language ability, word retrieval from long-term memory, and association of visual stimuli with language (Brownell, 2000b; Elliott, 1990; German, 1989; Sattler & Saklofske, 2001; Semel et al., 1995; Wechsler, 2002). It loads on the Verbal Comprehension factor. This subtest is a good measure of g and has adequate amount of specificity.

Composite Descriptions and Rationales

All Wechsler intelligence scales provide factor-based Index scores that measure major cognitive domains identified in contemporary theories of intelligence. The primary advantage of the Index scores is their measurement of relatively purer cognitive domains than traditional IQ scores. For example, the traditional Verbal IQ (VIQ) score summarizes an individual's performance on subtests designed to measure both Verbal Comprehension and Working Memory, and the traditional Performance IQ (PIQ) score summarizes an individual's performance on subtests that measure both Perceptual Organization and Processing Speed. An individual can obtain an average VIQ score because he or she performs at an average level on both domains, or at an above-average level on one domain and at a below-average level on the other domain. In the latest Wechsler scale (i.e., the WISC-IV and WPPSI-III, the VIQ and PIQ no longer coexist with the factor Index scores. Instead, the Index scores become the core composite scores in addition to the FSIQ. Because the Indexes represent an individual's functioning in more narrowly defined domains, the clinician is able to evaluate specific aspects of cognitive functioning more clearly. Below are brief descriptions of the common Wechsler factor Index scores.

Verbal Comprehension Index

The Verbal Comprehension Index (VCI) is a measure of verbal concept formation, verbal reasoning and comprehension, acquired knowledge, and attention to verbal stimuli. It measures a narrower domain of cognitive functioning than the traditional VIQ score and is less confounded with other cognitive functions (working memory). Therefore, the VCI is considered to be a purer measure of verbal reasoning than VIQ. In particular, it may be a more appropriate indicator of verbal reasoning ability for an individual with depressed memory functioning or in situations where there is a large amount of scatter among the subtests contributing to VIQ (Kaufman, 1994; Kaufman & Lichtenberg, 1999; Prifitera, Weiss, & Saklofske, 1998; Psychological Corporation, 1997; Sattler & Saklofske, 2001; Wechsler, 2002, 2003; Zhu et al., 2003).

Perceptual Reasoning Index

The Perceptual Reasoning Index (PRI; named the Perceptual Organization Index [POI] in WISC-III and WAIS-III) is a measure of fluid reasoning, spatial processing, attentiveness to detail, and visual–motor integration. It is less confounded with processing speed and may better reflect the true nonverbal reasoning ability of an individual with depressed processing speed ability (Kaufman, 1994; Kaufman & Lichtenberg, 1999; Prifitera et al., 1998; Psychological Corporation, 1997; Sattler & Saklofske, 2001; Wechsler, 2002, 2003; Zhu et al., 2003).

Working Memory Index

The Working Memory Index (WMI) measures mental capacity where incoming information is temporarily stored, where calculations and transformation processing occurs, and where the products/outputs of these calculations and transformations are held (Psychological Corporation, 1997; Wechsler, 2002, 2003; Zhu et al., 2003). Because working memory is a key component of learning, differences in working memory capacity may account for some variance of the individual differences related to attention, learning capacities, and fluid reasoning (Fry

& Hale; 1996; Sternberg, 1995; Kyllonen & Christal, 1989).

Processing Speed Index

Performance on the Processing Speed Index (PSI) is an indication of the rapidity with which an individual can process simple or routine information without making errors. Cognitive research indicates that the speed of information processing correlates significantly with g (Jensen, 1982, 1987; Neisser et al., 1996; Neubauer & Knorr, 1998; Kranzler & Jensen, 1989). Because learning often involves a combination of routine and complex information processing, a weakness in the speed of processing may make the task of comprehending novel information more time-consuming and difficult, and leave an individual with less mental energy for the complex task of understanding new material.

Full Scale Intelligence Quotient

The FSIQ is the overall composite score that estimates an individual's general level of intellectual functioning. It is the aggregate score of the core subtest scores. The FSIQ is usually considered to be the most representative of g, or global intellectual functioning.

PSYCHOMETRIC PROPERTIES

According to the criteria proposed by Flanagan and Alfonso (1995), Hammill, Brown, and Bryant (1992), and Bracken (1987), all the latest editions of the Wechsler intelligence scales have outstanding psychometric properties.

Standardization Samples

All the latest editions of the Wechsler scales have excellent standardization samples (Kaufman & Lichtenberger, 1999; Sattler, 2001). The sizes of the normative samples, recency of the normative data, and the stratification of the normative sample are all in the "good" category. The sizes of the normative samples are 1,700, 2,200, and 2,450 for the WPPSI-III, WISC-IV, and WAIS-III, respectively. The sample size for most norming age groups is usually 200 cases. As this book goes to press, the recency of the normative data is 7 years for the WAIS-III, 2 years for the WPPSI-III, and 1 year for the WISC-IV. The stratification of the normative samples matches recent U.S. census data closely on five key demographic variables: age, gender, race/ethnicity, educational level, and geographic region.

Reliability

The latest Wechsler scales have outstanding reliabilities (Kaufman & Lichtenberger, 1999; Sattler & Saklofske, 2001). First, the overall internal-consistency reliability coefficients for the normative sample are in the .90s for all Wechsler IQ and Index scores except the PSI. The internal-consistency reliability coefficients of the PSI are slightly lower, ranging from .87 to .89, because this Index consists of only two subtests. At subtest level, the overall internal-consistency reliability coefficients of the normative sample are in the .80s or .90s for most of the Wechsler core subtests. The coefficients of two of the WISC-IV and WAIS-III core subtests are in the .70s. In addition, the internal-consistency reliability coefficients of the Wechsler subtests calculated using clinical samples are very consistent with those using normative samples (Wechsler, 2002, 2003; Zhu, Tulsky, Price, & Chen, 2001). Second, the test–retest stability coefficients of the Wechsler scales are from .86 to .95 for IQ and Index scores, and mostly in the high .70s to low .90s for subtests. Third, the interscorer agreement of the Wechsler subtests are all in the high .90s for the non-verbal subtests and above .90 for the verbal subtests that require more judgment in scoring.

Validity

There is ample evidence to support the validity of the Wechsler scales. The exploratory and confirmatory factor-analytic studies reported in the test manuals provide strong evidence of construct validity. These studies clearly demonstrate that in addition to measuring an overall general intellectual ability, the Wechsler scales measure four cognitive domains: Verbal Comprehension, Perceptual Organization/Perceptual Reasoning, Working Memory, and Processing Speed (Wechsler,

1991, 1997b, 2002, 2003). Considerable evidence supporting the construct validity of the Wechsler scales has also been reported by some independent researchers. For instance, using both exploratory and confirmatory factor analyses on data obtained from a nationally representative sample of 1,118 cases, Roid, Prifitera, and Weiss (1993) successfully replicated the four-factor structure of the WISC-III. In separate confirmatory factor analyses of the WISC-III standardization sample, Kamphaus, Benson, Hutchinson, and Platt (1994) also found the fit of the four-factor model to be superior to alternative models for all age groups and major ethnic groups. Further confirmation of the four-factor model has been obtained in studies with such clinical populations as psychiatric inpatients (Tupa, Write, & Fristad, 1997) and children with traumatic brain injuries (Donders & Warschausky, 1997). In addition, subsequent adaptations in different countries have provided additional evidence supporting the construct validity of the Wechsler scales. For example, the four-factor solution has been independently replicated in Canada (Wechsler, 1995b), Australia (Wechsler, 1995a), Taiwan (Wechsler, 1997a), and Japan (Wechsler, 1998). In a factor analysis of WISC-III data from 15 nations ($N = 15,999$), Georgas, Van de Vijver, Weiss, and Saklofske (2003) replicated the four-factor structure, although in some countries Arithmetic loaded mostly on the Verbal Comprehension factor, producing a three-factor structure. Taken together, results from these studies indicate that the latent traits measured by the Wechsler scales appear consistently across different ages, ethnicities, cultures, and specific clinical populations.

Previous studies indicate that the Wechsler intelligence scales correlate highly with other measures of intelligence. Table 14.3 presents the correlation coefficients between the Wechsler scales and other measures of intelligence or cognitive ability. The magnitude of these coefficients is very high. For instance, the correlation between the FSIQ of the Wechsler intelligence scales and the GCA composite of the DAS is .84–.91 (Elliott, 1990), and the correlation between the FSIQ of the Wechsler scales and Stanford–Binet Intelligence Scale: Fourth Edition (SB-IV) composite is .80–.91 (Psychological Corporation, 1997; Thorndike, Hagen, & Sattler,

TABLE 14.3. Correlations between the Wechsler Scales and Other Scales

Other measures	Wechsler scales FSIQ	Source
Differential Ability Scales	.84–.91	Elliott (1990); Wechsler (2002)
Stanford–Binet Intelligence Scale: Fourth Edition and Stanford–Binet Intelligence Scales, Fifth Edition	.80–.91	Lavin (1996); Roid (2003); Psychological Corporation (1997); Thorndike, Hagen, and Sattler (1986)
Kaufman Adolescent and Adult Intelligence Test	.83–.88	Kaufman and Kaufman (1993)
Woodcock–Johnson Psycho–Educational Battery	.79–.83	Woodcock (1978)

1986). More interestingly, the correlations between the Wechsler scales and other measures are just slightly lower than the test–retest reliability of SB-IV.

Third, the Wechsler intelligence scales have very good predictive validity. The correlations between the FSIQ and academic achievement generally range from .65 to .75 (Psychological Corporation, 1992, 1997, 2001b; Wechsler, 2002, 2003).

INTERPRETATION

In addition to the basic interpretation steps and procedures suggested in the technical manuals of the latest Wechsler scales (Psychological Corporation, 1997; Wechsler, 2002, 2003), many interpretation strategies, methods, and procedures that were developed and refined by experienced clinicians and researchers for the previous versions of the Wechsler scales continue to be valid and useful (Kaufman, 1990, 1994; Kaufman & Lichtenberger, 1999; Prifitera & Saklofske, 1998; Sattler, 2001; Weiss, Saklofske, & Prifitera, 2003). Although a detailed discussion of interpretation strategies, methods, and procedures is beyond the scope of this chapter, we suggest a few basic interpretive considerations that may help readers understand the nature of clinical interpretation. However, these suggestions should not be used as a "cookbook" or comprehensive guideline for interpretation. Clinical interpretation is a very complicated hypothesis-testing process that varies from situation to situation. Therefore, no single approach will work for all scenarios.

The interpretation of test results is a systematic hypothesis-generating and hypothesis-testing process (Kamphaus, 1993; Prifitera et al., 1998). Results from the Wechsler intelligence scales provide important information regarding an individual's cognitive functioning, but they should never be interpreted in isolation. Four broad sources of information are typically available to the clinician conducting a psychological evaluation: (1) psychiatric, medical, educational, and psychosocial history; (2) direct behavioral observations; (3) quantitative test scores; and (4) qualitative aspects of test performance, such as motivation and test session compliance. The scores and item responses on the Wechsler intelligence scales provide quantitative and qualitative information that is best interpreted in conjunction with a thorough history and careful clinical observations of the individual. Results should always be evaluated within the context of the reasons for referral and all known collateral information.

Testing is different from assessment (Matarazzo, 1990; Prifitera et al., 1998; Robertson & Woody, 1997). Psychological *testing* is a data collection process in which an individual's behaviors are sampled and observed systematically in a standardized environment. Psychological *assessment* is a complicated problem-solving process that usually begins with psychological testing. Therefore, obtaining test scores is just the beginning of assessment, not the end.

Interpretation is an attempt to explain test results, which often includes a very complicated, multilevel, hypothesis-testing process—including profile, strengths and weaknesses, scatter, and discrepancy analysis. Interpretation converts the data collected through testing (such as a discrepancy score and behavior observation notes) into meaningful information, which may be used as evidence supporting certain conclusions. Each segment of information is like a puzzle piece. Clinicians must first gather all of the puzzle pieces and then assemble them in a meaningful way to draw appropriate conclusions. With this analogy in mind, it is clear that the identification of one puzzle piece is usually not sufficient to solve the whole puzzle, but it is a necessary and important step. It is similar to the physician's measurement of a patient's body temperature and blood pressure as the initial steps in forming a diagnosis. Temperature and blood pressure readings are universally performed procedures; however, in isolation, neither of them is conclusive for a final diagnosis. Similarly, scores on an intelligence test must be combined with scores on other measures, the examinee's demographic information (e.g., socioeconomic status, life history, educational background), and other information before any clinical decision can be made.

Basic Interpretation of Wechsler Intelligence Scales

Wechsler Scores

The Wechsler intelligence scales utilize two types of standard scores: scaled scores and composite scores (i.e., IQ and Index scores). The conversion of raw scores into standard scores allows clinicians to interpret scores within the Wechsler intelligence scales and between the Wechsler intelligence scales and other related measures. The scaled scores and composite scores are age-corrected standard scores that allow the test user to compare each individual's cognitive functioning with that of other individuals in the same age group.

Scaled scores are derived from the total raw scores on each subtest. They are scaled to a metric with a mean of 10 and a standard deviation (SD) of 3. A subtest scaled score of 10 reflects the average performance of a given age group. Scores of 7 and 13 correspond to 1 SD below and above the mean, respectively, and scaled scores of 4 and 16 deviate 2 SDs from the mean.

Composite scores (e.g., FSIQ and WMI) are standard scores based on various combinations of subtest scaled scores. They are scaled to a metric with a mean of 100 and an SD of 15. A score of 100 on any of composites defines the average performance of individuals of similar age. Scores of 85 and 115 correspond to 1 SD below and above the mean, respectively, and scores of 70 and 130 deviate 2 SDs from the mean. About 68% of all examinees obtain scores between 85 and 115; about 96% score in the 70–130 range; and nearly all examinees (about 99.9%) obtain scores between 55 and 145 (3 SDs on either side of the mean).

In general, standard scores provide the most accurate description of test data. However, for individuals who are unfamiliar with test interpretation, standard scores are often difficult to understand. Other methods, such as percentile ranks and test age equivalents are, are often used in conjunction with standard scores to describe an examinee's performance. Scores on the Wechsler intelligence scales should be reported in term of confidence intervals, so that each actual score is evaluated in light of the score's reliability. Confidence intervals assist the examiner in test interpretation by delineating a range of scores in which the examinee's true score is most likely to fall, and they remind the examiner that the observed score contains measurement error.

Level of Performance

The IQ, Index, and scaled scores can be characterized as falling within a certain level of performance (e.g., superior, high average, average, low average). The *level of performance* refers to the rank obtained by an individual on a given test, compared to the performance of an appropriate normative group. The descriptive classifications corresponding to scores on the Wechsler intelligence scales are presented in Table 14.4.

Test results on Wechsler intelligence scales can be described in a manner similar to the following example:

Relative to individuals of comparable age, this individual is currently functioning within the [descriptive classification] range of intelligence on a standardized measure of intellectual ability.

TABLE 14.4. Qualitative Descriptions of IQ and Index Scores

Score	Classification	Percent included in theoretical normal curve
130 and above	Very superior	2.2
120–129	Superior	6.7
110–119	High average	16.1
90–109	Average	50.0
80–89	Low average	16.1
70–79	Borderline	6.7
69 and below	Extremely low	2.2

Clinically speaking, the level of performance is important for estimating the presence and severity of any relative strength or weakness in an individual's performance. Clinical decisions can then be made if the individual's level of performance is significantly lower than that of the normative group. An alternative to this normative approach is that clinical decisions can also be made if a specific score is significantly lower than the individual's other scores (i.e., an intraindividual weakness).

In nonclinical settings (e.g., industrial and occupational settings), the emphasis on level of performance shifts slightly; more weight is placed on competency and the patterns of a person's strengths and weaknesses, without necessarily implying any type of impairment.

Analysis of Discrepancies among Domain Composite Scores

The IQ and Index scores are much more reliable measures than the subtest scaled scores, and in general, they are the first scores examined by the practitioner. Because the FSIQ summarizes an individual's performance across four different cognitive domains, and because individuals often show unbalanced development across these domains, it is good practice to evaluate the discrepancies among Index scores before interpreting the FSIQ. Such analysis may produce valuable information for clinical interpretation. Many clinical studies demonstrate that, compared with the normative sample, individuals diagnosed with certain clinical conditions (e.g., ADHD,

learning disability, epilepsy, and traumatic brain injury) are more likely to show certain patterns of discrepancies among Index scores (Brown, 1996; Donders & Warschausky, 1997; Prifitera & Dersh, 1993; Prifitera et al., 1998; Schwean, Saklofske, Yackulic, & Quinn, 1993; Wechsler, 1991). Clinicians should put less focus on the interpreting of the FSIQ if significant discrepancies among the Index scores are observed.

The first step of the discrepancy analysis is to determine the statistical significance of the discrepancy between a pair of composite scores. A *statistically significant difference* between scores—for example, between the VCI and the POI (or PRI) scores—refers to the likelihood that obtaining such a difference by chance is very low (e.g., $p < .05$) if the true difference between the scores is zero (Matarazzo & Herman, 1985). The level of significance reflects the level of confidence the clinician can have that the difference between the scores, called the *difference score*, is a true difference.

Often the difference between an individual's composite scores is significant in the statistical sense, but is not at all rare among individuals in the general population. The statistical significance of discrepancies between scores and the rarity of the difference are two separate issues and have different implications for test interpretation (Matarazzo & Herman, 1985; Payne & Jones, 1957; Sattler, 2001; Silverstein, 1981).

The Wechsler intelligence scales provide both critical values and base rate data in the manuals for evaluating whether a given discrepancy is statistically significant and how frequently such a discrepancy occurred in the normative sample. Because the discrepancies among Index scores are related to ability level, the base rate data are also provided by five ability levels. In addition, the base rates are provided by the direction of the discrepancy, because previous research has revealed that the frequencies of score differences vary with the direction of the difference (Sattler, 2001). For instance, the percentage of the WISC-IV normative sample with VCI scores greater than their PRI scores is not the same percentage of the normative sample with PRI scores greater than their VCI scores. Clinically speaking, the direction of VCI-PRI discrepancy is related to different patterns of cognitive strengths and weaknesses (Rourke,

1998). Data analysis of the WISC-IV norma-tive data revealed that about 62% of the His-panic children obtained higher PRI than VCI scores. On the other hand, only 48% of white non-Hispanic children obtained higher PRI than VCI scores. Therefore, social and cultural factors should be considered when one is interpreting the discrepancies among composite scores.

Interpreting IQ versus Index Scores

For the latest version of the Wechsler scales (i.e., the WPPSI-III and WISC-IV, the dual IQ (VIQ or PIQ) and Index score structure is no longer utilized. Such a change makes the in-terpretation of the composite scores easier. Currently, the WAIS-III is the only Wechsler instrument that has the dual IQ (VIQ or PIQ) and Index score structure. In the WAIS-III, the VIQ score summarizes an individual's performance on subtests that are designed to measure both Verbal Comprehension and Working Memory, and the PIQ score summarizes an individual's performance on subtests that measure Perceptual Organiza-tion and Processing Speed. An individual can obtain an average VIQ score because he or she performs at an average level on both do-mains, or at an above-average level on one domain and at a below-average level on the other domain. Therefore, VCI and POI are relatively purer measures of verbal and non-verbal reasoning, respectively, than VIQ and PIQ. The dual structure was used in WAIS-III for historical reasons and for the purpose of smooth transition from IQ to Index score. It is time now for practitioners to shift the fo-cus of interpretation from IQ scores to Index scores.

Examining the Scatter in Subtest Scaled Scores

IQ and Index scores are estimates of overall functioning in their respective areas and should always be evaluated within the con-text of the subtests that contribute to them (Kaufman & Lichtenberger, 1999; Wechsler 2002, 2003). It is good practice to evaluate the level of score consistency or variability (i.e., *scatter*) among subtest scaled scores before interpreting composite scores. Pro-files that have similar scaled scores indicate considerable consistency of an individual's

cognitive abilities. If the scaled scores are consistent, the composite is more likely to accurately summarize an individual's cogni-tive ability in the related area. However, the composite may not accurately summarize an individual's cognitive ability if the subtest scaled scores demonstrate significant vari-ability. Score variability is evident in scaled scores that range from very high to very low. The scatter score is calculated by subtracting the lowest score from the highest one. The Wechsler intelligence scales provide both critical values and base rate data in the man-uals for evaluating whether a given scatter is statistically significant and how frequently such a scatter occurred in the normative sample. The focus of interpretation should shift from composite to subtest scale scores if a significant scatter score is observed.

Analysis of Subtest Strengths and Weaknesses

If the subtest scaled scores demonstrate sig-nificant variability, it is a good practice to conduct an analysis of subtest strengths and weaknesses. Such an analysis is usually hy-pothesis- driven and focused on certain cog-nitive domains associated to the referral question (Kamphaus, 1993). The first step of a strengths-and-weaknesses analysis is to de-termine whether or not the differences be-tween each scaled score and the average of all scaled scores are statistically significant. The clinician should then examine whether such differences occur rarely. Score differ-ences can be statistically significant yet occur frequently within a general population. All the latest versions of the Wechsler intelli-gence scales provide tables of critical values and base rates that can be referred to for a strengths-and-weaknesses analysis.

Process Analysis

Another important step in interpretation is process analysis. The *process approach* to in-terpretation has been advocated by Kaplan and others (Kaplan, 1988; Kaplan, Fein, Morris, & Delis, 1991). This is a method for evaluating the nature of unusual responses and errors. Two individuals may obtain the same score on a given subtest or item for to-tally different reasons. On the Similarities subtest, for example, a scaled score of 10 points without any intrasubtest scatter may reflect an average reasoning ability. However, a scaled score of 10 points with considerable intrasubtest scatter may reflect an above-average reasoning ability depressed by language difficulty. Therefore, the interpretation of test results should go beyond the subtest scaled score level.

Similarly, paying attention to the response patterns of failed items and types of errors may reveal valuable information about the underlying process. Remember that an instrument that measures a single pure cognitive ability does not exist. All ecologically valid measures of cognitive ability invoke multiple cognitive functions that may affect the testing results. For instance, although Arithmetic is a ecologically valid test of working memory (Hitch, 1978; Sternberg, 1993), it also involves auditory verbal comprehension, mental manipulation, attention, concentration, long-term memory, processing speed, and numerical reasoning ability. Therefore, an individual might do poorly on this subtest due to many different reasons, such as language difficulty, inability to convert a verbal problem into a numerical one, poor working memory, poor math ability, slowness, or simply not trying hard enough. Experienced clinicians usually analyze the pattern and errors of an individual's performance first and then identify all the possible causes of the problem. Systematic hypothesis testing is then conducted to pinpoint the root causes.

A commonly used process analysis procedure is to compare an individual's performance under different testing conditions that involve different cognitive processes. For instance, poor performance on Coding might be caused by poor handwriting skills, poor incidental learning ability, or slow mental processing speed. By comparing an individual's score on coding, coding copy, and incidental learning, a clinician can test the hypothesis about each potential cognitive process and shorten the list of potential root causes. The latest version of the Wechsler scales provide some optional procedures and additional normative data to facilitate process analysis. For details about the process approach and the optional procedures, the reader is referred to the (WISC-III PI) manual (Kaplan, Fein, Kramer, Morris, & Delis, 1999).

Prediction of Premorbid Functioning

A difficult task faced by many clinicians is determining whether an individual's current test scores reflect a drop in performance from his or her previous ability before an accident occurred or illness began (Franzen, Burgess, & Smith-Seemiller, 1997). This process can help the clinician to infer whether the individual has sustained loss of functioning as a result of the accident or illness. Wechsler (1994) was the first person to propose that there was a "determination index" that could be derived by comparing performance on the so-called "hold" subtests of the Wechsler scales to that on the "don't hold" subtests. However, some research has demonstrated that basing the assessment of premorbid function on "hold" tests can underestimate premorbid IQ by as much as a full 1 SD (Larrabee, Largen, & Levin, 1985).

Alternative techniques include using scores that are obtained on vocabulary or reading tests, because the skills they reflect are believed to be relatively independent of general loss of functioning and can therefore be used as an index of premorbid functioning. Yates (1956) was the first person to hypothesize that one could estimate premorbid functioning with the WAIS Vocabulary score, because it is relatively independent of age-related decline in performance. Follow-up research by Russell (1972) and Swiercinsky and Warnock (1977) showed that individuals with brain damage did much more poorly than the general population on Vocabulary—a finding that contradicted Yates's hypothesis.

The more recent focus has been on using reading tests as indicators of premorbid functioning (Nelson, 1982; Nelson & McKenna, 1975; Nelson & O'Connell, 1978). Nelson and O'Connell (1978) introduced the National Adult Reading Test (subsequently named the New Adult Reading Test [NART]), which is a reading test using irregularly pronounced words. They developed a regression-based formula for estimating WAIS IQ scores from the scores on NART and concluded that predictions based on NART scores are fairly accurate.

Other alternative methods of determining premorbid functioning utilize the relationship between Wechsler IQ scores and demographic variables such as age, education, sex, race, and occupation. (Heaton, Ryan, Grant, & Mathews, 1996; Kaufman, McLean, & Reynolds, 1988). In general, two methods have prevailed. One method uses the correlation between the demographic variables and the IQ scores to develop prediction equations (e.g., Barona, Reynold, & Chastain, 1984; Wilson et al., 1978). The other method is to develop demographic-adjusted norms. During the standardization of the WAIS-III and WMS-III, additional effort was made to ensure that at least 30 individuals were sampled for each age × education level. In addition, a new word-reading test—the Wechsler Test of Adult Reading (WTAR; Psychological Corporation, 2001a)—was developed and conormed with the WAIS-III and WMS-III. The test uses words that are phonetically difficult to decode and would probably require previous learning. Regression analyses demonstrate that this reading test adds more incremental validity in predicting IQ and memory scores than do equations that just include demographic variables. Moreover, because it has been conormed directly with the Wechsler scales, the WTAR should provide invaluable information to the clinician who is trying to determine premorbid IQ.

CLINICAL APPLICATIONS

Because the Wechsler intelligence scales are reliable and valid instruments for comprehensive assessment of general cognitive functioning, clinicians have found many clinical applications of these instruments. Currently, each of the Wechsler scales is widely used as one of several key instruments for the assessment and diagnosis of (1) psychoeducational and developmental disorders, such as developmental delay, developmental risk, mental retardation, learning disability, ADHD, language disorders, motor impairment, and autistic; (2) cognitive giftedness; (3) neuropsychological disorders, such as traumatic brain injury, Alzheimer disease, Huntington disease, Parkinson disease, multiple sclerosis, and temporal lobe epilepsy; and (4) alcohol-related disorders, such as chronic alcohol abuse and Korsakoff syndrome. In addition, the Wechsler scales are frequently used for educational and vocational planning; qualification for private schools; and short-term and long-term social, educational, and psychological research. In addition to the many clinical validation studies reported in the technical manuals of the Wechsler scales (Psychological Corporation, 1997; Wechsler, 2002, 2003), please refer to Kaufman and Lichtenberger (1999), Prifitera and Saklofske (1998), Sattler (2001), and Tulsky and colleagues (2003) for more detailed discussion of the clinical utilities of the Wechsler scales.

INNOVATIONS IN MEASUREMENT OF COGNITIVE ABILITIES

Assessing Working Memory

As mentioned previously, inspired by recent cognitive and clinical research about mental capacity (i.e., working memory), the latest versions of Wechsler intelligence scales (e.g., WAIS-III and WISC-IV) lead the field of intellectual assessment by providing measurement of working memory. Although underemphasized by some modern intelligence theories, working memory is a key component to information processing, learning and fluid reasoning (Kyllonen, 1987; Kyllonen & Christal, 1989, 1990). Some recently published studies demonstrate the clinical utilities of the new WMI (Fry & Hale, 1996; Gussin & Javorsky, 1995; Perlow et al., 1997; Psychological Corporation, 1997; Swanson, 1999; Wechsler, 2002, 2003).

Assessing Processing Speed

Because measures of processing speed are usually simple visual scanning and tracking tasks, and they are not the best measures of g, they are often considered "minor" components of intellectual assessment instruments (Weiss et al., 2003). However, modern cognitive and clinical research has revealed that there is a dynamic relationship among processing speed, working memory, reasoning, and learning. More rapid processing of information may reduce demands on working memory and facilitate reasoning and learning. Therefore, all the latest Wechsler scales include subtests and a composite that assess processing speed. These measures were well received by clinicians in the field. Their clinical utilities are clearly demonstrated by several recent clinical studies (Brown, 1996; Donders, 1997; Donders & Warschausky, 1997; Donders, Zhu, & Tulsky, 2001; Hawkins, 1998; Prifitera & Dersh, 1993; Prifitera et al., 1998; Psychological Corporation, 1997; Schwean et al., 1993; Wechsler, 1991, 2002, 2003).

Optional Procedures for Process Analysis

The latest Wechsler scales have incorporated several optional procedures and additional normative information that can be used for a process evaluation. Optional procedures for a process evaluation are also available in a companion instrument of the WISC-IV designed for this purpose, the WISC-IV Integrated (Wechsler, 2004). The WISC-IV Integrated provides normative data for many optional procedures, based upon the process approach to interpretation advocated by Kaplan and others (e.g., Kaplan, 1988). These procedures and normative data provide a method for evaluating the nature of the errors made on the WISC-IV. For details of the process approach and the optional procedures, the reader is referred to the WISC-III PI manual (Kaplan et al., 1999).

Additional Normative Information

The Wechsler intelligence scales provide additional normative information for clinical evaluation, such as profile analysis (e.g., determining strengths and weaknesses, scatter, IQ and Index score discrepancies), memory–ability discrepancy, and achievement–ability discrepancy. To facilitate interpretation of assessment results, critical values and base rates are available in the test manual to determine the statistical significance of a given discrepancy and the frequency of its occurrence in the normative sample (base rate), respectively. The base rate data are also provided by ability levels and by the direction of the discrepancy. This normative information allows the clinician to determine whether a given score discrepancy is clinically meaningful. Previously, this type of normative data was only available in journal articles and related literature that appeared well after a test was published.

Conorming and Linkage to Other Measures

The Wechsler scales are often conormed with or linked to measures of memory and academic achievement. For instance, the WAIS-III has been conormed with the WMS-III (Wechsler, 1997c). Similarly, the WISC-IV has been linked to the Children's Memory Scale (CMS; Cohen, 1997). This linkage allows clinicians to examine IQ–memory discrepancy scores and assists them in the interpretation of additional domains of cognitive functioning that include both intelligence and memory assessment. The WAIS-III/WMS-III technical manual and the CMS manual both provide tables of critical values and base rates that allow clinicians to determine whether a given memory–IQ score discrepancy is statistically significant and how frequently it is observed in the normative sample. Discrepancies between intelligence and memory are sometimes used to evaluate memory impairment. With this approach, learning and memory are assumed to be underlying components of general intellectual ability and, as such, to be significantly related to an individual's performance on tests of intellectual functioning.

In addition, all the latest versions of the Wechsler scales are linked to the Wechsler Individual Achievement Test—Second Edition (WIAT–II; Psychological Corporation, 2001b). Such linkage provides a means of comparing an individual's general intellectual ability level to his or her level of academic achievement. Comparisons between intellectual ability and academic achievement have served as a primary criterion in determining eligibility for special educational services since the enactment of the 1997 amendments to the Individuals with Disabilities Education Act (IDEA, 1997).

BRIEF CASE STUDY

Report date: 11/18/2003
Examinee: Andy Ford
Age: 12 years
Date of birth: 11/13/91
Examinee ID: Not specified
Gender: Male
Grade: 6
Ethnicity: White non-Hispanic

Examiner: Paul Williams
Tests administered: WISC-IV (11/13/2003)
Age at testing: 12 years
Is this a retest? No

Reason for Referral

Andy was referred for an evaluation by his mother, Jane Ford. The reason for his referral is suspected hyperactivity.

Home

Andy is a 12-year-old who lives with his parents. There are two other children living in the home with Andy. His custodial arrangements have not changed in the last 3 years. Andy has been living in his present living arrangement since birth. Andy comes from a highly educated family. His mother completed 4 years of college. His father attended graduate school. Recently, there has been an event that has caused stress in his family; specifically, the family has experienced the death of a pet.

Language

Andy's dominant language is English. He has been exposed to English since birth. He has been speaking English since he began talking. Andy's speech during testing was clear and intelligible. Andy demonstrated English proficiency.

Development

According to his mother, Andy was born with no apparent complications. Andy's mother also reports that he reached the following milestones within the expected age ranges: sitting alone, crawling, standing alone, walking alone, and staying dry at night. He reached the following milestones later than expected: speaking first words and speaking short sentences. It is unknown whether the following milestone was accomplished early, typically, or late: using toilet when awake.

Health

According to his mother, Andy's vision screening results revealed that he has normal visual acuity. The results of his hearing screen revealed that he has normal auditory acuity. Andy's mother reports that he has no sensory or motor difficulties. During testing, Andy had no apparent sensory or motor difficulties. Andy's mother reports that he has no major medical or psychiatric diagnoses. According to Andy's mother, he had no signs of neurological concerns in the past, and he currently has no such signs. During the assessment, it was observed that Andy appeared to be in good health. Regarding Andy's use of medication, it is reported that he has taken medication for a cold; currently, he is not taking any prescription medications. It is also reported that he has no known past or current substance abuse. During testing, Andy did not appear under the influence of any medication or substance.

School

According to Andy's mother, his prekindergarten experience included an early childhood intervention program. His pre-first-grade experience included transitional kindergarten classes. Andy has been assigned to the same school since his initial enrollment. He currently attends classes full time, including special education classes. There is no information provided regarding Andy's retention history. In the past, Andy had an excellent attendance record, and he is currently maintaining good attendance. In the past, Andy had an exemplary conduct record; currently, he has only minor disciplinary problems. Both in the past and currently, however, Andy has had many academic difficulties. His past performance was below average in the following areas: reading, math, and language. Recently, his performance has been below average in the same three areas.

Behavior Observation

Andy appeared alert and oriented, shy, and well-groomed. It was observed that Andy required frequent encouragement and required frequent redirection.

Interpretation of WISC-IV Results

Andy was administered 10 subtests of the Wechsler Intelligence Scale for Children—Fourth Edition (WISC-IV), from which his composite scores are derived (see Tables 14.5

TABLE 14.5. Andy's WISC-IV Composite Scores

Scale	Sum of scaled scores	Composite score	Percentile rank	Confidence interval	Qualitative description
Verbal Comprehension Index (VCI)	25	91	27	85–98	Average
Perceptual Reasoning Index (PRI)	29	98	45	91–106	Average
Working Memory Index (WMI)	10	71	3	66–81	Borderline
Processing Speed Index (PSI)	11	75	5	69–87	Borderline
Full Scale IQ (FSIQ)	75	81	10	77–87	Low average

and 14.6 for his composite and subtest scores, respectively). The Full Scale IQ (FSIQ) is derived from a combination of 10 subtest scores and is considered the most representative estimate of global intellectual functioning. Andy's general cognitive ability is within the low average range of intellectual functioning, as measured by the FSIQ. His overall thinking and reasoning abilities exceed those of approximately 10% of children his age (FSIQ = 81; 95% confidence interval = 77–87). His ability to think with words is comparable to his ability to reason without the use of words. Both Andy's verbal and nonverbal reasoning abilities are also in the average range. He performed slightly better on nonverbal than on verbal reasoning tasks, but there is no significant meaningful

difference between his performance on the two types of tasks.

Andy's verbal reasoning abilities, as measured by the Verbal Comprehension Index (VCI), are in the average range but above those of approximately 27% of his peers (VCI = 91; 95% confidence interval = 85–98). The VCI is designed to measure verbal reasoning and concept formation. Andy performed comparably on the verbal subtests contributing to the VCI, suggesting that these verbal cognitive abilities are similarly developed.

Andy's nonverbal reasoning abilities, as measured by the Perceptual Reasoning Index (PRI), are in the average range and above those of approximately 45% of his peers (PRI = 98; 95% confidence interval = 91–

TABLE 14.6. Andy's WISC-IV Subtest Scores

Subtests	Raw score	Scaled score	Test age equiv.	Percentile rank
Similarities	23	9	11:6	37
Vocabulary	36	9	11:2	37
Comprehension	21	7	9:10	16
(Information)	17	8	10:6	25
(Word Reasoning)	13	7	9:6	16
Block Design	31	8	10:2	25
Picture Concepts	20	11	14:10	63
Matrix Reasoning	23	10	11:10	50
(Picture Completion)	20	6	8:2	9
Digit Span	11	5	6:2	5
Letter–Number Sequencing	12	5	7:6	5
(Arithmetic)	16	5	7:10	5
Coding	30	4	< 8:2	2
Symbol Search	20	7	9:6	16
(Cancellation)	67	7	9:2	16

106). The PRI is designed to measure fluid reasoning in the perceptual domain with tasks that assess nonverbal concept formation, visual perception and organization, simultaneous processing, visual–motor coordination, learning, and the ability to separate figure and ground in visual stimuli. Andy performed comparably on the performance subtests contributing to the PRI, suggesting that his visual–spatial reasoning and perceptual-organizational skills are similarly developed.

Andy's abilities to sustain attention, concentrate, and exert mental control, as measured by the Working Memory Index (WMI), are in the borderline range. He performed better than approximately 3% of his age-mates in this area (WMI = 71; 95% confidence interval = 66–81). Andy's abilities to sustain attention, concentrate, and exert mental control are weaknesses in relation to his nonverbal and verbal reasoning abilities. A weakness in mental control may make the processing of complex information more time-consuming for Andy, draining his mental energies more quickly as compared to other children his age, and may perhaps result in more frequent errors on a variety of learning tasks.

Andy was referred for this evaluation because it is suspected that he may be hyperactive. His score profile is consistent with this possibility. A pattern of weaker performance on mental control and processing speed tasks than on reasoning tasks occurs more often among students with attention deficits and hyperactive behavior than among children without these difficulties. Andy's active style of behavior may be related to difficulties in his home life, because his family is currently struggling with the death of a pet. Some children become overactive when they are having trouble coping with stressful circumstances in their lives. This possibility is worthy of further investigation, and Andy's activity level should be reevaluated when the stress is relieved.

Andy's abilities to process simple or routine visual material without making errors, as measured by the Processing Speed Index (PSI), are in the borderline range compared to those of his peers. He performed better than approximately 5% of his age-mates on these tasks (PSI = 75; 95% confidence interval = 69–87). Processing visual material

quickly is an ability that Andy performs poorly as compared to his nonverbal reasoning ability. Because learning often involves a combination of routine information processing (such as reading) and complex information processing (such as reasoning), a weakness in the speed of processing routine information may make the task of comprehending novel information more time-consuming and difficult for Andy. Thus this weakness in simple visual scanning and tracking may leave him less time and mental energy for the complex task of understanding new material.

Personal Strengths and Weaknesses

Andy's performance on the Picture Concepts subtest was significantly better than his own mean score. On the Picture Concepts subtest, Andy was presented with two or three rows of easily identifiable pictures and asked to choose one picture from each row to form a group with a common characteristic. This subtest is designed to measure fluid reasoning and abstract categorical reasoning ability. The task invokes verbal concepts, but does not require verbal responses (Picture Concepts scaled score = 11).

Summary

Andy is a 12-year-old who completed the WISC-IV. He was referred by his mother due to suspected hyperactivity. His general cognitive ability, as estimated by the WISC-IV, is in the low average range. Andy's verbal comprehension and perceptual reasoning abilities were both in the average range (VCI = 91, PRI = 98).

REFERENCES

Ackerman, P. L., Beier, M. E., & Bowen, K. R. (2000). Explorations of crystallized intelligence: Completion tests, cloze tests, and knowledge. *Learning and Individual Differences, 12*(1), 105–121.

Alexander, P. A., & Kulikowich, J. M. (1991). Domain knowledge and analogic reasoning ability as predictors of expository text comprehension. *Journal of Reading Behavior, 23*(2), 165–190.

Bannatyne, A. (1974). Diagnosis: A note on recategorization of the WISC scaled scores. *Journal of Learning Disabilities, 7,* 272–274.

Barona, A., Reynolds, C.R., & Chastain, R. (1984). A

demographically based index of premorbid intelligence for the WAIS-R. *Journal of Consulting and Clinical Psychology, 52*, 885–887.

Bate, A. J., Mathias, J. L., & Crawford, J. R. (2001). Performance on the test of everyday attention and standard tests of attention following severe traumatic brain injury. *The Clinical Neuropsychologist, 15*(3), 405–422.

Beres, K. A., Kaufman, A. S., & Perlman, M. D. (2000). Assessment of child intelligence. In G. Goldstein & M. Hersen (Eds.), *Handbook of psychological assessment* (3rd ed., pp. 65–96). New York: Elseiver Pergamon Press.

Berthier, N. E., DeBlois, S., Poirier, C. R., Novak, M. A., & Clifton, R. K. (2000). Where's the ball?: Two and three-year-olds reason about unseen events. *Developmental Psychology, 36*(3), 394–401.

Bracken, B. A. (1987). Limitations of preschool instruments and standards for minimal level of technical adequacy. *Journal of Psychoeducational Assessment, 4*, 313–326.

Brown, T. E. (1996). *Brown Attention-Deficit Disorder Scales.* San Antonio, TX: Psychological Corporation.

Brownell, R. (Ed.). (2000a). *Expressive One-Word Picture Vocabulary Test—Third Edition.* Novato, CA: Academic Therapy Press.

Brownell, R. (Ed.). (2000b). *Receptive One-Word Picture Vocabulary Test—Third Edition.* Novato, CA: Academic Therapy Press.

Carpenter, P. A., & Just, M. A. (1989). The role of working memory in language comprehension. In D. Klahr & K. Kotovsky (Eds.), *Complex information processing: The impact of Herbert A. Simon* (pp. 31–64). Hillsdale, NJ: Erlbaum.

Carpenter, P. A., Just, M. A., & Shell, P. (1990). What one intelligence test measures: A theoretical account of the processing in the Raven Progressive Matrices Test. *Psychological Review, 97*(3), 404–431.

Carroll, J. B. (1993). *Human cognitive abilities: A survey of factor-analytic studies.* New York: Cambridge University Press.

Cattell, R. B. (1943). The measurement of adult intelligence. *Psychological Bulletin, 40*(3), 153–159.

Cattell, R. B. (1963). Theory of fluid and crystallized intelligence: A critical experiment. *Journal of Educational Psychology, 54*(1), 1–22.

Cattell, R. B., & Horn, J. L. (1978). A check on the theory of fluid and crystallized intelligence with description of new subtest designs. *Journal of Educational Measurement, 15*(3), 139–164.

Cepeda, N. J., Kramer, A. F., & Gonzalez de Sather, J. C. M. (2001). Changes in executive control across the life span: Examination of task-switching performance. *Developmental Psychology, 37*(5), 715–730.

Cohen, J. (1952a). A factor-analytically based rationale for the Wechsler–Bellevue. *Journal of Consulting Psychology, 16*, 272–277.

Cohen, J. (1952b). Factors underlying Wechsler–Bellevue performance of three neuropsychiatric groups. *Journal of Abnormal and School Psychology, 47*, 359–364.

Cohen, J. (1957a). The factorial structure of the WAIS between early adulthood and old age. *Journal of Consulting Psychology, 21*, 283–290.

Cohen, J. (1957b). A factor-analytically based rationale for the Wechsler Adult Intelligence Scale. *Journal of Consulting Psychology, 6*, 451–457.

Cohen, J. (1959). The factorial structure of the WISC at ages 7-6, 10-6, and 13-6. *Journal of Consulting Psychology, 23*, 285–299.

Cohen, M. (1997). *Children's Memory Scale.* San Antonio, TX: Psychological Corporation.

Cooper, S. (1995). The clinical use and interpretation of the Wechsler intelligence scale for children (3rd ed.). Springfield, IL: Charles C. Thomas.

Crowe, S. F. (2000). Does the letter number sequencing task measure anything more than digit span? *Assessment, 7*(2), 113–117.

Daneman, M., & Carpenter, P. A. (1980). Individual differences in working memory and reading. *Journal of Verbal Learning and Verbal Behavior, 19*, 450–466.

Deak, G. O., & Maratsos, M. (1998). On having complex representations of things preschoolers use multiple words for objects and people. *Developmental Psychology, 34*(2), 224–240.

Deary, I. J., & Stough, C. (1996). Intelligence and inspection time: Achievements, prospects, and problems. *American Psychologist, 51*, 599–608.

de Jonge, P., & de Jonge, P. F. (1996). Working memory, intelligence and reading ability in children. *Personality and Individual Differences, 21*, 1007–1020.

Delis, D. C., Kaplan, E., & Kramer, J. H. (2001). *Delis–Kaplan Executive Function System.* San Antonio, TX: Psychological Corporation.

DeSanti, R. J. (1989). Concurrent and predictive validity of a semantically and syntactically sensitive cloze scoring system. *Reading, Research, and Instruction, 28*(2), 29–40.

Donders, J. (1997). Sensitivity of the WISC-III to injury severity in children with traumatic head injury. *Assessment, 4*(1), 107–109.

Donders, J., & Warschausky, S. (1997). WISC-III factor index score patterns after traumatic head injury in children. *Child Neuropsychology, 3*, 71–78.

Donders, J., Zhu, J., & Tulsky, D. S. (2001). Factor index score patterns in the WAIS-III standardization sample. *Assessment. 8*, 193–203.

Elliott, C. D. (1990). *Differential Ability Scales: Introductory and technical handbook.* San Antonio, TX: Psychological Corporation.

Flanagan, D. P., & Alfonso, V. C. (1995). A critical review of the technical characteristics of new and recently revised intelligence test for preschool children. *Journal of Psychoeducational Assessment, 13*, 66–90.

Flavell, J. H. (1985). *Cognitive development* (2nd ed.). Englewood Cliffs, NJ: Prentice-Hall.

Franzen, M. D., Burgess, E. J., & Smith-Seemiller, L. (1997). Methods of estimating premorbid functioning. *Archives of Clinical Neuropsychology, 12*(8), 711–738.

Fry, A. F., & Hale, S. (1996). Processing speed, working memory, and fluid intelligence: Evidence for a developmental cascade. *Psychological Science, 7,* 237–241.

Gauthier, L., Dehaut, F., & Joanette, Y. (1989). The Bells Test: A quantitative and qualitative test for visual neglect. *International Journal of Clinical Neuropsychology, 11,* 49–54.

Geldmacher, D. S. (1996). Effects of stimulus number and target-to-distractor ratio on the performance of random array letter cancellation tasks. *Brain and Cognition, 32,* 405–415.

Georgas, J., Van de Vijver, F., Weiss, L., & Saklofske, D. (2002). A cross-cultural analysis of the WISC-III. In J. Georgas, L. Weiss, F. Van de Vijver, & D. Saklofske (Eds.), *Cross-cultural analysis of the WISC-III: Cultural considerations in assessing intelligence* (pp. 277–313). San Diego, CA: Academic Press.

German, D. J. (1989). *Test of Word Finding.* Austin, TX: Pro-Ed.

Glasser, A. J., & Zimmerman, I. L. (1967). *Clinical interpretation of the WISC.* New York: Grune & Stratton.

Gold, J. M., Carpenter, C., Randolph, C., Goldberg, T. E., & Weinberger, D. R. (1997). Auditory working memory and Wisconsin Card Sorting Test performance in schizophrenia. *Archives of General Psychiatry, 54,* 159–165.

Groth-Marnat, G. (1997). *Handbook of psychological assessment* (3rd ed.). New York: Wiley.

Gussin, B., & Javorsky, J. (1995, Fall). The utility of the WISC-III Freedom from Distractibility in the diagnosis of youth with attention deficit hyperactivity disorder in a psychiatric sample. *Diagnostique, 21*(1), 29–42.

Hale, J. B., Hoeppner, J. B., & Fiorello, C. A. (2002). Analyzing digit span components for assessment of attention processes. *Journal of Psychoeducational Assessment, 20,* 128–143.

Halligan, P. W., Marshall, J. C., & Wade, D. T. (1989, October 14). Visuospatial neglect: Underlying factors and test sensitivity. *Lancet,* pp. 908–911.

Hammill, D. D., Brown, L., & Bryant, B. R. (1992). *A consumer's guide to tests in print* (2nd ed.). Austin, TX: Pro-Ed.

Harrison, P. L., Kaufman, A. S., Hickman, J. A., & Kaufman, N. L. (1988). A survey of tests used for adult assessment. *Journal of Psychoeducational Assessment, 6,* 188–198.

Hawkins, K. A. (1998). Indicators of brain dysfunction derived from graphic representations of the WAIS-III/WMS-III technical manual samples: A preliminary approach to clinical utility. *The Clinical Neuropsychologist, 12,* 535–551.

Heaton, R. K., Ryan, L., Grant, I., & Matthews, C. G. (1996). Demographic influences on neuropsychological test performance. In I. Grant & K. M. Adams (Eds.), *Neuropsychological assessment of neuropsy-*

chiatric disorders (pp. 141–163). New York: Oxford University Press.

Hitch, G. (1978). The role of short-term working memory in mental arithmetic. *Cognitive Psychology, 10,* 302–323.

Horn, J. L. (1985). Remodeling old models of intelligence. In B. B. Wolman (Ed.), *Handbook of intelligence: Theories, measurement, and applications* (pp. 267–300). New York: Wiley.

Horn, J. L. (1991). Measurement of intellectual capabilities: A review of theory. In K. S. McGrew, J. K. Werder, & R. W. Woodcock, *WJ-R technical manual* (pp. 197–232). Chicago: Riverside.

Horn, J. L. (1994). Theory of fluid and crystallized intelligence. In R. J. Sternberg (Ed.), *Encyclopedia of human intelligence* (pp. 443–451). New York: Macmillan.

Horn, J. L., & Noll, J. (1997). Human cognitive capabilities: Gf-Gc theory. In D. P. Flanagan, J. L. Genshaft, & P. L. Harrison (Eds.), *Contemporary intelligence assessment: Theories, tests, and issues* (pp. 53–91). New York: Guilford Press.

Individuals with Disabilities Education Act Amendments of 1997, Pub. L. 105-17, 20 U.S.C. 33, §§ 1431 *et seq.* (1997).

Jensen, A. R. (1982). Reaction time and psychometric *g.* In H. J. Eysenck (Ed.), *A model for intelligence* (pp. 93–132). New York: Sringer-Verlag.

Jensen, A. R. (1987). Process differences and individual difference in some cognitive tasks. *Intelligence, 11,* 107–136.

Kail, R. (2000). Speed of information processing: Developmental change and links to intelligence. *Journal of School Psychology, 38*(1), 51–61.

Kail, R., & Salthouse, T. A. (1994). Processing speed as a mental capacity. *Acta Psychologica, 86,* 199–225.

Kamphaus, R. W. (1993). *Clinical assessment of children's intelligence.* Needham Heights, MA: Allyn & Bacon.

Kamphaus, R. W., Benson, J., Hutchinson, S., & Platt, L. O. (1994). Identification of factor models for the WISC-III . *Educational and Psychological Measurement, 54*(1), 174 –186.

Kaplan, E. (1988). A process approach to neuropsychological assessment. In T. J. Boll & B. K. Bryant (Eds.), *Clinical neuropsychology and brain function: Research, measurement, and practice* (pp. 129–167). Washington, DC: American Psychological Association.

Kaplan, E., Fein, D., Kramer, J., Morris, R., & Delis, D. C. (1999). *Manual for WISC-III as a Process Instrument.* San Antonio, TX: Psychological Corporation.

Kaplan, E., Fein, D., Morris, R., & Delis, D. C. (1991). *Manual for WAIS-R as a Neuropsychological Instrument.* San Antonio, TX: Psychological Corporation.

Kaufman, A. S. (1990). *Assessing adolescent and adult intelligence.* Boston: Allyn & Bacon.

Kaufman, A. S. (1994). *Intelligent testing with the WISC-III.* New York: Wiley.

Kaufman, A. S., & Kaufman, N. L. (1993). *Kaufman*

Adolescent and Adult Intelligence Test. Circle Pines, MN: American Guidance Service.

Kaufman, A. S., & Lichtenberger, E. O. (1999). *Essentials of WAIS-III assessment.* New York: Wiley.

Kaufman, A. S., McLean, J. E., & Reynolds, C. R. (1988). Sex, race, residence, region, and education difference on the II WAIS-R subtests. *Journal of Clinical Psychology, 44*(2), 231–248.

Kranzler, J. H., & Jensen, A.R. (1989). Inspection time and intelligence: A meta-analysis. *Intelligence, 13,* 329–347.

Kyllonen, P. C. (1987). Theory-based cognitive assessment. In J. Zeidner (Ed.), *Human productivity enhancement: Organizations, personnel, and decision making* (Vol. 2, pp. 338–381). New York: Praeger.

Kyllonen, P. C., & Christal, R. E. (1989). Cognitive modeling of learning abilities: A status report of LAMP. In R. Dillon & J. W. Pelegrino (Eds.), *Testing: Theoretical and applied issues.* New York: Freeman.

Kyllonen, P. C., & Christal, R. E. (1990). Reasoning ability is (little more than) working-memory capacity?! *Intelligence, 14,* 389–433.

Larrabee, G. J., Largen, J. W., & Levin, H. S. (1985). Sensitivity of age-decline resistant ("hold") WAIS subtests to Alzheimer's disease. *Journal of Clinical and Experimental Neuropsychology, 7,* 497–504.

Lavin, C. (1996). The Wechsler Intelligence Scale for Children—Third Edition and the Stanford–Binet Intelligence Scale: Fourth Edition: A preliminary study of validity. *Psychological Report, 78,* 491–496.

Matarazzo, J. D. (1990). Psychological assessment versus psychological testing: Validation from Binet to the school, clinic, and courtroom. *American Psychologist, 45,* 999–1017.

Matarazzo, J. D., & Herman, D. O. (1985). Clinical uses of the WAIS-R: Base rates of differences between VIQ and PIQ in the WAIS-R standardization sample. In B. B. Wolman (Ed.), *Handbook of intelligence: Theories, measurements, and applications* (pp. 899–932). New York: Wiley.

McFie, J. (1975). *Assessment of organic intellectual impairment.* New York: Academic Press.

McKenna, M. C., & Layton, K. (1990). Concurrent validity of cloze as a measure of intersentential comprehension. *Journal of Educational Psychology, 82*(2), 372–377.

Neisser, U., Boodoo, G., Bouchard, T. J., Boykin, A. W., Brody, N., Ceci, S. J., et al. (1996). Intelligence: Knowns and unknowns, *American Psychologist, 51*(2) 77–101.

Nelson, H. E. (1982). *National Adult Reading Test (NART) manual.* Windsor, UK: NFER-Nelson.

Nelson, H. E., & McKenna, P. (1975). The use of current reading ability in the assessment of dementia, *British Journal of Social and Clinical Psychology, 14,* 259–267.

Nelson, H. E., & O'Connell, A. (1978). Dementia: The estimation of premorbid intelligence levels using the New Adult Reading Test. *Cortex, 14,* 234–244.

Neubauer, A. C., & Knorr, E. (1998). Three paper-and-pencil tests for speed of information processing: Psychometric properties and correlations with intelligence. *Intelligence, 26*(2), 123–151.

Newstead, S. E., Thompson, V., & Handley, S. J. (2002). Generating alternatives: A key component in human reasoning? *Memory and Cognition, 30*(1), 129–137.

Payne, R. W., & Jones, H. G. (1957). Statistics for the investigation of individual cases. *Journal of Clinical Psychology, 13,* 115–121.

Perlow, R., Jattuso, M., & Moore, D. D. (1997). Role of verbal working memory in complex skill acquisition. *Human Performance, 10*(3), 283–302.

Politano, P. M., & Finch, A. J. (1996). The Wechsler Intelligence Scale for Children—Third Edition. In C. S. Newmark (Ed.), *Major psychological assessment instruments* (pp. 294–319). Boston: Allyn & Bacon.

Prifitera, A., & Dersh, J. (1993). Base rates of WISC-III diagnostic subtest patterns among normal, learning-disabled, and ADHD samples. *Journal of Psychoeducational Assessment Monograph Series. Advances in Psychological Assessment: Wechsler Intelligence Scale for Children—Third Edition, 43–55.*

Prifitera, A., & Saklofske, D. H. (Eds.). (1998). *WISC-III clinical use and interpretation: Scientist-practitioner perspectives.* San Diego, CA: Academic Press.

Prifitera, A., Weiss, L. G., & Saklofske, D. H. (1998). The WISC-III in context. In A. Prifitera & D. H. Saklofske (Eds.), *WISC-III clinical use and interpretation: Scientist-practitioner perspectives* (pp. 1–38). San Diego, CA: Academic Press.

Psychological Corporation. (1992). *WIAT examiner's manual.* San Antonio, TX: Author.

Psychological Corporation. (1997). *WAIS-III–WMS-III technical manual.* San Antonio, TX: Author.

Psychological Corporation. (2001a). *Wechsler Test of Adult Reading.* San Antonio, TX: Author.

Psychological Corporation. (2001b). *WIAT-II examiner's manual.* San Antonio, TX: Author.

Psychological Corporation. (2002). *WAIS-III–WMS-III technical manual—updated.* San Antonio, TX: Author.

Reynolds, C. R. (1997). Forward and backward memory span should not be combined for clinical analysis. *Archives of Clinical Neuropsychology, 12*(1), 29–40.

Ridgeway, V. (1995). The use of cloze as a measure of the interactive use of prior knowledge and comprehension strategies. In W. M. Linek & E. G. Sturtevant (Eds.), *Generations of literacy: The seventeenth yearbook of the College Reading Association, 1995* (pp. 26–34). Commerce: East Texas State University.

Robertson, M. H., & Woody, R. H. (1997). *Theories and methods for practice of clinical psychology.* Madison, CT: International Universities Press.

Robinson, E. L., & Saxon, T. F. (1999, April). *Language and cognition: Examining the importance of early* language competence and subsequent intellectual ability. Poster session presented at the annual meeting of the National Association of School Psychologists, Las Vegas, NV.

Roid, G. H. (2003). *Stanford–Binet Intelligence Scale, Fifth Edition: Technical manual.* Itasca, IL: Riverside.

Roid, G. H., Prifitera, A., & Weiss, L. G. (1993). Replication of the WISC-III factor structure in an independent sample. *Journal of Psychoeducational Assessment Monograph Series. Advances in Psychological Assessment: Wechsler Intelligence Scale for Children–Third Edition,* 6–21.

Rourke, B. P. (1998). Significance of Verbal–Performance discrepancies for subtypes of children with learning disabilities: Opportunities for the WISC-III. In A. Prifitera & D. Saklofske (Eds.), *WISC-III clinical use and interpretation: Scientist-practitioner perspectives* (pp. 139–156). San Diego, CA: Academic Press.

Ryan, J. J., & Smith, J. W. (2003). Assessing the intelligence of adolescents with the Wechsler Adult Intelligence Scale—Third Edition. In C. R. Reynolds & R. W. Kamphaus (Eds.), *Handbook of psychological and educational assessment of children: Intelligence, aptitude, and achievement* (2nd ed., pp. 147–173). New York: Guilford Press.

Russell, E. (1972). WAIS factor analysis with brain-damaged subjects using criterion measures. *Journal of Consulting and Clinical Psychology, 39,* 133–139.

Sattler, J. M. (2001). *Assessment of children: Cognitive applications* (4th ed.). San Diego, CA: Jerome M. Sattler.

Sattler, J. M., & Ryan, J. J. (2001). WAIS-III subtests and interpreting the WAIS-III. J. M. Sattler, *Assessment of children: Cognitive applications* (4th ed., pp. 415–454). San Diego, CA: Jerome M. Sattler.

Sattler, J. M., & Saklofske, D. H. (2001). WISC-III subtests. In J. M. Sattler, *Assessment of children: Cognitive applications* (4th ed., pp. 266–297). San Diego, CA: Jerome M. Sattler.

Schatz, J., Kramer, J. H., Albin, A., & Matthay, K. K. (2000). Processing speed, working memory and IQ: A developmental model of cognitive deficits following cranial radiation therapy. *Neuropsychology, 14*(2), 189–200.

Schwean, V. L., Saklofske, D. H., Yackulic, R. A., & Quinn, D. (1993). WISC-III performance of ADHD children. *Journal of Psychoeducational Assessment Monograph Series. Advances in Psychological Assessment: Wechsler Intelligence Scale for Children—Third Edition,* 56–70.

Semel, E., Wiig, E. H., & Secord, W. A. (1995). *Clinical Education of Language Fundamentals—Third Edition.* San Antonio, TX: Psychological Corporation.

Shulman, C., Yirmiya, N., & Greenbaum, C. W. (1995). From categorization to classification: A comparison among individuals with autism, mental retardation,

and normal development. *Journal of Abnormal Psychology, 104*(4), 601–609.

Silverstein, A. B. (1981). Reliability and abnormality of test score differences. *Journal of Clinical Psychology, 37*(2), 392–394.

Sternberg, R. J. (1993). Rocky's back again: A review of the WISC-III. *Journal of Psychoeducational Assessment Monograph Series. Advances in Psychological Assessment: Wechsler Intelligence Scale for Children—Third Edition,* 161–164.

Sternberg, R. J. (1995). *In search of the human mind.* Fort Worth, TX: Harcourt Brace.

Swanson, H. L. (1999). What develops in working memory?: A life span perspective. *Developmental Psychology, 35,* 986–1000.

Swiercinsky, D. P., & Warnock, J. K. (1977). Comparison of the neuropsychological key and discriminate analysis approaches in predicting cerebral damage and localization. *Journal of Consulting and Clinical Psychology, 45,* 808–814.

Thorndike, R. L., Hagen, E. P., & Sattler, J. M. (1986). *Stanford–Binet Intelligence Scale: Fourth Edition: Technical manual.* Chicago: Riverside.

Tulsky, D. S., & Price, L. R. (2003). The joint WAIS-III and WMS-III factor structure: Development and cross-validation of a six-factor model of cognitive functioning. *Psychological Assessment, 15*(2), 149–162.

Tulsky, D. S., Saklofske, D. H., Chelune, G. J., Heaton, R. K., Ivnik, R. J., Bornstein, R., et al. (2003). *Clinical interpretation of the WAIS-III and WMS-III.* San Diego, CA: Academic Press.

Tulsky, D. S., Zhu, J., & Prifitera, A. (2000). Assessing adult intelligence with the WAIS–III. In G. Goldstein & M. Hersen (Eds.), *Handbook of psychological assessment* (3rd ed.). New York: Pergamon Press.

Tupa, D. J., Write, M. O., & Fristad, M. A. (1997). Confirmatory factor analysis of the WISC-III with child psychiatric inpatients. *Psychological Assessment, 9*(3), 302–306.

Wasserman, J. D., & Maccubbin, E. M. (2002). *Wechsler at The Psychological Corporation: Chorus girls and taxi drivers.* Paper presented at the 110th Annual Convention of the American Psychological Association, Chicago.

Watkins, C. E., Campbell, V. L., Nieberding, R., & Hallmark, R. (1995). Contemporary practice of psychological assessment by clinical psychologists. *Professional Psychology: Research and Practice, 26*(1), 54–60.

Wechsler, D. (1939). *Wechsler–Bellevue Intelligence Scale.* New York: Psychological Corporation.

Wechsler, D. (1944). *The measurement of adult intelligence* (3rd ed.). Baltimore: Williams & Wilkins.

Wechsler, D. (1945). *Wechsler Memory Scale.* New York: Psychological Corporation.

Wechsler, D. (1946). *Wechsler–Bellevue Intelligence Scale—Form II.* New York: Psychological Corporation.

Wechsler, D. (1949). *Wechsler Intelligence Scale for Children*. New York: Psychological Corporation.

Wechsler, D. (1950). Cognitive, conative, and non-intellective intelligence. *American Psychologist, 5,* 78–83.

Wechsler, D. (1955). *Wechsler Adult Intelligence Scale.* New York: The Psychological Corporation.

Wechsler, D. (1958). *The measurement and appraisal of adult intelligence* (4th ed.). Baltimore: Williams & Wilkins.

Wechsler, D. (1967). *Wechsler Preschool and Primary Scale of Intelligence*. New York: Psychological Corporation.

Wechsler, D. (1974). *Wechsler Intelligence Scale for Children—Revised Edition*. New York: Psychological Corporation.

Wechsler, D. (1975). Intelligence defined and undefined: A relativistic appraisal. *American Psychologist, 30,* 135–139.

Wechsler, D. (1981). *Wechsler Adult Intelligence Scale—Revised*. New York: Psychological Corporation.

Wechsler, D. (1987). *Wechsler Memory Scale—Revised.* San Antonio, TX: Psychological Corporation.

Wechsler, D. (1989). *Wechsler Preschool and Primary Scale of Intelligence—Revised*. San Antonio, TX: Psychological Corporation.

Wechsler, D. (1991). *Wechsler Intelligence Scale for Children—Third Edition*. San Antonio, TX: Psychological Corporation.

Wechsler, D. (1995a). *Manual for the Wechsler Intelligence Scale for Children—Third Edition: Australia edition*. Marrickville, Australia: Psychological Corporation.

Wechsler, D. (1995b). *Manual for the Wechsler Intelligence Scale for Children—Third Edition: Canadian edition*. Toronto: Psychological Corporation.

Wechsler, D. (1997a). *Manual for the Wechsler Intelligence Scale for Children—Third Edition: Taiwan edition*. Taipei, Taiwan: Chinese Behavior Science Corporation.

Wechsler, D. (1997b). *Wechsler Adult Intelligence Scale—Third Edition*. San Antonio, TX: Psychological Corporation.

Wechsler, D. (1997c). *Wechsler Memory Scale—Third Edition*. San Antonio, TX: Psychological Corporation.

Wechsler, D. (1998). *Manual for the Wechsler Intelligence Scale for Children—Third Edition: Japanese Edition*. Tokyo: Psychological Corporation.

Wechsler, D. (2002). *Wechsler Preschool and Primary Scale of Intelligence—Third Edition*. San Antonio, TX: Psychological Corporation.

Wechsler, D. (2003). *Wechsler Intelligence Scale for Children—Fourth Edition*. San Antonio, TX: Psychological Corporation.

Wechsler, D. (2004). *Wechsler Intelligence Scale for Children Fourth Edition—Integrated*. San Antonio, TX: Harcourt Assessment.

Weiss, L. G., Saklofske, D. H., & Prifitera, A. (2003). Clinical interpretation of the Wechsler Intelligence Scale for Children—Third Edition (WISC-III) Index scores. In C. R. Reynolds & R. W. Kamphaus (Eds.), *Handbook of psychological and educational assessment of children: Intelligence, aptitude, and achievement* (2nd ed., pp. 115–146). New York: Guilford Press.

Wilson, R. S., Rosenbaum, G., Brown, G., Rourke, D., Whitman, D., & Grissell, J. (1978). An index of premorbid intelligence. *Journal of Consulting and Clinical Psychology, 46,* 1554–1555.

Wojciulik, E., Husain, M., Clarke, K., & Driver, J. (2001). Spatial working memory deficit in unilateral neglect. *Neuropsychologia, 39,* 390–396.

Wolman, B. B. (Ed.). (1985). *Handbook of intelligence: Theories, measurements, and applications*. New York: Wiley.

Woltz, D. J. (1988). An investigation of the role of working memory in procedural skill acquisition. *Journal of Experimental Psychology: General, 117,* 319–331.

Woodcock, R. W. (1978). *Development and standardization of the Woodcock–Johnson Psycho-Educational Battery*. Allen, TX: DLM Teaching Resources.

Yates, A. (1956). The use of vocabulary in the measurement of intellectual deterioration: A review. *Journal of Mental Science, 102,* 409–440.

Zachary, R. A. (1990). Wechsler's intelligence scales: Theoretical and practical considerations. *Journal of Psychoeducational Assessment, 8,* 276–289.

Zhu, J., Tulsky, D. S., Price, L., & Chen, H. Y. (2001). WAIS-III reliability data for clinical groups. *Journal of International Neuropsychological Society, 7,* 862–866.

Zhu, J. J., Weiss, L. G., Prifitera, A., & Coalson, D. (2003). The Wechsler intelligence scales for children and adults. In M. Hersen (Series Ed.) & G. Goldstein & S. R. Beers (Vol. Eds.), *Comprehensive handbook of psychological assessment: Vol. 1. Intellectual and neuropsychological assessment* (pp. 51–75). New York: Wiley.

15

Interpreting the Stanford–Binet Intelligence Scales, Fifth Edition

GALE H. ROID
MARK POMPLUN

Following the long tradition begun by Binet and Simon (1908) and Terman (1916), the Stanford–Binet Intelligence Scales, Fifth Edition (SB5; Roid, 2003a) was recently published. The new edition combines the point scale format of the Fourth Edition (Thorndike, Hagen, & Sattler, 1986) with the age-level format of the Terman and Merrill (1937, 1960) editions. Also, the SB5 combines the use of routing subtests with functional levels. These functional levels were based on item response theory (IRT; Rasch, 1980). One of the routing subtests, Vocabulary, has been used in all editions to tailor the remainder of the testing to the functional level of the examinee. For the SB5, a nonverbal subtest, Object-Series/Matrices, was added as a second routing test.

The SB5 is a cognitive abilities battery, individually administered for the age range of 2 to 85+ years. It was constructed on a five-factor hierarchical model similar to the four-factor model of the Fourth Edition. Importantly, for the first time in cognitive testing history, these five cognitive factors—Fluid Reasoning, Knowledge, Quantitative Reasoning, Visual–Spatial Processing, and Working Memory—are measured in both Nonverbal and Verbal domains. Thus a full one-half of the new test battery is devoted to a reduced-language (Nonverbal) section. The Nonverbal section uses "hands-on" tasks involving brightly colored pictures, toys, and other objects that engage examinees, particularly young children and individuals with low cognitive functioning.[1] Some of the new features of the SB5 include the following:

- Brightly colored toys, blocks, and pictures have been restored in the new edition.
- Extended low-end and high-end items allow for early childhood and giftedness assessment.
- New composite scores have a mean of 100 and a standard deviation of 15, including Full Scale IQ (FSIQ), Nonverbal IQ (NVIQ), Verbal IQ (VIQ), and the five factor index scores.
- An Abbreviated Battery IQ (ABIQ) is formed from the routing tests.
- IRT-based *change-sensitive scores* (CSSs) are optional for criterion-referenced interpretation.
- The new Verbal and Nonverbal Working Memory subtests require two of the subsystems of short-term memory defined by Baddeley (1986), one for language and one for visual–spatial information. A nonverbal block-tapping task also requires the planning and motor control abilities within executive processing, in which the individual guides his or her own thinking pro-

cesses (Lezak, 1995). These new subtests provide new tools for the assessment of elderly individials, persons with neuropsychological disorders, and persons with learning disabilities (LDs).

- The SB5 is linked to the Woodcock–Johnson III (WJ III) Tests of Achievement (Woodcock, McGrew, & Mather, 2001a) for assessment of persons with LDs.

THEORY AND STRUCTURE

Based on the important research of Carroll (1993), the SB5 was constructed on a five-factor hierarchical cognitive model. The five factors were derived from the combined model of Carroll (1993), Cattell (1943), and Horn (1965, 1994). The combination of models, now called the *Cattell–Horn–Carroll* (CHC) theory (see McGrew, Chapter 8, this volume, for a detailed discussion), normally lists 8–10 factors. Many of the supplemental factors, such as processing speed, auditory processing, and long-term retrieval, require specialized timing or test apparatus (e.g., tape recorders). However, the selection of the SB5's five cognitive factors (see Figure 15.1) was based on research on school achievement and on expert ratings of the importance of these factors in the assessment of reasoning, especially in giftedness assessment. Expert ratings were obtained from several sources: from an advisory panel of prominent researchers and practitioners;

from contracted consultants; from a workshop on assessment of gifted individuals, held in Denver, Colorado; and from key advisors such as John Carroll (1993), John Horn (1994), Richard Woodcock, and Kevin McGrew (Woodcock et al., 2001a), at meetings in which all of these four experts were present. Also, the memory factor was shifted from an emphasis on short-term memory only, as in the Fourth Edition of the Stanford–Binet, to an emphasis on working memory.

Some expert consultants and advisors disagreed about the role of a hierarchical general factor (g) in CHC theory and the five-factor version in SB5. The consensus of the SB5 development staff and author, Gale Roid, was to emphasize the importance of the empirical studies of Carroll (1993) and the tradition of hierarchical models in previous versions of the Stanford–Binet. Therefore, the overall model shown in Figure 15.1 is a hierarchical g model, with five factors emphasizing reasoning abilities that can be easily administered within a 1-hour assessment.

The types of item content measured by the SB5 are shown in Table 15.1. The Verbal and Nonverbal domains include 5 subtests each, for a total of 10 subtests. The subtests each have raw score totals that are converted to various derived scores, such as the normalized scaled scores (mean = 10, standard deviation = 3) used to form the profile of 10 subtest scores used in the interpretation of

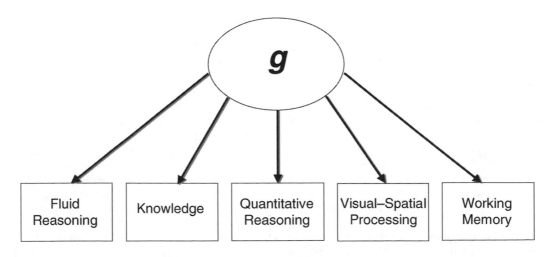

FIGURE 15.1. Theoretical model of SB5 cognitive factors.

TABLE 15.1. The Contents of SB5: The Activities That Compose the 10 Subtests (5 Nonverbal and 5 Verbal Subtests)

Cognitive factor	Nonverbal subtest activities	Verbal subtest activities
Fluid Reasoning	*Object-Series/Matrices	Early Reasoning Verbal Absurdities Verbal Analogies
Knowledge	Procedural Knowledge Picture Absurdities	*Vocabulary
Quantitative Reasoning	Nonverbal Quantitative Reasoning	Verbal Quantitative Reasoning
Visual–Spatial Processing	Form Board Form Patterns	Position and Direction
Working Memory	Delayed Response Block Span	Memory for Sentences Last Word

Note. Activities marked with an asterisk (*) are the initial routing tests used to tailor the assessment to the functional ability of the examinee.

the SB5. The Nonverbal subtests require a small degree of receptive language and allow for nonverbal responses such as pointing, moving blocks, or assembling pieces to indicate correct answers to problems presented in pictures, designs, or other illustrations. The Verbal subtests require facility with words and printed material (reading or speaking) to solve problems or indicate knowledge for each of the five cognitive factors covered by the test.

DESCRIPTION OF SUBTESTS

Table 15.1 shows contents of the SB5 subtests as reflected in the activities (tasks and types of items) that constitute each subtest. Testing begins with two subtests located in the first of three item books. Each item book (a spiral-bound book with a built-in easel) contains both the actual pictures and items of the test on one side of the page and examiner directions on the other side of the page. The Nonverbal Fluid Reasoning subtest is Object-Series/Matrices, an extension of the Matrices subtest of the Fourth Edition, which is one of the routing subtests presented in a point scale format in item book 1. The Verbal Knowledge subtest is Vocabulary—also a routing subtest in the point scale format in item book 1. These two subtests are administered first and are used to route the examinees to the proper functional ability level on the remaining subtests. The remaining subtests are organized into sets of

three to six items (called *testlets*), organized into functional ability levels based on the difficulty of the items. This structure of levels is similar to the classic design of the early editions of the Stanford–Binet. Item book 2 contains the four Nonverbal subtests—Knowledge, Quantitative Reasoning, Visual–Spatial Processing, and Working Memory. Nonverbal Knowledge includes an activity called Procedural Knowledge, in which the examinee expresses knowledge of objects shown in pictures by using gestures. Also, the classic Picture Absurdities (pointing and briefly explaining what is silly or unusual about a picture) is included in the more difficult levels of Nonverbal Knowledge.

Nonverbal Quantitative Reasoning includes items measuring numerical concepts and problems shown with counting rods (red plastic pieces designed as miniature rulers), blocks, or pictures. Nonverbal Visual–Spatial Processing tasks include the classic Form Board (a simple structured puzzle) and the new Form Patterns, in which pieces are used to form designs of animals, people, and objects. Nonverbal Working Memory is composed of an activity with plastic cups used to hide toys (Delayed Response) and a block-tapping task (Block Span).

Verbal Fluid Reasoning includes three types of tasks. Children and lower-functioning individuals begin with early reasoning tasks, such as identifying cause-and-effect relationships in pictures. Advanced examinees and adolescents progress to the Verbal Absurdities items (sentences expressing absurd contradictions), and finally, at the highest level, to difficult Verbal Analogy items ("*A* is to *B* as *C* is to *D*"). Verbal Quantitative Reasoning contains items containing numerical concepts and increasingly difficult word problems. The innovative Verbal Visual–Spatial Processing subtest employs some classic Binet items requiring understanding of verbal descriptions of spatial orientations ("Heading south, turn left, then right . . . ") and the explanation of directions on map-like displays. Finally, the Verbal Working Memory subtest includes the classic Binet task of remembering all the words in a given sentence, followed at the higher levels by a new task requiring memory of the last word in a series of sentences.

Two subtests (one Nonverbal and one Verbal) combine to form scores for each cognitive factor. Definitions of each of the factors are as follows:

• *Fluid Reasoning* is the ability to solve novel problems, whether with visual material in the Nonverbal domain or with words and print material in the Verbal domain.
• *Knowledge* is the fund of general information that is accumulated over time by the individual from experiences at home, in school, at work, or in the environment.
• *Quantitative Reasoning* is the ability to solve numerical problems, deal with fundamental number concepts, and solve word problems. In Quantitative Reasoning the emphasis is on general logical, numerical thinking, with reduced dependency on academic mathematical knowledge (such as the ability to solve specific algebraic equations).
• *Visual–Spatial Processing* is the ability to see relationships among figural objects, describe or recognize spatial orientation, identify the "whole" among a diverse set of parts, and generally see patterns in visual material.
• *Working Memory* is the ability to hold both visual and verbal information in short-term memory and then transform it or "sort it out." An example of a working memory task was studied by Baddeley, Logie, Nimmo-Smith, and Brereton (1985). They used a series of two, three, or more sentences presented one after the other. Some of the sentences made sense ("People eat food"), and some did not ("Cats sing water"). The examinee had to respond to each sentence, identifying the absurd sentences. Then, after

all sentences were presented, the examinee had to recall key words from the sentences (in the preceding examples, *food* and *water*). Thus the task required the examinee to overcome the interference of responding to each sentence so that the key words could be sorted out and recalled. In the SB5, a similar (but less complex) task is used, in which a series of sentences (in the form of questions, answered "yes" or "no") is presented and the examinee must recall the last word in each sentence; hence the subtest name, Last Word. Working memory is a very important clinical indicator of brain functioning, and difficulty with working memory is highly related to cognitive process deficits underlying LDs (Reid, Hresko, & Swanson, 1996). Some researchers believe that working memory is a central part of reasoning ability (e.g., Kyllonen & Christal, 1990).

TEST ADMINISTRATION AND SCORING

Background of the Examinee

The classic description of the role of the assessment professional given by Matarazzo (1990) is still highly relevant today. Matarazzo argued that assessment is quite different from measurement, and that intellectual assessment in particular requires experienced examiners who carefully evaluate the match between the instruments and the examinee. In terms of the SB5, the examiner should reflect on the cultural and linguistic background of the examinee. In particular, if the examinee has communication difficulties, has a hearing disability, comes from a nonmajority culture, or has a dominant language other than English, great caution should be taken in administering the SB5 and interpreting results. Half of the SB5 consists of Nonverbal subjects and can be considered for administration as a separate battery from the Verbal subtests. The Verbal subtests of the SB5 do require English-language expression and word knowledge. The Nonverbal subtests require only pointing responses or a small degree of receptive language in most subtests, or brief gestures and expressive language in Nonverbal Knowledge (Picture Absurdities).

The examiner not only should reflect on the cultural and linguistic background or disability of the examinee, but should also look at acculturation (Dana, 1993). *Acculturation* is the degree to which an individual has learned, adopted, or possibly rejected elements of mainstream North American culture. If there is a question about acculturation, perhaps one of the various questionnaires developed for this purpose should be employed (Paniagua, 1994). Issues include whether the examinee and his or her family read in English, socialize outside their own linguistic culture, attend school, or attended school before coming to North America.

Preparation for Administration

Because the SB5 is a standardized instrument, careful attention should be given to the exact directions detailed in the examiner's manual (Roid, 2003b). Conveniently for the examiner, all directions for the instrument are printed on the examiner pages of the easel booklets, called *item books* in the SB5. As always, best practices should be followed; these include establishing rapport with the examinee prior to testing, to practicing the administration of SB5 before using it in a clinical setting, and preparing all ma-

terials before testing. Also, the test environment should be controlled to minimize distractions. Variations in the order of administration, or various adaptations of the test or accommodations due to disabilities, need to be documented carefully. When accommodations are allowed, they should be described in the report, and normative scores based on the national standardization of the SB5 should be interpreted with caution. In these cases, the SB5 offers the possibility of qualitative interpretation or use of the alternative criterion-referenced scoring system.

Administration

Figure 15.2 shows the standard administration procedure for the SB5. Testing begins with the first section of item book 1. This Nonverbal section of item book 1 presents the Object-Series/Matrices subtest, which is one of the routing subtests, provided in a point scale format. Unless there is a nonstandard administration emphasizing only nonverbal subtests, the next step is to administer a Verbal subtest, Vocabulary, the second routing subtest in item book 1. Following the administration of these routing subtests,

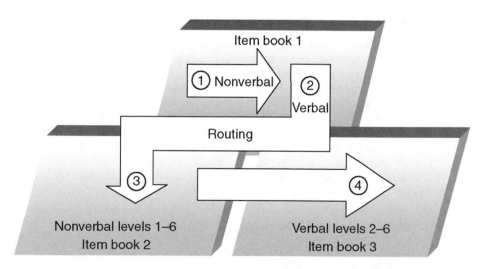

① Administer Object-Series/Matrices (Nonverbal Fluid Reasoning) routing subtest.

② Administer Vocabulary (Verbal Knowledge) routing subtest.

③ Route to Nonverbal levels section based on Object-Series/Matrices score.

④ Route to Verbal levels section based on Vocabulary score.

FIGURE 15.2. Standard administration of the SB5.

point scale scores from these subtests are then used to determine the proper functioning level where testing will continue in item book 2 (Nonverbal) and item book 3 (Verbal). Therefore, the third step in the standard administration is to enter item book 2 at the proper level, indicated by the score on the Object-Series/Matrices subtest. The final step (step 4) is to route the subject to the proper Verbal level in item book 3, based on the score on the Vocabulary subtest. In both item books 2 and 3 (steps 3 and 4), the examiner should employ the basal and ceiling rules that are clearly marked on each page of the record form. Most examiners find that they will begin at the starting level indicated by the routing tests and test two levels (two pages in the record form for each domain—Nonverbal and Verbal).

Several important features of the SB5 test administration should be highlighted. First, the SB5 employs routing subtests in item book 1 to define the level at which the examinee will continue the assessment. This routing procedure adds precision to the measurement by tailoring the level of difficulty of the items to the examinee's ability level. Second, the SB5 employs different basal and ceiling rules for the routing subtests in comparison to the level subtests. In item book 1 for the routing subtest, the basal and ceiling rules are the typical ones found in point scales, with an age-estimated start point and a ceiling at a certain number of consecutive errors. Within the level subtests, the basal and ceiling rules are different from those in other batteries, because they are based on sufficient (basal) or insufficient (ceiling) performance within a given level and subtest.

A second feature of the SB5 is that the level subtest sections in item books 2 and 3 are organized into smaller sections called *testlets*, as discussed previously. These testlets are designed to produce a maximum of 6 raw score points.[2] For example, the set of three Verbal Absurdity items (scored 0, 1, or 2 for different degrees of correctness) form a testlet for the Verbal Fluid Reasoning subtest, producing a maximum of 6 points. As the examinee is administered a series of testlets, the scores are accumulated to provide the total raw score for each subtest. When the examinee achieves too few points on a testlet, testing is stopped for that subtest, whereas testing of other subtests continues. Each subtest is consistently located in

one of the four corners of the record form. So, to continue testing for an individual subtest, the examiner should simply turn to the next page of the record form and continue by administering the testlet located in the appropriate corner for that subtest.

In the third feature to be highlighted, the SB5 employs very few time limits and does not use time bonuses. However, in order to encourage a quick and efficient assessment, a system of examiner prompts is also employed on the most difficult items. For the most difficult items in Object-Series/Matrices, Quantitative Reasoning, and Verbal Analogies, for example, an examiner prompt rule employs a liberal 3-minute signal to encourage the examinee to move forward. This should not be a rigid time limit, but rather used as a method of moving examinees forward when they are stymied.

One of the final features of the SB5 is the use of teaching items. At the beginning of testlets that contain a new type of task for the examinee, the first item is employed not only as a sample item, but also as a teaching task in which feedback is given to the examinee. For certain unique tasks that are administered to lower-functioning examinees, these teaching items reveal the correct answer to the examinees for purposes of fairness.

Record Form

The record form for the SB5 has a familiar format. The first page includes a section for converting raw scores to normative scores and includes various profile graphs. Additional pages present one of the routing subtests or the levels subtest. For subtests requiring a verbal response, such as Vocabulary or Verbal Absurdities, spaces are provided for the examiner to write verbatim answers given by the examinee. Most of the items of the SB5 are scored according to a dichotomous format—that is, 0 or 1. However, some items have multiple score points. For example, Vocabulary items are scored 0, 1, or 2 to allow for partially correct answers.

After completing the identifying information about the examinee, the examiner begins with the routing subtests in item book 1 and records responses on pages 3 through 5 of the record form. Once the raw scores for each routing subtest are obtained, the examiner uses the Nonverbal routing table on page 6 to identify the recommended starting level for the examinee in the record form. The examiner then finds the same level in item book 2 by noting the color-printed stripes at the bottom of each page that identify the levels. For example, if the raw score on the Object-Series/Matrices routing subtest is 20 points, the routing table tells the examiner to start at level 3 on page 8 of the record form. The examiner proceeds to page 8 and begins with the instructions for level 3 in item book 2 (page 26). The next page of the item book (page 27) presents the first item in the Nonverbal Knowledge subtest (the Procedural Knowledge activity). This testlet has 6 items in which the examinee demonstrates the motions characteristic of people, using the pictured object shown on the examinee's side of the item book. The examiner sums the number correct for that testlet, and continues with the other three testlets on that page (next will be Quantitative Reasoning, in the bottom left corner of the record form). Observing the basal and ceiling rules, the examiner continues on page 9 and beyond as needed in the Nonverbal section of the record form. Then the examiner goes to the level recommended by the Verbal routing table (on page 5), and administers the Verbal testlets indicated until the ceiling is reached for each of the four subtests being measured. In the case of a child or adult who does not speak English, or who has a documented, severe verbal communication disorder, a nonverbal administration may be chosen. This type of administration requires the examiner to begin with the Nonverbal routing subtest and complete the recommended Nonverbal testlets separately from the Verbal portions of the test to obtain the NVIQ and a profile of Nonverbal subtests.

Scoring

Once all the required subtests and testlets have been completed, the examiner copies all raw scores from the various pages of the record form to the summary tables on the front cover of the record form. First, the raw score totals for the routing subtests are entered in the section located in the upper left of the front cover of the record form. The routing subtests are each marked with a colored arrow labeled "Routing." For the testlet scores, the examiner begins entering the raw

scores for testlets at the starting level and continues entering testlet scores until the ceiling is reached. All levels above the ceiling can be marked with a dash or zero. Credit is given for testlet scores below the starting level by tracing over the lightly printed numbers printed in the boxes for the lower-level testlets. The examiner sums the testlet scores (including credit for lower-level testlets not administered) down each column and places the sum in the boxes provided. Then the examiner uses the norm tables in the appendix of the examiner's manual (Roid, 2003b) to convert raw scores to derived scores used in interpretation of results.

Two systems of scoring are provided in the SB5—*norm-referenced* and *criterion-referenced*. First, the traditional normative standard scores are used to compare the examinee's performance to age-level peers from the nationally representative norm sample. As noted earlier, IQ scores (mean of 100, standard deviation of 15) include the NVIQ, VIQ, and FSIQ. Also, an optional ABIQ is available from the two routing subtests (Object-Series/Matrices plus Vocabulary). Factor index scores are each composed of two subtests (one Nonverbal and one Verbal) and contrast performance on each of the five cognitive factors. For example, the Nonverbal Knowledge subtest scaled score is added to the Vocabulary (Verbal Knowledge) scaled score, and this sum is converted to the Knowledge factor index score. Because the factor index scores are expressed in the same metric as IQ scores (mean of 100, standard deviation of 15), they can be entered on the same type of profile as the IQ scores for visual comparison (located on the lower right of the front cover of the record form). The final set of normative scores is the set of 10 subtest profile scores (mean of 10, standard deviation of 3), including 5 Nonverbal and 5 Verbal subtests.

Also as noted earlier, a supplementary and optional scoring system employs CSSs, which convert raw scores into ability-level estimates from IRT analysis. Raw scores for each of the five factors and the three IQ scores are converted to Rasch-based scores (Rasch, 1980; Wright & Lineacre, 1999), in the same metric as the W scores of the WJ III Tests of Cognitive Abilities (Woodcock, McGrew, & Mather, 2001b). The average CSSs of SB5 and W-scores from the WJ III tests range from approximately 425 for 2-

year-olds to 525 for high-functioning adults. These scores, along with the *growth scores* of the Leiter International Performance Scale—Revised (Roid & Miller, 1997), are centered at 500—the average score for examinees who are 10 years, 0 months of age. As shown in the interpretive manual for the SB5 (Roid, 2003c), CSS for the Quantitative Reasoning factor, for example, can be related to increasingly complex mathematical concepts and problems as the scores progress from 425 to 525.[3] Thus the CSSs can be "anchored" to the criterion of developmental age level as well as to the level of task difficulty, demonstrating their criterion-referenced characteristics. Also, CSS measures can be recorded across multiple tests and retests to measure change across time, whether that change is improvement or decline in cognitive function. Such scores are highly useful in clinical intervention research and in documenting the improvement of individuals in special education programs.

PSYCHOMETRIC PROPERTIES

Extensive studies of reliability, validity, and fairness were conducted as part of the SB5 standardization. These studies are detailed in the technical manual (Roid, 2003e). The main technical features of SB5 are briefly outlined here. Additional statistical analyses, useful tables, and case studies are presented in the interpretive manual (Roid, 2003c) and in Roid and Barram (2004).

The normative sample for SB5 included 4,800 subjects, ages 2–96 years. The highest age grouping employed in the norm tables was 85+. The composition of the normative sample closely approximated the stratification percentages reported by the U.S. Bureau of the Census (2001). Stratification variables included sex, geographic region, ethnicity (African American, Asian American, European American, Hispanic, Native American, and other), and socioeconomic level (years of education completed or parents' educational attainment). In addition, subjects were tested ($N = 1,365$) from officially documented special groups, such as individuals with mental retardation, LDs, attention-deficit/hyperactivity disorder (ADHD), and speech or hearing impairments. Details of these special studies are provided in Roid (2003e).

Internal-consistency reliability ranged from .95 to .98 for IQ scores and from .90 to .92 for the five factor index scores.[4] For the 10 subtests, average reliabilities ranged from .84 to .89, providing a strong basis for profile interpretation. Test–retest and inter-examiner reliability studies were also conducted and showed the stability and consistency of SB5 scoring (Roid, 2003e). Test–retest data were collected on more than 80 subjects at four age levels: 2–5, 6–20, 21–59, and 60 years or older. Correlations between test and retest scores (stability coefficients) showed medians of .93 to .95 for IQ scores, .88 for factor index scores, and .82 for subtest scaled scores. The practice effect on scores, as measured by the size of the mean difference between test and retest scores, was smaller than expected, ranging from 2 to 5 points for IQ scores (with NVIQ shifting more than VIQ). However, the NVIQ practice effects on SB5 were small (2–5 points), compared to those for other prominent batteries such as the Wechsler Intelligence Scale for Children—Third Edition (WISC-III; Wechsler, 1991), where mean differences are often as high as 11–13 points on Performance IQ. Perhaps the stability of SB5 IQ scores is due to the complexity of tasks and the lack of time limits for most subtests.

IRT (Rasch, 1980; Wright & Lineacre, 1999) was used to design the routing procedure and levels, and to check the consistency among the items and tasks within each subtest. Thus the routing subtests (Object-Series/Matrices and Vocabulary in item book 1) are the first stage of a two-stage adaptive testing design. Ability is estimated from the Rasch-calibrated difficulties of the routing subtest items in order to place the examinee in the matching range of estimated ability in both the Nonverbal and Verbal levels. The levels sections of SB5 (item books 2 and 3) form the second stage of the two-stage assessment. For the subtests in this stage, testlets were chosen to create a stairstep design, with each testlet made increasingly difficult at each ascending level from level 1 to level 6. The Rasch analyses provide a verification that all items in a subtest, regardless of level or type of task, share communality with the underlying latent trait being measured collectively by the subtest items. Various indices of fit to the Rasch model were used to quantitatively verify fit to the unidimensional, underlying cognitive trait (Wright & Lineacre, 1999).

Evidence for content-, criterion-, and construct-related validity of SB5 is detailed in Roid (2003e), including extensive studies of concurrent, predictive, and factorial validity. Also, consequential validity and fairness of predicting achievement scores are reported in Roid (2003c). Examples of validity include correlations with other assessment batteries, as shown in Table 15.2. The technical manual for SB5 (Roid, 2003e) provides the details of these correlation studies, but some key descriptors of the samples employed are included in Table 15.2. The correlations shown in Table 15.2 are quite substantial and similar in magnitude to the concurrent correlations observed for other major intelligence batteries. The substantial predictive correlations between SB5 and two major achievement batteries (WJ III and the Wechsler Individual Achievement Test—Second Edition [WIAT-II]) provide a strong basis for comparing individuals' intellectual and achievement scores.

Extensive studies of the factor structure of SB5 were conducted and are summarized in Roid (2003e). Confirmatory factor analyses using LISREL 8.3 (Joreskog & Sorbom, 1999) were calculated for five successive age groups (2–5, 6–10, 11–16, 17–50, and 51+), and factor models with one, two, three, four, and five factors were compared. Split-half scores (scores for odd- and even-numbered

items in each of the 10 subtests) were employed to provide more stable estimates of each factor in the maximum-likelihood analyses. The five-factor models showed superior fit, including a non-normed fit index ranging from .89 to .93, a comparative fit index ranging from .91 to .93, and a root mean square error of approximation ranging from .076 to .088. A second series of confirmatory analyses was conducted with LISREL, using conventional full-length subtests across two batteries: the SB5 and the WJ III (Woodcock et al., 2001b). Again, the five-factor model showed the best fit, with all five factors aligning across the SB5 and WJ III as predicted.

GENERAL INTERPRETATION OF SB5 TEST SCORES

Roid (2003b, 2003c) has recommended a seven-step interpretive strategy for the SB5. Each step is briefly described as follows. First, in steps 1 and 2, the purpose of the assessment and the context of the examinee are evaluated in terms of language and cultural factors to assure that the SB5 is the appropriate instrument for the individual and the assessment purpose. For example, if the examinee is a recent immigrant to the United States and does not speak or read English well, the individual's language context must be taken into account. In such a case, either

TABLE 15.2. Correlations of SB5 FSIQ Scores with Full-Scale Scores on Other Intelligence Tests and with Multiple Subtests in Achievement Batteries

Test	N	Age range	% Minority	Correlations
Stanford–Binet Fourth Edition	104	3–20	35%	.90
Stanford–Binet L–M Edition	80	3–19	17%	.85
Wechsler scales: WISC–III	66	6–16	47%	.84
Wechsler scales: WAIS–III	87	16–84	7%	.82
Wechsler scales: WIAT–II	80	6–15	19%	.53 to .80
WJ III Cognitive	145	4–11	25%	.90*
WJ III Achievement	472	6–19	29%	.66 to .84

Note. N, number of subjects; % Minority, percentage of the sample that was Asian American, African American, Native American (Indian), multiple-ethnicity, or other nonwhite/non-European American ethnicity; WISC-III, Wechsler Intelligence Scale for Children—Third Edition; WAIS-III, Wechsler Adult Intelligence Scale—Third Edition; WIAT-II, Wechsler Individual Achievement Test—Second Edition; WJ III, Woodcock–Johnson III. Correlations are product–moment coefficients, and the correlation marked with an asterisk (*) is based on a special WJ III composite score consisting of the five cognitive factors measured by the SB5. Correlation of the SB5 FSIQ with the multifactor General Ability Index of the WJ III was .78.

accommodations in test administration (e.g., translation of items), or use of the nonverbal sections of SB5 alone may be necessary.

In the third step, the domains of Verbal and Nonverbal abilities, represented by VIQ and NVIQ, are contrasted and significant differences noted. Given the high reliability and five-factor comprehensiveness of each domain in the SB5, the contrast between VIQ and NVIQ becomes much more important for interpretation than the same distinction in other intellectual batteries. Thus the fourth step of evaluating the overall level of cognitive performance, reflected in the FSIQ, may have to be tempered when VIQ and NVIQ differ significantly. For example, for an examinee who is a recent immigrant to the United States and has Spanish as his or her dominant language, the VIQ may be only 85 while the NVIQ is 105, resulting in a difference that is both statistically significant and relatively rare in the normative sample (only 3.7% obtain a 20-point difference or greater). For these reasons, the NVIQ of 105 may be closer to the examinee's latent global ability than an FSIQ of 95, for example.

In the fifth step of interpretation, differences among the five factor index scores are evaluated through tables provided in Roid (2003e). *Ipsative* comparisons (those made within an individual's own set of five factor index scores) can be made by looking at the numerical differences between each pair of scores. Generally, differences of approximately 18–19 points are needed to show significance both statistically and practically (i.e., significance at the .05 level and rarity in the normative population). Because the five factors of SB5 were developed on the strong theoretical framework of the CHC model, the factor index profile should be valuable for cross-battery interpretation when other cognitive batteries have been administered to the examinee (Flanagan & Ortiz, 2001; McGrew & Flanagan, 1998).

In the sixth step of interpretation, the individual subtests (five Nonverbal and five Verbal) are compared and contrasted. Again, the statistical significance of score differences and the frequency of various magnitudes of difference in the normative population are examined. Several types of interpretive tables are provided in the technical manual (Roid, 2003e) and in the computer scoring software (Roid, 2003d). Subtest differences can be compared to the mean scaled score among all 10 subtests (the generally recommended procedure). Subtests should be compared to the mean of only the five Nonverbal subtests or only the Verbal subtests when there is a significant difference between NVIQ and VIQ. Tables to evaluate the differences between each pair of subtests within each factor (e.g., Nonverbal and Verbal Working Memory) are also provided, and are recommended especially for neuropsychological evaluations. Caution should be taken in comparing all possible pairwise combinations of subtests, because the repetition of repeated statistical tests multiplies the likelihood of chance differences' being overinterpreted. Fortunately, because the subtest reliability on SB5 is high (median internal consistency of .84 to .89), ipsative profile analysis on the SB5 (except as stated above) is on more solid ground than with tests having lower subtest reliability. Professional assessment practices always dictate, however, that multiple sources of information should be used to make diagnostic decisions about individuals. Therefore, diagnoses should not be made solely on the basis of a given individual's SB5 profile patterns.

In the final step of interpretation, various qualitative indicators of the examinee's performance should be considered. These include patterns of errors in the examinee's item responses (as seen in the record form). In addition, patterns of inattention or distractibility may be found, because all items are arranged in order of increasing difficulty within each subtest and testlet. Alternatively, "testing the limits" can be employed after the standardized administration is completed. For example, school-age children can be asked to explain their thinking or strategies for solving quantitative problems, or elderly examinees can be given more time on working memory tasks (e.g., repetition of the last word in a series of sentences) to test the limits of their memory capacity.

CLINICAL INTERPRETATIONS BASED ON GROUP DIFFERENCES

Professionals who work with children are sometimes faced with difficult clinical decisions. These difficult decisions include cases where a child displays behavioral and cognitive indicators that are diagnostic indicators for more than one clinical classification. Examples of these include distinguishing between low-functioning autism and mental retardation, or determining whether the weaknesses in the score profile of a student enrolled in an English-language learner (ELL) program are primarily due to a language deficit or to second-language status.

Discriminant-function analyses were used in a study conducted specifically for this chapter. The goal of the discriminant analyses was to distinguish group membership on the basis of factor index scores from the SB5 to aid in making difficult clinical decisions. After the discriminant functions were derived by the computer, any individual with a discriminant score above zero was assigned to one group, while an individual with a score below zero was assigned to the contrasting group.

Table 15.3 displays the group comparisons, including the number of subjects in each group, the SB5 FSIQ for each group, the variables in the prediction equation, the prediction coefficients including the constant, and the classification percentage. The tough clinical distinctions studied here were as follows: ADHD versus average-IQ autism, mental retardation versus low-IQ autism,

ELL status versus speech and language impairment, and mild mental retardation versus all autism. The second column of Table 15.3 shows the number of subjects in each group, and the next column shows the average SB5 FSIQ for these groups. Each pair of contrasting groups had very similar average FSIQ values, indicating one of the difficulties in making clinical distinctions between these categories. The results displayed for each pair of groups include the coefficients (weights applied to each factor index score) and the constant derived for the best-fitting prediction equation. In addition, the results include a measure of the accuracy of the function (i.e., the classification percentage). This statistic shows the percentage of the original cases that were correctly classified with the linear prediction equation provided.

For the ADHD versus average-IQ autism comparison, the Fluid Reasoning and Quantitative Reasoning factor index scores were the best predictor scores. For the original groups, this equation correctly classified 61% of the students. For the mental retardation versus low-IQ autism comparison, the Working Memory factor index score was the best predictor score, and the equation correctly classified 58% of the original students.

TABLE 15.3. Descriptive Statistics for Each Group, Prediction Variables, Discriminant Functions, and Classification Percentages for Four Comparisons with SB5 Factors as Predictors

Group comparison	Number in group	SB5 FSIQ	Prediction variables	Coefficients of discriminant function	Classification percentage
ADHD vs. average-IQ autism	94 (ADHD), 41 (autism)	93 (ADHD), 89 (autism)	Fluid Reasoning	−.065	
			Quantitative Reasoning	.099	
			Constant	−3.235	61%
MR vs. low-IQ autism	119 (MR), 42 (autism)	56 (MR), 53 (autism)	Working Memory	.081	
			Constant	−4.991	58%
ELL status vs. SLI	66 (ELL), 108 (SLI)	91 (ELL), 85 (SLI)	Knowledge	−.062	
			Quantitative Reasoning	.091	
			Constant	−2.819	64%
Mild MR vs. all autism	73 (MR), 83 (autism)	66 (MR), 70 (autism)	Knowledge	.087	
			Working Memory	−.065	
			Constant	−1.654	59%

Note. ADHD, attention-deficit/hyperactivity disorder; MR, mental retardation; ELL, English-language learner; SLI, speech and language impairment.

For the ELL status versus speech and language impairment comparison, the Knowledge and Quantitative Reasoning factor index scores were the best predictor scores, and the equation correctly classified 64% of the students. A subset of 73 individuals with mental retardation had mild delays (e.g., IQ in the range of 60–69), and these persons were compared to all the individuals with autism. For this final comparison, the Knowledge and Working Memory factor index scores were the best predictor scores. For the original groups, this equation correctly classified 59% of the students.

The results of these analyses may provide guidance for difficult clinical decisions in the following way. If the values in Table 15.3 are used to determine diagnostic classification, each factor index score should be multiplied by the coefficient listed. Then the results must be summed for all the factor index scores included in the prediction, and the constant must be added (or subtracted if it has a minus sign). If the grand total is a positive number, the examiner can then form a clinical hypothesis that this individual's score pattern is more similar to that for people in the first group listed in the comparison. Similarly, if the grand total is a negative number, the individual's score pattern is more similar to that for the second group in the comparison. The more the grand total differs from zero, the more the clinician can have confidence in the hypothesis.

INTERPRETATION BASED ON STUDIES OF ACHIEVEMENT PREDICTION

Another method of interpreting SB5 scores for school-age children and adolescents is to closely examine any scores related to academic achievement. School psychologists may find these achievement-related scores helpful in making recommendations to teachers and other school personnel who provide services to examinees.

The results presented in Table 15.4 are from a larger study of the predictive power of the SB5 Working Memory factor for reading and mathematics achievement (Pomplun, 2004). Establishing the nature of this relationship is important, because (1) many

TABLE 15.4. The Prediction of WJ III Mathematics Achievement by SB5 Quantitative Reasoning and Working Memory

WJ III criterion	SB5 predictors	Adjusted R^2	R^2 increase	Statistical significance
Calculation	Quantitative Reasoning	.370	—	.000
	+ Working Memory	.392	.022	.000
	+ Interaction	.391	.000	.623
Mathematics Fluency	Quantitative Reasoning	.149	—	.000
	+ Working Memory	.191	.042	.000
	+ Interaction	.196	.005	.054
Applied Problems	Quantitative Reasoning	.361		.000
	+ Working Memory	.384	.023	.000
	+ Interaction	.385	.001	.128
Quantitative Concepts	Quantitative Reasoning	.421	—	.000
	+ Working Memory	.457	.036	.000
	+ Interaction	.461	.004	.028
Mathematics Reasoning	Quantitative Reasoning	.448		.000
	+ Working Memory	.481	.033	.000
	+ Interaction	.489	.008	.003

Note. Data from Pomplun (2004).

modern theories of intelligence delineate specific cognitive abilities and school achievement variables (Carroll, 1993; Horn, 1994); (2) much of past research on specific abilities was based on tests with incomplete factorial coverage (McGrew, Flanagan, Keith, & Vanderwood, 1997); and (3) current models of cognitive processes involved in achievement deficits postulate specific abilities, such as working memory (Felton & Pepper, 1995).

Some researchers believe that working memory is a central part of reasoning ability (Jensen, 1998). Wilson and Swanson (2001) concluded that deficits in mathematics were mediated by both a domain-general and a domain-specific working memory system. The Pomplun (2003) study extended this research by using a working memory measure consisting of both verbal and nonverbal measures, and also testing the interaction of this measure with other important predictors of mathematics achievement.

Three hundred and thirty-eight students ages 6–19 (median age = 10) were administered the SB5 and the WJ III Tests of Achievement (Woodcock et al., 2001a). The score for the SB5 Quantitative Reasoning factor was used as the primary predictor of mathematics achievement. The score for the SB5 Working Memory factor was used as the second predictor of mathematics achievement.

Specifically, the achievement tests from WJ III were Calculation, a test of basic math computation skills; Mathematics Fluency, a timed test of basic computation skills; Applied Problems, a test of the proper selection and completion of computations for problems; Quantitative Concepts, a test of math concepts, symbols, and vocabulary through concepts and number series; and Mathematics Reasoning, a composite of Quantitative Concepts and Applied Problems (McGrew & Woodcock, 2001).

The predictive power of the Working Memory factor was studied through a series of three hierarchical least-squares regression models, with each WJ III achievement test score as a criterion. For the prediction of each achievement test score, the first regression model had three predictors: the score for the Quantitative Reasoning factor, the score for the Working Memory factor, and a term for the interaction between Quantita-

tive Reasoning and Working Memory (i.e., created by multiplying Quantitative Reasoning and Working Memory together). If the interaction term in this model was statistically significant, the sum of the two factors was conditional on the other predictor's score level. If the interaction term was nonsignificant, a second regression model (with two predictors, Quantitative Reasoning and Working Memory) was investigated. If the Working Memory variable was statistically significant, this indicated that the additivity of the two factors was constant across score levels for each predictor. A probability level of .05 was used for statistical significance for each term in these models.

Table 15.4 contains results from the hierarchical prediction models with the different achievement criterion variables for the mathematics tests. These tables show the WJ III criterion variables, the SB5 predictors, the adjusted R^2, the increase in R^2 when variables were added and the statistical significance of the increase in R^2. In Table 15.4, the Quantitative Reasoning score predicted from 15% to 45% of the variance (estimated from R^2) in the mathematics achievement test scores. Two of the five interaction terms were statistically significant at the .05 level, and another interaction term was nearly significant (.054). The interaction terms were statistically significant in the models for the prediction of Quantitative Concepts and Mathematics Reasoning, and near significance for the prediction of Mathematics Fluency. For the prediction of Mathematics Reasoning achievement scores, the interaction was disordinal, with the regression lines crossing in the region of 130. The differences became larger as the predictor scores decreased. For example at a Quantitative Reasoning score of 70, a Working Memory score difference of 40 points translated into a predicted Mathematics Reasoning score difference of more than 15 points. In contrast, at a Quantitative Reasoning score of 130, a Working Memory score difference of 40 points translated into a predicted Mathematics Reasoning score difference of only 1 point.

Across the five WJ III mathematics achievement scores, Working Memory added from 2% to 4% to the prediction over and above the contribution of Quantitative Reasoning, based on the increases in R^2. Also, Working Memory added significantly to the interaction term for three achievement scores. The nature of the significant interaction terms suggests that prediction of Mathematics Reasoning using Working Memory translates into practically significant score differences in Mathematics Reasoning only for those with below-average Quantitative Reasoning scores. For those with average or above-average Quantitative Reasoning scores, Working Memory does not add much to the predicted Mathematics Reasoning scores. The results demonstrate the predictive validity of the unique SB5 measure of Working Memory based on Verbal and Nonverbal subtests. These results suggest that the interpretation of Working Memory scores along with Quantitative Reasoning scores may need to go beyond simply adding these scores (i.e., in a composite). Instead, Working Memory should be used to predict Mathematics Reasoning scores only for the students with below-average Quantitative Reasoning scores.

INTERPRETATION OF SB5 PROFILE PATTERNS USING SUBTEST SPECIFICITY

Several methods of interpreting the 10-subtest profile of the SB5 have been described in the section "General Interpretation of SB5 Test Scores" above. These include the analysis of subtest score differences by the methods of (1) examining statistical significance of differences, (2) comparing the magnitude of the differences to those found in the normative populations, (3) comparing the subtest scores to the mean of all 10 subtest scores in the individual's profile, and (4) comparing the individual's Nonverbal versus Verbal subtest scores for a given cognitive factor. To supplement these methods, a further analysis of the SB5 subtest specificity was completed for this chapter. Subtest specificity is derived from factor analysis of the subtest scores by separating profile score variance into common, specific, and error variance. Cohen (1957, 1959) originally studied the specificity of the Wechsler scales, and nearly every major test battery has since been analyzed for specificity, including the Fourth Edition of the Stanford–Binet

(Reynolds, Kamphaus, & Rosenthal, 1988). When clinicians assess the cognitive strengths and weaknesses of individuals based on individual profile scores, the implicit assumption is that each subtest has reliable specific variance.

Table 15.5 presents the common, specific, and error variance for each of the SB5 subtests in each of five age groups (2–5, 6–10, 11–16, 17–50, and 51+ years). The values in Table 15.5 were derived as follows. First, the internal-consistency reliability coefficients from Roid (2003e), averaged for each age group, were used to define error variance (the quantity of 1.0 minus the reliability). Second, the common variance was obtained from factor analysis of the subtest scores at each age level and was the communality (degree of shared variance across all subtests) of each subtest score. The difference between common variance and true variance was the specific variance. Analyses for Table 15.5 were conducted on the SB5 standardization sample ($N = 4,800$).

The bottom right corner of Table 15.5 shows the overall averages of 64% common, 22% specific, and 14% error variance—a classic pattern of common variance > specific variance > error variance, meaning that the unique specificity of subtest variation is higher than error (Cohen, 1959). Also, the overall average common variance of 64% is similar to that for adult intelligence batteries (e.g., Wechsler Adult Intelligence Scale (WAIS), 66%; WAIS-R, 57%; see Roid & Gyurke, 1991). The age trend of increasing common variance across the preschool, school-age, and adult Wechsler scales can also be observed in Table 15.5. As shown in the bottom row of Table 15.5, average common variance ranged from 59% at ages 2–5, to 70% and 69% in the adult ranges. Presence of a substantial percentage of common variance provides evidence of construct validity for the composite IQ scores of the SB5, which summarize the overall level of cognitive ability across subtests.

Clinicians look for good specificity among subtests of a cognitive battery, in order to justify the interpretation of profile patterns and strengths and weaknesses. Cohen (1959) suggested 25% specificity that exceeds error variance as an ideal. As shown in the right column of Table 15.5, average specificity for the SB5 subtests ranged from 12% to 33%

TABLE 15.5. Percentages of Common, Specific, and Error Variance Derived from Factor Analysis for Each of the 10 SB5 Subtest Scaled Scores in Each of Five Age Groups

Subtest	Ages 2–5			Ages 6–10			Ages 11–16			Ages 17–50			Ages 51+			Average		
	C	S	E	C	S	E	C	S	E	C	S	E	C	S	E	C	S	E
NVFR	38	47	15	48	37	15	41	41	18	60	21	19	72	20	8	52	33	15
NVKN	59	27	14	64	15	21	63	21	16	73	15	12	75	12	13	67	18	15
NVQR	68	18	14	73	9	18	75	11	14	78	10	12	78	9	13	74	12	14
NVVS	54	34	12	60	23	17	45	36	19	66	23	11	68	24	8	59	28	13
NVWM	56	34	10	50	33	17	60	28	12	53	37	10	70	17	13	58	30	12
Nonverbal average	55	32	13	59	23	18	57	27	16	66	21	13	73	16	11	62	24	14
VFR	57	35	8	60	29	11	62	19	19	66	11	23	66	18	16	62	23	15
VKN	61	27	12	59	28	13	56	31	13	68	23	9	63	30	7	61	28	11
VQR	66	18	16	68	14	18	73	13	14	83	7	10	77	15	8	73	14	13
VVS	67	14	19	72	15	13	71	17	12	76	15	9	66	23	11	70	17	13
VWM	62	23	15	51	34	15	49	31	20	80	4	16	58	29	13	60	24	16
Verbal average	63	23	14	62	24	14	62	22	16	75	12	13	66	23	11	65	21	14
Overall average	59	28	13	60	24	16	59	25	16	70	17	13	69	20	11	64	22	14

Note. Based on $N = 4,800$. C, common; S, specific; E, error; NV, Nonverbal; V, Verbal; FR, Fluid Reasoning; KN, Knowledge; QR, Quantitative Reasoning; VS, Visual–Spatial Processing; WM, Working Memory.

across age groups (overall average 22%). All subtests except Nonverbal Quantitative Reasoning had specificity higher than error variance. The bottom row of Table 15.5 shows that average specificity was greater and in the ideal range for preschool and school-age ranges (28% for 2–5, 24% for 6–10, and 25% for 11–17), as compared to the adult age levels (17% and 20%). Because common variance increases in the adult range due to an apparent globalization of abilities, specificity naturally decreases from that of the younger age ranges (Roid & Gyurke, 1991).

In terms of profile analysis of strengths and weaknesses in individuals, Table 15.5 indicates that an excellent level of average specificity was found for four subtests: Nonverbal Fluid Reasoning (33%), Nonverbal Visual–Spatial Processing (28%), Nonverbal Working Memory (30%), and Verbal Knowledge (28%). Clinicians should exercise some caution in interpretation of individual profile scores for Quantitative Reasoning due to their lower specificity, which is similar to the level of their error variance. However, Quantitative Reasoning is lower in specificity because of its excellent contribution to common variance (74% Nonverbal, 73% Verbal), and thus to overall IQ. Nonverbal Knowledge and Verbal Visual–Spatial Processing are also similar in their high common variance and somewhat lower specificity than other subtests.

Examiners who make decisions about individuals (especially decisions that attach a label such as *mental retardation* to individuals) should be cautious in the interpretation of differences among subtest scores of SB5, given that some degree of difference is due to measurement error. Also, error of measurement is compounded in the subtraction of two scores and in the comparison of all possible pairs of scores. The number of pairwise comparisons among 10 subtests is 45 (a large number for one individual), increasing the possibilities of chance differences. Profile patterns of individuals should be used cautiously in diagnosis unless there are several sources of information showing consistency among diagnostic signs in an individual's cumulative folder of background information.

Also, some researchers have questioned the wisdom of profile analysis that compares scores within one individual (ipsative analysis) in tests of cognitive ability. For example, McDermott, Fantuzzo, and Glutting (1990) concluded that most of the variance in intelligence tests such as the Wechsler scales was due to general ability (*g*) reflected in the Wechsler FSIQ, because they were unable to identify differentiated profiles patterns from cluster analysis of normative data. They claimed that most of the profile patterns were "flat" (all scores low or all scores high), rather than differentiated profiles with scattered high and low scores. However, Roid (1994, 2003c), drawing on the recommendations of Aldenderfer and Blashfield (1984), showed that differentiated profile patterns can be found in 40–50% of individual profiles in large samples when sensitive cluster analysis methods are employed. Roid (1994) showed that the use of Pearson product–moment correlations (R. K. Blashfield, personal communication, February 22, 1992), rather than Euclidean distance, as a measure of profile similarity allowed differentiated profiles to emerge more clearly in large samples.

For these reasons, although interpretive caution is always recommended, clinicians should be encouraged that the subtest scores of the SB5 have good specificity for individual profile interpretation. The exceptions are profile patterns involving low or high scores for Quantitative Reasoning, for which more caution is needed. Also, the generally high level of subtest reliability in the SB5, as compared to many other cognitive batteries (average subtest reliabilities ranged from .84 to .89; Roid, 2003e), results in low error variance for all subtests throughout the age range and supports profile interpretation.

BRIEF CASE STUDY

Table 15.6 shows the SB5 subtest scores and composite IQ and Factor Index scores for a 7-year-old boy. Eduardo is from the southern region of the United States; his parents have some post-high school education. Although Eduardo has a Hispanic background, he was born in the United States and speaks English fluently, also being exposed to Spanish in his home environment. He has been identified as having documented LDs in writing and oral expression and shows some delays in reading. His LDs were identified with the WJ III (both cognitive and achievement tests), using the school district's regression discrepancy formulas. As was documented in research conducted by Roid (2003c, 2003e) and in

TABLE 15.6. SB5 Scores for the Case of a 7-Year-Old Male (Eduardo) with LD

IQ scores		Factor index scores		Subtest scaled scores[a]	
NVIQ	93	Fluid Reasoning	100	Nonverbal FR	11
VIQ	87			Verbal FR	9
FSIQ	90	Knowledge	97	Nonverbal KN	9
				Verbal KN	10
		Quantitative Reasoning	94	Nonverbal QR	10
				Verbal QR	8
		Visual–Spatial Processing	91	Nonverbal VS	9
				Verbal VS	8
		Working Memory	74	Nonverbal WM	6
				Verbal WM	5

Note. All scores are normalized standard scores. IQ and factor index scores have mean 100 based on the normative sample of 4,800 examinees with standard deviation 15. Subtest scaled scores have a mean of 10 and a standard deviation of 3.

[a]FR, Fluid Reasoning; KN, Knowledge; QR, Quantitative Reasoning; VS, Visual–Spatial Processing; WM, Working Memory.

this chapter (see "Interpretation Based on Studies of Achievement Prediction," above), the Working Memory factor index and the Working Memory subtests show significantly lower scores than other scores within his profile. The Working Memory score of 74 is significantly different from the other factor index scores, and this difference is relatively rare in the normative population (e.g., only 10.5% of subjects have a difference of 20 points or more between the Working Memory and Quantitative Reasoning factor index scores). At the individual subtest level, both the Nonverbal and the Verbal Working Memory scores are considerably lower than other scores in the profile (scores of 6 and 5 compared to the other subtests, which vary between 8 and 11; a 3-point difference between pairs of subtest scores is statistically significant). Not only are the low Working Memory factor and subtest scores lower than other scores, but they also reflect normative weaknesses of the individual in relation to the normative sample.

For these reasons, Eduardo's SB5 profile shows a pattern similar to other cases of LDs (Roid, 2003c). Also, research on working memory has shown the connection between deficits in the ability to process and transform information in short-term memory to deficits in learning (Reid et al., 1996). This case study demonstrates the possibility that the Working Memory factor index and subtest scores of the SB5, when they are significantly lower than other scores in the profile, can be used with other data to support or refute hypotheses that LDs are present in an individual. For example, in empirical studies comparing verified cases of LDs with normative cases, Roid (2003c) used composites of SB5 Working Memory and Knowledge subtest scores to classify individual cases of documented LDs in reading achievement. Sums of the two Nonverbal and the two Verbal Working Memory and Knowledge subtests were calculated and transformed into an IQ metric (mean of 100, standard deviation of 15) based on the SB5 norm sample for ages 5 to 7 years. To calculate the composite, the weight of 1.875 was multiplied by the sum of the four subtest scaled scores, and 25 points were added. For Eduardo, the rounded result for this composite was 81. When a cutoff score of 89 was used (desig-

nating LD cases as those with scores less than 89 on the new composite), 67% of the LD cases were correctly identified, although 17% of normative cases were falsely identified as LD cases. Thus the composite of Working Memory and Knowledge scores was accurate in about two-thirds of LD cases—high enough for clinical hypothesis testing, but too low for LD identification purposes. Such composites should only be used when further data on an individual, collected from classroom teachers, parents, other tests, and observations in multiple settings, are consistent with a diagnosis of an LD. For older students (age 8 years and older) and adults, the LD reading achievement composite should be calculated with a slightly different formula derived from an analysis of the SB5 norm sample (Roid & Barram, 2004). The composite should be calculated by multiplying the sum of the scaled scores (Working Memory and Knowledge) by 1.56 (instead of 1.875) and then adding 37.9 points (instead of 25) to the result. The adjustment to the formula will provide more predictive accuracy for older students and adults.

CONCLUSION: INNOVATIONS IN COGNITIVE ASSESSMENT

The newest edition of the Stanford–Binet, the SB5, provides some intriguing new innovations in cognitive assessment. Foremost is the development of a factorially comprehensive Nonverbal domain of subtests, measuring five cognitive factors. The SB5 NVIQ is quite innovative among IQ measures because of its coverage of five factors from the work of Cattell (1943), Horn (1994), and Carroll (1993). Second, the innovative use of IRT in the SB5 is notable. Rasch analysis (Rasch, 1980; Wright & Lineacre, 1999) was employed throughout the development of items and subtest scales, and in the design of the routing procedure. In the routing procedure, Rasch ability scores are estimated from two initial subtests used to assign a functional level for the remainder of the assessment. Also notable is the development of the criterion-referenced CSSs. The CSSs provide an innovative method of interpreting SB5 results and for tracking cognitive change (growth or decline) across time. Finally, the

SB5 combines the classic age-level (now called functional-level) format of earlier editions with the point scale format used in the Fourth Edition, preserves many classic toys and tasks, enhances the cognitive factor composition of the battery, and continues the long tradition (beginning with Terman, 1916) of the Stanford–Binet.

NOTES

1. Note that the Nonverbal section requires a small degree of receptive language for the examinee to understand brief instructions by the examiner and does not rely solely on pantomime instructions.
2. The exception is level 1 of Nonverbal item book 2, which has two testlets with a maximum of 4 points each.
3. Quantitative items, as well as other items on the SB5, are also scaled in the CSS metric, allowing the items of the test to be related to the ability level of the examinees. For example, according to the calibration procedures of Wright and Lineacre (1999), a math item with difficulty 500 has a 50% probability of being mastered by the average 10-year-old, whereas a math item with difficulty 480 has a 90% probability of being answered correctly by the average 10-year-old.
4. See Roid (2003e) for more details. Split-half reliability formulas were used for subtests, and composite reliabilities for IQ and factor scores. Coefficients reported in the text are the overall average reliabilities across age groups.

REFERENCES

Aldenderfer, M. S., & Blashfield, R. K. (1984). *Cluster analysis.* Beverly Hills, CA: Sage.

Baddeley, A. D. (1986). *Working memory.* Oxford: Clarendon Press.

Baddeley, A. D., Logie, R., Nimmo-Smith, I., & Brereton, N. (1985). Components of fluent reading. *Journal of Memory and Language, 24,* 119–131.

Binet, A., & Simon, T. (1908). Le development de l'intelligence chez les enfants. *L'Année Psychologique, 14,* 1–94.

Carroll, J. B. (1993). *Human cognitive abilities: A survey of factor-analytic studies.* New York: Cambridge University Press.

Cattell, R. B. (1943). The measurement of intelligence. *Psychological Bulletin, 40,* 153–193.

Cohen, J. (1957). The factorial structure of the WAIS between early adulthood and old age. *Journal of Consulting Psychology, 21,* 283–290.

Cohen, J. (1959). The factorial structure of the WISC at ages 7–6, 10–6, and 13–6. *Journal of Consulting Psychology, 23,* 285–299.

Dana, R. H. (1993). *Multicultural assessment perspectives for professional psychology.* Boston: Allyn & Bacon.

Felton, R. H., & Pepper, P. P. (1995). Early identification and intervention of phonological deficits in kindergarten and early elementary children at risk for reading disability. *School Psychology Review, 24,* 405–414.

Flanagan, D. P., & Ortiz, S. O. (2001). *Essentials of cross-battery assessment.* New York: Wiley.

Horn, J. L. (1965). *Fluid and crystallized intelligence.* Unpublished doctoral dissertation, University of Illinois, Urbana–Champaign.

Horn, J. L. (1994). Theory of fluid and crystallized intelligence. In R. J. Sternberg (Ed.), *Encyclopedia of human intelligence* (pp. 443–451). New York: Macmillan.

Jensen, A. R. (1998). *The g factor: the science of mental ability.* Westport, CT: Praeger.

Joreskog, K. G., & Sorbom, D. (1999). *LISREL 8: User's reference guide.* Chicago: Scientific Software.

Kyllonen, P. C., & Christal, R. E. (1990). Reasoning ability is (little more than) working-memory capacity. *Intelligence, 14*(4), 389–433.

Lezak, M. D. (1995). *Neuropsychological assessment* (3rd ed.). New York: Oxford University Press.

Matarazzo, J. D. (1990). Psychological assessment versus psychological testing: Validation from Binet to the school, clinic, and courtroom. *American Psychologist, 45*(9), 999–1017.

McDermott, P. A., Fantuzzo, J. W., & Glutting, J. J. (1990). Just say no to subtest analysis: A critique on Wechsler theory and practice. *Journal of Psychoeducational Assessment, 8,* 290–302.

McGrew, K. S., & Flanagan, D. P. (1998). *The intelligence test desk reference (ITDR): Gf-Gc cross-battery assessment.* Boston: Allyn & Bacon.

McGrew, K. S., Flanagan, D. P., Keith, T. Z., & Vanderwood, M. (1997). Beyond g: The impact of Gf-Gc specific abilities research on the future use and interpretation of intelligence test batteries in schools. *School Psychology Review, 26,* 189–210.

McGrew, K. S., & Woodcock, R. W. (2001). *Woodcock–Johnson III technical manual.* Itasca, IL: Riverside.

Paniagua, F. A. (1994). *Assessing and treating culturally diverse clients: A practical guide.* Thousand Oaks, CA: Sage.

Pomplun, M. (2004, August). *The importance of working memory in the prediction of academic achievement.* Paper presented at the annual meeting of the American Psychological Association, Honolulu.

Rasch, G. (1980). *Probabilistic models for some intelligence and attainment tests.* Chicago: University of Chicago Press.

Reid, D. K., Hresko, W. P., & Swanson, H. L. (Eds.). (1996). *Cognitive approaches to learning disabilities* (3rd ed.). Austin, TX: Pro-Ed.

Reynolds, C. R., Kamphaus, R. W., & Rosenthal, B. L. (1988). Factor analysis of the Stanford–Binet: Fourth Edition for ages 2 through 23 years. *Measurement and Evaluation in Counseling and Development, 21,* 52–63.

Roid, G. H. (1994). Patterns of writing skills derived from cluster analysis of direct-writing assessments. *Applied Measurement in Education, 7*(2), 159–170.

Roid, G. H. (2003a). *Stanford–Binet Intelligence Scales, Fifth Edition.* Itasca, IL: Riverside.

Roid, G. H. (2003b). *Stanford–Binet Intelligence Scales, Fifth Edition: Examiner's manual.* Itasca, IL: Riverside.

Roid, G. H. (2003c). *Stanford–Binet Intelligence Scales, Fifth Edition: Interpretive manual.* Itasca, IL: Riverside.

Roid, G. H. (2003d). *Stanford–Binet Intelligence Scales, Fifth Edition: Scoring Pro* [Computer software]. Itasca, IL: Riverside.

Roid, G. H. (2003e). *Stanford–Binet Intelligence Scales, Fifth Edition: Technical manual.* Itasca, IL: Riverside.

Roid, G. H., & Barram, A. (2004). *Essentials of Stanford–Binet Intelligence Scales (SB5) assessment.* New York: Wiley.

Roid, G. H., & Gyurke, J. (1991). General-factor and specific variance in the WPPSI-R. *Journal of Psychoeducational Assessment, 9,* 209–223.

Roid, G. H., & Miller, L. J. (1997). *Leiter International Performance Scale—Revised.* Wood Dale, IL: Stoelting.

Terman, L. M. (1916). *The measurement of intelligence: An explanation of and a complete guide for the use of the Stanford revision and extension of the Binet–Simon Scale.* Boston: Houghton Mifflin.

Terman, L. M., & Merrill, M. A. (1937). *Measuring intelligence.* Boston: Houghton Mifflin.

Terman, L. M., & Merrill, M. A. (Eds.). (1960). *Stanford–Binet Intelligence Scale: Manual for the Third Revision Form L-M.* Boston: Houghton Mifflin.

Thorndike, R. L., Hagen, E. P., & Sattler, J. M. (1986). *The Stanford–Binet Intelligence Scale: Fourth Edition. Guide for administering and scoring.* Itasca, IL: Riverside.

U.S. Bureau of the Census. (2001). *Census 2000 summary file 1: United States.* Washington, DC: Author.

Wechsler, D. (1991). *Wechsler Intelligence Scale for Children—Third Edition.* San Antonio, TX: Psychological Corporation.

Wilson, K. M., & Swanson, H. L. (2001). Are mathematics disabilities due to a domain-general or a domain-specific working memory deficit? *Journal of Learning Disabilities, 34*(3), 237–248.

Woodcock, R. W., McGrew, K. S., & Mather, N. (2001a). *Woodcock–Johnson III Tests of Achievement.* Itasca, IL: Riverside.

Woodcock, R. W., McGrew, K. S., & Mather, N. (2001b). *Woodcock–Johnson III Tests of Cognitive Abilities.* Itasca, IL: Riverside.

Wright, B. D., & Lineacre, J. M. (1999). *WINSTEPS: Rasch analysis for all two-facet models.* Chicago: MESA Press.

16

The Kaufman Assessment Battery
for Children—Second Edition
and the Kaufman Adolescent
and Adult Intelligence Test

JAMES C. KAUFMAN
ALAN S. KAUFMAN
JENNIE KAUFMAN-SINGER
NADEEN L. KAUFMAN

This chapter provides an overview of two comprehensive, individually administered Kaufman tests of cognitive ability: the recently revised and restandardized second edition of the Kaufman Assessment Battery for Children (K-ABC; Kaufman & Kaufman, 1983), known as the KABC-II (Kaufman & Kaufman, 2004a), and the Kaufman Adolescent and Adult Intelligence Test (KAIT; Kaufman & Kaufman, 1993). The KABC-II is discussed first, followed by the KAIT, with the following topics featured for each of these multisubtest batteries: theory and structure, description of subtests, administration and scoring, psychometric properties, interpretation, clinical applications, and innovations in measures of cognitive assessment. Due to space limitations, an illustrative case report is provided for the new KABC-II but not for the KAIT. However, illustrative KAIT case reports have appeared in several publications by Liz Lichtenberger and her colleagues (Kaufman & Lichtenberger, 2002; J. C. Kaufman, Lichtenberger,

& Kaufman, 2003; Lichtenberger, 2001; Lichtenberger, Broadbooks, & Kaufman, 2000), and in the KAIT chapter of the first edition of this book (Kaufman & Kaufman, 1997).

KAUFMAN ASSESSMENT BATTERY FOR CHILDREN—SECOND EDITION

Theory and Structure

Structure and Organization

The KABC-II (Kaufman & Kaufman, 2004a) measures the processing and cognitive abilities of children and adolescents between the ages of 3 years, 0 months and 18 years, 11 months (3:0 and 18:11). Like the original K-ABC (Kaufman & Kaufman, 1983), the second edition is an individually administered, theory-based, clinical instrument. However, the KABC-II represents a substantial revision of the K-ABC, with a greatly expanded age range (3:0–18:11 instead of 2:6–12:6) and the addition of 8 new subtests (plus a Delayed Recall scale) to the battery. Of the original 16 K-ABC subtests, 8 were eliminated and 8 were retained. Like the K-ABC, the revised battery provides examiners with a Nonverbal scale, composed of subtests that may be administered in pantomime and responded to motorically, to permit valid assessment of children who have hearing impairments, limited English proficiency, and so forth.

The KABC-II is grounded in a dual theoretical foundation: Luria's (1966, 1970, 1973) neuropsychological model, featuring three blocks or functional units, and the Cattell–Horn–Carroll (CHC) approach to categorizing specific cognitive abilities (Carroll, 1993; Flanagan, McGrew, & Ortiz, 2000; Horn & Noll, 1997; see also Horn & Blankson, Chapter 3, Carroll, Chapter 4, and McGrew, Chapter 8, this volume). In contrast, the K-ABC had a single theoretical foundation, the distinction between sequential and simultaneous processing.

The KABC-II includes both Core and Expanded Batteries, with only the Core Battery needed to yield the child's scale profile. Like that of the KAIT, the KABC-II Expanded Battery offers supplementary subtests to increase the breadth of the constructs measured by the Core Battery and to follow up hypotheses. Administration time for the Core Battery takes about 30–70 minutes, depending on the child's age and whether the examiner administers the CHC model of the KABC-II or the Luria model. One of the features of the KABC-II is the flexibility it affords the examiner in determining the theoretical model to administer to each child.

When interpreted from the Luria model, the KABC-II focuses on mental processing, excludes acquired knowledge to the extent possible, and yields a global standard score called the Mental Processing Index (MPI) with a mean of 100 and a standard deviation (SD) of 15. Like the original K-ABC, the Luria model measures *sequential processing* and *simultaneous processing*, but the KABC-II goes beyond this dichotomy to measure two additional constructs: *learning ability* and *planning ability*.

From the vantage point of the CHC model, the KABC-II Core Battery includes all scales in the Luria system, but they are interpreted from an alternative perspective; for example, the scale that measures sequential processing from the Luria perspective is seen as measuring the CHC ability of *short-term memory* (Gsm), and the scale that measures planning ability (Luria interpretation) aligns with Gf or *fluid reasoning* (CHC interpretation). The CHC model includes one extra scale that is *not* in the Luria model—namely, a measure of *crystallized ability* (Gc), which is labeled Knowledge/Gc. The global standard score yielded by the CHC model is labeled the Fluid–Crystallized Index (FCI), also with a mean of 100 and SD of 15.

Table 16.1 summarizes the dual-model approach, showing the Luria process and corresponding CHC ability measured by each scale. The use of two theoretical models allows examiners to choose the model that

TABLE 16.1. The Dual Theoretical Foundations That Underlie the KABC-II

	Interpretation of scale from Luria theory	Interpretation of scale from CHC theory	Name of KABC-II scale
	Learning ability	Long-term storage and retrieval (Glr)	Learning/Glr
	Sequential processing	Short-term memory (Gsm)	Memory/Gsm
	Simultaneous processing	Visual processing (Gv)	Simultaneous/Gv
	Planning ability	Fluid reasoning (Gf)	Planning/Gf
	—	Crystallized ability (Gc)	Knowledge/Gc
Name of global score	Mental Processing Index (MPI)	Fluid–Crystallized Index (FCI)	

Note. Knowledge/Gc is included in the CHC system for the computation of the FCI, but it is excluded from the Luria system for the computation of the MPI. The Planning/Gf scale is for ages 7–18 only. All other scales are for ages 4–18. Only the MPI and FCI are offered for 3-year-olds.

best meets the needs of the child or adolescent being evaluated. The dual labels for the scales reflect the complexity of what the cognitive tasks measure and how their scores are interpreted. Examiners must select either the Luria or CHC model *before* they administer the test, thereby determining which global score should be used—the MPI (Luria model) or FCI (CHC model).

• The CHC model is the model of choice—except in cases where including measures of acquired knowledge (crystallized ability) is believed by the examiner to compromise the validity of the FCI. In those cases, the Luria-based global score (MPI) is preferred.
• The CHC model is given priority over the Luria model, because we believe that knowledge/Gc is, in principle, an important aspect of cognitive functioning. Therefore, the CHC model (FCI) is preferred for children with known or suspected disabilities in reading, written expression, or mathematics; for children assessed for giftedness or mental retardation; for children assessed for emotional or behavioral disorders; and for children assessed for attentional disorders such as attention-deficit/hyperactivity disorder (ADHD).
• Situations in which the Luria model (MPI) is preferred include, but are not limited to, the following:

• A child from a bilingual background.
• A child from any nonmainstream cultural background that may have affected knowledge acquisition and verbal development.
• A child with known or suspected language disorders, whether expressive, receptive, or mixed receptive–expressive.
• A child with known or suspected autism.
• An examiner with a firm commitment to the Luria processing approach who believes that acquired knowledge should be excluded from any global cognitive score (regardless of reason for referral).

This set of recommendations does not imply that we consider one model to be theoretically superior to the other. Both theories are equally important as foundations of the KABC-II. The CHC psychometric theory emphasizes specific cognitive abilities, whereas the Luria neuropsychological theory emphasizes *processes*—namely, the way children process information when solving problems. Both approaches are valid for understanding how children learn and solve new problems, which is why each scale has two names, one from Luria theory and the other from CHC theory. Regardless of the model of the KABC-II that is *administered* (Luria or CHC), the way in which psychologists *interpret* the scales will undoubtedly be influenced by their theoretical preference.

On the original K-ABC, the Sequential and Simultaneous Processing scales were joined by a separate Achievement scale. That concept is continued with the Luria model of the KABC-II, although conventional kinds of achievement (reading, arithmetic) are excluded from the KABC-II Knowledge/Gc scale.

At age 3, only a global score is offered, either the MPI or FCI. For ages 4–18, the global scale is joined by an array of scales (see Table 16.1). The Planning/Gf scale is included only at ages 7–18, because a factor corresponding to the high-level set of abilities did not emerge for younger children. All KABC-II scales have a mean of 100 and *SD* of 15.

Theory: Luria and CHC

Luria (1970) perceived the brain's basic functions to be represented by three main blocks or functional systems, which are responsible for arousal and attention (block 1); the use of one's senses to analyze, code, and store information (block 2); and the application of executive functions for formulating plans and programming behavior (block 3). Within block 2, Luria (1966) distinguished between "two basic forms of integrative activity of the cerebral cortex" (p. 74), which he labeled *successive* and *simultaneous*. Despite Luria's interpretation of three blocks, each with separate functions, his focus was on *integration* among the blocks to be capable of complex behavior. Block 3 is very closely related to the functions of block 1, as both blocks are concerned with overall efficiency of brain functions; part of the role of block 2 is to establish connections with block 3 (Reitan, 1988). Indeed, "integration of these systems constitutes the real key to understanding how the brain mediates complex behavior" (Reitan, 1988, p. 333).

In the development of the KABC-II, we emphasized the integration of the three blocks, not the measurement of each block in isolation. The block 1 arousal functions are key aspects of successful test performance on any cognitive task, but attention and concentration per se do not fit our definition of high-level, complex, intelligent behavior. The Learning/Glr scale requires much sustained attention and concentration (block 1), but depends more on the integration of the three blocks than on any one in isolation. The Sequential/Gsm and Simultaneous/Gv scales are deliberately targeted to measure the block 2 successive and simultaneous functions, respectively, but again we have striven for complexity. Luria (1966) defined the block 2 functions of analysis and storage of incoming stimuli via successive and simultaneous processing as *coding* functions, not problem-solving functions. But because block 2 is responsible for establishing connections with block 3, the KABC-II measures of simultaneous processing require not just the analysis, coding, and storage of incoming stimuli, but also the block 3 executive functioning processes for success. In addition, block 2 requires the integration of the incoming stimuli; hence subtests like Word Order and Rover require synthesis of auditory and visual stimuli. Planning/Gf was intended to measure Luria's block 3—but, again, success on these complex tasks requires not just executive functioning, but also focused attention (block 1) and the coding and storage of incoming stimuli (block 2).

The CHC model is a psychometric theory that rests on a large body of research, especially factor-analytic investigations, accumulated over decades. The CHC theory represents a data-driven theory, in contrast to Luria's clinically driven theory. CHC theory has two separate psychometric lineages: (1) Raymond Cattell's (1941) original Gf-Gc theory, which was expanded and refined by Horn (1968, 1985, 1989) to include an array of abilities (not just Gf and Gc); and (2) John Carroll's (1943, 1993) half-century of rigorous efforts to summarize and integrate the voluminous literature on the factor analysis of cognitive abilities. Ultimately, Horn and Carroll agreed to merge their separate but overlapping models into the unified CHC theory. This merger was done in a personal communication to Richard Woodcock in July 1999; the specifics of CHC theory and its applications have been articulated by Dawn Flanagan, Kevin McGrew, and their colleagues (Flanagan, McGrew, & Ortiz, 2000; Flanagan & Ortiz, 2001; see also McGrew, Chapter 8, this volume).

Both the Cattell–Horn and Carroll models essentially started from the same point—Spearman's (1904) g factor theory. Though they took different paths, they ended up with remarkably consistent conclusions about the spectrum of broad cognitive abilities. Cattell built upon Spearman's g to posit two kinds of g: *fluid intelligence* (Gf), the ability to solve novel problems by using reasoning (believed by Cattell to be largely a function of biological and neurological factors), and *crystallized intelligence* (Gc), a knowledge-based ability that is highly dependent on education and acculturation.

Almost from the beginning of his collaboration with Cattell, Horn believed that the psychometric data, as well as neurocognitive and developmental data, were suggesting more than just these two general abilities. Horn (1968) quickly identified four additional abilities; by the mid-1990s, his model included 9–10 *broad abilities* (Horn, 1989; Horn & Hofer, 1992; Horn & Noll, 1997). The initial dichotomy had grown, but not in a hierarchy. Horn retained the name of Gf-Gc theory, but the diverse broad abilities were treated as equals, not as part of any hierarchy.

Carroll (1993) developed a hierarchical theory based on his in-depth survey of factor-analytic studies composed of three levels or strata of abilities: *Stratum III (general)*, a Spearman-like g, which Carroll considered to be a valid construct based on overwhelming evidence from factor analysis; *stratum II (broad)*, composed of eight broad factors that correspond reasonably closely to Horn's broad abilities; and stratum I (narrow), composed of numerous fairly specific abilities, organized by the broad factor with which each is most closely associated (many relate to level of mastery, response speed, or rate of learning).

To Horn, the g construct had no place in his Gf-Gc theory; consequently, Carroll's stratum III is not usually considered part of CHC theory. Nonetheless, the KABC-II incorporates stratum III in its theoretical model because it corresponds to the global measure of general cognitive ability, the FCI. However, the g level is intended more as a practical than a theoretical construct. The KABC-II scales correspond to 5 of the 10 broad abilities that make up CHC stratum II—Glr, Gsm, Gv, Gf, and Gc. The test authors chose not to include separate measures of Gq (*quantitative knowledge*) or Grw (*reading and writing*), because they believe that reading, writing, and mathematics fit in better with tests of academic achievement, like the Kaufman Test of Educational Achievement—Second Edition (KTEA-II; Kaufman & Kaufman, 2004b); however, Gq is present in some KABC-II tasks. The Gq ability measured, however, is considered secondary to other abilities measured by these subtests.

The KABC-II assesses 15 of the approximately 70 CHC narrow abilities. Table 16.2 shows the relationship of the KABC-II scales and subtests to the three strata. For the KABC-II, the broad abilities are of primary importance for interpreting the child's cognitive profile. In developing the KABC-II, the test authors did not strive to develop "pure" tasks for measuring the five CHC broad abilities. In theory, for example, Gv tasks should exclude Gf or Gs. In practice, however, the goal of comprehensive tests of cognitive ability is to measure problem solving in different contexts and under different conditions, with complexity being necessary to assess high-level functioning. Consequently, the test authors constructed measures that featured a particular ability while incorporating aspects

TABLE 16.2. General (Stratum III), Broad (Stratum II), and Narrow (Stratum I) CHC Abilities Measured by the KABC-II

CHC ability	Measured on KABC-II by:
General ability (stratum III in Carroll's theory)	**Mental Processing Index (MPI)**—Luria model of KABC-II (excludes acquired knowledge), ages 3–18
	Fluid–Crystallized Index (FCI)—CHC model of KABC-II (includes acquired knowledge), ages 3–18
Broad ability (stratum II in CHC theory)	
Long-term storage and retrieval (Glr)	**Learning/Glr Index** (ages 4–18)
Short-term memory (Gsm)	**Sequential/Gsm Index** (ages 4–18)
Visual processing (Gv)	**Simultaneous/Gv Index** (ages 4–18)
Fluid reasoning (Gf)	**Planning/Gf Index** (ages 7–18)
Crystallized ability (Gc)	**Knowledge/Gc Index** (ages 4–18)
Narrow ability (stratum I in CHC theory)	
Glr: Associative memory (MA)	*Atlantis, Rebus, Delayed Recall scale*
Glr: Learning abilities (L1)	*Delayed Recall scale*
Gsm: Memory span (MS)	*Word Order* (without color interference), *Number Recall, Hand Movements*
Gsm: Working memory (WM)	*Word Order* (with color interference)
Gv: Visual memory (MV)	*Face Recognition, Hand Movements*
Gv: Spatial relations (SR)	*Triangles*
Gv: Visualization (VZ)	*Triangles, Conceptual Thinking, Block Counting, Story Completion*
Gv: Spatial scanning (SS)	*Rover*
Gv: Closure speed (CS)	*Gestalt Closure*
Gf: Induction (I)	*Conceptual Thinking, Pattern Reasoning, Story Completion*
Gf: General sequential reasoning (RG)	*Rover, Riddles*
Gc: General information (K0)	*Verbal Knowledge, Story Completion*
Gc: Language development (LD)	*Riddles*
Gc: Lexical knowledge (VL)	*Riddles, Verbal Knowledge, Expressive Vocabulary*
Gq: Math achievement (A3)	*Rover, Block Counting*

Note. Gq, quantitative ability. KABC-II scales are in **bold**, and KABC-II subtests are in *italics*. All KABC-II subtests are included, both Core and supplementary. CHC stratum I categorizations are courtesy of D. P. Flanagan (personal communication, October 2, 2003).

of other abilities. To illustrate, Rover is primarily a measure of Gv, because of its visualization component, but it also involves Gf; Story Completion emphasizes Gf, but Gc is also required to interpret the social situations that are depicted.

Description of KABC-II Subtests

Sequential/Gsm Scale

• *Word Order (Core for ages 3:0 to 18:11).* The child touches a series of silhouettes of common objects in the same order as the examiner said the names of the objects; more difficult items include an interference task (color naming) between the stimulus and response.

• *Number Recall (supplementary for ages 3:0 to 3:11; Core for ages 4:0 to 18:11).* The child repeats a series of numbers in the same sequence as the examiner has said them, with series ranging in length from two to nine numbers; the numbers are digits, except that 10 is used instead of 7 to ensure that all numbers are one syllable.

• *Hand Movements (supplementary for ages 4:0 to 18:11; Nonverbal scale for ages 4:0 to 18:11).* The child copies the examiner's precise sequence of taps on the table with the fist, palm, or side of the hand.

Simultaneous/Gv Scale

• *Triangles (Core for ages 3:0 to 12:11; supplementary for ages 13:0 to 18:11; Nonverbal scale for ages 3:0 to 18:11).* For most items, the child assembles several identical rubber triangles (blue on one side, yellow on the other) to match a picture of an abstract design; for easier items, the child assembles a different set of colorful rubber shapes to match a model constructed by the examiner.

• *Face Recognition (Core for ages 3:0 to 4:11; supplementary for ages 5:0 to 5:11; nonverbal scale for ages 3:0 to 5:11).* The child attends closely to photographs of one or two faces that are exposed briefly, and then selects the correct face or faces, shown in a different pose, from a group photograph.

• *Conceptual Thinking (Core for ages 3:0 to 6:11; Nonverbal scale for ages 3:0 to 6:11).* The child views a set of four or five pictures and then identifies the one picture that does not belong with the others; some

items present meaningful stimuli, and others use abstract stimuli.

• *Rover (Core for ages 6:0 to 18:11).* The child moves a toy dog to a bone on a checkerboard-like grid that contains obstacles (rocks and weeds), and tries to find the "quickest" path—the one that takes the fewest moves.

• *Block Counting (supplementary for ages 5:0 to 12:11; Core for ages 13:0 to 18:11; Nonverbal scale for ages 7:0 to 18:11).* The child counts the exact number of blocks in various pictures of stacks of blocks; the stacks are configured so that one or more blocks are hidden or partially hidden from view.

• *Gestalt Closure (supplementary for ages 3:0 to 18:11).* The child mentally "fills in the gaps" in a partially completed "inkblot" drawing, and names (or describes) the object or action depicted in the drawing.

Planning/Gf Scale (Ages 7–18 Only)

• *Pattern Reasoning (Core for ages 7:0 to 18:11; Nonverbal scale for ages 5:0 to 18:11; Core for ages 5:0 to 6:11, but on the Simultaneous/Gv scale).* The child is shown a series of stimuli that form a logical, linear pattern, but one stimulus is missing; the child completes the pattern by selecting the correct stimulus from an array of four to six options at the bottom of the page (most stimuli are abstract, geometric shapes, but some easy items use meaningful shapes).

• *Story Completion (Core for ages 7:0 to 18:11; Nonverbal scale for ages 6:0 to 18:11; supplementary for ages 6:0 to 6:11, but on the Simultaneous/Gv scale).* The child is shown a row of pictures that tell a story, but some of the pictures are missing. The child is given a set of pictures, selects only the ones that are needed to complete the story, and places the missing pictures in their correct locations.

Learning/Glr Scale

• *Atlantis (Core for ages 3:0 to 18:11).* The examiner teaches the child the nonsense names for fanciful pictures of fish, plants, and shells; the child demonstrates learning by pointing to each picture (out of an array of pictures) when it is named.

• *Rebus (Core for ages 3:0 to 18:11).* The

examiner teaches the child the word or con-cept associated with each particular rebus (drawing), and the child then "reads" aloud phrases and sentences composed of these re-buses.

• *Delayed Recall (supplementary scale for ages 5:0 to 18:11).* The child demonstrates delayed recall of paired associations learned about 20 minutes earlier during the Atlantis and Rebus subtests (this requires the exam-iner to administer the Atlantis—Delayed and Rebus—Delayed tasks).

Knowledge/Gc Scale (CHC Model Only)

• *Riddles (Core for ages 3:0 to 18:11).* The examiner provides several characteris-tics of a concrete or abstract verbal concept, and the child has to point to it (early items) or name it (later items).

• *Expressive Vocabulary (Core for ages 3:0 to 6:11; supplementary for ages 7:0 to 18:11).* The child provides the name of a pic-tured object.

• *Verbal Knowledge (supplementary for ages 3:0 to 6:11; Core for ages 7:0 to 18:11).* The child selects from an array of six pic-tures the one that corresponds to a vocabu-lary word or answers a general information question.

Administration and Scoring

For the KABC-II, the Core Battery for the Luria model comprises five subtests for 3-year-olds, seven subtests for 4- and 5-year-olds, and 8 subtests for ages 6–18. The CHC Core Battery includes two additional sub-tests at each age, both measures of crystal-lized ability. Approximate average adminis-tration times for the Core Battery, by age, are given in Table 16.3. For the CHC test bat-tery, the additional two Core subtests add about 10 minutes to the testing time for ages 3–6 and about 15 minutes for ages 7–18 years.

Examiners who choose to administer the entire Expanded Battery—all Core and supplementary subtests, the Delayed Recall scale, and all measures of crystallized abil-ity—can expect to spend just under 60 minutes for 3- and 4-year-olds, about 90 minutes for ages 5 and 6, and about 100 minutes for ages 7–18. However, examiners who choose to administer supplementary

TABLE 16.3. Average Administration Times (in Minutes) for the KABC-II Core Battery

Ages =	MPI (Luria model)	FCI (CHC model)
3–4	30	40
5	40	50
6	50	60
7–18	55	70

subtests need not give all of the available subtests to a given child or adolescent—just the ones that are most pertinent to the rea-sons for referral.

Sample and teaching items are included for all subtests, except those that measure ac-quired knowledge, to ensure that children understand what is expected of them to meet the demands of each subtest. Scoring of all subtests is objective. Even the Knowledge/Gc subtests require pointing or one-word re-sponses rather than longer verbal responses, which often introduce subjectivity into the scoring process.

Psychometric Properties

Many of the analyses of standardization and validity data were being conducted when this chapter was written, so the data provided here are incomplete and focus on the KABC-II global scores (MPI and FCI) rather than the scale profile. For a thorough description of the normative sample and reliability, sta-bility, and validity data, see the KABC-II manual (Kaufman & Kaufman, 2004a) and *Essentials of KABC-II Assessment* (Kauf-man, Lichtenberger, Fletcher-Janzen, & Kaufman, in press).

Standardization Sample

The KABC-II standardization sample was composed of 3,025 children and adolescents. The sample matched the U.S. population on the stratification variables of gender, race/ethnicity, socioeconomic status (SES—parent education), region, and special education status. Each year of age between 3 and 18 was represented by 125–250 children, about equally divided between males and females, with most age groups consisting of exactly 200 children.

Reliability

KABC-II global scale (MPI and FCI) split-half reliability coefficients were in the mid-.90s for all age groups (only the value of .90 for the MPI at age 3 was below .94). The mean MPI coefficient was .95 for ages 3–6 and ages 7–18; the mean values for FCI were .96 (ages 3–6) and .97 (ages 7–18). Mean split-half reliability coefficients for the separate scales (e.g., Learning/Glr, Simultaneous/Gv) averaged .91–.92 for ages 3–6 and ranged from .88 to .93 (mean = .90) for ages 7–18. Similarly, the Nonverbal Index—the alternate global score for children and adolescents with hearing impairments, limited English proficiency, and the like—had an average coefficient of .90 for 3- to 6-year-olds and .92 for those ages 7–18. Mean split-half values for Core subtests across the age range were .82 (age 3), .84 (age 4), .86 (ages 5–6), and .85 (ages 7–18). Nearly all Core subtests had mean coefficients of .80 or greater at ages 3–6 and 7–18. Stability data over an interval of about 1 month for three age groups (total N = 203) yielded coefficients of .86–.91 for the MPI and .90–.94 for the FCI. Stability coefficients for the separate scales averaged .81 for ages 3–6 (range = .74–.93), .80 for ages 7–12 (range = .76–.88), and .83 for ages 13–18 (range = .78–.95).

Validity

Most data on the KABC-II's validity were in various stages of analysis when this chapter was written. Construct validity was given strong support by the results of confirmatory factor analysis (CFA). The CFA supported four factors for ages 4 and 5–6, and five factors for ages 7–12 and 13–18, with the factor structure supporting the scale structure for these broad age groups. The fit was excellent for all age groups; for ages 7–12 and 13–18, the five-factor solution provided a significantly better fit than the four-factor solution.

Correlation coefficients between the FCI and Wechsler Intelligence Scale for Children (WISC) Full Scale IQ, corrected for the variability of the norms sample, were .89 for the WISC-IV (N = 56, ages 7–16) and 77 for the WISC-III (N = 119, ages 8–13). The FCI also correlated .91 with KAIT Composite IQ (N = 29, ages 11–18), .78 with Woodcock–Johnson III (WJ III) General Intellectual Ability (N = 86, ages 7–16), .72 with K-ABC Mental Processing Composite (MPC) for preschool children (N = 67), and 84 with K-ABC MPC for school-age children (N = 48). Correlations with MPI were generally slightly lower (by an average of .05).

Fletcher-Janzen (2003) conducted a correlational study with the WISC-IV for 30 Native American children from Taos, New Mexico, who were tested on the KABC-II at an average age of 7:8 (range = 5–14) and on the WISC-IV at an average age of 9:3. As shown in Table 16.4, the two global scores correlated about .85 with WISC-IV Full Scale IQ. This strong relationship indicates that the KABC-II global scores and the WISC-IV global score measure the same construct; nevertheless, the KABC-II yielded global scores that were about 0.5 SD higher

TABLE 16.4. Means, SDs, and Correlations between KABC-II and WISC-IV Global Scores for 30 Native American Children and Adolescents from Taos, New Mexico

KABC-II and WISC-IV global scores	Mean	SD	r with WISC-IV FSIQ	Mean difference MPI vs. FSIQ	Mean difference FCI vs. FSIQ
KABC-II					
Mental Processing Composite (MPI)	95.1	13.3	.86	+8.4	—
Fluid–Crystallized Index (FCI)	94.1	12.5	.84	—	+7.4
WISC-IV					
Full Scale IQ (FSIQ)	86.7	12.3	—	—	—

Note. Children were tested first on the KABC-II (age range = 5–14, mean = 7:8) and second on the WISC-IV (age range = 6–15, mean = 9:3). Data from Fletcher-Janzen (2003).

than the Full Scale IQ for this Native American sample.

Correlations were obtained between KABC-II and achievement on the WJ III, Wechsler Individual Achievement Test—Second Edition (WIAT-2), and Peabody Individual Achievement Test—Revised/Normative Update (PIAT-R/NU) for six samples with a total N of 401. Coefficients between the FCI and total achievement for the six samples, corrected for the variability of the norms sample, ranged from .67 on the PIAT-R/NU for grades 1–4 to .87 on the WIAT-2 for grades 6–10 (mean $r = .75$). For these same samples, the MPI correlated .63 to .83 (mean $r = .71$).

Interpretation

What the Scales Measure

Sequential/Gsm (Ages 4–18)

- *CHC interpretation.* Short-term memory (Gsm) is the ability to apprehend and hold information in immediate awareness briefly, and then use that information within a few seconds, before it is forgotten.
- *Luria interpretation.* Sequential processing is used to solve problems, where the emphasis is on the serial or temporal order of stimuli. For each problem, the input must be arranged in a strictly defined order to form a chain-like progression; each idea is linearly and temporally related only to the preceding one.

Simultaneous/Gv (Ages 4–18)

- *CHC interpretation.* Visual processing (Gv) is the ability to perceive, manipulate, and think with visual patterns and stimuli, and to mentally rotate objects in space.
- *Luria interpretation.* Simultaneous processing demands a Gestalt-like, frequently spatial, integration of stimuli. The input has to be synthesized simultaneously, so that the separate stimuli are integrated into a group or conceptualized as a whole.

Learning/Glr (Ages 4–18)

- *CHC interpretation.* Long-term storage and retrieval (Glr) is the ability both to store information in long-term memory and to retrieve that information fluently and efficiently. The emphasis of Glr is on the *effi-*

ciency of the storage and retrieval, not on the specific nature of the information stored.

- *Luria interpretation.* Learning ability requires an integration of the processes associated with all three of Luria's functional units. The attentional requirements for the learning tasks are considerable, as focused, sustained, and selective attention are requisites for success. However, for effective paired-associate learning, children need to apply both block 2 processes, sequential and simultaneous. Block 3 planning abilities help them generate strategies for storing and retrieving the new learning.

Planning/Gf (Ages 7–18)

- *CHC interpretation.* Fluid reasoning (Gf) refers to a variety of mental operations that a person can use to solve a novel problem with adaptability and flexibility—operations such as drawing inferences and applying inductive or deductive reasoning. Verbal mediation also plays a key role in applying fluid reasoning effectively.
- *Luria interpretation.* Planning ability requires hypothesis generation, revising one's plan of action, monitoring and evaluating the best hypothesis for a given problem (decision making), flexibility, and impulse control. This set of high-level skills is associated with executive functioning.

Knowledge/Gc (Ages 4–18)—CHC Model Only

- *CHC interpretation.* Crystallized ability (Gc) reflects a person's specific knowledge acquired within a culture, as well as the person's ability to apply this knowledge effectively. Gc emphasizes the *breadth* and *depth* of the specific information that has been stored.
- *Luria interpretation.* The Knowledge/Gc scale is not included in the MPI, but may be administered as a supplement if the examiner seeks a measure of the child's acquired knowledge. From a Luria perspective, Knowledge/Gc measures a person's knowledge base, developed over time by applying block 1, block 2, and block 3 processes to the acquisition of factual information and verbal concepts. Like Learning/Glr, this scale requires an integration of the key processes, but unlike learning ability, acquired knowledge emphasizes the *content* more than the *process.*

Gender Differences

Analysis of KABC-II standardization data explored gender differences at four different age ranges: 3–4 years, 5–6 years, 7–12 years, and 13–18 years. At ages 3–4, females significantly outperformed males on the MPI, FCI, and Nonverbal Index by about 5 points (0.33 SD), but there were no other significant differences on the global scales at any age level (J. C. Kaufman, 2003). Consistent with the literature on gender differences, females tended to score higher than males at preschool levels. Females scored significantly higher than males at ages 3 and 4 years by about 3–4 points, with significant differences emerging on Learning/Glr (0.27 SD) and Simultaneous/Gv (0.34 SD). Also consistent with previous findings, males scored significantly higher than females on the Simultaneous/Gv scale at ages 7–12 (0.24 SD) and 13–18 (0.29 SD). Females earned significantly higher scores than males at ages 5–6 on the Sequential/Gsm scale (0.22 SD) and at ages 13–18 on the Planning/Gf scale (0.13 SD). In general, gender differences on the KABC-II were small and, even when significant, tended to be small in effect size (McLean, 1995).

Ethnicity Differences

Because the original K-ABC yielded considerably smaller ethnic differences than conventional IQ tests did, it was especially important to determine the magnitude of ethnic differences for the substantially revised and reconceptualized KABC-II. On the original K-ABC, the mean MPC for African American children ages 5:0 to 12:6 was 93.7 (Kaufman & Kaufman, 1983, Table 4.35). On the KABC-II, the mean MPI for African American children ages 7–18 in the standardization sample (N = 315) was 94.8, and the mean FCI was 94.0. On the two new KABC-II scales, African American children ages 7–18 averaged 94.3 (Planning/Gf) and 98.6 (Learning/Glr). At ages 3–6, African American children averaged 98.2 on Learning/Glr.

When standard scores were adjusted for SES and gender, European Americans scored 4.4 points higher than African Americans at 7–12 years on the MPI, smaller than an adjusted difference of 8.6 points on WISC-III

Full Scale IQ at ages 6–11 (J. C. Kaufman, 2003). At the 13- to 18-year level, European Americans scored 7.7 points higher than African Americans on the adjusted MPI (J. C. Kaufman, 2003), substantially smaller than the 14.1-point discrepancy on adjusted WISC-III Full Scale IQ for ages 12–16 (WISC-III data are from Prifitera, Weiss, & Saklofske, 1998). The adjusted discrepancies of 6.2 points (ages 7–12) and 8.6 points (ages 13–18) on the FCI—which includes measures of acquired knowledge—were also substantially smaller than WISC-III Full Scale IQ differences. The KABC-II thus seems to continue in the K-ABC tradition of yielding higher standard scores for African Americans than are typically yielded on other instruments. In addition, as shown in Table 16.4, the mean MPI and FCI earned by the 30 Native American children in Taos are about 7–8 points higher than this sample's mean WISC-IV Full Scale IQ.

Further ethnicity analyses of KABC-II standardization data were conducted for the entire age range of 3–18 years, which included 1,861 European Americans, 545 Hispanics, 465 African Americans, 75 Asian Americans, and 68 Native Americans. When adjusted for SES and gender, mean MPIs were 101.7 for European Americans, 97.1 for Hispanics, 96.0 for African Americans, 103.4 for Asian Americans, and 97.6 for Native Americans. Mean adjusted FCIs were about 1 point lower than the mean MPIs for all groups except European Americans (who had a slightly higher FCI) (J. C. Kaufman, 2003).

Clinical Applications

Like the original K-ABC, the KABC-II was designed to be a clinical and psychological instrument, not merely a psychometric tool. It has a variety of clinical benefits and uses:

1. The identification of process integrities and deficits for assessment of individuals with specific learning disabilities.
2. The evaluation of individuals with known or suspected neurological disorders, when the KABC-II is used along with other tests as part of a comprehensive neuropsychological battery.
3. The integration of the individual's profile of KABC-II scores with clinical behaviors

observed during the administration of each subtest (Fletcher-Janzen, 2003)— identified as Qualitative Indicators (QIs) on the KABC-II record form (see Kaufman & Kaufman, 2004a; Kaufman et al., in press).

4. The selection of the MPI to promote the fair assessment of children and adolescents from African American, Hispanic, Native American, and Asian American backgrounds (an application that has empirical support, as summarized briefly in the previous section on "Ethnicity Differences" and in Table 16.4).

5. Evaluation of individuals with known or suspected ADHD, mental retardation/developmental delay, speech/language difficulties, emotional/behavioral disorders, autism, reading/math disabilities, intellectual giftedness, and hearing impairment (KABC-II data on all of these clinical samples are presented and discussed in the KABC-II manual).

We believe that whenever possible, clinical tests such as the KABC-II should be interpreted by the same person who administered them—an approach that enhances the clinical benefits of the instrument and its clinical applications. The main goal of any evaluation should be to *effect change* in the person who was referred. Extremely competent and well-trained examiners are needed to best accomplish that goal; we feel more confident in a report writer's ability to effect change and to derive clinical benefits from an administration of the KABC-II when the professional who interprets the test data and writes the case report has also administered the test and directly observed the individual's test behaviors.

Innovations in Measures of Cognitive Assessment

Several of the features described here for the KABC-II are innovative relative to the Wechsler and Stanford–Binet tradition of intellectual assessment, which has century-old roots. However, some of these innovations are not unique to the KABC-II; rather, several of these innovations are shared by other contemporary instruments such as the KAIT (as discussed later in this chapter), the WJ III

(Woodcock, McGrew, & Mather, 2001), the Cognitive Assessment System (CAS; Naglieri & Das, 1997), and the most recent revisions of the Wechsler scales (Wechsler, 2002, 2003).

Integrates Two Theoretical Approaches

As discussed previously, the KABC-II utilizes a dual theoretical approach—Luria's neuropsychological theory and CHC theory. This dual model permits alternative interpretations of the scales, based on the examiner's personal orientation or based on the specific individual being evaluated One of the criticisms of the original K-ABC was that we interpreted the mental processing scales solely from the sequential–simultaneous perspective, despite the fact that alternative interpretations are feasible (Keith, 1985). The KABC-II has addressed that criticism and has provided a strong theoretical foundation for the test by building the test on a dual theoretical model.

Provides the Examiner with Optimal Flexibility

The two theoretical models that underlie the KABC-II not only provide alternative interpretations of the scales, but also give the examiner the flexibility to select the model (and hence the global score) that is better suited to the individual's background and reason for referral. As mentioned earlier, the CHC model is ordinarily the model of choice, but examiners can choose to administer the Luria model when exclusion of measures of acquired knowledge from the global score promotes fairer assessment of a child's general cognitive ability. The MPI that results is an especially pertinent global score, for example, for individuals who have a receptive or expressive language disability or who are from a bilingual background. This flexibility of choice permits fairer assessment for anyone referred for an evaluation.

The examiner's flexibility is enhanced as well by the inclusion of supplementary subtests for most scales, including a supplementary Delayed Recall scale to permit the evaluation of a child's recall of paired associations that were learned about 20 minutes earlier. Hand Movements is a supplementary Sequential/Gsm subtest for ages 4–18, and Gestalt Closure is a supplementary task across the entire 3–18 range. Supplementary subtests are not included in the computation of standard scores on any KABC-II scales, but they do permit the examiner to follow up hypotheses suggested by the profile of scores on the Core Battery, to generate new hypotheses, and to increase the breadth of measurement on the KABC-II constructs.

Promotes Fairer Assessment of Minority Children

As mentioned earlier, children and adolescents from minority backgrounds—African American, Hispanic, Asian American, and Native American—earned mean MPIs that were close to the normative mean of 100, even prior to adjustment for SES and gender. In addition, there is some evidence that the discrepancies between European Americans and African Americans are smaller on the KABC-II than on the WISC-III, and that Native Americans score higher on the KABC-II than the WISC-IV (see Table 16.4). These data suggest that the KABC-II, like the original K-ABC, will be useful for promoting fairer assessment of children and adolescents from minority backgrounds.

Offers a Separate Nonverbal Scale

Like the K-ABC, the KABC-II offers a reliable, separate Nonverbal scale composed of subtests that can be administered in pantomime and responded to nonverbally. This special global scale, for the entire 3–18 age range, permits valid assessment of children and adolescents with hearing impairments, moderate to severe speech/language disorders, limited English proficiency, and so forth.

Permits Direct Evaluation of a Person's Learning Ability

The KABC-II Learning/Glr scale allows direct measurement of a child's ability to learn new information under standardized conditions. These tasks also permit examiners to observe the child's ability to learn under different conditions; for example, Atlantis gives the child feedback after each error, but Re-

bus does not offer feedback. In addition, Rebus involves meaningful verbal labels for symbolic visual stimuli, whereas Atlantis involves nonsensical verbal labels for meaningful visual stimuli. When examiners choose to administer the supplementary Delayed Recall scale to children ages 5–18, they are then able to assess the children's ability to retain information that was taught earlier in the evaluation. The inclusion of learning tasks on the KABC-II (and on the WJ III and KAIT) reflects an advantage over the Wechsler scales, which do not directly measure learning ability.

KABC-II Illustrative Case Study

Name: Jessica T.
Age: 12 years, 3 months
Grade in school: 7
Evaluator: Jennie Kaufman-Singer, PhD

Reason for Referral

Jessica was referred for a psychological evaluation by her mother, Mrs. T., who stated that Jessica has been struggling at school; she appears to have particular problems with reading comprehension. Jessica also exhibits difficulty following instructions at home and acts in an oppositional manner at times. In addition, Mrs. T. is concerned that Jessica tends to act angry and irritable much of the time, and seems to be depressed.

Evaluation Procedures

- Clinical interview with Jessica
- Collateral interview with Mrs. T.
- Kaufman Assessment Battery for Children—Second Edition (KABC-II)
- Kaufman Test of Educational Achievement—Second Edition, Comprehensive Form (KTEA-II, Form A)
- Review of school records

Background Information

Mrs. T., a single mother, adopted Jessica when Jessica was 6 years old. Jessica's biological mother has a drug addiction; both Jessica and Jessica's younger sister (now age 9) were removed from the home by the Department of Social Services when the girls were ages 5 and 2. Jessica was living in a foster home when Mrs. T. adopted her. Jessica's biological mother did not show up to contest the adoption, nor did she respond to any attempt to reunite her family. Mrs. T. believes that Jessica may have been physically abused by her biological mother, but there is no evidence that Jessica was sexually abused. Another family that lives approximately 3 hours away from Mrs. T.'s home adopted Jessica's younger sister. Mrs. T. makes sure that the girls get to visit each other as frequently as possible, which is usually two to four times per year.

Jessica exhibited anger and behavioral problems for the first year that she lived with Mrs. T. By age 7 her behavior had calmed considerably, and she behaved in a generally compliant manner for several years. Mrs. T. describes her home as loving, and she spends her free time doting on her daughter, including spending many volunteer hours at Jessica's school. Despite a tight financial situation, Mrs. T. owns her own home, and the family owns two dogs and three cats. Mrs. T. described herself as being a fairly consistent and somewhat strict disciplinarian. She uses the removal or addition of privileges and treats to motivate her daughter to do her homework and to complete daily chores. Mrs. T. admitted that she does have a temper, however, and that she yells at her daughter when she herself becomes overwhelmed. In the past year, Jessica has been talking back to her and refusing to do requested tasks. In addition, Jessica has told Mrs. T. that she feels "cheated" because she does not have a father. Her sister was adopted into a two-parent family—a fact that Jessica has brought up to Mrs. T. on many occasions. Mrs. T. reported that on one occasion she saw a scratch on Jessica's arm, and that Jessica admitted that she had made the mark herself with an opened safety pin when she felt "bored" and "upset."

Mrs. T. reported that Jessica, a seventh-grade student, has also been having difficulty at school. Her grades, usually B's and C's, have dropped in the past semester. She has received D's in physical education and in English, and her usual B in math has been lowered to a C–. Her teachers report that Jessica is frequently late for classes, and that she occasionally has cut one or more classes

during the day. In general, her teachers report that she is very quiet and nonparticipatory in her classes.

Jessica did not wish to talk at length with this examiner. She admitted that she did not like school at times, and that she sometimes got into screaming fights with her mother. She described her mother as "bossy, but very nice." She said that her mother likes to sew dresses for her and was teaching her to sew. She stated that she was glad that she was adopted, but that she missed her sister a lot. She also stated that she felt sad a lot, but that she "hated" to talk about her feelings. She admitted that she did scratch her arm, and said that she did things to hurt herself "just a little" when she felt overwhelmed or upset. She denied any suicidal ideation in the past or at the current time.

Jessica was tested by the school psychologist at age 9, because her teacher thought Jessica was depressed and not giving her best effort in school, even though she was earning adequate grades. The school psychologist reported that Jessica had "good self-esteem and good relationships with others." At that evaluation, Jessica was administered the Wechsler Intelligence Scale for Children—Third Edition (WISC-III), the Woodcock–Johnson Psycho-Educational Battery—Revised (WJ-R) Tests of Achievement, and the Bender Visual–Motor Gestalt Test. Jessica earned WISC-III IQs that were in the average range (Verbal IQ = 97, Performance IQ = 94, Full Scale IQ = 95). Her scaled scores ranged from 5 (Picture Arrangement) to 12 (Object Assembly), with all other scaled scores 8 to 10. Supplementary WISC-III subtests were not administered, preventing the computation of a factor Index profile. Her Full Scale IQ of 95 corresponds to a percentile rank of 37. Scores on the WJ-R Tests of Achievement were basically consistent with her IQs: Broad Reading = 98 (45th percentile), Broad Mathematics = 112 (80th percentile), and Broad Written Language = 94 (34th percentile). The school psychologist did not report separate subtest scores on the WJ-R. On the Bender–Gestalt, Jessica earned a standard score of 83. She had difficulty with integration and a distortion of shape, mainly the angles. The school psychologist concluded that Jessica's achievement, based on WJ-R scores and grades in school, was commensurate with her intellectual abilities.

Behavioral Observations

Jessica presented as carefully groomed and dressed for both of her testing sessions. She appeared slightly younger than her chronological age of 12. She is a slim and attractive girl, with straight, shoulder-length blonde hair and a shy smile. She was very quiet during the testing and did not talk unless spoken to. She tended to personalize some of the test questions. For example, during a reading comprehension task on the KTEA-II, she was asked how a woman lost her son. Jessica did not remember the correct answer, but stated, "She had to give her child up—like an orphan for adoption."

On many tasks, Jessica appeared to be unsure of answers. For example, on a task of written expression, she asked that all instructions be repeated two times. She erased many of her answers, then wrote, and sometimes erased them again before writing down her answer a third time. However, there were many tasks, such as one where she was asked to answer riddle-like questions, where she concentrated very hard and appeared very motivated and calm. On a task that involved using reasoning ability to complete patterns, she appeared calm, but changed her answers a few times. She was also persistent. On a task where she was asked to copy a picture with triangle-shaped pieces, she attempted all items offered, even if the task was clearly too hard. On a game-like task where she was asked to get a dog named Rover to his bone in the fewest moves possible, she answered a difficult item correctly after the allotted time had elapsed. On a task of verbal knowledge, she was willing to guess at an answer, even if she was clearly unsure whether the answer was correct. This kind of risk-taking behavior characterized her response style on virtually all tasks administered to her. On a sequential memory test, she whispered to herself during the time period when she had to remember what she had seen.

Test Results and Interpretation

Assessment of Cognitive Ability

Jessica was administered the KABC-II, a comprehensive test of general cognitive abilities, to determine her overall level of functioning, as well as her profile of cognitive and processing abilities. The KABC-II per-mits the examiner to select the theoretical model that best fits assessment needs. The Cattell–Horn–Carroll (CHC) model includes tests of acquired knowledge (*crystallized ability*), whereas the Luria model excludes such measures. Jessica was administered the CHC model of the KABC-II, the model of choice for children from mainstream backgrounds who have learning problems in school.

She earned a KABC-II Fluid–Crystallized Index (FCI) of 103, ranking her at the 58th percentile and classifying her general cognitive ability in the average range. The chances are 90% that her "true" FCI is within the 99–107 range. However, that global score is not very meaningful in view of the high degree of variability among her KABC-II scale Indexes. On the five KABC-II scales, Jessica's standard scores ranged from a high of 120 (91st percentile, above average) on the Learning/Glr scale to a low of 88 on the Simultaneous/Gv scale (25th percentile, average range).

Both of her extreme Indexes not only deviated significantly from her own mean standard score on the KABC-II, but were unusually large in magnitude, occurring less than 10% of the time in normal individuals. In addition, Jessica demonstrated a personal strength on the Planning/Gf scale (Index = 111, 77th percentile, average range) and a personal weakness on the Sequential/Gsm scale (Index = 94, 34th percentile, average range). The most notable finding is her high score on the Learning/Glr scale, because it is a normative strength as well as a personal strength: She performed better than 91% of other 12-year-olds in her ability to learn new information, to store that information in long-term memory, and to retrieve it fluently and efficiently. For example, she was able to learn a new language with efficiency, as the examiner systematically taught her the words that corresponded to an array of abstract symbols. Importantly, she was also able to retain the new information over time, as she scored at a similarly high level on two supplementary delayed recall tasks (standard score = 118, 88th percentile, above average) that measured her retention of newly learned material over a 20- to 25-minute interval. Her learning and long-term retrieval strengths are assets suggesting that she has the ability to perform at a higher level in her schoolwork than she is currently achieving. That conclusion is supported by Jessica's other area of strength on the KABC-II: her planning (decision making) and fluid reasoning, which refer to her strong ability to be adaptable and flexible when applying a variety of operations (e.g., drawing inferences and understanding implications) to solve novel (not school-related) problems. For example, Jessica was able to "fill in" the missing pictures in a story so that the complete sequence of pictures told a meaningful story.

In contrast to Jessica's areas of strength on the KABC-II, her two significant weaknesses suggest that she has some difficulties (1) in her ability to process information visually, and (2) with her performance on short-term memory tasks in which the stimuli are presented in sequential fashion. She surpassed only 25% of other 12-year-olds in her visual processing—that is, in her ability to perceive, manipulate, and think with visual patterns and stimuli, and to mentally rotate objects in space. For example, she had difficulty assembling triangular blocks to match a picture of an abstract design; even when she was able to construct some of the more difficult designs correctly, she received no credit because she did not solve them within the time limit. Similarly, she performed better than only 34% of her age-mates on tasks of short-term memory, denoting a relative weakness in her ability to take in information, hold it in immediate awareness briefly, and then use that information within a few seconds (before it is forgotten). She had difficulty, for example, pointing in the correct order to pictures of common objects that were named by the examiner; as noted, she whispered to herself as an aid to recall the stimuli, but this compensatory technique could not be used for the more difficult items that incorporated an interference task (Jessica had to rapidly name colors before pointing to the sequence of pictures, so whispering was not possible), and she failed virtually all of the hard items.

Jessica's two areas of relative weakness (visual processing and short-term memory) are nonetheless within the average range compared to other 12-year-olds, and are not causes for special concern. However, one test result should be followed up with additional testing: She had unusual difficulty on a supplementary KABC-II subtest that requires *both* visual processing and short-term memory—a task that required Jessica to imitate a sequence of hand movements performed by the examiner. On that subtest, she only got the first series of three movements correct and missed all subsequent items, despite good concentration and effort. Her scaled score of 3 (1st percentile) was well below the mean of 10 for children in general, and also well below her scaled scores on the other 15 KABC-II subtests that were administered to her (range of 7–14, all classifying her ability as average or above average).

Of the five KABC-II scales, the only one that was neither a strength nor a weakness for Jessica was Knowledge/Gc. Her Index of 100 (50th percentile) indicated average crystallized ability, which reflects her breadth and depth of specific knowledge acquired within a culture, as well as her ability to apply this knowledge effectively. This KABC-II scale is also a measure of verbal ability, and her Index is consistent with the WISC-III Verbal IQ of 97 that she earned at age 9. Similarly, her WISC-III Performance IQ of 94, which is primarily a measure of visual processing, resembles her Index of 88 on the KABC-II Simultaneous/Gv scale. Her WISC-III Full Scale IQ of 95 is, however, 8 points (about half of a standard deviation) below her FCI of 103 on the KABC-II. It is possible that this difference is due to chance, but it also notable that Jessica's best abilities on the KABC-II (learning ability and fluid reasoning) are not measured in any depth on the WISC-III. In addition, the one unusually low score that Jessica obtained at age 9 (a scaled score of 5 on Picture Arrangement) is of no consequence, in view of her excellent performance on the similar KABC-II Story Completion subtest (scaled score of 14). Furthermore, on the KABC-II, Jessica performed significantly better on tasks involving meaningful stimuli (people and things) than on tasks utilizing abstract stimuli (symbols and designs)—standard scores of 119 and 104, respectively, corresponding to the 90th versus 61st percentile. Jessica's relative weakness in visual processing and her better performance on tasks with meaningful versus abstract stimuli are both consistent with the difficulties she had on the Bender–Gestalt design-copying test at age 9 (standard score of 83).

Assessment of Achievement

On the KTEA-II Comprehensive Form, Jessica scored in the average range on all composite areas of achievement, ranging from a standard score of 104 (61st percentile) on the Mathematics Composite to a standard score of 90 (25th percentile) on the Reading Composite. Her Reading Composite is a relative weakness for her, with her lowest performance on the test of Reading Comprehension (19th percentile), consistent with Mrs. T.'s specific concerns about Jessica's academic achievement. Neither Jessica's Oral Language Composite of 99 (47th percentile) nor her Written Language Composite of 102 (55th percentile) can be meaningfully interpreted, because of notable variability in her scores on the subtests that compose each of these composite scores. Within the domain of Oral Language, Jessica performed significantly better in her ability to express her ideas in words (Oral Expression = 79th percentile) than in her ability to understand what is said to her (Listening Comprehension = 21st percentile). Regarding Written Language, Jessica's ability to spell words spoken by the examiner (Spelling = 82nd percentile) is significantly higher than her ability to express her ideas in writing (Written Expression = 27th percentile).

Both the Reading Comprehension and Listening Comprehension subtests measure understanding of passages via different methods of presentation (printed vs. oral). Her performance was comparable on both subtests (standard scores of 87–88), indicating that she performed at the lower end of the average range in her ability to take in information, whether by reading or listening. Based on the KTEA-II Error Analysis (presented at the end of this report), Jessica displayed weakness on *both* the Reading Comprehension and Listening Comprehension subtests on those items measuring *literal* comprehension—questions that require a response containing explicitly stated information from a story. In contrast, on both comprehension subtests, she performed at an average level on items requiring *inferential* comprehension—questions that require a student to use reasoning to respond correctly (e.g., to deduce the central thought of a passage, make an inference about the content of the passage, or recognize the tone and mood of the passage). The results of the error analysis are consistent with the KABC-II cognitive findings: She has a strength in fluid reasoning and a weakness in short-term memory. Her difficulty with literal items relates directly to her relative weakness in short-term memory, whereas her ability to respond better to inferential items suggests that she is able to apply an area of strength (fluid reasoning) to enhance her performance on tasks that are more difficult for her (i.e., understanding what she reads and hears).

In contrast to the variability on some achievement composites, Jessica performed consistently on the Mathematics Computation and Mathematics Concepts and Applications subtests (58th and 68th percentiles, respectively). In addition, Jessica's achievement on all KTEA-II subtests (range = 87–114) all correspond to the average to above-average range, and are entirely consistent with her cognitive abilities as measured by the WISC-III when she was 9 years old, and by the KABC-II during the present evaluation. She displayed wide variability in both the ability and achievement domains, but when her performance is viewed as a whole, she is achieving at the level that would be expected from her cognitive abilities.

Her present KTEA-II achievement scores are also commensurate with her WJ-R achievement scores at age 9 (range of 94–112 on composites). Therefore, even her achievement on measures of Reading Comprehension, Listening Comprehension, and Written Expression (standard scores of 87–91) is not a cause for concern. However, the notable cognitive strengths that she displayed on measures of learning ability and fluid reasoning should be relied on to help her improve her academic achievement in her areas of relative weakness; in any case, she has too much ability to be earning grades such as her recent D in English or C- in math. Specific kinds of errors that Jessica made during the administration of the KTEA-II are listed in the Error Analysis at the end of this report. The categories listed as weaknesses suggest specific content areas to be targeted.

Diagnostic Impressions

Axis I: 300.4 (dysthymic disorder)
Axis II: None
Axis III: None

Axis IV: Adoption issues resurfacing at adolescence

Axis V: Global Assessment of Functioning (GAF) = 75

Summary

Jessica, age 12 and in the 7th grade, was referred for evaluation by her mother, Mrs. T., who has concerns about Jessica's reading comprehension, oppositional behavior, anger, irritability, and possible depression. During the evaluation, Jessica was quiet, persistent, and attentive. Although often unsure of her answers, she tried to answer virtually all items presented to her. On the KABC-II (see Table 16.5), Jessica earned an FCI of 103 (58th percentile, average range) and displayed considerable variability in her cognitive profile. She demonstrated strengths on two KABC-II scales—one that measures learning ability and long-term retrieval, and another that measures planning ability and fluid reasoning—but had relative weaknesses on measures of visual processing and short-term memory. On the KTEA-II (see Table 16.6), she performed in the average range on all achievement composites (ranging from 90 on Reading to 104 on Mathematics). However, she displayed relative weaknesses on tests of Reading Comprehension, Listening Comprehension, and Written Expression. Her abilities and achievement are commensurate with each other, and her relative weaknesses are not of special concern because they are all in the average range. Nonetheless, she can improve her achievement if she is shown how to use her cognitive strengths to facilitate school learning.

TABLE 16.5. Jessica's Scores on the KABC-II (CHC Model Interpretation)

Scale	Index (mean = 100, SD = 15)	Percentile rank
Learning/Glr	120	91st
Sequential/Gsm	94	34th
Simultaneous/Gv	88	25th
Planning/Gf	111	77th
Knowledge/Gc	100	50th
Fluid–Crystallized Index (FCI)	103	58th

Recommendations

1. Jessica will benefit from understanding her cognitive strengths and weaknesses, and learning how to use these strengths to help her to be more successful in school. A particularly pertinent and practical source is *Helping Children Learn: Intervention Handouts for Use in School and at Home* (Naglieri & Pickering, 2003).

2. Jessica would benefit from utilizing coping mechanisms in order to help her overcome her cognitive weaknesses. Many examples of coping mechanisms could be recommended. She could write notes while listening to a lecture or when reading a textbook, making sure to capture key words and phrases that she may be called upon to remember verbatim. Whenever information is presented in a sequential fashion, Jessica would benefit from making notes in order to restructure the material into a more holistic or Gestalt-oriented presentation, so that the material is more easily accessible to her learning style. She could benefit from a tutor or learning specialist in order to help her to learn how certain kinds of note-taking skills and figure drawing can help her to overcome deficits in sequential processing and in literal reading and listening comprehension. Finally, working with a tutor or learning specialist could help Jessica to improve her writing skills. This area is extremely important, as her areas of strength in learning ability, planning ability, and problem solving will be put to better use if Jessica is able to put her knowledge in writing.

3. Jessica would benefit from further testing that would focus more on her current intrapsychic issues. Instruments such as the Rorschach, the Minnesota Multiphasic Personality Inventory for Adolescents (MMPI-A), the Thematic Apperception Test (TAT), and self-report questionnaires would yield important information regarding her interpersonal issues, as well as further diagnostic input.

4. Jessica would benefit from individual therapy at this time. As she is reluctant to talk openly at first, the therapist would benefit from the results of the personality tests mentioned above. The therapist could focus on adoption issues, adolescent issues, and skill building in the areas of modulating emotions in an appropriate manner, commu-

TABLE 16.6. Jessica's Scores on the KTEA-II, Form A

Scale	Standard score	Percentile rank
Reading Composite	90	25th
Letter and Word Recognition	94	34th
Reading Comprehension	87	19th
(Nonsense Word Decoding)	(93)	(32nd)
Mathematics Composite	104	61st
Mathematics Concepts and Applications	107	68th
Mathematics Computation	103	58th
Oral Language Composite	99	47th
Listening Comprehension	88	21st
Oral Expression	112	79th
Written Language Composite	102	55th
Written Expression	91	27th
Spelling	114	82nd

Note. Nonsense Word Decoding appears in parentheses because it is a supplementary subtest that does not contribute to the reading composite.

nication, and exploring the causes of her anger. In addition, it is important that Jessica's self-injurious behavior be examined and stopped from progressing into potential suicide attempts.

5. Mrs. T. would benefit from counseling to help support her as a single parent during this difficult time. In addition, a counselor could help her with anger management and parenting skills for the adolescent.

6. Family therapy may be indicated, if Jessica's individual therapist is in agreement.

7. It is recommended that Jessica be referred to a child psychiatrist in order to evaluate a possible need for medication.

KTEA-II Error Analysis

Jessica's responses on several KTEA-II subtests were further examined to identify possible specific strengths and weaknesses. First, her errors on each subtest were totaled according to skill categories. Then the number of errors Jessica made in each skill category was compared to the average number of errors made by the standardization sample students, similar in age, who attempted the same items. As a result, Jessica's performance in each skill category could be rated as strong, average, or weak. *Illustrative* diag-

nostic information obtained from Jessica's error analysis is summarized below.

Letter and Word Recognition

The following skill category was identified as a strength for Jessica:

• *Prefixes and word beginnings.* Common prefixes such as *in-*, *un-*, *pre-*; Greek and Latin morphemes used as word beginnings, such as *micro-*, *hyper-*, *penta-*. Examples: *progressive, hemisphere.*

The following skill category was identified as a weakness for Jessica:

• *Consonant blends.* Common blends that occur in the initial, medial, and final positions of words, such as *bl, st, nd, sw.* Examples: *blast, mist, send, swipe.*

Reading Comprehension

The following skill category was identified as a weakness for Jessica:

• *Literal comprehension items.* Questions that require a response containing explicitly stated information from a story. Examples: "Who is the story about? What is the animal doing? Where are the kids going?"

Nonsense Word Decoding

The following skill categories were identified as weaknesses for Jessica:

- *Vowel diphthongs.* The vowel sound in a diphthong is made by gliding or changing continuously from one vowel sound to another in the same syllable. Examples: *doubt, how, oil.*
- *Consonant–le conditional rule.* The final *e* of the consonant–*le* pattern corresponds to a schwa sound directly preceding an /l/ sound. Examples: *bumble, apple, couple, trouble.*

Mathematics Concepts and Applications

The following skill category was identified as a strength for Jessica:

- *Geometry, shape, and space.* Problems involving geometric formulas, shapes, or computing the space contained within them. Example: "Determine the length of the diameter of a circle, given the radius."

Listening Comprehension

The following skill category was identified as a weakness for Jessica:

- *Literal comprehension items.* Questions that require a response containing explicitly stated information from a story. Examples: "Who is the story about? What is the person doing? What happened at the end of the story?"

KAUFMAN ADOLESCENT AND ADULT INTELLIGENCE TEST

Theory and Structure

The KAIT (Kaufman & Kaufman, 1993) is based on the theoretical model of Horn and Cattell (1966, 1967; Horn, 1985, 1989) and assesses adolescents and adults from ages 11 to more than 85 years old with Fluid, Crystallized, and Composite IQs, each with a mean of 100 and *SD* of 15. The KAIT uses the original, dichotomous Horn–Cattell model of Gf-Gc (Horn & Cattell, 1966,

1967). As noted earlier, crystallized intelligence (Gc) represents acquired knowledge and concepts, whereas fluid intelligence (Gf) measures problem-solving ability with novel stimuli, adaptability, and flexibility. In Horn's expanded theory (and from the perspective of CHC theory), the KAIT Fluid scale also measures Glr (with the Rebus Learning subtest), and the Crystallized scale also measures Gsm (with the Auditory Comprehension subtest).

The KAIT is organized into a six-subtest Core Battery and a 10-subtest Expanded Battery.

Description of Subtests

The 10 subtests that compose the KAIT Expanded Battery are described here, along with an 11th, supplementary subtest (Mental Status). The number preceding each subtest indicates the order in which it is administered. Subtests 1–6 constitute the Core Battery; subtests 1–10 comprise the Expanded Battery. Each subtest except Mental Status yields age-based scaled scores with a mean of 10 and *SD* of 3.

Crystallized Scale

1. *Definitions.* Figuring out a word based both on the configuration of the word (it is presented with some of its letters missing) and on a clue about its meaning (e.g., "It's awfully old. What word goes here?" (" _ N T   Q _____ " Answer: *antique*).

4. *Auditory Comprehension.* Listening to a recording of a news story, and then answering literal and inferential questions about the story.

6. *Double Meanings.* Studying two sets of word clues, and then thinking of a word with two different meanings that relates closely to both sets of clues (e.g., *bat* goes with "animal and vampire" and also with "baseball and stick"). This subtest has a Gf component in addition to Gc, especially at ages 11–19 (Kaufman & Kaufman, 1993, Table 8.8).

10. *Famous Faces (alternate subtest).* Naming people of current or historical fame, based on their photographs and a verbal clue about them (e.g., pictures of Lucille Ball and Bob Hope are shown; the person is asked to "name either one of these comedians"). As

an alternate subtest, Famous Faces is not included in the computation of Crystallized IQ.

Fluid Scale

2. *Rebus Learning.* Learning the word or concept associated with numerous rebus drawings, and then "reading" phrases and sentences composed of these rebuses.

3. *Logical Steps.* Attending to logical premises presented both visually and aurally, and then responding to a question by making use of the logical premises (e.g., "Here is a staircase with seven steps. Bob is always one step above Ann. Bob is on step 6. What step is Ann on?"). This verbal test is a strong measure of Gf across the age range (overall loading of .66). It involves Gc only to a small extent (overall loading of .13) (Kaufman & Kaufman, 1993, Table 8.8), consistent with Horn's findings for common word analogies.

5. *Mystery Codes.* Studying the identifying codes associated with a set of pictorial stimuli, and then systematically figuring out the code for a novel pictorial stimulus by using deductive reasoning. Harder items are highly speeded to assess speed of planning ability, so the test involves Gs as well as Gf.

9. *Memory for Block Designs (alternate subtest for Fluid scale).* Studying a printed abstract design that was exposed briefly, and then copying the design from memory, using six cubes and a formboard. In addition to Gf, this task requires short-term apprehension and retrieval (SAR) and broad visualization (Gv). It does not, however, contribute to Fluid IQ because of its status as an alternate subtest. Although it involves coordination for success, and has a 45-second time limit, individuals who are working slowly but accurately are given an extra 45 seconds of response time without penalty.

Additional Subtests

7. *Rebus Delayed Recall.* "Reading" phrases and sentences composed of rebus drawings whose meaning was taught previously during subtest 2, Rebus Learning. These items include different phrases and sentences from the ones in subtest 2, but they are composed of the same symbols that correspond to the words or concepts that were taught during that task (the symbols are not retaught). This delayed-recall subtest is administered, without prior warning, about 45 minutes after Rebus Learning, following the "interference" of subtests 3 through 6.

8. *Auditory Delayed Recall.* Answering literal and inferential questions about the mock news stories that were presented by cassette during subtest 4, Auditory Comprehension. The questions are different from the ones asked in subtest 4, but they are based on the same news stories (which are not repeated). This task is administered without any warning about 25 minutes after Auditory Comprehension. Subtests 5 through 7 serve as interference tasks.

Administration and Scoring

The KAIT is organized into an easel format. Easel 1 includes the six Core subtests; easel 2 includes the additional four subtests from the Expanded Battery plus Mental Status. Directions for administration and scoring appear on the easel pages facing the examiner and/or on the individual test record. Administration is straightforward, with objective scoring for nearly all subtests. Some subjectivity is needed for scoring some items on Auditory Comprehension and Auditory Delayed Recall.

Sample and teaching items are included for most subtests, to ensure that examinees understand what is expected of them to meet the demands of each subtest. Specific wording is provided for much of the teaching to encourage uniformity, especially for a learning task such as Mystery Codes, which requires individuals to master basic concepts before they can apply these concepts to higher-level items. Mystery Codes requires practice to administer correctly, whereas another learning task (Rebus Learning) requires practice to score correctly as the examinee is responding.

An administration and scoring training video for the KAIT, available from the publisher, demonstrates each subtest with "clients" who span the age range and include a variety of presenting problems (Kaufman, Kaufman, Grossman, & Grossman, 1994). The video provides administration and scoring clues and hints and highlights most of the potential administration and scoring pitfalls for new examiners.

Psychometric Properties

Standardization Sample

The KAIT normative sample, composed of exactly 2,000 adolescents and adults between the ages of 11 and 94, was stratified on the variables of gender, racial/ethnic group, geographic region, and SES (educational attainment). For the SES variable, parents' education was used for ages 11–24, and self-education was used for ages 25–94. Gender distributions matched U.S. census proportions for 13 age groups between 11 and 75–94 years (Kaufman & Kaufman, 1993, Table 7.1). The matches between the census and sample were close for the educational attainment variable for the total sample and for separate racial/ethnic groups (Kaufman & Kaufman, 1993, Tables 7.3 and 7.5). The geographic region matches were close for the North Central and South regions, but the sample was underrepresented in the Northeast and overrepresented in the West (Kaufman & Kaufman, 1993, Table 7.2).

Reliability

For the KAIT, mean split-half reliability coefficients for the total normative sample were .95 for Crystallized IQ, .95 for Fluid IQ, and .97 for Composite IQ (Kaufman & Kaufman, 1993, Table 8.1). Mean test–retest reliability coefficients, based on 153 identified nondisabled individuals in three age groups (11–19, 20–54, 55–85+) who were retested after a 1-month interval, were .94 for Crystallized IQ, .87 for Fluid IQ, and .94 for Composite IQ (Kaufman & Kaufman, 1993, Table 8.2). Mean subtest split-half reliabilities for the four Gc subtests ranged from .89 for Auditory Comprehension and Double Meanings to .92 for Famous Faces (median = .90). Mean values for the four Gf subtests ranged from .79 for Memory for Block Designs to .93 for Rebus Learning (median = .88) (Kaufman & Kaufman, 1993, Table 8.1). Median test–retest reliabilities for the eight subtests ranged from .72 on Mystery Codes to .95 on Definitions (median = .78). An additional study of 120 European Americans found slightly lower test–retest reliabilities, in the .80s, but concluded that the KAIT was a reliable measure (Pinion, 1995).

Validity

Factor analysis, both exploratory and confirmatory, gave strong construct validity support for the Fluid and Crystallized scales and for the placement of each subtest on its designated scale. This support was provided in the KAIT manual for six age groups ranging from 11–14 to 70–94 years and for a mixed clinical sample (Kaufman & Kaufman, 1993, Ch. 8). Crystallized IQs correlated .72 with Fluid IQs for the total normative group of 2,000 (Kaufman & Kaufman, 1993, Table 8.4), supporting the use of the oblique rotated solutions reported in the KAIT manual.

Two-factor solutions corresponding to distinct Gc and Gf factors were also identified for separate groups of European Americans, African Americans, and Hispanics included in the standardization sample (Kaufman, Kaufman, & McLean, 1995) and for males and females within these three racial/ethnic groups (Gonzalez, Adir, Kaufman, & McLean, 1995). In addition, Caruso and Jacob-Timm (2001) applied CFA to the normative group of 375 adolescents aged 11–14 years and a cross-validation sample of 60 sixth and eighth graders. They examined three factor models: a single-factor general intelligence (g) model, an orthogonal Gf-Gc model, and an oblique Gf-Gc model. The orthogonal model fit poorly for both samples, while the g model only fit the cross-validation sample. The oblique model, however, fit both samples (and fit significantly better than the g model in both samples).

In a recent investigation, Cole and Randall (2003) applied CFA to the KAIT standardization data and found that the dichotomous Horn–Cattell Gf-Gc model on which the KAIT is based provided a significantly better fit than either Spearman's g model or Carroll's hierarchical model.

KAIT Composite IQ has consistently correlated highly with other measures of intelligence, such as the Wechsler scales, with values typically in the .80s (Kaufman & Kaufman, 1993, Ch. 8). For these same samples, KAIT Fluid IQ and Crystallized IQ also correlated substantially (and about equally well) with the various global scores, typically correlating in the mid-.70s to low .80s. Other studies have also supported the construct and criterion-related validity of the three KAIT IQs (e.g., Vo, Weisenberger, Becker, & Jacob-Timm, 1999; Woodrich & Kush, 1998).

Interpretation

Age-Related Differences on the KAIT

Crystallized abilities have been noted to be fairly well maintained throughout the life-span, but fluid abilities are not as stable, peaking in adolescence or early adulthood before dropping steadily through the lifespan (Horn, 1989; Kaufman & Lichtenberger, 2002). To analyze age trends in the KAIT standardization data, a separate set of so-called "all-adult" norms was developed to provide the means with which to compare performance on the KAIT subtests and IQ scales (Kaufman & Kaufman, 1993). Data from 1,500 individuals between ages 17 and 85+ were merged to create the all-adult norms. The IQs from this new all-adult normative group were also adjusted for years of education, so that this would not be a confounding variable in analyses.

Analyses of the Crystallized and Fluid scales across ages 17 to 85+ produced results that generally conformed to those reported in previous investigations. Crystallized abilities generally increased through age 50, but did not drop noticeably until ages 75 and older. The fluid abilities, on the other hand, peaked in the early 20s, then reached a plateau from the mid-20s through the mid-50s, and finally began to drop steadily after age 55. These findings were consistent for males and females (Kaufman & Horn, 1996). In the first edition of this book, Kaufman and Kaufman (1997) hypothesized that the fluid aspects of some of the KAIT Crystallized subtests may have contributed to the accelerated age-related decline in scores on these subtests.

Gender Differences

Gender differences on Crystallized and Fluid IQ for ages 17–94 on the KAIT were examined for 716 males and 784 females. When adjustments were made for educational attainment, less than 1 IQ point separated males and females on both IQs (J. C. Kaufman, Chen, & Kaufman, 1995;

Kaufman & Horn, 1996; Kaufman & Lichtenberger, 2002, Table 4.1). However, several KAIT subtests did produce gender differences that were large enough to be meaningful: Memory for Block Designs, Famous Faces, and Logical Steps. On each of these subtests, males scored higher than females by about 0.2 to 0.4 SD. However, even those subtests that yielded the largest gender differences reflected small (or, at best, moderate) effect sizes (McLean, 1995)—discrepancies that are too small to be of much clinical use.

Ethnicity Differences

Differences between European Americans and African Americans on the KAIT were examined in a sample of 1,547 European Americans and 241 African Americans. Without educational adjustment, European Americans scored approximately 11–12 IQ points higher than African Americans ages 11–24 years; at ages 25–94 years, the discrepancy was approximately 13–14 IQ points (Kaufman, McLean, & Kaufman, 1995). When adjustments were made for educational attainment, these differences were reduced to about 8–9 points for ages 11–24 years and 10 points for ages 25–94 (Kaufman, McLean, & Kaufman, 1995).

Without educational adjustment, European Americans scored approximately 12–13 points higher on Crystallized IQ than Hispanics ages 11–24 years, and 9 points higher on Fluid IQ. At ages 25–94 years, European Americans scored approximately 17 points higher than Hispanics on Crystallized IQ, and 10 points higher on Fluid IQ (Kaufman, McLean, & Kaufman, 1995). When adjustments were made for educational attainment, these differences reduced to approximately 6 points for ages 11–24 years and 9 points for ages 25–94.

It is worth noting that Hispanics scored about 4 points higher on Fluid IQ than Crystallized IQ at ages 11–24 and almost 6 points higher at ages 25–94, without an adjustment for education (Kaufman, McLean, & Kaufman, 1995). These differences resemble the magnitude of Performance > Verbal differences on the Wechsler scales, although Fluid IQ is not the same as Performance IQ; they load on separate factors (Kaufman,

Ishikuma, & Kaufman, 1994), and the Fluid subtests require verbal ability for success (Kaufman & Lichtenberger, 2002).

Clinical Applications

Clinical validity and applications of the KAIT were explored in the manual by examining the profiles obtained by several small samples of individuals with neurological impairment to the left hemisphere (n = 18), neurological impairment to the right hemisphere (n = 25), clinical depression (n = 44), Alzheimer-type dementia (n = 10), and reading disabilities (n = 14). Each subsample was matched with a control group of individuals from the standardization sample on the variables of gender, racial/ethnic group, age, and educational attainment (Kaufman & Kaufman, 1993, Ch. 8). The KAIT IQs and subtests discriminated effectively between the control samples and the samples of individuals with neurological impairment and Alzheimer-type dementia. Auditory Comprehension, Famous Faces, Rebus Learning, Mental Status, and the Delayed Recall tasks tended to be the most discriminating subtests.

When the KAIT profiles of neurologically impaired patients with right- versus left-hemisphere brain damage were compared, the most discriminating subtests were Rebus Learning, Rebus Delayed Recall, Famous Faces, and Memory for Block Designs; patients with right-hemisphere damage scored higher on the first three tasks and lower on Memory for Block Designs. Most of the noteworthy differences in the clinical validity studies were on the subtests that are excluded from the Core Battery but are administered as part of the Expanded Battery. These results support our contention that the Expanded Battery should prove especially useful for neuropsychological assessment.

The sample of patients with clinical depression, most of whom were hospitalized with major depression, averaged about 102 on the three KAIT IQs, and did not differ significantly from their matched control group on any subtest (Grossman, Kaufman, Mednitsky, Scharff, & Dennis, 1994). One significant difference was noted, however, and again it involved the Expanded Battery. When the mean difference between scaled scores earned on Auditory Comprehension and Auditory Delayed Recall (a comparison of immediate and delayed memory) was evaluated, the discrepancy was significantly larger for the depressed than for the control group. (The depressed sample performed considerably higher on the delayed than on the immediate task.) Also, virtually every KAIT subtest discriminated significantly between the total group of patients with neurological impairment and those with depression (Kaufman & Kaufman, 1993).

The good performance by depressed patients on the KAIT is contrary to some research findings that have pinpointed deficiencies by depressed individuals in memory, both primary (Gruzelier, Seymour, Wilson, Jolley, & Hirsch, 1988) and secondary (Henry, Weingartner, & Murphy, 1973); in planning and sequential abilities (Burgess, 1991); and, more generally, in cognitive tests that demand sustained, effortful responding (Golinkoff & Sweeney, 1989). The KAIT subtests require good skills in planning ability and memory, and clearly require effortful responding for success. The ability of patients with depression to cope well with the demands of the various KAIT subtests, and to excel on measures of delayed recall, suggests that some of the prior research may have reached premature conclusions about these patients' deficiencies—in part because of weaknesses in experimental design (such as poor control groups) and inappropriate applications of statistics (Grossman et al., 1994; Miller, Faustman, Moses, & Csernansky, 1991). This notion is given support by the results of other investigations of patients with depression, which have shown their intact performance on the Luria–Nebraska Neuropsychological Battery (Miller et al., 1991) and on a set of tasks that differed in its cognitive complexity (Kaufman, Grossman, & Kaufman, 1994).

The one area of purported weakness that may characterize depressed individuals is the so-called "psychomotor retardation" (Blatt & Allison, 1968) that is sometimes reflected in low Performance IQs. As noted, the KAIT minimizes visual–motor speed for responding, and only Memory for Block Designs places heavy demands on coordination. Perhaps consistent with the "psychomotor retardation" of depressed patients is the finding that the depressed patients in Grossman and colleagues' (1994) study earned their lowest KAIT scaled score on Memory for Block Designs. However, speed per se was not a weak area for depressed patients, as they performed intactly on tests requiring quick mental (as opposed to motor) problem-solving speed (Grossman et al., 1994; Kaufman, Grossman, & Kaufman, 1994).

Innovations in Measures of Cognitive Assessment

As we have noted concerning the features described for the KABC-II, the points mentioned here for the KAIT are innovative relative to the Wechsler and Stanford–Binet tradition of intellectual assessment, but some of these innovations are not unique to the KAIT. Several of these innovations are shared by other contemporary instruments, such as the KABC-II (as discussed earlier in this chapter), the WJ III (Woodcock et al., 2001), the CAS (Naglieri & Das, 1997), and the most recent revisions of the Wechsler scales (Wechsler, 2002, 2003).

Integrates Several Theoretical Approaches

The KAIT benefits from an integration of theories that unite developmental (Piaget), neuropsychological (Luria), and experimental–cognitive (Horn–Cattell) models of intellectual functioning. The theories interface well with each other and do not compete; the Piaget (1972) and Luria approaches provided the rationale for task selection, whereas the Horn–Cattell model offered the most parsimonious explanation for the co-variation among the subtests, and hence of the resultant scale structure. The Gc-Gf distinction measures a difference in human abilities that has been widely validated by Horn and his colleagues, and that relates to a person's skill at solving problems rooted in education and acculturation versus solving novel problems. This distinction bears an important relationship to how individuals learn best, and how much they may have benefited or been handicapped by their cultural environments and formal education experiences. Taken together, the theories give the KAIT a solid theoretical foundation that facilitates test interpretation across the broad age range (11–94 years) on which the battery was normed.

Offers Flexibility to Examiner

The inclusion of Core and Expanded Batteries of the KAIT gives examiners a choice whenever they evaluate an adolescent or adult. The Core Battery is all that is needed for mandatory reevaluations when diagnostic issues are not involved, or for any type of evaluation for which possible neurological impairment or memory problems are not at issue. The 90-minute Expanded Battery has special uses for elderly clients, for anyone whose memory processes are suspect, and for individuals referred for possible neurological disorders.

Provides a Bridge between Intellectual and Neuropsychological Batteries

As is true for the KABC-II, the inclusion of Delayed Recall subtests in the KAIT Expanded Battery, and the concomitant ability to compare statistically a person's immediate versus delayed recall of semantic information (Auditory tasks) and of verbally coded symbols (Rebus tasks), resembles the kinds of memory functions that are tapped by subtests included in neuropsychological batteries. The supplementary Crystallized (Famous Faces) and Fluid (Memory for Block Designs) subtests both resemble tests that have rich neurological research histories, and the supplementary Mental Status task provides a well-normed alternative to the mental status exams that are routinely administered by neurologists and neuropsychologists. The KAIT was found to be a useful tool for evaluating adults' cognitive functioning while they were undergoing electroencephalography to measure their visual and auditory evoked brain potentials (J. L. Kaufman, 1995).

The KAIT Expanded Battery includes sets of tasks that resemble both conventional intelligence tests and neuropsychological batteries. Furthermore, the KAIT was conormed with two brief tests that are particularly useful for neuropsychological assessment: the Kaufman Short Neuropsychological Assessment Procedure (K-SNAP; Kaufman & Kaufman, 1994b) and the Kaufman Functional Academic Skills Test (K-FAST; Kaufman & Kaufman, 1994a). The K-SNAP measures neurological intactness, and the K-FAST assesses functional reading and functional math ability (e.g., understanding the words and numbers in recipes and newspaper ads). The joint norming aids interpretation of the K-SNAP and K-FAST within the context of the Gf and Gc constructs.

Permits Direct Evaluation of a Person's Learning Ability

Unlike the Wechsler scales, the KAIT, WJ III, and KABC-II all include several subtests that assess a person's ability to learn new information and apply this information to new, more complex problems. In the KAIT, Rebus Learning, Mystery Codes, and Logical Steps all offer good assessment of a person's ability to learn new material and to apply that learning in a controlled learning situation. Because most KAIT tasks include teaching items with prescribed words to say, the KAIT tasks also enable examiners to observe individuals' ability to benefit from structured feedback. When this teaching occurs on a learning task, an examiner can obtain much clinical information about a person's learning ability.

The best example is Mystery Codes, which requires an examiner to explain several initial answers, even when the person gets the items right (to ensure that the person did not answer correctly by chance, and to ensure that all examinees have equal amounts of instruction). A few experienced KAIT examiners have told us during KAIT workshops that they have found the administration of Mystery Codes to resemble the test–teach–test model that characterizes Feuerstein's work on dynamic assessment (e.g., Feuerstein & Feuerstein, 2001). In addition, the focused attention and concentration that are necessary to solve the hypothetico-deductive items in tasks such as Mystery Codes and Logical Steps present special problems for individuals with ADHD; clinical observations during these tasks can be quite useful for the assessment of individuals suspected of having ADHD (N. L. Kaufman, 1994).

REFERENCES

Blatt, S. J., & Allison, J. (1968) The intelligence test in personality assessment. In A. I. Rabin (Ed.), Projective techniques in personality assessment (pp. 421–460). New York: Springer.

Burgess, J. W. (1991). Neurocognition in acute and chronic depression: Personality disorder, major depression, and schizophrenia. Biological Psychiatry, 30, 305–309.

Carroll, J. B. (1943). The factorial representation of mental ability and academic achievement. Educational and Psychological Measurement, 3, 307–332.

Carroll, J. B. (1993). Human cognitive abilities: A survey of factor analytic studies. New York: Cambridge University Press.

Caruso, J. C., & Jacob-Timm, S. (2001). Confirmatory factor analysis of the Kaufman Adolescent and Adult Intelligence Test with young adolescents. Psychological Assessment, 8, 11–17.

Cattell, R. B. (1941). The measurement of adult intelligence. Psychological Bulletin, 40, 153–193.

Cole, J. C., & Randall, M. K. (2003). Comparing the cognitive ability models of Spearman, Horn and Cattell, and Carroll. Journal of Psychoeducational Assessment, 21, 160–179.

Feuerstein, R., & Feuerstein, R. S. (2001). Is dynamic assessment compatible with the psychometric model? In A. S. Kaufman & N. L. Kaufman (Eds.), Specific learning disabilities and difficulties in children and adolescents: Psychological assessment and evaluation (pp. 218–246). Cambridge, UK: Cambridge University Press.

Flanagan, D. P., McGrew, K. S., & Ortiz, S. (2000). The Wechsler intelligence scales and Gf-Gc theory: A contemporary approach to interpretation. Boston: Allyn & Bacon.

Flanagan, D. P., & Ortiz, S. O. (2001). Essentials of cross-battery assessment. New York: Wiley.

Fletcher-Janzen, E. (2003, August). Neuropsychologically-based interpretations of the KABC-II. In M. H. Daniel (Chair), KABC-II: Theory, content, and interpretation. Symposium presented at the annual meeting of the American Psychological Association, Toronto.

Golinkoff, M., & Sweeney, J. A. (1989). Cognitive impairments in depression. Journal of Affective Disorders, 17, 105–112.

Gonzalez, J., Adir, Y., Kaufman, A. S., & McLean, J. E. (1995, February). Race and gender differences in cognitive factors: A neuropsychological interpretation. Paper presented at the meeting of the International Neuropsychological Society, Seattle, WA.

Grossman, I., Kaufman, A. S., Mednitsky, S., Scharff, L., & Dennis, B. (1994). Neurocognitive abilities for a clinically depressed sample versus a matched control group of normal individuals. Psychiatry Research, 51, 231–244.

Gruzelier, J., Seymour, K., Wilson, L., Jolley, A., & Hirsch, S. (1988). Impairments on neuropsychologic tests of temporohippocampal and frontohippocampal functions and word fluency in remitting schizophrenia and affective disorders. Archives of General Psychiatry, 45, 623–629.

Henry, G. M., Weingartner, H., & Murphy, D. L. (1973). Influence of affective states and psychoactive drugs on verbal learning and memory. *American Journal of Psychiatry, 130,* 966–971.

Horn, J. L. (1968). Organization of abilities and the development of intelligence. *Psychological Review, 75,* 242–259.

Horn, J. L. (1985). Remodeling old models of intelligence. In B. B. Wolman (Ed.), *Handbook of intelligence: Theories, measurements, and applications* (pp. 267–300). New York: Wiley.

Horn, J. L. (1989). Cognitive diversity: A framework of learning. In P. L. Ackerman, R. J. Sternberg, & R. Glaser (Eds.), *Learning and individual differences* (pp. 61–116). New York: Freeman.

Horn, J. L., & Cattell, R. B. (1966). Refinement and test of the theory of fluid and crystallized intelligence. *Journal of Educational Psychology, 57,* 253–270.

Horn, J. L., & Cattell, R. B. (1967). Age differences in fluid and crystallized intelligence. *Acta Psychologica, 26,* 107–129.

Horn, J. L., & Hofer, S. M. (1992). Major abilities and development in the adult period. In R. J. Sternberg & C. A. Berg (Eds.), *Intellectual development* (pp. 44–99). New York: Cambridge University Press.

Horn, J. L., & Noll, J. (1997). Human cognitive capabilities: Gf-Gc theory. In D. P. Flanagan, J. L. Genshaft, & P. L. Harrison (Eds.), *Contemporary intellectual assessment: Theories, tests, and issues* (pp. 53–91). New York: Guilford Press.

Kaufman, A. S., Grossman, I., & Kaufman, N. L. (1994). Comparison of hospitalized depressed patients and matched normal controls on tests differing in their level of cognitive complexity. *Journal of Psychoeducational Assessment, 12,* 112–125.

Kaufman, A. S., & Horn, J. L. (1996). Age changes on tests of fluid and crystallized ability for females and males on the Kaufman Adolescent and Adult Intelligence Test (KAIT) at ages 17 to 94 years. *Archives of Clinical Neuropsychology, 11,* 97–121.

Kaufman, A. S., Ishikuma, T., & Kaufman, N. L. (1994). A Horn analysis of the factors measured by the WAIS-R, KAIT, and two brief tests for normal adolescents and adults. *Assessment, 1,* 353–366.

Kaufman, A. S., Kaufman, J. C., & McLean, J. E. (1995). Factor structure of the Kaufman Adolescent and Adult Intelligence Test (KAIT) for whites, African-Americans, and Hispanics. *Educational and Psychological Measurement, 55,* 365–376.

Kaufman, A. S., & Kaufman, N. L. (1983). *K-ABC interpretive manual.* Circle Pines, MN: American Guidance Service.

Kaufman, A. S., & Kaufman, N. L. (1993). *Manual for the Kaufman Adolescent and Adult Intelligence Test (KAIT).* Circle Pines, MN: American Guidance Service.

Kaufman, A. S., & Kaufman, N. L. (1994a). *Manual for the Kaufman Functional Academic Skills Test (K-FAST).* Circle Pines, MN: American Guidance Service.

Kaufman, A. S., & Kaufman, N. L. (1994b). *Manual for the Kaufman Short Neuropsychological Assessment Procedure (K-SNAP).* Circle Pines, MN: American Guidance Service.

Kaufman, A. S., & Kaufman, N. L. (1997). The Kaufman Adolescent and Adult Intelligence Test (KAIT). In D. P. Flanagan, J. L. Genshaft, & P. L. Harrison (Eds.), *Contemporary intellectual assessment: Theories, tests, and issues* (pp. 209_229). New York: Guilford Press.

Kaufman, A. S., & Kaufman, N. L. (2004a). *Manual for the Kaufman Assessment Battery for Children— Second Edition (KABC-II), Comprehensive Form.* Circle Pines, MN: American Guidance Service.

Kaufman, A. S., & Kaufman, N. L. (2004b). *Manual for the Kaufman Test of Educational Achievement— Second Edition (KTEA-II), Comprehensive Form.* Circle Pines, MN: American Guidance Service.

Kaufman, A. S., Kaufman, N. L., Grossman, D., & Grossman, I. (1994). *KAIT administration and scoring video* [Videotape]. Circle Pines, MN: American Guidance Service.

Kaufman, A. S., & Lichtenberger, E. O. (2002). *Assessing adolescent and adult intelligence* (2nd ed.). Boston: Allyn & Bacon.

Kaufman, A. S., Lichtenberger, E. O., Fletcher-Janzen, E., & Kaufman, N. L. (in press). *Essentials of KABC-II assessment.* New York: Wiley.

Kaufman, A. S., McLean, J. E., & Kaufman, J. C. (1995). The fluid and crystallized abilities of white, black, and Hispanic adolescents and adults, both with and without an education covariate. *Journal of Clinical Psychology, 51,* 637–647.

Kaufman, J. C. (2003, August). Gender and ethnic differences on the KABC-II. In M. H. Daniel (Chair), *The KABC-II: Theory, content, and administration.* Symposium presented at the annual meeting of the American Psychological Association, Toronto.

Kaufman, J. C., Chen, T., & Kaufman, A. S. (1995). Race, education, and gender differences on six Horn abilities for adolescents and adults. *Journal of Psychoeducational Assessment, 13,* 49–65.

Kaufman, J. C., Lichtenberger, E. O., & Kaufman, A. S. (2003). Assessing the intelligence of adolescents with the Kaufman Adolescent and Adult Intelligence Test (KAIT). In C. R. Reynolds & R. W. Kamphaus (Eds.), *Handbook of psychological and educational assessment of children: Intelligence, aptitude, and achievement* (2nd ed., pp. 174–186). New York: Guilford Press.

Kaufman, J. L. (1995). *Visual and auditory evoked brain potentials, the Hendricksons' pulse train hypothesis, and the fluid and crystallized theory of intelligence.* Unpublished doctoral dissertation, California School of Professional Psychology, San Diego.

Kaufman, N. L. (1994, September). *Behavioral and educational issues in childhood ADD: Psychoeducational assessment of ADD/ADHD.* Invited address presented at Attention Deficit Disorder in Childhood and Adulthood, a workshop sponsored by the San Diego Psychiatric Society, San Diego, CA.

Keith, T. Z. (1985). Questioning the K-ABC: What does it measure? *School Psychology Review, 14,* 9–20.

Lichtenberger, E. O. (2001). The Kaufman tests—K-ABC and KAIT. In A. S. Kaufman & N. L. Kaufman (Eds.), *Specific learning disabilities and difficulties in children and adolescents: Psychological assessment and evaluation* (pp. 97–140). Cambridge, UK: Cambridge University Press.

Lichtenberger, E. O., Broadbooks, D. A., & Kaufman, A. S. (2000). *Essentials of cognitive assessment with the KAIT and other Kaufman measures.* New York: Wiley.

Luria, A. R. (1966). *Human brain and psychological processes.* New York: Harper & Row.

Luria, A. R. (1970). The functional organization of the brain. *Scientific American, 222,* 66–78.

Luria, A. R. (1973). *The working brain: An introduction to neuropsychology.* Harmondsworth, UK: Penguin.

McLean, J. E. (1995). *Improving education through action research: A guide for administrators and teachers.* Thousand Oaks, CA: Corwin Press.

Miller, L. S., Faustman, W. O., Moses, J. A., Jr., & Csernansky, J. G. (1991). Evaluating cognitive impairment in depression with the Luria–Nebraska Neuropsychological Battery: Severity correlates and comparisons with nonpsychiatric controls. *Psychiatry Research, 37,* 219–227.

Naglieri, J. A., & Das, J. P. (1997). *Das–Naglieri Cognitive Assessment System (CAS).* Itasca, IL: Riverside.

Naglieri, J. A., & Pickering, E. B. (2003). *Helping children learn: Intervention handouts for use in school and at home.* Baltimore: Brookes.

Piaget, J. (1972). Intellectual evolution from adolescence to adulthood. *Human Development, 15,* 1–12.

Pinion, G. A. (1995). *Test–retest reliability of the Kaufman Adolescent and Adult Intelligence Test.* Unpublished doctoral dissertation, Oklahoma State University.

Prifitera, A., Weiss, L. G., & Saklofske, D. H. (1998). The WISC-III in context. In A. Prifitera & D. H. Saklofske (Eds.), *WISC-III clinical use and interpretation* (pp. 1–38). San Diego, CA: Academic Press.

Reitan, R. M. (1988). Integration of neuropsychological theory, assessment, and application. *The Clinical Neuropsychologist, 2,* 331–349.

Spearman, C. (1904). "General intelligence," objectively determined and measured. *American Journal of Psychology, 15,* 201–293.

Vo, D. H., Weisenberger, J. L., Becker, R., & Jacob-Timm, S. (1999). Concurrent validity of the KAIT for students in grade six and eight. *Journal of Psychoeducational Assessment, 17,* 152–162.

Wechsler, D. (2002). *Wechsler Preschool and Primary Scale of Intelligence—Third Edition.* San Antonio, TX: Psychological Corporation.

Wechsler, D. (2003). *Wechsler Intelligence Scale for Children—Fourth Edition.* San Antonio, TX: Psychological Corporation.

Woodcock, R. W., McGrew, K. S., & Mather, N. (2001). *Woodcock–Johnson III.* Itasca, IL: Riverside.

Woodrich, D. L., & Kush, J. C. (1998). Kaufman Adolescent and Adult Intelligence Test (KAIT): Concurrent validity of fluid ability for preadolescents and adolescents with central nervous system disorders and scholastic concerns. *Journal of Psychoeducational Assessment, 16,* 215–225.

17

Woodcock–Johnson III Tests of Cognitive Abilities

FREDRICK A. SCHRANK

The Woodcock–Johnson III (WJ III; Woodcock, McGrew, & Mather, 2001a) includes 31 cognitive tests for measuring (in various combinations) general intellectual ability, broad and narrow cognitive abilities, and aspects of executive functioning. The Woodcock–Johnson III Tests of Cognitive Abilities (WJ III COG; Woodcock, McGrew, & Mather, 2001c) includes 20 tests. Two easels house the Standard Battery (tests 1–10) and the Extended Battery (tests 11–20). The Woodcock–Johnson III Diagnostic Supplement to the Tests of Cognitive Abilities (Diagnostic Supplement; Woodcock, McGrew, Mather, & Schrank, 2003) includes an additional 11 tests. Some of the tests are appropriate for individuals as young as 24 months; all of the tests can be used with individuals from 5 to 95 years of age.

The WJ III provides measures of multiple intelligences. Each of the 31 tests measures one or more narrow, or specific, cognitive abilities as informed by the independent research efforts of Horn (1965, 1988, 1989, 1991), Horn and Stankov (1982), Cattell (1941, 1943, 1950), and Carroll (1987, 1990, 1993, 2003; see also Carroll, Chapter 4, this volume). Each of the tests can also be thought of as a single measure of a broad cognitive ability, or domain of intellectual functioning. Table 17.1 identifies the broad and narrow cognitive abilities measured by

each test; it also includes brief test descriptions. The tests are organized into clusters for interpretive purposes. These clusters are outlined in Table 17.2. The cognitive abilities measured by the WJ III COG and Diagnostic Supplement can have instructional implications and can be used as the basis for making recommendations.

ADMINISTRATION AND SCORING

Administration and scoring of the WJ III COG and the Diagnostic Supplement require knowledge of the exact administration and scoring procedures, as well as an understanding of the importance of adhering to standardized procedures. The WJ III COG examiner's manual (Mather & Woodcock, 2001) and the Diagnostic Supplement manual (Schrank, Mather, McGrew, & Woodcock, 2003) provide guidelines for this purpose. The test books contain instructions for administering and scoring items on each test. These are found on the introductory page of each test (the first printed page after the tab page). Additional instructions appear on the test pages, such as in boxes with special instructions.

Administration of the WJ III COG requires the examiner to use an audio recording and a subject response booklet. Exam-

TABLE 17.1. WJ III COG Tests, Broad and Narrow Abilities Measured, and Brief Test Descriptions

Test name	Broad/narrow abilities measured[a]	Brief test description
Test 1: Verbal Comprehension	Comprehension–knowledge (Gc) *Lexical knowledge* (VL) *Language development* (LD)	Measures aspects of language development in English, such as knowledge of vocabulary or the ability to reason using lexical (word) knowledge.
Test 2: Visual–Auditory Learning	Long-term retrieval (Glr) *Associative memory* (MA)	Measures the ability to learn, store, and retrieve a series of rebuses (pictographic representations of words).
Test 3: Spatial Relations	Visual–spatial thinking (Gv) *Visualization* (VZ) *Spatial relations* (SR)	Measures the ability to identify the two or three pieces that form a complete target shape.
Test 4: Sound Blending	Auditory processing (Ga) *Phonetic coding* (PC)	Measures skill in synthesizing language sounds (phonemes) through the process of listening to a series of syllables or phonemes and then blending the sounds into a word.
Test 5: Concept Formation	Fluid reasoning (Gf) *Induction* (I)	Measures categorical reasoning ability and flexibility in thinking.
Test 6: Visual Matching	Processing speed (Gs) *Perceptual speed* (P)	Measures speed in making visual symbol discriminations.
Test 7: Numbers Reversed	Short-term memory (Gsm) *Working memory* (WM)	Measures the ability to hold a span of numbers in immediate awareness (memory) while performing a mental operation on it (reversing the sequence).
Test 8: Incomplete Words	Auditory processing (Ga) *Phonetic coding* (PC)	Measures auditory analysis and auditory closure, aspects of phonemic awareness, and phonetic coding.
Test 9: Auditory Working Memory	Short-term memory (Gsm) *Working memory* (WM)	Measures the ability to hold information in immediate awareness, divide the information into two groups, and provide two new ordered sequences.
Test 10: Visual–Auditory Learning—Delayed	Long-term retrieval (Glr) *Associative memory* (MA)	Measures ease of relearning a previously learned task.
Test 11: General Information	Comprehension–knowledge (Gc) *Verbal information* (V)	Measures general verbal knowledge.
Test 12: Retrieval Fluency	Long-term retrieval (Glr) *Ideational fluency* (FI)	Measures fluency of retrieval from stored knowledge.
Test 13: Picture Recognition	Visual–spatial thinking (Gv) *Visual memory* (MV)	Measures visual memory of objects or pictures.
Test 14: Auditory Attention	Auditory processing (Ga) *Speech sound discrimination* (US) *Resistance to auditory stimulus distortion* (UR)	Measures the ability to overcome the effects of auditory distortion in discrimination of speech sounds.
Test 15: Analysis–Synthesis	Fluid reasoning (Gf) *General sequential reasoning* (RG)	Measures the ability to reason and draw conclusions from given conditions (or deductive reasoning).

(continued)

TABLE 17.1. (*continued*)

Test name	Broad/narrow abilities measured[a]	Brief test description
Test 16: Decision Speed	Processing speed (Gs) *Semantic processing speed* (R4)	Measures the ability to make correct conceptual decisions quickly.
Test 17: Memory for Words	Short-term memory (Gsm) *Memory span* (MS)	Measures short-term auditory memory span.
Test 18: Rapid Picture Naming	Processing speed (Gs) *Naming facility* (NA)	Measures speed of direct recall of names from acquired knowledge.
Test 19: Planning	Visual–spatial thinking (Gv)/ Fluid reasoning (Gf) *Spatial scanning* (SS) *General sequential reasoning* (RG)	Measures use of forethought to determine, select, or apply solutions to a series of problems presented as visual puzzles.
Test 20: Pair Cancellation	Processing speed (Gs) *Attention and concentration* (AC)	Measures the ability to control interferences, sustain attention, and stay on task in a vigilant manner by locating and marking a repeated pattern as quickly as possible.
Test 21: Memory for Names	Long-term retrieval (Glr) *Associative memory* (MA)	Measures ability to learn associations between unfamiliar auditory and visual stimuli.
Test 22: Visual Closure	Visual–spatial thinking (Gv) *Closure speed* (CS)	Measures the ability to identify a picture of an object from a partial drawing or representation.
Test 23: Sound Patterns—Voice	Auditory processing (Ga) *Sound discrimination* (U3)	Measures speech sound discrimination (whether pairs of complex voice-like sound patterns, differing in pitch, rhythm, or sound content, are the same or different).
Test 24: Number Series	Fluid reasoning (Gf) *Quantitative reasoning* (RQ)	Measures the ability to reason with concepts that depend upon mathematical relationships by completing sequences of numbers.
Test 25: Number Matrices	Fluid reasoning (Gf) *Quantitative reasoning* (RQ)	Measures quantitative reasoning ability by completing two-dimensional displays of numbers.
Test 26: Cross Out	Processing speed (Gs) *Perceptual speed* (P)	Measures the ability to scan and compare visual information quickly.
Test 27: Memory for Sentences	Short-term memory (Gsm) *Auditory memory span* (MS) *Listening ability* (LS)	Measures the ability to remember and repeat single words, phrases, and sentences.
Test 28: Block Rotation	Visual–spatial thinking (Gv) *Visualization* (Vz) *Spatial relations* (SR)	Measures the ability to view a three-dimensional pattern of blocks and then identify the two sets of blocks that match the pattern, even though their spatial orientation is rotated.
Test 29: Sound Patterns—Music	Auditory processing (Ga) *Sound discrimination* (U3)	Measures the ability to indicate whether pairs of musical patterns are the same or different.
Test 30: Memory for Names—Delayed	Long-term retrieval (Glr) *Associative memory* (MA)	Measures the ability to recall associations that were learned earlier.
Test 31: Bilingual Verbal Comprehension— English/Spanish	Comprehension–knowledge (Gc) *Lexical knowledge* (VL) *Language development* (LD)	Measures aspects of language development in Spanish, such as knowledge of vocabulary or the ability to reason using lexical (word) knowledge.

[a]Full names of narrow abilities are given in italics.

TABLE 17.2. WJ III COG Clusters and Brief Cluster Descriptions

Cluster	Brief cluster description
General Intellectual Ability	A measure of psychometric g. Selected and different mixes of narrow cognitive abilities constitute the GIA—Standard, GIA—Extended, GIA—Early Development, and GIA—Bilingual scales.
Broad Cognitive Ability—Low Verbal	A special-purpose, broad measure of cognitive ability that has relatively low overall receptive and expressive verbal requirements.
Brief Intellectual Ability	A brief measure of intelligence consisting of three tests measuring acquired knowledge, reasoning, and cognitive efficiency.
Verbal Ability	Higher-order language-based acquired knowledge and the ability to communicate that knowledge.
Thinking Ability	A sampling of four different thinking processes (long-term retrieval, visual–spatial thinking, auditory processing, and fluid reasoning).
Cognitive Efficiency	A sampling of two different automatic cognitive processes—processing speed and short-term memory.
Comprehension–Knowledge (Gc)	The breadth and depth of a person's acquired knowledge, the ability to communicate this knowledge (especially verbally), and the ability to reason using previously learned experiences or procedures.
Long-Term Retrieval (Glr)	The ability to store information and fluently retrieve it later.
Visual–Spatial Thinking (Gv)	The ability to perceive, analyze, synthesize, and think with visual patterns, including the ability to store and recall visual representations.
Auditory Processing (Ga)	The ability to analyze, synthesize, and discriminate auditory stimuli, including the ability to process and discriminate speech sounds that may be presented under distorted conditions.
Fluid Reasoning (Gf)	The ability to reason, form concepts, and solve problems using unfamiliar information or novel procedures.
Processing Speed (Gs)	The ability to perform automatic cognitive tasks, an aspect of cognitive efficiency.
Short-Term Memory (Gsm)	The ability to apprehend and hold information in immediate awareness and then use it within a few seconds.
Phonemic Awareness (PC)	The ability to attend to the sound structure of language through analyzing and synthesizing speech sounds (phonetic coding).
Working Memory (WM)	The ability to hold information in immediate awareness while performing a mental operation on the information.
Numerical Reasoning (RQ)	The ability to reason with mathematical concepts involving the relationships and properties of numbers.
Associative Memory (MA)	The ability to store and retrieve associations.
Visualization (Vz)	The ability to envision objects or patterns in space by perceiving how they would appear if presented in an altered form.
Sound Discrimination (U3)	The ability to distinguish between pairs of voice-like or musical patterns.
Auditory Memory Span (MS)	The ability to listen to a presentation of sequentially ordered information and then recall the sequence immediately.
Perceptual Speed (P)	The ability to rapidly scan and compare visual symbols.
Broad Attention	A global measure of the cognitive components of attention.
Cognitive Fluency	A measure of cognitive automaticity, or the speed with which an individual performs simple to complex cognitive tasks.
Executive Processes	Measures selected aspects of central executive functions, such as response inhibition, cognitive flexibility, and planning.
Delayed Recall	Measures the ability to recall and relearn previously presented information.
Knowledge	Measures general information and curricular knowledge.

iners will need to learn how to establish a basal and a ceiling for several tests. They will also need to learn how to score items and calculate the raw score for each test.

The audio recording is used to ensure standardized presentation of certain auditory and short-term memory tasks (test 4, Sound Blending; test 7, Numbers Reversed; test 8, Incomplete Words; test 9, Auditory Working Memory; test 14, Auditory Attention; test 17, Memory for Words; test 23, Sound Patterns—Voice; test 27, Memory for Sentences; and test 29, Sound Patterns—Music). The audio equipment must have a good speaker, be in good working order, and produce a faithful, clear reproduction of the test items. Using headphones is recommended, as they were used in the WJ III standardization. Examiners can wear a monaural earphone or wear only one headphone over one ear to monitor the audio recording while the subject is also listening through his or her headphones.

Directions for using the subject response booklet are provided in the test book. Three tests (test 16, Decision Speed; test 19, Planning; and test 20, Pair Cancellation) require the use of the subject response booklet for administration. Test 6, Visual Matching (Version 2), and test 26, Cross Out, require the subject to use test material that is located in the corresponding test record.

Many of the tests require the examiner to establish a basal and a ceiling. Basal and ceiling criteria are included in the test book for each test requiring them. For some tests, subjects begin with item 1 and test until they reach their ceiling level; these tests do not require a basal. When administering a test with items arranged in groups, the basal criterion is met when the subject correctly responds to the three consecutive lowest-numbered items in a group. If a subject fails to meet the basal criterion for any test, the examiner is directed to test backward, full page by full page, until the subject has met the basal criterion or until item 1 has been administered.

Individual test items are scored during test administration. The majority of tests use a 1 (correct) or 0 (incorrect) scoring rule for determining raw scores. Three tests (test 2, Visual–Auditory Learning; test 10, Visual–Auditory Learning—Delayed; and test 19, Planning) have a different scoring procedure,

in that raw scores are determined by counting the number of errors.

Generally, raw scores are determined by adding the number of correctly completed items to the number of test items below the basal. Scores for sample or practice items should not be included when calculating raw scores. The correct and incorrect keys in the test books are intended to be guides to demonstrate how certain responses are scored. Not all possible responses are included in the keys. In cases where the subject's response does not fall clearly in either the correct or incorrect category, the examiner should write down the response and come back to it later. Completion of the scoring procedure requires using the WJ III Compuscore and Profiles Program (WJ III CPP; Schrank & Woodcock, 2003), a computer software program that is included with each WJ III COG kit.

Examiners should use the selective testing table (Figure 17.1) to determine which tests to administer. Rarely would it be advisable to administer all 31 tests. Testing time will vary, depending on the number of tests that are administered. In general, an examiner should allow 5–10 minutes per test. Very young subjects or individuals with unique learning patterns may require more time. The tests may be administered in any order deemed appropriate and testing may be discontinued after completion of any test.

PSYCHOMETRIC PROPERTIES

Median reliability coefficients (r_{11}) and the standard errors of measurement (SEM) are reported for the WJ III COG and Diagnostic Supplement tests in Table 17.3. The SEM values are in standard score (SS) units. The reliabilities for all but the speeded tests and tests with multiple-point scoring systems were calculated with the split-half procedure (odd and even items) and corrected for length with the Spearman–Brown correction formula. The reliabilities for the speeded tests (test 6, Visual Matching; test 12, Retrieval Fluency; test 16, Decision Speed; test 18, Rapid Picture Naming; test 20, Pair Cancellation; and test 26, Cross Out) and tests with multiple-point scored items (test 3, Spatial Relations; test 12, Retrieval Fluency; test 13, Picture Recognition; and test 19,

Tests of Cognitive Abilities

Standard Battery:
- Test 1: Verbal Comprehension
- Test 2: Visual–Auditory Learning
- Test 3: Spatial Relations
- Test 4: Sound Blending
- Test 5: Concept Formation
- Test 6: Visual Matching
- Test 7: Numbers Reversed
- Test 8: Incomplete Words
- Test 9: Auditory Working Memory
- Test 10: Visual–Auditory Learning—Delayed

Extended Battery:
- Test 11: General Information
- Test 12: Retrieval Fluency
- Test 13: Picture Recognition
- Test 14: Auditory Attention
- Test 15: Analysis–Synthesis
- Test 16: Decision Speed
- Test 17: Memory for Words
- Test 18: Rapid Picture Naming
- Test 19: Planning
- Test 20: Pair Cancellation

Diagnostic Supplement:
- Test 21: Memory for Names
- Test 22: Visual Closure
- Test 23: Sound Patterns—Voice
- Test 24: Number Series
- Test 25: Number Matrices
- Test 26: Cross Out
- Test 27: Memory for Sentences
- Test 28: Block Rotation
- Test 29: Sound Patterns—Music
- Test 30: Memory for Names—Delayed
- Test 31: Bilingual Verbal Comprehension—English/Spanish

Column groupings:

- Intellectual ability: General Intellectual Ability—Std; General Intellectual Ability—Ext; General Intellectual Ability—EDev; General Intellectual Ability—Bil; Broad Cognitive Ability—Low Verbal; Brief Intellectual Ability; Verbal Ability—Std; Verbal Ability—Ext
- Cognitive performance model clusters: Thinking Ability—Std; Thinking Ability—Ext; Cognitive Efficiency—Std; Cognitive Efficiency—Ext
- Broad CHC clusters: Comprehension–Knowledge (Gc); Long-Term Retrieval (Glr); Visual–Spatial Thinking (Gv); Visual–Spatial Thinking 3 (Gv3); Auditory Processing (Ga); Fluid Reasoning (Gf); Fluid Reasoning 3 (Gf3); Processing Speed (Gs); Short-Term Memory (Gsm); Phonemic Awareness (PC); Phonemic Awareness 3; Working Memory (WM); Numerical Reasoning (RQ); Associative Memory (MA); Associative Memory—Delayed; Visualization (Vz); Sound Discrimination (U3); Auditory Memory Span (MS); Perceptual Speed (P)
- Narrow CHC clusters: Broad Attention; Cognitive Fluency; Executive Processes
- Clinical clusters: Delayed Recall; Knowledge

Footnotes:

^{1} Test 31: Bilingual Verbal Comprehension is not required for calculation of this cluster. If administered, items answered correctly on test 31 are added to the raw score for test 1, Verbal Comprehension.

^{2} Also includes test 12, Story Recall–Delayed, from the WJ III Tests of Achievement.

^{3} Also includes test 19, Academic Knowledge, from the WJ III Tests of Achievement.

^{4} Also includes test 21, Sound Awareness, from the WJ III Tests of Achievement.

FIGURE 17.1. Complete WJ III COG selective testing table (includes Diagnostic Supplement).

TABLE 17.3. Median Test Reliability Statistics

Test	Median r_{11}	Median SEM (SS)
Standard Battery		
Test 1: Verbal Comprehension	.92	4.24
Test 2: Visual–Auditory Learning	.86	5.56
Test 3: Spatial Relations	.81	6.51
Test 4: Sound Blending	.89	5.04
Test 5: Concept Formation	.94	3.64
Test 6: Visual Matching	.91	4.60
Test 7: Numbers Reversed	.87	5.38
Test 8: Incomplete Words	.81	6.61
Test 9: Auditory Working Memory	.87	5.37
Test 10: Visual–Auditory Learning—Delayed	.94	3.73
Extended Battery		
Test 11: General Information	.89	4.97
Test 12: Retrieval Fluency	.85	5.87
Test 13: Picture Recognition	.76	7.36
Test 14: Auditory Attention	.88	5.21
Test 15: Analysis–Synthesis	.90	4.74
Test 16: Decision Speed	.87	5.33
Test 17: Memory for Words	.80	6.63
Test 18: Rapid Picture Naming	.97	2.47
Test 19: Planning	.74	7.65
Test 20: Pair Cancellation	.81	6.56
Diagnostic Supplement		
Test 21: Memory for Names	.88	5.10
Test 22: Visual Closure	.82	6.41
Test 23: Sound Patterns—Voice	.94	3.64
Test 24: Number Series	.89	5.09
Test 25: Number Matrices	.91	4.60
Test 26: Cross Out	.76	7.33
Test 27: Memory for Sentences	.89	4.90
Test 28: Block Rotation	.82	6.39
Test 29: Sound Patterns—Music	.90	4.85
Test 30: Memory for Names—Delayed	.90	4.74
Test 31: Bilingual Verbal Comprehension–English/Spanish	.92	4.24

Planning) were calculated via Rasch analysis procedures. Most reliabilities reported in Table 17.3 are .80 or higher. Table 17.4 reports median reliabilities and standard errors of measurement for the WJ III COG and Diagnostic Supplement clusters across their range of intended use. Note that most reliabilities in this table are .90 or higher.

Validity is inextricably tied to theory. John Horn and John Carroll served as consultants in the development of the WJ III. A synthesis of their research, now called Cattell–Horn–Carroll (CHC) theory, provided guidance for the blueprint of constructs to be measured. Identification of the broad CHC abilities in the WJ III is historically and primarily linked to the Gf-Gc research of Cattell (1941, 1943, 1950), Horn (1965, 1988, 1989, 1991), and their associates (Horn & Stankov, 1982; Horn & Noll, 1997; Horn & Masunaga, 2000; see also Horn & Blankson, Chapter 3, and McGrew, Chapter 8, this volume). The specification of the narrow abilities and general intellectual ability (g) construct was heavily influenced by Carroll's (1993, 2003; see also Chapter 4, this volume) research.

The WJ III COG is supported by several sources of validity evidence, as documented in the WJ III technical manual (McGrew & Woodcock, 2001) and Diagnostic Supplement manual (Schrank, Mather, McGrew, &

TABLE 17.4. Median Cluster Reliability Statistics

Test	Median r_{11}	Median SEM (SS)
Standard Battery		
General Intellectual Ability—Std	.97	2.60
Brief Intellectual Ability	.95	3.35
Verbal Ability—Std	.92	4.24
Thinking Ability—Std	.95	3.35
Cognitive Efficiency—Std	.92	4.24
Phonemic Awareness (PC)	.90	4.86
Working Memory (WM)	.91	4.50
Extended Battery		
General Intellectual Ability—Ext	.98	2.12
Verbal Ability—Ext	.95	3.35
Thinking Ability—Ext	.96	3.00
Cognitive Efficiency—Ext	.93	3.97
Comprehension–Knowledge (Gc)	.95	3.35
Long-Term Retrieval (Glr)	.88	5.20
Visual–Spatial Thinking (Gv)	.81	6.54
Auditory Processing (Ga)	.91	4.50
Fluid Reasoning (Gf)	.95	3.35
Processing Speed (Gs)	.92	4.24
Short-Term Memory (Gsm)	.88	5.20
Broad Attention	.92	4.24
Cognitive Fluency	.96	3.00
Executive Processes	.93	3.97
Delayed Recall		
Knowledge	.94	3.67
Phonemic Awareness 3 (PC)	.91	4.62
Diagnostic Supplement		
General Intellectual Ability—Bilingual	.96	3.00
General Intellectual Ability—Early Development	.94	3.67
Broad Cognitive Ability—Low Verbal	.96	3.00
Thinking Ability—Low Verbal	.95	3.18
Visual–Spatial Thinking 3 (Gv3)	.85	5.81
Fluid Reasoning 3 (Gf3)	.96	3.00
Associative Memory (MA)	.92	4.24
Associative Memory—Delayed (MA)	.94	3.67
Visualization (Vz)	.83	6.18
Sound Discrimination (U3)	.96	3.00
Auditory Memory Span (MS)	.88	5.20
Perceptual Speed (P)	.91	4.50
Numerical Reasoning (RQ)	.94	3.82

Woodcock, 2003). Much of this evidence is reviewed and discussed by Floyd, Shaver, and McGrew (2003). Subsequent to publication, other research supporting the validity of the WJ III was conducted.

A review of the WJ III technical manual suggests that the ecological validity of the tests is supported by reviews of content experts, psychologists, and teachers who reviewed items and made suggestions for item revision. A description of the response pro-

cesses assumed to be requisite for each test is outlined in Table 4-2 of the technical manual and in Table 6-1 of the Diagnostic Supplement manual. Each of these manuals also presents a series of divergent growth curves to support the construct of unique abilities. A number of confirmatory factor analyses presented in the technical manual provide evidence that the CHC model upon which the WJ III is based is not implausible. The WJ III COG provides scores that are both similar and dissimilar to scores from other intelligence batteries. Some of the differences may exist because no other intelligence battery provides measures of as many broad and narrow cognitive abilities. Measures of long-term retrieval *(Glr)* and auditory processing *(Ga)*, in particular, are lacking in other intelligence tests.

Additional studies have been conducted that support the differential validity of the CHC factor scores in the prediction of reading and mathematics (Evans, Floyd, McGrew, & Leforgee, 2002; Floyd, Evans, and McGrew, 2001). Also, Taub and McGrew (2004) have demonstrated that the WJ III COG measures the same CHC constructs from age 6 through adulthood.

INTERPRETATION

Intelligence is impossible to describe in concrete terms. The abilities defined by CHC theory are not static properties, but dynamic processes and capacities that people possess differentially. Horn (1991) stated this most clearly:

> Ability, cognitive capability, and cognitive processes are not segments of behavior but abstractions that we have applied to an indivisible flow of behavior. One cannot distinguish between reasoning, retrieval, perception, and de-

tection. The behavior one sees indicates all of these, as well as motivation, emotion, drive, apprehension, feeling, and more. Specifying different features of cognition is like slicing smoke—dividing a continuous, homogeneous, irregular mass of gray into . . . what? Abstractions. (p. 199)

The processes or capacities we observe and measure in the WJ III are not entities but abstractions, or ways we organize our perceptions. Figure 17.2 displays an abstraction step ladder to describe how different levels of interpretation can be applied to understanding the nature of intelligence. The abstraction step ladder is based on the principles of general semantics, particularly as applied to the advancement of scientific thinking (Korzybski, 1933).

The process of abstracting helps us understand the nature of human intelligence. The WJ III provides scores representing intellectual or cognitive ability at four different levels of abstraction. The lowest level of the step ladder represents the *narrow abilities*—the abilities that are as close to operational definitions as practicable. The WJ III COG and Diagnostic Supplement tests are examples of operational definitions of the narrow abilities they measure. As operational definitions, each test explains "what to do" and "what to observe" to bring about its effects.

To infer that an individual has a defined

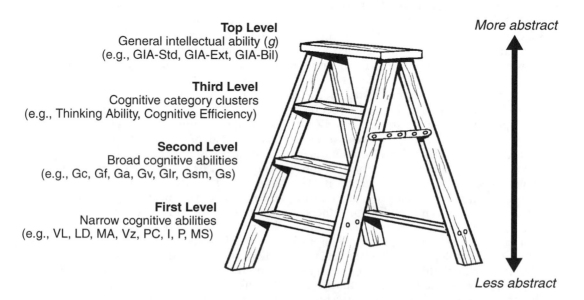

Top Level
General intellectual ability (*g*)
(e.g., GIA-Std, GIA-Ext, GIA-Bil)

Third Level
Cognitive category clusters
(e.g., Thinking Ability, Cognitive Efficiency)

Second Level
Broad cognitive abilities
(e.g., Gc, Gf, Ga, Gv, Glr, Gsm, Gs)

First Level
Narrow cognitive abilities
(e.g., VL, LD, MA, Vz, PC, I, P, MS)

More abstract

Less abstract

FIGURE 17.2. Four levels of abstraction applied to WJ III COG test and cluster score interpretation.

level of a specified type of *broad ability*, we must leap across a huge chasm. That is, we must infer a relatively static concept from a dynamic process or processes. To bridge that chasm, the CHC broad abilities are defined so as to combine two or more dynamic processes that are similar in some way. The commonality between the two dynamic processes helps define an ability of a higher level. Consequently, the WJ III clusters representing the CHC broad abilities—Comprehension–Knowledge *(Gc)*, Long-Term Retrieval *(Glr)*, Visual–Spatial Thinking *(Gv)*, Auditory Processing *(Ga)*, Fluid Reasoning *(Gf)*, Short-Term Memory *(Gsm)*, and Processing Speed *(Gs)*—are abstractions that describe broad classes of narrow abilities, based on two or more operational definitions of the capacities.

Moving up a step on a step ladder has a purpose and a benefit. It allows us to extend our reach to grasp entities that we otherwise could not. Moving up one level on the CHC step ladder also has a purpose: It allows us to describe a class of processes. As a benefit, we can make generalizations about a broad, although still circumscribed, category of cognition.

As we move further up the step ladder of abstraction, several of the WJ III COG tests can be combined into logically derived clusters that provide another level of interpretive information about an individual's performance. Each of these clusters (Verbal Ability, Thinking Ability, and Cognitive Efficiency) represents a general category of broad cognitive abilities that influence, in a similar way, what we observe in an individual's cognitive or academic performance.

At the top of the abstraction step ladder, the General Intellectual Ability (GIA) scores are first-principal-component measures. General intellectual ability, or *g*, represents a very high level of abstraction, because its nature cannot be described in terms of information content. Some scholars of intelligence, notably Horn, posit that evidence of a singular *g* construct has not been established. Others, such as Jensen (1998), refer to *g* as a distillate of cognitive processing, rather than an ability. For example, Jensen has said that *g* "reflects individual differences in information processing as manifested in functions such as attending, selecting, searching,

internalizing, deciding, discriminating, generalizing, learning, remembering, and using incoming and past-acquired information to solve problems and cope with the exigencies of the environment" (p. 117).

The different levels of WJ III scores allow professionals to move up and down the step ladder of abstraction to describe the nature of an individual's cognitive functioning. The terms used by a professional can vary, based on the level of abstraction or generalization required by the purpose of the assessment. Further up the step ladder, higher-level abstractions can be properly and uniformly made from starting points in operational definitions of narrow cognitive abilities. From the top level, general intellectual ability can be described in terms of its component processes. Further down the step ladder, abilities at any level can be described as members of a broad class of abilities defined by the next higher level.

Level 1: Narrow Cognitive Abilities

Each test in the WJ III COG and the Diagnostic Supplement measures one or more of the narrow abilities defined by CHC theory. The narrow abilities represent the lowest level on the ladder of abstraction.

Test 1, Verbal Comprehension, primarily measures *lexical knowledge* (VL; vocabulary knowledge) and *language development* (LD; general development in spoken English-language skills). Test 31, Bilingual Verbal Comprehension—English/Spanish, provides a procedure for measuring aspects of lexical knowledge and language development in Spanish.

Test 2, Visual–Auditory Learning, measures *associative memory* (MA; paired-associate learning). Test 21, Memory for Names, also measures this narrow ability. An Associative Memory cluster score may also be obtained by administering these two tests together. The narrow ability of associative memory may be particularly useful when the ability to store and retrieve associations is of interest. A measure of the ability to recall previously learned associations (Associative Memory—Delayed) may be obtained by administering test 10, Visual–Auditory Learning—Delayed, and test 30, Memory for Names—Delayed.

Test 3, Spatial Relations, measures the ability to use *visualization* (Vz; the ability to apprehend spatial forms or shapes, often through rotation or manipulation of the objects in the imagination) in thinking. A narrow-ability Visualization (Vz) cluster can be obtained by administering test 28, Block Rotation, in addition to test 3.

Test 4, Sound Blending, measures *phonetic coding* (PC; phonological awareness or the ability to code phonetic data in memory). A two-test phonetic coding cluster may be obtained by administering test 8, Incomplete Words, in conjunction with test 4. This cluster is called Phonemic Awareness and measures the ability to attend to the sound structure of language through analyzing and synthesizing speech sounds. A phonetic coding cluster with greater content coverage (Phonemic Awareness 3) can be obtained by conjointly administering test 21, Sound Awareness, from the Woodcock–Johnson III Tests of Achievement (WJ III ACH; Woodcock, McGrew, & Mather, 2001b).

Test 5, Concept Formation, primarily measures the narrow ability of *induction* (I; to educe or infer). Although the task is primarily inductive in nature, the process of solving each item on this test also involves a final deductive step to arrive at the correct response. The ability to educe relations also requires flexibility in thinking.

Test 6, Visual Matching, is a measure of the narrow ability of *perceptual speed* (P; speeded clerical ability in which a perceived configuration is compared to a remembered one). Perceptual speed involves peripheral motor behavior in the form of eye movements in making rapid visual searches. A two-test narrow-ability Perceptual Speed cluster may be obtained by administering test 26, Cross Out, in conjunction with test 6.

Test 7, Numbers Reversed, is a measure of *working memory* (WM; ability to temporarily store and perform a cognitive operation on information). A narrow-ability Working Memory cluster may be obtained by administering test 9, Auditory Working Memory, in conjunction with test 7.

Test 11, General Information, primarily measures *general verbal information* (V; general information). This test samples an individual's store of general knowledge, or information that can be readily accessed without any particular kind of integrative mental process. The information is expressed verbally.

Test 12, Retrieval Fluency, measures *ideational fluency* (FI; divergent production in thinking). This test measures the rate and extent to which subjects are able to think of, or recall, examples of a given category.

Test 13, Picture Recognition, is a task of *visual memory* (MV; iconic memory). The nature of this task requires the subject to form and remember (over a few seconds) mental images or representations of visual stimuli, or icons, that cannot easily be encoded verbally.

Test 14, Auditory Attention, measures the narrow abilities of *speech sound discrimination* (US; perception of speech sounds) and *resistance to auditory stimulus distortion* (UR; the ability to process and discriminate speech sounds that have been presented under distorted conditions).

Test 15, Analysis–Synthesis, primarily measures the narrow ability of *general sequential reasoning* (RG; the ability to draw correct conclusions from stated conditions or premises, often from a series of sequential steps). The test also measures the narrow ability of *quantitative reasoning* (RQ; reasoning based on mathematical properties and relations) because the task involves learning and using symbolic formulations used in mathematics, chemistry, and logic. Test 24, Number Series, and test 25, Number Matrices, also provide measures of the narrow ability of quantitative reasoning.

Test 16, Decision Speed, is a measure of *speed of semantic processing* (R4; speed of encoding or mental manipulation of stimulus content).

Test 17, Memory for Words, is a test of verbal *memory span* (MS; attention to a temporally ordered stimulus, registration of the stimulus sequence in immediate memory, and repetition of the sequence). A cluster measuring the narrow ability of Auditory Memory Span may be obtained by administering test 27, Memory for Sentences, in addition to test 17.

Test 18, Rapid Picture Naming, measures the narrow ability of *naming facility* (NA; speed of producing names for objects or certain attributes of objects). This test measures the speed of direct recall of names of pictured objects from acquired knowledge.

Test 19, Planning, measures the narrow ability of *spatial scanning* (SS; speed in visually surveying a complicated spatial field). This test also measures general sequential reasoning, as it requires use of forethought.

Test 20, Pair Cancellation, measures attention and concentration. It is not clear, however, whether attention and concentration are cognitive abilities or facilitators/inhibitors of cognitive performance. The test also measures the ability to control interference, which can facilitate or inhibit cognitive performance.

Test 22, Visual Closure, measures the narrow ability of *closure speed* (CS; recognition of a visual stimulus that has been obscured in some way).

Test 23, Sound Patterns—Voice, and test 29, Sound Patterns—Music, each measure the narrow ability of *sound discrimination* (U3; the ability to discriminate tones or patterns of tones with respect to pitch, intensity, duration, and temporal relations). When both tests are administered, a Sound Discrimination cluster is obtained.

Test 24, Number Series, and test 25, Number Matrices, combine to form a Numerical Reasoning cluster. The cluster measures quantitative reasoning but requires *mathematics knowledge* (KM; knowledge of mathematics), particularly knowledge of mathematical relationships.

Level 2: Broad Cognitive Abilities

The WJ III tests combine to form clusters for interpretive purposes. Several of these clusters are markers of the broad cognitive abilities identified by CHC theory. The broad-cognitive-ability clusters represent the second level on the step ladder of abstraction. Two or more similar, but qualitatively different, narrow-ability tests combine to form a cluster representing a higher level construct. These clusters are useful in that they allow professionals to make generalizations about broad psychological constructs. The clusters representing these broad abilities often provide the most important information for analysis of within-individual variability and the best level of interpretive information for determining patterns of edu-

cationally and psychologically relevant strengths and weaknesses.

Comprehension–knowledge (*Gc*), sometimes called *crystallized intelligence*, includes the breadth and depth of a person's acquired knowledge, the ability to communicate one's knowledge (especially verbally), and the ability to reason using previously learned experiences or procedures. This broad ability is also called *verbal ability*. The WJ III Comprehension–Knowledge cluster combines the narrow abilities of lexical knowledge, language development, and general verbal information into one broad construct.

Long-term retrieval (*Glr*) is a broad category of cognitive processing that represents the ability to store information and retrieve it fluently at a later point. The WJ III Long-Term Retrieval cluster includes two different aspects of long-term storage and retrieval: associative memory and ideational fluency.

Visual–spatial thinking (*Gv*) is the ability to perceive, analyze, synthesize, and think with visual patterns, including the ability to store and recall visual representations. The WJ III Visual–Spatial Thinking cluster includes three narrow aspects of visual–spatial thinking: visualization, spatial relationships, and visual memory. If test 22, Visual Closure, is administered, a three-test Visual–Spatial Thinking 3 cluster is obtained. Inclusion of test 22 adds greater breadth to the measurement of visual–spatial thinking by incorporating the narrow ability of closure speed into the broad construct.

Auditory processing (*Ga*) is the ability to analyze, synthesize, and discriminate auditory stimuli, including the ability to process and discriminate speech sounds that are presented under distorted conditions. The WJ III Auditory Processing cluster combines three narrow abilities into the broad-ability score: phonetic coding, speech sound discrimination, and resistance to auditory stimulus distortion.

Fluid reasoning (*Gf*) is the ability to reason, form concepts, and solve problems using unfamiliar information or novel procedures. The WJ III Fluid Reasoning cluster includes two narrow aspects of fluid reasoning: induction and general sequential reasoning. A three-test Fluid Reasoning 3 cluster is obtained by administering test 25, Number Series. The three-test cluster provides greater breadth of fluid reasoning abilities by including the narrow ability of quantitative reasoning.

Processing speed (Gs) is the ability to perform automatic cognitive tasks. The WJ III Processing Speed cluster includes tests of the narrow abilities of perceptual speed and semantic processing speed.

Short-term memory (Gsm) is the ability to apprehend and hold information in immediate awareness and then use it within a few seconds. The WJ III Short-Term Memory cluster includes measures of working memory and memory span.

Two other clusters may be obtained when certain tests in the WJ III ACH are also administered. A Delayed Recall cluster may be obtained when test 10, Visual–Auditory Learning—Delayed, is combined with test 12, Story Recall—Delayed, from the WJ III ACH. This cluster provides a measure of the ability to both recall and relearn associations that were previously learned. A two-test Knowledge cluster, measuring both general information and curricular knowledge, can be obtained when WJ III ACH test 19, Academic Knowledge, is combined with WJ III COG test 11, General Information.

Level 3: Cognitive Category Clusters

Three categories of broad cognitive abilities represent the next level up on the abstraction step ladder. These clusters organize cognitive abilities into functional categories in the following way: Each of the three categories is composed of abilities that contribute in a common way to performance, but contribute differently from the common contributions of the other categories.

The *Verbal Ability* cluster represents higher-order, language-based acquired knowledge and the ability to communicate that knowledge. This cluster correlates highly with verbal scales from other intelligence batteries. Verbal Ability—Standard is the same as test 1, Verbal Comprehension, which includes four subtests (Picture Vocabulary, Synonyms, Antonyms, and Verbal Analogies). The Verbal Ability—Extended cluster is the same as the Comprehension–Knowledge cluster.

The *Thinking Ability* cluster is a sampling of different abilities (long-term retrieval, visual–spatial thinking, auditory processing, and fluid reasoning) that may be involved in cognitive processing when information

placed in short-term memory cannot be processed automatically. Comparisons among the component thinking ability scores may provide clues to any preferred learning styles or evidence of specific difficulties. Thinking Ability—Standard includes four tests: test 2, Visual–Auditory Learning; test 3, Spatial Relations; test 4, Sound Blending; and test 5, Concept Formation. Thinking Ability—Extended includes these same four tests, together with test 12, Retrieval Fluency; test 13, Picture Recognition; test 14, Auditory Attention; and test 15, Analysis–Synthesis.

The *Cognitive Efficiency* cluster is a sampling of two different automatic cognitive processes—processing speed and short-term memory, both of which are needed for complex cognitive functioning. Cognitive Efficiency—Standard includes test 6, Visual Matching, and test 7, Numbers Reversed. Cognitive Efficiency—Extended includes these two tests in addition to test 16, Decision Speed, and test 17, Memory for Words.

Top Level: General Intellectual Ability

The top level of the step ladder, indicating the highest level of abstraction—general intellectual ability—is represented by the WJ III GIA scores. There are several GIA scores available, including General Intellectual Ability—Standard (GIA-Std), General Intellectual Ability—Extended (GIA–Ext), General Intellectual Ability—Early Development (GIA-EDev), and General Intellectual Ability–Bilingual (GIA-Bil). The GIA scores are measures of psychometric *g*, one of psychology's oldest and most solidly established constructs, and the first authentic latent variable in the history of psychology. Each GIA score is an index of the common variance among the broad and narrow cognitive abilities measured by the component tests. Each is a distillate of several cognitive abilities and the primary source of variance that is common to all of the tests included in its calculation.

In the WJ III COG, computer scoring makes calculation of general intellectual ability, or *g*, possible. Each test included in a WJ III GIA score is differentially weighted, as a function of age, to provide the best estimate of *g*. In contrast, all other intelligence batteries use a simple arithmetic averaging of test scores to obtain an estimate of *g* (or full-scale intelligence). In the WJ III COG, the tests that measure *Gc* (test 1, Verbal Comprehension, and test 11, General Information) and *Gf* (test 5, Concept Formation, and test 15, Analysis–Synthesis) are among the highest *g*-weighted tests; this finding is consistent with the extant factor-analytic research on *g* (e.g., Carroll, 1993). Figure 17.3 is a graphic representation of the average relative test contributions comprising the GIA-Std scale. Figure 17.4 shows the average relative cluster and test contributions to the GIA–Ext scale. The relative contributions of the individual tests do not vary much by age. Also, note the relatively low contribution of the *Gv* tests to *g*. This information is of interest, because many other intelligence batteries emphasize tests of *Gv* (R. W. Woodcock, personal communication, July 15, 2003).

Two special-purpose GIA scores may be obtained, the GIA-Bil and the GIA-EDev. Each of these scales is also a first-principal-component *g* measure. The tests that contribute to each scale were selected as the most appropriate for use with the purpose of the scale.

The GIA-Bil scale was designed to measure the construct of general intellectual ability using an alternate set of seven cognitive tests that measure the same seven broad CHC factors that are included in the GIA-Std scale. Component tests were selected to

represent the most linguistically, developmentally, and diagnostically useful alternatives for assessment of bilingual individuals from within the WJ III COG and Diagnostic Supplement. The relative contributions of each of the component broad abilities to the GIA-Bil scale are represented in Figure 17.5.

The GIA-Bil scale is intended for use with English-dominant bilingual individuals. Spanish-dominant bilingual individuals should be assessed with the parallel GIA-Bil scale on the *Bateria III Woodcock–Muñoz: Pruebas de habilidades cognitivas* (Muñoz-Sandoval, Woodcock, McGrew, & Mather, 2005) and the *Bateria III Woodcock–Muñoz: Suplemento diagnóstico par alas pruebas de habilidades cognitivas* (Muñoz-Sandoval, Woodcock, McGrew, Mather, & Schrank, 2005).

To measure Gc, the GIA-Bil scale includes a procedure for measuring verbal comprehension in English and another language. The WJ III COG includes test 1, Verbal Comprehension and the Diagnostic Supplement includes test 31, Bilingual Verbal Comprehension—English/Spanish. For Spanish-speaking bilingual individuals, any items answered incorrectly (in English) on test 1 are to be subsequently administered in Spanish using test 31. The resulting Verbal Comprehension score represents knowledge in English and Spanish combined. Alternatively, examiners can use the Bilingual Verbal Ability

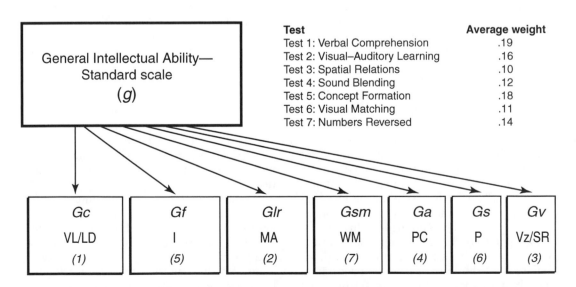

Test	Average weight
Test 1: Verbal Comprehension	.19
Test 2: Visual–Auditory Learning	.16
Test 3: Spatial Relations	.10
Test 4: Sound Blending	.12
Test 5: Concept Formation	.18
Test 6: Visual Matching	.11
Test 7: Numbers Reversed	.14

FIGURE 17.3. Average relative cluster and test contributions to the GIA-Std scale.

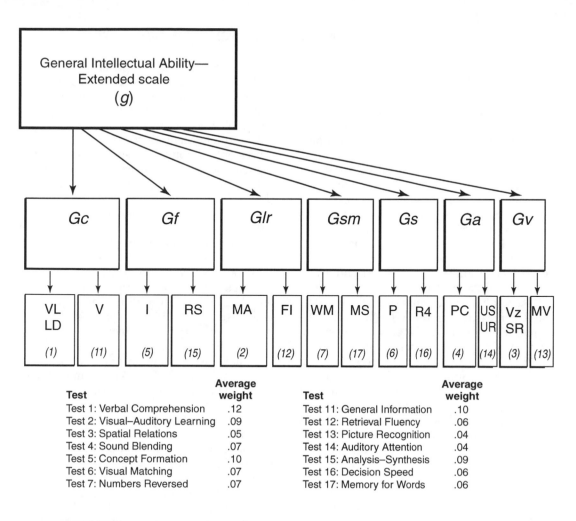

Test	Average weight	Test	Average weight
Test 1: Verbal Comprehension	.12	Test 11: General Information	.10
Test 2: Visual–Auditory Learning	.09	Test 12: Retrieval Fluency	.06
Test 3: Spatial Relations	.05	Test 13: Picture Recognition	.04
Test 4: Sound Blending	.07	Test 14: Auditory Attention	.04
Test 5: Concept Formation	.10	Test 15: Analysis–Synthesis	.09
Test 6: Visual Matching	.07	Test 16: Decision Speed	.06
Test 7: Numbers Reversed	.07	Test 17: Memory for Words	.06

FIGURE 17.4. Average relative cluster and test contributions to the GIA–Ext scale.

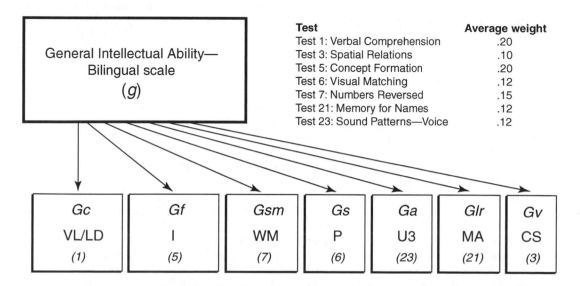

Test	Average weight
Test 1: Verbal Comprehension	.20
Test 3: Spatial Relations	.10
Test 5: Concept Formation	.20
Test 6: Visual Matching	.12
Test 7: Numbers Reversed	.15
Test 21: Memory for Names	.12
Test 23: Sound Patterns—Voice	.12

FIGURE 17.5. Average relative cluster and test contributions to the GIA-Bil scale.

Tests (BVAT; Muñoz-Sandoval, Cummins, Alvarado, & Ruef, 1998) to obtain a measure of verbal comprehension in several other languages for English-dominant bilingual individuals. The WJ III CPP automatically incorporates BVAT scores for this purpose.

Many of the component GIA-Bil tests require a relatively low level of receptive and/or expressive English language ability, such as test 3, Spatial Relations (a measure of Gv); test 6, Visual Matching (a measure of Gs); test 7, Numbers Reversed (a measure of Gsm); test 21, Memory for Names (a measure of Glr); and test 23, Sound Patterns—Voice (a measure of Ga).

Test 5, Concept Formation, is included as the Gf measure in the GIA-Bil scale. Although test 5 requires language comprehension of a series of sentences in the introductions, the constituent words are not linguistically complex (e.g., "same," "different," "rule"). In general, English-dominant bilingual individuals with receptive English oral-language abilities at the age of 4 years, 0 months and above typically possess the English language vocabulary required to attempt this test. The level of expressive vocabulary required includes the pronunciation of simple words such as "red," "yellow," "one," "two," "little," "small," "big," "large," "round," and "square."

A discussion of the receptive and expressive language requirements required in test 5 can be found in Read and Schrank (2003). Test items progress in terms of conceptual complexity, but not verbal complexity. For example, some of the more difficult items require an understanding of the concept of "and" as it infers partial inclusion among a set of attributes and an understanding of "or" as an exclusionary concept. It has been suggested that the ability to recognize and form concepts is one of the most important cognitive abilities necessary for language development (R. W. Woodcock, personal communication, August 26, 2004).

The GIA-EDev includes measures of six, rather than seven, broad cognitive abilities. This cluster does not include a measure of fluid reasoning (Gf). Confirmatory factor-analytic studies of the WJ III COG for children under 7 years old suggest that there is insufficient evidence for measuring fluid reasoning in young children (League, 2000;

Teague, 1999). The six tests constituting the GIA-EDev cluster were selected based on the developmental appropriateness of each task and adequacy of the test floors with young children. For example, testing may begin with test 21, Memory for Names, which requires only a pointing response. This ordering may be helpful in overcoming any initial shyness or hesitance to respond verbally (Ford, 2003).

The GIA-EDev scale includes test 1, Verbal Comprehension (a measure of Gc); an early development form of test 6, Visual Matching (Version 1; a measure of Gs); test 8, Incomplete Words (a measure of Ga); test 21, Memory for Names (a measure of Glr); test 22, Visual Closure (a measure of Gv); and test 27, Memory for Sentences (a measure of Gsm). Items from test 31, Bilingual Verbal Comprehension—English/Spanish, may also be administered to English-dominant Spanish-speaking individuals, providing an additional use for the scale for young, bilingual children. The scale is also useful for individuals of any age who function at a preschool level. The relative contributions of each of the component broad abilities to the GIA-EDev scale are represented in Figure 17.6.

There are two other special-purpose intellectual ability clusters, but these clusters are not first-principal-component g measures. The Broad Cognitive Ability—Low Verbal cluster is an alternative to so-called "nonverbal" scales on other intelligence batteries. It includes all of the tests in the GIA-Bil cluster, with the exception of test 1, Verbal Comprehension, and test 31, Bilingual Verbal Ability—English/Spanish. The Brief Intellectual Ability cluster is intended as a screening measure. It includes test 1, Verbal Comprehension; test 5, Concept Formation; and test 6, Visual Matching.

CLINICAL APPLICATIONS

CHC theory provides the basis for interpretation of the seven broad cognitive abilities measured in the WJ III COG. Strengths and weaknesses among these ability scores may be particularly useful for understanding the nature of a learning problem (Floyd, Shaver, & Alfonso, 2004; Gregg, Coleman, & Knight, 2003; Gregg et al., in press; Mather &

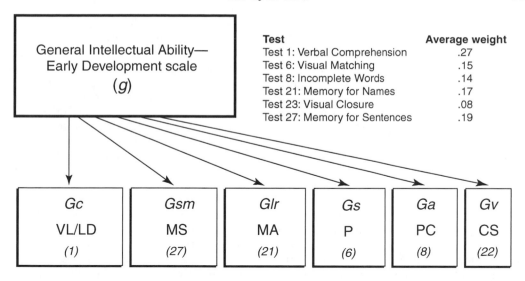

Test	Average weight
Test 1: Verbal Comprehension	.27
Test 6: Visual Matching	.15
Test 8: Incomplete Words	.14
Test 21: Memory for Names	.17
Test 23: Visual Closure	.08
Test 27: Memory for Sentences	.19

FIGURE 17.6. Average relative cluster and test contributions to the GIA-EDev scale.

Schrank, 2003; Proctor, Floyd, & Shaver, in press; see also Mather & Wendling, Chapter 13, this volume). According to the American Academy of School Psychology (2003), assessment of strengths and weaknesses in cognitive processes is important because limitations in cognitive processing may provide the necessary documentation required for legal protection and/or the provision of special services or accommodations. A statement by the National Association of School Psychologists (2002) entitled *Learning Disabilities Criteria: Recommendations for Change in IDEA Reauthorization* suggests that cognitive assessment measures should be used for "identifying strengths and weaknesses on marker variables (e.g., phonological processing, verbal short-term memory) known to be related to reading or other academic areas" (p. 1).

Many current theories of learning disabilities focus on the relevant contributions of specific cognitive processes and highlight the assessment of multiple cognitive abilities and how they vary (Mather & Schrank, 2003). Gregg and colleagues (2003) suggest that the characteristic profile of a student with learning disabilities is marked by significant scatter of scores within and between cognitive, linguistic, and achievement abilities. They recommend using the WJ III COG and WJ III ACH as two of the most comprehensive batteries available for documenting scatter

among these abilities, particularly within the context of clinical decision making. They suggest that an individual's unique pattern of cognitive and achievement strengths and weaknesses on the WJ III may inform diagnostic decisions and prescriptive teaching. Gregg and colleagues (in press) showed that students with dyslexia scored significantly lower than their normally achieving peers on WJ III COG measures of processing speed, short-term memory, working memory, and auditory processing.

Proctor and colleagues (in press) studied the cognitive profiles of children with mathematics weaknesses using the WJ III COG and WJ III ACH. They found that approximately half of the children with mathematics weaknesses on the WJ III ACH showed commensurate weaknesses in one or more cognitive abilities on the WJ III COG. In particular, they noted that children with low mathematics reasoning performance scored lower on fluid reasoning and comprehension knowledge than their average-performing peers. Similarly, Floyd and colleagues (2004) studied the cognitive profiles of children with weaknesses in reading comprehension. Although their review of the profiles of the children with poor reading comprehension revealed no consistent pattern of weaknesses in cognitive abilities, the children with poor reading comprehension scored significantly lower than their average-performing peers on many cognitive abilities. Evans and colleagues (2002) noted that, in particular, comprehension–knowledge demonstrates a strong and consistent relationship with reading comprehension ability across the lifespan.

Gregg and colleagues (2003) suggest a use for the *Cognitive Fluency* cluster. The Cognitive Fluency cluster measures several of the significant lexical processes that research has identified as important predictors of fluency in reading. Cognitive Fluency is an aggregate measure of *cognitive automaticity*, or the speed with which an individual performs simple to complex cognitive tasks. The three tests that constitute this cluster (test 12, Retrieval Fluency; test 16, Decision Speed; and test 18, Rapid Picture Naming) are all measures of rate of performance rather than level of ability. Gregg and colleagues suggest that an individual's score on Cognitive Fluency may provide a useful comparison to his or her scores on tests requiring processing of connected text.

Some WJ III tests and clusters may be helpful in understanding one or more of the executive functioning correlates of attention-deficit/hyperactivity disorder (ADHD). Ford, Keith, Floyd, Fields, and Schrank (2003) examined the WJ III *Executive Processes, Working Memory*, and *Broad Attention* clusters and tests as indicators of executive functioning for the diagnosis of ADHD. Parent and teacher checklists from the Report Writer for the WJ III (Schrank & Woodcock, 2002) were used to document behavioral indicators of this condition.

The Executive Processes cluster measures three aspects of executive functioning: strategic thinking, proactive interference control, and the ability to shift one's mental set. It includes three tests. Test 5, Concept Formation, requires mental flexibility when shifting mental sets, particularly in items 30-40 (see Read & Schrank, 2003). Test 19, Planning, requires the subject to determine, select, and apply solutions to visual puzzles using forethought. Test 20, Pair Cancellation, requires attention and concentration, two qualities that are important to higher-order information processing and task completion. An individual's performance on this test provides information about interference control and the ability to sustain his or her attention.

The four-test Broad Attention cluster provides a multidimensional index of the cognitive requisites of attention. Each of the four tests included in the cluster measures a different aspect of attention. Test 7, Numbers Reversed, requires *attentional capacity*, or the ability to hold information while performing some action on the information. Test 20, Pair Cancellation, requires *sustained attention*, or the capacity to stay on task in a vigilant manner. Test 14, Auditory Attention, requires *selective attention*, or the ability to focus attentional resources when distracting stimuli are present. Test 9, Auditory Working Memory, measures the ability to rearrange information placed in short-term memory to form two distinct sequences.

Ford and colleagues (2003) showed that the Executive Processes, Working Memory, and Broad Attention clusters and most of their component tests (with the exception of test 14, Auditory Attention) predict ADHD status at a statistically significant level. Additionally, both the parent and teacher checklists were statistically significantly related to ADHD status. Their study provided validity evidence for the WJ III Report Writer parent and teacher checklists; the WJ III Broad Attention, Working Memory, and Executive Processes clusters; and the Auditory Working Memory, Planning, Pair Cancellation, Numbers Reversed, and Concept Formation tests in the diagnosis of ADHD.

The WJ III also includes tests that are useful for understanding the cognitive development of young children (Tusing, Maricle, & Ford, 2003) and for understanding the unique sets of cognitive talents and knowledge possessed by gifted children (Gridley, Norman, Rizza, & Decker, 2003) or children with mental retardation (Shaver & Floyd, 2003).

Tusing and colleagues (2003) suggest that the WJ III can be used to contribute to a comprehensive evaluation of a young child's abilities. They provide a rationale for selective application of the WJ III COG at various ages, based on the psychometric characteristics of the tests, the developmental nature of the abilities, and their relationship to early learning. The WJ III COG can provide useful norm-referenced scores when information about a young child's level of a specific cognitive ability (such as verbal ability) is desired. Selected tests can also elicit information about the development or delay of specific cognitive abilities. Because not all of the WJ III tests and clusters measure the CHC abilities at a very low level, these authors have provided guidelines for test selection.

Gridley and colleagues (2003) describe how to use the WJ III for assessing gifted students. The empirical evidence provided by CHC theory and the measurement tools available in the WJ III COG support a multidimensional definition of giftedness. They suggest using the WJ III to promote a broad view of giftedness that allows for identifying students of outstanding specific cognitive abilities and/or superior general intellectual ability.

Similarly, Shaver and colleagues (2003) showed that children with mental retardation demonstrated a range of average-to-below average performance across the CHC broad cognitive abilities measured by the WJ III COG. These authors suggest that individuals with mental retardation should not be presumed to be deficient in all cognitive abilities and that the WJ III COG can be useful in identifying a pattern of cognitive strengths and weaknesses in individuals with mental retardation.

INNOVATIONS IN MEASUREMENT OF COGNITIVE ABILITIES

Although the WJ III includes several innovations in the measurement of cognitive abilities (Woodcock, 2002), this section describes only two unique contributions: (1) the measurability of a wide array of CHC broad and narrow abilities, including discrepancies among abilities, based on a single normative sample; and (2) an application of the Rasch single-parameter logistic test model (Rasch, 1960; Wright & Stone, 1979) to the interpretation of an individual's proficiency in the broad and narrow CHC abilities measured by the WJ III.

Measurability of Broad and Narrow CHC Abilities Based on a Single Normative Sample

The WJ III COG measures 7 broad and 25 or more narrow CHC abilities, based on a nationally representative standardization sample of over 8,000 carefully selected individuals. No other battery measures as many broad and narrow cognitive abilities. As a result of the single normative sample, professionals can accurately compare scores between and among an individual's cognitive abilities.

The WJ III includes several procedures that can be used to evaluate the presence and severity of discrepancies among an individual's measured broad and narrow CHC abilities. Elsewhere (Mather & Schrank, 2003), the WJ III discrepancy procedures are described in detail. The intracognitive discrepancy procedures (standard and extended) can be used to help identify an individual's relative cognitive strengths and weaknesses and may reveal factors intrinsic or related to learning difficulties. The intracognitive (extended) discrepancy procedure includes the seven WJ III clusters measuring broad CHC abilities (Comprehension–Knowledge, Long-Term Retrieval, Visual–Spatial Thinking, Auditory Processing, Fluid Reasoning, Processing Speed, and Short-Term Memory). This procedure contrasts a person's performance in each CHC broad ability to a predicted score based on the average of his or her performance in the other six broad abilities. Eight narrow CHC abilities can also be included in the intracognitive (extended) discrepancy procedure (phonemic awareness, working memory, perceptual speed, associative memory, visualization, sound discrimination, auditory memory span, and numerical reasoning). This procedure may be particularly useful in identifying information-processing strengths and weaknesses.

Professionals can use one or more of several available discrepancy procedures to provide other types of information to address a referral question. Because the WJ III COG was conormed with the WJ III ACH, psychometrically sound comparisons can be made between cognitive and achievement areas. In particular, the predicted-achievement/achievement discrepancy procedure can be used to determine whether the individual's performance in an academic area is at a level that would be expected, based on his or her levels of associated cognitive abilities. Although the predicted-achievement/achievement discrepancy procedure was not designed to estimate a person's potential for future academic success, it can be useful for describing whether an individual's current level of academic achievement is expected or unexpected.

The predicted-achievement/achievement procedure produces unique predictions of achievement in each of 14 achievement and oral language clusters measured by the WJ III ACH. Each prediction of achievement is used to predict an individual's near-term performance in the academic area. Each prediction of achievement is based on test weights that vary developmentally. The weights represent the best statistical relationship between the broad and narrow cognitive abilities measured by WJ III COG tests 1 through 7. The heaviest weights are assigned to the tests that are most closely related to an area of academic achievement at any given point in development. For example, in the prediction of reading, the relative weights utilized at the first-grade level differ from the relative weights used during the secondary school years. In this procedure, when a significant discrepancy exists between predicted and actual achievement, the observed difference suggests that the measured CHC abilities are not a principal factor inhibiting performance. In some cases, extrinsic factors (e.g., lack of proper instruction or opportunity to learn, lack of interest, and/or poor motivation) may be causing or contributing to the observed discrepancy.

Interpretation of Proficiency in the CHC Broad and Narrow Abilities

For many applications, proficiency-level information may provide the most useful information about an individual's test performance. The interpretation plans for many tests do not contain this level of information. Most cognitive batteries limit interpretation to peer comparison scores. Although standard scores may be used to describe relative standing in a group (and even then they must be understood in terms of their equivalent percentile ranks), they provide no direct information about an individual's level of cognitive proficiency.

The ability to make proficiency statements is based on a unique application of objective measurement called the W scale. The Rasch-derived W scale allows the professional to provide a criterion-referenced interpretation of an individual's level of actual task proficiency. On the W scale, item difficulties and

ability scores are on the same scale (Woodcock & Dahl, 1971). The difference between an individual's ability and the ability of the average person at his or her age or grade is called the W Diff (difference). This difference provides a direct and quantifiable implication of performance for the task. Figure 17.7 illustrates the relationship between a person's ability and task difficulty on the W scale. If an individual is presented with tasks whose difficulty level on the W scale is of the same value as the person's ability, then there is a 50% probability that the individual will succeed with those tasks. If the individual is presented with tasks that are lower on the W scale than his or her ability, then the probability of success is greater than 50%. On the other hand, if the tasks are above the individual's ability on the scale, the probability of success is less than 50%. In psychometrics, the W Diff is an example of the person-characteristic function defined by Carroll (1987, 1990). This function predicts the individual's probability of success as items or tasks increase in difficulty. Carroll referred to this concept as *behavioral scaling*. Because the W scale is an equal-interval scale of measurement, any given distance between two points on the W scale has the same interpretation for any area measured by the WJ III. This is true whether the W Diff represents a person's ability to solve problems involving novel reasoning or the person's verbal ability.

On the WJ III, the difference between an individual's ability on each scale and the difficulty of the task can be directly translated into a set of descriptive labels and probabilistic implications about the individual's expected level of success with tasks similar to those on the scale (Woodcock, 1999). Table 17.5 contains a set of alternative descriptive labels and task implications corresponding to the W Diff. For example, this interpretive system can be used with the WJ III to predict functional outcomes of localized brain damage (Dean, Decker, Schrank, & Woodcock, 2003). The W scale provides the basis for this criterion-referenced interpretation of an individual's functional level of cognitive abilities. This scale allows a psychologist to describe broad categories of functional level ranging from "very advanced" to "severely impaired" that describe how proficient an individual is with tasks that are of average difficulty for others of the same age or grade.

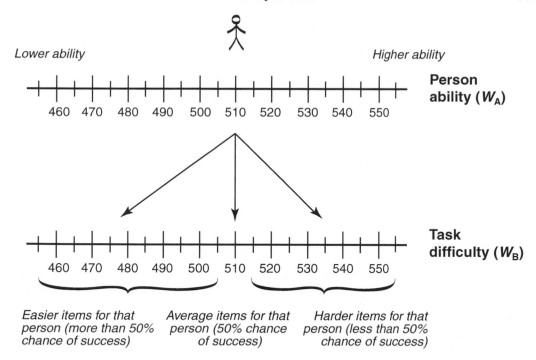

FIGURE 17.7. Relationship between a person's ability and task difficulty on the W scale.

TABLE 17.5. Descriptive Labels and Implications Corresponding to *W* Diff

W Diff	Proficiency	Functionality	Development	Implications
+31 and above	Very advanced	Very advanced	Extremely easy	
+14 to +30	Advanced	Advanced	Advanced	Very easy
+7 to +13	Average to advanced	Within normal limits to advanced	Age-appropriate to advanced	Easy
−6 to +6	Average	Within normal limits	Age-appropriate	Manageable
−13 to −7	Limited to average	Mildly impaired to within normal limits	Mildly delayed to age-appropriate	Difficult
−30 to −14	Limited	Mildly impaired	Mildly delayed	Very difficult
−50 to −31	Very limited	Moderately impaired	Moderately delayed	Extremely difficult
−51 and below	Negligible	Severely impaired	Severely delayed	Impossible

In addition, the interpretation system allows the evaluator to make criterion-referenced, probabilistic statements about how easy or difficult the individual will find similar tasks. These probabilities range from "impossible" for individuals whose functional level is "severely impaired" to "extremely easy" for individuals whose functional level is "very advanced." These descriptive labels can be useful for describing the presence and severity of any impairment.

CASE STUDY

The following case study is based on an administration and interpretation of 28 cognitive tests from the WJ III COG and the Diagnostic Supplement, and several reading and reading-related tests from the WJ III ACH. Qualitative information, relative cognitive strengths and weaknesses identified by the WJ III intracognitive discrepancy procedure, limitations in proficiency in several related abilities, and an identified predicted-achievement/achievement discrepancy combine to substantiate a diagnosis of a specific reading disability.

The case includes background information as reported by the child's mother. The intracognitive (extended) discrepancy procedure reveals significant relative weaknesses in processing speed and perceptual speed. The predicted-achievement/achievement discrepancy procedure suggests that Keith's negligible reading abilities are unexpected, based on his levels of associated cognitive abilities. Note also the description of the individual's level of proficiency in each measured area. These are discussed in the narrative and/or listed on the table of scores (see Figure 17.8). The levels of proficiency are based on the W Diff, as described earlier in this chapter. Very importantly, note how the instructional recommendations follow directly from interpretation of test performance.

Cognitive and Educational Evaluation

Name: Keith Groeschel
Date of Birth: 12/03/90
Age: 12 years, 7 months
Sex: Male
School: JFK Academy
Teacher: Mr. Brewster

Grade: 6.9
Examiner: Fredrick A. Schrank

Reason for Referral

Elizabeth Groeschel, Keith's mother, referred him for an evaluation of his reading difficulties. Keith has a history of reading problems beginning in first grade. Now Keith attempts reading, but gives up easily when confronted with difficult reading tasks and is easily distracted. When required to read, he often fidgets with his hands or feet, or sometimes squirms in his seat.

Mother's Report

Mrs. Groeschel reported that Keith lives with his mother and father, along with one brother, age 6. Over the last 10 years, the family has moved around the country five times.

According to his mother, Keith is usually in good health and is physically fit. Mrs. Groeschel reported that Keith's vision and hearing are normal, although she indicated that he has not had a recent vision or hearing test.

During pregnancy, Keith's mother had no significant health problems. Keith's delivery was normal. Immediately after birth, Keith was healthy. His mother remembers him as an affectionate and active infant and toddler, but also a demanding one. Keith's early motor skills, such as sitting up, crawling, and learning to walk, developed normally. His early language development, such as first words, asking simple questions, and talking in sentences, seemed to be typical. Keith attended preschool, beginning at age 2. In preschool, he seemed to learn things later or with more difficulty than other children did. However, his social skills developed at about the same rate as the other children's.

Because he was not ready for first grade, Keith repeated kindergarten. In first grade and thereafter, he had extreme difficulties learning to read, and consequently received special reading instruction beginning at age 8. Now he attends a special school for children with learning disabilities. He has small classes and a lot of one-on-one instruction.

At the time of this assessment, Mrs. Groeschel described Keith as intelligent, caring, and determined. She said that Keith is

TABLE OF SCORES

Woodcock–Johnson III Tests of Cognitive Abilities (including Diagnostic Supplement) and Tests of Achievement; COG norms based on age 12-6; DS norms based on age 12-7; ACH norms based on age 12-6.

CLUSTER/Test	W	AE	Proficiency	RPI	PR	SS (68% band)	GE
GIA-Ext	492	8-7	Limited	56/90	5	75 (73–77)	2.9
VERBAL ABILITY—Ext	498	9-7	Limited	64/90	16	85 (82–89)	4.2
THINKING ABILITY—Ext	497	8-11	Lmtd to avg	78/90	13	83 (80–86)	3.4
THINKING ABILITY—LV	494	8-2	Lmtd to avg	75/90	14	84 (81–87)	2.9
COG EFFICIENCY—Ext	487	8-6	Limited	28/90	3	72 (69–76)	3.1
COMP-KNOWLEDGE (Gc)	498	9-7	Limited	64/90	16	85 (82–89)	4.2
L-T RETRIEVAL (Glr)	496	8-5	Lmtd to avg	81/90	10	81 (77–85)	2.7
VIS–SPATIAL THINK (Gv)	500	10-0	Average	85/90	33	93 (89–98)	4.9
VIS–SPA THINK 3 (Gv3)	508	13-10	Average	92/90	60	104 (99–108)	8.3
AUDITORY PROCESS (Ga)	508	14-0	Average	92/90	59	104 (98–109)	9.3
FLUID REASONING (Gf)	482	7-5	Limited	35/90	4	74 (71–78)	2.1
FLUID REASON 3 (Gf3)	483	7-11	Limited	32/90	6	77 (74–80)	2.5
PROCESS SPEED (Gs)	476	8-1	V limited	6/90	0.4	60 (57–63)	2.6
SHORT-TERM MEM (Gsm)	498	9-6	Lmtd to avg	69/90	26	90 (85–95)	4.2
PHONEMIC AWARE	501	10-5	Average	85/90	32	93 (88–99)	5.0
PHONEMIC AWARE 3	494	8-2	Lmtd to avg	70/90	10	81 (77–85)	2.5
WORKING MEMORY	489	8-4	Limited	44/90	9	79 (75–84)	2.9
BROAD ATTENTION	497	9-8	Lmtd to avg	71/90	12	82 (78–86)	4.2
COGNITIVE FLUENCY	507	11-3	Average	84/90	35	94 (92–97)	6.2
EXEC PROCESSES	494	9-0	Lmtd to avg	70/90	10	81 (78–84)	3.6
ASSOCIATIVE MEMORY	491	7-0	Lmtd to avg	74/90	8	79 (75–82)	1.6
ASSOC MEM—DELAY	488	4-7	Limited	62/90	1	67 (63–71)	<K.0
VISUALIZATION	496	8-4	Average	82/90	21	88 (82–93)	3.2
SOUND DISCRIMINATION	507	15-8	Average	93/90	69	107 (100–115)	10.4
AUDITORY MEM SPAN	516	15-8	Average	95/90	65	106 (100–111)	9.7
PERCEPTUAL SPEED	484	8-8	V limited	12/90	1	66 (62–69)	3.2
BROAD READING	423	6-7	Negligible	0/90	.1	44 (41–46)	1.3
BASIC READING SKILLS	434	6-11	Negligible	0/90	0.2	57 (55–60)	1.6
READING COMP	446	6-5	Negligible	1/90	.1	40 (36–44)	1.2
PHON/GRAPH KNOW	473	7-3	V limited	15/90	2	70 (66–74)	1.8
Verbal Comprehension	489	8-7	Limited	46/90	9	80 (76–85)	3.2
Visual–Auditory Learning	487	6-10	Limited	60/90	4	74 (70–78)	1.4
Spatial Relations	500	9-6	Average	84/90	33	93 (89–98)	4.6
Sound Blending	509	13-4	Average	92/90	54	102 (96–107)	8.4
Concept Formation	478	7-0	V limited	24/90	6	77 (73–80)	1.8
Visual Matching	456	7-5	Negligible	0/90	<0.1	47 (43–50)	1.8
Numbers Reversed	476	6-11	V limited	18/90	6	76 (71–82)	2.0
Incomplete Words	493	7-3	Lmtd to avg	75/90	10	81 (73–89)	1.8
Auditory Work Memory	503	10-5	Lmtd to avg	75/90	28	91 (87–95)	4.9
Vis–Aud Learn—Delayed	487	5-0	Limited	54/90	0.1	54 (49–59)	<K.0
General Information	507	10-10	Lmtd to avg	79/90	31	93 (87–98)	5.5
Retrieval Fluency	506	19	Average	93/90	82	114 (108–119)	12.9
Picture Recognition	501	10-7	Average	86/90	40	96 (91–101)	5.1
Auditory Attention	506	17-3	Average	92/90	64	105 (97–113)	12.3
Analysis–Synthesis	487	7-9	Limited	48/90	11	82 (77–86)	2.4
Decision Speed	496	9-6	Limited	51/90	13	83 (79–87)	4.1
Memory for Words	520	17-6	Avg to adv	96/90	66	106 (99–114)	10.4
Rapid Picture Naming	519	12-9	Average	91/90	51	101 (99–103)	7.7

(continued)

FIGURE 17.8. Table of scores on the WJ III for Keith Groeschel. W, W score; AE, age equivalent in years/months (12-6 is 12 years, 6 months); RPI, relative proficiency index; PR, percentile rank; SS, standard score; GE, grade equivalent (2.9 is the ninth month of grade 2); SD, standard deviation; SEE, standard error of the estimate; z, z score.

CLUSTER/Test	W	AE	Proficiency	RPI	PR	SS (68% band)	GE
Planning	501	11-10	Average	90/90	47	99 (86–111)	7.0
Pair Cancellation	503	11-3	Average	82/90	35	94 (92–96)	5.9
Memory for Names	495	7-5	Average	85/90	30	92 (88–97)	2.2
Visual Closure	523	>22	Advanced	98/90	87	117 (111–124)	>18.0
Sound Patterns—Voice	503	12-2	Average	89/90	48	99 (93–106)	6.7
Cross Out	512	11-8	Average	83/90	38	96 (90–101)	6.4
Memory for Sentences	512	14-4	Average	93/90	61	104 (99–109)	8.6
Block Rotation	492	6-10	Lmtd to avg	81/90	14	84 (74–94)	1.4
Sound Patterns—Music	511	24	Avg to adv	95/90	92	121 (109–134)	16.4
Mem Names—Delayed	489	4-0	Lmtd to avg	69/90	10	81 (75–86)	<K.0

Form B of the following Achievement tests was administered:

	W	AE	Proficiency	RPI	PR	SS (68% band)	GE
Letter–Word Identification	413	6-11	Negligible	0/90	<0.1	47 (44–50)	1.6
Reading Fluency	420	6-2	Negligible	0/90	0.1	55 (51–59)	1.0
Passage Comprehension	437	6-5	Negligible	0/90	<0.1	42 (37–46)	1.1
Word Attack	454	7-0	Negligible	2/90	3	71 (67–75)	1.6
Reading Vocabulary	455	6-6	Negligible	2/90	<0.1	53 (48–58)	1.3
Spelling of Sounds	491	7-10	Limited	61/90	9	80 (75–84)	2.3
Sound Awareness	479	6-11	Limited	29/90	2	70 (66–74)	1.5

Discrepancies: Intracognitive	Standard scores			Discrepancy		Significant at ± 1.50 SD (SEE)
	Actual	Predicted	Difference	PR	SD	
COMP–KNOWLEDGE (Gc)	85	86	−1	48	−0.04	No
L–T RETRIEVAL (Glr)	81	85	−4	37	−0.33	No
VIS–SPATIAL THINK (Gv)	93	89	4	63	+0.34	No
VIS–SPA THINK 3 (Gv3)	104	89	15	86	+1.07	No
AUDITORY PROCESS (Ga)	104	86	18	91	+1.35	No
FLUID REASONING (Gf)	74	87	−13	14	−1.09	No
FLUID REASON 3 (Gf3)	77	86	−9	20	−0.85	No
PROCESS SPEED (Gs)	60	92	−32	1	−2.26	Yes
SHORT–TERM MEM (Gsm)	90	87	3	61	+0.29	No
PHONEMIC AWARE	93	86	7	71	+0.54	No
WORKING MEMORY	79	86	−7	30	−0.52	No
ASSOCIATIVE MEMORY	79	87	−8	26	−0.64	No
VISUALIZATION	88	88	0	49	−0.02	No
SOUND DISCRIMINATION	107	87	20	91	+1.36	No
AUDITORY MEM SPAN	106	87	19	93	+1.51	Yes
PERCEPTUAL SPEED	66	92	−26	1	−2.25	Yes

Discrepancies: Predicted achievement/achievement	Standard scores			Discrepancy		Significant at ± 1.50 SD (SEE)
	Actual	Predicted	Difference	PR	SD	
BROAD READING	44	71	−27	0.3	−2.79	Yes
BASIC READING SKILLS	57	77	−20	3	−1.88	Yes
READING COMP	40	79	−39	<0.1	−4.14	Yes

*These discrepancies compare predicted achievement scores with Broad, Basic, and Applied ACH clusters.

Discrepancies: Measures of delayed recall*	Discrepancy		Significant at ± 1.50 SD (SEE)	Interpretation
	PR	SD (or z)		
ASSOC MEM—DELAY	13	−1.10	No	Within normal limits
Vis–Aud Learn—Delayed	17	−0.94	No	Within normal limits
Mem Names—Delayed	14	−1.06	No	Within normal limits

*These discrepancies are based on predicted difference between initial and delayed scores.

FIGURE 17.8. *(continued)*

usually happy and that his social interaction skills are typical for boys his age. She also said that Keith generally likes school and tries very hard to succeed at schoolwork. At home, Keith exhibits many positive behaviors. He is extremely attentive to details when helping or working at home, and he is highly organized. Keith always (or almost always) listens when spoken to directly, keeps his personal belongings in order, follows instructions, and finishes his homework.

Tests Administered

- WJ III Tests of Cognitive Abilities (WJ III COG; administered on 06/13/03)
- WJ III Diagnostic Supplement to the Tests of Cognitive Abilities (Diagnostic Supplement; administered on 06/25/03)
- WJ III Tests of Achievement (WJ III ACH; administered on 06/13/03)

Test Session Observations

Keith's conversational proficiency seemed advanced for his age level. He was exceptionally cooperative throughout the examinations. He seemed attentive to the tasks. Although Keith was very motivated to succeed throughout testing, he showed different behaviors during reading tasks compared to the cognitive tasks. He seemed to be much more aware of his limitations during reading activities. For example, he appeared fidgety or restless at times during the reading tasks. In contrast, his activity level seemed typical for his age on the cognitive tasks. During administration of the cognitive tests, Keith appeared confident and self-assured. Then, during the reading tests, Keith appeared tense or worried. In general, he responded promptly but carefully, to all test questions, but he gave up easily after attempting difficult reading tasks.

General Intellectual Ability

Keith's general intellectual ability, as measured by his WJ III GIA-Ext standard score, is in the low range for others his age. There is a 68% probability that his true GIA score would be included in the range of scores from 73 to 77.

Broad and Narrow Cognitive Abilities

Among the WJ III COG clusters measuring broad cognitive abilities, Keith shows a relative strength on Auditory Memory Span. Auditory Memory Span measures the ability to listen to a presentation of sequentially ordered information and then recall the sequence immediately. His auditory memory span is average; Keith will probably find age-level tasks such as remembering just-imparted instructions or information manageable.

Keith's performance is also average on the clusters of Sound Discrimination, Visual–Spatial Thinking, Visualization, and Auditory Processing. It is limited to average on the Long-Term Retrieval, Short-Term Memory, Associative Memory, and Phonemic Awareness 3 clusters. In contrast, Keith's performance on the Comprehension–Knowledge, Fluid Reasoning, and Working Memory clusters is limited.

Keith shows relative weaknesses on the Processing Speed and Perceptual Speed clusters. Processing Speed measures Keith's ability to perform simple and automatic cognitive tasks rapidly, particularly when under pressure to maintain focused attention. Perceptual Speed measures the ability to rapidly scan and compare visual symbols. Although his overall processing speed and perceptual speed are very limited, he performs differently on two types of speeded tasks. Keith's performance is limited on tasks requiring speed in correctly processing simple concepts. His performance is negligible on tasks requiring visual perceptual speed.

Under delayed conditions, Keith's Associative Memory performance is very limited. However, when his retest performance is compared to his initial test performance, his ability is within normal limits.

Clinical Interpretation of Cognitive Fluency and Executive Processing

Overall, Keith's cognitive fluency is average. On tasks requiring fluency of retrieval from stored knowledge, he gave examples very rapidly. Although he was able to specify names for pictures rapidly, instances of naming inaccuracy were observed. His performance on tasks requiring speed of direct recall of simple vocabulary is average. Although he worked extremely quickly, he appeared unable to "move on" when he couldn't recall a word. Instead, he persevered until he found the answer. This hampered his overall performance. Although he makes decisions quickly, Keith's performance on tasks requiring speed of forming simple concepts is limited.

Keith's overall ability to plan, monitor, and arrive at solutions to problems is limited to average. For example, on tasks measuring his ability to plan and implement solutions to problems, his performance was average. His ability to maintain focus on a task amid visual distractors is average, even though he appeared to be highly vigilant. Keith kept his face very close to the test page and used a verbalization strategy to maintain his attention. During testing, his ability to focus his attention on relevant stimuli for information processing purposes was limited to average. However, Keith appears to have difficulty shifting concepts; his performance on tasks requiring adaptive learning and flexibility in thinking is very limited. He does not appear to benefit from or use feedback and instructions to improve his performance.

Achievement

The WJ III ACH Basic Reading Skills cluster includes sight vocabulary, phonics, and structural analysis skills. Keith's basic reading skills are comparable to those of the average individual at age 6 years, 11 months (6-11). When compared to scores for others of his age, his standard score is within the very low range (percentile rank of <1; standard score of 57). His basic reading skills are negligible; tasks requiring reading skills above the age 7-2 level will be quite difficult for him. He did not appear to possess any strategies to decode words that he didn't know by sight.

The Reading Comprehension cluster measures Keith's reading vocabulary and his ability to comprehend connected discourse while reading. His reading comprehension is comparable to that of the average individual at age 6-5. His standard score is within the very low range (percentile rank of; standard score of 40) for his age. Keith's reading comprehension is negligible; reading comprehension tasks above the age 6-9 level will be quite difficult for him. During the passage

comprehension task, he had more difficulties if a picture was not presented with the printed material. During the reading vocabulary task, he appeared fidgety and restless.

Keith reads very slowly. His knowledge of phoneme–grapheme relationships is very limited. In particular, his ability to spell nonwords is limited. His ability to pronounce nonwords is negligible. On sound awareness tasks, Keith required extra time on all items; he didn't seem to "catch on" to the task requirements (rhyming words, deleting, substituting, or reversing sounds).

Case Summary, Integration, and Recommendations

Keith was referred for an evaluation of a reading disability. Although Keith's general intellectual ability is limited, his proficiency with various types of cognitive tasks ranges from average to very limited. He has significant cognitive weaknesses in processing speed, perceptual speed, and auditory memory span. Based on a mix of the cognitive tasks associated with and most relevant to reading, Keith's reading achievement is significantly lower than predicted. When compared to others at his age level, his reading performance is negligible. His knowledge of phoneme–grapheme relationships is very limited. These findings (reading achievement lower than predicted; identified and relevant cognitive weaknesses amid other average cognitive abilities; negligible reading ability; very limited phoneme–grapheme knowledge) are consistent with a diagnosis of a specific reading disability.

Because Keith has limitations in knowledge, cognitive efficiency, perceptual speed, fluid reasoning, working memory, basic reading skills, reading comprehension, and phoneme–grapheme knowledge, an individualized program of instruction and educational accommodations are required to meet his educational needs.

Keith does not have a solid foundation of lexical and general knowledge. This may be one barrier to the development of his basic reading skills and reading comprehension. His limited verbal comprehension may be related to his very limited ability to work effectively with abstract connections and concept formulations. It may also be a product of inconsistent instructional and educational experiences related to his family's frequent moves. Keith's limited verbal comprehension and limited visual–auditory learning suggest that he will be expected to show weaknesses with encoding/recalling, and that he will require greater than average explicit teaching and practice before he will be able to master and apply new words. Inferential learning should not be assumed. Keith may benefit from multisensory study techniques when he is studying fact-based information (e.g., science), or when the teacher's testing formats tend to focus on events and details rather than concepts. An example of a multisensory technique might be using a combination of a categorization strategy to organize the information, and then paired visual and auditory activities to practice it.

When Keith is required to mentally reorganize information, he may be at risk for difficulties and inaccuracies. As Keith progresses through the upper grades of middle and high school, such task requirements will become more prevalent. Note taking, oral presentations, construction of complex sentences and paragraphs, time management, and mathematics will all require a considerable amount of mental reorganization. Keith's teachers should be alerted to the potential for difficulty and should not wait until he has failed or performed poorly before considering accommodations.

As for other students who demonstrate difficulties with prediction, inference, and hypothesis, it may be helpful for Keith to use strategies that organize prior knowledge about a topic or task before starting. Keith needs to organize what he already knows and what he needs to learn about a topic. If he is not cognizant of what he needs to learn, he may confine his learning to his personal knowledge or frame of reference, and this may inhibit his ability to be flexible in considering alternate hypotheses or other points of view.

Overall, Keith's retrieval of previously learned information is limited. This suggests that sustaining cumulative new learning will be very difficult for him. Retention and durability of newly learned information will be severely affected over time without use of repetition, review, and overlearning techniques. Keith should be taught to use strategies for on-demand recall. For example, he should be able to articulate an understanding of the content of what he is required to remember. This may need to be done through verbalizing and expounding on what he has learned. For example, if Keith is taught the numerical notation for the current date (e.g., 6/7/03), he not only should be able to state that the "6" represents June, but also should know why June can be represented by a "6" (i.e., it's the sixth month of the year). Keith may also benefit from visual cues paired with verbal concepts to learn new material and grasp the logic for associations.

Keith's negligible reading ability may be related to his limited awareness of sounds. He has not mastered the phonics skills needed for reading and spelling. Keith will benefit from intensive instruction in phonics skills, in immediate recognition of common letter patterns, in reading/spelling rules, and in syllabication and structural analysis skills. Keith will benefit from a highly structured synthetic approach to phonics for at least 15 minutes daily. For example, he can alternate between pronouncing rows of words and then spelling the same words from dictation. When these lessons have been completed, he can focus on building structural analysis skills. To practice the sequencing of sounds, he can use a series of activities along with regular writing activities. For example, Keith can be provided with predetermined sets of six to eight letters that he can use to make 12–15 words. The activities should begin with short, easy words and then progress to larger words that use successively more letters from the set. Games can be used to increase knowledge of sound–symbol correspondences. For example, a teacher or other adult can number a paper from 1 to 10 (or any other number); write a short, phonically regular word; pass the paper to Keith; and ask him to form a new word by changing just one letter. Letters may be inserted, omitted, or rearranged. If Keith cannot think of a word, the adult can provide as much assistance as needed. After he writes a word, he returns the paper to the adult. This can continue until 10 words are written. When finished, Keith should read the list of words aloud as rapidly as he can.

Because Keith does not easily perceive and remember the letter patterns in words, he should be taught spelling rules explicitly. Activities should be designed to draw his attention to letter patterns, such as color coding, circling, or searching for specific letter patterns in text. For practice in learning how to spell irregular words, a multisensory procedure can be used. For example, an adult can write a word neatly in large, bold, cursive letters (1½ to 2 inches high) on a strip of paper or index card. Then Keith should repeatedly trace the letters of the word as he says each sound (not the letter name). When he thinks he can write the word from memory, he should write it without looking and then check the accuracy. Covering up his previous attempt, the adult can have him write the word correctly three times. If Keith makes a mistake at any point, he should repeat the tracing procedure.

Keith's negligible reading fluency is probably a result of negligible reading decoding skills. Until his decoding skills are better developed, his instructional program should limit the amount of required reading. Keith would also benefit from a program of reading rate building activities with progress monitoring. Other techniques for building reading fluency should also be used, including repeated readings, choral reading, using decodable texts, speed drills, and daily practice.

As Keith develops basic reading skills, he will need to learn strategies for reading comprehension. Comprehension strategies that promote or activate his prior knowledge of a topic to be read will be important. Techniques that allow for the previewing of vocabulary, key ideas, events, and characters will be critical components that will give Keith the opportunity to build meaningful associations to his prior knowledge as he reads. Self-questioning strategies should also be developed.

Keith's educational program should be structured to limit activities that require him to work under time pressure. Emphasis should be placed on accuracy rather than speed. Because Keith will have difficulties learning and demonstrating his knowledge under time pressure, he should be provided with extended time for activities that require reading, including any mandated district-wide testing. Tests that involve significant timed formats will not be effective ways to assess what he has learned or what he understands. Also, tests that require isolated recall of facts or events will be an ineffective way

of prompting his knowledge of a topic. Test formats such as multiple-choice questions or matching questions may not be as easy for Keith to work with, because these formats place too much emphasis on isolated fact recall and decoding.

Finally, Keith should undergo a functional vision examination to examine the possibility that any visual problems may be contributing to his negligible reading ability.

CHAPTER SUMMARY

The 31 tests included in the WJ III COG and Diagnostic Supplement provides measures of multiple intelligences. A single normative sample provides a psychometrically sound basis for measuring many of the broad and narrow abilities described by CHC theory.

The abilities identified by CHC theory and measured by the WJ III are not static properties; rather, they are constructs that have been abstracted by theorists in attempts to describe dynamic cognitive processes. The available scores on the WJ III COG and the Diagnostic Supplement can be described in terms of their relative level on a step ladder of abstraction. The 31 tests each measure one or more narrow, or specific, cognitive abilities. Because scores from the 31 tests can be described in terms of operational definitions of the narrow abilities they are intended to measure, they represent the lowest level of abstraction. The CHC broad cluster scores represent the next level up on the step ladder of abstraction, because they are inferences, or postulates, about a commonality between two or more narrow abilities. General intellectual ability, or g, is represented by the top level on the step ladder. The construct of general intellectual ability is the highest level of abstraction on the step ladder. It is impossible to describe general intellectual ability in concrete terms without reference to lower levels of abstraction. The four levels of scores on the WJ III COG and the Diagnostic Supplement allow professionals to describe the nature of an individual's intellectual abilities at any level (or levels) of abstraction to teachers, parents, and other professionals.

Interpretation of an individual's scores on the broad and narrow abilities measured by the WJ III can be particularly useful for assisting with the formulation and interpretation of diagnostic hypotheses, and can lead to instructional implications and recommendations (Mather & Jaffe, 2002; Mather & Wendling, 2003; Read & Schrank, 2003). Because of the breadth of cognitive abilities measured, the intracognitive discrepancy procedures are well suited to help specify relative strengths and weaknesses among several broad and narrow cognitive abilities identified by CHC theory. Such patterns of strengths and weaknesses may be helpful in determining a specific learning disability (Gregg et al., 2003; Mather & Schrank, 2003) or identifying general and specific domains of intellectual giftedness (Gridley et al., 2003). The W scale that underlies each of the tests and clusters provides the basis for criterion-referenced interpretation of an individual's proficiency with tasks similar to those measured on the WJ III (Dean et al., 2003).

The WJ III (WJ III COG and WJ III ACH combined) has been positively reviewed. Cizek (2003) has stated, "Of the batteries available to users such as school psychologists and others who require individual norm-referenced ability and achievement measurement, the WJ III is clearly a superior instrument." Sandoval (2003) adds, "The WJ III must be considered the premier battery for measuring both cognitive abilities and school achievement of school-aged children and young adults."

ACKNOWLEDGMENTS

Appreciation is extended to Krista Smart, Nancy Mather, Barbara Wendling, and Barbara Read for their assistance in the development of the case study included in this chapter. Appreciation is also extended to Richard Woodcock for his review and suggestions for the development of the principal thesis of this chapter—the step ladder of abstraction applied to interpretation of the WJ III Tests of Cognitive Abilities.

REFERENCES

American Academy of School Psychology (AASP). (2003, February). *Statement on comprehensive evaluation for learning disabilities.* Retrieved from *http://espse.ed.psu.edu/spsy/aasp/AASPstateLD.pdf*

Carroll, J. B. (1987). New perspectives in the analysis of abilities. In R. R. Ronning, J. A. Glover, J. C. Conoley, & J. C. Witt (Eds.), *The influence of cognitive psychology on testing* (pp. 267–284). Hillsdale. NJ: Erlbaum.

Carroll, J. B. (1990). Estimating item and ability parameters in homogeneous tests with the person characteristic function. *Applied Psychological Measurement, 14*(2), 109–125.

Carroll, J. B. (1993). *Human cognitive abilities: A survey of factor-analytic studies.* New York: Cambridge University Press.

Carroll, J. B. (2003). The higher stratum structure of cognitive abilities: Current evidence supports g and about ten broad factors. In H. Nyborg (Ed.), *The scientific study of general intelligence: Tribute to Arthur R. Jensen* (pp. 5–22). Amsterdam: Pergamon Press.

Cattell, R. B. (1941). Some theoretical issues in adult intelligence testing. *Psychological Bulletin, 38,* 592.

Cattell, R. B. (1943). The measurement of adult intelligence. *Psychological Bulletin, 40,* 153–193.

Cattell, R. B. (1950). *Personality: A systematic theoretical and factoral study.* New York: McGraw-Hill.

Cizek, G. J. (2003). Review of the Woodcock–Johnson III. From B. S. Plake, J. C. Impara, & R. A. Spies (Eds.), *The fifteenth mental measurements yearbook* [Electronic version]. Retrieved from *http://www.unl.edu/buros*

Dean, R. S., Decker, S. L., Schrank, F. A., & Woodcock, R. W. (2003). A cognitive neuropsychological assessment system. In F. A. Schrank & D. P. Flanagan (Eds.), *WJ III clinical use and interpretation: Scientist-practitioner perspectives* (pp. 345–376). San Diego, CA: Academic Press.

Evans, J. J., Floyd, R. G., McGrew, K. S., & Leforgee, M. H. (2002). The relations between measures of Cattell–Horn (CHC) cognitive abilities and reading achievement during childhood and adolescence. *School Psychology Review, 31,* 246–262.

Floyd, R. G., Evans, J. J., & McGrew, K. S. (2001). Relations between measures of Cattell–Horn–Carroll (CHC) cognitive abilities and mathematics achievement across the school-age years. *Psychology in the Schools, 40*(2), 155–171.

Floyd, R. G., Shaver, R. B., & Alfonso, V. C. (2004). *Cognitive ability profiles of children with reading comprehension difficulties.* Manuscript submitted for publication.

Floyd, R .G., Shaver, R. B., & McGrew, K. S. (2003). Interpretation of the Woodcock–Johnson III Tests of Cognitive Abilities: Acting on evidence. In F. A. Schrank & D. P. Flanagan (Eds.), *WJ III clinical use and interpretation: Scientist-practitioner perspectives* (pp. 1–46). San Diego, CA: Academic Press.

Ford, L. (2003). Assessment of young children. In F. A. Schrank, N. Mather, K. S. McGrew, & R. W. Woodcock, *Manual: Woodcock–Johnson III Diagnostic Supplement to the Tests of Cognitive Abilities* (pp. 37–46). Itasca, IL: Riverside.

Ford, L., Keith, T. Z., Floyd, R. G., Fields, C., & Schrank, F. A. (2003). Using the Woodcock–Johnson Test of Cognitive Abilities with students with attention deficit/hyperactivity disorder. In F. A. Schrank & D. P. Flanagan (Eds.), *WJ III clinical use and interpretation: Scientist-practitioner perspectives* (pp. 319–344). San Diego, CA: Academic Press.

Gregg, N., Coleman, C., & Knight, D. (2003). Use of the Woodcock–Johnson III in the diagnosis of learning disabilities. In F. A. Schrank & D. P. Flanagan (Eds.), *WJ III clinical use and interpretation: Scientist-practitioner perspectives* (pp. 125–174). San Diego, CA: Academic Press.

Gregg, N., Hoy, C., Flaherty, D. A., Norris, P., Coleman, C., et al. (in press). Documenting decoding and spelling accommodations for postsecondary students demonstrating dyslexia—it's more than processing speed. *Learning Disabilities: A Contemporary Journal.*

Gridley, B. E., Norman, K. A., Rizza, M. A., & Decker, S. L. (2003). Assessment of gifted children with the Woodcock–Johnson III. In F. A. Schrank & D. P. Flanagan (Eds.), *WJ III clinical use and interpretation: Scientist-practitioner perspectives* (pp. 285–317). San Diego, CA: Academic Press.

Horn, J. L. (1965). *Fluid and crystallized intelligence.* Unpublished doctoral dissertation, University of Illinois, Urbana–Champaign.

Horn, J. L. (1988). Thinking about human abilities. In J. R. Nesselroade & R. B. Cattell (Eds.), *Handbook of multivariate psychology* (2nd ed., pp. 645–865). New York: Academic Press.

Horn, J. L. (1989). Models for intelligence. In R. Linn (Ed.), *Intelligence: Measurement, theory and public policy* (pp. 29–73). Urbana: University of Illinois Press.

Horn, J. L. (1991). Measurement of intellectual capabilities: A review of theory. In K. S. McGrew, J. K. Werder, & R. W. Woodcock, *WJ-R technical manual* (pp. 197–232). Itasca, IL: Riverside.

Horn, J. L., & Noll, J. (1997). Human cognitive capabilities: Gf-Gc Theory. In D. P. Flanagan, J. L. Genshaft, & P. L. Harrison (Eds.), *Contemporary intellectual assessment: Theories, tests, and issues* (pp. 53–91). New York: Guilford Press.

Horn, J. L., & Masunaga, H. (2000). New directions for research into aging and intelligence. The development of expertise. In T. J. Perfect & E. A. Maylor (Eds.), *Models of cognitive aging* (pp. 125–159). Oxford: Oxford University Press.

Horn, J. L., & Stankov, L. (1982). Auditory and visual factors of intelligence. *Intelligence, 6,* 165–185.

Jensen, A. R. (1998). *The g factor.* Wesport, CT: Praeger.

Korzybski, A. (1933). *Science and sanity: An introduction to non-Aristotelian systems and general semantics.* New York: Institute of General Semantics.

League, S. (2000). *Joint factor analysis of the Woodcock–Johnson III and the Wechsler Preschool and Primary Scale of Intelligence—Revised.* Unpublished doctoral dissertation, University of South Carolina.

Mather, N., & Jaffe, L. E. (2002). *Woodcock–Johnson III: Reports, recommendations, and strategies.* New York: Wiley.

Mather, N., & Schrank, F. A. (2003). Using the Woodcock–Johnson III discrepancy procedures for diagnosing learning disabilities. In F. A. Schrank & D. P. Flanagan (Eds.), *WJ III clinical use and interpretation: Scientist-practitioner perspectives* (pp. 175–198). San Diego, CA: Academic Press.

Mather, N., & Wendling, B. J. (2003). Instructional implications from the Woodcock–Johnson III. In F. A. Schrank & D. P. Flanagan (Eds.), *WJ III clinical use and interpretation: Scientist-practitioner perspectives* (pp. 93–124). San Diego, CA: Academic Press.

Mather, N., & Woodcock, R. W. (2001). Examiner's manual. *Woodcock–Johnson III Tests of Cognitive Abilities.* Itasca, IL: Riverside.

McGrew, K. S., & Woodcock, R. W. (2001). *Technical manual. Woodcock–Johnson III.* Itasca, IL: Riverside.

Muñoz-Sandoval, A. F, Cummins, J., Alvarado, C. G., & Ruef, M. L. (1998). *Bilingual Verbal Ability Tests.* Itasca: IL: Riverside.

Muñoz-Sandoval, A. F., Woodcock, R. W., McGrew, K. S., & Mather, N. (2005). *Bateria III Woodcock–Muñoz: Pruebas de habilidades cognitivas.* Itasca, IL: Riverside.

Muñoz-Sandoval, A. F., Woodcock, R. W., McGrew, K. S., Mather, N., & Schrank, F. A. (2005). *Bateria III Woodcock–Muñoz: Suplemento diagnóstico para las pruebas de habilidades cognitivas.* Itasca, IL: Riverside.

National Association of School Psychologists (NASP). (2002). *Position statement: Learning disabilities criteria: Recommendations for change in IDEA reauthorization.* Retrieved from *http:// www.nasponline.org/advocacy/NASP_IDEA.html*

Proctor, B., Floyd, R. G., & Shaver, R. B. (in press). CHC broad cognitive ability profiles of low math achievers. *Psychology in the Schools.*

Rasch, G. (1960). *Probabilistic models for some intelligence and attainment tests.* Chicago: MESA Press.

Read, B. G., & Schrank, F. A. (2003). Qualitative analysis of Woodcock–Johnson III test performance. In F. A. Schrank & D. P. Flanagan (Eds.), *WJ III clinical use and interpretation: Scientist-practitioner perspectives* (pp. 47–91). San Diego, CA: Academic Press.

Sandoval, J. (2003). Review of the Woodcock–Johnson III. From B. S. Plake, J. C. Impara, & R. A. Spies (Eds.), *The fifteenth mental measurements yearbook* [Electronic version]. Retrieved from *http:// www.unl.edu/buros*

Schrank, F. A., Mather, N., McGrew, K. S., & Woodcock, R. W. (2003). *Manual. Woodcock–Johnson III Diagnostic Supplement to the Tests of Cognitive Abilities.* Itasca, IL: Riverside.

Schrank, F. A., & Woodcock, R. W. (2002). *Report Writer for the WJ III* [Computer software]. Itasca, IL: Riverside.

Schrank, F. A., & Woodcock, R. W. (2003). *WJ III*

Compuscore and Profiles Program [Computer software]. Itasca, IL: Riverside.

Shaver, R. B., & Floyd, R. G. (2003, March). *Children with mental retardation: CHC broad cognitive ability profiles.* Paper presented at the annual meeting of the National Association of School Psychologists, Toronto.

Taub, G. E., & McGrew, K. S. (2004). A confirmatory factor analysis of CHC theory and cross-age invariance of the Woodcock–Johnson Tests of Cognitive Abilities III. *School Psychology Quarterly, 19*(1), 72–87.

Teague, T. (1999). *Confirmatory factor analysis of Woodcock–Johnson—Third Edition and the Differential Ability Scales with preschool age children.* Unpublished doctoral dissertation, University of South Carolina.

Tusing, M. E., Maricle, D. E., & Ford, L. (2003). Assessment of young children with the Woodcock–Johnson III. In F. A. Schrank & D. P. Flanagan (Eds.), *WJ III clinical use and interpretation: Scientist-practitioner perspectives* (pp. 243-283). San Diego, CA: Academic Press.

Woodcock, R. W. (1999). What can Rasch-based scores convey about a person's test performance? In S. E. Embretson & S. L. Hershberger (Eds.), *The new rules of measurement: What every psychologist and educator should know* (pp. 105–128). Mahwah, NJ: Erlbaum.

Woodcock, R. W. (2002). New looks in the assessment of cognitive ability. *Peabody Journal of Education, 77*(2), 6–22.

Woodcock, R. W., & Dahl, M. N. (1971). *A common scale for the measurement of person ability and test item difficulty* (AGS Paper No. 10). Circle Pines, MN: American Guidance Service.

Woodcock, R. W., McGrew, K. S., & Mather, N. (2001a). *Woodcock–Johnson III.* Itasca, IL: Riverside.

Woodcock, R. W., McGrew, K. S., & Mather, N. (2001b). *Woodcock–Johnson III Tests of Achievement.* Itasca, IL: Riverside.

Woodcock, R. W., McGrew, K. S., & Mather, N. (2001c). *Woodcock–Johnson III Tests of Cognitive Abilities.* Itasca, IL: Riverside.

Woodcock, R. W., McGrew, K. S., Mather, N., & Schrank, F. A. (2003). *Woodcock–Johnson III Diagnostic Supplement to the Tests of Cognitive Abilities.* Itasca, IL: Riverside.

Wright, B. D., & Stone, M. H. (1979). *Best test design.* Chicago: MESA Press.

18

The Differential Ability Scales

COLIN D. ELLIOTT

The Differential Ability Scales (DAS; Elliott, 1990a) battery, developed and standardized in the United States, has become widely used for cognitive assessment in recent years. It has a longer history than its publication date suggests, however, as it is based on a predecessor, the British Ability Scales (BAS; Elliott, 1983a, 1983b). In its turn, the BAS incorporated new features from the DAS in its second edition (BAS II; Elliott, 1996), and at the time of this writing, a second edition of the DAS (DAS II) is being standardized and will be published in 2006.

This chapter primarily describes the existing DAS, because no data have yet been gathered on the DAS II. However, later in the chapter there is a brief description of the DAS II's expected form under the main heading "Organization and Format" (see "The DAS II: Changes in Content and Structure"). As its name suggests, the DAS was developed with a primary focus on specific abilities rather than on general "intelligence."

STRUCTURE OF THE DAS

The DAS consists of (1) a cognitive battery of 17 subtests divided into two overlapping age levels; and (2) a short battery of three school achievement tests, conormed with the cognitive battery. The Preschool and School-Age levels of the cognitive battery were conormed on children ages 5 years, 0 months through 6 years, 11 months (5:0 through 6:11), with most preschool subtests also conormed through 7:11.

The total age range covered by the instrument is 2:6 through 17:11. The DAS cognitive battery yields a composite score—General Conceptual Ability (GCA)—focused on reasoning and conceptual abilities; a Special Nonverbal Composite; and lower-level composite scores called *cluster scores*. These composites are derived from the core subtests, which are highly g-saturated. Diagnostic subtests measure other specific abilities that do not contribute to the composites. The overall structure is summarized in Table 18.1.

THEORETICAL UNDERPINNINGS

Two principles—self-evident truths to many practitioners—drove the development of the DAS. The first is that professionals assessing children with learning disabilities (LDs) and developmental disabilities need information at a finer level of detail than an IQ score. IQ tests in the past have had a primary, disproportionate focus on global composite scores. The second principle is that psychometric assessment has much to offer the practitioner. Psychometric tests of cognitive abilities not only have well-established qualities of reliability, validity, time efficiency, objectivity, and lack of bias, but often provide informa-

TABLE 18.1. Number of DAS Subtests and Composites at Each Age Level

Age level	Number of subtests	General composite	Cluster scores
Lower Preschool level Age 2:6–3:5 (Extended age 2:6–4:11)	4 core 2 diagnostic	1. GCA 2. Special Nonverbal	
Upper Preschool level Age 3:6–5:11 (Extended age 3:6–6:11)	6 core 5 diagnostic	1. GCA 2. Special Nonverbal	1. Verbal Ability 2. Nonverbal Ability
School-Age level Age 6:0–17:11 (Extended age 5:0–17:11)	6 core 4 diagnostic 3 achievement	1. GCA 2. Special Nonverbal	1. Verbal Ability 2. Nonverbal Reasoning Ability 3. Spatial Ability

tion critical to an understanding of a child's learning styles and characteristics.

The first principle led to the major priority in the development of the DAS: to produce a battery in which subtests would be sufficiently reliable and measure sufficiently distinct cognitive functions to make them individually interpretable. Although it was expected that meaningful composites would be derived from the subtests, the primary focus in test development was at the subtest level. This emphasis distinguishes the DAS from most other batteries.

The DAS was not developed solely to reflect a single model of cognitive abilities but may be interpreted from a number of theoretical perspectives. It is designed to address processes that often underlie children's difficulties in learning and what we know about neurological structures underlying these abilities. As Carroll (1993, 2003) has shown, there are considerable similarities in the factor structures of cognitive batteries. A general factor (*g*) is an inescapable reality. It pervades all measures of ability and all relationships between cognitive abilities of any kind. It must therefore be represented in any test battery structure and in its theoretical model. When the many theories of the structure of abilities were reviewed at the time of the DAS's development, it was apparent that no single theory was entirely persuasive, and certainly no single theory had universal acceptance among theoreticians or practitioners.

During the years since publication of the DAS, there has developed what appears to be a growing consensus among factor theorists of human abilities. This centers on what has

become widely referred to as Gf-Gc theory (Carroll, 1993; Cattell, 1971; Cattell & Horn, 1978; Horn & Noll, 1997). The term Gf-Gc is something of a misnomer, because the factors of *fluid reasoning* (Gf) and *crystallized intelligence* (or *verbal ability*; Gc) form only a part of a hierarchical structure of abilities consisting of numerous first-order, narrow abilities, and 8–10 second-order, broad abilities, with *g* at the apex of the hierarchy as a third-order factor. An alternative name for Gf-Gc theory is Cattell–Horn–Carroll (CHC) theory (McGrew & Woodcock, 2001; see McGrew, Chapter 8, this volume). Even well over a decade after publication of the DAS, it is evident that the originators of CHC theory do not agree on (1) the number of factors representing independent abilities in the model or (2) the precise nature of each factor (see Horn & Blankson, Chapter 3, and Carroll, Chapter 4, this volume). Moreover, it remains open to debate whether and to what extent subtests from different test batteries that purport to measure a given factor actually do so (Alfonso, Flanagan, & Radwan, Chapter 9, this volume).

Despite the fact that no single theory or model has universal acceptance, there is a common core of theory and research that supports a number of propositions on which the development of the DAS was based:

- Human abilities are not explainable solely in terms of a single cognitive factor (*g*), or even in terms of two or three lower-order factors.
- Human abilities form multiple dimensions on which individuals show reliably ob-

servable differences (Carroll, 1993), and which are related in complex ways with how children learn, achieve, and solve problems.

- Human abilities are interrelated but not completely overlapping, thus making many of them distinct (Carroll, 1993).
- The wide range of human abilities represents a number of interlinked subsystems of information processing.
- Subsystems of information processing have structural correlates in the central nervous system, in which some functions are localized and others are integrated.

The relationship between cognitive abilities and neurological structure has long exercised the discipline of psychology, because although it has been known for many years that there are cause-and-effect relationships, their nature has not been clear. The following section outlines some links between the factor structure of abilities and neuropsychological structures in the areas of verbal and spatial abilities, fluid reasoning abilities, and some aspects of memory. DAS measures (both subtests and composites) are mapped onto this structure.

Broad Verbal and Visual–Spatial Abilities

Two of the major ability clusters in the DAS and other cognitive batteries reflect two major systems through which we receive, perceive, remember, and process information. These systems are linked to the auditory and visual modalities. Factorially, the systems are represented by *crystallized intelligence* (or *verbal ability* and *visual* (or *visual–spatial*) *processing*—Gc and Gv, respectively, in Gf-Gc theory. Neuropsychologically, there is strong evidence for the existence of these systems. They tend to be localized in the left and right cerebral hemispheres, respectively, although there are individual differences in areas of localization of function. Moreover, the systems are doubly dissociated; that is, they represent two distinct, independent systems of information processing (McCarthy & Warrington, 1990; Springer & Deutsch, 1989). In the DAS, crystallized intelligence or verbal ability (Gc) is measured by the Verbal cluster in both the Preschool and School-Age cognitive batteries. At the Preschool level, the Verbal cluster is formed by the

Naming Vocabulary and Verbal Comprehension subtests, and at the School-Age level it is formed by Similarities and Word Definitions. Visual or visual–spatial processing (Gv) is measured by the Spatial cluster at the School-Age level (consisting of the Pattern Construction and Recall of Designs subtests), and by the Pattern Construction, Block Building, and Copying subtests at the Preschool level.

Integration of Complex Information Processing

For normal cognitive functioning, the auditory–verbal and visual–spatial systems operate in an integrated fashion. Integration of the visual and auditory information-processing systems (and information from all subsystems) is probably a necessary underpinning for complex mental activity. Factorially, this integrative system is represented by the broad ability of *fluid reasoning* (Gf) in Gf-Gc theory. It seems likely that the best measures of Gf require integrated analysis of both verbal and visual information. Neuropsychologically, it seems that the integrative function of frontal lobe systems is central to complex mental functioning (Luria, 1973; discussed by McCarthy & Warrington, 1990, pp. 343–364), and it is therefore reasonable to hypothesize that it provides a structural correlate for Gf. In the DAS, the Gf factor is measured in the School-Age battery by the Nonverbal Reasoning cluster. Both subtests require integrated analysis and complex transformation of both visual and verbal information. For example, in the Matrices subtest, verbal mediation is critical for the solution of visually presented problems for most individuals. Precisely the same process consideration applies to the Sequential and Quantitative Reasoning subtest, and also to Picture Similarities, which provides a measure of fluid reasoning at the Preschool level.

There is evidence that Gf is highly correlated with *g*, the higher-order general factor (Carroll, 2003; Gustafsson, 1988, 1989, 2001; Härnqvist, Gustafsson, Muthén, & Nelson, 1994). Although many factors at a lower order of generality are also related to *g*, the three that have the greatest contribution to defining *g* are the Gf, Gv, and Gc factors, discussed earlier. Carroll (1993) puts it this way: "There is abundant evidence for a factor of general intelligence . . . that dominates factors or variables that can be mastered in performing induction, reasoning, visualization, and language comprehension tasks" (p. 624). The hierarchical factor analyses of the DAS standardization data by Keith (1990) provide further support for this position. At the School-Age level, the subtests with the highest loadings on *g* are those forming the Verbal (Gc), Nonverbal Reasoning (Gf), and Spatial (Gv) clusters. In the DAS, *g* is measured by an overall composite, General Conceptual Ability (GCA; so named because it provides a brief description of *g*). Because it is estimated from only those subtests that are the best estimators of *g* (i.e., those that measure Gf, Gc, and Gv), the GCA is a purer measure of *g* than the composites of most other batteries—which include all cognitive subtests in the composite, regardless of their *g* loading.

Verbal and Visual Short-Term Memory Systems

Some cognitive tests, such as the Woodcock–Johnson III Tests of Cognitive Abilities (WJ III COG; Woodcock, McGrew, & Mather, 2001b), represent memory by a single factor. Supporting this position, Gf-Gc theory does not distinguish at the second-order, group factor level between separate, modality-related memory systems. Proponents of the theory, however, admit uncertainty. On the one hand, Carroll (1993) included the first-order *visual memory* (MV) factor in a primarily auditory–verbal second-order *short-term memory* (Gsm) factor. On the other hand, Flanagan, McGrew, and Ortiz (2000) place MV under the second-order factor of *visual processing* (Gv). Evidence from the fields of cognitive psychology and neuropsychology shows clearly, however, that verbal and visual short-term memory systems are distinct and are doubly dissociated (Hitch, Halliday, Schaafstal, & Schraagen, 1988; McCarthy & Warrington, 1990, pp. 275–295). The DAS therefore keeps visual and auditory short-term memory tasks as distinct measures and does not treat short-term memory as unitary. Visual short-term memory is represented at the Preschool level by Recognition of Pictures, and at the School-Age level by Recall of Designs and Recogni-

tion of Pictures (out-of-level for ages 8 and over; a reliable and valid measure for older children of average to below-average ability). Auditory short-term memory is represented across the entire age range by Recall of Digits, a subtest designed to be a purer measure of this function than the Digit Span subtest of a number of other batteries.

The *intermediate-term memory* (Glr) factor in the Gf-Gc model (called *long-term retrieval* by Carroll, 2003, and *long-term storage and retrieval* by Flanagan et al., 2000) is typically measured by tests that have both visual and verbal components. In the DAS Recall of Objects subtest, for example, pictures are presented, but they have to be recalled verbally. McCarthy and Warrington (1990, p. 283) call this *visual–verbal short-term memory* and conclude that it is underpinned by another distinct information-processing system. In the DAS, the Recall of Objects subtest, which provides a measure of this factor, is for children 4 years of age and older.

ORGANIZATION AND FORMAT

Test Structure

The DAS has three major groups of component tests: the Preschool level of the cognitive battery, the School-Age level of the cognitive battery, and the brief achievement battery. These are listed in Tables 18.2, 18.3, and 18.4. In each table for the cognitive battery, the subtests are grouped according to whether they are designated *core* subtests or *diagnostic* subtests. Each subtest has a brief description of the abilities it measures, including its relation to the Gf-Gc factors. The core subtests are relatively strongly *g*-related and therefore measure complex processing and conceptual ability. The diagnostic subtests have a lower *g* saturation and measure such less cognitively complex functions as short-term memory and speed of information processing. Subtests have normative scores in a *T*-score metric (mean = 50; standard deviation [*SD*] = 10).

Tables 18.2 and 18.3 also show the composites that can be derived from the core subtests, and the subtests that contribute to those composites. Two types of composites are provided, all in a standard score metric (mean = 100, *SD* = 15). First are lower-order cluster scores. There are two of these at the Upper Preschool level (Verbal and Nonverbal), for children ages 3:6 to 5:11. There are three cluster scores at the School-Age level (Verbal, Nonverbal Reasoning, and Spatial). Note that at the Lower Preschool level (ages 2:6 to 3:5), there are no cluster scores.

Second are the higher-order composites. For most children, the most general composite will be the GCA score. For children for whom it is judged that the verbal component of that score is inappropriate, a Special Nonverbal Composite is provided. For the Upper Preschool age level, this is identical to the lower-order Nonverbal composite, formed from three subtests. For the School-Age battery, this is formed from the four subtests in

the Nonverbal Reasoning and Spatial clusters.

Table 18.4 lists the three achievement tests. The normative scores on these tests are in a standard score metric (mean = 100, SD = 15), to facilitate comparison with composite scores from the cognitive battery. The achievement and cognitive batteries were fully conormed. Discrepancies between ability (as measured by GCA or the Special Nonverbal Composite) and achievement may be evaluated by taking either (1) the simple difference between the achievement score and the composite, or (2) the difference between predicted and observed achievement, with predicted achievement being based on the GCA or Special Nonverbal Composite score.

TABLE 18.2. Subtests of the DAS Preschool Cognitive Battery, Showing Abilities Measured (and Relation of Measures to Gf-Gc Factors) and Their Contribution to Composites

Subtest	Abilities measured	Contribution to composite
Core subtests		
Block Building[a]	Visual-perceptual matching, especially of spatial orientation, in copying block patterns (Gv)	GCA
Verbal Comprehension	Receptive language: Understanding oral instructions using basic language concepts (Gc)	Verbal, GCA
Naming Vocabulary	Expressive language: Knowledge of names (Gc)	Verbal, GCA
Picture Similarities	Nonverbal reasoning: Matching pictures that have a common element or concept (Gf)	Nonverbal, GCA
Pattern Construction	Nonverbal, spatial visualization in reproducing designs with colored blocks and flat squares (Gv)	Nonverbal, GCA
Copying	Visual–spatial matching and fine motor coordination in copying line drawings (Gv)	Nonverbal, GCA
Early Number Concepts[b]	Knowledge of prenumerical and numerical quantitative concepts (Gq)	GCA
Diagnostic subtests		
Matching Letter-Like Forms	Visual discrimination of spatial relationships among similar shapes (Gv)	N/A
Recall of Digits	Short-term auditory–sequential memory for sequences of numbers (Gsma)	N/A
Recall of Objects	Short-term and intermediate-term learning and verbal recall of a display of pictures (Glr)	N/A
Recognition of Pictures	Short-term, nonverbal visual memory measured through recognition of familiar objects (Gsmv, Gv)	N/A

Note. N/A, not applicable. The DAS Preschool cognitive battery includes Verbal and Nonverbal and clusters, as well as the GCA and Special Nonverbal Composite. Gf-Gc factors: Gv, visual–spatial processing; Gc, crystallized intelligence or verbal ability; Gf, fluid reasoning; Gsma, auditory short-term memory; Gsmv, visual short-term memory; Glr, intermediate-term memory; Gq, quantitative. See text and see Carroll (1993), p. 626.
[a]Used only for the GCA at the Lower Preschool level. Used as a diagnostic subtest at the Upper Preschool level.
[b]Not used for either cluster score, because it has similar factor loadings on both the Verbal and Nonverbal factors.

TABLE 18.3. Subtests of the DAS School-Age Cognitive Battery, Showing Abilities Measured (and Relation of Measures to Gf-Gc Factors) and Their Contribution to Composites

Subtest	Abilities measured	Contribution to composite
Core subtests		
Word Definitions	Expressive language: Knowledge of word meanings (Gc)	Verbal, GCA
Similarities	Verbal, inductive reasoning and verbal knowledge (Gc)	Verbal, GCA
Matrices	Nonverbal, logical reasoning: Perception and application of relationships among abstract figures (Gf)	Nonverbal Reasoning, GCA, Special Nonverbal
Sequential and Quantitative Reasoning	Detection of sequential patterns or relationships in figures or numbers (Gf)	Nonverbal Reasoning, GCA, Special Nonverbal
Recall of Designs	Short-term recall of visual–spatial relationships through drawing abstract figures (Gv, Gsmv)	Spatial, GCA, Special Nonverbal
Pattern Construction	Nonverbal, spatial visualization in reproducing designs with colored blocks and flat squares (Gv)	Spatial, GCA, Special Nonverbal
Diagnostic subtests		
Recall of Digits	Short-term auditory–sequential memory for sequences of numbers (Gsma)	N/A
Recall of Objects	Short-term and intermediate-term learning and verbal recall of a display of pictures (Glr)	N/A
Speed of Information Processing	Speed in performing simple mental operations (Gs)	N/A

Note. N/A, not applicable. The DAS school-age cognitive battery contains Verbal, Nonverbal Reasoning, and Spatial clusters, as well as the GCA and Special Nonverbal composite. Gf-Gc factors: Gv, visual–spatial processing; Gc, crystallized intelligence or verbal ability; Gf, fluid reasoning; Gsma, auditory short-term memory; Gsmv, visual short-term memory; Glr, intermediate-term memory; Gs, cognitive speed. See text and see Carroll (1993), p. 626.

TABLE 18.4. DAS Achievement Tests

Achievement test	Skills measured
Basic Number Skills	Recognition of printed numbers and performance of arithmetic operations. Includes diagnostic performance analysis of errors.
Spelling	Knowledge and written recall of spellings. Includes diagnostic performance analysis on items.
Word Reading	Recognition and decoding of printed words.

The DAS handbook provides information on both the statistical significance (or reliability) of discrepancies, and their frequency of occurrence (or unusualness) in the standardization sample.

Overlapping Preschool and School-Age Levels

The Preschool and School-Age levels of the cognitive battery were fully conormed for children in the age range of 5:0 to 7:11. This provides a major advantage for the professional examiner, who has the option of choosing which battery is most developmentally appropriate for a given child in this age range. Both the DAS handbook and an independent study by Keith (1990) demonstrated that the *g* factors measured at the Preschool and School-Age levels are identical.

Test Content

Developmental Appropriateness

The two levels of the DAS cognitive battery were deliberately designed to be developmentally appropriate and engaging for preschool and school-age children, respectively. By contrast, the practice of other test developers (e.g., in the Wechsler and WJ III scales) to push tasks originally designed for adults or older children into the preschool domain was considered undesirable. Such a practice leads to tasks that are less intrinsically interesting for preschoolers, resulting in poorer motivation and greater difficulty for the examiner in maintaining rapport.

Subtests as Specific Ability Measures

The chief aim in designing the content of the DAS was to produce subtests that are individually interpretable and can stand technically as separate, specific measures of various abilities. Once a specification was made of the desired tasks and dimensions to be measured, each subtest was designed to be unidimensional and homogeneous in content and distinct from other subtests, thus aiding the interpretation of children's performance. If a subtest score is to be interpreted as a measure of a specific, identifiable ability, the items within that subtest must be of similar content and must require the examinee to perform similar operations. In each item of the Naming Vocabulary subtest, a child is asked to name an object in a picture. All items are therefore homogeneous. Naming Vocabulary is distinct from Verbal Comprehension, another verbal subtest, because the former requires a verbal response and the latter does not.

In addition to having homogeneous content that focuses on a distinct ability, each subtest should also be reliable. Because the DAS emphasizes the identification of cognitive strengths and weaknesses, subtests must have a sufficient amount of reliable specificity to be separately interpretable (see "Accuracy, Reliability, and Specificity," below).

Verbal Content

Although it was considered important to include measures of verbal ability in the DAS cognitive battery, too many verbal tasks would present problems for examiners wishing to assess children from multicultural or culturally disadvantaged backgrounds. In particular, my colleagues and I considered and rejected the inclusion of measures of general knowledge (either verbally or pictorially presented, as in the Wechsler Information subtest or the Faces and Places subtest in the original Kaufman Assessment Battery for Children [K-ABC; Kaufman & Kaufman, 1983]). In developing verbal items, considerable attention was paid to whether items and language would be usable throughout the English-speaking world. Colloquialisms or words with a specific meaning in the United States were eliminated as far as possible.

Because verbal abilities are a major component of cognition, it is certainly necessary to have some subtests, particularly at the School-Age level, that are purely verbally presented. However, getting the balance right in a test battery is important, too. In developing the DAS content, only two core subtests were included with entirely verbal presentation and response (both at the School-Age level), plus the verbally administered Recall of Digits subtest as a measure of auditory short-term memory. Other than those subtests, the aim was to have subtests with varied tasks and materials. The "Test Materials" section below shows the range and variety of DAS stimulus materials.

Timed or Speeded Items

The DAS content minimizes the use of timed or speeded items. The Speed of Information Processing subtest is an obvious exception, as the nature of the task is to process information as speedily as possible. Apart from that subtest, only one subtest—Pattern Construction—gives extra points for correct completion of the designs within specified time limits. Of course, this feature of the subtest, which is appropriate for most individuals, is inappropriate for some children. Speed of response to the Pattern Construction items may not produce a valid measure for a child with a physical disability such as cerebral palsy, or one with an attentional problem, or one who takes an extremely deliberate approach to a task. For such children, an alternative procedure is provided, in which the score is based solely on accuracy within very liberal time limits. Confirmatory factor analyses reported in the DAS handbook demonstrated the factorial equivalence of the standard and alternative versions of Pattern Construction.

Teaching Procedures

Finally, a major focus in the development of DAS subtest content was to ensure as far as possible that children who are being assessed understand what they are supposed to be doing. Young children, and children with developmental disabilities and LDs, often have difficulty in "warming up" to a task and initially understanding the task requirements. For this reason, most of the DAS subtests have demonstration and teaching procedures built into the administration.

Test Materials

The DAS test kit includes two informational volumes: an administration and scoring manual (Elliott, 1990a), and an introductory and technical handbook (Elliott, 1990b). Separate record forms are provided for the Preschool and School-Age levels of the cognitive battery. The kit contains three stimulus books, as well as a variety of consumable booklets and manipulable materials. Materials vary for each subtest. The materials were specifically designed to be varied and engaging for children and students of all

developmental levels. To this end, uniform presentation of subtests (e.g., in an easel format) was not considered acceptable in the design. As a result, the materials are colorful, manipulable, and varied, while being also easy to administer.

At the Preschool level, only one subtest, Recall of Digits, is purely verbally presented, with no additional stimulus materials. At the School-Age level, three subtests are purely verbally presented, with no additional stimulus materials. These are Word Definitions and Similarities, which constitute the Verbal cluster, and Recall of Digits.

The DAS II: Changes in Content and Structure

The basic organizational structure and features of the DAS, outlined above, will be retained in the DAS II, which is currently in development. The following summary states the currently planned differences between the two editions, which are of course subject to revision on the basis of psychologists' feedback and data.

Normative Age Ranges

There is one change of note. The norm overlap for the Upper Preschool and School-Age levels of the DAS will be extended by 1 year. Thus both levels will be administered to all children in the age range 5:0 through 8:11, in contrast with a 2-year norm overlap from 5:0 through 7:11 in the first edition. This will enable psychologists to obtain full normative scores for any 8-year-old for whom Upper Preschool level is considered to be developmentally appropriate.

Existing Subtests

The three brief achievement tests (Basic Number Skills, Spelling, Word Reading) will be dropped in favor of linking the DAS II to the Wechsler Individual Achievement Test—Second Edition (WIAT-II; Psychological Corporation, 2001). To make this possible, 750 students from the DAS II standardization sample will also take the WIAT-II. In addition, correlational data will be obtained between the DAS and two other achievement batteries: the Woodcock–Johnson III Tests of Achievement (WJ III ACH; Woodcock,

McGrew, & Mather, 2001a) and the Kaufman Tests of Educational Achievement—Second Edition (KTEA-II; Kaufman & Kaufman, 2004).

All existing cognitive subtests will be retained. Many subtests will have some item changes or scoring changes as are considered necessary. Such changes will be designed to produce the following, where required: (1) better floors with easier items for younger, less able children; (2) better ceilings with more difficult items for older, more able students; or (3) improvements of *item gradients* (i.e., the progression of item difficulties) including the removal of ambiguous or outdated questions.

A number of other changes are noteworthy:

1. Some subtests will have new artwork, with color rather than black-and-white art being used in Picture Similarities, and in the first set of items for Matrices.

2. The first set of items in Sequential and Quantitative Reasoning will no longer require a disposable booklet on which the child draws his or her responses to each item. Instead, children will be presented with conceptually similar items in color and in a multiple-choice format.

3. Verbal Comprehension, a Preschool subtest whose norms currently stop at age 6:11, will have its ceiling extended so it may be used with children through 8:11.

4. Block Building, a subtest for young children between ages 2:6 and 4:0, will be merged with Pattern Construction. The original DAS standardization item response data for Block Building and Pattern Construction were analyzed in preparation for the DAS II development. These data showed that the Block Building and Pattern Construction subtests measure the same ability dimension. The present Block Building items will form the first item set in DAS II Pattern Construction, thereby giving the new subtest a wider age range and a low floor for young children.

It is planned to prepare a Spanish translation of the subtests contributing to the Special Nonverbal Composite, which includes the Spatial and Nonverbal Reasoning clusters. In addition, pantomimed instructions for these subtests will be developed and validated on a sample of children with hearing impairments.

New DAS II Subtests

1. An additional Nonverbal Reasoning (Gf) subtest will be included at the Upper Preschool level (age range 3:6 through 8:11). This subtest will be a downward extension of Matrices, with all items being pictorial and in color.

2. A Phonological Processing subtest will be included at the School-Age level (age range 5:0 through 21:11). This will consist of items measuring an examinee's ability in segmenting syllables and beginning phonemes, in rhyming, and in blending syllables and phonemes to form words. Colorful pictures will be used to maintain interest in the tasks.

3. A Rapid Naming subtest will be included at the School-Age level (age range 5:0 through 21:11). This task assesses the speed with which a child can access common, previously learned names held in long-term memory. The subtest will present the child with cards showing colored dots, shapes, or pictures in semirandom order. Children will be required to name the colors, shapes, or pictures in the order shown on the card as quickly as possible under timed conditions. Evidence is strong that some poor readers are slow in retrieving names and words from memory.

4. Two new subtests measuring working memory will be included at the School-Age level (age range 5:0 through 21:11). Items such as digits reversed are used in the BAS II, the Wechsler batteries, and the WJ III as measures of working memory. The Wechsler batteries also include Letter–Number Sequencing, and the WJ III has a similar measure including numbers and words. The essential feature of working memory tasks is that they require some transformation, usually in the order, of a list of stimulus words presented to the individual. The DAS II will have two working memory subtests. One will be the familiar Recall of Digits Backward, providing a measure of verbal working memory. The other is a new subtest, Recall of Body Parts. This will require the child to recall verbally lists of names of body parts

(e.g., neck, foot, mouth) in order from the uppermost to the lowest. This novel task is expected to provide a measure of visual-verbal working memory, because visualization of the body and verbal recall are both required.

Factor Structure of DAS II

The inclusion of a pictorial version of Matrices for preschool children is expected to change the factor structure of the DAS at the Upper Preschool level. Currently, the DAS yields two cluster scores (Verbal and Nonverbal) at this level. The inclusion of Matrices, which is expected to form a pair with Picture Similarities, should produce a similar structure of cluster scores for preschool children as for those at school age—namely, Verbal (Gc), Nonverbal Reasoning (Gf), and Spatial (Gv). These clusters at the School-Age level are not expected to change.

The inclusion of the Phonological Processing subtest is expected to provide a measure of *auditory processing* (Ga) in terms of Gf-Gc theory. This subtest will thereby fill a gap in the coverage of Gf-Gc second-order factors that McGrew (1997, p. 160) noted in the DAS. Perhaps more importantly, it will also meet a clinical need for such a test that is relevant to reading acquisition and reading disability.

The new Rapid Naming subtest, a task that is also clearly related to reading acquisition (according to the literature), may cluster with Speed of Information Processing rather than with Phonological Processing when the final data are analyzed, as did similar subtests in the WJ III (McGrew & Woodcock, 2001).

Finally, the two working memory subtests (Recall of Digits Backward and Recall of Body Parts) may form a cluster with Recall of Digits Forward to form a working memory factor, as happened with two similar subtests in the Wechsler Intelligence Scale for Children-Fourth Edition (WISC-IV; Wechsler, 2003). Alternatively, it seems possible that the standardization data may show that Recall of Digits Forward and Recall of Digits Backward form a *verbal* working memory cluster, but that Recall of Body Parts clusters with Recall of Objects to form a *visual–verbal* working memory factor.

PSYCHOMETRIC PROPERTIES

The DAS standardization sample, the norming procedures, and data on the reliability and validity of the battery are by now well known, and are described elsewhere (Elliott, 1990b, 1990c, 1997). The same procedures in sampling and in obtaining a substantial bias oversample will be followed in the standardization of the DAS II.

Accuracy and Reliability

The DAS uses what is termed an *item set* approach to test administration. This is a form of tailored testing that makes the assessment time-efficient while maintaining a high level of accuracy. This approach, and the procedures used in the DAS to achieve accuracy and reliability are described in the DAS handbook (Elliott, 1990b) and in the first edition of this volume (Elliott, 1997).

Specificity

The variance of test scores can be partitioned into a number of components. As described earlier, the *proportion of error variance* may be estimated and is defined as the value of 1 minus the reliability of a test. The *proportion of reliable variance* (i.e., the reliability of the test) may itself be partitioned into two components: *reliable common variance*, which is shared or overlapping with other tests in the battery, and *reliable specific variance*, which is not shared and does not overlap with other tests.

The proportion of common variance (often termed *communality*) may be estimated by the squared multiple correlation between a subtest and all others in the battery (Kaufman, 1979; Silverstein, 1976). The proportion of specific reliable variance is usually termed the *specificity* of a test and is estimated by subtracting the communality from the reliability coefficient of the test.

McGrew and Murphy (1995) consider test specificity to be high when it is (1) .25 or more (indicating that it accounts for 25% or more of the total variance of the test), and (2) greater than the proportion of error variance. Analyses of the specificity of the DAS (Elliott, 1990b, 1997) showed every subtest in the DAS to have high specificity. All specificity values were above .25, the lowest being .30 and the highest .82. Moreover, all subtest specificities substantially exceeded the proportion of error variance. Similarly, the specificities of the cluster scores were high. For the Preschool cognitive battery, the specificities for the Verbal and Nonverbal clusters were .45 and .35, respectively. For the School-Age cognitive battery, the specificities were .47 for the Verbal cluster, .39 for Nonverbal Reasoning, and .49 for the Spatial cluster.

To compare the DAS with other popular cognitive batteries, precisely the same procedure was applied to the analysis of specificity in the following batteries: the BAS II; the Revised version and Third Edition of Wechsler Preschool and Primary Scale of Intelligence (WPPSI-R and WPPSI-III; Wechsler, 1989, 2002); the Revised version, Third Edition, and Fourth Edition of the Wechsler Intelligence Scale for Children (WISC-R, WISC-III, and WISC-IV; Wechsler, 1974, 1991, 2003); the K-ABC (Kaufman & Kaufman, 1983) at preschool and school-age levels; the Kaufman Adolescent and Adult Intelligence Test (KAIT; Kaufman & Kaufman, 1993) for ages 11–19; the Stanford–Binet Intelligence Scale: Fourth Edition (SB-IV; Thorndike, Hagen, & Sattler, 1986) at ages 3–5, 7–11, and 12–17 years; the Woodcock–Johnson Psycho-Educational Battery—Revised Tests of Cognitive Ability (WJ-R COG; Woodcock & Johnson, 1989) at age 4 and at ages 6, 9, and 13 combined; and, finally, the WJ III COG (Woodcock et al., 2001b) at ages 4–5 and 6–13 years. Internal-reliability coefficients and correlation matrices were obtained from the published manuals for the purpose of doing the analyses. In addition to the batteries listed above, results for the Stanford–Binet Intelligence Scales, Fifth Edition (SB5; Roid, 2003) are shown; data provided by Roid and Pomplun (Chapter 15, this volume) were used.

Results are shown in Table 18.5. Those for the WJ-R COG are much the same as results reported in a similar study by McGrew and Murphy (1995). The estimated specificities for the WJ III COG are higher than for the

TABLE 18.5. Specificity of Various Cognitive Batteries

Battery	Mean h^2	Mean e	Mean s	Range of s
DAS Preschool	.34	.19	.47	.31 to .65
DAS School-Age	.34	.16	.50	.30 to .82
BAS II Preschool	.33	.20	.47	.38 to .57
BAS II School-Age	.36	.14	.50	.24 to .82
WPPSI-R	.42	.21	.37	.24 to .47
WPPSI-III	.54	.12	.34	.16 to .51
WISC-R	.42	.22	.36	.22 to .54
WISC-III	.42	.21	.37	.21 to .63
WISC-IV	.47	.15	.38	.18 to .60
K-ABC (preschool)	.44	.19	.37	.23 to .53
K-ABC (school-age)	.48	.17	.35	.22 to .47
KAIT (ages 11–19)	.48	.14	.38	.29 to .47
SB-IV (ages 3–5)	.51	.14	.35	.22 to .45
SB-IV (ages 7–11)	.46	.13	.41	.23 to .55
SB-IV (ages 12–17)	.56	.12	.32	.15 to .42
SB5[a] (ages 2–5)	.59	.13	.28	.14 to .47
SB5[a] (ages 6–10)	.60	.16	.24	.09 to .37
SB5[a] (ages 11–16)	.59	.16	.25	.11 to .41
WJ-R COG (age 4)	.53	.12	.35	.07 to .61
WJ-R COG (ages 6, 9, 13)	.46	.19	.35	.12 to .59
WJ III COG (ages 4–5)	.45	.12	.43	.11 to .63
WJ III COG (ages 6–13)	.40	.15	.44	.00 to .76

Note. h^2, proportion of variance shared with other subtests (communality); e, error variance; s, specificity (proportion of reliable specific variance).
[a]The figures for the SB5 are based on Roid and Pomplun (Chapter 15, this volume).

WJ-R COG, due to a mean increase in reliability combined with a mean decrease in common (shared) variance, the causes of which are unknown. Overall, the results strongly support the conclusion that the DAS and its sister battery, the BAS II, have approximately one-third more reliable specificity than the other batteries. The other batteries show remarkably similar mean specificities—mostly about 35–38% of the total variance (with the exception of two more recently published batteries: the WJ III COG at 43% and 44%, and the SB5 at 24% and 25%). In comparison, the DAS mean specificities of .47 for the Preschool cognitive battery and .50 for the School-Age battery are very high. The lowest values of specificity for the DAS subtests are not much lower than the mean specificities for the other test batteries. These results show the DAS to have about one-third greater specificity than other batteries, and they strongly suggest that the original development goal of a battery with reliable, specific, individually interpretable subtests has been achieved.

Validity

The DAS handbook contains extensive information on the validity of the instrument, using data collected prior to publication in 1992. The chapter on the DAS in the first edition of this volume (Elliott, 1997) presented subsequently published data on (1) an independent confirmatory factor analysis of the DAS standardization data by Keith (1990), (2) joint factor analyses of the DAS and WISC-R, and (3) data on the relationship between the DAS and WISC-III. The present section reports some additional confirmatory factor analyses and correlational data published since 1997. The section concludes with a report and discussion of substantial data on samples of students with LDs or specific reading disabilities.

Confirmatory Factor Analysis of the DAS

We (Keith, Quirk, Schartzer, & Elliott, 1999) examined the question of construct bias in the DAS, using the standardization sample and the bias oversample. The study tested for construct bias for black, Hispanic, and white children through hierarchical, multisample confirmatory factor analysis. Results showed that the DAS measures the same constructs across all three ethnic groups across all age levels of the battery. We concluded that the DAS shows no construct bias, and that users of the battery can have confidence that they are assessing the same abilities for black, Hispanic, or white children and youth.

Dunham, McIntosh, and Gridley (2002) conducted an independent confirmatory factor analysis on DAS data gathered from 130 nondisabled school-age children. Their analyses strongly supported the factorial structure of the battery. The study also found a reasonably good fit with Keith's (1990) model, which included both core and diagnostic subtests.

Relationship of the DAS to the WISC-III, WISC-IV, and WJ-R

Readers are referred to the first edition's chapter on the DAS (Elliott, 1997), which presented data on the relation between the DAS and WISC-III. Data to be reviewed below suggests that students with LDs tend to achieve low scores on the DAS Nonverbal Reasoning (Gf) subtests. The Wechsler scales until recently have not contained measures of fluid reasoning (see Carroll, 1993; Elliott, 1997). With the publication of the WPPSI-III and WISC-IV, they have included a Matrix Reasoning subtest that may provide a single-subtest measure of Gf, even though the subtest is still included in the Perceptual Reasoning factor and appears to load substantially on it. The change of name for that factor from Perceptual Organization to Perceptual Reasoning is perhaps intended to reflect that it represents a mixture of Gv and Gf. Time will tell whether this subtest will enable the Wechsler batteries to pick up the Gf processing difficulty of students with LDs.

No information is provided in the WISC-IV manual (Wechsler, 2003) concerning the relationship between that battery and the DAS.

A small-scale study on the relationship between the DAS and the WJ-R COG standard battery (Woodcock & Johnson, 1989) was reported by Dumont, Willis, Farr, McCarthy, and Price (2000). Eighty-one students who had been referred for a special education evaluation were administered the seven-subtest WJ-R COG battery and the six-subtest

DAS core battery, plus two DAS diagnostic subtests. Both the mean GCA and the mean Nonverbal Reasoning cluster score on the DAS were significantly lower than the WJ-R COG Broad Cognitive Ability score. Correlations between subtests measuring related constructs were low to moderate. In particular, the WJ-R Gv subtest (Visual Closure) bore virtually no relationship to students' scores on the DAS Spatial ability cluster. Although the results of comparisons of the DAS and Wechsler scales suggest the presence of strong common factors, the results from the study of the WJ-R COG and DAS do not. Caution therefore needs to be exercised in comparing results for individuals who have been given these two instruments. Of course, the WJ-R COG has been superseded by the WJ III COG. In the absence of studies, it is presently unknown whether the same conclusions apply to comparisons between the DAS and the WJ III.

INTERPRETATION

Recommendations for Interpreting General, Broad, and Specific Cognitive Abilities

Chapters 4 and 5 in the DAS handbook (Elliott, 1990b) give detailed suggestions about cognitive processes underlying scores on the various DAS subtests and composites, and give a systematic procedure for test interpretation. The procedure is partly based on the identification of scores that are significantly high or low at the .05 probability level. This is greatly facilitated by the design of the summary page of the record form, which shows significant differences at the $p <$ .05 level between achievement tests, composites, and subtest scores.

Other comparisons are made possible by tables in the DAS handbook. In particular, the handbook provides tables enabling discrepancies between observed and predicted achievement to be evaluated, as well as tables showing the frequency or unusualness of discrepancies. Because the development of interpretable subtests was a primary goal of the DAS, the handbook contains extensive interpretive guidelines for subtest scores. (Note: In the DAS standardization sample, 60% of children had one or more subtest scores that were significantly different from the mean core subtest T score, and 7% had 3 or more significantly high or low subtests.)

The chapter on the DAS in the first edition of this volume (Elliott, 1997) also gives an overview of the strategy used in the interpretation of DAS scores, together with some basic interpretations of composite and subtest scores.

Studies Conducted with Samples of Students with LDs

The DAS, with its emphasis on cognitive processes and high subtest specificity, appears well suited to the identification of students with LDs. Federal regulations define an LD as "a disorder in one or more of the basic psychological processes involved in understanding or in using language, spoken or written" (Individuals with Disabilities Education Act [IDEA], 1997).

In practice, students are often identified as having LDs if they show a combination of low achievement and a severe ability–achievement discrepancy (IDEA, 1997). If these were the sole criteria for identifying students with LDs (without additional evidence of any psychological processing deficit), a significant proportion of such students would have relatively flat cognitive profiles, indicating few, if any, specific strengths or weaknesses in cognitive abilities. For such students, ability–achievement discrepancies may have noncognitive causes, perhaps related to motivational or environmental factors. As a result, mixed samples of students with LDs would be expected to contain one or more subgroups with flat cognitive profiles, reflecting noncognitive causative factors. This is so for each of the samples of students with LDs reported below.

A number of studies have been reported on students from the DAS standardization sample, and on those classified as having LDs or specific reading disabilities. These earlier studies all used cluster analysis as the method by which different subgroups of students could be identified, each subgroup having a similar profile of DAS or BAS subtest or composite scores (Elliott, 1989, 1990b; Glutting, McDermott, Konold, Snelbaker, & Watkins, 1998; Holland & McDermott, 1996; Kercher & Sandoval, 1991; McIntosh, 1999; McIntosh & Gridley, 1993; Shapiro, Buckhalt & Herod, 1995;

Tyler & Elliott, 1988). Similar earlier studies on subtest profiles for students assessed on the BAS had been reported (Tyler & Elliott, 1988; Elliott, 1989). Readers are referred to previous reviews of these studies (Elliott, 1997, 2001). All studies using cluster analysis have two problems in common with exploratory factor analysis: (1) They are atheoretical, being purely data-driven; and (2) there is no objective means to determine how many clusters (or factors) to extract. A further problem specific to cluster analysis is that such analyses typically identify several subgroups with flat subtest profiles, the groups being distinguished from each other only by the altitude of subtest scores. Thus one typically finds a subgroup with low scores, one with low average scores, one with high average scores, and so on. This is hardly enlightening! One might as well just use composites such as GCA scores to describe the subgroups.

The following analyses took a different approach to examining patterns of test scores. In this case, different profiles of DAS cluster scores (Verbal, Nonverbal Reasoning, and Spatial) were identified among students with LDs or specific reading disabilities. Four major sources of data were used, as follows:

1. *DAS standardization sample.* This consisted of 2,400 children, ages 6:0 through 17:11. A total of 353 poor readers were identified in this total sample. *Poor readers* were defined as those with DAS Word Reading standard scores below 85. These poor readers were further subdivided into two subsamples: (a) poor readers with no significant discrepancy (86 poor readers whose observed Word Reading score was not significantly lower than that predicted from their GCA), and (b) poor readers with significant discrepancy (267 poor readers whose observed Word Reading score was significantly lower than that predicted from their GCA). This sample provided base rate data (recommended by Glutting, McDermott, Watkins, Kush, & Konold, 1997) against which results from the other two samples could be evaluated.

2. *Clinical sample A: Children with dyslexia.*[1] This sample comprised 160 children with dyslexia by psychologists of the Dyslexia Institute in Great Britain. This sample

had the major advantage from a research perspective that the DAS had not been used in the original diagnostic process to identify these individuals with dyslexia. No information was available as to how much time elapsed between their initial identification and the subsequent DAS assessment. It seems likely that many would have received a considerable period of intervention for their reading difficulties before their DAS assessment. The sample was divided into two subsamples: (a) children with dyslexia whose DAS Word Reading standard scores were below 85, and (b) children with dyslexia whose DAS Word Reading scores were between 85 and 100.

3. *Clinical sample B: Children identified as having LDs.*[2] This sample comprised 53 children identified as having LDs, with the WISC-III used as the initial assessment battery. Once again, this sample had the major advantage that the DAS had not been used in the original diagnostic process to identify these individuals as having LDs. The children in the sample were reevaluated on the DAS 3 years after their initial assessment. Full details of the sample, the procedure, and initial findings are reported by Dumont, Cruse, Price, and Whelley (1996).

4. *Clinical sample C: Children identified as having LDs.*[3] This sample comprised 46 children from Pennsylvania identified as having LDs.

Definition of Subgroups

Children in all three clinical samples were placed into subgroups according to the presence or absence of significant discrepancies between DAS scores that were significant at the 5% confidence level, adjusted for multiple comparisons. The differences were obtained from Tables B.4 and B.5 in the DAS handbook (Elliott, 1990b), and are similar to the 16-point differences indicated on the record form.

The subgroups were defined according to the possible combinations of high and low scores that may be found among the three DAS School-Age clusters, and also included subgroups with flat cluster profiles. Even among poor readers with a significant discrepancy between GCA and Word Reading (or, more properly, between observed Word Reading and Word Reading predicted from the GCA), it would be expected that there would be a proportion of children with flat cognitive test profiles. Poor reading has many causes, and there is no reason to believe that children who have failed to read because of lack of exposure to teaching through absences from school, or because of poor teaching, or because of poor motivation, should have anything other than normal (i.e., flat) cognitive profiles. Other poor readers may have Verbal or Spatial disabilities, both of which are amply reported in the literature (e.g., Snow, Burns, & Griffin, 1998; Rourke, Del Dotto, Rourke, & Casey, 1990). Finally, there may be some whose Nonverbal Reasoning ability is lower than both their Verbal and Spatial abilities. Such a group was identified through cluster analysis by McIntosh and Gridley (1993). I myself have also received many questions and comments during the past several years from psychologists who have observed children with LDs showing this profile pattern. Finally, there may be some individuals who show the reverse pattern, with Nonverbal Reasoning scores higher than both Verbal and Spatial scores, although no research studies have identified such a subgroup. The subgroups in the analyses reported here were therefore as follows:

- *Flat cluster profile*: There were no statistically significant differences among the three DAS cluster scores.
- *Low Spatial, High Verbal*: The Verbal cluster score was significantly higher than the Spatial cluster. This pattern might possibly suggest a nonverbal LD.
- *Low Verbal, High Spatial*: The Verbal cluster score was significantly lower than the Spatial cluster. This has been a typically reported pattern for poor readers (e.g., British Psychological Society, 1999; Snow et al., 1998).
- *High Nonverbal Reasoning*: The Nonverbal Reasoning cluster score was higher than both the Verbal and Spatial scores, and significantly higher than at least one of them. This pattern might signify good ability to process complex auditory–visual information.
- *Low Nonverbal Reasoning*: The Nonverbal Reasoning cluster score was lower than both the Verbal and Spatial scores, and significantly lower than at least one

of them. This might suggest difficulty in processing complex auditory–visual information.

Results

The frequency and percentage of children with each profile are shown in Table 18.6 for the standardization sample, and in Table 18.7 for the three clinical samples of children with dyslexia or LDs. As might be expected from inspection of these two tables, there was a highly significant difference between the frequencies for each profile for the combined clinical samples on the one hand, and the standardization sample on the other. Comparison of the frequencies for each profile for the combined clinical samples and the poor readers with discrepancy, taken from the standardization sample, yielded a chi-square (χ^2) of 49.15 ($df = 4$, $p < .001$). Similarly, comparison of the combined clinical sample and total standardization sample yielded $\chi^2 = 109.49$ ($df = 4$, $p < .001$). The differences accounting for the highest chi-square values were for children with the Low and High Nonverbal Reasoning profiles. Among children identified as having dyslexia or LDs, substantially more than expected had the Low Nonverbal Reasoning profile. Conversely, fewer than expected in these samples had the High Nonverbal Reasoning profile.

Table 18.6 shows estimated base rates of each profile in the school-age population. Fifty percent of the total standardization sample had a flat cluster profile. About 10% fell into the Low Verbal, High Spatial and the Low Spatial, High Verbal groups, respectively. And about 14% of the total sample were in the Low Nonverbal Reasoning and High Nonverbal Reasoning groups, respectively.

As the columns for poor readers indicate, only 3.6% of the total standardization sample were poor readers who had no discrepancy between observed and predicted reading, and 66.3% of them had a flat cluster profile. With a restricted range of GCA scores (54–84), there were relatively few children in this group who showed any significant differences between cluster scores.

Eleven percent of the standardization sample were classified as poor readers with a significant discrepancy between observed and

TABLE 18.6. Number of Students drawn from DAS Standardization Sample with Various Profiles: Normative Data on Base Rates

Type of profile	Poor readers with no discrepancy	Poor readers with discrepancy	Total DAS standardization sample
Flat profile	57	121	1,203
	66.3	**45.3**	**50.1**
Low Spatial, High Verbal	6	16	257
	7.0	**6.0**	**10.7**
Low Verbal, High Spatial	8	63	239
	9.3	**23.6**	**10.0**
High NVR	8	28	355
	9.3	**10.5**	**14.8**
Low NVR	7	39	346
	8.1	**14.6**	**14.4**
Sample sizes	86	267	2,400

Note. NVR, Nonverbal Reasoning. Column percentages are shown in bold type. The term *discrepancy* refers to the presence or absence of a statistically significant difference ($p < .05$) between obtained and predicted Word Reading scores (the prediction was based on the GCA score). The subsamples in the first two columns formed 14.7% of the total standardization sample. Of the 178 poor readers with flat cluster profiles, 35 (19.7%) showed significant differences between their mean core T score and scores on the DAS diagnostic subtests.

predicted reading. As might be expected, this subgroup had a large spread of GCA scores, ranging from 46 to 118. Compared with the total standardization sample, a slightly smaller percentage (45.3%) of these poor readers with a discrepancy showed flat profiles. About a quarter of this subgroup (23.6%), as might be expected, had significantly lower Verbal than Spatial ability, but only 6% of them had the Low Spatial, High Verbal profile. More of these children had the Low Nonverbal Reasoning profile (14.6%) than the High Nonverbal Reasoning profile (10.5%).

Table 18.7 shows the results for the samples with dyslexia and LDs. They are remarkably similar for the three samples, despite the fact that the data were gathered in different countries and in different settings. About one-third to nearly one-half of these samples had flat cluster profiles—fewer than in the standardization sample, but still a substantial proportion. The sample with dyslexia and Word Reading scores below 85 and the Dumont and Kurie samples had 11–15% in the Low Verbal, High Spatial subgroup. This is at least 10% fewer than the number of Low Verbal children in the comparable subgroup from the standardization sample

who were poor readers with ability–achievement discrepancies. One wonders whether Low Verbal children tend not to be identified as having dyslexia or LDs. It seems possible that many such children may be found in inner-city and low socioeconomic environments. They may thereby get special educational services from other sources, such as Title 1 funding. Such children may often be considered to be "garden-variety" poor readers, to use Stanovich's (1988) term, rather than children with dyslexia or LDs. In the Low Spatial, High Verbal subgroup, the clinical samples showed a similar proportion, compared to the base rate, of students with this profile. It is possible that a number of children with this profile have a nonverbal LD (Rourke et al., 1990).

Few children with dyslexia or LDs had a High Nonverbal Reasoning profile—considerably fewer than the proportion in the total DAS sample. However, more than one-third of the children with reading difficulties fell into the Low Nonverbal Reasoning subgroup. Considering the different times and settings when these data were gathered, the results are remarkably similar, providing mutual cross-validation of these findings. The mean profile for the children in this

TABLE 18.7. Number of Students Identified as Having Dyslexia or LDs with Various Profiles

Type of profile	Sample A: Dyslexia, Word Reading below 85	Sample A: Dyslexia, Word Reading 85–100	Sample B: LDs	Sample C: LDs, Word Reading below 85	Sample C: LDs, Word Reading 85–100
Flat profile	28 **34.5**	28 **35.5**	20 **37.7**	8 **29.6**	7 **36.8**
Low Spatial, High Verbal	4 **4.9**	12 **15.2**	5 **9.4**	1 **3.7**	3 **15.8**
Low Verbal, High Spatial	10 **12.3**	7 **8.9**	6 **11.3**	4 **14.8**	3 **15.8**
High NVR	5 **6.2**	4 **5.1**	1 **1.9**	3 **11.1**	0 **0.0**
Low NVR	34 **42.0**	28 **35.4**	21 **39.6**	11 **40.7**	6 **31.6**
Sample sizes	81	79	53	27	19

Note. NVR, Nonverbal Reasoning. Column percentages are shown in bold type. For a description of clinical samples A, B and C, see text. The term *discrepancy* refers to the presence or absence of a statistically significant difference ($p < .05$) between obtained and predicted Word Reading scores (the prediction was based on the GCA score). Of the 56 students in sample A who had flat cluster profiles, 27 (48.2%) showed significant differences between their mean core T score and scores on the DAS diagnostic subtests. Data on children in samples B and C did not include scores for all students on the diagnostic subtests. There was no significant difference in the numbers in each profile group between the two subgroups of sample A (Word Reading below 85 and Word Reading 85–100, $\chi^2 = 5.13$ (*df* = 4, N.S.). There was no significant difference in the numbers in each profile group between the combined subgroups of sample A on the one hand, and the combined groups of samples B and C on the other, $\chi^2 = 0.71$ (*df* = 4, N.S.).

subgroup—those with dyslexia and LDs who had Word Reading scores below 85 (*n* = 66)—is shown in Figure 18.1. The differences between the mean scores were dramatic: Nonverbal Reasoning was lower than both the Verbal and Spatial means by more than 1 *SD*.

Why should children with reading disabilities score poorly on the two DAS subtests measuring Nonverbal Reasoning? The answer seems most plausibly to lie in the nature of the tasks of reading and "nonverbal" reasoning. Reading requires a high level of visual–verbal integration in order to convert visual printed codes into sounds and words. For fluent reading, and for recognition of common words or letter strings, an individual needs information in the auditory–verbal and visual processing systems to be effectively integrated. Similarly, to perform well on the DAS Nonverbal Reasoning tasks (or indeed any good measures of fluid reasoning), one needs good integration of the visual and verbal processing systems. These tasks are presented visually—hence the term *nonverbal* that describes them—but to solve the

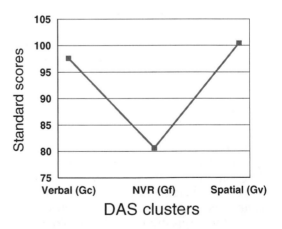

FIGURE 18.1. Mean scores on DAS clusters for 66 students in the Low Nonverbal Reasoning (NVR) subgroup. Note that 34 of the students were from clinical sample A (all with Word Reading scores below 85), 21 were from clinical sample B, and 11 were from clinical sample C (all with Word Reading scores below 85).

problems effectively, the use of internal language to label and to mediate the solution of the problems is generally essential. In the case of an individual who has excellent verbal and spatial abilities, if the two brain processing systems specialized for those abilities do not "talk" to each other effectively, this may have an adverse effect on performance both in reasoning and in reading acquisition.

The findings reported above provide clear evidence of the ability of the DAS to identify distinctive profiles in individuals and groups of students with particular learning difficulties. Readers may wonder why these striking findings, on two independent samples, have not been reported previously for other test batteries. The simple and short answer (because there is insufficient space to elaborate on it) is that no other psychometric battery used with children, with one exception, has three separate measures of Verbal (Gc), Spatial (Gv), and Nonverbal Reasoning (Gf) abilities. The exception is the WJ III, whose Gf measures are described by Mather and Woodcock (2001) as *controlled learning* tasks, and as such differ in a number of important respects from the DAS Nonverbal Reasoning subtests.

INNOVATIONS IN MEASUREMENT OF COGNITIVE ABILITIES

This chapter has presented evidence on the advances in cognitive assessment represented by the DAS. The innovations in the DAS are summarized below.

Innovations in Conceptualization

- The DAS estimates the g factor only by those subtests that are the best estimators of *g*, in contrast to virtually all other cognitive batteries. The DAS does not refer to *g* by the terms *intelligence* and *IQ*, but by the descriptive term *General Conceptual Ability* (GCA).
- The DAS composites reflect three major information-processing systems: Verbal, Spatial (or visual–spatial processing), and Nonverbal Reasoning (Gc, Gv, and Gf in the CHC structure).
- In terms of Gf-Gc theory, the DAS contains measures of auditory short-term memory (Gsm), processing speed (Gs), and intermediate-term visual–verbal memory (Glr), in addition to the core subtest measures of Gc, Gv, and Gf.
- The DAS II will have additional measures of phonological processing (Ga), rapid naming, and working memory, thus completing the representation of the most important group factors in Gf-Gc theory.

Innovations in Content

- The DAS has separate but conormed Preschool and School-Age cognitive batteries that are developmentally appropriate for their respective age levels.
- Materials vary considerably in content, including plenty of manipulables for younger children. The result is a range of appealing and engaging subtests that recapture the child-centered approach and appeal of the old Stanford–Binet Form L-M (Terman & Merrill, 1960).
- The DAS brief achievement battery is completely conormed with the Preschool and School-Age cognitive batteries. This makes the evaluation of ability–achievement discrepancies both easy and objective.
- The relative importance of purely verbal tests has been reduced in the DAS. There are no core subtests for preschool children that are purely verbal (requiring only verbal input and an oral response). At the School-Age level, there are only two such subtests, Similarities and Word Definitions, that form the Verbal cluster. There are no tests of general knowledge, consistent with the aim of reducing culture-specific knowledge.
- The DAS Special Nonverbal Composite provides an estimate of *g* for children with limited verbal abilities, perhaps due to limited English-language experience, hearing impairments, or other difficulties that may have a negative effect on the administration of a verbal test.

Innovations in Technical Quality

- The DAS standardization sample was unusually accurate (Elliott, 1997). No weighting was required to adjust the norms for lack of representativeness.

- The use of the Rasch item response theory model enabled the development of unidimensional, focused subtests of specific abilities. The Rasch model also enabled realistic assessment to be made of the reliability of DAS subtests and composites, with emphasis on assessing the accuracy of individual scores.
- The DAS subtests and cluster scores have higher specificity than those of other batteries, thus supporting their interpretation as measures of specific abilities.
- Extensive additional data were collected to address bias issues. The DAS handbook (Elliott, 1990b) and subsequent research (Keith et al., 1999) provide excellent evidence of the lack of bias of the DAS against minorities.

Innovations in Assessment Procedures

- The item set approach to test administration is a major innovation. It makes the DAS relatively quicker and more time-efficient to administer than scales that require traditional basals and ceilings. It also helps with rapport, because it enables subtests to be discontinued while the child is still succeeding.
- The DAS contains a large number of teaching and unscored items, with modeling of correct responses. This enables children who are inexperienced or unsure of the task requirements to be encouraged to develop an appropriate "set" for the task and minimizes the number of children who fail because they do not understand the nature of the task.
- Out-of-level testing procedures and an extended GCA (taking the lowest GCA score down to 25) are provided for children with LDs and developmental disabilities. Thus a school-age child may be assessed using the Preschool materials if these are considered by the examiner to be more developmentally appropriate.
- The design of scoring procedures on the record form enables statistically significantly high and low scores to be identified immediately. Thus an examiner can have immediate knowledge of significant discrepancies between cluster scores, and between subtests. The handbook also provides frequency information, so the examiner can evaluate the unusualness of discrepancies.
- Ability–achievement discrepancy analysis includes both simple differences between the GCA (or Special Nonverbal Composite) and each of the achievement tests, and also differences between obtained and predicted achievement scores. In this case, predicted achievement is based on the child's GCA or Special Nonverbal Composite score.

BRIEF CASE STUDY

Nico (age 6:11) was referred for assessment because of difficulties and avoidance tendencies he was showing in early reading tasks. He appeared to be bright verbally, and held a good conversation for his age. Also, he had good skills in art and constructional activities for his age. Because of his difficulties, it was decided to administer the Upper Preschool battery, as this was age-appropriate and would probably give him plenty of items on which he could be successful. Because he obtained a high raw score on Verbal Comprehension (which is an out-of-level subtest at this age level), Similarities was also administered from the School-Age battery. In addition, the School-Age subtest Matrices was given to supplement the Gf measure from Picture Similarities in the Upper Preschool battery. His scores on the DAS are shown in Table 18.8.

Although the Upper Preschool battery was administered, cluster scores at the School-Age level were estimated for Spatial ability by using Pattern Construction and Copying (as a substitute for Recall of Designs), and for Nonverbal Reasoning ability by using Picture Similarities (as a substitute for Sequential and Quantitative Reasoning). There are no significant differences between Nico's scores on the two Verbal, the two Nonverbal Reasoning, or the two Spatial subtests. However, his Nonverbal Reasoning cluster score is significantly lower than his Verbal and Spatial cluster scores, thereby making his profile fit that of the Low Nonverbal Reasoning subgroup. His Nonverbal Reasoning and Verbal scores are also significantly lower and higher than his GCA score, respectively, and are consequently marked (L) and (H). His Recall of Objects score is also signifi-

TABLE 18.8. DAS Subtest and Cluster Scores for Nico (Age 6:11).

DAS subtest or cluster	Score
Core subtests (upper preschool battery)	
Verbal Comprehension	54 (replaced by Similarities)
Naming Vocabulary	57
Picture Similarities	40
Pattern Construction	50
Copying	51
Early Number Concepts	52
Additional core subtests (School-Age battery)	
Similarities	60
Matrices	36
Diagnostic subtests	
Recall of Digits	47
Recall of Objects (Immediate)	38 (L)
Recognition of Pictures	49
Clusters (Upper Preschool battery)	
Verbal	114 (H)
Nonverbal	93
GCA	103
Clusters (School-Age battery)	
Nonverbal Reasoning	79 (L)
Spatial	100

Note. In the score column, (L) denotes a statistically significant low score, and (H) a statistically significant high score. Subtest scores have a mean of 10 and *SD* of 15; clusters and composites have a mean of 100 and *SD* of 15.

cantly below the mean of his scores on the core subtests, and is therefore marked (L). As discussed earlier, it seems probable that while Nico has good verbal abilities and average spatial abilities, he has problems in auditory–visual integration that arguably have influenced his acquisition of reading skills.

The question now arises about appropriate intervention methods for students with Low Nonverbal Reasoning profiles. For many years, teachers of children with dyslexia have actively advocated multi-sensory teaching methods, despite research evidence that appeared to discredit auditory–visual integration as a cause of poor reading acquisition (e.g., Bryant, 1968). Teachers appear to have long held to the view that children with dyslexia have difficulty integrating visual and verbal information. The reader will recall the hypothesis that a relative weakness in this ability underlies the Low Nonverbal Reasoning profile found in the samples of children identified as having dyslexia and LDs, reported earlier. Thus it has been recommended that multisensory teaching methods should be used as much as possible in teaching Nico basic literacy skills. Useful references to multisensory teaching approaches are given by Thomson and Watkins (1998), Augur and Briggs (1992), Walker and Brooks (1993), Birsh (1999), and Walker (2000).

CONCLUSION

This chapter has outlined various ways in which the DAS represents an advance in cognitive assessment. In a review of the BAS, the forerunner of the DAS, Embretson (1985) stated: "The BAS is an individual intelligence test with greater scope and psychometric sophistication than the major American individual tests. The test development procedures and norms are laudatory" (p. 232). In another review, Wright and Stone (1985) described the BAS as "a significant advance in mental measurement. . . . Its form and function are a model for contemporary test builders and a preview of the future of test construction" (p. 232). The future, in the form of the DAS, has now arrived! Kamphaus (1993) summarized his account of the battery thus: "There is every indication that the developers of the DAS erred in the direction of quality at every turn. The manual is extraordinarily thorough, the psychometric properties are strong, and the test materials are of high quality" (pp. 320–321). Anastasi and Urbina (1997), reviewing the DAS, wrote that "the DAS is a 'state of the art' instrument of its type, as yet unsurpassed in the possibilities and advantages it affords to users" (p. 232). Sound theory, technical sophistication, and high-quality norms all characterize the DAS and are essential qualities in a good cognitive assessment instrument. Perhaps even more important, the DAS is also engaging for children and time-efficient for the examiner, and it yields a range of subtest and composite scores that are reliable, interpretable, and relevant to children's learning and development. The DAS II, when published, will not only maintain but augment these advances.

NOTES

1. The data for this sample, gathered before 1997, were kindly provided by Martin Turner, Head of Psychology, Dyslexia Institute, Staines, England.
2. The data for this sample, reported by Dumont and colleagues (1996), are used by kind permission of Ron Dumont, Director, MA and PsyD Programs in School Psychology, Fairleigh Dickinson University, Teaneck, New Jersey.
3. The data for this sample, gathered before 2001, were kindly provided by George Kurie, school psychologist, Pennsylvania.

REFERENCES

Anastasi, A., & Urbina, S. (1997). *Psychological testing* (7th ed.). Upper Saddle River, NJ: Prentice Hall.

Augur, J., & Briggs, S. (Eds.). (1992). *The Hickey multisensory language course* (2nd ed.). London: Whurr.

Birsh, J. R. (1999). *Multisensory teaching of basic language skills.* Baltimore: Paul H. Brookes.

British Psychological Society. (1999). *Dyslexia, literacy and psychological assessment* (Report by a working party of the Division of Educational and Child Psychology). Leicester, UK: Author.

Bryant, P. E. (1968). Comments on the design of developmental studies of cross-modal matching and cross-modal transfer. *Cortex, 4,* 127–137.

Carroll, J. B. (1993). *Human cognitive abilities: A survey of factor-analytic studies.* New York: Cambridge University Press.

Carroll, J. B. (2003). The higher-stratum structure of cognitive abilities: Current evidence supports *g* and about ten broad factors. In H. Nyborg (Ed.), *The scientific study of general intelligence: Tribute to Arthur R. Jensen* (pp. 5–22). Amsterdam: Pergamon Press.

Cattell, R. B. (1971). *Abilities: Their structure, growth, and action.* Boston: Houghton Mifflin.

Cattell, R. B., & Horn, J. L. (1978). A check on the theory of fluid and crystallized intelligence with description of new subtest designs. *Journal of Educational Measurement, 15,* 139–164.

Dumont, R. P., Cruse, C. L., Price, L., & Whelley, P. (1996). The relationship between the Differential Ability Scales (DAS) and the Wechsler Intelligence Scale for Children, Third Edition (WISC-III) for students with learning disabilities. *Psychology in the Schools, 33,* 203–209.

Dumont, R. P., Willis, J. O., Farr, L. P., McCarthy, T., & Price, L. (2000). The relationship between the Differential Ability Scales (DAS) and the Woodcock–Johnson Tests of Cognitive Ability—Revised (WJ-R COG) for students referred for special education evaluations. *Journal of Psychoeducational Assessment, 18,* 27–38.

Dunham, M., McIntosh, D., & Gridley, B. E. (2002). An independent confirmatory factor analysis of the Differential Ability Scales. *Journal of Psychoeducational Assessment, 20,* 152–163.

Elliott, C. D. (1983a). *The British Ability Scales: Manual 1. Introductory handbook.* Windsor, UK: NFER-Nelson.

Elliott, C. D. (1983b). *The British Ability Scales: Manual 2. Technical handbook.* Windsor, UK: NFER-Nelson.

Elliott, C. D. (1989). Cognitive profiles of learning disabled children. *British Journal of Developmental Psychology, 7,* 171–178.

Elliott, C. D. (1990a). *Differential Ability Scales.* San Antonio, TX: Psychological Corporation.

Elliott, C. D. (1990b). *Differential Ability Scales: Introductory and technical handbook.* San Antonio, TX: Psychological Corporation.

Elliott, C. D. (1990c). The nature and structure of children's abilities: Evidence from the Differential Ability Scales. *Journal of Psychoeducational Assessment, 8,* 376–390.

Elliott, C. D. (1996). *British Ability Scales—Second Edition.* Windsor, UK: NFER-Nelson.

Elliott, C. D. (1997). The Differential Ability Scales. In D. P. Flanagan, J. L. Genshaft, & P. L. Harrison (Eds.), *Contemporary intellectual assessment: Theories. tests, and issues* (pp. 183–208). New York: Guilford Press.

Elliott, C. D. (2001). Application of the Differential Ability Scales (DAS) and the British Ability Scales, Second Edition (BAS II), for the assessment of learning disabilities. In A. S. Kaufman & N. L. Kaufman (Eds.), *Specific learning disabilities and difficulties in children and adolescents: Psychological assessment and evaluation* (pp. 178–217). New York: Cambridge University Press.

Embretson, S. (1985). Review of the British Ability Scales. In J. V. Mitchell (Ed.), *Ninth mental measurements yearbook* (pp. 231–232). Lincoln: University of Nebraska Press.

Flanagan, D. P., McGrew, K. S., & Ortiz, S. O. (2000). *The Wechsler intelligence scales and Gf-Gc theory.* Boston: Allyn & Bacon.

Glutting, J. J., McDermott, P. A., Konold, T. R., Snelbaker, A. J., & Watkins, M. W. (1998). More ups and downs of subtest analysis: Criterion validity of the DAS with an unselected cohort. *School Psychology Review, 27,* 599–612.

Glutting, J. J., McDermott, P. A., Watkins, M. W., Kush, J. C., & Konold, T. R. (1997). The base rate problem and its consequences for interpreting children's ability profiles. *School Psychology Review, 26,* 176–188.

Gustafsson, J.-E. (1988). Hierarchical models of individual differences in cognitive abilities. In R. J. Sternberg (Ed.), *Advances in the psychology of human intelligence* (Vol. 4, pp. 35–71). Hillsdale, NJ: Erlbaum.

Gustafsson, J.-E. (1989). Broad and narrow abilities in research on learning and instruction. In R. Kanfer, P. L. Ackerman, & R. Cudeck (Eds.), *Abilities, motivation, and methodology: The Minnesota Symposium on Learning and Individual Differences* (pp. 203–237). Hillsdale, NJ: Erlbaum.

Gustafsson, J.-E. (2001). On the hierarchical structure of ability and personality. In J. M. Collis & S. Messick (Eds.), *Intelligence and personality: Bridging the gap in theory and measurement* (pp. 25–42). Mahwah, NJ: Erlbaum.

Härnqvist, K., Gustafsson, J.-E., Muthén, B. O., & Nelson, G. (1994). Hierarchical models of ability at individual and class levels. *Intelligence, 18,* 165–187.

Hitch, G. J., Halliday, S., Schaafstal, A. M., & Schraagen, J. M. C. (1988). Visual working memory in young children. *Memory and Cognition, 16,* 120–132.

Holland, A. M., & McDermott, P. A. (1996). Discovering core profile types in the school-age standardization sample of the Differential Ability Scales. *Journal of Psychoeducational Assessment, 14,* 131–146.

Horn, J. L., & Noll, J. (1997). Human cognitive capabilities: Gf-Gc theory. In D. P. Flanagan, J. L. Genshaft, & P. L. Harrison (Eds.), *Contemporary intellectual assessment: Theories. tests, and issues* (pp. 53–91). New York: Guilford Press.

Individuals with Disabilities Education Act Amendments of 1997, Pub. L. 105-17, 20 U.S.C. 33 (1997). (Department of Education Regulations for IDEA, to be codified at 34 C.F.R. § 300)

Kamphaus, R. W. (1993). *Clinical assessment of children's intelligence: A handbook for professional practice.* Boston: Allyn & Bacon.

Kaufman, A. S. (1979). *Intelligent testing with the WISC-R.* New York: Wiley.

Kaufman, A. S., & Kaufman, N. L. (1983). *Kaufman Assessment Battery for Children.* Circle Pines, MN: American Guidance Service.

Kaufman, A. S., & Kaufman, N. L. (1993). *Kaufman Adolescent and Adult Intelligence Test.* Circle Pines, MN: American Guidance Service.

Kaufman, A. S., & Kaufman, N. L. (2004). *Kaufman Test of Educational Achievement—Second Edition.* Circle Pines, MN: American Guidance Service.

Keith, T. Z. (1990). Confirmatory and hierarchical confirmatory analysis of the Differential Ability Scales. *Journal of Psychoeducational Assessment, 8,* 391–405.

Keith, T. Z., Quirk, K. J., Schartzer, C., & Elliott, C. D. (1999). Construct bias in the Differential Ability Scales?: Confirmatory and hierarchical factor structure across three ethnic groups. *Journal of Psychoeducational Assessment, 17,* 249–268.

Kercher, A. C., & Sandoval, J. (1991). Reading disability and the Differential Ability Scales. *Journal of School Psychology, 29,* 293–307.

Luria, A. R. (1973). *The working brain.* New York: Basic Books.

Mather, N., & Woodcock, R. W. (2001). *Woodcock–Johnson III Tests of Cognitive Abilities: Examiner's manual.* Itasca, IL: Riverside.

McCarthy, R. A., & Warrington, E. K. (1990). *Cognitive neuropsychology: An introduction.* San Diego, CA: Academic Press.

McGrew, K. S. (1997). Analysis of the major intelligence batteries according to a proposed comprehensive Gf-Gc framework. In D. P. Flanagan, J. L. Genshaft, & P. L. Harrison (Eds.), *Contemporary intellectual assessment: Theories, tests, and issues* (pp. 151–179). New York: Guilford Press.

McGrew, K. S., & Murphy, S. (1995). Uniqueness and general factor characteristics of the Woodcock–Johnson Tests of Cognitive Ability—Revised. *Journal of School Psychology, 33,* 235–245.

McGrew, K. S., & Woodcock, R. W. (2001). *Woodcock–Johnson III: Technical manual.* Itasca, IL: Riverside.

McIntosh, D. E. (1999). Identifying at-risk preschoolers: The discriminant validity of the Differential Ability Scales. *Psychology in the Schools, 36,* 1–10.

McIntosh, D. E., & Gridley, B. E. (1993). Differential Ability Scales: Profiles of learning-disabled subtypes. *Psychology in the Schools, 30,* 11–24.

Psychological Corporation. (2001). *Wechsler Individual Achievement Test—Second Edition.* San Antonio, TX: Author.

Roid, G. H. (2003). *Stanford–Binet Intelligence Scales, Fifth Edition.* Itasca, IL: Riverside.

Rourke, B. P., Del Dotto, J. E., Rourke, S. B., & Casey, J. E. (1990). Nonverbal learning disabilities: The syndrome and a case study. *Journal of School Psychology, 28,* 361–385.

Shapiro, S. K., Buckhalt, J. A., & Herod, L. A. (1995). Evaluation of learning disabled students with the Differential Ability Scales (DAS). *Journal of School Psychology, 33,* 247–263.

Silverstein, A. B. (1976). Variance components in the subtests of the WISC-R. *Psychological Reports, 39,* 1109–1110.

Snow, C. E., Burns, M. S., & Griffin, P. (Eds.). (1998). *Preventing reading difficulties in young children.* Washington, DC: National Academy Press.

Springer, S. P., & Deutsch, G. (1989). *Left brain, right brain* (3rd ed.). New York: Freeman.

Stanovich, K. E. (1988). Explaining the differences between the dyslexic and the garden-variety poor reader: The phonological–core variable–difference model. *Journal of Learning Disabilities, 21,* 590–604.

Terman, L. M., & Merrill, M. A. (1960). *Stanford–Binet Intelligence Scale, Form L-M.* Boston: Houghton Mifflin.

Thomson, M. E., & Watkins, E. J. (1998). *Dyslexia: A teaching handbook* (2nd ed.). London: Whurr.

Thorndike, R. L., Hagen, E. P., & Sattler, J. M. (1986). *Stanford–Binet Intelligence Scale: Fourth Edition.* Chicago: Riverside.

Tyler, S., & Elliott, C. D. (1988). Cognitive profiles of groups of poor readers and dyslexic children on the British Ability Scales. *British Journal of Psychology, 79,* 493–508.

Walker, J. (2000). Teaching basic reading and spelling. In J. Townend & M. Turner (Eds.), *Dyslexia in practice: A guide for teachers* (pp. 93–129). New York: Kluwer Academic/Plenum.

Walker, J., & Brooks, L. (1993). *Dyslexia Institute literacy programme.* London: James & James.

Wechsler, D. (1974). *Wechsler Intelligence Scale for Children—Revised.* San Antonio, TX: Psychological Corporation.

Wechsler, D. (1989). *Wechsler Preschool and Primary Scale of Intelligence—Revised.* San Antonio, TX: Psychological Corporation.

Wechsler, D. (1991). *Wechsler Intelligence Scale for Children—Third Edition.* San Antonio, TX: Psychological Corporation.

Wechsler, D. (2002). *Wechsler Preschool and Primary Scale of Intelligence—Third Edition.* San Antonio, TX: Psychological Corporation.

Wechsler, D. (2003). *Wechsler Intelligence Scale for Children—Fourth Edition.* San Antonio, TX: Psychological Corporation.

Woodcock, R. W., & Johnson, M. B. (1989). *Woodcock–Johnson Psycho-Educational Battery—Revised.* Chicago: Riverside.

Woodcock, R. W., McGrew, K. S., & Mather, N. (2001a). *Woodcock–Johnson III Tests of Achievement.* Itasca, IL: Riverside.

Woodcock, R. W., McGrew, K. S., & Mather, N. (2001b). *Woodcock–Johnson III Tests of Cognitive Abilities.* Itasca, IL: Riverside.

Wright, B. D., & Stone, M. H. (1985). Review of the British Ability Scales. In J. V. Mitchell (Ed.), *Ninth mental measurements yearbook* (pp. 232–235). Lincoln: University of Nebraska Press.

19

The Universal Nonverbal Intelligence Test

A Multidimensional Measure of Intelligence

R. STEVE McCALLUM
BRUCE A. BRACKEN

The Universal Nonverbal Intelligence Test (UNIT; Bracken & McCallum, 1998) is a language-free test of cognitive ability; that is, it requires no receptive or expressive language from the examiner or the examinee for administration. The need for nonverbal assessment in the United States is obvious. According to the U.S. Bureau of the Census (2000), 31,844,979 people did not speak English as their primary language, and almost 2,000,000 had no English-speaking ability. According to estimates from the reauthorization of the Individuals with Disabilities Act (IDEA, 1997), nearly one of three (of the nation's 275,000,000 people at that time) was a member of a minority group—either African American, Hispanic, Asian American, or Native American—as of 2000. And, taken together, minority children constitute an ever larger percentage of public school children, particularly in many large cities. For example, minorities constitute an overwhelming percentage of the school population in Miami (approximately 84%), Chicago (89%), and Houston (88%). In addition, the population with limited English proficiency (LEP) population is the fastest-growing in the nation. There are over 200 languages spoken in the greater Chicago area (Pasko, 1994), 140 in California (Unz,

1997), and 61 in Knoxville, Tennessee (S. Forrester, personal communication, March 12, 2002). In fact, in the nation's largest two school districts, students with LEP make up almost half of all students at the kindergarten level. A fact causing concern is that there are discrepancies in the levels of referral and placement of minority children in special education (e.g., although African Americans make up 16% of the population, they constitute 21% of the enrollment in special education). These statistics prompted the framers of the 1997 reauthorization of IDEA to state that "greater efforts are needed to prevent the intensification of problems connected with mislabeling . . . minority children with disabilities" (p. 4). In most U.S. school systems, IQ tests are used as part of the referral-to-placement process. Because existing tests cannot be translated to accommodate all of the languages spoken, nonverbal assessment of these at-risk childrens' intelligence seems like the best and most viable solution. And consistent with this recommendation, IDEA admonishes educators to select and administer technically sound tests that will *not* result in discriminatory practices based on racial or cultural bias.

Similar assessment-related problems exist for children with limited hearing abilities or

425

receptive and expressive language disabilities. Children with severe language-related disabilities are at an unfair disadvantage when assessed by means of spoken language. Consequently, children with such impairments may be more fairly assessed with a comprehensive nonverbal intelligence test.

THEORY AND STRUCTURE OF THE UNIT

The UNIT contains six subtests designed to assess functioning according to a *two-tier model of intelligence* (memory and reasoning), which incorporates *two organizational strategies* (symbolic and nonsymbolic organization). Within each of the two fundamental organizational strategies, the two cognitive abilities of memory and reasoning are assessed in a hierarchical arrangement (see Bracken & McCallum, 1998). The three memory subtests include Object Memory, Spatial Memory, and Symbolic Memory. Similarly, three subtests were developed to assess reasoning; these subtests are Cube Design, Mazes, and Analogic Reasoning. Five of the subtests require minor motoric manipulation, and the remaining subtest (Analogic Reasoning) requires only a pointing response. With two exceptions (Cube Design and Mazes), the subtests that require motoric manipulation can be adapted to allow for a pointing response only, if necessary.

Symbolic organization strategies require the use of concrete and abstract symbols to conceptualize the environment; these symbols are typically language-related (e.g., words), although the symbols may take on any form (e.g., numbers, statistical equations, rebus characters, flags). Symbols are eventually internalized and come to label, mediate, connote, and (over time) make meaningful our experiences. *Nonsymbolic* strategies require the ability to perceive and

make meaningful judgments about the physical relationships within our environment; this ability is symbol-free, or relatively so, and is closer to fluid-like intellectual abilities.

Within each of the two fundamental organizational categories included in the UNIT (nonsymbolic and symbolic), problem solution requires one of two types of abilities—*memory* or *reasoning*. That is, some of the items require primarily symbolic organization and rely heavily on memory (e.g., those included on the Symbolic Memory subtest). Other items require considerable symbolic organization and reasoning skills, but less memory (e.g., those included on the Analogic Reasoning subtest). Some items seem to require nonsymbolic organization strategies and memory primarily (e.g., those on the Spatial Memory subtest). Finally, others may require nonsymbolic organization and reasoning, but *little* memory (Cube Design). Consequently, the UNIT assesses four basic cognitive abilities operationalized by the six subtests (see Figure 19.1).

An existing body of literature supports the rationale for using the four strategies operationalized by the UNIT to assess intelligence. For example, Wechsler (1939) emphasized the importance of distinguishing between highly symbolic (verbal) and nonsymbolic perceptual (performance) means of expressing intelligence. Jensen (1980) provided rationale for a two-tiered hierarchical conceptualization of intelligence, consisting of the two subconstructs of memory (level I) and reasoning (level II). However, in contrast to many of the low-*g*-loaded level I memory tasks designed to require reproduction or recall of simple content, the UNIT memory tasks were developed to require more complex memory functioning.

The theoretical organization of the UNIT is consistent with a number of newly developed instruments that adopt the Gf-Gc

	Memory	Reasoning
Symbolic	Symbolic Memory Object Memory	Analogic Reasoning
Nonsymbolic	Spatial Memory	Cube Design Mazes

FIGURE 19.1. Conceptual model of the UNIT

model of fluid and crystallized abilities (more recently known as the *Cattell–Horn–Carroll* [CHC] model), as described by Cattell (1963), Horn (1968), Carroll (1993), and others (e.g., Woodcock, 1990; Woodcock, McGrew, & Mather, 2001). (See also Horn & Blankson, Chapter 3, Carroll, Chapter 4, and McGrew, Chapter 8, this volume.) UNIT subtests tap components of strata I and II within this model, including *fluid reasoning, general sequential reasoning, visual processing, visual memory, spatial scanning, spatial relations,* and *induction.*

Intelligence consists primarily of a pervasive and fundamental ability, g, which provides a base for the development of somewhat unique specialized skills. Although there are many means of determining intelligence, it makes little sense to conceptualize intelligence as being either verbal or nonverbal. Rather, there are verbal and nonverbal means available to assess intelligence. Consequently, the UNIT should be considered a nonverbal measure of intelligence, not a measure of nonverbal intelligence, and was designed to be a strong measure of g.

DESCRIPTION OF THE UNIT SUBTESTS

As a result of the 2 × 2 structural scheme, several scores can be calculated for the UNIT total test, including a Full Scale IQ (FSIQ), Memory Quotient, Reasoning Quotient, Symbolic Quotient, and Nonsymbolic Quotient. Finally, individual subtest scores can be derived for each of the six subtests for further analysis of examinee's performance. UNIT subtests are described below. The first three subtests are designed to assess memory, the second three reasoning.

1. *Symbolic Memory.* The examinee recalls and recreates sequences of visually presented universal symbols (e.g., green boy, black woman).
2. *Spatial Memory.* The examinee must remember and recreate the placement of black and/or green chips on a 3 × 3 or 4 × 4 cell grid.
3. *Object Memory.* The examinee is shown a visual array of common objects (e.g., shoe, telephone, tree) for 5 seconds, after which he or she identifies the pictured ob-

jects from a larger array of pictured objects.
4. *Cube Design.* The examinee completes a three-dimensional block design task, using between one and nine green and white blocks.
5. *Analogic Reasoning.* The examinee completes a matrix analogies task using common objects (e.g., hand/glove, foot/_____?) and novel geometric figures.
6. *Mazes.* The examinee completes a maze task by tracing a path through each maze from the center starting point to an exit.

ADMINISTRATION AND SCORING

Administration

Completion of all six subtests requires approximately 45–50 minutes. UNIT norms allow for two- and four-subtest short-form batteries, in addition to the full six subtest battery. The shorter batteries require approximately one-third to two-thirds less time.

Although administration of the UNIT subtest is 100% nonverbal, the examiner may communicate with the examinee (if they have a common language) to establish rapport, discuss extratest issues, and the like, as well as to reduce the awkwardness that may otherwise occur with a nonverbal interaction. The examiner must present the UNIT stimuli nonverbally, using eight nonverbal gestures that were used during standardization and are presented in the manual (as well as on a training video available from the publisher). To aid in teaching task demands, the examiner is instructed to make liberal use of demonstration items, sample items, and so-called "checkpoint" items; checkpoint items allow feedback, but are scored.

For the Symbolic Memory subtest, stimulus plates are presented on an easel. The easel contains plates showing pictures of one or more of the following universal human figures, in a particular order: a green baby, a black baby, a green girl, a black girl, a green boy, a black boy, a green woman, a black woman, a green man, a black man. The examinee is presented the stimulus plate and then is instructed through gestures to replicate the order shown on the stimulus plate. The examinee uses 1½" × 1½" response cards, each containing one of the universal human figures, to reproduce the array depicted on the stimulus plate. The task has no time limits other than a 5-second exposure time. Each correct item is assigned 1-point credit, and color, gender, and size are critical variables for scoring.

For the Spatial Memory subtest, the examiner briefly presents a series of grids on stimulus plates located on an administration easel. The grids show one or more green or black polka dots placed within cells (on the grid). The less difficult items use a 3×3 grid; the more difficult items require a 4×4 grid. The stimulus plate is shown for 5 seconds and then is removed from view. The examinee places response chips on a blank grid that is placed on the table top in front of him or her. Spatial Memory has no time limits, except for the 5-second exposure. Each correct response is assigned 1-point credit.

The Object Memory subtest requires presentation of pictures of common objects arranged on stimulus plates located on an administration easel. The easel is laid flat on the table, and the examinee is shown a plate containing pictures of one or more objects for 5 seconds; then the examinee is shown a second plate containing pictures from the first plate *and* pictures of distractor objects. The examinee identifies pictures on the second plate that were shown on the first plate; to create a semipermanent response, the examinee places black chips on the pictures selected. This memory task is not timed, other than the 5-second exposure. Each correct object identified on the response place is assigned 1-point credit.

The Cube Design subtest requires the examinee to use up to nine cubes to replicate three-dimensional designs shown on a stimulus plate. Each cube has six facets: two white sides, two green sides, and two sides that contain diagonals (triangles), one green and one white. These cubes can be arranged to replicate the three-dimensional figures depicted on the stimulus plates. This task is timed, but the time limits are liberal, to emphasize assessment of ability rather than speed. Except for the very early items, which are scored either correct or incorrect and yield a maximum of 1 point per item, examinees may earn up to 3 points (per item). Each facet of the three-dimensional construction is judged to be either correct or in-

correct. Each correct facet is assigned 1-point credit.

The Analogic Reasoning subtest requires the examinee to solve analogies presented in a matrix format. The examinee is directed to indicate which one of several options best completes a two-cell or a four-cell analogy. Task solution requires the examinee to determine the relationships between objects. For example, in a four-cell matrix, the first cell may depict a fish and the second water; the third cell may show a bird, and the fourth cell is blank. The examinee selects from several options the picture that best completes the matrix. In this case, a picture of the sky is a correct response. This reasoning subtest is not timed. Each correct response is assigned 1-point credit.

The Mazes subtest requires the examinee to complete a maze using a #2 lead pencil, minus the eraser. The examinee is presented with a maze showing a mouse in the center and one or more pieces of cheese on the outside of the maze. The cheese depicts one or more possible exits from the maze. The task is to determine the correct path from the center to the (correct) piece of cheese. The examinee is stopped after the first error. The task is timed, though the time limits are quite liberal. Each decision point is scored, and correct decisions are assigned 1-point credit.

Materials and Scoring

General materials required to administer the UNIT include a stopwatch, a #2 lead pencil, two test booklets (one for the Mazes subtest and one for recording the student's performance on the remaining five subtests), and relevant demographic information. Except for Mazes and Object Memory (optional subtests, to be administered as part of the Extended Battery only), the stimulus plates for all subtests are contained in one stand-up easel. Object Memory stimuli are presented on a small separate easel, if needed. The larger easel containing the four Standard Battery subtests contains subtest stimuli printed on front and back for efficiency and economy; colored tabs are provided to inform the examiner as to the direction of administration (e.g., tabs with subtest names in green alert the examiner that the book is oriented in the correct direction for those subtests).

Scoring is simple and straightforward. Raw scores for each item are summed to provide a subtest total raw score. Raw scores are easily transformed to standard scores with either the tables provided in the UNIT manual (Bracken & McCallum, 1998) or the UNIT Compuscore software (Bracken & McCallum, 2001). The Abbreviated Battery is used for screening purposes (Symbolic Memory and Cube Design); the Standard Battery for most purposes that include placement decisions (the Abbreviated Battery subtests, plus Spatial Memory, Matrix Analogies); and the Extended Battery for diagnostic purposes (the Standard Battery subtests, plus Object Memory and Mazes).

PSYCHOMETRIC PROPERTIES

Norming Procedures, Standardization Characteristics, and Technical Data

Standardization data were collected from a representative sample of 2,100 children and adolescents ranging in age from 5 years, 0 months to 17 years, 11 months. These children and adolescents were carefully selected to represent the U.S. population in terms of age, sex, race, parent educational attainment, community size, geographic region, and ethnicity (see sample-to-population match data in the UNIT manual). Importantly, children and adolescents from special education categories were included to the extent that these individuals were present in the school population.

Readers are urged to consult the UNIT manual for results of numerous special studies conducted to assess UNIT technical adequacy, including reliability, validity, and fairness data for a variety of populations. We summarize some of the most important data from the manual in the next paragraph, followed by summaries of results of studies conducted after the manual was published.

According to the manual, UNIT reliability data are strong; the average composite scale reliability coefficients average range from .86 to .96 for the typical and clinical/exceptional samples across all batteries. The FSIQ reliability coefficients range from .91 to .93. Test–retest stability coefficients (corrected for restriction in range) range from .79 to .84 for IQs for a sample of 197 participants. Average test–retest practice effects (approximately 3 weeks) are 7.2 for the Abbreviated Battery, 5.0 for the Standard Battery, and 4.8 for the Extended Battery. Validity data are supportive of the model as well. For example, expected raw score age progressions for Cube Design are 13, 19, 26, and 33 for the groups ages 5–7, 8–10, 11–13, and 14–17 years, respectively. Exploratory and confirmatory factor-analytic data have provided evidence to support the UNIT model. Using the standardization data, an exploratory analysis yielded a large first eigenvalue, 2.33; other values were below 1.0. These findings suggest the presence of a strong first factor, commensurate with the interpretation of the FSIQ as a good overall index of global intellectual ability, or g. The factor structure also supports the two-factor memory and reasoning model, particularly for the Standard Battery. When the Extended Battery subtests were factor-analyzed, all subtests loaded appropriately, although the Mazes subtest yielded a borderline low loading on the reasoning factor. Confirmatory factor-analytic procedures were equally supportive, showing strong fit statistics for a two-factor memory and reasoning model. Strong concurrent data are also reported in the manual. For example, data from a sample of 61 children with learning disabilities yielded correlation coefficients (corrected for restriction in range) between the FSIQs from the three UNIT batteries and the Wechsler Intelligence Scale for Children—Third Edition (WISC-III; Wechsler, 1991) FSIQ; from .78 to .84, and from .84 to .88 for a sample of 59 children with mental retardation. Strong coefficients were obtained, showing the relationship between UNIT and other instruments for various populations (e.g., Native Americans). Coefficients between the UNIT IQs and scores from the Bateria-R (Woodcock & Muñoz-Sandoval, 1996) are more variable. Corrected coefficients between the three UNIT FSIQs and the Bateria-R Broad Cognitive Ability score (Standard Battery) ranged from .30 to .67 for 27 Spanish-speaking bilingual education students. Additional current validity data are available from the manual (e.g., correlations with Raven's [1960] Progressive Matrices). In general, predictive validity coefficients obtained between the UNIT and various achievement tests are relatively strong, and comparable to those between language-loaded tests and achievement measures. An interesting finding from the studies reported in the UNIT manual is that the magnitude of the coefficients between the UNIT global Symbolic Quotient and measures of language-based achievement (e.g., reading subtests) is often higher than the magnitude of coefficients between the UNIT Nonsymbolic Quotient and these language-loaded achievement measures. In fact, this pattern is found in 21 out of 36 comparisons (58%). This pattern would be predicted from the nature of the symbolic–nonsymbolic distinction, and provides some additional evidence of predictive and construct validity of the test model.

Since the publication of the UNIT, results from several independent studies have become available showing relevant technical data. For example, Hooper (2002) has explored the relationship between the Leiter International Performance Scale—Revised (Leiter-R; Roid & Miller, 1997) and the UNIT for 100 elementary and middle school students. Correlation coefficients obtained from the comparison of the Leiter-R FSIQ and Fluid Reasoning scale and all UNIT global scales (Memory, Reasoning, Symbolic, and Nonsymbolic Quotients) are statistically significant ($p < .01$) and range from .33 for the UNIT Memory Quotient versus Leiter-R Fluid Reasoning comparison to .72 for the UNIT FSIQ versus Leiter-R FSIQ comparison. Importantly, global scale means for the two tests are similar generally, although the UNIT FSIQ is approximately 5 points higher than the Leiter-R FSIQ. The other mean global scores are more similar in magnitude across the two tests; the UNIT means range from 101.54 to 103.67, and the Leiter-R Fluid Reasoning score is 99.07.

Hooper (2002) has also reported correlation coefficients ranging from .49 to .72 between the four UNIT global scores and end-of-the-year scores from the Total Reading, Total Math, and Total Language scores of the Comprehensive Test of Basic Skills (CTBS/McGraw-Hill, 1996) for 100 elementary and middle school children. Using stepwise multiple-regression analyses, Hooper found that the UNIT FSIQ predicted all three academic areas from the CTBS better than the Leiter-R FSIQ; the UNIT FSIQ entered the multiple-regression equation first, accounting for 39–55% of the variance in the three criterion scores, and the Leiter-R contributed an additional 1–2% for each.

Farrell and Phelps (2000) have compared scores from the Leiter-R and the UNIT for 43 elementary and middle school children with severe language disorders. Correlation coefficients between the UNIT quotients and Leiter-R Fluid Reasoning scale scores range from .65 to .67; the coefficients between UNIT quotients and Leiter-R Visualization Reasoning scale scores range from .73 to .80. For this sample, Leiter-R mean scores are 65.07 and 66.33 for the Fluid Reasoning and Visualization Reasoning scales, respectively. UNIT global scale scores range from 66.71 (FSIQ) to 70 (Symbolic Quotient). The authors conclude that both tests show promise for providing fair and valid assessment of cognitive functioning for children with severe language impairments, and that both should be considered superior to conventional language-loaded tests (e.g., the Kaufman Assessment Battery for Children and WISC-III) for use with this population.

Scardapane, Egan, Torres-Gallegos, Levine, and Owens (2002) have investigated the relationship among the UNIT, the Wide Range Intelligence Test (WRIT; Glutting, Adams, & Sheslow, 2000), and the Gifted and Talented Evaluation Scales (GATES; Gilliam, Carpenter, & Christensen, 1996) for English-speaking children and English-language learners. The correlation coefficient obtained between the WRIT Visual scale and the UNIT FSIQ of .59 can be compared to the coefficient between the UNIT FSIQ and the WRIT Verbal scale of .11. Contrary to the authors' predictions, the coefficients showing the relationship between the GATES scores and the WRIT Verbal scale are not higher than the coefficients showing relationships between the UNIT FSIQ and the four GATES scores. The coefficients between the UNIT FSIQ and the GATES scales of Intellectual Ability, Academic Skills, Creativity, Leadership, and Artistic Talent range from .50 to .57 ($p < .05$); the coefficients between the WRIT Verbal scale and these GATES scores range from .004 to .10 ($p > .05$). The authors conclude that their data support the use of the UNIT as a nonverbal measure of intelligence.

Fairness

Because of an increasingly diverse society and the need to ensure sensitive and equally valid assessment for a wide variety of populations, authors of new instruments are charged with ensuring that their instruments are as fair as possible. The UNIT manual includes an entire chapter entitled "Fairness," and describes extensive efforts to ensure that the test is appropriate for use for all children in the United States (i.e., that construct-irrelevant variance is minimized for all relevant populations). (Also see McCallum, 1999, for additional descriptions of efforts to ensure fairness for the UNIT.)

The test model was formulated, and the test was developed, on the basis of five core fairness concepts: (1) A language-free test is less susceptible to bias than a language-loaded test; (2) A multidimensional measure of cognition is fairer than a unidimensional one; (3) a test that minimizes the influence of acquired knowledge (i.e., crystallized ability) is fairer than one that does not; (4) a test that minimizes speeded performance is fairer than one with greater emphasis on speed; and (5) a test that relies on a variety of response modes is more motivating and thereby fairer than one relying on a unidimensional response mode. Several other steps were taken to ensure fairness. For example, in the initial item development phase, items were submitted to a panel of "bias experts"—individuals sensitive to inclusion of items that might be offensive to or more difficult for individuals within certain populations (e.g., Native Americans, Hispanics). Items identified by these individuals, and those identified via statistical item bias analyses, were removed.

A number of statistical procedures were undertaken to help ensure fairness, including calculation of separate reliabilities, factor structure statistics, mean-difference analyses, and so forth. for subpopulations. Reliabilities for FSIQs for females, males, African Americans, and Hispanic Americans were all greater than .91 (uncorrected) and .94 (corrected) for the Abbreviated Battery, and greater than .95 for the Standard and Extended Battery. Separate confirmatory factor analyses for these subpopulations have provided evidence for "a single general intelli-gence factor as well as the primary and secondary scales," as well as "evidence supporting the construct validity of the UNIT across sex, race, and ethnic groups" (Bracken & McCallum, 1998, p. 182).

Mean IQ difference analyses using matched groups from the UNIT standardization data have also provided evidence of fairness, as reported in the manual. The mean scores of males and females matched on age, parent educational level, and ethnicity were very similar, with effect sizes ranging from .02 to .03 across all three batteries. Mean differences, estimated via effect sizes, ranged from .22 to .43 for FSIQs across all batteries for Native Americans matched on age, sex, and parent educational levels; the largest mean difference, 6.50, was obtained from the Standard Battery. Mean differences of FSIQs, reflected via effect sizes, ranged from .10 to .14 for matched Hispanic Americans across all batteries; the largest difference, 2.13, occurred on the Standard Battery. Effect sizes for matched African Americans ranged from .51 to .65; a mean FSIQ difference of 8.63 between African Americans and European Americans was obtained using the Standard Battery. A mean FSIQ Standard Battery difference of 6.20 was found between examinees with deafness/hearing impairments and a matched nonimpaired sample; a Standard Battery FSIQ mean difference of 5.33 was found between Ecuadorian and matched non-Ecuadorian examinees. Evidence that prediction is not a function of gender and racial membership was provided by using the regression slope as a measure of the strength of the relationships between UNIT scores and achievement on the Woodcock–Johnson Psycho-Educational Battery—Revised Achievement Battery subtests in a regression equation; race and sex did not contribute significantly to the prediction ($p > .05$).

In a recent study using UNIT standardization data but applying a matching strategy more refined than the one reported in the manual, Upson (2003) found a further reduction of mean difference scores between Hispanic Americans and European Americans (i.e., white non-Hispanics). Matching on all relevant variables reported in the manual *and* community size *and* the educational level of both parents, rather than just one, reduced the mean differences between matched Hispanic Americans and European Americans considerably for the Standard Battery FSIQ, from 2.13 to 0.47. Although further refinement reduced the African American and European Americans differences slightly, the reductions were not as pronounced. The Standard Battery FSIQ difference of 8.51 for 168 matched African Americans and European Americans is only slightly smaller than the 8.63 reported in the manual.

Additional data generated after the UNIT was developed also have relevance for UNIT fairness. For example, Maller (2000) conducted a sophisticated item analysis, using the Mantel–Haenszel (MH) procedure and item response theory (IRT), to detect differential item functioning (DIF) for 104 children and adolescents with deafness/hearing impairments. Using a group of children from the UNIT standardization sample matched on age, gender, and ethnicity to these 104 youngsters, she concluded that no items in the UNIT exhibited DIF when either the MH procedure or IRT was used; that is, the probability of a correct response on the UNIT items does not seem to be affected by hearing status. Consequently, she notes that the UNIT seems appropriate for this population, and there may be no need to develop special norms for children with deafness/hearing impairments. Additional evidence for this conclusion is provided by Krivitski (2000). She compared children with deafness to a matched sample of hearing children from the UNIT standardization sample; the children were matched on age, race/ethnicity, socioeconomic status, and gender. Results of a profile analysis showed that the children with deafness displayed similar patterns of UNIT subtest performance. Krivitski concludes that the data support use of the UNIT for children with deafness.

Although the preponderance of data from the literature is supportive of the use of the UNIT for non-English-speaking children, not all the studies are so positive. Jimenez (2001) reports that the internal consistency reliability for five of the six UNIT subtests "failed to show acceptable internal consistency" and did not reach "the recommended coefficient of .90" (p. 5424B) for test–retest stability for 60 Puerto Rican children. The UNIT correlation coefficients with the Bateria-R Reading cluster were "moderate to low" for these children. Finally, they scored almost one-half standard deviation lower than a matched control group of non-Hispanic children. Jimenez concludes that although the UNIT may be a fair instrument to measure cognitive abilities of Puerto Rican children, it may not be optimal when used in isolation, and should be part of a multifaceted assessment process.

Athanasiou (2000) has compared five nonverbal assessment instruments for psychometric integrity and fairness, including the UNIT. She concludes that all have unique strengths and weaknesses. Although she notes that the UNIT fails to meet Bracken's (1987) criterion for test–retest stability (.90) at all ages, her assessment of the UNIT is mostly favorable. For example, she comments that the UNIT's reliance on only nonverbal directions is likely to reduce the potential for cultural bias in administration; the use of checkpoint items allows for periodic assessment of understanding during the administration; presentation of psychometric properties of subpopulations enhances the confidence users can have that the test is appropriate for a variety of examinees; and the floors, ceilings, and item gradients for the UNIT Standard and Extended Batteries exceed minimum recommendations. But perhaps the most important observation Athanasiou offers regarding the UNIT addresses the extent to which the manual provides evidence of test fairness. She notes that all five of the tests she reviewed are generally impressive in terms of their technical adequacy, but "as a whole they present much less statistical evidence of test fairness. The UNIT appears to be an unqualified exception to this statement," and the UNIT is the only test "to provide evidence of consistent factor structure across subgroups" (p. 227).

Fives and Flanagan (2002) conclude their extensive review of the UNIT by noting that the test is well constructed, theoretically driven, psychometrically sound, and highly useful, and that its use will permit more effective assessment of some traditionally difficult to assess populations. They conclude their review by presenting a case study illustrating use of the UNIT for a 12-year-old Hispanic female. Her UNIT IQ scores were higher than those obtained from more language-loaded tests, even those typically considered to assess nonverbal performance and fluid abilities; the authors conclude, "Had this particular youngster not been given the UNIT, an error might have been made and she might not have been classified learning disabled and received appropriate services" (p. 445).

Additional reviews by Bandalos (2001), Kamphaus (2001), and Sattler (2001) are generally positive, particularly regarding basic technical properties (e.g., reliability, floors, ceilings). Bandalos concludes a review reported in the Buros Institute's *Mental Measurement Yearbook* by noting that the UNIT provides a "much needed means of obtaining reliable and valid assessments of intelligence for children with a wide array of disabilities who cannot be tested accurately with existing instruments. It is a carefully developed instrument with excellent reliability and impressive evidence of validity for use as supplement to or substitute for more traditional measures such as the WISC-III" (p. 1298). All these reviewers note the need for certain types of validity studies, particularly those investigating the construct validity of symbolic and nonsymbolic processing and the ability of the UNIT to predict grades and/or classroom achievement.

INTERPRETING THE UNIT

Multidimensional test interpretation is complicated, partly because it is requires that examiners engage in a number of steps, consult numerous tables, consider a variety of cognitive models, consider carefully the limitations of the instruments they use, and (finally and most importantly) make the test results relevant for real-world application. In addition to traditional normative interpretation, there are at least three other interpretive models available: *traditional ipsative strategies*, *subtest profile base rate analyses*, and *cross-battery assessment* (CBA). Traditional ipsative interpretation is controversial, but is still used by practitioners who want to get more from the instruments they use than the good predictive capabilities of an FSIQ. The goal of ipsative interpretation is to uncover relationships between cognitive strengths and weaknesses and these important academic and work-related skills. Consequently, we first describe traditional ipsative strategies, followed by brief descriptions of subtest

base rate profile analyses and CBA. Citations are provided for more specific guidelines for all three methods.

Ipsative Interpretation

Because the UNIT is multidimensional, interpretation requires multiple steps. General steps for interpretation are discussed below, followed by a discussion of three specific interpretive procedures. The following guidelines are based on the psychometric strengths expressed in the UNIT manual, and detailed guidelines are provided there and on the Compuscore scoring and interpretation software (Bracken & McCallum, 2001), available from the publisher. Because of space limitations, the guidelines are presented in brief form here.

1. First, the UNIT composite or global scores should be interpreted within a normative context. The most global score, the FSIQ, should be interpreted according to its relative standing in the population, using standard scores, percentile ranks, age equivalents, and so on as indications of performance. For multidimensional tests like the UNIT, it is useful to provide some statement regarding the representativeness of the score; that is, does the FSIQ represent the examinee's overall intellectual functioning well, as operationalized by the test? Then the examiner should consider the next level of global scores, the scale scores (i.e., Reasoning Quotient, Memory Quotient, Symbolic Quotient, or Nonsymbolic Quotient). Are these scores comparable, or do they deviate significantly from one another? If these scores show considerable variability, the most global score may not represent the examinee's overall intellectual functioning very well. Considerable scatter in global and subtest scores reveals a profile with peaks and valleys, and corresponding cognitive strengths and weaknesses. These weaknesses should be determined by examining the magnitude of differences, using statistical significance and frequency-of-occurrence data.

2. The band of error of the UNIT FSIQ should be communicated next. Typically, the most reliable single score from *any* multidimensional test is the total or composite score. This global score should be considered within a band of confidence framed by one

or more standard errors of measurement, determined by the level of significance desired.

3. Step 3 provides elaboration of step 1 and a transition to the more specific interpretative procedures described below. In step 3, all UNIT standard scores should be compared *systematically*. As stated above in step 1, if UNIT scale (global) scores are highly variable (i.e., if there are statistically significant differences among them), the composite score cannot be considered to be representative of the examinee's overall intellectual functioning. On the other hand, if there is little variability (i.e., nonsignificant amounts of variability), the composite score may be considered as a reasonable estimate of the examinee's overall functioning.

Further description of the examinee's performance should be given at this point. For example, the examiner may provide additional information about the nature of the UNIT, and the abilities presumed to be measured by the instrument; in addition, the examiner may indicate that the examinee's abilities in particular areas as measured by the test (e.g., short-term memory, reasoning) are uniformly developed (or not, as the case may be). The examinee's overall level of ability should be described, and inferences about the examinee's prognosis for achievement can be made. If qualitative (e.g., intrasubtest scatter) and quantitative (i.e., variable scores) data show variability in the examinee's performance, further analyses should be performed to determine unique intrachild (ipsative) strengths and weaknesses.

More specific interpretation is possible with three other procedures (after McCallum & Whitaker, 2000), depending on the nature of the score variability. These three interpretive procedures include (1) the *pooled procedure*, (2) the *independent-factors procedure*, and (3) the *rational–intuitive procedure*. The pooled procedure is the first of the three techniques discussed. It requires computing the mean of all six UNIT subtests and individually comparing each subtest score to that mean to identify so-called "outliers" (i.e., scores which differ significantly from the overall subtest mean). The independent-factors procedure is so named because it relies on interpretation based on the (independent-factor) factor-analytic structure of the UNIT. More specifically, it is based on

the factor structure obtained by maximizing the independence of the factors constituting the test. For the UNIT, the best factor-analytic solution from currently available data shows a good two-factor model (i.e., the best factor solution appears to reveal a three-subtest memory factor and a three-subtest reasoning factor). Thus the examiner should first look for the pattern of consistently higher memory (over reasoning) subtests, or the reverse, assuming little within-factor variance. The rational–intuitive procedure is so named because it relies on the interpretation of a multidimensional test based on the theoretical model that underpins the development of a test, or on other theoretical models of which the examiner is aware. In this case, users of the UNIT may find that some children will perform well on all the symbolic subtests relative to the nonsymbolic subtests, or vice versa. Examiners should keep in mind that other cognitive models can be applied to ipsative interpretation.

Base Rate Interpretation

Glutting, McDermott, and Konold (1997) presented a model of interpretation using subtest profile base rate analysis as a beginning point to interpret WISC-III performance. That is, they described procedures that allow an examiner to determine the extent to which an examinee's profile of subtest scores is rare in the population. First, they applied sophisticated statistical techniques to calculate common profiles in the WISC-III standardization data, and then made those profiles available to test users. Next, they provided examiners with a set of relatively straightforward calculations allowing them to determine the likelihood that a particular profile matches one or more of these common profiles. Glutting and colleagues argued that unusual profiles are more likely to have clinical significance than those that occur often in the population.

Following the logic described by Glutting and colleagues (1997), Wilhoit and McCallum (2002) have provided the information examiners need to apply the base rate method to analysis of UNIT scores. Although the base rate analysis is not particularly complicated to use, deriving the data necessary to obtain common or typical profiles is. Wilhoit and

McCallum describe the lengthy cluster analysis procedures used to provide those profiles from the UNIT standardization data. Via cluster analyses, six common profiles were identified for the Standard Battery (i.e., delayed, low average, average, above average with high Memory and Symbolic Quotients, above average with high Reasoning and Nonsymbolic Quotients, and superior) and seven for the Extended Battery (i.e., delayed, low average with higher Memory and Symbolic than Reasoning and Nonsymbolic Quotients, low average with higher Reasoning and Nonsymbolic than Memory and Symbolic Quotients, average with higher Memory and Symbolic than Reasoning and Nonsymbolic Quotients, average, high average, and superior). Specific demographics are associated with each of these profiles (e.g., percentage of females, males, African Americans, European Americans, family educational levels). Because these profiles are considered typical, profiles of examinees that "fit" one of them may not be diagnostic, according to the logic from Glutting and colleagues. Examiners can determine the fit by following a few easy steps. First, each of the examinee's subtest scores is subtracted from the like subtest scores provided from the profiles in the relevant table with the closest FSIQ. These scores are squared and summed to produce a score that can be compared to a critical value (i.e., 272 for the Standard Battery and 307 for the Extended Battery). This procedure is repeated for the three profiles with FSIQs closest to the examinee's obtained FSIQ. If the obtained score from any one of these comparisons is equal to or larger than the critical value, the obtained profile is considered rare in the population, and thus potentially diagnostic. To obtain the FSIQs and subtest scores for the common profiles for both Standard and Extended Batteries, see Tables 2, 3, 5, and 6 in the Wilhoit and McCallum (2002) article in the *School Psychology Review*.

Cross-Battery Assessment

McGrew and Flanagan (1998) first described the rationale and procedures required to use the CBA process. One important assumption of CBA is that subtests can be selected from different batteries and used to assess particular cognitive constructs, thereby increasing assessment precision and efficiency. This technique is particularly useful when there is no need to administer and interpret a particular test in its entirety (e.g., the referral question does not require that an FSIQ be obtained from a specific cognitive test)

To aid in the application of CBA, McGrew and Flanagan have provided a cognitive nomenclature based on the work of several researchers, particularly Cattell (1963), Horn (1968, 1994), and Carroll (1993). This nomenclature—referred to in recent years as the CHC system or model as noted earlier—is embedded in a three-tier hierarchical model. Stratum III represents g, the general cognitive energy presumed to underlie performance across all tasks individuals undertake. Stratum II represents relatively broad abilities that can be operationalized fairly well as factors from a factor analysis (e.g., short-term memory, long-term memory, fluid ability, acquired knowledge, visual processing, auditory processing, processing speed). Stratum I represents abilities at a more specific level, and can be assessed relatively purely by many existing subtests; two or more of these subtests can be used to operationalize stratum II abilities. Using this system, McGrew and Flanagan characterized subtests from most existing batteries as measures of stratum I and stratum II abilities, provided several caveats about the use of these operationalizations, and even provided models of worksheets to aid examiners in using CBA.

Wilhoit and McCallum (2003) have recently extended the McGrew and Flanagan (1998) model to assessment of cognitive constructs via only nonverbal tests, including the UNIT. Application of CBA is somewhat detailed, requiring the use of worksheets containing the names of tests and subtests, and the broad stratum II and stratum III abilities those subtests measure. Using the worksheets, an examiner can determine strengths and weaknesses according to operationalization of the CHC model by subtests from various nonverbal measures. Assessment of stratum II abilities is the primary focus. Typically, each subtest from nonverbal tests assesses a narrow stratum I ability, and two or more can be used to provide a good assessment of stratum II. The six stratum II abilities assessed by nonverbal tests include fluid intelligence (Gf), crystallized intelligence (Gc), visual processing (Gv), short-term memory (Gsm), long-term memory (Glr), and processing speed (Gs). The other ability typically included in CBA, auditory processing (Ga), is not assessed by nonverbal tests and is not included on the worksheets. The worksheets allow an examiner to calculate the mean performance by averaging scores from all subtests. Each stratum II ability score (determined by averaging two or more stratum I measures within that stratum II ability) can be compared to the overall stratum II average in an ipsative fashion. Assuming that all subtests use a mean of 100 and a standard deviation of 15 (or have been converted accordingly), each average stratum II ability score that is more than 15 points from the overall mean is considered a strength or a weakness, depending upon the direction of the difference. Wilhoit and McCallum provide the worksheets for this application of the UNIT (and other nonverbal tests), modified from the procedure originally described by Flanagan and McGrew (1997). Importantly, the stratum II abilities have been linked to several important real-world products (e.g., processing speed and short-term memory underpin the ability to learn to decode words quickly, according to Mather & Jaffe, 2002). Consequently, using CBA can aid in diagnosing academic and other problems.

ADDITIONAL CLINICAL APPLICATIONS

The UNIT can be employed easily with non-English-speaking populations, without the traditional language demands of conventional intelligence tests or costly translations. The UNIT gestures (e.g., affirmative head nods, pointing) were chosen because they seem to be ubiquitous modes of communication across cultures. Also, an effort was made to employ universal item content (i.e., objects found in all industrialized cultures). Thus use of the UNIT with children who come into the United States from other countries is facilitated. In addition, the format is appropriate for children with deafness/hearing impairments and for those who have other types of language deficits (e.g., selective mutism, severe dyslexia, speech articula-

tion difficulties). Additional clinical applications of the UNIT as well as other nonverbal tests are described by McCallum, Bracken, and Wasserman (2001). For example, they provide information describing how members of various populations compare on the UNIT scores; technical data such as reliability coefficients for those examinees who earn scores close to typical "cutoff points" of 70 and 130; a case study illustrating use of the test for a child with language delays; and a UNIT interpretive worksheet showing step by step interpretation guidelines. Also, a recent book by McCallum (2003) provides a discussion of procedures/techniques to help examinees choose technically appropriate and fair(est) tests for assessing a range of nonverbal abilities, including nonverbally functional behaviors, academic skills, personality, cognition, and neurological functioning. This book provides chapters focusing on the nonverbal assessment of all these abilities, plus chapters describing best practices in eliminating bias in item selection for nonverbal tests; contextual and within-child influences on nonverbal performance (including pharmacological agents); and brief treatment of the history and current sociological context for nonverbal assessment.

INNOVATIONS IN THE MEASUREMENT OF COGNITIVE ABILITIES

Several features set the UNIT apart from all or most existing nonverbal scales.

1. The UNIT is administered solely through the use of examiner demonstrations and gestures. The liberal use of sample, demonstration, and (unique) checkpoint items ensures that the examinee understands the nature of each task prior to attempting the subtest for credit.

2. The test comprises a battery of subtests that will provide the opportunity for both motoric and motor-reduced (i.e., pointing) responses. Administration of UNIT subtests can be modified so that only a pointing response is required on four of the six subtests. The use of motoric and motor-reduced subtests facilitates administration by optimizing motivation and rapport. For example, a very

shy child may be encouraged initially to point only; later, as rapport is gained, other, more motorically involved responses may be possible. Also, use of the motor-reduced subtests may be indicated for children with limited motor skills.

3. Subtests contain items that are as culturally fair as possible. We have included line drawings and objects that are recognizable to most individuals from all cultures.

4. The test is model-based. That is, we have included subtests designed to assess reasoning—a higher-order mental processing activity—as well as complex memory. Also, we have included symbolically loaded subtests as well as less symbolically laden ones. Interpretation of the UNIT is facilitated because of these theoretical underpinnings.

5. Samples of non-English-speaking individuals have been included for UNIT validation studies, collected by Riverside during the UNIT norming. Children from other cultures and children residing in the United States who had limited English facility and/or special education diagnoses were included in the norming and validation of the UNIT.

6. Administration time can be controlled by the examiner, depending on the number of subtests administered. The UNIT includes three administration formats: a two-subtest version, a four-subtest (standard) version, and a six-subtest (extended) version.

7. Reliability estimates were calculated for two critical cut points (i.e., for those with FSIQs around 70 and those with FSIQs around 130).

8. There is an unprecedented array of support resources for a nonverbal test, including a training video, a university training manual, and a computerized scoring and interpretation software program.

BRIEF CASE STUDY

Name: Sean Steven Sanders
Age: 7 years, 7 months
Date of Birth: 12/07/93
Grade: Entering 1
School: Hillside Elementary
Date(s) of Assessment: 07/07/01; 07/22/01; 08/06/01
Examiner: Sherry Mee Bell, PhD, NCSP

Reason for Referral and Background Information

Sean was referred to determine his current functioning and to obtain information useful in planning his educational program. He lives with both parents and an older sister. Parents report a healthy pregnancy and delivery. Birth weight was within normal limits, although developmental milestones were somewhat delayed. Sean walked independently at age 1 year, 4 months (1:4) and talked at 3:0; speech and language development was significantly delayed. Sean was toilet-trained for urination at 3:0 and for bowels between 4:0 and 5:0. He had his tonsils and adenoids removed at 4:6. Chronic middle ear infections reportedly stopped after the tonsillectomy.

Due to apparent delays in speech and language skills, Sean was evaluated at the University Hearing and Speech Center at age 4:6. Sean exhibited a communication disorder characterized by delayed receptive and expressive language skills. He exhibited difficulty naming and identifying objects and following directions; in addition, he exhibited echolalia. Spontaneous speech was characterized by strings of unintelligible reduplicative utterances, interspersed with some intelligible words.

Testing in October 2000 yielded a standard score of 59 on the Peabody Picture Vocabulary Test—Third Edition (PPVT-III; population mean = 100). In addition, he achieved a raw score of 23 (population mean = 39) on the Templin–Darley Articulation Test. Hearing was evaluated and reported to be normal. Sean has been receiving special education services through the local school system and was identified as eligible for special education services (because of developmental delays) in April 1999.

Relevant Test Behaviors

Sean is short for his chronological age, and is slender, with dark hair and large brown eyes. He presented as somewhat shy, but he separated from his parents upon request. Sean seemed to put forth good effort during assessment and responded well to praise and encouragement, although he had difficulty following oral directions at times. At times he whispered his answers, especially when he seemed unsure of himself. Results are considered to represent a valid estimate of his current functioning level.

Assessment Test Results

On the Universal Nonverbal Intelligence Test (UNIT), Sean achieved a Memory Quotient of 100, Reasoning Quotient of 98, Symbolic Quotient of 95, and Nonsymbolic Quotient of 104. His Full Scale IQ (FSIQ) was 98. The range of scores from 92 to 104 is believed to capture Sean's true score with 90% confidence. The Quotient and FSIQ scores of the UNIT have a mean of 100 and a standard deviation of 15, similar to many other intelligence tests. The subtests of the UNIT have a mean of 10 and a standard deviation of 3. Sean scored as follows on the subtests: Symbolic Memory, 10; Analogic Reasoning, 8; Cube Design, 11; Object Memory, 9; Spatial Memory, 11; and Mazes, 10.

Sean displayed relatively little variability on these nonverbal cognitive tasks. He performed somewhat more strongly (a little more than half a standard deviation) on nonsymbolic versus symbolic tasks. There was no difference in his performance on reasoning versus memory tasks. The slight relative strength in nonsymbolic versus symbolic abilities is consistent with Sean's deficits in language, because language requires symbolic thinking/problem solving. Results of the UNIT indicate average cognitive abilities overall.

Further assessment of cognitive abilities was accomplished by administration of selected subtests from the Stanford–Binet Intelligence Scale: Fourth Edition. These subtests have a mean of 50 and a standard deviation of 8. On the Stanford–Binet, Sean achieved a standard score of 36 on the Vocabulary subtest. This score is in the borderline range of intellectual functioning. In contrast, Sean achieved a standard score of 58 on the Pattern Analysis subtest. This score is in the high average range of intellectual functioning. The Vocabulary subtest measures expressive vocabulary, whereas the Pattern Analysis subtest measures nonverbal, visual–spatial reasoning. Sean's performance on the Pattern Analysis subtest is consistent with his performance on Cube Design from the UNIT, indicating well-developed nonverbal,

visual–spatial abilities. His performance on the Vocabulary subtest is consistent with previous assessments indicating significant delays or deficits in language skills.

Sean was also administered the screener portion of the Wechsler Individual Achievement Test (WIAT). Standard scores were calculated based on grade norms, because Sean will be entering first grade this month. The WIAT subtests have a mean of 100 and a standard deviation of 15. Sean scored as follows on the WIAT subtests: Basic Reading, 104 (61st percentile, grade equivalent of K.7); Mathematics Reasoning, 89 (23rd percentile, grade equivalent of K.3); Spelling, 94 (34th percentile, grade equivalent of K.9).

Some caution should be used in interpreting these scores, because the WIAT has a limited floor for children Sean's age. Sean performed in the average range on tasks measuring beginning reading and spelling skills. Performance was slightly weaker on tasks measuring mathematics reasoning. However, this relative weakness is most likely to be explained by Sean's difficulty with language. The WIAT Mathematics Reasoning subtest uses questions involving language rather than math calculation only.

Sean was administered the PPVT-III, Form L. Results yielded a standard score of 77, which is at the 6th percentile, and an age equivalent of 5:6. Results indicate that Sean's receptive language skills continue to be somewhat delayed, approximately 2 years below his chronological age.

Parents responded to the Vineland Adaptive Behavior Scales. Results yielded an overall Adaptive Behavior Composite standard score of 53 and age equivalent of 4:5. Domain standard scores were as follows: Communication, 60; Daily Living, 46; and Socialization, 71. The following age equivalents were calculated for the domains: Communication, 4:6; Daily Living, 3:5; and Socialization, 4:6. In addition, though no standard score could be calculated for the Motor Skills domain, an age equivalent was calculated: 3:5.

Mrs. Sanders responded to the Behavior Assessment System for Children (BASC). Validity scales were acceptable. Results yielded an overall Behavioral Symptoms Index in the average range, with scores on the Externalizing Problems, Internalizing Problems, and Adaptive Skills composites all in the average range. In addition, results on the following subscales were in the average range: Hyperactivity, Aggression, Conduct Problems, Anxiety, Depression, Atypicality, Withdrawal, Attention Problems, Adaptability, Social Skills, and Leadership. The only elevated BASC score was Somatization, which was probably elevated because Sean requires medication on a routine basis for asthma and allergies. Scores do *not* indicate atypical social development/functioning.

Summary and Recommendations

Assessment results tentatively suggest a *Diagnostic and Statistical Manual of Mental Disorders*, fourth edition, text revision (DSM-IV-TR) diagnosis of mixed receptive–expressive language disorder (Axis I, 315.32). Sean is also referred for a neurological evaluation to assist in determining the exact nature of his developmental delay. Participation in a regular classroom with special educational support is recommended. Sean continues to be eligible for rather intensive speech and language services. In addition, he is likely to need support from the school resource teacher, either in an inclusion format or in a pull-out format. Modifications and adaptations in assignments will be needed. A multisensory approach to instruction should be most beneficial for Sean. Grading modifications may be needed, and teachers are encouraged to conduct error analysis (with Sean) to determine which kinds of tasks give him more difficulty. In the classroom, Sean may benefit from being paired with a "study buddy" who can prompt Sean on how to complete tasks and assignments. Sean's progress should be monitored routinely. A thorough reevaluation of academic progress using informal assessment strategies is recommended in 1 year.

REFERENCES

Athanasiou, M. S. (2000). Current nonverbal assessment instruments: A comparison of psychometric integrity and test fairness. *Journal of Psychoeducational Assessment, 18*, 211–299.

Bandalos, D. L. (2001). Review of the Universal Nonverbal Intelligence Test. In B. S. Plake & J. C. Impara (Eds.), *Fourteenth mental measurements yearbook* (pp. 1296–1298). Lincoln, NE: Buros Institute.

Bracken, B. A. (1987). Limitations of preschool instruments and standards for minimal levels of technical adequacy. *Journal of Psychoeducational Assessment, 5*, 313–326.

Bracken, B. A., & McCallum, R. S. (1998). *The Universal Nonverbal Intelligence Test*. Itasca, IL: Riverside.

Bracken, B. A., & McCallum, R. S. (2001). *UNIT Compuscore*. Itasca, IL: Riverside.

Carroll, J. B. (1993). *Human cognitive abilities: A survey of factor-analytic studies*. New York: Cambridge University Press.

Cattell, R. B. (1963). Theory for fluid and crystallized intelligence: A critical experiment. *Journal of Educational Psychology, 54*, 1–22.

CTBS/McGraw-Hill. (1996). *Comprehensive Test of Basic Skills*. Monterey, CA: Author.

Farrell, M. M., & Phelps, L. (2000). A comparison of the Leiter-R and the Universal Nonverbal Intelligence Test (UNIT) with children classified as language impaired. *Journal of Psychoeducational Assessment, 18*, 268–274.

Fives, C. J., & Flanagan, R. (2002). A review of the Universal Nonverbal Intelligence Test (UNIT): An advance for evaluating youngsters with diverse needs. *School Psychology International, 23*, 425–448.

Flanagan, D. P., & McGrew, K. S. (1997). A cross-battery approach to assessing and interpreting cognitive abilities: Narrowing the gap between practice and cognitive science. In D. P. Flanagan, J. L. Genshaft, & P. L. Harrison (Eds.), *Contemporary intellectual assessment: Theories, tests, and issues* (pp. 314–325). New York: Guilford Press.

Gilliam, J. E., Carpenter, B. O., & Christensen, J. R. (1996). *Gifted and Talented Evaluation Scales: A norm referenced procedure for identifying gifted and talented students*. Austin, TX: Pro-Ed.

Glutting, J., Adams, W., & Sheslow, D. (2000). *Wide Range Intelligence Test manual*. Wilmington, DE: Wide Range.

Glutting, J., McDermott, P. A., & Konold, T. R. (1997). Ontology, structure, and diagnostic benefits of a normative subtest taxonomy from the WISC-III standardization sample. In D. P. Flanagan, J. L. Genshaft, & P. L. Harrison (Eds.), *Contemporary intellectual assessment: Theories, tests, and issues* (pp. 349–372). New York: Guilford Press.

Hooper, V. S. (2002). *Concurrent and predictive validity of the Universal Nonverbal Intelligence Test and the Leiter International Performance Scale—Revised*. Unpublished doctoral dissertation, University of Tennessee, Knoxville.

Horn, J. L. (1968). Organization of abilities and the development of intelligence. *Psychological Review, 75*, 242–259.

Horn, J. L. (1994). Theory of fluid and crystallized intelligence. In R. J. Sternberg (Ed.), *Encyclopedia of human intelligence* (pp. 443–451). New York: Macmillan.

Individuals with Disabilities Education Act Amendments of 1997, Pub.L. No. 105–17, 20 U.S.C.33 (1997).

Jensen, A. R. (1980). *Bias in mental testing*. New York: Free Press.

Jimenez, S. (2001). An analysis of the reliability and validity of the Universal Nonverbal Intelligence Test (UNIT) with Puerto Rican children (Doctoral dissertation, Texas A&M University, 2001). *Dissertation Abstracts International, 62*, 5424B.

Kamphaus, R. W. (2001). *Clinical assessment of child and adolescent intelligence* (2nd ed.). Boston: Allyn & Bacon.

Krivitski, E. C. (2000). Profile analysis of deaf children using the Universal Nonverbal Intelligence Test (Doctoral dissertation, State University of New York at Albany, 2000). *Dissertation Abstracts International, 61*, 2593B.

Maller, S. J. (2000). Item invariance in four subtests of the Universal Nonverbal Intelligence Test (UNIT) across groups of deaf and hearing children. *Journal of Psychoeducational Assessment, 18*, 240–254.

Mather, N., & Jaffe, L. E. (2002). *Woodcock–Johnson III: Reports, recommendations, and strategies*. New York: Wiley.

McCallum, R. S. (1999). A "baker's dozen" criteria for evaluating fairness in nonverbal testing. *The School Psychologist, 53*, 40–43.

McCallum, R. S. (Ed.). (2003). *Handbook of nonverbal assessment*. New York: Kluwer Academic/Plenum.

McCallum, R. S., Bracken, B. A., & Wasserman, J. (2001). *Essentials of nonverbal assessment*. New York: Wiley.

McCallum, R. S., & Whitaker, D. A. (2000). Using the Stanford–Binet: FE to assess preschool children. In B. A. Bracken (Ed.), *The psychoeducational assessment of preschool children* (3rd ed.). Boston: Allyn & Bacon.

McGrew, K. S., & Flanagan, D. P. (1998). *The intelligence test desk reference (ITDR): Gf-Gc cross-battery assessment*. Boston: Allyn & Bacon.

Pasko, J. R. (1994). Chicago—don't miss it. *Communique, 23*, 2.

Raven, J. C. (1960). *Guide to standard progressive matrices*. London: Lewis.

Roid, G. H., & Miller, L. J. (1997). *Leiter International Performance Scale—Revised*. Wood Dale, IL: Stoelting.

Sattler, J. M. (2001). *Assessment of children: Cognitive applications* (4th ed.). San Diego, CA: Jerome M. Sattler.

Scardapane, J. R., Egan, A., Torres-Gallegos, M., Levine, N., & Owens, S. (2002, March). *Relationships among WRIT, UNIT, and GATES scores and language proficiency*. Paper presented at the meeting of the Council for Exceptional Children, New York.

Unz, R. (1997). Perspective on education: Bilingual is a damaging myth, a system that ensures failure is kept alive by the flow of federal dollars. A 1998 initiative would bring change. *Los Angles Times*, Section M, p. 5.

Upson, L. M. (2003). *Effects of an increasingly precise socioeconomic match on mean score differences in nonverbal intelligence test scores*. Unpublished doctoral dissertation, University of Tennessee, Knoxville.

U.S. Bureau of the Census. (2000). *Language use*. Retrieved from http://www.census.gov/population.www.socdemo/lang_use.html

Wechsler, D. (1939). *The measurement of adult intelligence*. Baltimore: Williams & Wilkins.

Wechsler, D. (1991). *Wechsler Intelligence Scale for Children—Third Edition*. San Antonio, TX: Psychological Corporation.

Wilhoit, B. E., & McCallum, R. S. (2002). Profile analysis of the Universal Nonverbal Intelligence Test standardized sample. *School Psychology Review, 31*, 263–281.

Wilhoit, B. E., & McCallum, R. S. (2003). Cross-battery analysis of the UNIT. In R. S. McCallum (Ed.), *Handbook of nonverbal assessment* (pp. 63–83). New York: Kluwer Academic/Plenum.

Woodcock, R. W. (1990). Theoretical foundations of the WJ-R measures of cognitive ability. *Journal of Psychoeducational Assessment, 8*, 231–258.

Woodcock, R. W., & Muñoz-Sandoval, A. F. (1996). *Bateria Woodcock–Muñoz Pruebas de habilidad cognoscitiva—Revisada*. Itasca, IL: Riverside.

Woodcock, R. W., McGrew, K. S., & Mather, N. (2001). *Woodcock–Johnson III Tests of Cognitive Abilities*. Itasca, IL: Riverside.

20

The Cognitive Assessment System

JACK A. NAGLIERI

THEORY AND STRUCTURE

Theory

The Cognitive Assessment System (CAS; Naglieri & Das, 1997a) is built strictly on the Planning, Attention, Simultaneous, and Successive (PASS) theory (see Naglieri & Das, Chapter 7, this volume). This theory describes four basic psychological processes, following largely from the neuropsychological work of A. R. Luria (1966a, 1966b, 1973, 1980, 1982). The PASS theory had a strong empirical base prior to the publication of the CAS (see Das, Kirby, & Jarman, 1979; Das, Naglieri, & Kirby, 1994), and its research foundation remains strong (see Naglieri, 1999a; Naglieri & Das, 1997c). The PASS theory places emphasis on cognitive processes that are related to performance, rather than on a general intelligence verbal–nonverbal model. The four PASS scales represent the kinds of basic psychological processes described in the Individuals with Disabilities Education Act amendments of 1997 (IDEA '97; see Naglieri & Sullivan, 1998) and its current reauthorization—processes that are used, for example, in the definition of a specific learning disability. The four basic psychological processes can be used to (1) gain an understanding of how well a child thinks; (2) discover the child's strengths and needs, which can then be used for effective differential diagnosis; (3) con-duct fair assessment; and (4) select or design appropriate interventions.

The PASS cognitive processes are the basic building blocks of human intellectual functioning (Naglieri, 1999a). These processes form an interrelated system of cognitive processes or abilities that interact with an individual's base of knowledge and skills, and are defined below (see Chapter 7 for a fuller discussion).

- *Planning* is a mental activity that provides cognitive control, use of processes, knowledge and skills, intentionality, and self-regulation. Planning is critical to all activities where the child or adult has to determine how to solve a problem. This includes selfmonitoring and impulse control, as well as generation, evaluation, and execution of a plan. This process provides the means to solve problems of varying complexity and may involve control of attention, simultaneous, and successive processes, as well as acquisition of knowledge and skills. Planning is measured with tests that require the child to develop a plan of action, evaluate the value of the method, monitor its effectiveness, revise or reject a plan to meet the demands of the task, and control the impulse to act without careful consideration.
- *Attention* is a mental activity that provides focused, selective cognition over time, as well as resistance to distraction. Attention occurs when a person selectively focuses on

particular stimuli and inhibits responses to competing stimuli. The process is involved when the child must demonstrate focused, selective, sustained, and effortful activity. *Focused* attention involves concentration directed toward a particular activity, and *selective* attention is important for the inhibition of responses to distracting stimuli. *Sustained* attention refers to the variation of performance over time, which can be influenced by the different amount of effort required to solve the test. An effective measure of attention presents children with competing demands on their attention and requires sustained focus.

• *Simultaneous processing* is a mental activity by which the child integrates separate stimuli into groups or into a whole. An essential aspect of simultaneous processing is the organization of interrelated elements into a whole. Simultaneous processing tests have strong spatial aspects for this reason. Simultaneous processing can be used to solve tasks with both nonverbal and verbal content, as long as the cognitive demand of the task requires integration of information. Simultaneous processing underlies the use and comprehension of grammatical statements, because they demand comprehension of word relationships, prepositions, and inflections, so that the person can obtain meaning based on the whole idea. Simultaneous processing is measured with tasks that require integration of parts into a single whole and understanding of logical and grammatical relationships.

• *Successive processing* is a mental activity by which the person works with stimuli in a specific serial order to form a chain-like progression. This processing is required when a child arranges things in a strictly defined order, where each element is only related to those that precede it and these stimuli are not interrelated. Successive processing involves both the perception of stimuli in sequence and the formation of sounds and movements in order. For this reason, successive processing is involved with activities such as phonological skills (Das et al., 1994) and the syntax of language. This process is measured with tests that demand use, repetition, or comprehension of information based on order.

• *PASS processes.* The four PASS processes are interrelated constructs that func-

tion as a whole. Luria (1973) stated that "each form of conscious activity is always a complex functional system and takes place through the combined working of all three brain units, each of which makes its own contribution" (p. 99). This means that the four PASS processes are a "working constellation" (Luria, 1966b, p. 70) of cognitive activity and therefore *not* uncorrelated. In fact, Luria's description specifies that the processes are related and at the same time distinct. This means that most cognitive tasks involve many if not all of the PASS processes, even though not every process is equally involved in every task. For example, tests like math calculation may be heavily weighted toward planning, while reading decoding tasks may be heavily weighted toward successive processing (Naglieri, 1999a). Because of the interrelated nature of the processes and their interaction with achievement based upon the particular demands of a task, a thorough understanding of a child's competence in all these areas is important for addressing educational problems.

Structure

The CAS (Naglieri & Das, 1997a) is an individually administered measure of ability designed for children and adolescents ages 5 through 17 years. The 12 regularly administered subtests are organized into four scales that represent the PASS theory of psychological processing. The PASS scale scores and a total score called the Full Scale (FS) are expressed as standard scores (mean of 100, standard deviation [SD] of 15). There are two forms of the test: the Basic Battery (8 subtests, 2 per PASS scale), and the Standard Battery (all 12 subtests). The scales and subtests are briefly described below.

• *Full Scale.* The FS score is an overall measure of cognitive processing based on the combination of either 8 or 12 subtests from the four PASS scales.

• *PASS scales.* The PASS scale scores are computed on the basis of the sum of subtest scaled scores included in each respective scale. These scales represent a child's cognitive processing in specific areas and are used to examine cognitive strengths and/or weaknesses.

- *Subtests*. Each of the 12 subtests measures the specific PASS process corresponding to the scale on which it is found. The subtests are not considered to represent their own sets of specific abilities, but rather are measures of one of the four types of processes. They vary in content (some are verbal, some involve memory, etc.), but each is an effective measure of a specific PASS process. A fuller description of the subtests follows.

DESCRIPTION OF SUBTESTS

Development of Subtests

Subtests for the CAS were developed specifically to operationalize the PASS theory over a period of about 25 years (summarized in three sources: Das et al., 1979, 1994; Naglieri & Das, 1997c). Each subtest's correspondence to the theoretical framework of the PASS theory, and the relationships between that subtest and others, formed the basis of selection and modification during construction. Development of the subtests was accomplished following a carefully prescribed sequence of item generation, experimental research, test revision, and reexamination until the instructions, items, and other dimensions were refined over a series of pilot tests, research studies, national tryouts, and national standardization. This allowed for the identification of subtests that provide an efficient way to measure each of the processes (Das et al., 1994; Naglieri & Das, 1997c). Descriptions of the experimental tasks that became the CAS subtests used to measure the PASS processes, and efforts to evaluate their practical utility and validity, are contained in more than 100 published papers and several books (see Naglieri & Das, 1997c, for references). Each subtest is more completely described below.

The Planning Subtests

All of the CAS Planning subtests require the child to create and apply some plan, verify that the approach achieves the original goal, and modify the plan as needed. These subtests contain tasks that are relatively easy to perform, but require the individual to make a decision (or decisions) about how to solve the novel tasks.

- *Matching Numbers* consists of four pages, each consisting of eight rows of numbers with six numbers per row. Children are instructed to underline the two numbers in each row that are the same. Numbers increase in length across the four pages from one digit to seven digits, with four rows for each digit length. Each item (defined as a page of eight rows) has a time limit. The subtest score is based on the combination of time and number correct for each page.
- *Planned Codes* contains two pages, each with a distinct set of codes and arrangement of rows and columns. A legend at the top of each page shows how letters correspond to simple codes (e.g., A, B, C, and D correspond to OX, XX, OO, and XO, respectively). Each page contains seven rows and eight columns of letters without codes. Children fill in the appropriate codes in empty boxes beneath each letter. On the first page, all the A's appear in the first column, all the B's in the second column, all the C's in the third column, and so on. On the second page, letters are configured in a diagonal pattern. Children are permitted to complete each page in whatever fashion they desire. The subtest score is based on the combination of time and number correct for each page.
- *Planned Connections* contains eight items. The first six items require children to connect numbers appearing in a quasi-random order on a page in sequential order. The last two items require children to connect both numbers and letters in sequential order alternating between numbers and letters (e.g., 1-A-2-B-3-C). The items are constructed so that children never complete the sequence by crossing one line over the other. The score is based on the total amount of time in seconds used to complete the items.

The Attention Subtests

The Attention subtests require the focus of cognitive activity, detection of a particular stimulus, and inhibition of responses to irrelevant competing stimuli. These subtests always involve examination of the features of the stimulus, as well as a decision to respond to one feature and not to other competing features in a complex environment.

- *Expressive Attention* consists of two different sets of items, depending on the age of the child. Children 5 though 7 years of age are asked to identify whether each animal depicted in the item is big or small. In the first item, the animals are the same size (approximately 1 inch high and 1 inch wide). In the second item, the animals are sized appropriately (big animals are approximately 1 inch high and 1 inch wide, and small animals are about ½ inch by ½ inch). In the third item, where selective attention is being measured, the realistic sizes of the animals usually differ from the relative sizes they appear to be in the item. In each instance, the child responds based upon the size of these animals in real life, ignoring their relative size on the page. For children 8 years of age and older, the stimuli are color words. On the first item children are asked to read 40 words (BLUE, YELLOW, GREEN, and RED) from the stimulus page. In the next item children are asked to name the colors of a series of rectangles (printed in blue, yellow, green, and red). In the final item the words BLUE, YELLOW, GREEN, and RED are printed in ink of a different color from the colors the words name. The child is instructed to name the color the word is printed in, rather than to read the word. The last item administered at each age is used as the measure of selective attention. The raw score on this subtest is the ratio of the accuracy (total number correct) and time on the final item.

• *Number Detection* is comprised of a page of specially formatted numbers. Children are asked to underline specific numbers when they are printed in an outlined typeface. There are 18 rows of 10 numbers with 45 targets (25% targets) in each of the first two pages (treated as one item each), and 15 rows of 12 numbers in the third and fourth pages (items), with a total of 45 targets (25% targets) in each item. Children must complete each page by working from left to right and top to bottom, and may not go back to check the page upon completion. The raw score for Number Detection is the ratio of the accuracy (total number correct minus the number of false detections) and the total time for each item, summed across the items.

• *Receptive Attention* is a two-page paper-and-pencil subtest written in two versions, depending on the age of the child. The version for children ages 5 through 7 is contained on four pages of pictures arranged in pairs. In the first condition (item 1), a child is asked to underline pairs of drawings that are identical in appearance. In the second condition (item 2), the child is required to underline the pairs of pictures that are the same from a lexical perspective (i.e., they have the same name). Children ages 8 years and above are also presented with two conditions (items 1 and 2). One page contains 200 pairs of letters with 50 targets (25% targets), and the second page also has 200 pairs of letters with 50 targets (25% targets). Although the targets are different on these two pages, the distractors are the same. In the first condition, a child underlines pairs of letters that are identical in appearance (e.g., AA, not Aa). In the second condition, the child circles all the pairs of letters that have the same name (e.g., Aa, not Ba). At all ages, the child must complete the subtest by working from left to right and top to bottom. The child may not go back to check the page upon completion. The raw score is the ratio of the accuracy (total number correct minus the number of false detections) and the total time for each item, summed across the items.

The Simultaneous Subtests

• *Nonverbal Matrices* is a 33-item progressive matrix test; it utilizes shapes and geometric elements that are interrelated through spatial or logical organization. Children are required to comprehend the relationships among the parts of the item and respond by choosing the best of six options. Items are scored as correct or incorrect (1, 0). The raw score is the total number of items answered correctly.

• *Verbal–Spatial Relations* is composed of 27 items that require the comprehension of logical and grammatical descriptions of spatial relationships. Children are shown items that depict six drawings and a printed question at the bottom of each page. The items involve both objects and shapes that are arranged in a specific spatial configuration. The examiner reads the question aloud, and the child is required to select the option that matches the verbal description. The raw score is the total number of items correctly answered.

• *Figure Memory* is a 27-item subtest where a child is shown a page that contains a two- or three-dimensional geometric figure for 5 seconds. The figure is then removed and the child is presented with a response page that contains the original design embedded in a larger, more complex geometric pattern. Children are required to identify the original design that it is embedded within the larger figure by tracing over the appropriate lines with a red pencil. For a response to be scored correct, all lines of the design have to be indicated without any additions or omissions. Items are scored as either correct or incorrect (1, 0).

The Successive Subtests

• *Word Series* consists of 27 items, each of which uses from two to nine single-syllable, high-frequency words. The child is asked to repeat the words in the same order as stated by the examiner. Each series is read at the rate of one word per second. Each item is scored as either correct or incorrect (1, 0). The child must reproduce the entire word series in the order presented to receive credit for the item. The raw score is the total number of items repeated correctly.

• *Sentence Repetition* consists of 20 sentences composed of color words (e.g., "The blue is yellowing") that are read to the child. The child is required to repeat each sentence verbatim. Each item is scored as either correct or incorrect (1, 0).

• *Speech Rate* is an eight-item, timed subtest used at ages 5–7 years. In each item, children are required to repeat a three-word series of high-imagery, single- or double-syllable words in order, 10 times in a row. The examiner begins timing when the child says the first word in the series and stops timing when the child finishes repeating the last word in the 10th repetition. The total time taken to repeat the eight items 10 times each is the total raw score.

• *Sentence Questions* is a 21-item subtest that is used in place of Speech Rate for children ages 8–17 years. The subtest uses the same type of sentences as those in Sentence Repetition. Children are read a sentence and then asked a question about it (e.g., "The blue is yellowing," "Who is yellowing?") Each item is scored as either correct or incorrect (1, 0), based upon rules defined on the record form. The raw score is the total number of questions answered correctly.

ADMINISTRATION AND SCORING

Administration

The directions for administration are provided in the CAS administration and scoring manual (Naglieri & Das, 1997c). These instructions include both verbal statements and nonverbal actions to be used by the examiner. The combination of oral and nonverbal communication is designed to ensure that all children understand each task.

CAS subtests were carefully sequenced to ensure the integrity of the subtests and to reduce the influence of extraneous variables on a child's performance. The Planning tests are administered first, because the child is given flexibility to solve the subtest in any manner. Attention subtests must be completed in the prescribed order (i.e., left to right, top to bottom), so they are given later in the test.

All Planning subtests include strategy assessment, which is conducted during and after the administration of each Planning subtest. Observed strategies are those seen by the examiner through careful observation of the child completing the items. Reported strategies are obtained following completion of an item. The examiner obtains this information by saying, "Tell me how you did these," or "How did you find what you were looking for?" or some similar statement. The child can communicate the strategies by either verbal or nonverbal (gesturing) means. Strategies are recorded in the "Observed" and "Reported" sections of the Strategy Assessment Checklist included in the record form.

Several methods have been used to ensure that a child understands what is being requested. These include sample and demonstration items, as well as opportunities for the examiner to clarify the requirements of the task. If, however, the child does not understand the demands of the subtest or appears in any way confused or uncertain, the examiner is instructed to "provide a brief explanation if necessary" (Naglieri & Das, 1997c, p. 8). This instruction gives the examiner the freedom to explain what the child must do in whatever terms are considered necessary to ensure that the child understands the task. This type of instruction can be given in any form—including gestures, as well as the use of a language other than English. However, it is important to remember that these alternative instructions are meant to ensure that the child understands what to do; they are not intended to teach the child how to do the test.

Scoring

The CAS is scored via a standard method of subtest raw scores to subtest scaled scores to composite (PASS scale and CAS FS) standard scores. The CAS subtest raw scores are calculated in various ways: the total number correct (Nonverbal Matrices, Verbal–Spatial Relations, Figure Memory, Word Series, Sentence Repetition, and Sentence Questions); time in seconds (Planned Connections and Speech Rate); and ratio scores that combine time and number correct (Matching Numbers, Planned Codes, and Expressive Attention) or time, number correct, and number of false detections (Number Detection and Receptive Attention). *False detections* are defined as the number of times a child underlines a stimulus that is not a target.

The CAS subtest scaled scores are obtained by using the appropriate age-based ta-ble for the child's chronological age in years, months, and days. The PASS and FS standard scores are obtained from the sum of the subtests on either the Standard (12-subtest) or Basic (8-subtest) Battery. Conversions from raw to standard scores are made easier by use of the CAS Rapid Score (Naglieri, 2002). This program computes the ratio scores (where applicable), sums the raw scores for each subtest, sums the subtest scores, calculates all subtest scaled scores, and calculate PASS as well as FS standard scores. In addition, the CAS Rapid Score computes all the values needed to make comparisons among CAS scores and to compare CAS and achievement test scores.

The CAS Rapid Score is a record-form-based program designed on the premise that computer scoring, interpretation, and report generation should be managed in a clear and easily understood environment. When the program is opened, the first page that appears is one that looks very much like the first page of the CAS record form (see Figure 20.1). Data entry requires the examiner to enter actual item data. For example, when

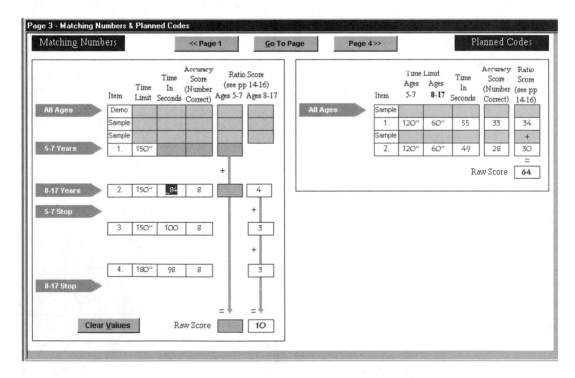

FIGURE 20.1. Data entry windows for CAS Rapid Score. From Naglieri (2002). Copyright 2002 by NL Associates. All rights reserved. Reprinted with permission.

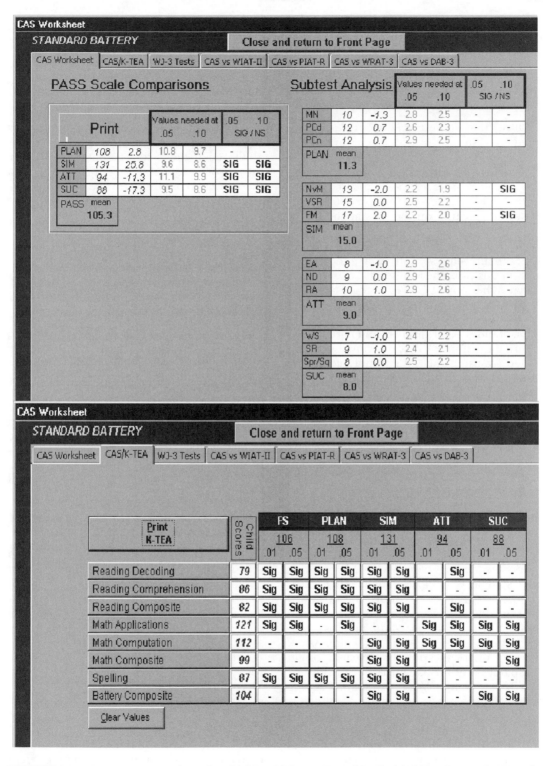

FIGURE 20.2. Interpretive windows for CAS Rapid Score. From Naglieri (2002). Copyright 2002 by NL Associates. All rights reserved. Reprinted with permission.

time scores and number correct are entered for each Matching Numbers page, the program computes the ratio score, and then the sum of the ratio scores is calculated automatically. Alternatively, subtest raw scores can be entered directly on the front of the record form.

Once the subtest raw scores are entered, the subtest scaled scores and PASS Scale standard scores are computed. The "PASS Scale Comparisons" button (see Figure 20.2) provides PASS scale comparisons to the child's mean, as well as subtest comparisons. Clicking on the tabs at the top of the window (e.g., "CAS/KTEA") will yield another window that will compare all CAS scales to any subtest score from another battery (in this case, the Kaufman Test of Educational Achievement [K-TEA]) that is entered. A click of the "Narrative" button yields a five-paragraph written report of the CAS results. Handouts for teachers and parents that describe the four PASS scales can also be obtained by using the CAS Rapid Score. The program performs all the interpretive tasks described by Naglieri (1999a) and provides some of the intervention handouts included in the book *Helping Children Learn: Intervention Handouts for Use in School and at Home* (Naglieri & Pickering, 2003).

PSYCHOMETRIC PROPERTIES

Standardization

The CAS was standardized on a sample of 2,200 children ages 5–17 years. A stratified random sampling plan was used, resulting in a sample that closely matched the U.S. population. The CAS sample was stratified on the following variables: age (5 years, 0 months through 17 years, 11 months); gender (female, male); race (black, white, Asian, Native American, other); Hispanic origin (Hispanic, non-Hispanic); region (Midwest, Northeast, South, West); community setting (urban/suburban, rural); classroom placement (full-time regular classroom, part-time special education resource, full-time self-contained special education); educational classification (learning disability, speech/language impairment, social-emotional disability, mental retardation, giftedness, and non-special-education); and parental educational attainment level (less than high school de-

gree, high school graduate or equivalent, some college or technical school, 4 or more years of college).

Reliability

The CAS subtests and scales have high reliability and meet or exceed minimum values suggested by Bracken (1987). The FS reliability coefficients for the Standard Battery range from a low of .95 to a high of .97, and the average reliabilities for the Standard Battery PASS scales are .88 (Planning and Attention scales) and .93 (Simultaneous and Successive scales). The Basic Battery reliabilities are as follows: FS, .87; Planning, .85; Simultaneous, .90; Attention, .84; and Successive, .90.

Validity

Elsewhere (Naglieri & Das, 1997c; Naglieri, 1999a, 1999b), considerable information is provided about the validity of the PASS theory as operationalized by the CAS. In this part of the chapter, several validity issues are covered: the relationships between PASS and achievement; race differences; examination of PASS profiles for children with reading disabilities and attention-deficit/hyperactivity disorders (ADHD); the relevance of the PASS scores to intervention; and factorial studies.

Relationships to Achievement

An examination of the relationships between several tests of ability and achievement (Naglieri, 1999a) found that the correlation between the CAS FS and achievement was highest among the major intelligence tests. This summary only involved large-scale investigations. The median correlation between the Wechsler Intelligence Scale for Children—Third Edition (WISC-III; Wechsler, 1991) Full Scale IQ (FSIQ) and all Wechsler Individual Achievement Test (WIAT; Wechsler, 1992) achievement scores was .59 for a sample of 1,284 children ages 5–19 years from all regions of the country, each parental educational level, and different racial and ethnic groups. A similar correlation of .60 was found between the Differential Ability Scales (Elliott, 1990) General Conceptual Ability and achievement for a sample of 2,400 children included in the standardization sample. The median correlation between the Woodcock–Johnson Psycho-Educational Battery Revised (WJ-R) Broad Cognitive Ability Extended Battery score and the WJ-R Tests of Achievement (ACH) (reported by McGrew, Werder, & Woodcock, 1991) was .63 (N = 888 children ages 6, 9, and 13 years). The median correlation between the Kaufman Assessment Battery for Children (K-ABC; Kaufman & Kaufman, 1983) Mental Processing Composite and achievement was .63 for 2,636 children ages 2½ through 12½ years. Finally, the median correlation between the CAS FS and the WJ-R ACH (Naglieri & Das, 1997c) was .70 for a representative sample of 1,600 children ages 5–17 years who closely matched the U.S. population. These results suggested that a cognitive processing approach to ability has great utility for the prediction of achievement. This study had one limitation, however: In no case did investigators give children two tests of ability and then correlate the values obtained with the same achievement scores.

We (Naglieri, Goldstein, & DeLauder, 2003) compared the WISC-III and CAS with the Woodcock–Johnson III (WJ III) ACH, using a sample of children ages 6–16 (N = 119) who were referred for evaluation due to learning problems. The children earned the following mean standard scores: WISC-III FSIQ of 104.5 (SD = 13.2), CAS FS of 97.2 (SD = 11.6), and WJ III ACH Academic Skills Cluster of 98.5 (SD = 12.0). The obtained correlations and those corrected for restriction in range between the WJ III ACH cluster and the WISC-III were .52 and .63, respectively; between the WJ III ACH and CAS, these correlations were .69 and .83, respectively. These results suggest that when the WISC-III, CAS, and WJ III ACH were given to the same children, the correlations between the CAS and achievement were substantially higher than those between the WISC-III and achievement.

The accumulating evidence continues to demonstrate that the PASS theory as operationalized by the CAS is related strongly to academic skills. This finding is especially important for two reasons. First, one of the most important dimensions of validity for a test of cognitive ability is its relationship to achievement (Brody, 1992; Cohen, Swerdlik,

& Smith, 1992). The purpose of a test like the CAS is to determine a child's level of cognitive functioning and to use this information to anticipate academic performance. High scores on the CAS suggest that a child should do well academically, while low scores indicate that learning problems are possible. Second, because the CAS, unlike traditional IQ tests, does not have subtests that are highly reliant on acquired knowledge (e.g., Arithmetic, Information, Vocabulary), it offers a way of measuring ability that is not influenced by limited academic success. This is quite important for children who come from disadvantaged environments, as well as those who have had a history of academic failure. The inclusion of verbal and quantitative tests on intelligence tests serves to lower scores for minority groups (Wasserman & Becker, 2000). This is discussed further in the following section.

Race Differences

There is little doubt that race differences are among the most emotionally and politically charged topics in the study of intelligence. As the characteristics of the U.S. population have become more diverse, the issues of race differences in general, and the fair assessment of children from different racial groups in particular, have become increasingly important. Most of the discussion of racial differences has centered on the widely used Wechsler scales. However, these scales have been criticized for being biased against minority children (e.g., Hilliard, 1979), for a variety of reasons. Of considerable concern is that black students have consistently earned lower Wechsler FSIQ mean scores than whites (Kaufman, Harrison, & Ittenbach, 1990; Prifitera & Saklofske, 1998). Most psychometric experts, however, reject the use of mean score differences as evidence of test bias (Reynolds & Kaiser, 1990). Yet the differences in mean scores appear to have some influence in the overrepresentation of black students in special education classes for children with mental retardation (Naglieri & Rojahn, 2001; Reschly & Bersoff, 1999).

Some researchers have argued that mean score differences should be considered test bias. The perspective is that bias is found in elements of any IQ test scores that (1) are irrelevant to the construct being measured and (2) systematically cause differences between groups. Messick (1995) has argued that because the consequences of the test scores may contribute to issues such as overrepresentation of minorities in classes for children with mental retardation and underrepresentation of minorities in programs for the gifted, the validity of the instruments should be questioned. In a recent study, Wasserman and Becker (2000) examined the differences between race groups on commonly used intelligence tests and addressed the question of whether such differences are influenced by the nature of the ability test that is used.

Wasserman and Becker (2000) summarized several studies of race differences for nearly all the major intelligence tests, including the WISC-III (Wechsler, 1991); the Stanford–Binet Intelligence Scale: Fourth Edition (SB-IV; Thorndike, Hagen, & Sattler, 1986); the Universal Nonverbal Intelligence Test (UNIT; Bracken & McCallum, 1998); the WJ-R Tests of Cognitive Ability (Woodcock & Johnson, 1989b; Woodcock, McGrew, & Mather, 2001); and the CAS (Naglieri & Das, 1997a). I have added results for the K-ABC (Kaufman & Kaufman, 1983; Naglieri, 1986), the KABC-II (J. C. Kaufman, 2003), and the Naglieri Nonverbal Ability Test (NNAT; Naglieri, 1997), all of which measure ability without inclusion of traditional verbal and arithmetic tests. Each of the investigations used a matched group design. This means that samples of black and white children who were similar on as many demographic variables as available (e.g., age, sex,

parent education, community setting, and region) were compared. Group mean scores were then examined and effect sizes (differences between the means divided by the groups' average standard deviation) were computed. The results of this summary are presented in Table 20.1.

The magnitude of the black–white differences shown in Table 20.1 varied considerably as a function of the instrument used. Those tests that include verbal and quantitative subtests (most achievement-like) showed the largest differences (Wasserman & Becker, 2000). Tests that include verbal subtests (the WISC-III, WJ-R, and SB-IV) yielded larger race differences than those that do not include verbal subtests and those that measure cognitive processing (e.g., the CAS and K-ABC). Similarly, nonverbal tests (e.g., the NNAT and UNIT) that also require minimal achievement showed smaller race differences than the more achievement-oriented tests. The most salient conclusion that may be drawn from the findings presented in Table 20.1 is the fact that the content and methods used to conceptualize and measure intelligence across these tests are very different, and that these differences appear to be related to the size of black–white differences.

It may be argued that those tests of ability that do not contain verbal achievement tests are somehow less valid measures of ability, and therefore that the differences between race groups are reduced for this reason. However, as addressed earlier, tests like the K-ABC and CAS correlate very well with achievement, even though they do not con-

TABLE 20.1. Differences between Mean Scores for Black and White Samples on Several Ability Tests

Test	Blacks	Whites	N	Difference	Effect size
WJ-R Cognitive	90.9	102.6	854	11.7	0.69
WISC-III FSIQ	89.9	100.9	252	11.0	0.73
Stanford–Binet IV	98.0	106.1	364	8.1	0.54
UNIT	91.6	99.1	222	7.5	0.54
K-ABC	91.5	97.6	172	6.1	0.59
KABC-II	96.0	101.7	465	5.7	—
NNAT	99.3	95.1	4,612	4.2	0.25
CAS	95.3	98.8	238	3.5	0.26

Note. Sample sizes are for both groups combined except in the case of the KABC-II, which is for blacks only. All comparisons include samples that were either matched or controlled on demographic variables.

tain verbal and quantitative subtests. It is therefore reasonable to conclude that redefining intelligence without verbal and quantitative tests is a viable option both for prediction to achievement and for fair assessment. The shortcoming of using nonverbal tests is that such tests do not measure multiple forms of ability—something that is very important for differential diagnosis and treatment planning.

PASS Profiles

Several researchers have examined the profiles of PASS scores obtained for populations of children with ADHD, mental retardation, and reading disabilities. The important finding among the various studies was that differences in PASS profiles between groups emerged in predictable ways. Children with mental retardation earned similarly low PASS scores; children with reading disabilities generally evidenced average Planning, Attention, and Simultaneous scores, but low Successive scores; and those with ADHD (combined type) generally earned average Attention, Simultaneous, and Successive scores, but low Planning scores. The finding of low Planning scores in children with ADHD is a seemingly contradictory result, because ADHD is thought to be a failure of *attention*. However, as Barkley (1997, 1998) and others have suggested, ADHD is a failure of control related to frontal lobe functioning intimately involved in regulating and self-monitoring performance, which is con-

sistent with the *planning* part of the PASS theory.

Paolitto (1999) was the first to study the cognitive performance of matched samples of children with ADHD and no disability on the CAS. He found that the children with ADHD earned significantly lower scores on the Planning scale. Two subsequent studies (Dehn, 2000; Naglieri, Goldstein, Iseman, & Schwebach, 2003) found that groups of children who met diagnostic criteria for ADHD earned significantly lower mean scores on the Planning scale of the CAS than matched controls. Importantly, we (Naglieri, Goldstein, Iseman, et al., 2003) also found that children with ADHD had a different PASS profile (lowest in Planning [87] and highest in Simultaneous [99]) from those with anxiety disorders, whose four PASS scores were all in the average range (94 [Planning] to 105 [Simultaneous]). These results support the view of Barkley (1997, 1998) that ADHD involves problems with behavioral inhibition and self-control, which is associated with poor executive control (assessed by the Planning scale). These findings are in contrast to those reported for children with reading disabilities, who earned low scores on the CAS Successive scale (Naglieri & Das, 1997a), and for children with mental retardation, who had similar low PASS scores (Naglieri & Rojahn, 2001).

The various studies involving special populations are summarized in Figure 20.3. This figure provides a graph of the differences between each group's average PASS score and

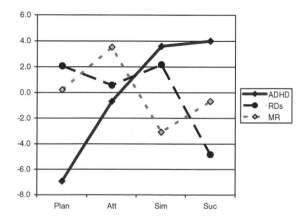

FIGURE 20.3. PASS profiles for children with attention-deficit/hyperactivity disorder (ADHD), reading disabilities (RDs), and mental retardation (MR).

each PASS scale. The ADHD means were computed on the basis of all the samples described in the previous paragraph. The results illustrate that the group with mental retardation showed minimal variation among the four PASS scales (about ±2 standard score points). In contrast, the profiles of the children with ADHD and reading disabilities are quite disparate. The children with reading problems showed a Successive weakness (about 5 points), whereas the children with ADHD evidenced a Planning deficit (about 7 points). These findings are consistent with Das's view (see Das et al., 1994) of reading failure as a deficit in sequencing of information (successive), as well as with Barkley's view of ADHD as a failure in control (planning). These findings suggest that the PASS processing scores may have utility for differential diagnosis and, by implication, intervention. This is discussed in the next section.

Intervention Relevance and Clinical Applications

Two methods have been used successfully that relate PASS theory to interventions for children who have learning problems. The first is the PASS Remedial Program (PREP; Das, 1999), and the second is the Planning Facilitation Method (Naglieri & Gottling, 1997). In addition, a recent book (Naglieri & Pickering, 2003) describes academic interventions based on the PASS theory. These approaches to intervention vary from formal (PREP) to less formal (Planning Facilitation), but both are based on the PASS theory and help relate information about a student's processing levels to cognitively based intervention methods.

PASS Remedial Program

The PREP is based on the PASS theory and supported by a line of research beginning with Brailsford, Snart, and Das (1984), D. Kaufman and P. Kaufman (1979), and Krywaniuk and Das (1976). These researchers demonstrated that students could be trained to use successive and simultaneous processes more efficiently, and thereby improve "their performance on that process and some transfer to specific reading tasks also occurred" (Ashman & Conway, 1997, p. 169). The most current version of PREP

(Das, 1999) makes the connection of successive and simultaneous processes with reading more explicit. The focus of PREP is on successive processing, even though it includes tasks that involve simultaneous processing. The tasks teach children to focus their attention on the sequential nature of many tasks, including reading. This helps the children better utilize successive processing, which is important in reading decoding.

Studies of the effectiveness of PREP for children with reading decoding problems have provided support for the instructional method. Carlson and Das (1997) studied Chapter 1 children who received PREP (n =22) in comparison to a regular reading program (control n = 15). The samples were tested before and after intervention, using two reading tests (WJ-R Word Attack and Word Identification). The intervention was conducted in two 50-minute sessions each week for 12 weeks. Das, Mishra, and Pool's (1995) study involved 51 children with reading disabilities who were divided into PREP (n = 31) and control (n =20) groups. There were 15 PREP sessions given to small groups of four children. The WJ-R Word Attack and Word Identification tests were administered pre- and posttreatment. In both studies, the PREP groups significantly outperformed the control groups.

Boden and Kirby (1995) studied a group of children with learning disabilities who were randomly assigned to PREP training and to a control group that received regular classroom instruction. As in previous studies, the results showed significant differences between the two groups in reading decoding of real words and pseudowords. Similarly, Das, Parrila, and Papadopoulos (2000) found that children who were taught with PREP (n = 23) improved significantly more in pseudoword reading than did a control group (n = 17). All of these experimental studies of the value of PREP "suggest that process training can assist in specific aspects of beginning reading" (Ashman & Conway, 1997, p. 171). In addition, they illustrate the connection between PASS theory and instruction.

Planning Facilitation

The connection between planning and intervention has been examined in several studies involving both math and reading. These intervention studies focused on the concept that children can be encouraged to be more planful when they complete academic tasks, and that the facilitation of plans has a positive impact on academic performance. The initial concept for the Planning Facilitation Method was based on the work of Cormier, Carlson, and Das (1990) and Kar, Dash, Das, and Carlson (1992). These authors taught children to discover the value of strategy use without being specifically instructed to do so. The children were encouraged to examine the demands of the task in a strategic and organized manner. They demonstrated that students *differentially* benefited from the techniques that facilitated planning. Children who performed poorly on measures of planning demonstrated significantly greater gains than those with higher planning scores. These first results indicated that a relationship between PASS theory and instruction might be possible.

We (Naglieri & Gottling, 1995, 1997) demonstrated that Planning Facilitation could improve children's performance in math calculation. All participants in these studies attended a special school for children with learning disabilities. In the investigations, students completed mathematics worksheets in sessions over about a 2-month period. The method designed to teach planning indirectly was applied in individual, one-on-one tutoring sessions (Naglieri & Gottling, 1995) or in the classroom by the teacher (Naglieri & Gottling, 1997) about two to three times per week in 30-minute blocks of time. In the intervention phase, the students were given a 10-minute period to complete a page of math problems; a 10-minute period was then used for facilitating planning; and, finally, another 10-minute period was allotted for completing the math problems. All students were exposed to the intervention sessions that involved these three 10-minute segments (mathematics, discussion, and mathematics) in 30-minute instructional periods. During the baseline period the discussion was unrelated to the task, but during the intervention period the students were encouraged to recognize the need to plan and use strategies when completing math problems. The teachers provided probes that facilitated discussion and encouraged the children to consider various ways to be more successful. When a student

provided a response, this often became the beginning point for discussion and further development of the strategy. More details about the method are provided elsewhere (Naglieri & Gottling, 1995, 1997; Naglieri & Pickering, 2003).

We (Naglieri & Johnson, 2000) further studied the relationship between Planning Facilitation and PASS profiles for a class of children with learning disabilities and mild mental impairments. The purpose of this study was to determine whether children with a cognitive weakness in one of the four PASS processes would show different rates of improvement as a function of their processing disorder when given the same group Planning Facilitation instruction. Children with a cognitive weakness (an individual score significantly lower than the child's mean and below 85 on either the Planning, Attention, Simultaneous, or Successive scale of the CAS) were used to form contrast groups. A group with no cognitive weakness was also identified. We found that children with a cognitive weakness on the Planning scale improved considerably over baseline rates, while those with no cognitive weakness improved only marginally. Similarly, children with cognitive weaknesses on the Simultaneous, Successive, and Attention scales showed substantially lower rates of improvement than either the group with a Planning weakness or the group with no cognitive weakness. The importance of this study was that the five groups of children responded very differently to the same intervention. Thus PASS scale scores on the CAS were predictive of the children's response to this math intervention. This technique can also be applied in other academic areas.

In the most recent study of the effects of Planning Facilitation (Haddad et al., 2003), researchers examined whether an instruction designed to facilitate planning would have differential benefit on reading comprehension and whether improvement was related to the PASS processing scores of each child. We used a sample of general education children sorted into three groups based on their PASS scale profiles from the CAS. Even though the groups did not differ by CAS FS scores or pretest reading comprehension scores, children with a Planning scale weakness benefited substantially (effect size of 1.52) from the instruction designed to facilitate planning. In contrast, children with no PASS scale weakness or a Successive scale weakness did not benefit as much (effect sizes of 0.52 and 0.06, respectively). These results further supported previous research suggesting that PASS profiles are relevant to instruction.

The results of these studies of Planning Facilitation, using nonacademic as well as academic (reading and math) tasks, suggest that changing the way aptitude is conceptualized (i.e., in terms of PASS theory rather than traditional IQ) and measured (with the CAS) increases the probability of detecting an aptitude × treatment interaction (ATI). Past ATI research suffered from inadequate conceptualizations of aptitudes based on the general intelligence model. That approach is different from the basic psychological processing view represented by the PASS theory and operationalized by the CAS. The summary of studies summarized here are particularly different from previous ATI research, which found that students with low general ability improved little, whereas those with high general ability improved a lot with instruction. In contrast, children with a weakness in one of the PASS processes (i.e., planning) benefited *more* from instruction than did children who had no weakness or a weakness in a different PASS process. The results of these studies also suggests that PASS profiles can help predict which children will respond to the academic instruction called Planning Facilitation and which will not. This offers an important opportunity for researchers and practitioners to use PASS profiles for the design of instruction, as suggested elsewhere (Naglieri, 1999; Naglieri & Pickering, 2003).

Factor Analysis

Factor structure of the CAS, and by implication the PASS theory, has been a topic of some discussion. In the CAS Interpretive Handbook, Naglieri and Das (1997c) reported information about the factor structure of the CAS using both exploratory and confirmatory factor-analytic methods. They provided evidence that the PASS four-factor solution was the best solution based on the convergence of both factor-analytic results, clinical utility of the four separate scores, evidence of strategy use, and theoretical interpretation of the subtests. Keith and Kranzler

(1999) challenged this position and argued that there was not sufficient support for the PASS structure. Naglieri (1999b) responded with considerable evidence and rational arguments in defense of the structure of the test and the validity of the theory. The issue has again been examined using an alternative to the methods used by both Naglieri and Das and Keith and Kranzler. This factor technique is considered more objective than the statistical approaches previously used (Blaha, 2003).

Blaha (2003) conducted an examination of the CAS subtest assignment using an exploratory hierarchical factor-analytic method described by Blaha and Wallbrown (1996). This method is less subjective and follows the data more closely, allowing for the most probable factor-analytic model (Carroll, 1993). Blaha found a general factor that he equated to the CAS Full Scale and interpreted as a general intelligence factor. This represents the overlap among the diverse PASS scales. After removal of the variance caused by the general factor, two factors emerged. The first was comprised of the Simultaneous and Successive and the second included the Planning and Attention subtests. At the third level four primary factors were found that consisted of each of the four PASS scales. He concluded that the results "provide support for maintaining the Full Scale as well as Planning, Attention, Simultaneous, and Successive standard scores of the CAS" (p. 1).

It is important to recognize that the technique of factor analysis is far from objective. In fact, Carroll (1994) wrote that "analyzing factor-analytic data is in many respects an art rather than a science" (p. 49). Even his important work, based on factor analysis, illustrates the problem with the method. For example, Carroll noted that not all the analyses included in his book were conducted with the same methodologies. He noted that

in the course of the project, over more than five years, various refinements in techniques were discovered or devised, but it was not deemed feasible to go back and apply these refinements uniformly to all datasets that had already been analyzed at a given stage of the work. . . . Perhaps partly for this reason, but mostly because of characteristics inherent in the data, the reanalyses resulted in many indeterminacies and questions that the data left unresolved. (Carroll, 1993, p. 113)

Variety in the exact methods, assumptions, and decisions made by investigators can lead to different results. Factor-analytic methods are therefore far from decisive, and factor analysis should not be given inordinate weight as a method for establishing or discrediting the validity of any instrument. At best, it provides one piece of evidence that must be part of a balanced examination of validity. Other types of validity evidence—such as relationships to achievement, diagnostic utility, issues of fair assessment, and relevance to instructional interventions—should also be considered.

INTERPRETATION

A summary of CAS interpretation methods is provided in this section, but a complete discussion can be found in Naglieri (1999a). These interpretive steps should be applied within the context of all available information about a child, so that a comprehensive assessment (diagnosis and treatment planning) of the child is achieved. All the values needed to conduct interpretation of CAS are provided by the CAS Rapid Score (Naglieri, 2002).

Interpretation of CAS scores involves four essential steps that may be modified according to the specific purposes of the assessment. The two steps described here involve examination of the PASS scales and subtests; the others are comparison of CAS results with tests of achievement, and comparisons of CAS scores obtained over time.

Step 1

The first step in any ability test evaluation includes an examination of the child's levels of performance, in terms of descriptive categories, confidence intervals, and percentile ranks. Each of these scores is interpreted according to the PASS theory (see Naglieri, 1999a). The CAS FS score is intended to be an overall estimate of processing based on the combination of the four PASS scales. This score is intended to be a convenient summary of performance. It will be a good overall description of a child's cognitive processing when the four PASS scale scores are similar. However, when there is significant variability among the PASS scale standard scores, the FS will not show important relative strengths and weaknesses; it should be deemphasized in such cases.

Step 2

The examination of differences in the four PASS scale scores for an individual child is conducted next, to determine whether cognitive strengths or weaknesses are found. This is an essential component of the CAS interpretation. Variation in PASS scores is accomplished by examining the statistical significance of the profile of scores, using an intraindividual or ipsative method. The approach provides a way to determine when the variation in PASS scores is meaningful. When the variation is not significant, any differences are assumed to reflect measurement error. Meaningful, or reliable, variation can be (1) interpreted within the context of the theory, (2) related to strategy use, (3) evaluated in relation to achievement tests, and (4) used for treatment planning.

When a PASS score is significantly above the child's mean score, then a cognitive processing strength is found. When a PASS score is significantly lower than the child's mean score, then a weakness is detected. Strengths and weaknesses determined relative to the child's own average level of performance tell us about relative strengths or weaknesses. The substeps needed to determine whether a child's PASS profile is significant are shown below. The values needed for significance at different levels of significance and for the Standard and Basic Batteries are provided elsewhere (Naglieri, 1999a; Naglieri & Das, 1997b).

1. Calculate the average of the four PASS standard scores.
2. Subtract the mean from each of the PASS standard scores to obtain the intraindividual difference scores.
3. Compare the difference scores (ignore the sign) to the values in the CAS administration and scoring manual (Naglieri & Das, 1997b). When the difference score is equal to or greater than the values, the score differs significantly from the child's average PASS scale standard score.

4. Label any significant score that is above the mean as a *strength*, and any significant score that is below the mean as a *weakness*. Any variation from the mean that is not significant should be considered chance fluctuation.

There is an important distinction between a relative weakness and a cognitive weakness (Naglieri, 2000). A *relative weakness* is found when at least one PASS scale standard score is significantly lower than the child's mean PASS score. Because the PASS scores are compared to the individual child's average (and not the normative mean of 100), this tells us about relative strengths or weaknesses. For example, if a child has scores of 114 (Planning), 116 (Simultaneous), 94 (Successive), and 109 (Successive), the Successive score—which is 14.25 points below the child's mean of 108.25—is a relative weakness.

A *cognitive weakness* is found when there is significant PASS variability (a relative weakness) *and* the lowest score is below average (<85). The child with a cognitive weakness is likely to have significantly lower achievement scores and more likely to have been identified as exceptional (Naglieri, 2000). Using this method ensures that the deficit in basic psychological processing is found in relation to peers, not just in relation to the child him- or herself. A child who has a cognitive weakness has evidence of a disorder in one of the four PASS basic psychological processes—evidence that, when paired with a deficit in achievement can form the basis of eligibility determination according to IDEA '97. This will be discussed further in the case study that appears later in this chapter.

INNOVATIONS IN MEASUREMENT OF COGNITIVE ABILITIES

What is innovative about the CAS—and, by extension, the PASS theory? First, CAS represents a substantial change from the general intelligence approach that has dominated the field of intellectual assessment. By rejecting the verbal–nonverbal dichotomy and eliminating achievement-like content (e.g., Vocabulary and Arithmetic subtests), the CAS provides a very different view of ability. The new understanding represented by the CAS is based on neuropsychology and cognitive psychology rather than on traditional IQ, which was developed largely on methods used by the U.S. military in the early 1900s (Yoakum & Yerkes, 1920). This new understanding provides a number of important advantages that have been summarized in the "Validity" section of this chapter—most notably fairer assessment of minority children, identification of the cognitive deficits that interfere with academic success, and an opportunity for differential diagnosis. Perhaps most importantly, the shift from general intelligence to a cognitive processing approach as represented by PASS theory and the CAS provides a clear connection to instructional intervention, as shown by a number of research studies also summarized in this chapter.

The connection between PASS theory and the CAS on the one hand, and intervention on the other, extends beyond the research on PREP and Planning Facilitation described earlier. The concept of using a cognitive approach to instruction (Ashman & Conway, 1997) forms the basis of several books (Ashman & Conway, 1993; Kirby & Williams, 1991; Mastropieri & Scruggs, 1991; Minskoff & Allsopp, 2003; Pressley & Woloshyn, 1995; Scheid, 1993). Our (Naglieri & Pickering, 2003) book of instructional handouts exemplifies the connection between PASS and the application of cognitive instructional methods. The relationship between cognition as measured by PASS and learning is a strong one, and therefore utilization of PASS information by practitioners for instructional (as well as eligibility) purposes is supported by the scientific research cited here.

BRIEF CASE STUDY: THE CASE OF BEN

The following is a case abstracted from one described in the book *Helping Children Learn: Intervention Handouts for Use in School and at Home* (Naglieri & Pickering, 2003). I provide this case to illustrate how the PASS constructs can be used to identify a cognitive processing weakness, how that weakness can be related to academic failure, how these two findings interface with issues of eligibility for special education, and how the information can be used for instructional planning. The approach is intentionally limited to CAS and achievement results for the purpose of efficiency and length. In actuality, a complete assessment should include more than is presented in this illustration.

Ben is an energetic but frustrated third-grade student who likes his teachers, is popular with his peers, and socially fits in well at school. He reports, however, that he does not like school at all. Even though he puts forth much effort, Ben earns poor grades and is getting more and more frustrated each year. Ben struggles to perform well because he has a lot of trouble following directions, and he does not appear to read very well or understand what he reads. He has considerable trouble with spelling and makes many errors in the sequence of letters in words. Ben's written work is also problematic. He does not express his ideas in a logical order, and he sometimes uses incorrect tense or plurals and conjugates incorrectly. After reading short stories and books for reading class, he does not remember the sequence of events, and therefore often comes to illogical conclusions. Ben has considerable trouble with math as well, particularly with remembering basic math facts. Ben reports that even though he tries to learn his math facts by writing them repeatedly every day, he still does not know them. Ben's parents note that he does not do things around the house in a logical and efficient order. Ben's mother reports that he cannot remember phone numbers and has had to write the combination for his bike lock on his hand. In addition, he has trouble finding words in a dictionary, because he does not seem to know the order of letters.

It is not hard to anticipate that Ben probably has difficulty with successive processing. In fact, a complete assessment has revealed that Ben is an emotionally healthy young man with anxiety about his problems with learning. He has about average scores on many measures of achievement, but especially poor scores on Spelling, Reading Decoding, and Math Calculation. Ben also has a cognitive weakness on the Successive scale of the CAS (see Table 20.2), because this score is 11.1 standard score points below his PASS average of 98.0, *and* it is considerably below normal. Ben has adequate scores on

TABLE 20.2. Selected Standard Scores from Ben's Psychoeducational Assessment, in Order of Magnitude

CAS of achievement test scale	Score
Spelling	79
Reading Decoding	81
Successive	81
Math Calculation	83
Math Reasoning	90
Reading Comprehension	91
Simultaneous	93
Attention	106
Planning	112

the CAS Simultaneous, Attention, and Planning scales, as well as Reading Comprehension. His adequate score in Reading Comprehension may seem counterintuitive, given the description of his school problems, but a careful analysis of the reading comprehension questions included on the test indicted that few were based on ordering of information. How would this portion of Ben's assessment relate to eligibility determination?

Ben's academic failure and cognitive weakness in successive processing fit with the IDEA '97 definition of a specific learning disability (SLD). His CAS Successive score and achievement scores provide evidence of "a disorder in one or more of the basic psychological processes involved in understanding or in using language, spoken or written, that may manifest itself in an imperfect ability to listen, think, read, write, spell, or to do mathematical calculations" (Naglieri & Sullivan, 1998, p. 27). Ben's disorder in successive processing underlies his academic failure in reading and spelling (and math calculation as well). The disorder in basic psychological processing and achievement has been documented with reliable and valid standardized instruments, and there is clear evidence of variability in his levels of ability and achievement. Ben's difficulty with successive processing has made attempts to teach him ineffective and the need for of specialized instruction clear. What types of instruction would be likely to work best for Ben?

The Naglieri and Pickering (2003) book provides academic instructional handouts and other methods that illustrate ways Ben's teachers and his parents can help him overcome his problem with successive tasks. The aim of the intervention is to focus on specific strategies for dealing with academic problems related to the successive weakness. Ben's successive weakness limits his ability to acquire serially ordered information. Instruction, therefore, should provide alternative ways of learning that do not rely heavily on this weakness. For example, to reduce the successive demands of letter sequences, Ben can be taught to use the "Chunking for Spelling" and "Strategies for Spelling" handouts (see Naglieri & Pickering, 2003, pp. 89 and 95–96, respectively). These utilize plans for remembering order, thereby reducing the importance of successive processing. To help Ben better remember the sequence of events in a story, he can use simultaneous and planning processes to create *story maps*" (see Naglieri & Pickering, 2003, p. 97). A story map is a plan that uses graphic representations of the facts of a story, so that Ben can organize what he reads into discrete steps and can thus better understand the story's order. The instructional handout titled "Story Grammar" (see Naglieri & Pickering, 2003, p. 101) can also be used to help him write in an order that makes sense.

Ben's difficulty with math calculation can be addressed with methods such as the "Plans for Basic Math Facts" handout, which will allow him to learn his basic facts through a logical method rather than relying on recall of the sequence of facts (see Naglieri & Pickering, 2003, p. 113). In addition, the "Number Squares" handout (see Naglieri & Pickering, 2003, p. 111) helps the child understand the relationships between numbers (simultaneous) and relies less on sequencing.

The instructional methods described above are intended to provide practitioners with illustrations of how a teacher can more effectively teach a child with a learning disability, as well as a child with mild cognitive problems. For example, using a collaborative consultation approach, a school psychologist can work with teachers to develop additional methods that address the problems created by a child's cognitive weakness. Through a better understanding of the particular cognitive strengths and weakness of the child and how these interface with academic performance, a child like Ben (as well as other children with specific learning disorders) can be more successful.

CONCLUSIONS

This chapter is based on the assumption that a cognitive approach to conceptualizing and measuring basic psychological processes offers a better solution than traditional IQ tests to the demands for efficient diagnosis and treatment that are placed on today's school and clinical psychologist. Advances in cognitive psychology and neuropsychology have provided the opportunity for change, and the PASS theory, as represented by the CAS, reflects this modern view of ability. The research summarized in this chapter demonstrates that the CAS offers a strong alternative to traditional tests, as evidenced by four major findings. First, children with disabilities (particularly reading disabilities and ADHD) have PASS profiles that are relevant to diagnosis. Second, the CAS is an excellent predictor of achievement, despite the fact that it does not contain verbal and achievement-based tests like those found in traditional IQ tests. Third, the CAS yields the smallest difference between white and black children among the tests of ability described in this chapter. And fourth, the PASS theory provides information that is relevant to intervention and instructional planning. The advantages offered by the CAS are timely, given the demands placed on practitioners today, and important to help children maximize academic success.

ACKNOWLEDGMENTS

Preparation of this chapter was supported in part by Grant No. R215K010121 from the U.S. Department of Education.

REFERENCES

Ashman, A. F., & Conway, R. N. F. (1993). *Using cognitive methods in the classroom*. London: Routledge.
Ashman, A. F., & Conway, R. N. F. (1997). *An introduction to cognitive education: Theory and applications*. London: Routledge.
Barkley, R. A. (1997). *ADHD and the nature of self-control*. New York: Guilford Press.
Barkley, R. A. (1998). *Attention-deficit hyperactivity*

disorder: A handbook for diagnosis and treatment (2nd ed.). New York: Guilford Press.

Blaha, J. (2003). *What does the CAS really measure?: An exploratory hierarchical factor analysis of the Cognitive Assessment System*. Paper presented at the annual convention of the National Association of School Psychologists, Chicago.

Blaha, J., & Wallbrown, F. H. (1996). Hierarchical factor structure of the Wechsler Intelligence Scale for Children—III. *Psychological Assessment, 8,* 214–218.

Boden, C., & Kirby, J. R. (1995). Successive processing, phonological coding and the remediation of reading. *Journal of Cognitive Education, 4,* 19–31.

Bracken, B. A. (1987). Limitations of preschool instruments and standards for minimal levels of technical adequacy. *Journal of Psychoeducational Assessment, 5,* 313–326.

Bracken, B. A., & McCallum, R. S. (1998). *The Universal Nonverbal Intelligence Test*. Itasca, IL: Riverside.

Brailsford, A., Snart, F., & Das, J. P. (1984). Strategy training and reading comprehension. *Journal of Learning Disabilities, 17,* 287–290.

Brody, N. (1992). *Intelligence*. San Diego, CA: Academic Press.

Carlson, J., & Das, J. P. (1997). A process approach to remediating word decoding deficiencies in Chapter 1 children. *Learning Disabilities Quarterly, 20,* 93–102.

Carroll, J. B. (1993). *Human cognitive abilities: A survey of factor-analytic studies*. New York: Cambridge University Press.

Carroll, J. B. (1994). Cognitive abilities: Constructing a theory from data. In D. K. Detterman (Ed.), *Current topics in human intelligence: Vol. 4. Theories of intelligence* (pp. 43–63). Norwood, NJ: Ablex.

Cohen, R. J., Swerdlik, M. E., & Smith, D. K. (1992). *Psychological testing and assessment*. Mountain View, CA: Mayfield.

Cormier, P., Carlson, J. S., & Das, J. P. (1990). Planning ability and cognitive performance: The compensatory effects of a dynamic assessment approach. *Learning and Individual Differences, 2,* 437–449.

Das, J. P. (1999). *PASS Reading Enhancement Program*. Deal, NJ: Sarka Educational Resources.

Das, J. P., Kirby, J. R., & Jarman, R. F. (1979). *Simultaneous and successive cognitive processes*. New York: Academic Press.

Das, J. P., Mishra, R. K., & Pool, J. E. (1995). An experiment on cognitive remediation or word-reading difficulty. *Journal of Learning Disabilities, 28,* 66–79.

Das, J. P., Naglieri, J. A., & Kirby, J. R. (1994). *Assessment of cognitive processes*. Needham Heights, MA: Allyn & Bacon.

Das, J. P., Parrila, R., & Papadopoulos, R. (2000). Cognitive education and reading disability. In A. Kozulin & Y. Rand (Eds.), *Experiences of mediated learning* (pp. 274–291). Amsterdam: Pergamon Press.

Dehn, M. (2000). *Cognitive assessment system performance of children with ADHD*. Poster presented at the annual convention of the National Association of School Psychologists, New Orleans, LA.

Elliott, C. D. (1990). *Differential ability scales: Introductory and technical handbook*. San Antonio, TX: Psychological Corporation.

Haddad, F. A., Garcia, Y. E., Naglieri, J. A., Grimditch, M., McAndrews, A., & Eubanks, J. (2003). Planning facilitation and reading comprehension: Instructional relevance of the PASS theory. *Journal of Psychoeducational Assessment, 21,* 282–289.

Hilliard, A. G. (1979). Standardization and cultural bias as impediments to the scientific study and validation of "intelligence." *Journal of Research and Development in Education, 12,* 47–58.

Kar, B. C., Dash, U. N., Das, J. P., & Carlson, J. S. (1992). Two experiments on the dynamic assessment of planning. *Learning and Individual Differences, 5,* 13–29.

Kaufman, A. S., & Kaufman, N. L. (1983). *Kaufman Assessment Battery for Children*. Circle Pines, MN: American Guidance Service.

Kaufman, A. S., Harrison, P. L., & Ittenbach, R. F. (1990). Intelligence testing in the schools. In T. B. Gutkin & C. R. Reynolds (Eds.), *Handbook of school psychology* (pp. 289–327). New York: Wiley.

Kaufman, D., & Kaufman, P. (1979). Strategy training and remedial techniques. *Journal of Learning Disabilities, 12,* 63–66.

Kaufman, J. C. (2003). *Race differences on the KABC-II*. Paper presented at the Gender and Ethnic Differences on the KABC-II convention, Toronto.

Keith, T. Z., & Kranzler, J. H. (1999). Independent confirmatory factor analysis of the Cognitive Assessment System (CAS): What does the CAS measure? *School Psychology Review, 28,* 117–144.

Kirby, J. R., & Williams, N. H. (1991). *Learning problems: A cognitive approach*. Toronto: Kagan & Woo.

Krywaniuk, L. W., & Das, J. P. (1976). Cognitive strategies in native children: Analysis and intervention. *Alberta Journal of Educational Research, 22,* 271–280.

Luria, A. R. (1966a). *Higher cortical functions in man*. New York: Basic Books.

Luria, A. R. (1966b). *Human brain and psychological processes*. New York: Harper & Row.

Luria, A. R. (1973). *The working brain: An introduction to neuropsychology*. New York: Basic Books.

Luria, A. R. (1980). *Higher cortical functions in man* (2nd ed.). New York: Basic Books.

Luria, A. R. (1982). *Language and cognition*. New York: Wiley.

Mastropieri, M. A., & Scruggs, T. E. (1991). *Teaching students ways to remember: Strategies for learning mnemonically*. Cambridge, MA: Brookline Books.

McGrew, K. S., Werder, J. K., & Woodcock, R. W. (1991). *WJ-R technical manual*. Chicago: Riverside.

Messick, S. (1995). Validity of psychological assessment: Validation of inferences from persons' responses and performances as scientific inquiry into score meaning. *American Psychologist, 50,* 741–749.

Minskoff, E., & Allsopp, D. (2003). *Academic success*

strategies for adolescents with learning disabilities and ADHD. Baltimore: Brookes.

Naglieri, J. A. (1986). WISC-R and K-ABC comparison for matched samples of black and white children. Journal of School Psychology, 24, 81–88.

Naglieri, J. A. (1997). Naglieri Nonverbal Ability Test. San Antonio, TX: Psychological Corporation.

Naglieri, J. A. (1999a). Essentials of CAS assessment. New York: Wiley.

Naglieri, J. A. (1999b). How valid is the PASS theory and CAS? School Psychology Review, 28, 145–162.

Naglieri, J. A. (2000). Can profile analysis of ability test scores work?: An illustration using the PASS theory and CAS with an unselected cohort. School Psychology Quarterly, 15(4), 419–433.

Naglieri, J. A. (2002). CAS Rapid Score [Computer software]. Centreville, VA: NL Associates.

Naglieri, J. A., & Das, J. P. (1997a). Cognitive Assessment System. Itasca, IL: Riverside.

Naglieri, J. A., & Das, J. P. (1997b). Cognitive Assessment System: Administration and scoring manual. Itasca, IL: Riverside.

Naglieri, J. A., & Das, J. P. (1997c). Cognitive Assessment System: Interpretive handbook. Itasca, IL: Riverside.

Naglieri, J. A., Goldstein, S., & DeLauder, B. (2003). A comparison of WISC-III and CAS correlations with WJ-III Achievement scores. Manuscript submitted for publication.

Naglieri, J. A., Goldstein, S., Iseman, J. S., & Schwebach, A. (2003). Performance of children with attention deficit hyperactivity disorder and anxiety/depression on the WISC-III and Cognitive Assessment System (CAS). Journal of Psychoeducational Assessment, 21, 32–42.

Naglieri, J. A., & Gottling, S. H. (1995). A cognitive education approach to math instruction for the learning disabled: An individual study. Psychological Reports, 76, 1343–1354.

Naglieri, J. A., & Gottling, S. H. (1997). Mathematics instruction and PASS cognitive processes: An intervention study. Journal of Learning Disabilities, 30, 513–520.

Naglieri, J. A., & Johnson, D. (2000). Effectiveness of a cognitive strategy intervention to improve math calculation based on the PASS theory. Journal of Learning Disabilities, 33, 591–597.

Naglieri, J. A., & Pickering, E. (2003). Helping children learn: Instructional handouts for use in school and at home. Baltimore: Brookes.

Naglieri, J. A., & Rojahn, J. (2001). Evaluation of African-American and white children in special education programs for children with mental retardation using the WISC-III and Cognitive Assessment System. American Journal on Mental Retardation, 106, 359–367.

Naglieri, J. A., & Sullivan, L. (1998). IDEA and identification of children with specific learning disabilities. Communiqué, 27, 20–21.

Paolitto, A. W. (1999). Clinical validation of the Cognitive Assessment System with children with ADHD. ADHD Report, 7, 1–5.

Pressley, M. P., & Woloshyn, V. (1995). Cognitive strategy instruction that really improves children's academic performance (2nd ed.). Cambridge, MA: Brookline Books.

Prifitera, A., & Saklofske, D. (Eds.). (1998). WISC-III clinical use and interpretation: Scientist-practitioner perspectives. San Diego, CA: Academic Press.

Reschly, D. J., & Bersoff, D. N. (1999). Law and school psychology. In C. R. Reynolds & T. B. Gutkin (Eds.), The handbook of school psychology (3rd ed., pp. 1077–1112). New York: Wiley.

Reynolds, C. R., & Kaiser, S. M. (1990). Bias in assessment of aptitude. In C. R. Reynolds & R. W. Kamphaus (Eds.), Handbook of psychological and educational assessment of children: Intelligence and achievement (pp. 611–653). New York: Guilford Press.

Thorndike, R. L., Hagen, E. P., & Sattler, J. M. (1986). The Stanford–Binet Intelligence Scale: Fourth Edition. Guide for administering and scoring. Chicago: Riverside.

Wasserman, J. D., & Becker, K. A. (2000, August). Racial and ethnic group mean score differences on intelligence tests. In J. A. Naglieri (Chair), Making assessment more fair: Taking verbal and achievement out of ability tests. Symposium conducted at the annual convention of the American Psychological Association, Washington, DC.

Wechsler, D. (1991). Wechsler Intelligence Scale for Children—Third Edition. San Antonio, TX: Psychological Corporation.

Wechsler, D. (1992). Wechsler Individual Achievement Test. San Antonio, TX: Psychological Corporation.

Woodcock, R. W., & Johnson, M. B. (1989a). Woodcock–Johnson Psycho-Educational Battery Revised Tests of Achievement: Standard and supplemental batteries. Itasca, IL: Riverside.

Woodcock, R. W., & Johnson, M. B. (1989b). Woodcock–Johnson Psychoeducational Battery, Tests of Cognitive Abilities. Itasca, IL: Riverside.

Woodcock, R. W., McGrew, K. S., & Mather, N. (2001). Woodcock–Johnson III Test of Cognitive Abilities. Itasca, IL: Riverside.

Yoakum, C. S., & Yerkes, R. M. (1920). Army mental tests. New York: Holt.

21

Introduction to
the Reynolds Intellectual Assessment Scales
and the Reynolds Intellectual Screening Test

CECIL R. REYNOLDS
RANDY W. KAMPHAUS

This chapter provides the reader with an extensive introduction to the Reynolds Intellectual Assessment Scales (RIAS; Reynolds & Kamphaus, 2003), a recently published measure of intelligence for children and adults. A brief overview of the subtests is provided, followed by a review of the theory and structure of the RIAS, framed primarily around its goals for development. A more extensive description is then provided, of the subtests and their administration and scoring. Psychometric characteristics of the RIAS are next presented, along with guidelines for interpretation and clinical applications. The chapter closes with a case study using the RIAS as the featured measure of intelligence.

The RIAS is an individually administered test of intelligence appropriate for ages 3 years through 94 years, with a conormed, supplemental measure of memory. The RIAS includes a two-subtest Verbal Intelligence Index (VIX) and a two-subtest Nonverbal Intelligence Index (NIX). The scaled sums of T scores for the four subtests are combined to form the Composite Intelligence Index (CIX), which is a summary estimate of global intelligence. Administration of the four intelligence scale subtests by a trained, experienced examiner requires approximately 20–25 minutes. A Composite Memory Index (CMX) is derived from the two supplementary memory subtests, which require approximately 10–15 minutes of additional testing time. The CIX and the CMX represent combinations of verbal and nonverbal subtests. Table 21.1 provides an overview of the Indexes and subtests of the RIAS.

The Reynolds Intellectual Screening Test (RIST; Kamphaus & Reynolds, 2003) is a two-subtest screening version of the RIAS that covers the same age range. The RIST is designed to allow users to make the decision regarding the need for a full RIAS evaluation in about 10 minutes or less (see Reynolds & Kamphaus, 2003, for complete RIST administration, scoring, and interpretation procedures).

THEORY AND STRUCTURE

The RIAS was designed to meld practical and theoretical aspects of the assessment of intelligence. Although the models of

---

Portions of this chapter are based on Reynolds and Kamphaus (2003).

TABLE 21.1. RIAS Composite Scores and Subtests

Composite Intelligence Index (CIX)

Subtests of the Verbal Intelligence Index (VIX)

Guess What. Examinees are given a set of two or three clues, and are asked to deduce the object or concept being described. This subtest measures verbal reasoning in combination with vocabulary, language development, and overall fund of available information.

Verbal Reasoning. Examinees listen to a propositional statement that essentially forms a verbal analogy, and are asked to respond with one or two words that complete the idea or proposition. This subtest measures verbal-analytical reasoning ability, but with fewer vocabulary and general knowledge demands than Guess What.

Subtests of the Nonverbal Intelligence Index (NIX)

Odd-Item Out. Examinees are presented with a picture card containing five to seven pictures or drawings, and are asked to designate which one does not belong or go with the others. This subtest measures nonverbal reasoning skills, but also requires the use of spatial ability, visual imagery, and other nonverbal skills on various items. It is a form of reverse nonverbal analogy.

What's Missing. A redesign of a classic task present on various ability measures. Examinees are shown a picture with some key element or logically consistent component missing, and are asked to identify the missing essential element. This subtest assesses nonverbal reasoning: The examinee must conceptualize the picture, analyze its Gestalt, and deduce what essential element is missing.

Composite Memory Index (CMX)

Subtests

Verbal Memory. In this verbal memory subtest, depending upon the examinee's age, a series of sentences or brief stories are read aloud by the examiner and then recalled by the examinee. This task assesses the ability to encode, store briefly, and recall verbal material in a meaningful context where associations are clear and evident.

Nonverbal Memory. This visual memory subtest contains a series of items in which a stimulus picture is presented for 5 seconds, following which an array of pictures is presented. The examinee must identify the target picture from the new array of six pictures. It assesses the ability to encode, store, and recognize pictorial stimuli that are both concrete and abstract or without meaningful referents.

Note. From Reynolds and Kamphaus (2003). Copyright 2003 by Psychological Assessment Resources, Inc. Adapted by permission.

Carroll (1993) and Cattell and Horn (Horn & Cattell, 1966; Kamphaus, 2001) were the primary theoretical guides, the RIAS also followed closely the division of intelligence into verbal and nonverbal domains, due to the practical benefits of assessing verbal and nonverbal intelligence. Memory was included as a separate scale on the RIAS, due to the growing importance of working memory in models of intelligence and the practical aspects of memory to everyday diagnostic questions faced by the practitioner (see, e.g., Bigler & Clement, 1997; Goldstein & Reynolds, 1999; Reynolds & Bigler, 1994; Reynolds & Fletcher-Janzen, 1997). To clarify the theoretical underpinnings of the RIAS as well as its practical aspects and structure, a review of the goals for development of the test provides a strong heuristic.

Development Goals

We (Reynolds & Kamphaus, 2003) described a set of eight primary goals for development of the RIAS. These goals were derived from our experiences over the years in teaching intelligence testing, our use of many different intelligence tests in clinical practice, and the current literature surrounding theoretical models of intelligence and research on intelligence test interpretation (for more extensive review and discussion, see Reynolds & Kamphaus, 2003, especially Chs. 1 and 6).

1. Provide a reliable and valid measurement of *g* and its two primary components, verbal and nonverbal intelligence, with close correspondence to crystallized and fluid intelligence.

2. Provide a practical measurement device

in terms of efficacies of time, direct costs, and information needed from a measure of intelligence.

3. Allow continuity of measurement across all developmental levels from ages 3 years through 94 years for both clinical and research purposes.

4. Substantially reduce or eliminate dependence on motor coordination and visual–motor speed in the measurement of intelligence.

5. Eliminate dependence on reading in the measurement of intelligence.

6. Provide for accurate prediction of basic academic achievement, at levels that are at least comparable to that of intelligence tests twice the length of the RIAS.

7. Apply familiar, common concepts that are clear and easy to interpret, coupled with simple administration and scoring.

8. Eliminate items that show differential item functioning, or DIF, associated with gender or ethnicity.

In addition to tasks targeting g and its two primary components, the RIAS was designed to assess basic memory functions in the verbal and nonverbal domains. Brief assessments of the integrity of memory have appeared on intelligence tests since Binet first asked children to recall a single picture and repeat a sentence of 15 words (Binet & Simon, 1905). Traditionally, scores on these tasks have been included as a component of IQ; the RIAS assesses memory function in a separate scale. The RIAS includes assessment of memory function because it is crucial to the diagnostic process for numerous disorders of childhood (Goldstein & Reynolds, 1999; Reynolds & Fletcher-Janzen, 1997) and adulthood, particularly later adulthood (Bigler & Clement, 1997). The RIAS CMX does not provide a comprehensive memory assessment, but it does cover the two areas of memory that are historically assessed by intelligence tests and are considered by many to be the two most important memory functions to assess (e.g., Bigler & Clement, 1997; Reynolds & Bigler, 1994): memory for meaningful verbal material and visual memory. Memory assessment conorming presents the best possible scenario for contrasting test scores (Reynolds, 1984–1985), allowing the clinician to compare general intelligence directly with key memory functions.

Theory

The RIAS is a measure of intelligence that focuses on the measurement of g, or general intelligence (the CIX), and the two major components of general intelligence: verbal intelligence (the VIX) and nonverbal intelligence (the NIX). As with any measure of intelligence, many other basic but subsidiary cognitive processes, such as auditory and visual perception, logical reasoning, language processing, spatial skills, visual imagery, attention, and the like, play a role in performance on the RIAS. These skills are the building blocks of the primary intellectual functions assessed by the RIAS. The RIAS CMX is offered as a basic overall measure of short-term memory skills, with the Verbal Memory subtest measuring recall in the verbal associative domain, and the Nonverbal Memory subtest measuring ability to recall pictorial stimuli in both concrete (i.e., meaningful) dimensions and abstract dimensions (where concrete referents are not provided or easily derived).

The RIAS was designed to measure four important aspects of intelligence: *general intelligence* (of which the major component is *fluid* or *reasoning abilities*); *verbal intelligence* (sometimes referred to as *crystallized abilities*, a closely related though not identical concept); *nonverbal intelligence* (referred to in some theories as *visualization* or *spatial abilities*, and closely allied with fluid intelligence); and *memory* (subtests measuring this ability have been labeled variously as assessing *working memory*, *short-term memory*, or *learning*). These four constructs are measured by combinations of the six RIAS subtests (see Table 21.1).

The RIAS subtests were selected and designed to measure intelligence constructs that have a substantial history of scientific support. In addition, Carroll's (1993) seminal and often-cited three-stratum theory of intelligence informed the creation of the RIAS by demonstrating that many of the latent traits tapped by intelligence tests were test-battery-independent. He clearly demonstrated, for example, that numerous tests measured the same crystallized, visual-perceptual, and memory abilities. However, Kamphaus (2001) concluded that these same test batteries did not measure fluid abilities to a great extent.

The RIAS focuses on the assessment of stratum III and stratum II abilities from Carroll's three-stratum theory (1993; see also Carroll, Chapter 4, this volume). Stratum III is composed of one construct only, *g*. Psychometric *g* accounts for the major portion of variance assessed by intelligence test batteries. More important, however, is the consistent finding that the correlations of intelligence tests with important outcomes, such as academic achievement and occupational attainment, are related to the amount of *g* measured by the test battery. In other words, so-called "*g*-saturated" tests are better predictors of important outcomes than are tests with low *g* saturation. One theory posits that *g* is actually a measure of working memory capacity (Kyllonen, 1996), whereas another theory posits that it is a measure of reasoning ability (Gustafsson, 1999). Regardless of the theory that will eventually be supported, the utility of psychometric *g* remains, much in the same way that the usefulness of certain pharmaceutical drugs will continue before their mechanisms of action are fully understood. For these reasons, the RIAS places great emphasis on the assessment of psychometric *g* and on the assessment of its theorized main components (i.e., verbal and nonverbal reasoning and working memory).

The second stratum in Carroll's (1993) hierarchy consists of traits that are assessed by combinations of subtests, or stratum I measures. There are, however, several stratum II traits to choose from. These second-stratum traits include fluid intelligence, crystallized intelligence, general memory and learning, broad visual perception, broad auditory perception, broad retrieval ability, broad cognitive speed, and processing speed (i.e., reaction time or decision speed). Of importance, however, is the suggestion (from the findings of hundreds of investigations) that these abilities are ordered by their assessment of *g* (Kamphaus, 2001). Specifically, subtests that tap fluid abilities are excellent measures of *g*, whereas tests of psychomotor speed are the weakest. If one accepts the aforementioned finding that *g* saturation is related to predictive validity, then the first few stratum II factors become the best candidates for inclusion in an intelligence test battery like the RIAS, especially one that seeks to be a time-efficient test. This logic informed subtest selection as well as item writing throughout the RIAS developmental process.

Any test of *g* must measure so-called "higher-order" cognitive abilities—those associated with fluid abilities, such as general sequential reasoning, induction, deduction, syllogisms, series tasks, matrix reasoning, analogies, quantitative reasoning, and so on (Carroll, 1993). Kamphaus (2001) has advocated the following definition of *reasoning*: "that which follows as a reasonable inference or natural consequence; deducible or defensible on the grounds of consistency; reasonably believed or done" (*New Shorter Oxford English Dictionary*, 1993). This definition emphasizes a central cognitive requirement to draw inferences from knowledge. This characteristic of general intelligence is measured best by two RIAS subtests, Verbal Reasoning and Odd-Item Out, although all of the subtests have substantial *g* saturation (see Reynolds & Kamphaus, 2003, especially Ch. 6).

First-order factors of crystallized ability typically have one central characteristic: They involve language abilities (Vernon, 1950). These language abilities range from vocabulary knowledge to spelling to reading comprehension. On the other hand, it is not possible to dismiss this type of intelligence as a general academic achievement factor (see Reynolds & Kamphaus, 2003, for a discussion of this point). Kamphaus (2001) has proposed that the *verbal* factor be defined as "oral and written communication skills that follow the system of rules associated with a language" (p. 45), including comprehension skills.

Nonverbal tests have come to be recognized as measures of important spatial and visual-perceptual abilities; abilities that may need to be assessed for a variety of clients including those with brain injuries. In the 1963 landmark Educational Testing Service Kit of Factor-Referenced Cognitive Tests, *spatial ability* was defined as "the ability to manipulate or transform the image of spatial patterns into other visual arrangements" (cited in Carroll, 1993, p. 316). The RIAS What's Missing and Odd-Item Out subtests follow in this long tradition of tasks designed to measure visual–spatial abilities.

Digit recall, sentence recall, geometric design recall, bead recall, and similar measures loaded consistently on a *general memory and learning* stratum II factor identified by Carroll (1993) in his numerous analyses. The RIAS Verbal Memory and Nonverbal Memory subtests are of this same variety, although they are more complex than simple confrontational memory tasks such as pure digit recall. Carroll's findings suggest that the RIAS Verbal Memory and Nonverbal Memory subtests should be good measures of the memory construct that has been identified previously in so many investigations of a diverse array of tests. Memory is typically considered a complex trait with many permutations, including visual, verbal, long term, and short term. Carroll's analysis of hundreds of data sets supports the organization of the RIAS, in that he found ample evidence of a general memory trait that may be subdivided further for particular clinical purposes.

Description of Subtests

Subtests with a familiar look and feel with essentially long histories in the field of intellectual assessment—were chosen for inclusion on the RIAS. There are a total of four intelligence subtests and two memory subtests. The intelligence subtests were also chosen because of their complex nature: Each assesses many intellectual functions and requires their integration for successful performance (see also a later section of this chapter, "Evidence Based on Response Processes"). The memory subtests were chosen not only for complexity, but also due to their representation of the primary content domains of memory.

• *Guess What.* This subtest measures vocabulary knowledge in combination with reasoning skills that are predicated on language development and fund of information. For each item, the examinee listens to a question containing clues presented orally by the examiner and then gives a verbal response (one or two words) consistent with the clues. The questions pertain to physical objects, abstract concepts, and well-known places and historical figures from a variety of cultures, geographic locations, and disciplines.

• *Verbal Reasoning.* The second verbal subtest measures analytical reasoning abilities. More difficult items also require advanced vocabulary knowledge. For each item, the examinee is asked to listen to an incomplete sentence presented orally by the examiner, and then to give a verbal response, typically one or two words, that completes the sentence (most commonly completing a complex analogy). Completion of the sentences requires the examinee to evaluate the various conceptual relationships that exist between the physical objects or abstract ideas contained in the sentences.

• *Odd-Item Out.* This subtest measures general reasoning skills emphasizing nonverbal ability. For each item, the examinee is presented with a picture card containing from five to seven figures or drawings. One of the figures or drawings on the picture card has a distinguishing characteristic, making it different from the others. For each item, the examinee is given two chances to identify the figure or drawing that is different from the others. Two points are awarded for a correct response given on the first attempt. One point is awarded for a correct response given on the second attempt (i.e., if the first response was incorrect).

• *What's Missing.* This subtest measures nonverbal reasoning skills through the presentation of pictures in which some important component of the pictured object is missing. Examinees must understand or conceptualize the pictured object, assess its Gestalt, and distinguish essential from nonessential components. For each item the examinee is shown a picture card, asked to examine the picture, and then asked to indicate (in words or by pointing) what is missing from the picture. Naming the missing part correctly is not required, so long as the examinee can indicate the missing component correctly. For each item, the examinee is given two chances to identify what is missing from the picture.

• *Verbal Memory.* This subtest measures the ability to encode, briefly store, and recall verbal material in a meaningful context. Young children (ages 3–4 years) are asked to listen to sentences of progressively greater length read aloud by the examiner, and then asked to repeat each sentence word for word immediately after it is read aloud. Older children and adults listen to two stories read aloud by the examiner, and then repeat each story back to the examiner immediately after it is read aloud. The sentences and stories were written to provide developmentally appropriate content and material of interest to the targeted age group. Specific stories are designated for various age groups.

• *Nonverbal Memory.* This subtest measures the ability to encode, briefly store, and recall visually presented material, whether the stimuli represent concrete objects or abstract concepts. For each item, the examinee is presented with a target picture for 5 seconds, and then with a picture card containing the target picture and an array of similar pictures. The examinee is asked to identify the target picture among the array of pictures presented on the picture card. For each item, the examinee is given two chances to identify the target picture. The pictures are primarily abstract at the upper age levels, and pictures of common objects at the lower age levels. The use of naming and related language strategies is not helpful, however, due to the design of the distractors.

ADMINISTRATION AND SCORING

The RIAS was specifically designed to be easy to administer and objective to score. For all subtests except Verbal Memory, there are clear, objective lists of correct responses for each test item, and seldom are any judgment calls required. Studies of the interscorer reliability of these five subtests produced interscorer reliability coefficients of 1.00 by trained examiners (Reynolds & Kamphaus, 2003). On Verbal Memory, some judgment is required when examinees do not give verbatim responses; however, the scoring criteria provide clear examples and guidelines for such circumstances, making the Verbal Memory subtest only slightly more difficult to score. The interscorer reliability study of this subtest produced a coefficient of .95.

The time required to administer the entire RIAS (including both the intelligence and the memory subtests) averages 30–35 minutes once the examiner has practiced giving the RIAS and has become fluent in its administration. The RIST averages about 10–12 minutes. As with most tests, the first few administrations are likely to take longer. The four intelligence subtests alone (i.e., Guess What, Odd-Item Out, Verbal Reasoning, and What's Missing) can be administered to most examinees in about 20–25 minutes. The two memory subtests can typically be

administered in about 10 minutes. However, significant time variations can occur as a function of special circumstances (e.g., very low-functioning individuals will probably take much less time to complete the battery, and very bright individuals may take longer). Basal and ceiling rules along with age-designated starting points were employed to control the administration time, and each was derived empirically from the responses of the standardization sample. Also, to facilitate ease and efficiency of administration, the RIAS and RIST record forms contain all of the necessary instructions and examiner guides necessary to administer the tests.

PSYCHOMETRIC PROPERTIES

Due to the length restrictions in a single book chapter, a discussion of the developmental process of the tests simply cannot be provided. However, the RIAS underwent years of development, including tryout and review of the items on multiple occasions by school psychologists, clinical psychologists, neuropsychologists, and others. Items were written to conform to clear specifications consistent with the goals for development of the test as given previously in this chapter. Items were reviewed by panels of expert psychologists for content and construct consistency, and by expert minority psychologists to ascertain the cultural saliency of the items and any potential problems of ambiguity or offensiveness. The developmental process speaks directly to the psychometric characteristics of the tests, and is described in far more detail in Reynolds and Kamphaus (2003). It should be considered carefully in any full evaluation of the instrument.

Standardization

The RIAS was normed on a sample of 2,438 participants residing in 41 states between the years of 1999 and 2002. U.S. Bureau of the Census projected characteristics of the U.S. population projected initially to the year 2000, and then updated through 2001, were used to select a population-proportionate sample. Age, gender, ethnicity, educational level (parent educational level was used for ages 3 years through 16 years, and the participants' actual educational level was used at all other ages), and region of residence were used as stratification variables. The resulting norms for the RIAS and the RIST were calculated on a weighted sampling that provided a virtually perfect match to the census data. The overall sample was a close match to the population statistics in every regard (see Reynolds & Kamphaus, 2003, especially Tables 4.2–4.5).

Norm Derivation and Scaling

All standard scores for the RIAS were derived via a method known as *continuous norming*. Continuous norming is a regression-based methodology used to mitigate the effects of any sampling irregularities across age groupings and to stabilize parameter estimation. An important feature of continuous norming is that it uses information from all age groups, rather than relying solely on the estimates of central tendency, dispersion, and the shape of the distributions of a single age grouping for producing the norms at each chosen age interval in the normative tables for a particular test. As such, the continuous-norming procedure maximizes the accuracy of the derived normative scores and has become widespread in its application to the derivation of test norms over the last 20 years (see, e.g., Reynolds, 2003; Roid, 2003). Calculation of normative scores via continuous norming essentially involves calculating these things, sequentially: the lines or curves of best fit for the progression of means and standard deviations across age groupings of the norming variables (using polynomial regression); the mean, standard deviation, skewness, and kurtosis of the distribution of scores for each normative age group; and percentiles and scaled scores based on the estimates obtained from the prior steps.

For the RIAS and the RIST, census-weighted means and standard deviations of the subtest raw scores for the 52 age groups in the normative sample were analyzed separately to determine the best-fitting polynomial regression equations. Mean subgroup age and its powers up to the sixth power were used as predictors. Visual inspection of the polynomial curves derived from the group standard deviations, and those previously derived from the individuals' raw scores, showed considerable congruence.

Means and standard deviations were then calculated for each normative age group, using the polynomial regression equations derived above. The method of continuous norming assumes that the best estimate of distribution shape is derived from the composite skewness and kurtosis aggregated across groupings of the normative variables (Angoff & Robertson, 1987). Composite estimates of skewness and kurtosis were thus calculated from the averages of these respective values in the 52 age groups. Percentiles and normalized standardized scores corresponding to raw scores were calculated for every normative age group, using the respective mean and standard deviation values obtained in step 2. *T* scores were derived to have a mean of 50 and a standard deviation of 10 for each of the RIAS subtests. These scores were then combined into the various composite and index scores described previously (see Table 21.1) and scaled via a similar procedure to a mean of 100 and standard deviation of 15.

T scores were chosen for the RIAS subtests over the more traditional scaled scores (mean = 10) popularized by Wechsler (e.g., Wechsler, 1949), due to the higher reliability coefficients obtained for the RIAS subtest scores. With high degrees of reliability of test scores, the use of scales that make finer discriminations among individuals is possible, producing a more desirable range of possible scores. For the convenience of researchers and examiners who wish to use other types of scores for comparative, research, or other purposes, the RIAS manual (Reynolds & Kamphaus, 2003, Appendix B) provides several other common types of scores for the RIAS and RIST indexes, including percentiles, *T* scores, *z* scores, normal curve equivalents, and stanines, along with a detailed explanation of each score type.

Score Reliability

Since the RIAS is a power test (i.e., items are presented in order of difficulty, from least to most difficult, and individuals' scores depend entirely on how many items they respond to correctly), the internal-consistency reliability of the items on the RIAS subtests was investigated by using Cronbach's coefficient alpha. Alpha reliability coefficients for the RIAS subtest scores and the Nunnally reliability estimates for the index scores are presented in Tables 21.2 and 21.3, respectively, for 16 age groups from the total standardization sample. The reliability estimates are rounded to two decimal places and represent the lower limits of the internal-consistency reliability of the RIAS scores.

According to the tables, 100% of the alpha coefficients for the RIAS subtest scores reach .84 or higher for every age group. As the data in Table 21.2 show, the median alpha reliability estimate for each RIAS subtest across age equals or exceeds .90. This point is important, because many measurement experts recommend that reliability estimates above .80 are necessary and those above .90 are highly desirable for tests used to make decisions about individuals. All RIAS subtests meet these recommended levels. As shown in Table 21.3, the reliability estimates for all RIAS indexes have median values across age that equal or exceed .94. These reliability estimates are viewed as excellent and often exceed the reliability values presented for the composite indexes or IQs of tests two or three times the length of the RIAS.

TABLE 21.3. Reliability Estimates of the RIAS Indexes by Age Group

Age (years)	Index			
	VIX	NIX	CIX	CMX
3	.91	.92	.94	.94
4	.94	.93	.95	.95
5	.94	.92	.96	.95
6	.94	.94	.96	.94
7	.94	.95	.97	.95
8	.94	.94	.96	.93
9	.94	.95	.97	.95
10	.93	.95	.95	.95
11–12	.94	.95	.96	.93
13–14	.95	.95	.97	.95
15–16	.95	.95	.97	.95
17–19	.95	.94	.96	.93
20–34	.96	.96	.97	.96
35–54	.97	.96	.98	.97
55–74	.95	.95	.97	.95
75–94	.96	.96	.98	.97
Median	.94	.95	.96	.95

Note. VIX, verbal intelligence index; NIX, nonverbal intelligence index; CIX, composite intelligence index; CMX, composite memory index. From Reynolds and Kamphaus (2003). Copyright 2003 by Psychological Assessment Resources, Inc. Reprinted by permission.

TABLE 21.2. Reliability Coefficients of the RIAS Subtests by Age Group

Age (years)	Subtest					
	Guess What (GWH)	Verbal Reasoning (VRZ)	Odd-Item Out (OIO)	What's Missing (WHM)	Verbal Memory (VRM)	Nonverbal Memory (NVM)
3	.89	.84	.93	.84	.93	.93
4	.92	.87	.91	.89	.94	.93
5	.95	.86	.90	.85	.95	.94
6	.93	.86	.94	.92	.89	.96
7	.93	.89	.95	.94	.93	.96
8	.92	.88	.94	.92	.90	.95
9	.92	.90	.95	.93	.92	.96
10	.91	.88	.94	.93	.92	.96
11–12	.89	.90	.94	.93	.90	.95
13–14	.90	.92	.94	.93	.91	.96
15–16	.91	.92	.95	.92	.93	.95
17–19	.92	.92	.94	.90	.94	.90
20–34	.92	.94	.95	.93	.94	.95
35–54	.95	.94	.95	.93	.94	.96
55–74	.91	.93	.95	.91	.93	.95
75–94	.94	.93	.95	.92	.94	.96
Median	.92	.90	.94	.92	.93	.95

Note. From Reynolds and Kamphaus (2003). Copyright 2003 by Psychological Assessment Resources, Inc. Reprinted by permission.

One cannot always assume that because a test is reliable for a general population, it will be equally reliable for every subgroup within that population. Therefore, test developers should demonstrate whenever possible that their test scores are indeed reliable for subgroups, especially those subgroups that, because of gender, ethnic, or linguistic differences, might experience test bias (Reynolds, 2000). As noted in the *Standards for Educational and Psychological Testing* (American Educational Research Association [AERA], American Psychological Association [APA], & National Council on Measurement in Education [NCME], 1999) these values may also provide information relevant to the consequences of test use. When calculated separately for male and female examinees, the reliability coefficients are high and relatively uniform (see Table 5.4 of Reynolds & Kamphaus, 2003, for the full table of values), with no significant differences in test score reliability at any age level as a function of gender. For male and female examinees, the RIAS subtests and the indexes are highly comparable across groups. Reliability estimates were also calculated separately for European American and African American ethnic/racial group members (see Reynolds & Kamphaus, 2003).

The stability of RIAS scores over time was investigated via the test–retest method with 86 individuals ages 3 years through 82 years. The intervals between the two test administrations ranged from 9 to 39 days, with a median test–retest interval of 21 days. The correlations for the two testings, along with mean scores and standard deviations, are reported in detail in the RIAS manual (Reynolds & Kamphaus, 2003) in Tables 5.7 through 5.11 for the total test–retest sample and for four age groups: 3–4 years, 5–8 years, 9–12 years, and 13–82 years. The obtained coefficients are of sufficient magnitude to allow confidence in the stability of RIAS test scores over time. In fact, the values are quite good for all of the subtests, but especially for the index scores. The uncorrected coefficients are all higher than .70, and 6 of the 10 values are in the .80s. The corrected values are even more impressive, with all but 2 values ranging from .83 to .91. When viewed across age groups, the values are generally consistent with the values obtained for the total test–retest sample.

Validity of RIAS Test Scores as Measures of Intelligence

The *Standards* volume (AERA et al., 1999, pp. 11–17) suggests a five-category scheme for organizing sources of evidence to evaluate proposed interpretations of test scores, although clearly recognizing that other organizational systems may be appropriate. The RIAS manual (Reynolds & Kamphaus, 2003) provides a thorough analysis of the currently available validity evidence associated with the RIAS/RIST scores as measures of intelligence organized according to the recommendations just noted.

Evidence Based on Test Content

Evidence with respect to the content validity of the RIAS subtests may be gleaned from the item review and item selection processes. As the *Standards* volume (AERA et al., 1999) notes, expert judgments may be used to assess agreement with test specifications and constructs in evaluating validity based on test content. During the first item tryout, a panel of minority psychologists, all with experience in assessment, reviewed all RIAS items for appropriateness as measures of their respective constructs and for applicability across various U.S. cultures. Another panel of five psychologists with doctoral degrees in school psychology, clinical psychology, clinical neuropsychology, and measurement also reviewed all items in the item pool for appropriateness. Items questioned or found faulty were either eliminated outright or modified. The RIAS items in the published version thus passed a series of judgments by expert reviewers. Final items were then chosen on the basis of traditional item statistics derived from true-score theory. Analyses of item characteristics across age, gender, and ethnicity were also undertaken to ensure appropriateness of content across various nominal groupings.

Evidence Based on Response Processes

Evidence based on the response processes of the tasks is concerned with the fit between the nature of the performance or actions in which the examinee is actually engaged and the constructs being assessed. For heavily *g*-loaded and memory tasks on the RIAS, the best evidence related to the response process is gleaned from an examination of these tasks themselves, as well as from their correlates (see the later section on relations to external variables).

The four RIAS intelligence subtests are designed to measure general intelligence in the verbal and nonverbal domains. As such, the tasks are complex and require the integration of multiple cognitive skills, thereby avoiding contamination by irrelevant, noncognitive response processes.

Because of their relationship to crystallized intelligence, the two verbal subtests invoke vocabulary and language comprehension. However, clearly academic or purely acquired skills such as reading are avoided. The response process requires integration of language and some general knowledge to deduce relationships; only minimal expressive language is required. One- or two-word responses are acceptable for virtually all items. The response process also is not contaminated by nonintellectual processes, such as motor acuity, speed, and coordination. Rather, problem solving through the processes of deductive and inductive reasoning is emphasized.

Likewise, the two nonverbal tasks avoid contamination by extraneous variables such as motor acuity, speed, and coordination. Examinees have the response options of pointing or giving a one- or two-word verbal indication of the correct answer. As with any nonverbal task, some examinees may attempt to use verbal encoding to solve these tasks, and some will do so successfully. However, the tasks themselves are largely spatial and are known to be more affected by right-than by left-hemisphere impairment (e.g., Joseph, 1996; Reynolds & French, 2003)—a finding that supports the lack of verbal domination in strategies for solving such problems.

Response processes of the two RIAS memory subtests also avoid contamination from reading and various aspects of motor skills. Although good language skills undoubtedly facilitate verbal memory, they are not the dominant skills involved. The RIAS memory tasks are very straightforward, with response processes that coincide with their content domain—verbal in the Verbal Memory subtest and nonverbal in the Nonverbal Memory subtest. Even so, in the latter case,

examinees who have severe motor problems may give a verbal indication of the answer they have selected.

Evidence Based on Internal Structure

The RIAS provides an index score (CIX) that purports to be a measure of *g*. The RIAS additionally provides indexes that focus on verbal ability (VIX), a construct closely related to crystallized intelligence, and nonverbal ability (NIX), a construct closely related to fluid intelligence. A separate memory index (CMX) is also provided. The CIX, which is derived from the four intelligence subtests of the RIAS, presupposes a common underlying construct that reflects overall intelligence. The other index scores likewise presuppose some meaningful, identifiable dimension underlying their construction. The extent to which a composite score can be evaluated internally is directly related to the dimensionality of the scores that make up the composite. Therefore, evidence based on the internal structure of the RIAS is provided from two sources: item coherence (or internal consistency), and factor analyses of the intercorrelations of the subtests. The internal-consistency evidence has been reviewed in the section on the reliability of test scores derived from the RIAS. Factor analysis is another method of examining the internal structure of a scale that lends itself to assessing the validity of recommended score interpretations.

Factor analysis is a common method of examining the patterns of relationships among a set of variables. It is a commonly recommended analytical approach to evaluating the presence and structure of any latent constructs among a set of variables, such as subtest scores on a test battery (see Cronbach, 1990; Kamphaus, 2001). Two methods of factor analysis have been applied to the intercorrelation matrix of the RIAS subtests, first with only the four intelligence subtests examined, and then with all six subtests examined under both techniques of analysis. Exploratory analyses were undertaken first and were followed by a set of confirmatory analyses to assess the relative goodness of fit of the chosen exploratory results to mathematically optimal models. For the exploratory factor analyses, the method of *principal factors* was chosen. In such analyses, the first unrotated factor to be extracted is commonly interpreted as *g*. The correlations of each subtest with this factor (i.e., the factor loadings) are indicators of the degree to which each subtest measures general intelligence as opposed to more specific components of ability.

For purposes of factor analyses of the RIAS subtest's intercorrelations, the sample was divided into five age groups (rather than 1-year interval groups) to enhance the stability and the generalizability of the factor analyses of the RIAS scores. These age groupings reflect common developmental stages. The five age groupings were early childhood, ages 3 years through 5 years; childhood, ages 6 years through 11 years; adolescence, ages 12 years through 18 years; adulthood, ages 19 years through 54 years; and senior adulthood, ages 55 years through 94 years. A Pearson correlation between each possible pair of RIAS subtest scores within each age level was determined, and factor analyses were performed.

When the two-factor and three-factor solutions were subsequently obtained, the two-factor varimax solution made the most psychological and psychometric sense for both the set of four intelligence subtests and for all six RIAS subtests. In the four-subtest three-factor solution, no variables consistently defined the third factor across the four age groupings. In the six-subtest three-factor solutions, singlet factors (i.e., factors with a single salient loading) appeared, commonly representing a memory subtest; What's Missing tended to behave in an unstable manner as well. Summaries of the two-factor varimax solutions are presented for the four-subtest and six-subtest analyses in Table 21.4. In each case, the first, unrotated factor is a representation of *g* as measured by the RIAS.

The *g* factor of the RIAS is quite strong. Only the intelligence subtests have loadings that reach into the .70s and .80s. All four intelligence subtests are good measures of *g*; however, of the four, the verbal subtests are the strongest. Odd-Item Out and What's Missing follow, the latter being the weakest measure of *g* among the four intelligence subtests. The strength of the first unrotated factor is, however, indisputable; it indicates that first and foremost, the RIAS intelligence subtests are measures of *g*, and that the

strongest interpretive support is given in these analyses to the CIX. At the same time, the varimax rotation of the two-factor solution clearly delineates two components of the construct of *g* among the RIAS intelligence subtests. For every age group, the verbal and nonverbal subtests clearly break into two distinct factors that coincide with their respective indexes, VIX and NIX. The six-subtest solution also breaks along content dimensions, with Verbal Memory joining the two verbal intelligence subtests on the first rotated factor and Nonverbal Memory joining the two nonverbal intelligence subtests on the second rotated factor. However, in view of the analysis of the content and response processes as well as other evidence presented throughout the RIAS manual (Reynolds & Kamphaus, 2003), we continue to believe that the separation of the Verbal Memory and Nonverbal Memory subtests into a separate memory index (i.e., CMX) is more than justified. Memory is clearly a component of intelligence. The two memory tasks that were chosen for the RIAS are relatively complex, and both are strong predictors of broader composites of verbal and nonverbal memory (Reynolds & Bigler, 1994)—characteristics that are at once an asset and a liability. Although these two memory tasks are good measures of overall or general memory skill, they tend to correlate more highly with intelligence test scores than do very simple, confrontational measures of working memory, such as digit repetition. Given the purpose of providing a highly reliable assessment of overall memory skill, such a compromise is warranted.

The stability of the two-factor solution across other relevant nominal groupings and the potential for cultural bias in the internal structure of the RIAS were also assessed. For this purpose, the factor analyses were also calculated separately for males and females and for European Americans and African Americans, according to recommendations and procedures outlined in detail by Reynolds (2000). Tables 6.3 through 6.6 in Reynolds and Kamphaus (2003) present these results for each comparison. The similarity of the factor-analytic results across gender and across ethnicity was also assessed. Two indexes of factorial similarity were calculated for the visually matched rotated factors and for the first unrotated fac-

TABLE 21.4. Two-Factor Solutions for the Four-Subtest and Six-Subtest Analyses of the RAIS

Subtest	g^a					Factor 1					Factor 2				
	3–5 years	6–11 years	12–18 years	19–54 years	55–94 years	3–5 years	6–11 years	12–18 years	19–54 years	55–94 years	3–5 years	6–11 years	12–18 years	19–54 years	55–94 years
RIAS intelligence subtest loadings from a principal-factors solution by age group															
Guess What	.71	.77	.88	.87	.82	.66	.73	.78	.74	.65	.34	.32	.44	.48	.50
Verbal Reasoning	.78	.81	.85	.84	.85	.69	.74	.78	.73	.80	.40	.37	.39	.45	.38
Odd-Item Out	.70	.60	.60	.73	.74	.36	.32	.30	.42	.50	.63	.57	.58	.62	.55
What's Missing	.60	.49	.63	.66	.69	.30	.21	.32	.36	.33	.58	.53	.60	.60	.67
RIAS intelligence and memory subtest loadings from a principal-factors solution by age group															
Guess What	.70	.77	.84	.82	.82	.66	.74	.77	.77	.68	.29	.33	.38	.35	.47
Verbal Reasoning	.79	.79	.86	.83	.83	.78	.70	.83	.78	.76	.29	.39	.34	.36	.40
Odd-Item Out	.67	.63	.58	.71	.74	.41	.26	.23	.44	.48	.57	.67	.64	.58	.57
What's Missing	.59	.44	.57	.64	.68	.37	.21	.38	.46	.32	.47	.44	.43	.45	.66
Verbal Memory	.54	.48	.41	.58	.60	.51	.48	.40	.49	.56	.22	.18	.15	.31	.28
Nonverbal Memory	.49	.48	.57	.66	.61	.16	.23	.26	.28	.31	.59	.47	.59	.71	.56

Note. From Reynolds and Kamphaus (2003). Copyright 2003 by Psychological Assessment Resources, Inc. Adapted by permission.
[a]g, or general intelligence factor, reported as the subtests' loadings on the first unrotated principal factor. Loadings for both factor 1 and factor 2 are those following varimax rotation.

tor—the coefficient of congruence (r_c) and Cattell's (1978) salient variable similarity index—as recommended in several sources (e.g., Reynolds, 2000). In all cases, the factor structure of the RIAS was found to be highly consistent across gender and ethnicity.

Subsequent to the exploratory factor analyses, several confirmatory factor analyses were conducted to examine the fit of our choice of exploratory analyses to a more purely mathematical model (see Reynolds & Kamphaus, 2003, for table values and a thorough discussion). Based on the theoretical views of the structure of the RIAS discussed earlier in this chapter, three theoretical models were tested. The models were defined as follows: (1) The RIAS is a measure of general intellectual abilities; (2) the RIAS is a measure of verbal and nonverbal abilities; and (3) the RIAS is a measure of verbal, nonverbal, and memory abilities.

The resulting chi-square (χ^2), residuals, root mean square error of approximation (RMSEA), and other model-fitting statistics were then compared; the LISREL-VI program (Joreskog & Sorbom, 1987) was used to test the relative fit of the three models. Model 1, general intelligence, clearly fit better when only the four intelligence subtests were included ($\chi^2 = 8.17$ to 20.57 and RMSEA ranging from .10 to .14, depending on the age range studied) than when six subtests were included. Although these models suggested, much in the same way as the exploratory factor analyses showed, that the RIAS is dominated by a large first factor, the RMSEAs were still high enough to suggest that models 2 and 3 should be explored.

Model 2 was a very good fit to the data, particularly when four subtests were included in the model versus six subtests. For the model that included four subtests, the chi-square values were between .22 and 1.49. Similarly, the RMSEAs were less than .01 for the first four age groups (i.e., 3 years to 54 years) and .04 for ages 55 years and older—values suggesting that two factors explained virtually all of the variance between the four subtests. These findings indicated that the fit of a three-factor model was not likely to be as good.

In fact, model 3 with six subtests included ($\chi^2 = 14.14$ to 37.48, and RMSEA ranging from .01 to .09) did not fit nearly as well as model 2. There were some indications that

the six-subtest two-factor model was also plausible for the population 19 years and older. Although the four-subtest two-factor model is recommended, these results suggest that use of all six subtests for assessing verbal and nonverbal intelligence may be defensible for adults as well. In cases where memory problems are part of the referral question for adults, the use of six subtests may be beneficial; however, integrating the memory subtests into the VIX and NIX is not recommended. With clinical populations, we continue to prefer the division of the RIAS subtests into the VIX, NIX, and CMX, even though placing the memory subtests into the VIX and NIX may have a reasonable mathematical foundation in the confirmatory factor analyses.

In summary, the results of the confirmatory factor analyses suggest that the CIX, VIX, and NIX possess evidence of factorial validity. The CMX, in particular, requires further research with a variety of clinical and nonclinical samples. Although factor-analytic results are often open to alternate interpretations, it is our opinion, based on the findings just described as well as the conceptual distinctions we have drawn previously, that it is best not to use all six subtests to measure general intelligence.

Evidence Based on Relations with Other (External) Variables

Another important area in the validation process is the evaluation of the relationship of scores on the instrument of interest to variables that are external to the test itself. This evaluation may include, for example, relationships with other tests that measure similar or dissimilar constructs, diagnostic categorizations, and relationships with developmental constructs such as age. The standards emphasize that a wide range of variables are of potential interest, and that different relationships will have different degrees of importance to examiners who work in different settings or are using the test for different purposes. As with other areas of evidence, test users ultimately have the responsibility of evaluating the evidence and determining its saliency and adequacy for their own intended use of the instrument. Several different external variables were chosen for investigation with the RIAS, including devel-

opmental variables (i.e., age), demographic
variables, relations with other tests, and clinical status.

Developmental Trends

As a developmental construct, intellectual
ability grows rapidly in the early years, begins to plateau in the teens but shows some
continued growth (particularly in verbal domains), and eventually declines in the older
years. This decline generally begins sooner
and is more dramatic for nonverbal, or fluid,
intelligence (Kaufman, McLean, Kaufman-
Packer, & Reynolds, 1991; Kaufman,
Reynolds, & McLean, 1989; Reynolds,
Chastain, Kaufman, & McLean, 1987). If
raw scores on the tasks of the RIAS reflect
such a developmental process or attribute,
then relationships with age should be evident. The relationship between age (a variable external to the RIAS) and performance
on the RIAS was investigated in two ways.

First, the correlation between age and raw
score for each subtest was calculated for the
primary developmental stage, ages 3 years
through 18 years. The correlations for all
groups were uniformly large, typically exceeding .80 and demonstrating that raw
scores on the RIAS increase with age and in a
relatively constant manner across subtests
(see Reynolds & Kamphaus, 2003). To examine the issue in more detail, lifespan developmental curves were generated for each
subtest from ages 3 years through 94 years.
These curves are presented in the RIAS
manual (Reynolds & Kamphaus, 2003) and
show a consistent pattern of score increases
and declines (with aging) across all groups.

Correlations with the Wechsler Scales

The RIAS indexes all correlated highly with
the Wechsler Intelligence Scale for Children—
Third Edition (WISC-III; Wechsler, 1991)
Full Scale IQ (FSIQ), with correlations ranging from a low of .60 (NIX to FSIQ) to a
high of .78 (VIX to FSIQ). The relatively
lower correlations between the RIAS NIX
and the WISC-III IQs are probably attributable to the increased emphasis on motor and
language skills on the WISC-III Performance
IQ (PIQ) relative to that in the RIAS. The
WISC-III PIQ subtests also rely on sequencing (e.g., Picture Arrangement and Coding),

whereas the RIAS has no subtest in which sequencing is crucial to the task. Speed of
performance is also less important in the
RIAS. With this one exception, the pattern of
correlations was much as predicted; namely,
the highest correlations were between those
aspects of the tests most closely associated
with g (from their respective factor analyses).

A group of 31 adults were administered
the RIAS and the Wechsler Adult Intelligence
Scale—Third Edition (WAIS-III; Wechsler,
1997) in a counterbalanced design. All but
two of the correlations exceeded .70; the
VIX-PIQ correlation was the lowest at .61.
All of the RIAS indexes correlated at or
above .70 with the WAIS-III FSIQ. There
were no significant differences among any of
the correlations. This finding is most likely a
function of the g saturation of the various
scales.

Correlations with Measures
of Academic Achievement

One of the major reasons for the development of the early, individually administered
intelligence tests was to predict academic
achievement levels. Intelligence tests have
done well as predictors of school learning,
with typical correlations in the mid-.50s and
.60s (for summaries, see Kamphaus, 2001;
Sattler, 2001). To evaluate the relationship
between the RIAS and academic achievement, 78 children and adolescents were administered the RIAS and the Wechsler Individual Achievement Test (WIAT; Wechsler,
1992).

School learning is fundamentally a
language-related task, and this fact is
clearly evident in these data. Although all
of the RIAS indexes correlated well with all
of the WIAT composite scores, the highest
correlations were consistently between the
VIX and CIX and the WIAT composites.
These correlations were predominantly in
the .60s and .70s, indicating that the RIAS
has strong predictive value for educational
achievement.

Evidence Based on the Consequences
of Testing

The final area of the validation process is the
most controversial of all the aspects of this

process as presented in the *Standards* volume (AERA et al., 1999). It is most applicable to tests designed for selection and may deal with issues of bias or loss of opportunity. How these applications should be evaluated for clinical diagnostic tests is largely unclear. However, accurate diagnosis might be one anticipated consequence of testing and should be the key to evaluating the "consequential" validity of a clinical instrument. The evidence reviewed in the preceding sections demonstrates the ability of the RIAS to provide an accurate estimate of intellectual ability and certain memory skills, and to do so accurately across such nominal groupings as gender and ethnicity. Cultural biases in the format and content of tests, when apparent, have also been found to produce undue consequences of testing. Evidence pointing toward a lack of cultural bias in the RIAS is extensive for male and female examinees, as well as for European Americans, African Americans, and Hispanic Americans. This evidence has been provided previously in this chapter and in Chapter 4 of the RIAS manual (Reynolds & Kamphaus, 2003), where results of item bias studies are reported. The studies of potential cultural bias in the RIAS items were extensive in both objective and subjective formats and resulted in the removal of many items and modification of others, as described in detail in the manual. Evidence based on consequences is thus supportive, but work remains to be done in this arena, particularly with as yet unstudied ethnic groups.

In evaluating evidence for test score interpretations, examiners must always consider their purposes for using objective tests. Evidence clearly supports the use of the constructs represented on the RIAS. The potential consequences of knowing how an individual's performance compares to that of others are many and complex, and are not always anticipated. The RIAS was designed to eliminate or minimize any cultural biases in the assessment of intelligence and memory for individuals reared and educated in the United States (who are fluent in the English language). The data available to date indicate that the RIAS precludes undue consequences toward diverse individuals who fit the target population. Examiners must nevertheless act wisely, consider the need for ob-

jective testing of intelligence and memory, and work to minimize or eliminate unsupported interpretations of scores on such tests.

APPLICATIONS OF THE RIAS

As a measure of intelligence, the RIAS is appropriate for a wide array of purposes and should be useful when assessment of an examinee's intellectual level is needed. The RIAS will be useful with preschool and school-age children for purposes of educational placement, as well as for diagnosis of various forms of childhood psychopathology (especially developmental disorders) where intellectual functioning is an issue. Diagnosis of specific disorders—such as mental retardation, learning disabilities, the various dementias, and the effects of central nervous system (CNS) injury or compromise—most often calls for the use of an intelligence test as a component of patient evaluation, and the RIAS is appropriate for such applications. Clinicians who perform general clinical and neuropsychological evaluations will find the RIAS very useful when a measure of intelligence is needed. Practitioners will also find the RIAS useful in disability determinations under various state and federal programs, such as the Social Security Administration's disability program and Section 504 regulations. Although only published in February 2003, the RIAS is already being used consistently in such disability exams (M. Shapiro, personal communication, April 2003).

Although the RIAS is rapid to administer, relative to the majority of other comprehensive measures of intelligence, it is not an abbreviated measure or a short form of intellectual assessment. The RIAS is a comprehensive measure of verbal and nonverbal intelligence and of general intelligence, providing the same level of useful information often gleaned from much longer intelligence tests. When the memory subtests are also administered, the RIAS can provide even more useful information than typical intelligence tests currently used.

The major clinical uses of intelligence tests are generally classification (most commonly, diagnostic) and selection. The RIAS has broad applicability in each of these areas. Some of the more common uses in these areas are discussed here.

Learning Disability

For the evaluation of a learning disability, assessment of intelligence is a common activity. However, when a child or adult is evaluated for the possible presence of a learning disability, both verbal and nonverbal intelligence should be assessed. Individuals with learning disabilities may have spuriously deflated IQ estimates in one or the other domain, due to the learning disabilities themselves. Lower verbal ability is the more common type of learning disability in the school population and among adjudicated delinquents (Kaufman, 1994). However, the concept of nonverbal learning disabilities is gaining momentum. For individuals with such disabilities, verbal ability will often exceed nonverbal ability. The assessment of functioning in both areas is important, and the RIAS provides a reliable assessment of these domains, as well as a composite intelligence index.

Mental Retardation

Most definitions—including those of the American Association on Mental Retardation (2002) and the *Diagnostic and Statistical Manual of Mental Disorders*, fourth edition, text revision (DSM-IV-TR; American Psychiatric Association, 2000)—require the administration of an individually administered test of intelligence for diagnosis of mental retardation. The RIAS is applicable to the diagnosis of mental retardation, for which the evaluation of verbal and nonverbal intelligence as well as adaptive functioning is necessary. Mental retardation is a pervasive intellectual problem and not limited to serious problems in only the verbal or nonverbal domain. The range of scores available on the RIAS will also make it useful in distinguishing levels of severity of mental retardation. Lower levels of functioning, such as profound mental retardation, are difficult to assess accurately on nearly all tests of intelligence; this is likewise true of the RIAS. Although normed on children as young as 3 years of age, the RIAS also has limited discriminative ability below mild levels of

mental retardation in the 3-year-old age group.

Intellectual Giftedness

Many definitions of giftedness include reference to superior levels of performance on measures of intelligence. Here again, measures of both the verbal and nonverbal domains are useful, due to the influences of schooling and educational opportunity on verbal intelligence. The range of index scores available on the RIAS is adequate at all ages for identifying persons with significantly above-average levels of overall intellectual functioning, as well as in the verbal and nonverbal domains.

Physical/Orthopedic Impairment

The RIAS will be particularly useful in the evaluation of intellectual functioning among individuals with any significant degree of physical or motor impairment. The RIAS has no real demands for speed or accuracy of fine motor movements. If necessary, the pointing responses by the examinee on the RIAS nonverbal tasks can all be replaced with simple verbal responses, designating the location of the chosen response. It is, however, very important for an examiner to have knowledge of the physical impairments of any examinee and to make any necessary modifications in the testing environment, doing so in a manner consistent with appropriate professional standards (e.g., the *Standards for Educational and Psychological Testing*; AERA et al., 1999).

Neuropsychological and Memory Impairment

The information gleaned from evaluating memory functions can provide valuable clinical information above and beyond what is traditionally obtained with IQ measures. Memory is generally recognized as a focal or discreet subset of cognitive functions, and as such is often quite vulnerable to CNS trauma and various other CNS events. Disturbances of memory and attention are the two most frequent complaints of children and adults following traumatic brain injury at all levels of severity, as well as other forms of CNS compromise (e.g., viral meningitis, AIDS dementia complex, and other systemic insults). Therefore, it is not unusual for memory functioning to be affected, even when there is little or no impact on general intellectual ability. The memory measures on the RIAS offer clinicians valuable assessment tools with which to evaluate recent or more immediate memory functioning in both the auditory (i.e., verbal memory) and visual (i.e., nonverbal memory) modalities.

Emotional Disturbance

Individuals with various forms of emotional and/or psychotic disturbance (e.g., depression, schizophrenia) may exhibit cognitive impairments to varying degrees. Often clinicians do not assess the intelligence of such individuals because of the time required to do so. The RIAS offers clinicians a more efficient means of gathering information on the psychometric intelligence of individuals with emotional problems.

Job Performance

In personnel settings, IQ tests are sometimes used to predict success in job training programs; in other instances, lower limits are set on IQ levels for specific jobs. The RIAS and the RIST are strong predictors of academic performance, and the tasks involved and constructs assessed on these instruments match up well with known predictors of job performance in the form of other IQ tests. When intelligence level is a question in such situations, the RIAS and the RIST are appropriate choices.

CASE STUDY (ABBREVIATED)

Carl Last, age 6, was referred to the clinic by his parents, Jamie and Harold Last, for a psychoeducational evaluation. Carl's parents are concerned about his behavioral, emotional, and academic functioning. Six months prior to the current evaluation, Carl was diagnosed with attention and anxiety disorders. The Lasts are interested in verifying these diagnoses and hope to find out whether Carl is experiencing learning problems. Mr. and Mrs. Last are interested in receiving a better understanding of his difficul-

ties, so that they can help him be successful in school and at home.

Parent Interview

Carl's past medical history includes colic, occasional constipation, and complaints of itchy skin. Currently, Carl is in good physical health and wears glasses for corrective vision while reading. Mr. Last reported that results of Carl's previous hearing screenings have been within normal limits, but that his hearing has not been checked recently. Family history is significant for a variety of health problems.

According to Mr. Last, Carl has always been a hyperactive child. He reported that Carl "learned to hop before he could walk" and frequently bounces when he is excited. Furthermore, he noted that Carl has not taken naps since the age of 2 and is overly active, such as rocking back and forth and fidgeting with things in his hands. Mr. Last also noted that Carl often waves his fingers back and forth, especially when he is frustrated or doing an undesirable activity. Mr. Last indicated that Carl's rocking and finger waving could be due to anxiety related to school, as he often engages in these behaviors when doing school activities. Mrs. Last indicated that in addition to hyperactivity, Carl is easily distracted and pays too much attention to minute details. She described Carl as making many careless mistakes and answering questions impulsively.

In addition, Mr. Last reported that Carl displays atypical and compulsive behaviors. Carl has specific places for all of his belongings; he is disturbed when things are misplaced and must immediately return them to their desired place. Moreover, Mrs. Last indicated that Carl is "anal" at times about organization and neatness, and insists on placing his belongings (such as his trophies) in a perfect line. She noted that Carl engages in cleaning rituals one or two times a month. Mrs. Last described the cleaning as repetitive, with Carl frequently moving objects as if they are "just not quite right." Mr. Last also indicated that Carl says phrases repetitively, such as muttering a phrase he has heard to himself over and over.

In addition to difficulties with hand washing, cleaning, and repetitive speech patterns,

Mr. Last noted that Carl has unusual feelings and spells where he stares blankly. Specifically, Carl often claims, "Here comes that feeling. I don't like that feeling." At this point, Carl closes his eyes and is still for a couple of seconds until the feeling passes. He describes the experience as feeling "all shivery in my body and my brain." These experiences have occurred since Carl was 2 or 3 years old; they currently fluctuate from happening a couple of times a week to a couple of times a day. Mr. Last also reported that a couple of times a month, Carl appears to lose touch with reality and stares blankly for a few minutes. When he comes out of the stares, he does not rejoin the conversation in a normal matter; instead, he frequently asks about details from the past.

The Lasts reported that during kindergarten and first grade, Carl has experienced difficulties with inattention and concentration—specifically, problems with following directions and staying focused. The Lasts indicated that, due to these problems, Carl has had difficulty with reading comprehension and formerly received tutoring services after school. They are currently not concerned about his reading performance. Carl is currently receiving B's and C's.

Behavioral Observations

Carl appeared for the evaluation well groomed and appropriately dressed on both days of testing. Consistent with the reports from his parents, Carl was hyperactive. He frequently rocked back and forth repetitively in his seat and moved about the testing room on occasion. He fidgeted with his hands during most of the 2-day evaluation, often rolling a pencil back and forth on his legs. At times, Carl seemed focused on the breaks that he was allowed during testing; he frequently asked to take a break. He engaged in age-appropriate social interaction and was generally well behaved throughout the sessions. He seemed comfortable with the examiners, and rapport was easily established. Carl required frequent redirection to the task at hand, but upon redirection he could maintain focus. He answered questions impulsively and was talkative throughout the evaluation.

Overall, Carl presented himself as well behaved and cooperative during testing. He seemed engaged in most testing procedures

and appeared to put forth his best effort. Results of the evaluation are viewed as valid estimates of Carl's intellectual abilities, academic achievement, and social-emotional adjustment.

Teacher Interview

Carl's teacher, Mrs. Taylor, provided information regarding his overall functioning in the school setting. She noted that Carl is having learning problems, specifically with reading and reading comprehension. During the teacher interview, Mrs. Taylor noted that Carl has made adequate progress throughout the school year, but still seems to be having difficulties with reading. She indicated that Carl was hyperactive in the beginning of the year, but appears to have calmed down somewhat. However, she noted that he often does not seem relaxed and appears to feel "uncomfortable in his own body." Mrs. Taylor indicated that Carl's attention is variable, depending on the nature of the task; however, she noted that he often fails to give close attention to his assignments, such as failing to go back and check his work. Mrs. Taylor noted that Carl is well liked by his peers and does not have any behavior problems.

Intelligence Testing

The Reynolds Intellectual Assessment Scale (RIAS) and the Wechsler Abbreviated Scale of Intelligence (WASI) were given to evaluate Carl's intelligence. As Table 21.5 indicates, Carl earned a low average to average RIAS Verbal Intelligence Index (VIX) score of 89 (23rd percentile) and an average Nonverbal

TABLE 21.5. Carl's Composite Scores on the RIAS

Composites	Standard score	Confidence interval	Percentile
VIX	89	84–95	23rd
NIX	105	99–110	63rd
CIX	95	90–109	37th
CMX	107	101–112	68th

Note. The RIAS yields standard scores with a mean of 100 and a standard deviation of 15. Standard scores between 85 and 115, which include 68% of the general population, are considered to be within the average range.

Intelligence Index (NIX) score of 105 (63rd percentile). Taken together, the VIX and NIX scores yielded a Composite Intelligence Index (CIX) score of 95 (37th percentile), which falls in the average range. There was significant scatter within RIAS subtests, with scores ranging from high average to below average (see Table 21.6). For example, Carl had difficulty on a verbal subtest requiring him to complete verbal analogies, earning a below-average score. There is a significant discrepancy between Carl's verbal and performance intellectual ability scores, suggesting that his nonverbal reasoning skills as measured by the RIAS are more highly developed. Carl earned an average Composite Memory Index (CMX) score of 107, indicating that he has an average ability to learn and remember material.

Due to the considerable scatter on the subtests of the RIAS, Carl was administered the WASI as a second measure of cognitive ability. This instrument is an abbreviated version of the Wechsler Intelligence Scale for Children—Third Edition (WISC-III). Carl earned a Verbal composite score of 98 (45th percentile), which falls in the average range. His score of 78 (7th percentile, significantly below-average range) on the Performance component was significantly different from his Verbal IQ. Again, Carl's performance was variable and produced significant subtest scatter. Carl's Performance IQ was negatively affected by the timed nature of the Block Design task. Qualitatively, it was noticed that Carl was not interested by the blocks and was inattentive and off task during this subtest. He earned a significantly below-average score on this subtest, which affected his overall Performance IQ. Verbal and Performance IQ scores combined to yield an overall Full Scale IQ of 86, which is

TABLE 21.6. Carl's Subtest Scores on the RIAS

Subtest	Age-adjusted T score
Guess What	49
Odd Item Out	57
Verbal Reasoning	33
What's Missing	47
Verbal Memory	48
Nonverbal Memory	59

considered to be low average when compared to that of his same-age peers.

Overall, Carl appears to be functioning in the average to low average range of intelligence and conceptual reasoning skills. His performance seems to be adversely affected by difficulties with attention and off-task behaviors. During administration of both the RIAS and the WASI, Carl answered questions impulsively, failing to listen to detailed directions for the tasks. His scores on both verbal and performance tasks were variable, depending on the nature of each task. In general, however, Carl should be able to make age-appropriate progress in learning and remembering new information, given his cognitive abilities.

Parent and Teacher Rating Scales

Carl's mother and father both completed the Behavior Assessment System for Children—Parent Rating Scales (BASC-PRS), and Mr. Last completed the Conners Parent Rating Scale—Revised: Long Version (CPRS-R:L). On the BASC-PRS, they rated him as having attention problems in the at-risk range. Specifically, they indicated that Carl is easily distracted and sometimes has difficulties with listening to directions, completing work on time, listening attentively, and forgetfulness. In order to help clarify the results of the BASC-PRS, Carl's father also completed the CPRS-R:L. Although ratings were within the average range, Mr. Last endorsed items indicative of inattention and cognitive problems, such as failing to give close attention to details and making careless mistakes. This is consistent with information obtained during the parent interview.

Mrs. Taylor, Carl's first-grade teacher, completed the Behavior Assessment System for Children—Teacher Rating Scales (BASC-TRS) to evaluate his attentional skills. Mrs. Taylor did not rate him as having any clinically significant problems with attention on the BASC-TRS. However, she noted that Carl is easily distracted from classwork and often has trouble concentrating. Furthermore, during her interview, she noted (as indicated earlier) that Carl often does not pay close attention to his assignments, failing to check over his work for any potential errors. It should be noted that both the parents and the teacher completed their rating scales after Carl had been on medication for a sub-stantial amount of time. Therefore, it is possible that ratings of attention, which were below the clinically significant level, were influenced by the positive effects noticed since Carl has been taking atomoxetine hydrochloride (Strattera). Carl's parents and teacher indicated that they have noticed an increased ability to sustain attention and concentrate since he began taking Strattera. Based on conversations with the teachers, the parents, and the rating scales, however, it seems that Carl is still having difficulty with inattention. These difficulties are interfering with his ability to perform in the classroom and at home.

ACHIEVEMENT TESTING

Broad reading, basic reading skills, and reading comprehension were assessed by the Woodcock–Johnson III Tests of Achievement (WJ III ACH). Carl's overall reading achievement was commensurate with his overall intellectual functioning as measured by the RIAS and the WASI. Carl demonstrated average letter–word identification skills, average passage comprehension skills, and low average skills on a subtest measuring reading fluency or speed. These scores combined to form a WJ III Broad Reading Composite of 89 (24th percentile), which is in the average to low average range. Carl's decoding skills were assessed through a portion of the WJ III ACH. He was asked to pronounce nonwords to further measure phonic and structural analysis skills in the Word Attack subtest. This subtest assessed Carl's ability to match sound blends to letter combinations. Carl was asked to read such nonwords as *zoop* and *rox*. He earned a standard score of 102 (55th percentile), a score in the average range of functioning. These scores suggest that Carl's overall reading achievement falls within age-appropriate limits.

Carl's basic writing skills, such as spelling, sentence construction, and writing fluency, were also assessed by the WJ III ACH. The spelling subtest measured Carl's ability to write orally presented words correctly. Carl earned an average to low average standard score of 88. The Writing Fluency subtest measured his skill in formulating and writing short, simple sentences quickly. He earned a standard score of 91, which is in the average range. Carl was also asked to produce writing samples consisting of a sentence describing a given picture or using specific words. On this Writing Samples subtest, Carl earned an 84, in the low average range. He did not appear to be paying attention to the task or directions. When asked to write sentences, he frequently wrote fragments or single words. Overall, Carl demonstrated average to low average writing abilities. His lack of attention to the directions of the task had an adverse impact on his writing scores.

Carl's mathematical skills, such as calculation, applied problems, and math fluency, were likewise assessed with the WJ III ACH. Carl earned a significantly below-average score on the Calculation subtest (72, 3rd percentile); a below-average score on the Math Fluency subtest (77, 6th percentile); and a low-average score on the Applied Problems subtest (84, 15th percentile). When these subtests were examined, it was noticed that Carl failed to give close attention to detail, specifically regarding the addition or subtraction signs. For example, on the Math Fluency portion, which required him to do simple addition and subtraction quickly, Carl added all of the numbers. He was given oral instructions to pay attention to the signs, but Carl did not take notice of the changing signs.

Overall, achievement testing indicates that Carl's academic achievement is in the average to low average range and is consistent with his general cognitive ability. Carl demonstrated age-appropriate reading, writing, and mathematics skills. However, he failed to pay close attention to details and listen attentively to directions. Again, Carl's inattention seems to be having a negative impact on his academic performance.

Behavioral, Social, and Emotional Functioning

In order to better understand Carl's functioning across behavioral, social, and emotional domains, several measures of social and emotional functioning were given. As noted earlier, Mr. and Mrs. Last completed the BASC-PRS, and Mr. Last completed the CPRS-R:L. Also as noted earlier, Carl's teacher, Mrs. Taylor, was interviewed and completed the BASC-TRS to provide information regarding Carl's social, emotional, and behavioral functioning at school.

Finally, Carl himself was interviewed and completed two self-report measures—the Revised Children's Manifest Anxiety Scale (RCMAS) and the Children's Depression Inventory (CDI)—to discern his thoughts and feelings regarding numerous issues. The results of these latter two measures suggested that Carl generally perceives himself as a well-adjusted child. He reported that he is happy with himself, his family, and his friends. He further indicated that he enjoys school and likes his teacher. He does not indicate any significant problems with depression or anxiety. However, during the child interview, Carl noted that he is sometimes afraid of nightmares, blood, and skulls.

Mr. and Mrs. Last indicated that Carl demonstrates problems with hyperactivity, attention, perfectionism, and atypicality. Mrs. Taylor, Carl's first-grade teacher, also endorsed items indicative of difficulties with hyperactivity, attention, and atypicality. In the area of hyperactivity, Mr. Last indicated that Carl often talks excessively, is overly active, fidgets with his hands, and has difficulty playing in leisure activities quietly. Furthermore, the Lasts noted that Carl often interrupts others when they are speaking and occasionally blurts out answers to questions before the questions have been completed. Mrs. Taylor rated Carl as being overly active and often tapping his foot or pencil. She further indicated that at times he hurries through assignments, is unable to wait his turn, and acts without thinking. These symptoms of hyperactivity and impulsivity are consistent with information obtained during the parent interview and with observations of Carl during testing.

Carl's parents and teacher all also noted that Carl is displaying atypical behaviors. For example, they indicated that Carl will repeat one activity or thought over and over, and that he stares blankly at times. Furthermore, they noted that Carl often rocks back and forth and waves his fingers repeatedly when he seems excited. During time spent at the clinic, Carl indeed frequently rocked back and forth in his seat during testing. The Lasts also indicated that Carl complains about being unable to block out unwanted thoughts and feelings. For example, Carl often claims that he gets "shivery" feelings that he does not like and that he cannot block out. Moreover, the Lasts described Carl as having an acute sense of hearing and as often

hearing sounds that they do not hear. They also described Carl as "particular" and endorsed items suggesting that he displays perfectionistic behaviors. Specifically, Mr. Last noted that everything has to be just right, that he gets upset if someone rearranges his things, and that things must be done the same way every time. This information is consistent with that obtained during the parent interview, when Mr. Last described obsessive–compulsive behaviors. In addition, the Lasts described Carl as repetitively cleaning and lining up his belongings, and they indicated past difficulties with hand washing. During time spent at the clinic, Carl was observed going to the bathroom to wash his hands after playing with bubbles that made his hands "smell like throw-up." Furthermore, Mrs. Taylor indicated that Carl went to the bathroom more frequently than his classmates, approximately six times a day. The teacher also noted that Carl's desk is very organized, but that she did not see this neatness or his trips to the bathroom as interfering with his schoolwork. Similarly, the Lasts noted that Carl's compulsive behaviors are not having a significant impact on his functioning at home. Overall, Carl appears to be experiencing problems with hyperactivity and inattention, and is displaying some atypical behaviors.

Summary

The results of this evaluation reveal that Carl's developed intelligence is in the average to low average range. This suggests that Carl will be able to benefit from instruction, although difficulties with attention, impulsivity, and off-task behaviors are affecting his daily school performance. Carl is demonstrating average perceptual and visual–motor skills commensurate with cognitive functioning. Carl is functioning in the average to significantly below-average range on tests of attention and executive functioning measuring his ability to plan, organize, and regulate his mental activity. Specifically, Carl appears to have difficulty paying attention to speech sounds and using attention to hold and process information. Carl's difficulties with attention and executive functioning are likely to impede his academic progress.

Overall, Carl is achieving academically at a level that is expected for his cognitive abilities. Specifically, his reading, writing, and mathematics achievement skills are in the average to low average range. Consistent with his cognitive profile, his test performance was adversely affected by his difficulties with attention. He often failed to pay close attention to details, such as mathematical signs, and did not attend to the specific directions of the task. In all, Carl is achieving in the average to low average range, which is commensurate with his cognitive abilities. Therefore, Carl does not meet diagnostic criteria for a specific learning disability in any area.

Behaviorally, Carl appears to be experiencing significant problems with inattention, hyperactivity, and impulsivity. Parent and teacher reports indicate that Carl fails to give close attention to details in schoolwork and is easily distracted. Furthermore, they noted that he fails to finish schoolwork and chores, dislikes tasks that require sustained mental effort, and is often forgetful. This pattern of inattention was likewise observed during testing in the clinic.

Mr. and Mrs. Last and Mrs. Taylor also reported that Carl is hyperactive and impulsive. Specifically, he often talks excessively, is overly active, fidgets with his hands, and has difficulty playing in leisure activities quietly. In addition, he often interrupts others when they are speaking and occasionally blurts out answers to questions before the questions have been completed. During his evaluation at the clinic, Carl was overactive, frequently rocking back and forth in his seat, and answered questions impulsively. The Lasts and Mrs. Taylor indicated that Carl's ability to concentrate and attend has improved since he began taking Strattera. However, this pattern of behavior is still consistent with a *Diagnostic and Statistical Manual of Mental Disorders*, fourth edition, text revision (DSM-IV-TR) diagnosis of attention-deficit/hyperactivity disorder, combined type (314.01).

According to the Lasts and Mrs. Taylor, Carl displays a pattern of atypical behaviors. Mr. Last described Carl as often staring blankly and not making sense when he comes out of his stares. The Lasts noted that Carl often complains of unwanted "shivery" feelings and is extremely sensitive to sounds, hearing things that others do not hear. Furthermore, he often does not seem to listen when he is spoken to and has occasional days where he does not act like his usual self. On one occasion, Mr. Last noted that Carl seemed completely sedated and lethargic all day, and at times talked in nonsensical, incomplete thoughts.

Moreover, Carl has a history of engaging in obsessive–compulsive, repetitive behaviors. Carl engaged in repetitive hand-washing and lining-up behaviors as a toddler. He currently has occasional days, a couple of times a month, where he engages in repetitive cleaning rituals. Specifically, he must line up his toys and trophies in his room over and over as if they are not exactly right. Carl also engages in repetitive body rocking and often waves his fingers back and forth. Mr. Last indicated that these behaviors are worse when Carl is frustrated or when he is doing undesirable activities. He further indicated that these behaviors could be related to anxiety about school. In addition, Carl uses repetitive speech patterns, such as muttering a specific phrase over and over. Hand washing was noticed during the clinic evaluation, and the Lasts indicated that there are occasions when he feels that he must wash his hands due to smells. These behaviors are indicative of compulsions; however, it is unclear at this time whether Carl feels driven to perform these actions to reduce anxiety or distress. In addition, Carl's parents and teachers do not report that these behaviors significantly interfere in his daily life, and it is unclear at this time whether these behaviors cause Carl marked distress. Furthermore, Carl's compulsions are not time-consuming, lasting less than 1 hour a day.

DSM-IV-TR Diagnosis

314.01 Attention-deficit/hyperactivity disorder, combined type
307.6 Enuresis, nocturnal only
300.3 Obsessive–compulsive disorder (rule out)

REFERENCES

American Association on Mental Retardation. (2002). *Mental retardation: Definition, classification, and systems of supports* (10th ed.). Washington, DC: Author.

American Educational Research Association (AERA), American Psychological Association (APA), and National Council on Measurement in Education (NCME). (1999). *Standards for educational and psychological testing.* Washington, DC: AERA.

American Psychiatric Association. (2000). *Diagnostic and statistical manual of mental disorders* (4th ed., text rev.). Washington, DC: Author.

Angoff, W. H., & Robertson, G. R. (1987). A procedure for standardizing individually administered tests, normed by age or grade level. *Applied Psychological Measurement, 11*, 33–46.

Bigler, E. D., & Clement, P. F. (1997). *Diagnostic clinical neuropsychology* (3rd ed.). Austin: University of Texas Press.

Binet, A., & Simon, T. (1905). New methods for the diagnosis of the intellectual level of subnormals. *L'Année Psychologique, 11*, 191–244.

Carroll, J. B. (1993). *Human cognitive abilities: A survey of factor-analytic studies.* New York: Cambridge University Press.

Cattell, R. B. (1978). Matched determiners vs. factor invariance: A reply to Korth. *Multivariate Behavioral Research, 13*(4), 431–448.

Cronbach, L. J. (1990). *Essentials of psychological testing* (5th ed.). New York: Harper & Row.

Goldstein, S., & Reynolds, C. R. (Eds.). (1999). *Handbook of neurodevelopmental and genetic disorders in children.* New York: Guilford Press.

Gustafsson, J. E. (1999). Measuring and understanding g: Experimental and correlational approaches. In P. L. Ackerman, P. C. Kyllonen, & R. D. Roberts (Eds.), *Learning and individual differences: Process, trait, and content determinants* (pp. 275–291). Washington, DC: American Psychological Association.

Horn, J. L., & Cattell, R. B. (1966). Refinement and test of the theory of fluid and crystallized general intelligences. *Journal of Educational Psychology, 57*(5), 253–270.

Joreskog, K. G., & Sorbon, D. (1987). *LISREL 6.13: User's reference guide.* Chicago: Scientific Software.

Joseph, R. (1996). *Neuropsychiatry, neuropsychology, and clinical neuroscience: Emotion, evolution, cognition, language, memory, brain damage, and abnormal behavior* (2nd ed.). Baltimore: Williams & Wilkins.

Kamphaus, R. W. (2001). *Clinical assessment of child and adolescent intelligence* (2nd ed.). Boston: Allyn & Bacon.

Kamphaus, R. W., & Reynolds, c. R. (2003). *Reynolds Intellectual Screening Test.* Lutz, FL: Psychological Assessment Resources.

Kaufman, A. S. (1994). *Intelligent testing with the WISC-III.* New York: Wiley.

Kaufman, A. S., McLean, J. E., Kaufman-Packer, J., & Reynolds, C. R. (1991). Is the pattern of intellectual growth and decline across the adult lifespan different for men or women? *Journal of Clinical Psychology, 47*(6), 801–812.

Kaufman, A. S., Reynolds, C. R., & McLean, J. E. (1989). Age and WAIS-R intelligence in a national sample of adults in the 20 to 74 year range: A cross-sectional analysis with education level controlled. *Intelligence, 13*(3), 235–253.

Kyllonen, P. C. (1996). Is working memory capacity Spearman's g? In Dennis & P. Tapsfield (Eds.), *Human abilities: Their nature and measurement* (pp. 49–75). Mahwah, NJ: Erlbaum.

New shorter Oxford English dictionary. (1993). Portsmouth, NH: Oxford University Press.

Reynolds, C. R. (1984–1985). Critical measurement issues in learning disabilities. *Journal of Special Education, 18*, 451–476.

Reynolds, C. R. (2000). Methods for detecting and evaluating cultural bias in neuropsychological tests. In E. Fletcher-Janzen, T. Strickland, & C. R. Reynolds (Eds.), *Handbook of cross-cultural neuropsychology* (pp. 249–286). New York: Plenum Press.

Reynolds, C. R. (2003, August). *Twenty years of continuous norming: An author's perspective.* Paper presented at the annual meeting of the American Psychological Association, Toronto.

Reynolds, C. R., & Bigler, E. D. (1994). *Test of Memory and Learning.* Austin, TX: Pro-Ed.

Reynolds, C. R., & Kamphaus, R. W. (2003). *Reynolds Intellectual Assessment Scales.* Lutz, FL: Psychological Assessment Resources.

Reynolds, C. R., Chastain, R. L., Kaufman, A. S., & McLean, J. E. (1987). Demographic influences on adult intelligence at ages 16 to 74 years. *Journal of School Psychology, 25*(4), 323–342.

Reynolds, C. R., & Fletcher-Janzen, E. (Eds.). (1997). *Handbook of clinical child neuropsychology* (2nd ed.). New York: Plenum Press.

Reynolds, C. R., & French, C. L. (2003). The neuropsychological basis of intelligence. In A. M. Horton & L. C. Hartlage (Eds.), *Handbook of forensic psychology* (pp. 35–92). New York: Springer.

Sattler, J. M. (2001). *Assessment of children: Cognitive applications* (4th ed.). San Diego, CA: Jerome M. Sattler.

Vernon, P. E. (1950). *The structure of human abilities.* New York: Wiley.

Wechsler, D. (1949). *Wechsler Intelligence Scale for Children.* New York: Psychological Corporation.

Wechsler, D. (1991). *Wechsler Intelligence Scale for Children—Third Edition.* San Antonio, TX: The Psychological Corporation.

Wechsler, D. (1992). *Wechsler Individual Achievement Test.* San Antonio, TX: Psychological Corporation.

Wechsler, D. (1997). *Wechsler Adult Intelligence Scale—Third Edition.* San Antonio, TX: Psychological Corporation.

Zachary, R., & Gorsuch, R. (1985). Continuous norming: Implications for the WAIS-R. *Journal of Clinical Psychology, 41*, 86–94.

V

Use of Intelligence Tests in Different Populations

Part V, "Use of Intelligence Tests in Different Populations," is another new section for the second edition of this text. The chapters in Part V focus on the psychometric quality of intelligence tests for use with special populations, including preschool children and individuals with specific learning disabilities, with gifted abilities, and from diverse backgrounds. In Chapter 22, "Use of Intelligence Tests in the Assessment of Preschoolers," Laurie Ford and V. Susan Dahinten discuss how past events have influenced current instrumentation and practice in this field, and provide the reader with suggestions and recommendations regarding the most appropriate uses of these instruments in light of their stated limitations with preschool children. David E. McIntosh and Felicia A. Dixon's chapter, "Use of Intelligence Tests in the Identification of Giftedness" (Chapter 23), summarizes the historical foundation and current issues in using intelligence tests in identifying and planning for children with superior abilities. In Chapter 24, "Psychoeducational Assessment and Learning Disability Diagnosis," Jennifer T. Mascolo and Dawn P. Flanagan review issues concerning the use of intelligence tests in diagnosis of learning disabilities, and propose an operational definition of specific learning disabilities that accommodates but does not require the use of ability–achievement discrepancy analysis. The focus of their operational definition is on the identification of below-average cognitive processing and academic ability deficits within an otherwise normal ability profile.

In Chapter 25, "The Use of Intelligence Tests with Culturally and Linguistically Diverse Populations," Samuel O. Ortiz and Agnieszka M. Dynda outline best practices in nondiscriminatory assessment and methods for evaluations and interpretations of cognitive abilities.

Jeffery P. Braden and Michelle S. Athanasiou conclude Section V with Chapter 26, "A Comparative Review of Nonverbal Measures of Intelligence." The chapter authors provide a critical review of contemporary nonverbal tests. Following their review, these authors provide a summary of issues and recommendations regarding the proper use of nonverbal tests of intelligence.

22

Use of Intelligence Tests in the Assessment of Preschoolers

LAURIE FORD
V. SUSAN DAHINTEN

Cognitive assessment provides insights into a child's developmental strengths and limitations. Although the importance of the early years of life has long been recognized, more recent interdisciplinary research on brain–behavior relationships, the role of early environmental experiences in development, and the impact of early intervention on long-term success has solidified the importance of understanding early cognitive development (Brooks-Gunn et al., 1994; McLloyd, 1998; Shonkoff & Phillips, 2000; West, Denton, & Reaney, 2000; Willms, 2002; Zaslow et al., 2001). Accompanying the research advances in areas such as medicine, epidemiology, health, and child development have been advances in the measurement and assessment of cognitive or intellectual abilities in preschool-age children. Meisels and Atkins-Burnett (2001) note that "early childhood assessment is a field in transition" (p. 231). Although the field has long been dominated by psychometric models and approaches best used with older students and adults, approaches more appropriate for younger children have begun to be incorporated. Recent changes in policies and laws affecting professional practice, advances in psychometrics and measurement, and better conceptualiza-

tions of theory and its applications to test interpretation have all contributed to an increasing interest in understanding cognitive abilities in preschool children.

Although use of the term *intelligence* or *intelligence testing* is common with school-age children and adults, given many misunderstandings of the term *intelligence* and its potential use, most professionals working with young children prefer the broader term *cognitive ability* to *intelligence*. There are some differences between the two terms, but for the purposes of this chapter, *intelligence* and *cognitive ability* will be used interchangeably. Furthermore, what constitutes the preschool years is often not clear. In this chapter, *preschool age* will include the years from approximately 2 to 8. *Infancy and toddlerhood* will refer to the ages between birth and 2 years. The preschool years typically begin between 2 and 3. Although most children enter school and the primary years at about age 6 or 7, students with developmental delays at ages 6, 7, and 8 demonstrate many characteristics of preschool-age students. As a result, in our discussion of cognitive assessment procedures in this chapter, we deem the age range of 2–8 most appropriate.

487

HISTORICAL AND LEGISLATIVE INFLUENCES ON THE ASSESSMENT OF PRESCHOOL CHILDREN

The assessment of young children in their preschool years has been influenced by many of the major events and major figures (e.g., Binet, Terman, Merrill, Gesell, Cattell) common to the history of intellectual assessment with older populations. The child study movement of the early 1900s sparked the search for an understanding of the characteristics of both typically and atypically developing young children, and thus for improved assessment instruments. However, only in the years since the mid-1960s have laws addressing the assessment of young children have been passed (Anastasi & Urbina, 1997; Nuttall, Romero, & Kalesnik, 1992).

The Child Study Movement

During the early 1900s, researchers from major universities began searching for an understanding of the characteristics and determinants of typical and atypical preschool development. They sought to understand the causal influences of heredity versus environment, and wanted to know how the instruments for assessment with young children could be improved (Kelley & Surbeck, 2000). Gesell's (1925) work, which was based on normative data, was very crucial in describing developmental milestones in cognitive, motor, language, adaptive, and personal–social behaviors (Meisels & Shonkoff, 1990). The work of Gesell and colleagues at the Yale Clinic for Child Development, and their explorations of developmental change and a maturational perspective in typically developing young children, influenced debates on intellectual abilities in young children for the greater part of the 1900s. In addition, Wellman's (1932a, 1932b, 1934) and Goodenough's (1928, 1939, 1949) research sparked debates over the influence of genetics versus environment on the cognitive development of young children (Kelley & Surbeck, 2000). The nature–nurture controversy on the development process in early childhood continues to this day (Meisels & Shonkoff, 1990); it has encouraged the examination of cognitive abilities in young children, as well as the production of new measures of cognitive ability for these children (Kelley & Surbeck, 2000).

Head Start

The 1960s brought with them a new perspective on the early lives of children. This decade marked the beginning of the modern era of early intervention—the development of early childhood programs, and a sharp increase in public support for investing in such programs (Meisels & Shonkoff, 1990). Rather than simply waiting until a child was ready for school, researchers, educators, and parents began to look for ways to enhance school readiness (Peterson, 1987). In particular, efforts were directed toward children who were disadvantaged, disabled, or at risk.

Project Head Start had its roots in the Lyndon B. Johnson administration's War on Poverty (Meisels & Shonkoff, 1990; Peterson, 1987). It was set up during the 1960s as a national preschool intervention program for selected low-income families ito prepare their children for successful entry into school (Peterson, 1987). In 1972, the Economic Opportunity Amendments (P.L. 92-424) required that Head Start also serve children with disabilities. This mandate contributed greatly to the growth of early assessment and intervention services. Head Start was based on the premises that the intellectual development of young children was influenced by their early experiences and quality of care; that the poor nutrition and lack of educational opportunities associated with poverty interfered with children's intellectual growth and achievement; and that early education could facilitate the successful entry of disadvantaged children into school, (Peterson, 1987). The Head Start philosophy supported the use of multidisciplinary approaches to working with young children, and advocated for children with disabilities (Meisels & Shonkoff, 1990). This movement toward early intervention also brought with it an increased need for valid and reliable preschool assessment to document the anticipated gains in intelligence and program outcomes, in order to secure continued funding for the intervention programs.

Early Education Programs for Children with Disabilities

P.L. 90-538, the Handicapped Children's Early Education Assistance Act of 1968, provided further federal support for early identification and intervention (Paget & Nagle, 1986). This law sparked the development of model early intervention programs for preschoolers and infants with special needs and their families (Meisels & Shonkoff, 1990; Peterson, 1987). However, instead of focusing on alternative early childhood special education interventions for disadvantaged children (as had been the focus with other programs such as Head Start), this law focused on children with disabilities from birth to 8 years of age. P.L. 90-538 provided grants to projects to develop model *early education programs* for children with disabilities (Peterson, 1987); these served as the precursor to *early childhood special education*, as it became known under the Education for All Handicapped Children Act (EHA; P.L. 94-142).

Legislation

In addition to the contributions made by early education programs to the growth and need for assessment and other services to young children, many education laws have had a tremendous impact on this area. Perhaps the greatest influences on preschool assessment have been legal mandates in the area of special education, beginning with passage of the EHA in 1975. The EHA and the amendments that followed greatly increased the need for the assessment of young children. The EHA mandated free, appropriate public education for qualified children with disabilities between the ages of 3 and 21 (Yell, 1998). Although the provision of services for preschool children was encouraged, the EHA allowed states to choose whether they were going to serve preschool children. Legislation since 1975 has provided clarification and extension of the EHA requirements into the preschool years (Yell, 1998). The 1986 amendments of the EHA (P.L. 99-457, the Infants and Toddlers with Disabilities Act), and especially the Part B requirement to provide a free and appropriate public education for preschool children ages

3 through 5 with disabilities, had important implications for the assessment of young children. The addition of Part H, which established incentives for states to provide special education and related services to infants and toddlers from birth through age 2, stimulated an increase in the development of new measures to assess the abilities of infants, toddlers, and preschool-age children (Yell, 1998). P.L. 99-457 required that multidisciplinary evaluation and assessment of children be conducted, and that the assessment must include all information needed for an individual family service plan (Fewell, 1991).

The reauthorization of the EHA as the Individuals with Disabilities Education Act (IDEA) in 1990–1991 emphasized the currently preferred "people first" terminology and used the term *disability* rather than *handicap* (McLean, 1996). Part H and Part B were amended to allow states, at their discretion, to incorporate a *developmental delay* disability category for children ages 3 through 5 (Danaher, 1998). IDEA was reauthorized again in 1997 (PL 107-15); Part B of this reauthorization retained the original disability categories of IDEA for children ages 3 through 5, and expanded the definition for service eligibility called *developmental delay* to children ages 3 through 9. This allowed for "noncategorical" services to children through age 9. The amended acts of IDEA reorganized the original Part H, which authorized the early intervention programs for infants and toddlers, as Part C. As stated above, Part C (originally Part H) extended Part B protections to infants and toddlers with disabilities. It also strengthened incentives for states to develop a statewide system of multidisciplinary agency programs to provide early intervention services to infants and toddlers experiencing delays in one or more of the following areas: cognitive development; physical development, including hearing and vision; language and speech development; psychosocial development; and/or self-help skills (Yell, Drasgow, & Ford, 2001).

In summary, the expansion of early childhood special education programs, school readiness programs, and other early intervention programs contributed to the growth and need for reliable and valid assessment and other services to young children. Many young children currently receive developmental evaluations in their preschool years to help providers determine their current levels of developmental functioning, to determine eligibility for special intervention services, and to serve as a basis in planning appropriate early intervention programs.

Most recently, the No Child Left Behind Act of 2001 (P.L. 107-110), with its emphasis on greater accountability for the early identification of those children in need of support, points to the important role of early assessment of cognitive abilities—particularly those related to success in reading. As an increasing number of states implement school readiness programs and early school readiness assessment for a wide array of preschool-age children, there is an enhanced need for well-validated, theoretically grounded, empirically supported procedures to assess the cognitive abilities of such children.

THE PROCESS OF ASSESSMENT WITH PRESCHOOL-AGE CHILDREN

Although it is easy to focus exclusively on the characteristics of the tests themselves, a number of examiner, examinee, and environmental characteristics present special challenges that must also be considered as part of an effective cognitive assessment. The assessment of a young child can be an enjoyable experience for both the examiner and the child. However, the examiner experienced in the cognitive assessment of older students and adults must appreciate that preschool-age children's unique characteristics and behaviors will differ considerably from those of the school-age children and/or adults they typically assess. An error made frequently by examiners new to testing young children is a reliance on procedures more appropriate for older children (Bagnato, Neisworth, & Munson, 1997; McLean, 1996). A young child's spontaneity, activity level, wariness of strangers, inconsistent performance in new environments, and other developmental characteristics pose challenges for even the most experienced examiner. However, with awareness and practice, as well as knowledge of the predictable sequence of development in early childhood, reliable and valid assessment information may be obtained.

Examiner Characteristics

The level of expertise brought to the assessment process by an examiner can have a significant impact on the usefulness of child-specific information gained from any test (Flanagan, McGrew, & Ortiz, 2000). Perhaps the most common challenge for many examiners is the lack of training and supervised experience in the assessment of young children. Until the mid-1990s, few training programs in school or child clinical psychology offered formal training in the assessment of preschool children, and what was offered typically followed models more commonly used with older populations. Even fewer early childhood educators received training in assessment, and what was received did not emphasize standardized, norm-referenced procedures (Dudley, 2000; Ford & Rivera, 1995). However, given the increased need and opportunities for the assessment of preschool-age children that have arisen during recent years, increasing numbers of psychologists and educators are acquiring expertise in the assessment of such children (Dudley, 2000; Ford, Dudley, & Lapointe, 2004). Examiners new to the assessment of young children are encouraged to seek opportunities for supervision as they begin assessment with this new population.

Examinee Characteristics

It is important that an examiner become comfortable with the behaviors typical and appropriate for young children, and work with those behaviors to ensure reliable test results. Several developmental aspects of young children pose challenges to assessment. In their national survey of psychologists working with preschool children, Bagnato and Neisworth (1994) reported that nearly one-half of the young children referred for assessment were untestable with traditional, standardized measures. Short attention span, high activity levels, separation issues, and lack of concern with pleasing examiners through their responses are common examinee characteristics reported by examiners testing young children. A child's limited experience with unfamiliar adults may also have an impact on testing. The language level of the young child, and particularly the intelligibility of the child's speech, can likewise prove challenging to an examiner administering standardized tests.

When getting ready to test a young child, an examiner should allow extra time to set up the testing situation and to observe and establish rapport with the child. Young children are often not accustomed to the more structured atmosphere of a standardized testing situation. To accommodate the young child's needs, the examiner may need to adjust the order of administration, alter the pace of administration, or take frequent breaks. The appropriate accommodations allowable for the assessment of preschool-age children are discussed in the manuals for most cognitive tests. As is typical of most standardized measures of cognitive abilities, the examiner must be very familiar with the test and administration rules. This is even more essential in the preschool assessment situation, since once the test session begins, there is little time or opportunity to review administration procedures.

Environmental Characteristics

The room in which testing occurs may pose a challenge to the assessment of young children. Many examiners believe that a colorful and engaging testing room is useful in attracting young children to the testing situation. Others attempt to test a child in a corner of the child's own preschool classroom, because of its familiarity to the examinee. However, the distractions of the room, colorful pictures on the wall, and materials in the room may prove more interesting to the child than the testing situation.

When an examiner is setting up the testing environment, distractions should be kept to a minimum. If there are windows in the room, the windows and shades should be closed to limit visual and auditory distractions, and the child should be seated with his or her back to the window when possible. Only the materials being used in testing should be on the table. Other materials (e.g., pencils, response booklets, additional easel books) should be out of the child's reach. A table appropriate for the child's size and age should be used. The child should be able to sit in a chair with his or her feet on the ground and arms comfortably on the table. It is generally not appropriate to test young children on the floor. To help limit the child's

movement and maintain management, it may be helpful to seat the child in the corner of the room with the table at an angle across the corner, and the examiner at the end of the table. Good lighting is also important.

Because the young child may be uncomfortable separating from the parent, caregiver, or teacher, it is helpful to spend some time with the child before he or she is brought to the location where the testing will occur. This may include working with the child in his or her preschool classroom, reading a book to the child in a waiting area, or other ways of getting to know the child. The examiner should let the child know that the other adult is nearby and will be available when the testing is complete.

A parent (or other caregiver) may need to remain in the testing room if separation problems do occur, although this is not optimal. The goal of the parent's presence will be to help the child adjust to the test situation and to increase his or her comfort with the examiner. If a parent remains in the room, it is best to have the child sit on his or her own chair with the parent to one side and slightly behind the child, so that it is not easy for the child to interact with the parent. The reasons for and importance of standardized procedures should be explained to the parent. The parent should be reminded that he or she should not provide assistance on any items, even if the parent believes that the child knows the correct response but is not responding. It is helpful to let the parent know that some items may be easy and that others will be difficult, and that it is not anticipated that the student will know the answer to all items.

It is important for the examiner to interact in a friendly and engaging, yet professional, manner to help facilitate the session. Although simpler vocabulary that is developmentally appropriate for a preschool-age child should be used, the examiner should avoid "baby talk" and the tendency to be overly chatty and playful. Such behaviors may work against optimal testing, because the standardized testing situation requires the child to comply with a series of instructions. If the child views the test session as a game, he or she may be less likely to comply with examiner requests. With practice, the typical examiner who is firm and direct yet friendly can have a successful testing session.

Familiarity with a wide array of assessment instruments and procedures will help optimize the information available to the examiner. For example, if the child is initially shy and prefers not to respond verbally, the examiner can begin with a test that requires only a pointing response or involves manipulating materials, such as blocks or form boards. As the child becomes more familiar with the examiner, he or she may become less hesitant, and the examiner can administer the tests that require verbal responses. Adjusting the pace of the assessment is especially important in the case of young children, who fatigue and are distracted easily. Some young children will respond to a brisk, quick pace; others will respond best to a slower pace. The examiner should watch the child for fatigue and carefully monitor the need for breaks. Young children typically need more frequent breaks during the testing session than do older children or adults, because of their shorter attention spans and higher activity levels. Breaks should be short, with an understanding that the child will come back to the test situation when each break is completed. Breaks that have a clear beginning and end, such as taking a short walk, getting a drink of water or snack, tossing a ball, or doing stretches, are desirable. Young children may require more frequent praise than older students. Although verbal praise will be sufficient for most children, some may require additional reinforcement, such as touch or tangible reinforcers (such as stickers and stamps). The examiner should be careful to praise effort and not to correct the child's responses. Patience and flexibility are central to the effective assessment of a young child. It is important to remain not only calm and relaxed, but also alert and aware of the young child's behavior.

TECHNICAL CONSIDERATIONS FOR PRESCHOOL COGNITIVE MEASURES

The Standards for Educational and Psychological Testing (American Educational Research Association, American Psychological Association, & National Council on Measurement in Education, 1999) outline dimensions that should be considered for all testing procedures. These standards apply not only to measures of cognitive ability for preschool-age children, but to tests for individuals of all ages. The breadth and depth of areas (both psychometric and more practical) addressed by these standards provide a valuable starting point in considering the utility of preschool measures of intelligence. In addition to the examiner, examinee, and environment considerations discussed above, the technical adequacy of preschool cognitive measures must be carefully considered. A number of researchers have provided frameworks useful for examining the technical aspects of cognitive ability measures for preschoolers (and other age groups) (Alfonso & Flanagan, 1999; Bracken, 1987, 2000; Flanagan, Ortiz, Alfonso, & Mascolo, 2002; McGrew & Flanagan, 1998).

Traditional psychometric aspects of tests (i.e., reliability and validity); other technical characteristics, such as stability, item gradients, test floors and ceilings, specificity, and *g* loadings; and features often considered more qualitative in nature, such as construct validity, cultural influence, linguistic demand, and the role of basic concepts, must all be considered. Bracken (1987, 2000) has identified minimal standards for the technical adequacy of preschool tests. Flanagan and colleagues (Alfonso & Flanagan, 1999; Flanagan, Mascolo, & Genshaft, 2000; Flanagan & Ortiz, 2000; Flanagan et al., 2002; McGrew & Flanagan, 1998) have outlined additional important considerations when examiners are selecting and interpreting preschool measures of cognitive ability, especially when they are taking a cross-battery approach to interpretation. Although these considerations are important in interpreting all measures of cognitive abilities, some aspects warrant special attention in preschool cognitive measures.

The test–retest validity or stability of the preschool cognitive measure must be considered. Evidence of scores no lower than .80 for screening and .90 for instructional planning should be provided (Alfonso & Flanagan, 1999; Lehr, Ysseldyke, & Thurlow, 1987). Floors and ceilings are important to consider, given that the developmental level of many young children referred for evaluation at the preschool age level may fall outside the age range of a test. Floors so that a raw score of 1 is at least 2 standard deviations (2 SDs) below the mean, and the total score is at least 2 SDs below the mean, are considered most acceptable (Alfonso & Flanagan, 1999). At the other end of the scale, as preschool children get older, they may not reach a ceiling on many preschool measures of cognitive abilities. Tests with inadequate floors and/or ceilings will probably not discriminate children who are developing typically from those with significant delays or strengths (Bracken & Walker, 1997). In regard to the item gradient, only small standard score changes per raw score changes (no more than 0.33 SD alteration per single raw score) are considered acceptable (Bracken, 2000). Alfonso and Flanagan (1999) outline considerations beyond psychometric characteristics—including a description of the theoretical basis for the test, basic concepts needed to understand test tasks, clear descriptions of the abilities that the test assesses, and guidelines for interpretation—that are important for preschool cognitive measures.

Although many test manuals do not provide all the details suggested by researchers, a number of published reviews provide detailed characteristics of widely used measures of preschool cognitive abilities. Most of these reviews indicate good or adequate psychometric characteristics of the most widely used tests for children 4 years of age and older and/or children without significant cognitive delays (Alfonso & Flanagan, 1999; Bracken, 1987, 2000; Bracken & Walker, 1997; Bradley-Johnson, 2001; Flanagan & Alfonso, 1995; Ford, Tusing, Merkel, & Morgan, 2004; Lidz, 2003; Tusing, Maricle, & Ford, 2003).

CONTROVERSY OVER THE USE OF STANDARDIZED MEASURES WITH PRESCHOOL CHILDREN

One of the requirements of successful early identification is assessment. Assessment practices should not only aid in the identification of strengths and limitations, but also provide a means of measuring the success of early intervention and/or education programs. What constitutes best practice in the intellectual assessment of preschool-age children is fraught with controversy. In particular, the intellectual assess-

ment of this age group with standardized, norm-referenced instruments is a hotly debated topic (Bagnato & Neisworth, 1994; Bracken, 1994; Flanagan & Alfonso, 1995; Flanagan, Sainato, & Genshaft, 1993; Gyurke, 1994; Meisels & Atkins-Burnett, 2001; Neisworth & Bagnato, 1992; Paget & Nagle, 1986). Given the controversy that has plagued standardized, norm-referenced instruments, play-based and other alternative methods (which may or may not be standardized) have been proposed as viable and more developmentally suitable options (Bond, Creasey, & Abrams, 1990; Fewell, 1991; Lifter, 1996; Linder, 1993).

A great deal of research on the assessment of young children has examined the relationship between performance on early measures of cognitive development and later child performance (Brooks-Gunn et al., 1994; Konold, Juel, & McKinnon, 1999; Lonigan, Burgess, & Anthony, 2000; Whitehurst & Lonigan, 1998; Zaslow et al., 2001). The ability of standardized cognitive tests to predict future performance and to prescribe specific interventions in a reliable and valid manner has been criticized (Bagnato & Neisworth, 1994; Barnett, MacMann, & Carey, 1992; Greenspan & Meisels, 1996; Meisels & Atkins-Burnett, 2001). Indeed, concern over the treatment utility of standardized cognitive assessments and the ability of such measures to predict future academic or cognitive performance is not unique to preschool assessment (Reschly, 1997). Given strong position statements by a number of professional organizations (the National Association of School Psychologists, Zero to Three, and several others) on the need for developmentally appropriate assessment, including the use of such alternative approaches as dynamic and play-based approaches to assessment, the use of standardized measures of preschool cognitive abilities should be considered only one aspect of a comprehensive assessment. However, despite the challenges and criticisms, other commentators point to the utility of standardized, norm-referenced measures when they are used as part of a holistic approach to assessing cognitive abilities in preschool-age children (Bracken, 1994; Gyurke, 1994; Lidz, 2003). Bracken (1994) encourages the use of standardized measures as complementary to alternative assessment procedures, because both provide unique information in the assessment process.

The poor technical qualities of many cognitive measures for children younger than 4, and the behavioral and linguistic challenges associated with completing standardized assessment tools, may further limit the utility of norm-referenced assessment techniques with young children (Bracken, 1994; Flanagan & Alfonso, 1995; Meisels & Atkins-Burnett, 2001). However, reviews of the technical adequacy of assessment tools for young children suggest that there have been continued improvement and increased sophistication in test construction in recent years (Bradley-Johnson, 2001; Flanagan & Alfonso, 1995; Ford, Tusing, et al., 2004). Indeed, what is perhaps most striking in the reviews of studies conducted during the past 15 years is the steady improvement in the technical qualities of new and recently revised cognitive tests for preschoolers. Although most measures do still have some limitations that should be considered, this recent improvement—resulting from attention by test authors and publishers to a breadth of test characteristics—provides a reason for optimism that contemporary measures of intelligence for preschoolers will offer good utility and may yield less controversy.

Therefore, in spite of challenges to the use of standardized cognitive tests with preschool children, there does appear to be a recent trend toward more developmentally appropriate and technically adequate tests of cognitive abilities in young children (Coalson, Weiss, Zhu, Spruill, & Crockett, 2002; Korkman, Kirk, & Kemp, 1998; Mullen, 1995; Roid, 2003; Roid & Miller, 1997). The trend toward improved assessment tools coincides with the ever-increasing need for reliable and valid assessment practices with young children. As the relationships between specific cognitive abilities and later learning continue to be better defined (Evans, Floyd, McGrew, & LeForgee, 2003; Konold et al., 1999; Lonigan et al., 2000; Whitehurst & Lonigan, 1998), it is anticipated that assessment tools that reliably differentiate young children's abilities into specific predictive domains may also bridge the gap between assessment findings and treatment determination.

CONTEMPORARY PRESCHOOL INTELLECTUAL ASSESSMENT MEASURES

A detailed examination of the technical characteristics of all the major preschool measures of cognitive abilities is beyond the scope of this chapter. For more detailed reviews, the reader is referred to Alfonso and Flanagan (1999), Bracken (1987), Bradley-Johnson (2001), Flanagan and Alfonso (1995), Tusing and colleagues (2003), and Ford, Tusing, and colleagues (2004). One interesting challenge in selecting measures of cognitive abilities for preschool-age children is the age range of the tests. Tests for use with young children are typically designed for infants/toddlers (e.g., the Bayley Scales of Infant Development—Second Edition, or BSID-II) or preschoolers (e.g., the Wechsler Preschool and Primary Scale of Intelligence—Third Edition, or WPPSI-III). Given the rapid changes in development that occur during the period from birth through approximately 6 years of age, it is difficult to find one test that is developmentally appropriate for children across this entire age range. Historically, the ceiling problems of infant/toddler tests and floor problems of preschool tests presented examiners with challenges when they were assessing preschool-age children with developmental delays. However, recent revisions of several measures have attempted to address these concerns. For example, the upper age limit of the original BSID was extended in the BSID-II. The floors of the WPPSI-III, the Woodcock–Johnson III Tests of Cognitive Abilities (WJ III COG), and the Stanford–Binet Scales of Intelligence, Fifth Edition (SB5) were improved during recent revisions. Furthermore, the Mullen Scales for Early Learning cover the age range from infancy to the early elementary years. An overview of measures of cognitive abilities commonly used with preschool-age children is presented below. Although each test has numerous strengths as well as certain limitations, the tests discussed here represent the best and most widely used measures of cognitive abilities or intelligence for preschool children. The examiner is encouraged to review not only the information provided here, but also the reviews cited above and the manuals of these tests, to determine which tool is most appropriate—given the age of the child, the reason for referral, and the unique characteristics of the testing situation.

Bayley Scales of Infant Development— Second Edition

The BSID-II (Bayley, 1993) is the most widely used measure of infant development in both applied and research settings. It is designed to assess the developmental functioning of children from birth through 42 months of age. Although the test consists of three scales—the Mental Scale, the Motor Scale, and the Behavior Rating Scale—the Mental Scale is the one primarily used to assess what are considered cognitive abilities. The Mental Scale examines memory, habituation, problem solving, early number concepts, generalization, classification, vocalization, language, and social skills. However, only a global or Mental Development Index (MDI) score is reported. As a result, the *BSID-II* is useful primarily as a global indicator of cognitive functioning in young children. Although this may be useful at the youngest ages (birth through age 2), most other instruments provide scores in at least two primary areas by age 3 or 4. The BSID-II does provide so-called "facet results" in several additional domains (social, language, cognitive, motor); however, no scores are provided for these. While the facet results have some potential in helping the examiner better interpret BSID-II data, most commentators conclude that these results are confusing without scores provided, and there is limited empirical evidence to support their use (Bradley-Johnson, 2001; Fugate, 1998; Nellis & Gridley, 1994; Schock & Buck, 1995).

In spite of some concerns about the BSID-II, both Flanagan and Alfonso (1995) and Bradley-Johnson (2001) point to a number of strong technical characteristics of the test, most notably the extensive standardization sample. Another concern, however, is the limited discussion of the theoretical underpinnings of the test beyond an eclectic developmental approach. This makes interpretation difficult. Interestingly, though many in the field use the BSID-II in an effort to gain some sense of future cognitive and academic performance, adequate predictive validity has been difficult to obtain for children at the youngest ages (Bradley-Johnson, 2001), and no evidence of predictive validity is reported in the manual. Despite this limited predictive validity, the BSID-II has good technical properties as a measure of current overall developmental functioning.

Mullen Scales of Early Learning

The Mullen Scales of Early Learning (Mullen, 1995) constitute a comprehensive measure of cognitive functioning for infants and preschool children through age 5 years, 8 months (5:8). This battery assesses the child's abilities in visual, linguistic, and motor areas, and distinguishes between receptive and expressive language functioning. The instrument consists of five scales: Gross Motor, Visual Perception, Fine Motor, Receptive Language, and Expressive Language. It yields a single composite score, the Early Learning Composite, that (according to the author) represents general intelligence.

Although the Mullen Scales have a great deal of appeal to those working in early childhood, given the attractive and engaging materials (which have a developmentally appropriate feel about them), the technical characteristics of the test are not as strong as those of several other instruments considered in this chapter. The theoretical underpinnings of the test are difficult to ascertain from the manual and appear to be largely based on the clinical experience of its author (Bradley-Johnson, 2001; Ford, Tusing, et al., 2004). There may be some face validity to this approach, but the lack of clear theoretical underpinning makes interpretation difficult. Furthermore, the date of the test publication and the date of norming are nearly 8 years apart; this is an area of concern, especially considering that this makes the norms approximately 20 years old. In her review of the technical characteristics of cognitive assessment tools for the youngest children, Bradley-Johnson (2001) points to a number of other concerns with the Mullen Scales, in addition to those already mentioned. These other concerns include problems with the concurrent, construct, and content validity, with item gradients, with item bias, and with the lack of predictive validity. However, given the limited choices of instruments appropriate for children in the infant/toddler years, the opportunity for lower-functioning preschool-age children to take items at the lower end of the scale, and the untimed nature of the test, the Mullen Scales may provide the best alternative for some referrals.

Wechsler Preschool and Primary Scale of Intelligence—Third Edition

The WPPSI-III (Wechsler, 2002) is the current preschool version of the Wechsler scales. Historically, the WPPSI has been one of the most widely used measures of preschool intelligence. Previous editions of the test were critiqued for their psychometric shortcomings (Bracken, 1987; Flanagan & Alfonso, 1995). Of concern to many in the field was the practicality of the test, given its length and its strong emphasis on expressive language and fine motor abilities.

The WPPSI-III is a measure of intelligence for children ages 2:6 through 7:3. (For a full description, see Zhu & Weiss, Chapter 14, this volume.) Although it still provides a global measure of intelligence in the Full Scale IQ (FSIQ) score, as well as functioning in both Verbal (VIQ) and Performance (PIQ) domains, a number of revisions have resulted in a more developmentally appropriate measure of preschool cognitive abilities. In addition to an expanded age range and updated norms, new subtests, new composite scores, and (according to the test publisher) a more "developmentally appropriate structure based on contemporary developmental theory" (Wechsler, 2002, p. 1) have been incorporated. The combination of core subtests needed to obtain global scores such as the FSIQ, VIQ, and PIQ with supplemental subtests that provide additional diagnostic information enhances the utility of the WPPSI-III. For children ages 2:6 to 3:11, there are only four core subtests (much more appropriate than the 10 needed to get a FSIQ at age 3 on the WPPSI-R), and for children ages 4:0 to 7:3, seven core tests are administered at a minimum. An additional composite score for Processing Speed is provided for these ages. By using the WPPSI-III along with the Children's Memory Scale (CMS; Cohen, 1997), the test user can gain even more information on memory functioning. This pro-

vides information in a considerable breadth of cognitive areas for a preschool child. Although previous editions of the WPPSI have demonstrated some technical inadequacies (Bracken, 1987; Flanagan & Alfonso, 1995), preliminary investigations of the WPPSI-III indicate improvements in a number of areas over the past versions (e.g., test floors, construct validity, user-friendliness, item gradients) (Ford, Tusing, et al., 2004).

Differential Ability Scales

While developed for use with children ages 2:5 through 17:11, the Differential Ability Scales (*DAS*; Elliott, 1990) battery has been one of the most widely used measures of preschool intelligence in recent years. The DAS consists of School-Age and Preschool levels. Within the Preschool level are two sublevels, Upper and Lower Preschool. This division provides for a more developmentally responsive battery and was one of the first cognitive tests to set the stage for this approach, now used in other cognitive tests (e.g., the WPPSI-III). The design of the test as a strong measure of general intellectual abilities is demonstrated by the subtests that constitute the core battery, along with a number of diagnostic subtests designed to provide additional information regarding the child's strengths and limitations. Reviews of the test in the preschool age range consistently point to a number of strong technical characteristics (Bracken & Walker, 1997; Flanagan & Alfonso, 1995; Keith, 1990). Although the test has had a loyal following of professionals assessing cognitive abilities in preschool-age children, it is becoming old by intelligence-testing standards; many of the newer tests discussed here have features similar to those of the DAS with more recent standardization samples. However, Elliott (Chapter 18, this volume) notes that a second edition of the DAS will be published in the near future.

Stanford–Binet Scales of Intelligence, Fifth Edition

The SB5 (Roid, 2003) is the latest revision of the Stanford–Binet. Those familiar with the SB-IV should be aware that the most recent edition is a very different test from its most recent predecessor, as described in detail by

Roid and Pomplun (Chapter 15, this volume). For use with individuals 2 years though senior adulthood, the theoretical foundation of the SB5 is in the Cattell–Horn–Carroll (CHC) model. The engaging materials and developmentally appropriate tasks enhance its strengths as a measure of cognitive ability in preschoolers. Although independent studies of the use of the SB5 were not available at the time this chapter was written, because the test has only recently been published, the manual reports excellent psychometric properties for the test at the preschool ages. With its division into Verbal and Nonverbal domains, the opportunity to administer a number of subtests across five cognitive factors (Knowledge, Quantitative Reasoning, Working Memory, Visual–Spatial Processing, and Fluid Reasoning) is an advantage when examiners are assessing young children with early learning difficulties. The opportunity to obtain a number of area scores with children who have limited language development at the preschool age through the tests in the Nonverbal domain will also be of help to psychologists struggling for a valid cognitive measure to use with these children. A preliminary independent technical review rates the SB5 as adequate or above in most dimensions considered in the preschool age range (e.g., floors, ceilings, item gradients), and the well-articulated theoretical foundation, along with the young-child-friendly format, provides support for the SB5 as a good choice for those assessing the cognitive abilities of preschool children (Ford, Tusing, et al., 2004).

Woodcock–Johnson III Tests of Cognitive Abilities

Several WJ III COG (Woodcock, McGrew, & Mather, 2001) tests are useful for children as young as 2:0, depending on a child's ability level. The utility of the WJ III COG is enhanced with the use of the WJ III Diagnostic Supplement (Woodcock, McGrew, Mather, & Schrank, 2003) and a number of special tests appropriate for use with preschool-age children. The General Intellectual Ability—Early Development (GIA-EDev) score is specifically designed for use with preschool children or individuals of any age who function at a very low level. The Pre-Academic Skills

and Pre-Academic Knowledge and Skills clusters on the WJ III Tests of Achievement (WJ III ACH; Woodcock et al., 2001) can provide additional useful benchmarks for preacademic functioning when these are needed.

In their review of technical characteristics of preschool tests, Flanagan and Alfonso (1995) rated the previous edition of the Woodcock–Johnson (the WJ-R; Woodcock & Johnson, 1989) as technically adequate on the majority of dimensions considered. A considerable number of tests from the WJ-R were retained on the WJ III. Similar findings are reported in preliminary investigations of the technical adequacy of the WJ III (Ford, Tusing, et al., 2004; Tusing et al., 2003). In a preliminary investigation, Alfonso (2004) found some diagnostic difficulty of select WJ III COG tests (not including the Diagnostic Supplement tests) in a sample of preschoolers with developmental delays.

As Schrank (Chapter 17. this volume) describes, the WJ III has an interpretive advantage that may be particularly useful for determining the presence and severity of developmental delay in assessment of young children. This is accomplished through criterion-referenced interpretation of a child's W score. The difference between a child's measured ability and the ability of the median individual at his or her age (W Diff) may be particularly useful because it describes quality of performance, not relative standing in a group. The presence and severity of developmental delay are determined through criterion-referenced interpretation of the subject's performance on the underlying W scale. The W score is interpreted with the resulting Relative Proficiency Index (RPI) score. For example, a subject who obtained a W Diff of −20 would obtain an RPI of 50/90, meaning that he or she is only performing with 50% success on those tasks that typical age-mates would perform with 90% success.

Unfortunately, the WJ III examiner's and technical manuals do not provide much detail on the use of the WJ III with preschool-age children. However, for those considering the use of the WJ III COG, the manual for the Diagnostic Supplement (Schrank, Mather, McGrew, & Woodcock, 2003), contains a chapter on the use of the WJ III COG with preschool children. Additional details on the use of the WJ III with preschool children, including the floors and ceilings of individual tests, are provided by Tusing and colleagues (2003). Although many of the *WJ III* tests can be used with children as young as 24 months, this does not necessarily mean that they are appropriate for a 2-year-old child with severe developmental delays. Those examiners who are experienced in using the WJ III should carefully select the tests used with preschool children.

Kaufman Assessment Battery for Children—Second Edition

The Kaufman Assessment Battery for Children—Second Edition (KABC-II; Kaufman & Kaufman, 2004) is among the newest measures of cognitive ability. Although it is appropriate for use with school-age children, the test has subtests appropriate for children as young as 3 years of age, according to the test publisher. Unfortunately, the test had just become available at the time this chapter was written, so additional studies beyond those reported by the test authors were not available. The previous version of the test, the K-ABC, was popular with practitioners working with young children from culturally and linguistically diverse backgrounds, due to the efforts to minimize the effect of cultural differences. The earlier version received generally good reviews as a technically adequate measure of cognitive abilities in older preschool-age children (Bracken, 1997; Kamphaus & Reynolds, 1987; Lichtenberger & Kaufman, 2000), and initial review indicates that this tradition is likely to continue (Ford, Tusing, et al., 2004).

The engaging format of the original K-ABC continues with this edition, which is likely to help maintain its popularity with preschool-age children. One advantage of the KABC-II not found in many preschool cognitive measures is its strong theoretical foundation, as described by the Kaufmans in Chapter 16 of this volume. The test provides for interpretation from both a Luria information-processing perspective and a CHC model perspective, depending on the reason for referral. A nonverbal option is also provided for those students with limited verbal language proficiency. Although limited information specific to the use of the KABC-II with preschool-age children is available at this time, preliminary information and previous reviews of the early edition suggest that the KABC-II appears to have great promise for use in the assessment of cognitive abilities in older preschool-age students.

Leiter International Performance Scale—Revised

The Leiter International Performance Scale—Revised (*Leiter-R*; Roid & Miller, 1997) is a completely nonverbal measure for use with individuals ages 2:0 to 20:11. Like several other measures highlighted in this chapter, the Leiter-R is not exclusively a measure of cognitive abilities for preschoolers, but it has strong utility with preschool-age children. With 20 subtests in four domains (Reasoning, Visualization, Memory, and Attention), an FSIQ composite and a Brief IQ Screener score are provided. A separate set of six subtests is recommended for use with children ages 2–5 years; this yields an FSIQ score. Additional subtests for diagnostic purposes from the Attention and Memory batteries are available for preschool children ages 4 and older (Lidz, 2003).

A technical review by Bradley-Johnson (2001) gave the Leiter-R generally strong ratings in most areas. The Leiter-R is well standardized and has a strong theoretical foundation guided by Carroll's (1993) three-stratum model. Because it is a battery designed primarily for special-purpose use, those using the Leiter-R should interpret findings with caution in spite of the strong technical properties, since it does not measure a broad array of cognitive abilities. Its greatest strength—the usefulness with nonverbal populations, and especially the opportunity to use pantomime instructions—is also potentially its greatest limitation. Because the test relies only on nonverbal means to assess cognitive skills, other measures of communication should be administered when appropriate (Bradley-Johnson, 2001).

NEPSY: A Developmental Neuropsychological Assessment

The NEPSY: A Developmental Neuropsychological Assessment (NEPSY; Korkman et al., 1998), with an age range of 3–12 years, it is another specialized measure of cognitive ability useful for preschool-age children. The NEPSY was developed to provide (1) a tool standardized on a single sample of children that would provide a valid and reliable instrument for investigating both typical and atypical neurological development; (2) an instrument capable of identifying deficits in functioning that might lead to difficulties in learning within the five primary domains (attention/executive functioning/problem solving/planning, language, sensory–motor functioning, visual–spatial processing, and memory/learning); (3) an instrument able to assess brain damage or dysfunction and the extent to which it affects the ongoing development and functioning of the domain or domains under investigation; and (4) a tool with which clinicians and researchers could study typical and atypical neurological development longitudinally (Korkman et al., 1998). Clearly, the NEPSY was designed for use as a neuropsychological and not just a basic measure of intellectual abilities. As such, the NEPSY has its theoretical foundation in the information-processing approach of Luria and is most useful for clinicians with some training in neuropsychology. This approach is dynamic, with a focus not only on the individual subtests in the battery, but also on the interactions of the tasks on the individual subtests.

Few published reviews of the NEPSY are available, and none focus specifically on its use with preschoolers. Most point to the developmentally appropriate nature of the NEPSY tasks for the children in the age range of the test, and particularly to its strength as a developmentally appropriate measure of neuropsychological functioning (Miller, 1998; Wyckoff, 1999). In contrast, Stinnett, Oehler-Stinnett, Fuqua, and Palmer (2002) provided a mixed review of the psychometric properties of the NEPSY. Most subtests were found to have adequate to excellent specificity, but Stinnett and colleagues suggested that these results do not indicate that subtest data reflect unique neuropsychological processing skills, and therefore these reviewers raised questions regarding the content validity of the NEPSY. In addition, Kozey and Phillips (2004) pointed out that an exploratory factor analysis indicated that a one-factor solution best fit the core domain structure of the NEPSY, and that the five theoretical core domains may actually overdefine the structure of the NEPSY. Although the NEPSY appears to hold some promise as a valuable tool in measuring neuropsychological abilities in preschool-age children, much more information is needed before examiners using the NEPSY can be comfortable interpreting results.

TRENDS AND FUTURE DIRECTIONS

Although recent years have seen not only an increase in the number of reliable and valid measures of cognitive abilities for preschool children, but also an improvement in the technical characteristics of preschool cognitive measures, more work is needed. McGrew and Flanagan (1998) point to the theory-to-practice deficits that occur in the field of cognitive assessment. This is particularly noticeable in the present review of widely used preschool measures of cognitive abilities. Although some test developers report a strong theoretical foundation, many of the theories described have not been examined at the preschool level. One good example is the CHC model and the work of John Carroll (1993). CHC theory has revolutionized the interpretation of intelligence tests in the last decade, but surprisingly little work has been done to examine the validity of the model with preschool-age students. As with intelligence tests used with older populations, the CHC model holds great promise as a framework for interpreting preschool measures of intelligence, but more work is needed to understand the nuances of the model with preschool children (Ford, Tusing, et al., 2004; Tusing & Ford, 2004; Tusing et al., 2003). Continued work is needed in developing appropriate interpretive frameworks for preschool cognitive measures, as well as more developmentally appropriate, ecologically valid, and culturally responsive measures with strong treatment utility.

It was formerly asserted that young children's cognitive abilities are less differentiated than those of older children (Garrett, 1946). However, new questions and approaches to developmental cognitive research (Grannot, 1998) have resulted in evidence for the presence of specific cognitive abilities at much younger ages than was once believed (Chen & Siegler, 2000). Although most psychometric research investigating the developmental nature of cognitive abilities has typically included only children 6 years of age and older, evidence from factor-analytic research for a greater differentiation of specific cognitive abilities in younger children exists (Horn & Noll, 1997; Tusing et al., 2003; Tusing & Ford, 2004). Recent psychometric studies have identified multiple latent factors—including reasoning, memory, processing speed, visual and auditory processing, and acquired knowledge—from preschool assessment tools for children as young as age 4 (Ford, 2002; Hooper, 2000; League, 2000; Stone, Gridley, & Gyurke, 1991; Teague, 1999; Tusing, 1998; Tusing & Ford, 2004).

The field of preschool assessment is indeed in a time of transition. Several well-standardized, technically well-supported instruments are available, and more are on the way. With a better understanding of contemporary developmental and cognitive theories and their application to the assessment of preschool children, the future of preschool assessment is now, and it is a future with great promise to help us best meet the needs of our young children today.

ACKNOWLEDGMENTS

We would like to thank Lori Dudley, Susan League, Terri Teague, Mary Beth Tusing, Carla Merkel, and Michelle Kozey for their assistance, both direct and indirect, in the preparation of this chapter.

REFERENCES

Alfonso, V. (2004, August). *Use of the WJ III with a referred sample of preschool children*. Paper presented at WJ III Train the Trainers, Itasca, IL.

American Educational Research Association, American Psychological Association, & National Council on Measurement in Education. (1999). *Standards for educational and psychological testing*. Washington, DC: American Educational Research Association.

Alfonso, V. C., & Flanagan, D. P. (1999). Assessment of cognitive abilities in preschoolers. In E. V. Nuttall, I. Romero, & J. Kalisnik (Eds.), *Assessing and screening preschoolers: Psychological and educational dimensions* (pp. 186–217). Boston: Allyn & Bacon.

Anastasi, A., & Urbina, S. (1997). *Psychological testing* (7th ed.). Upper Saddle River, NJ: Prentice Hall.

Bagnato, S. J., & Neisworth, J. T. (1994). A national study of the social and treatment "invalidity" of intelligence testing for early intervention. *School Psychology Quarterly, 9*(2), 81–_108.

Bagnato, S. J., Neisworth, J. T., & Munson, S. M. (1997). *LINKing assessment and early intervention: An authentic curriculum-based approach*. Baltimore: Brookes.

Barnett, D. W., MacMann, G. M., & Carey, K. T. (1992). Early intervention and the assessment of developmental skills: Challenges and directions. *Topics in Early Childhood Special Education, 12*, 21–43.

Bayley, N. (1993). *Bayley Scales of Infant Development—Second Edition*. San Antonio, TX: Psychological Corporation.

Bond, L. A., Creasey, G. L., & Abrams, C. L. (1990). Play assessment: Reflecting and promoting cognitive competence. In E. D. Gibbs & D. M. Teti (Eds.), *Interdisciplinary assessment of infants: A guide for early intervention professionals* (pp. 113–128). Baltimore: Brookes.

Bracken, B. A. (1987). Limitations of preschool instruments and standards for minimal levels of technical adequacy. *Journal of Psychoeducational Assessment, 4*, 313–326.

Bracken, B. A. (1994). Advocating for effective preschool assessment practices: A comment on Bagnato and Neisworth. *School Psychology Quarterly, 9*(2), 103–_108.

Bracken, B. A. (2000). Maximizing construct relevant assessment: The optimal preschool testing situation. In B. A. Bracken (Ed.), *The psychoeducational assessment of preschool children* (3rd ed., pp. 33–44). Boston: Allyn & Bacon.

Bracken, B. A., & Walker, K. C. (1997). The utility of intelligence tests for preschool children. In D. P. Flanagan, J. L. Genshaft, & P. L. Harrison (Eds.), *Contemporary intellectual assessment: Theories, tests, and issues* (pp. 484–505). New York: Guilford Press.

Bradley-Johnson, S. (2001). Cognitive assessment for the youngest children: A critical review of tests. *Journal of Psychoeducational Assessment, 19*, 19–44.

Brooks-Gunn, J., McCarton, C. M., Casey, C. R., McCormick, J. C. ., Bauer, J., Bernhaum, M., et al. (1994). Early intervention of low birth weight premature infants: Results through age 5 years from the Infant Health Developmental Program. *Journal of the American Medical Association, 272*(16), 1257–1262.

Carroll, J. B. (1993). *Human cognitive abilities: A survey of factor-analytic studies*. New York: Cambridge University Press.

Chen, Z., & Siegler, R. S. (2000). Across the great divide: Bridging the gap between and understanding of toddlers and other children's thinking. *Monographs of the Society for Research in Child Development, 65*(2, Serial No. 261).

Coalson, D., Weiss, L., Zhu, J., Spruill, J., & Crockett, D. (2002, February). *Development of the WPPSI-III*. Paper presented at the annual meeting of the National Association of School Psychologists, Chicago.

Cohen, M. J. (1997). *Children's Memory Scale.* San Antonio, TX: Psychological Corporation.

Danaher, J. (1998). Eligibility policies and practices for young children under part B of IDEA. *National Early Childhood Technical Assistance System (NECTAS) Notes, 6,* 1–4.

Dudley, L. (2000). *A national investigation of the use of play as an assessment procedures with preschool children.* Unpublished doctoral dissertation, University of South Carolina.

Elliott, C. D. (1990). *Differential Ability Scales.* San Antonio, TX: Psychological Corporation.

Evans, J. J., Floyd, R. G., McGrew, K. S., & Leforgee, M. H. (2003). The relations between measures of Cattell–Horn–Carroll (CHC) cognitive abilities and reading achievement during childhood and adolescence. *School Psychology Review, 31*(2), 246–262.

Fewell, R. R. (1991). Trends in the assessment of infants and toddlers with disabilities. *Exceptional Children, 28,* 166–172.

Flanagan, D. P., & Alfonso, V. C. (1995). A critical review of the technical characteristics of new and recently revised intelligence tests for preschool children. *Journal of Psychoeducational Assessment, 13,* 66_90.

Flanagan, D. P., Mascolo, J., & Genshaft, J. L. (2000). A conceptual framework for interpreting preschool intelligence tests. In B. A. Bracken (Ed.), *The psychoeducational assessment of preschool children* (3rd ed., pp. 428–473). Boston: Allyn & Bacon.

Flanagan, D. P., McGrew, K. S., & Ortiz, S. O. (2000). *The Wechsler intelligence scales and Gf-Gc theory: A contemporary approach to interpretation.* Boston: Allyn & Bacon.

Flanagan, D. P., & Ortiz, S. O. (2000). *Essentials of cross-battery assessment.* New York: Wiley.

Flanagan, D. P., Ortiz, S, O., Alfonso, V, C., & Mascolo, J. (2002). *The achievement test desk reference (ATDR): Comprehensive assessment and learning disabilities.* Boston: Allyn & Bacon.

Flanagan, D. P., Sainato, D., & Genshaft, J. L. (1993). Emerging issues in the assessment of young children with disabilities: The expanding role of school psychologists. *Canadian Journal of School Psychology, 9,* 192–203.

Ford, L. (2002). Understanding cognitive abilities in young children: Exploring abilities beyond *g.* In R. Floyd (Chair), *Beyond* g*: Implications from research with contemporary tests of cognitive abilities.* Symposium presented at the annual meeting of the National Association of School Psychologists, Chicago.

Ford, L., Dudley, L., & Lapointe, V. (2004). *A national survey of the use of play as an assessment approach.* Manuscript submitted for publication.

Ford, L., & Rivera, B. D. (1995). *School psychologist and early childhood special educator training in culturally and linguistically diverse infants, toddlers, and young children.* Paper presented at the annual

meeting of the National Association of School Psychologists, Chicago.

Ford, L., Tusing, M. E., Merkel, C., & Morgan, J. (2004). *A reexamination and critical review of the technical characteristics of measures of cognitive abilities for young children.* Manuscript submitted for publication.

Fugate, M. H. (1998). Review of the Bayley Scales of Infant Development—Second Edition. In J. C. Impara & B. S. Plake (Eds.), *The eleventh mental measurements yearbook* (pp. 93–96). Lincoln: University of Nebraska.

Garrett, H. E. (1946). A developmental theory of intelligence. *American Psychologist, 1,* 372–378.

Gesell, A. (1925). *The mental growth of the preschool child: A psychological outline of normal development from birth to the sixth year.* New York: Macmillan.

Goodenough, F. L. (1928). A preliminary report on the effects of nursery school training upon intelligence test scores of young children. *Twenty-Seventh Yearbook of the National Society for the Study of Education,* pp. 361–369.

Goodenough, F. L. (1939). Look to the evidence: A critique of recent experiments on raising the IQ. *Educational Methods, 19,* 73–79.

Goodenough, F. L. (1949). *Mental testing.* New York: Rinehart.

Grannot, N. (1998). A paradigm shift in the study of development: Essay review of *Emerging minds* by R. S. Siegler. *Human Development, 41,* 360–365.

Greenspan, S. L., & Meisels, S. J. (1996). Toward a new vision for the developmental assessment of infants and young children. In S. J. Meisels & E. Fenichel (Eds.), *New visions for the developmental assessment of infants and young children* (pp. 11–26). Washington, DC: Zero to Three.

Gyurke, J. S. (1994). A reply to Bagnato and Neisworth: Intelligent versus intelligence testing of preschoolers. *School Psychology Quarterly, 9*(2), 109–_112.

Hooper, S. R. (2000). Neuropsychological assessment of the preschool child. In B. A. Bracken (Ed.), *The psychoeducational assessment of preschool children* (pp. 383–398). Boston: Allyn & Bacon.

Horn, J. L., & Noll, J. (1997). Human cognitive abilities: Gf-Gc theory. In D. P. Flanagan, J. L. Genshaft, & P. L. Harrison (Eds.), *Contemporary intellectual assessment: Theories, tests, and issues* (pp. 53–91). New York: Guilford Press.

Kamphaus, R. W., & Reynolds, C. R. (1987). *Clinical and research applications of the K-ABC.* Circle Pines, MN: American Guidance Service.

Kaufman, A. S., & Kaufman, N. L. (2004). *Kaufman Assessment Battery for Children—Second Edition.* Circle Pines, MN: American Guidance Service.

Keith, T. Z. (1990). Confirmatory and hierarchical confirmatory analysis of the Differential Ability Scales. *Journal of Psychoeducational Assessment, 8,* 391–405.

Kelley, M. F., & Surbeck, E. (2000). History of preschool assessment. In B. A. Bracken (Ed.), *The psychoeducational assessment of preschool children* (3rd ed., pp. 1–18). Boston: Allyn & Bacon.

Konold, T. R., Juel, C., & McKinnon, M. (1999). *Building an integrated model of early reading acquisition* (Tech. Rep. No. 1-003). Ann Arbor, MI: University of Michigan, Center for the Improvement of Early Reading Achievement. Retrieved from *http://www.ciera.org*

Korkman, M., Kirk, U., & Kemp, S. (1998). *NEPSY: A Developmental Neuropsychological Assessment.* San Antonio, TX: Psychological Corporation.

Kozey, M., & Phillips, L. (2004). *Review of the NEPSY.* Unpublished review.

League, S. (2000). *Joint factor analysis of the Woodcock–Johnson III and the Wechsler Preschool and Primary Scale of Intelligence—Revised.* Unpublished doctoral dissertation, University of South Carolina.

Lehr, C. A., Ysseldyke, J. E., & Thurlow, M. L. (1987). Assessment practices in model early childhood special programs. *Psychology in the Schools, 24,* 390–399.

Lichtenberger, E. O., & Kaufman, A. S. (2000). The assessment of preschool children with the Kaufman Assessment Battery for Children. In B. A. Bracken (Ed.), *The psychoeducational assessment of preschool children* (3rd ed., pp. 103–123). Boston: Allyn & Bacon.

Lidz, C. S. (2003). *Early childhood assessment.* New York: Wiley.

Lifter, K. (1996). Assessing play skills. In M. McLean, D. B. Bailey, Jr., & M. Wolery (Eds.), *Assessing infants and preschoolers with special needs* (2nd ed., pp. 428–448). Englewood Cliffs, NJ: Merrill.

Linder, T. W. (1993). *Transdisciplinary play-based assessment: A functional approach to working with young children.* Baltimore: Brookes.

Lonigan, C. J., Burgess, S. R., & Anthony, J. L. (2000). Development of emergent literacy and early reading skills in preschool children: Evidence from a latent-variable longitudinal study. *Developmental Psychology, 36*(5), 596–613.

McGrew, K. S., & Flanagan, D. P. (1998). *The intelligence test desk reference (ITDR): Gf-Gc cross-battery assessment.* Boston: Allyn & Bacon.

McLean, M. (1996). Assessment and its importance in early intervention/early childhood special education. In M. McLean, D. B. Bailey, Jr., & M. Wolery (Eds.), *Assessing infants and preschoolers with special needs* (2nd ed.). Englewood Cliffs, NJ: Merrill.

McLloyd, V. (1998). Socioeconomic disadvantage and child development. *American Psychologist, 53,* 185–204.

Meisels, S. J., & Atkins-Burnett, S. (2001). The elements of early childhood assessment. In J. P. Shonkoff & S. J. Meisels (Eds.), *Handbook of early childhood intervention* (2nd ed., pp. 231–257). New York: Cambridge University Press.

Meisels, S. J., & Shonkoff, J. P. (1990). Early childhood intervention: The evolution of a concept. In S. J. Meisels & J. P. Shonkoff (Eds.), *Handbook of early childhood intervention.* New York: Cambridge University Press.

Miller, A. (2001). The NEPSY. In B. S. Plake & J. C. Impara (Eds.), *The fourteenth mental measurements yearbook* (pp. 834–838). Lincoln: Buros Institute of Mental Measurements.

Mullen, E. M. (1995). *Mullen Scales of Early Learning.* Circle Pines, MN: American Guidance Service.

Neisworth, J. T., & Bagnato, S. J. (1992). The case against intelligence testing in early intervention. *Topics in Early Childhood Special Education, 12*(1), 1–20.

Nellis, L., & Gridley, B. E. (1994). Review of the Bayley Scales of Infant Development—Second Edition. *Journal of School Psychology, 32,* 201–209.

Nuttall, E. V., Romero, I., & Kalesnik, J. (1992). *Assessing and screening preschoolers: Psychological and educational dimensions.* Boston: Allyn & Bacon.

Paget, K. D., & Nagle, R. J. (1986). A conceptual model of preschool assessment. *School Psychology Review, 15*(2), 154–165.

Peterson, N. L. (1987). *Early intervention for handicapped and at-risk children: An introduction to early childhood special education.* Denver, CO: Love.

Reschly, D. J. (1997). Diagnostic and treatment utility of intelligence tests. In D. P. Flanagan, J. L. Genshaft, & P. L. Harrison (Eds.), *Contemporary intellectual assessment: Theories, tests, and issues* (pp. 437–456). New York: Guilford Press.

Roid, G. (2003). *The Stanford–Binet Intelligence Scales, Fifth Edition.* Itasca, IL: Riverside.

Roid, G. H., & Miller, L. J. (1997). *Leiter International Performance Scale—Revised.* Wood Dale, IL: Stoelting.

Schock, H. H., & Buck, K. (1995). Review of the Bayley Scales of Infant Development—Second Edition. *Child Assessment News, 5,* 12.

Schrank, F. A., Mather, N., McGrew, K. S., & Woodcock, R. W. (2003). *Manual for the Woodcock–Johnson III Diagnostic Supplement to the Tests of Cognitive Abilities.* Itasca, IL: Riverside.

Shonkoff, J. P., & Phillips, D. A. (2000). *From neurons to neighborhoods:The science of early childhood development.* Washington, DC: National Academy Press.

Stinnett, T. A., Oehler-Stinnett, J., Fuqua, D. R., & Palmer, L. S. (2002). Examination of the underlying structure of the NEPSY: A Developmental Neuropsychological Assessment. *Journal of Psychoeducational Assessment, 20,* 66–82.

Stone, B. J., Gridley, B. E., & Gyurke, J. S. (1991). Confirmatory factor analysis of the WPPSI-R at the extreme end of the age range. *Journal of Psychoeducational Assessment, 9,* 263–270.

Teague, T. (1999). *Confirmatory factor analysis of Woodcock–Johnson Third Edition and the Differential Ability Scales with preschool-age children.* Unpublished doctoral dissertation, University of South Carolina.

Tusing, M. E. (1998). *Validation studies with the Woodcock–Johnson Psycho-Educational Battery—Revised Tests of Cognitive Ability: Early Development Scale and the Differential Ability Scales: Preschool Level.* Unpublished doctoral dissertation, University of South Carolina.

Tusing, M. E., & Ford, L. (2004). Linking ability measures for young children to contemporary theories of cognitive ability. *International Journal of Testing, 4,* 283–299.

Tusing, M. E., Maricle, D., & Ford, L. (2003). Assessment of young children with the WJ III. In F. Schrank & D. P. Flanagan (Eds.), *WJ III clinical use and interpretation: Scientist-practitioner perspectives* (pp. 243–283). San Diego, CA: Academic Press.

Vacc, N. A., & Ritter, S. H. (1997). *Assessment of preschool children.* (ERIC Digest No. ED289964)

Wechsler, D. (2002). *Wechsler Preschool and Primary Scale of Intelligence—Third Edition.* San Antonio, TX: Psychological Corporation.

Wellman, B. L. (1932a). The effects of preschool attendance upon the IQ. *Journal of Experimental Education, 1,* 48–49.

Wellman, B. L. (1932b). Some new bases for interpretation of the IQ. *Journal of Genetic Psychology, 41,* 116–126.

Wellman, B. L. (1934). Growth of intelligence under different school environments. *Journal of Experimental Education. 3,* 59–83.

West, J., Denton, K., & Reany, L. M. (2000). *The kindergarten year: Findings from the Early Childhood Longitudinal Study kindergarten class of 1998–1999* (NCES Publication No. 2001-023). Washington, DC: U.S. Department of Education, National Center for Educational Statistics.

Whitehurst, G. J., & Lonigan, C. J. (1998). Child development and emergent literacy. *Child Development, 69,* 848–872.

Willms, J. D. (Ed.). (2002). *Vulnerable children: Findings from Canada's National Longitudinal Survey of Children and Youth.* Edmonton, AB, Canada: University of Alberta Press.

Woodcock, R. W., & Johnson, M. B. (1989). *The Woodcock–Johnson Psychoeducational Battery—Revised, Tests of Cognitive Ability.* Itasca, IL: Riverside.

Woodcock, R. W., McGrew, K. S., & Mather, N. (2001). *Woodcock–Johnson III.* Itasca, IL: Riverside.

Woodcock, R. W., McGrew, K. S., Mather, N., & Schrank, F. J. (2003). *Woodcock–Johnson III: Diagnostic Supplement to the Tests of Cognitive Abilities.* Itasca, IL: Riverside.

Wyckoff, P. (1999). *NEPSY: Cognitive assessment with a neurodevelopmental emphasis.* Retrieved from http://www.masspsy.com/leading/9904_testreview.html

Yell, M. L. (1998). *The law and special education.* Upper Saddle River, NJ: Merrill.

Yell, M. L., Dragsow, E., & Ford, L. (2001). The Individuals with Disabilities Education Act amendments of 1997: An introduction. Implications for school-based teams. In C. Telzrow & M. Tanskersly (Eds.), *IDEA amendments of 1997: Practice guidelines for school-based teams.* Silver Spring, MD: National Association of School Psychologists.

Zaslow, M., Reidy, M., Moorehouse, M., Halle, T., Calkins, J., & Margie, N. G. (2001, June). *Progress and prospects in the development of indicators of school readiness.* Paper presented at Child and Youth Indicators: Accomplishments and Future Directions, a workshop sponsored by the National Institutes of Health, Bethesda, MD.

23

Use of Intelligence Tests in the Identification of Giftedness

DAVID E. McINTOSH
FELICIA A. DIXON

This chapter begins by providing a brief historical overview of giftedness, with an emphasis on identifying the major figures in the field. The theoretical formulation of intelligence and the conceptual links between intelligence and giftedness are also discussed from a historical perspective. The evolution of multitrait theories of intelligence, the impact of advances in psychometrics on gifted assessment, and the increase in the number of theory-based cognitive measures are examined.

A significant portion of the chapter focuses on the definition of *giftedness*. The distinction between the terms *gifted* and *talented* is made. The most recent definition of *gifted and talented* provided by the U.S. Department of Education (1993) is presented and discussed. Renzulli's (1978) multitrait definition, Tannenbaum's (1983) conception of giftedness as a psychosocial construct, and Sternberg's implicit theory of giftedness (Sternberg & Zhang, 1995) are reviewed. The implicit links among definitions, cognitive theory, and cognitive assessment are explored.

The issues of multiple intelligences versus many factors of intelligence are considered. Specifically, Sternberg's triarchic theory of intelligence (Sternberg & Williams, 2002) and Gardner's theory of multiple intelli-

gences (Gardner, 1999) are reviewed. An extensive review of factor-analytic research is provided, exploring the multidimensional abilities of gifted children with commonly used measures of intelligence. Although factor-analytic research with gifted samples has for the most part supported Kaufman's (1975, 1979) two-factor model, there is a growing body of confirmatory factor-analytic research studying more complex models of intelligence. The methodological and statistical issues contributing to differences across studies are also examined.

The process of gifted identification is then reviewed. Clark's (1997) and Borland's (1989) recommended approaches for identification are discussed. The importance of demonstrating links among a school's definition of giftedness, the identification process, and educational programming is considered. In addition, important issues to consider during the identification of cognitively gifted minority children are explored within the chapter. Alternative approaches are provided for identifying gifted children with learning disabilities.

A major portion of the chapter focuses on discussing special issues related to the intellectual assessment of gifted children. The importance of considering the theoretical differences among intelligence measures, and the importance of using theory-based measures, are discussed. The need for a better understanding of the relationships between screening procedures and the final decision outcomes based upon intelligence tests is emphasized. Implications of using a single composite IQ score and setting specific IQ "cutoff" scores when making identification decisions are examined. The chapter concludes with specific recommendations on the effective use of intelligence measures in the identification of giftedness.

HISTORICAL OVERVIEW OF INTELLIGENCE AND GIFTEDNESS

Although America's interest in giftedness has been magnified since the late 1800s, giftedness has been of general interest to virtually all societies in recorded history (Colangelo & Davis, 1997). However, until Francis Galton (1822–1911) established the conceptual link between intelligence and giftedness, there had been little research studying intellectual differences among humans (Clark, 1997). Based upon the work of his cousin Charles Darwin (1859), Galton developed the theory of *fixed intelligence*, which essentially ignored the effects of the environment and emphasized the hereditary basis of intelligence. This theory of fixed intelligence dominated the literature for nearly half a century. Not until the mid-1950s, when research conducted by Jean Piaget, Maria Montessori, Beth Wellman, G. Stanley Hall, Arnold Gesell, and others was published, did researchers begin to question the fixed-intelligence model and begin to consider an interactive view of intelligence.

Along with the theoretical formulation of intelligence came the need to develop ways to assess intelligence. Interestingly, Francis Galton was credited with developing the first intelligence test, but Alfred Binet is more widely known for developing the first intelligence test in 1905, with the specific goal of differentially placing children in special education or regular classrooms. Binet has also been credited with establishing the concepts of *mental age* and *intelligence quotient* (IQ). As Colangelo and Davis (1997) deftly point out, it was Binet's concept of mental age that had implications for the identification of giftedness. Essentially, the concept of mental age implied that children demonstrate growth in intelligence; therefore, children may be behind, consistent with, or ahead of their peers intellectually (Colangelo & Davis, 1997). Consequently, some children identified will demonstrate advanced levels of intelligence.

In 1916, Lewis Terman published the famous Stanford–Binet Intelligence Scale, which has seen four revisions to date. Not only was Terman recognized for developing one of the most popular measures of intelligence, but he also was instrumental in one of the most significant longitudinal studies on giftedness of the 20th century, earning him the distinction as the "father of gifted education" (Clark, 1997; Colangelo & Davis, 1997). Soon after the development of the Stanford–Binet Intelligence Scale, the popularity of intelligence testing soared. In fact, it soared so greatly that many schools based educational placement decisions solely on IQ scores. Unfortunately, many schools continue to identify gifted students by using a single measure of cognitive ability. The benefits and limitations of such an approach are discussed later.

Another landmark event that was instrumental in the public's interest in giftedness occurred in 1957, when the Soviet Union launched the world's first human-made satellite, Sputnik. The fact that the Soviets had both the scientific and technological power to accomplish this feat was viewed by some Americans as a shocking defeat to U.S. education. The results were an increase in the focus on educating gifted children in more advanced classes, especially in science and mathematics, and a call to action for a "total talent mobilization" (Davis & Rimm, 1998). In the United States, Sputnik was a wake-up call; new programs and schools were designed for high-ability students, with the purpose of keeping ahead globally.

Over the last 30 years, new theories of intelligence, advances in psychometrics, and advances in technology have resulted in a renewed focus on the identification of gifted individuals. The focus on neurobiological data and mental processes has resulted in the development of new theories of intelligence. Gardner (1983, 1993, 1999; see also Chen & Gardner, Chapter 5, this volume) has proposed a theory of *multiple intelligences*, which focuses on eight areas of intellect (with a ninth one, *existential*, proposed): *linguistic*, *musical*, *logical–mathematical*, *spatial*, *bodily–kinesthetic*, *interpersonal*, *intrapersonal*, and *naturalistic*. The significance of his theory lies not so much in the eight identified areas of intellect as in the underlying assumptions that form the basis of his theory. To be specific, Gardner has emphasized the neurobiological influences on intelligence and the importance of better understanding the interaction between genetics and environment in the development of intelligence. Likewise, the *triarchic theory* of intelligence developed by Sternberg (1985; see also Sternberg, Chapter 6, this volume) and Sternberg and Williams (2002) has focused on better understanding three kinds of mental processes related to giftedness: *analytic*, *synthetic*, and *practical*. The difficulty with both these theories of intelligence has been in determining how to assess and apply the various constructs presented by the authors. However, there have been several attempts to apply Gardner's multiple-intelligences theory and Sternberg's triarchic theory within the school setting, with varying results (Coleman & Cross, 2001).

Long before Gardner and Sternberg developed their theories, L. L. Thurstone (1938) proposed his theory of *primary mental abilities*. According to Thurstone's theory, seven primary intelligence factors or abilities were measured in tests of intelligence: (1) *word fluency*, the ability to think of a lot of words, given a specific stimulus; (2) *verbal comprehension*, the ability to derive meaning from words; (3) *number* or *numerical ability*, the ability involved in all arithmetic tasks; (4) *memory*, the ability to use simple or rote memory of new material, both in verbal and in pictorial form; (5) *induction*, the ability to examine verbal, numerical, or pictorial material and derive from it a generalization, rule, concept, or principle; (6) *spatial perception*, the ability to see objects in space and to visualize varying arrangements of those objects; and (7) *perceptual speed*, the ability to discern minute aspects of elements of pictures, letters, and words as rapidly as possible. Feldhusen (1998) has suggested that close examination of these seven abilities reveals some parallels to the currently popular multiple intelligences of Gardner in the types of abilities mentioned. Thurstone's theory of primary mental abilities proposed that students' achievement in school could best be understood by their relative amount of ability in these seven areas.

Advancements in psychometrics and technology have led to the development of cognitive measures that are theory-driven and reflect the multitrait nature of intelligence. In the past, cognitive measures were developed with little or no consideration of intelligence theory. Consequently, there was an overreliance on the unitary construct of intelligence, *g* (Flanagan & Ortiz, 2002). However, an increasing number of published theory-based cognitive measures now exist: the Woodcock–Johnson III (WJ III; Woodcock, McGrew, & Mather, 2001); the Cognitive Assessment System (CAS; Naglieri & Das, 1997); the Stanford–Binet Intelligence Scales, Fifth Edition (SB5; Roid, 2003); and the Wechsler Intelligence Scale for Children—Fourth Edition (WISC-IV; Wechsler, 2003). These are discussed in more detail later.

There is a renewed interest in providing gifted students with specific programming to meet their educational needs. At the heart of this renewed interest is an often hotly debated issue: How should children be identified for these special programs? What should guide the process of identification? Central to this issue is the importance of establishing a clear definition of *giftedness* to guide the development of services for the population defined.

THE ISSUE OF DEFINITION

The terms *gifted* and *talented* have been used in a variety of ways to describe individuals who perform at a superior intellectual level. *High-ability* or *high-functioning* have been terms frequently used in order to avoid using either the term *gifted* or the term *talented*, because these terms have been problematic over the years. Borland (1989) has stated that there is a rupture between the word *gifted* in its various usages and a clearly and consensually defined group of children in schools. Hence the dichotomy between what the term actually means and how it is frequently used has caused some confusion about how to regard the dimensions of giftedness. Similarly, people have often disagreed over what *gifted* and *talented* mean in terms of individual characteristics, behaviors, and need for services.

Tannenbaum (1997) has defined *giftedness* as potential for becoming acclaimed producers. Gagne (1999) has differentiated between *gifts*, which he calls *aptitudes*, and *talents*, which he calls *expressions of systematically developed abilities or skills* in at least one field of human activity. According to Gagne, catalysts—environmental, intrapersonal, and motivational—transform intellectual, creative, socioaffective, and sensory-motor gifts (abilities, aptitudes) into talents (performances) in the academic, technical, artistic, interpersonal, and athletic areas (see also Davis & Rimm, 1998). Cox, Daniel, and Boston (1985) have avoided the term *gifted*, preferring to call these students *able learners*. Renzulli and Reis (1997) prefer *gifted behaviors*, which can be developed in certain students at certain times and in certain circumstances. Treffinger (1995) likes the term *talent development*, calling the shift a fundamentally new orientation to the nature of the field. Many others have used the terms *gifted* and *talented* synonymously. If one standard definition were always used, the confusion would be nonexistent. This confusion in definitions has indeed been a major issue to both those concerned with studying gifted individuals and those concerned with educating them.

The most recent definition of *gifted and talented* provided by the U.S. Department of Education (1993) is as follows:

> Children and youth with outstanding talent perform or show the potential for performing at remarkably high levels of accomplishment when compared with others of their age, experience, or environment. These children and youth exhibit high capability in intellectual, creative, and/or artistic areas, possess an unusual leadership capacity, or excel in specific academic fields. They require services or activities not ordinarily provided by the schools. Outstanding talents are present in children and youth from all cultural groups, across all economic strata, and in all areas of human endeavor. (p. 26)

Although this definition has served the purpose of informing schools of what areas should be considered in serving gifted students, it really does not inform anyone of specific ways to find these people and is perhaps too broad for most school corporations to operationalize effectively. In contrast, it does demonstrate the current trend in widening the perspective in order to allow more people to be served. Indeed, multitrait definitions tend to be the norm today.

Renzulli (1978) has proposed a multitrait definition of giftedness that focuses on three interlocking clusters of traits: above-average, but not necessarily superior, ability; motivational traits that Renzulli calls *task commitment*; and creativity. According to Renzulli, "it is the interaction among the clusters that . . . [is] the necessary ingredient for creative/ productive accomplishment" (p. 182). The form of giftedness characterized by high scores on standardized tests and model classroom behavior has been termed *schoolhouse giftedness* by Renzulli and Reis (1997).

Tannenbaum (1983) has defined *giftedness* as a psychosocial construct. He states that gifted individuals are those "with the potential for becoming critically acclaimed performers or exemplary producers of ideas in spheres of activity that enhance the moral, physical, emotional, social, intellectual, or aesthetic life of humanity" (p. 86). The key to this definition is the focus on the gifted individual as a producer of ideas.

Sternberg and Zhang (1995) have developed an implicit theory of giftedness that embodies five criteria: *excellence*, *rarity*, *productivity*, *demonstrability*, and *value*. Stating that implicit theories are relativistic because what is perceived as giftedness is based on the values of the particular time period or place in existence, Sternberg and Zhang have argued for the need for implicit theories to fill in the gaps left by explicit theories (i.e., those that specify the content of what it means to be gifted). "The problem is that in the science of understanding human gifts, we do not have certainties. There are no explicit theories known to be totally and absolutely correct, nor are there likely to be any in the foreseeable future" (p. 91).

In contrast to multitrait or all-encompassing definitions of giftedness are the group of definitions centering around the cognitive aspects of reasoning and judgment that can be found in a test score. To this end, the Binet–Simon test (Binet & Simon, 1905) was developed as an early paper-and-pencil test that attempted to measure intelligence. A revision of this test later became known as the Stanford–Binet Intelligence Scale (Terman, 1916), and this IQ-based definition is still widely accepted today (Coleman & Cross, 2001). Terman (1925a), the father of the gifted movement in this country, was perfectly content with defining giftedness as the possession of a very high IQ.

Using the Stanford–Binet to identify a population of gifted children, Lewis Terman and his research team were interested in investigating intelligence and achievement in a group of high-functioning children in the 1920s. Terman (1925b) wrote the following about gifted children:

> When the sources of our intellectual talent have been determined, it is conceivable that means may be found which would increase our supply. When the physical, mental and character traits of gifted children are better understood, it will be possible to set about their education with better hope of success. . . . In the gifted child, Nature has moved far back the usual limits of educability, but the realms thus thrown open to the educator are still *terra incognita*. It is time to move forward, explore, and consolidate. (pp. 16–17)

Specifically, Terman's team asked the following questions: Do precocious children become exceptional adults? Do high-IQ adults exhibit a disproportionate degree of mental health problems? Are brilliant children also physically superior? Does having a high IQ correlate with excellent school performance? Can gifted children be expected to display exceptional adult career achievements as eminent scientists, scholars, artists, and leaders? If high-ability children become extraordinary adults, what can be learned from the personal and educational antecedents that seem to nurture their development? (Sabotnik & Arnold, 1994). Terman's group's research focused on the lives of those high-functioning individuals who had scored in the top 1% on the Stanford–Binet Intelligence Scale, and on what could be learned about their lives to create educational opportunities that would serve similar people. They concluded from their research that superior children apparently became superior adults (Oden, 1968).

Leta Hollingworth's work with high-IQ students (i.e., children with IQs over 180) at the Speyer School in New York City was also important in informing researchers about the impact of an enrichment program for gifted students on their adult achievement and values (Hollingworth, 1942). In 1981, several adults who had formerly attended the school were interviewed concerning the school's impact on their lives (White & Renzulli, 1987). Among those interviewed, three were from the group in Hollingworth's early study. They stated that the school provided lifelong love for learning, pleasure in independent work, and joy in interacting with similar high-ability students (Sabotnik & Arnold, 1994). Hence both Terman's and Hollingworth's noteworthy research depended in large part on the IQ score measured for each individual and on what these high-ability individuals became later in life.

Gridley, Norman, Rizza, and Decker (2003) have proposed a definition of giftedness based on the *Cattell–Horn–Carroll* (CHC) theory of intelligence. This theory combines Cattell and Horn's model of Gf (fluid) and Gc (crystallized) intelligence with Carroll's standard multifactorial model. Carroll's model (see also Carroll, Chapter 4, this volume) suggests that cognitive abilities exist at three levels or *strata*: (1) a lower or first stratum composed of numerous narrow abilities; (2) a second stratum consisting of about 8–10 broad abilities; and (3) a third stratum comprising a single general intellectual ability, commonly called *g*. Gridley and colleagues' definition is as follows:

> Intellectually gifted students are those who have demonstrated 1) Superior potential or performance in general intellectual ability (Stratum III) and/or 2) Exceptional potential or performance in specific intellectual abilities (Stratum II) and/or 3) Exceptional general or specific academic aptitudes (Strata I and II). (p. 291)

The practicality of Gridley and colleagues' definition is that it suggests that giftedness can be measured by a test. The authors state that they do not "focus on the genetic causes of gifts, but rather . . . on gifts as intellectual abilities and talents as special academic aptitudes being of equal value in their need for nurturing and development" (pp. 290–291).

Most professionals regard giftedness in school as an academic need to be served (e.g., Coleman & Cross, 2001; Rizza, McIntosh, & McCunn, 2001). In order to be served appropriately, students must be identified, and standardized tests are the major method used for identification purposes. Although a standardized test is available to measure each dimension in the federal definition, most programs for gifted individuals are particularly interested in intelligence tests, because most gifted programs focus on serving students of high cognitive ability.

Gallagher (1995) has stated that IQ tests are merely one measure of the development of intellectual abilities at a given time. They give an indication of a child's current development, so that children can be compared to one another on such characteristics as their store of knowledge, reasoning ability, and ability to associate concepts—all of which are important predictors of academic success. IQ tests still remain the single most effective predictor of academic success that we have today. Pyryt (1996) agrees with this focus on the best measure currently available, stating that IQ tests are very useful for making legal decisions regarding the eligibility for participation in gifted programs. IQ tests still serve as important tools for recognizing the special education needs of intellectually gifted students.

THE ISSUE OF ONE VERSUS MANY FACTORS IN INTELLIGENCE

Defining Intelligence(s)

The IQ score, a unidimensional construct used for many purposes, has been historically very important in identifying and understanding giftedness. In fact, the idea that a child is intellectually precocious has often been synonymous with a high IQ score. Those arguing against the idea of an IQ score have stated that this measure leads to a narrow view of intelligence that is tied to the skills most valued in schools—linguistic and logical–mathematical skills (Ramos-Ford & Gardner, 1997). In addition, Ramos-Ford and Gardner note that a majority of children are still admitted to specialized educational programs for gifted students on the basis of an IQ score of 130, or 2 standard deviations above the mean on an intelligence test. A score of 129, virtually the same score, will keep another student out of such a program. This cutoff score process is problematic and all too prevalent in school programming for gifted students.

Arguing for a theory of multiple intelligences, Gardner (1999) has defined *intelligence* as an ability or set of abilities that permits an individual to solve problems or fashion products that are of consequence in a particular cultural setting. Ramos-Ford and Gardner (1997) conclude that "A multiple intelligences approach to assessment and instruction strives toward identifying and supporting the 'gifts' in every individual" (p. 65).

Sternberg's triarchic theory of intelligence suggests that intelligence includes "applying component processes to novel tasks for the purposes of adaptation to, shaping of, and selection of environments" (Sternberg & Williams, 2002, p.148). Sternberg has described both his triarchic theory of intelligence and Gardner's theory of multiple intelligences by using a systems metaphor. Sternberg's metaphor suggests that to understand the various aspects of intelligence working together as a system, one needs to understand the integration within the system itself (Sternberg & Williams, 2002). Although these theories have gained popularity in recent years, they lack empirical data to support their effectiveness (Sternberg & Williams, 2002).

Sternberg and Williams (2002) state, "Perhaps the most difficult challenge in the study of intelligence is figuring out the criteria for labeling a thought process or a behavior as intelligent" (p. 1). One must establish criteria to use in trying to decide what constitutes intelligence. Early experts suggested that intelligence is based on adaptation to the environment (e.g., Colvin, 1921; Pintner, 1921; Thurstone, 1921; all cited in Sternberg & Kaufman, 2001). Later, Boring (1923, cited in Sternberg & Kaufman, 2001) suggested that intelligence could and should be defined operationally as that which intelligence tests test. Current definitions by both experts and laypersons suggest that adaptation to the environment, whether with practical problem-solving ability or academic skills, is still the essential theme in defining intelligence. Sternberg and Williams have further suggested three criteria to understand the mental processes and behaviors that can be labeled intelligent: correlation of a target thought or behavior with cultural success, or *cultural adaptation*; mental skills development, or *cultural and biological adaptation*;

and evolutionary origins and development, or *biological adaptation.*

With these emphases in mind, then, individuals who are called gifted will be those who can best adapt to their environments, and the purpose of finding these individuals through identification processes in schools will be to maximize their abilities in doing so.

Factor-Analytic Research

Extensive factor-analytic research has been conducted with the goal of exploring the multidimensional nature of intellectual abilities among gifted children. The majority of this research has used the Wechsler Intelligence Scale for Children—Revised (WISC-R; Wechsler, 1974) (Brown & Yakimowski, 1987; Macmann, Plasket, Barnett, & Siler, 1991; Mishra, Lord, & Sabers, 1989; Reams, Chamrad, & Robinson, 1990; Watkins, Greenwalt, & Marcell, 2002). In general, factor-analytic studies have consistently found support for the Verbal Comprehension and the Perceptual Organization two-factor model (Karnes & Brown, 1980; Sapp, Chissom, & Graham, 1985; Watkins, Greenwalt, & Marcell, 2002) proposed by Kaufman (1975, 1979). Among the two-factor models, the Verbal Comprehension factor was typically composed of the Similarities, Vocabulary, Comprehension, and Information subtests. More variability was displayed across studies in the composition of the Perceptual Organizational factor. The majority of the studies found that the Block Design and Object Assembly subtests loaded on the Perceptual Organizational factor, while the Picture Completion and Picture Arrangement subtests were found to load inconsistently across studies on this factor.

Although factor-analytic studies generally have supported a two-factor model, there has been varying support for a three-factor model (Brown, Hwang, Baron, & Yakimowski, 1991; Brown & Yakimowski, 1987; Karnes & Brown, 1980; Macmann et al., 1991). Specifically, the composition of the third factor has varied significantly across studies. For example, several studies found that the Information, Arithmetic, and Coding subtests primarily composed the third factor (Brown & Yakimowski, 1987; Brown et al., 1991), whereas Sapp and colleagues (1985) found that the Information, Arithmetic, Vocabulary, and Block Design subtests primarily composed the third factor. In addition, Karnes and Brown (1980) noted that the Arithmetic and Picture Completion subtests composed the third factor (Freedom from Distractibility).

Only limited factor-analytic research has been conducted among gifted children with cognitive measures other than the WISC (Cameron et al., 1997). Cameron and colleagues (1997) conducted a confirmatory factor analysis using the Kaufman Assessment Battery for Children (K-ABC; Kaufman & Kaufman, 1983). Although they compared four models of intelligence, they determined that Horn and Cattell's theory of fluid–crystallized intelligence provided the broadest understanding of the cognitive functioning of children referred for gifted services (Cameron et al., 1997).

The factor structures of cognitive measures have also been studied among gifted ethnic minorities (Greenberg, Stewart, & Hansche, 1986; Masten & Morse, 1995; Mishra et al., 1989). Factor-analytic research conducted by Greenberg and colleagues (1986) supported the WISC-R Verbal Comprehension and Perceptual Organizational two-factor model with a sample of gifted black children. Another study, which examined the factor structure of the WISC-R with Mexican American children referred for intellectually gifted assessment (Masten & Morse, 1995), was unable to adequately replicate the factor structure proposed by Kaufman (1975). In contrast, the cognitive constructs of gifted Navajo children were similar to the Freedom from Distractibility and Perceptual Organization factors identified based upon the standardization sample of the WISC-R (Mishra et al., 1989).

The variability in results among factor-analytic studies appears to stem primarily from methodological and statistical differences. Macmann and colleagues (1991) noted that restriction in variance due to sample selection might have contributed to differences in the composition of factors. There also appears to be great disparity across studies related to sample sizes. Although the majority of studies used large samples (e.g., Macmann et al., 1991; Watkins et al., 2002), several studies used samples with fewer than 150 participants. Factor-analytic research using gifted ethnic minorities utilized the smallest samples, with some using fewer than 100 participants (e.g., Masten & Morse, 1995; Mishra et al., 1989).

A lack of consistency across studies in the criteria used for determining giftedness also made it difficult to compare factors across studies. The criteria for inclusion ranged from a WISC Full Scale IQ of 120 and higher to 130 and higher. In addition, it was not uncommon for the criteria for inclusion to include participants with a WISC Full Scale IQ, Verbal IQ, and/or Performance IQ of 130 or higher. Gifted eligibility for some studies included children who did not meet the stated IQ criteria but did demonstrate advanced academic performance. The study conducted by Brown and Yakimowski (1987) demonstrates how selection criteria can influence the composition and the number of factors identified. They studied the WISC-R scores for three different groups of children: children who scored in the average range (IQ score between 85 and 115), children who scored 120 or higher (high-IQ group), and children in gifted programs (gifted group). The average group displayed the two-factor model commonly associated with the WISC-R; however, a four-factor solution was identified for the gifted group, and a five-factor solution was identified for the high-IQ group. The additional factors suggested that children in the high-IQ and gifted groups processed information differently from the children with average cognitive abilities (Brown & Yakimowski, 1987). Thus the composition of the sample appears to have had an influence on the number and types of factors generated.

The use of different combinations of WISC subtests in factor analyses also contributed to the different composition of the factors and whether two- or three-factor models were generated. The 10 regularly administered WISC-R subtests were consistently utilized in the factor analyses, while the Digit Span and Mazes subtests were often excluded. Studies that included the Digit Span subtest found it to load consistently on the same factor with the Arithmetic subtest (Brown & Yakimowski, 1987; Watkins et al., 2002).

The type of extraction method used, the criteria used to determine the number of factors to interpret, and the criteria used to determine the composition of factors also varied greatly across studies. The type of extraction method used (e.g., maximum-

likelihood, principal-components, principal-axis) could have influenced the number of factors generated and the composition of those factors. In addition, a vast array of criteria was used across studies for determining the number of factors to interpret. Specifically, the scree test, the chi-square statistic, eigenvalues greater than 1.0, and various combinations of these techniques were used by researchers for making this determination. Differences were also found across studies in the type of rotation methods (e.g., varimax, oblique), resulting in differences among factors. There were considerable differences in the criteria used to determine whether a subtest loaded on a specific factor. Although some studies failed to indicate the criteria used for identifying significant factor loadings, the studies that did provide criteria for significant loadings tended to range from .30 to .50. Given these differences in methodology and statistical techniques across the factor-analytic studies, it is not surprising to find some differences in the cognitive constructs of gifted children on intelligence measures.

In summary, factor-analytic research using gifted samples has for the most part confirmed the presence of Kaufman's two-factor model. In addition, the WISC-R subtests that compose the Verbal Comprehension factor have been replicated across numerous studies, suggesting significant stability of this factor with gifted children. Less stability has been shown related to the composition of the Perceptual Organization factor, and even less stability has been shown related to a third factor. Although the majority of the research has been exploratory, a few confirmatory factor-analytic studies have been published (Brown et al., 1991; Cameron et al., 1997). However, there is a continued need to study hierarchical models of intelligence with gifted samples. There is also a need to demonstrate the utility of considering multiple cognitive constructs in identifying giftedness.

THE ISSUE OF IDENTIFICATION

The Process of Identification as Related to the Definition

Several authors previously mentioned have discussed the importance of cognitive ability measures for the identification process. A very controversial part of serving gifted students is the process of locating the population to be served—a process known as *identification*. Clark (1997) has suggested the following considerations in a comprehensive identification program:

- Evidence that students demonstrate extraordinary ability in relationship to their age-level peers.
- Evidence of the range of capabilities and needs.
- Processes that measure potential as well as achievement.
- Methods that seek out and identify students from varying linguistic, economic, and cultural backgrounds, and special populations.
- Implications for educational planning.

This comprehensive list of services has opened the door to much controversy as to what a school should do for this special population. Borland (1989) has cautioned that defining the target population is the first and most important step in programming for gifted students. In other words, if a school selects a narrow definition or one based exclusively on cognitive ability, then the school's program should reflect this definition. On the other hand, if the school chooses to adopt the U.S. Department of Education (1993) definition, then a very comprehensive array of services should be available. A major issue in identification of gifted and talented youth has been the validity of the identification process with respect to program goals and services (Feldhusen & Jarwan, 1993). Since placement decisions are the goal of identification, all measures used are very important.

Identification generally begins with a screening procedure, where students are selected first on the basis of their performance on a group achievement test. Students who score the highest on this general group test, according to the school's criteria, form a talent pool. Next, the talent pool's members take a more selective test (perhaps a more precise instrument with a lower standard error of measurement). High-ability students often score very highly on group tests, and a *ceiling effect* may occur, in which their scores cluster near the very top of possible scores on the test. It is sometimes incorrectly assumed that all of these children are equally talented

and need a similar program. However, this is not always the case. More precise tests that address this ceiling effect are preferred, so that those identified for the program are truly those students most capable (if that is the definition of the target population). After this second screening step, all measures to be considered in identification are added, and the top students are identified for the program. One approach to addressing the ceiling effect common with group measures may be to use individually administered intelligence tests (e.g., the WISC-IV, SB5, or WJ III). However, whatever test is administered, the ceiling effect must be considered in selecting tests that truly measure the abilities to be served.

Identification of Gifted Minority Students

A major issue in identification of gifted students relates to the representation of minority students in gifted programs. According to Ford and Harris (1999), projections are that minority students will comprise almost half (46%) of all public school students by the year 2020. This increase in minority students at the national level has not been reflected in gifted education. In fact, according to Gallagher (2002), national surveys indicate that only 10% of students performing at the highest levels are culturally, linguistically, and ethnically diverse students, even though these diverse students represent 33% of the school population. A major focus of attention in gifted education is the goal of parity in gifted programs among all members of society, but this parity has not been easy to achieve. Although the Jacob Javits Act of 1988 has helped initiate programs for gifted racial minority students from economically disadvantaged areas, the problem of finding and/or developing useful tools to identify these students still exists. Efforts to find more valid, reliable, and useful instruments to assess giftedness and potential among minority students, and to increase teacher training in identification and assessment so as ultimately to increase the referral of minority students to gifted services, are paramount in helping to find and serve these underrepresented students (Ford & Harris, 1999).

In July 1997, the National Association for Gifted Children (NAGC) adopted a policy statement on testing and assessment of gifted students, in which it called for more equitable identification and assessment instruments and procedures. The notions of fairness and accountability underlie the proposal. In this position paper on the use of tests in the identification and assessment of gifted students, the following issues were addressed:

> Given the limitations of all tests, no single measure should be used to make identification and placement decisions. That is, no single test or instrument should be used to include a child in or exclude a child from gifted education services. The most effective and equitable means of serving gifted students is to assess them—to identify their strengths and weaknesses, and to prescribe services based on these needs. Testing situations should not hinder students' performance. Students must feel comfortable, relaxed, and have a good rapport with the examiner. Best practices indicate that multiple measures and different types of indicators from multiple sources must be used to assess and serve gifted students. Information must be gathered from multiple sources (caregivers/families, teachers, students, and others with significant knowledge of the students), in different ways (e.g., observations, performances, products, portfolios, interviews) and in different contexts (e.g., in-school and out-of-school settings). (NAGC, 1997, p. 52)

This call for a different, more inclusive way to find and serve gifted minority students is a call for diversity in programs that have typically been labeled "elitist" by many. To widen the representation, school personnel must be educated to use multiple measures to find these underrepresented students. A change in identification practices must encourage the examination of gifted individuals in cultural and environmental contexts, and must provide a basis for recognizing talents without penalizing students for certain learning styles and expressions (Frasier et al., 1995).

Assessments used to identify gifted and talented students may represent a clash between cultures, in which the mainstream culture is unable to recognize or underestimates the abilities of underrepresented minority students (Briggs & Reis, 2004). One issue that has prevented the identification of gifted minority students is that of test bias. Reynolds and Kaiser (1990), in discussing the issue of content validity and its relation to test bias, have stated:

> An item or subscale of a test is considered to be biased in content when it is demonstrated to be relatively more difficult for members of one group than for members of another in a situation where the general ability level of the groups being compared is held constant and no reasonable theoretical rationale exists to explain groups' differences on the item (or subscale) in question. (p. 625)

Items on tests often tap experiences that are relevant to middle-class students. Those from impoverished families may simply not comprehend such items, and therefore may miss questions because of environmental deficiencies rather than actual lack of intelligence. Such problems point to the bias that underlies *content validity* in both achievement and intelligence tests.

In addition, bias in *construct validity* is of concern. The fact that different groups define giftedness and intelligent behaviors in a variety of ways makes the measurement of these constructs difficult and often invites bias. Again, if the construct in question is always defined in middle-class terms, impoverished students may not be found and served.

Finally, bias is also seen in terms of *predictive validity*—the extent to which an instrument predicts the future success of a person in various situations. If teachers read the results of an intelligence test and therefore judge a person's future worth on the basis of these results, the student may not fare well. In fact, teachers' expectations may diminish because of perceived deficiencies that may not be accurate indicators of a student's ability. For these reasons, assessment issues with minority students are of major concern in the identification of students for programs.

Ford and Harris (1999) have suggested the following options when evaluators are considering how best to assess ability and potential in linguistically, racially, and culturally diverse students:

- Adapt instruments (e.g., modify the instruments in terms of their language demands).
- Renorm the selected instruments based on local norms and needs.
- Modify predetermined cutoff scores for minority students.
- Use alternative nonverbal cognitive measure thought to assess the same construct.

The issue of diversity in membership in gifted programs is currently a major issue. Educators must understand its importance and must respond to the need for alternative identification tools if they desire to provide high-quality education for all.

Identification of Gifted Students with Learning Disabilities

Another group of students who are often missed in the identification process is the group of those who are gifted but have learning disabilities. Although this description seems to be an oxymoron, Davis and Rimm (1985) stated that estimates of the number of such students in U.S. schools range from 120,000 to 180,000. Identification of students with both talents and disabilities is problematic and challenges educators (Olenchak & Reis, 2002; Sternberg & Grigorenko, 1999). Most school personnel rely on discrepancy formulas between intelligence and ability test scores; analyses of intelligence test results for differences across subtests (*scatter*); and multidimensional approaches that incorporate qualitative data, such as structured interviews and observations (Lyon, Gray, Kavanagh, & Krasnegor, 1993).

Furthermore, the identification of these students is complicated because their gifted abilities often mask their disabilities, or, conversely, their disabilities may disguise their giftedness. These problems may exclude students from inclusion in either programs for gifted individuals or programs for those with learning disabilities (Baum, Owen, & Dixon, 1991; Olenchak & Reis, 2002). This also is true for students with other exceptionalities, such as attention-deficit/hyperactivity disorder and Asperger syndrome. Astute educators are aware of these major issues in identification and search for ways to include rather than exclude all gifted students.

Multiple Means of Assessment

For these reasons, multiple means of assessing students are often used. Test scores are one determinant. Others include nominations by teachers, students, parents, and peers. In addition, checklists often tap areas of strength in students. Performance assessments, such as portfolios and auditions, are often valuable in the identification of gifted and talented students for programs. Of course, the parameters of the program must be considered in the design of any identification criteria. In addition, determining a reasonable formula that takes into account all the criteria and determines the students who then emerge as those who qualify for the program is a difficult and challenging problem for educators who manage gifted programs in schools.

SPECIAL ISSUES IN THE INTELLECTUAL ASSESSMENT OF GIFTED CHILDREN

Atheoretical versus Theoretical Approach

Although a lack of consideration of theory when evaluators are selecting cognitive measures is a concern in intellectual assessment with all children (Flanagan & Ortiz, 2002), an atheoretical approach appears to predominate within the schools when cognitive measures to identify gifted children are being chosen. The selection of cognitive measures is often based upon ease of administration, cost, or a lack of familiarity with theory-based tests. Part of the problem has been the lack of theory-based measures of intelligence; however, within the last 5–10 years, a dramatic increase in well-constructed tests has occurred. Examples include the WJ III (Woodcock et al., 2001) and the CAS (Naglieri & Das, 1997). The WJ III is based upon the CHC theory of intelligence, and the CAS is based upon the *planning, attention, simultaneous, sequential* (PASS) model. More recently, the SB5 (Roid, 2003) has been published, and it too is based on CHC theory. Even the new WISC-IV (Wechsler, 2003) has discarded the dichotomous verbal–nonverbal format and become a more theory-driven instrument.

Although the current advances in instrument development have led to a plethora of choices, this plethora can create additional confusion when evaluators are trying to select a measure for identifying cognitively gifted children. The problem is that different measures of intelligence, theory-based or not, assess different skills; the result is that some children are not offered opportunities to participate in gifted programs (Simpson,

Carone, Burns, Seidman, & Sellers, 2002; Tyler-Wood & Carri, 1991). The implications of using a specific measure of intelligence should be considered prior to its selection. Characteristics of the gifted children identified, available programming that addresses the specific characteristics of the children identified, and the extent to which nonmodal gifted children (e.g., children from impoverished backgrounds, gifted children with disabilities) are excluded should all be considered when a specific measure of intelligence is chosen. Therefore, it is essential that the theoretical differences in intelligence measures be considered—and, more important, that theory-based measures be utilized during the identification process. This view is consistent with that of Flanagan and Ortiz (2002), who advocate theory as the center of all intellectual assessment activities. The process of identifying cognitively gifted children is complex enough without starting the identification process with an atheoretical or outdated measure of intelligence.

Linking Screening Procedures with Intelligence Measures

The majority of schools have developed some type of system for identifying gifted children, albeit some systems are better than others. Usually included within the system is a procedure for screening children and thus reducing the number who are eventually referred for more comprehensive testing. Unfortunately, the comprehensive testing typically includes the administration of a single standardized measure of intelligence. And in any case, many evaluators fail to study the accuracy of screening procedures related to the final decision on whether children receive gifted programming, which is often based upon individualized measures of intelligence.

Although many would consider screening to be the crucial point in the identification process, predictive validity must be established between the screening procedure and the intellectual measure(s) used to ensure the accuracy and utility of the identification process. The difficulty with demonstrating predictive validity is that screening procedures can vary from teacher nominations to the use of group intelligence tests (Coleman & Cross, 2001). Considering the wide variety of screening methods used, relationships between screening procedures and intellectual measures can range from very low to very high. To be clear, a screening procedure that is more highly related to a selected intelligence test will result in a higher level of agreement at different points in the identification process. Coleman and Cross (2001) recommend using a fairly liberal screening threshold, to avoid missing children who may qualify for gifted programming. This approach seems advisable, given the lack of research exploring the relationships between many of the screening procedures used and the final decision outcomes based upon intelligence tests.

Use of a Single Test Composite Score

The use of a single cognitive test composite score as the primary criterion for determining giftedness is highly common within schools. In the past, the Wechsler Intelligence Scale for Children—Third Edition (WISC-III; Wechsler, 1991) and the Stanford–Binet IV (SB-IV; Thorndike, Hagen, & Sattler, 1986) were the most commonly used cognitive measures in the schools (Coleman & Cross, 2001). Coleman and Cross (2001) also note that one of these measures was commonly used as the final decision criterion for determining giftedness. In fact, school districts and states have defined giftedness solely on cutoff levels of WISC IQ scores (Fox, 1981; Karnes, Edwards, & McCallum, 1986). Others have suggested that the use of strict IQ cutoff scores is too restrictive and does not consider other characteristics of giftedness (Renzulli & Delcourt, 1986; Renzulli, Reis, & Smith, 1981). However, due to the overwhelming use of intelligence tests, there is a need to discuss the implications of using a single IQ score for making decisions on giftedness.

Implications of Using Cutoff Scores

One of the crucial decisions made by any school system is where to set the IQ "cutoff" score. It is clear from reviewing the literature that there is little, if any, consensus on where the cutoff score should be set. This not only makes it extremely difficult to evaluate decision outcomes across studies, but also makes it extremely difficult to interpret research on giftedness in general. In the literature, the inconsistency is quite evident. For example, Karnes and Brown (1980) used a cutoff score of 119; Hollinger (1986) used a cutoff score of 130; and Fishkin, Kampsnider, and Pack (1996) used a cutoff score of 127. However, most studies use an overall IQ score that is at least 2 standard deviations above the mean. Currently, this would translate to a WISC-IV and an SB5 Full Scale IQ of 130. It should be noted that the newly revised SB5 has a standard deviation of 15. The point of this lengthy review of cutoff scores is that regardless of where a school system sets the cutoff score, it is still too rigid an approach.

Many school systems fail to understand the basic psychometric process of how scores are derived, and the pitfalls of placing so much weight on a single score. To be specific, when placement decisions are being made, it is important to consider the standard error of measurement (SEM), which allows an evaluator to estimate a range of scores based upon the obtained score. For example, suppose a child obtains a Full Scale IQ of 129 on a test with an SEM of ±4 points. The examiner can be 68% confident that the next time the child is administered the same test, the child's score will fall somewhere within the range from 125 to 133. Therefore, if the criterion for placement into a gifted program is rigidly set at 130, this child will be denied services. However, if the child is later administered the same intelligence test and obtains a Full Scale IQ score of 131, the child will then be recommended for gifted services.

It also is important to note that many test manuals now report confidence intervals using the method of regression to the mean, instead of rigidly applying the ±1 SEM. Although many might suggest that in considering the SEM, all that is being proposed is to lower the cutoff score, in fact that is not what is being proposed. What is being suggested is to allow for flexibility in making identification decisions, even when cutoff scores are being used. Therefore, identification decisions should be made with a proper understanding of the underlying psychometric characteristics of standardized intelligence tests, and also with consideration of other performance variables (e.g., academic achievement).

Beyond the Composite IQ Score

Interpretation of intelligence test results beyond the test composite score is also a recommended practice in identifying gifted children. Depending on an intelligence test's theoretical model, it can provide a multiple-cluster (e.g., verbal ability, thinking ability) index (e.g., Verbal Comprehension Index, Perceptual Reasoning Index) or composite scores (e.g., Verbal IQ, Nonverbal IQ) beyond the global composite score. Ignoring a child's performance on these other indices may preclude him or her from receiving gifted services. As an example, if a child attains a WISC-IV Full Scale IQ of 127, a Verbal Comprehension Index of 142, a Perceptual Reasoning Index of 117, a Working Memory Index of 121, and a Processing Speed Index of 100, the child may be overlooked for gifted services if the sole criterion is based upon the Full Scale IQ. Here is a child who obviously displays verbal abilities within the gifted range, and the Full Scale IQ fails to account for these specific cognitive skills.

Moreover, it is important to consider the demands and skills required by specific subtests that contribute to index, cluster, or composite scores. In the aforementioned example, the child's lowest WISC-IV Index score is in Processing Speed. The subtests that contribute to the Processing Speed Index rely on speed, short-term visual memory, cognitive flexibility, and concentration. Although this child demonstrates an average level of processing speed (which is considerably lower than his or her Verbal Comprehension Index score), the score may be more a function of how the child has approached each specific subtest contributing to the Processing Speed Index.

Many gifted children have learned to sacrifice speed for accuracy and perform less well on speed-related tasks than on others. Kaufman (1992) has noted that the highly reflective and perfectionistic nature of many gifted children affects their performance on measures of intelligence where speed is rewarded. Also, variances between composite scores are fairly common among gifted individuals (Malone, Brock, Brounstein, & Shaywitz, 1991). The key issue here is not to rely solely on the overall composite score in understanding the cognitive skills of gifted children, but to extend interpretation to the next level and ultimately to the subtest level when making identification decisions.

Lack of Ceilings

With many measures of intelligence, there are not enough items at the upper end of subtests to fully discriminate the cognitive abilities of gifted individuals. Although individual items used within specific subtests are selected for their ability to discriminate between children at different levels of cognitive ability, for many subtests it is difficult to establish a ceiling, which makes it difficult to obtain an accurate estimate of cognitive ability with gifted children. When gifted children are assessed, it is common for them not to obtain a ceiling on several subtests of a specific cognitive measure. When this occurs, the overall test composite score is likely to be an underestimate of their true level of cognitive functioning. Many would suggest that this does not matter, because their level of cognitive functioning is so high that they would qualify for gifted services anyway. Here the issue is not so much one of identification as of matching children with appropriate gifted programming. It is important to accurately assess the unique cognitive skills of even highly gifted students, to meet their educational needs and interests.

RECOMMENDATIONS ON THE EFFECTIVE USE OF INTELLIGENCE TESTS

A few general recommendations regarding the use of intelligence tests in the identification of giftedness are warranted. First, it is recommended that school systems develop an operational definition of giftedness that incorporates the term *cognitively gifted*. The use of this term is suggested if a school system's primary criterion for placement in its gifted program is based upon an individualized measure of intelligence. If other measures (e.g., rating scales, nominations, achievement tests) or characteristics (e.g., leadership skills, motivation) are considered along with results on an intelligence test, the definition should address the role of the intelligence test in relation to the other measures and characteristics tapped during the identification process. Second, it is recommended that the school system develop specific procedures related to the referral, screening, testing, and placement of gifted children. Again, if the school's primary identification criterion is based upon an individualized measure of intelligence and the goal is to identify cognitively gifted children, then the screening measure should be highly correlated with the selected intelligence test.

Third, it is recommended that school systems become thoroughly aware of the specific advantages and limitations of using standardized intelligence tests to identify giftedness. Coleman and Cross (2001) note that intelligence tests are highly reliable, are individually administered, allow the examiner to observe a child's behavior directly, and allow for a broader sampling of behavior than screening or group intelligence tests do. Other advantages of intelligence tests are their abilities to identify exceptionally gifted individuals with special educational needs (Gross, 1993); children who do not display the stereotypical high verbal ability, high achievement, and high motivation often associated with giftedness (Pyryt, 1996); and children who are "twice exceptional" (e.g., children identified as gifted and with learning disabilities). As for limitations, this chapter has primarily focused on assisting schools in making informed decisions regarding the use and limitations of intelligence tests with gifted students.

Fourth, it is recommended that school systems use theory as a primary guide in selecting intelligence tests. As Flanagan and Ortiz (2002) astutely note, the use of a modern and valid theory of intelligence at the beginning of the assessment process is critical in facilitating accurate measurement and interpretation. Given the recent theoretical advances in intelligence testing, there is no excuse for ignoring theory and blindly selecting intelligence tests to identify giftedness. To be specific, understanding that one measure of intelligence assesses the constructs of verbal comprehension and perceptual organization while another assesses verbal ability, working memory, and processing speed is important to consider when evaluators are choosing intelligence measures for making identification decisions. Without an understanding of the underlying theory behind the aforementioned constructs, it would be difficult to interpret an individual's results on an intellectual measure. Also, if a cognitive measure is primarily found to assess verbal ability, it is likely that only gifted children with strong verbal skills will be identified, while children with excellent perceptual organization skills, strong speed-of-information-processing skills, or excellent working memory skills will be missed during the identification process.

Lastly, it is recommended that school systems consider using a cross-battery approach when assessing for giftedness. Specifically, the CHC cross-battery approach (Flanagan, Ortiz, Alfonso, & Mascolo, 2002; McGrew & Flanagan, 1998) should be considered. This approach is a method for utilizing separate batteries of tests and ensuring a broader range of theoretical constructs in the assessment of children. Although research is needed to support using the CHC cross-battery approach in the identification of gifted children, it does demonstrate how multiple batteries can be used to decrease the reliance on the use of one measure of cognitive ability.

SUMMARY

This chapter has explored some of the central issues related to using intelligence tests in the identification of giftedness. Although identification of giftedness is complex and has been richly debated, our goal has been to advocate for school systems' making informed decisions about the role of intelligence tests in the identification process. Although many strategies exist for identifying gifted and talented children for services, it appears that the use of a specific measure of cognitive ability dominates the identification process within the schools. It is important to design programs that begin with a definition of giftedness and build from there. The definition precedes and guides the identification process and provides the rationale for what instruments to use in order to find and then to serve the appropriate students. This chapter has focused on the need for precision in choosing effective theory-driven intelligence tests for the identification process. Many

programs for gifted students are focused on cognitive ability, and yet misuse test data making critical decisions. The current availability of cognitive assessments for identifying superior cognitive ability is better now than ever before. It remains to be seen whether those who administer the programs will choose instruments wisely, in order to obtain the information needed to identify those students who are in need of a different type of program because of their demonstrated cognitive ability.

REFERENCES

Baum, S., Owen, S. V., & Dixon, J. (1991). *To be gifted and learning disabled: From definitions to practical intervention strategies.* Mansfield Center, CT: Creative Learning Press.

Binet, A., & Simon, T. (1905). New methods for the diagnosis of intelligence in the child. *L'Année Psychologique, 11,* 191–244.

Borland, J. H. (1989). *Planning and implementing programs for the gifted.* New York: Teachers College Press.

Briggs, C. J., & Reis, S. M. (2004). An introduction to the topic of cultural diversity and giftedness. In C. Tomlinson, D. Ford, S. Reis, C. Briggs, & C. Strickland (Eds.), *In search of the dream: Designing schools and classrooms that work for high potential students from diverse cultural backgrounds* (pp. 5–32). Washington, DC: National Association for Gifted Children.

Brown, S. W., Hwang, M. T., Baron, M., & Yakimowski, M. E. (1991). Factor analysis of responses to the WISC-R for gifted children. *Psychological Reports, 69,* 99–107.

Brown, S. W., & Yakimowski, M. E. (1987). Intelligence scores of gifted students on the WISC-R. *Gifted Child Quarterly, 31,* 130–134.

Cameron, L. C., Ittenbach, R. F., McGrew, K. S., Harrison, P. L., Taylor, L. R., & Hwang, Y. R. (1997). Confirmatory factor analysis of the K-ABC with gifted referrals. *Educational and Psychological Measurement, 57,* 823–840.

Clark, B. (1997). *Growing up gifted.* Upper Saddle River, NJ: Prentice Hall.

Colangelo, N., & Davis, G. A. (1997). Introduction and overview. In N. Colangelo & G. A. Davis (Eds.), *Handbook of gifted education* (2nd ed., pp. 3–9). Boston: Allyn & Bacon.

Coleman, L. J., & Cross, T. L. (2001). *Being gifted in school* Waco, TX: Prufrock Press.

Cox, J., Daniel, N., & Boston, B. O. (1985). *Educating able learners.* Austin: University of Texas Press.

Darwin, C. (1859). *On the origin of species.* London: Murray.

Davis, G. A., & Rimm, S. (1985). *Education of the*

gifted and talented. Englewood Cliffs, NJ: Prentice-Hall.

Davis, G. A., & Rimm, S. (1998). *Education of the gifted and talented* (4th ed.). Boston: Allyn & Bacon.

Feldhusen, J. F. (1998). A conception of talent and talent development. In R. C. Friedman & K. B. Rogers (Eds.), *Talent in context: Historical and social perspectives on giftedness* (pp. 193–209). Washington, DC: American Psychological Association.

Feldhusen, J. F., & Jarwan, F. A. (1993). Identification of gifted and talented youth for educational programs. In K. A. Heller, F. J. Monks, & A. H. Passow (Eds.), *International handbook of research and development of giftedness and talent* (pp. 233–251). New York: Pergamon Press.

Fishkin, A. S., Kampsnider, J. J., & Pack, L. (1996). Exploring the WISC-III as a measure of giftedness. *Roeper Review, 18,* 226–231.

Flanagan, D. P., & Ortiz, S. O. (2002). Best practices in intellectual assessment: Future directions. In A. Thomas & J. Grimes (Eds.), *Best practices in school psychology IV* (pp. 1351–1372). Bethesda, MD: National Association of School Psychologists.

Flanagan, D. P., Ortiz, S. O., Alfonso, V. C., & Mascolo, J. (2002). *The achievement test desk reference (ATDR): Comprehensive assessment and learning disability.* Boston: Allyn & Bacon.

Ford, D. Y., & Harris, J. J. (1999). *Multicultural gifted education.* New York: Teachers College Press.

Fox, L. H. (1981). Identification of the academically gifted. *American Psychologist, 36,* 1103–1111.

Frasier, M. M., Hunsaker, S. L., Lee, J., Finely, V. S., Frank, E., Garcia, J. H., et al. (1995). *Educators' perceptions of barriers to the identification of gifted children from economically disadvantaged and limited English proficient backgrounds* (Report No. RM95216). Storrs: University of Connecticut, National Research Center on the Gifted and Talented.

Gagne, F. (1999). My convictions about the nature of abilities, gifts, and talents. *Journal for the Education of the Gifted, 22,* 109–136.

Gallagher, J. J. (1995). Education of gifted students: A civil rights issue? *Phi Delta Kappan, 76*(5), 408–410.

Gallagher, J. J. (2002). *Society's role in educating gifted students: The role of public policy* (Report No. RM02162). Storrs: University of Connecticut, National Research Center on the Gifted and Talented.

Gardner, H. (1983). *Frames of mind: The theory of multiple intelligences.* New York: Basic Books.

Gardner, H. (1993). *Multiple intelligences: The theory in practice.* New York: Basic Books.

Gardner, H. (1999). Are there additional intelligences?: The case for naturalist, spiritual, and existential intelligences. In J. Kane (Ed.), *Education, information, and transformation* (pp. 111–131). Upper Saddle River, NJ: Prentice Hall.

Greenberg, R. D., Stewart, K. J., & Hansche, W. J. (1986). Factor analysis of the WISC-R for white and black children evaluated for gifted placement. *Journal of Psychoeducational Assessment, 4,* 123–130.

Gridley, B. E., Norman, K. A., Rizza, M. G., & Decker, S. L. (2003). Assessment of gifted children with the Woodcock–Johnson III. In F. A. Schrank & D. P. Flanagan (Eds.), *WJ III clinical use and interpretation: Scientist-practitioner perspectives* (pp. 285–317). San Diego, CA: Academic Press.

Gross, M. U. M. (1993). Nurturing the talents of exceptionally gifted individuals. In K. A. Heller, F. J. Monks, & A. H. Passow (Eds.), *International handbook of research and development of giftedness and talent* (pp. 473–490). New York: Pergamon Press.

Hollinger, C. L. (1986). Beyond the use of full scale IQ scores. *Gifted Child Quarterly, 30,* 74–77.

Hollingworth, L. S. (1942). *Children above 180 IQ.* Yonkers, NY: World Book.

Karnes, F. A., & Brown, K. E. (1980). Factor analysis of the WISC-R for the gifted. *Journal of Educational Psychology, 72,* 197–199.

Karnes, F. A., Edwards, R. P., & McCallum, R. S. (1986). Normative achievement assessment of gifted children: Comparing the K-ABC, WRAT, and CAT. *Psychology in the Schools, 23,* 346–352.

Kaufman, A. S. (1975). Factor structure of the WISC-R at eleven age levels between 6½ to 16½ years. *Journal of Consulting and Clinical Psychology, 43,* 135–147.

Kaufman, A. S. (1979). WISC-R research: Implications for interpretation. *School Psychology Digest, 18,* 5–27.

Kaufman, A. S. (1992). Evaluation of the WISC-III and WPPSI-R for gifted children. *Roeper Review, 14,* 154–158.

Kaufman, A. S., & Kaufman, N. L. (1983). *Kaufman Assessment Battery for Children.* Circle Pines, MN: American Guidance Service.

Lyon, G. R., Gray, D. B., Kavanagh, J. F., & Krasnegor, N. A. (Eds.). (1993). *Better understanding learning disabilities: New views from research and their implications for education and public policies.* Baltimore: Brookes.

Macmann, G. M., Plasket, C. M., Barnett, D. W., & Siler, R. F. (1991). Factor structure of the WISC-R for children of superior intelligence. *Journal of School Psychology, 29,* 19–36.

Malone, P. S., Brock, V., Brounstein, P. J., & Shaywitz, S. S. (1991). Components of IQ scores across levels of measured ability. *Journal of Applied Social Psychology, 21,* 15–28.

Masten, W. G., & Morse, D. T. (1995). Factor structure of the WISC-R for Mexican-American students referred for intellectually gifted assessment. *Roeper Review, 18,* 2, 130.

McGrew, K. S., & Flanagan, D. P. (1998). *The intelligence test desk reference (ITDR): Gf-Gc cross battery assessment.* Boston: Allyn & Bacon.

Mishra, S. P., Lord, J., & Sabers, D. L. (1989). Cognitive processes underlying WISC-R performance of gifted and learning disabled Navajos. *Psychology in the Schools, 26,* 31–36.

Naglieri, J. A., & Das, J. P. (1997). *Das–Naglieri Cognitive Assessment System.* Itasca, IL: Riverside.

National Association for Gifted Children (NAGC). (1997). *The use of tests in the identification and assessment of gifted students.* Washington, DC: Author.

Oden, M. H. (1968). The fulfillment of promise: 40 year follow-up of the Terman gifted group. *Genetic Psychology Monographs, 77,* 3–93.

Olenshak, F. R., & Reis, S. M. (2002). Gifted students with learning disabilities. In M. Neihart, S. Reis, N. Robinson, & S. Moon (Eds.), *The social and emotional development of gifted children* (pp. 177–191). Waco, TX: Prufrock Press.

Pyryt, M. C. (1996). IQ: Easy to bash, hard to replace. *Roeper Review, 18,* 255–258.

Ramos-Ford, V., & Gardner, H. (1997). Giftedness from a multiple intelligences perspective. In N. Colangelo & G. Davis (Eds.), *Handbook of gifted education* (pp. 54–66). Boston: Allyn & Bacon.

Reams, R., Chamrad, D., & Robinson, N. (1990). The race is not necessarily to the swift: Validity of the WISC-R bonus points for speed. *Gifted Child Quarterly, 34,* 108–110.

Renzulli, J. S. (1978). What makes giftedness: Reexamining a definition. *Phi Delta Kappan, 60,* 18–24.

Renzulli, J. S., & Delcourt, M. A. (1986). The legacy and logic of research on the identification of gifted persons. *Gifted Child Quarterly, 30,* 20–23.

Renzulli, J. S., & Reis, S. M. (1997). *The schoolwide enrichment model: A how-to guide for educational excellence.* Mansfield Center, CT: Creative Learning Press.

Renzulli, J. S., Reis, S. M., & Smith, L. H. (1981). *The revolving door identification model.* Mansfield Center, CT: Creative Learning Press.

Reynolds, C. R., & Kaiser, S. M. (1990). Bias in assessment of attitude. In C. R. Reynolds & R. W. Kamphaus (Eds.), *Handbook of psychological and educational assessment of children: Intelligence and achievement.* New York: Guilford Press.

Rizza, M. G., McIntosh, D. E., & McCunn, A. (2001). Profile analysis of the Woodcock–Johnson III Tests of Cognitive Abilities with gifted students. *Psychology in the Schools, 38,* 447–455.

Roid, G. H. (2003). *Stanford–Binet Intelligence Scales, Fifth Edition.* Itasca, IL: Riverside.

Sabotnik, R. F., & Arnold, K. D. (1994). *Beyond Terman: Contemporary longitudinal studies of giftedness and talent.* Norwood, NJ: Ablex.

Sapp, G. L., Chissom, B., & Graham, E. (1985). Factor analysis of the WISC-R for gifted students: A replication and comparison. *Psychological Reports, 57,* 947–951.

Simpson, M., Carone, D. A., Jr., Burns, W. J., Seidman, D. M., & Sellers, A. (2002). Assessing giftedness with the WISC-III and the SB-IV. *Psychology in the Schools, 39,* 515–524.

Sternberg, R. J. (1985). *Beyond IQ: A triarchic theory of human intelligence.* Cambridge, UK: Cambridge University Press.

Sternberg, R. J., & Grigorenko, E. I. (1999). *Our labeled children.* Reading, MA: Perseus Books.

Sternberg, R. J., & Kaufman, J. D. (2001). *The evolution of intelligence.* Mahwah, NJ: Erlbaum.

Sternberg, R. J., & Williams, W. (2002). *Educational psychology.* Boston: Allyn & Bacon.

Sternberg, R. J., & Zhang, L. (1995). What do we mean by giftedness?: A pentagonal implicit theory. *Gifted Child Quarterly, 39,* 88–94.

Tannenbaum, A. J. (1983). *Gifted children: Psychological and educational perspectives.* New York: Macmillan.

Tannenbaum, A. J. (1997). The meaning and making of giftedness. In N. Colangelo & G. Davis (Eds.), *Handbook of gifted education* (pp. 27–42). Boston: Allyn & Bacon.

Terman, L. M. (1916). *The measurement of intelligence.* Boston: Houghton Mifflin.

Terman, L. M. (1925a). *Genetic studies of genius: Mental and physical traits of a thousand gifted children* (Vol. 1). Stanford, CA: Stanford University Press.

Terman, L. M. (1925b). *Genetic studies of genius: Mental and physical traits of a thousand gifted children* (Vol. 4). Stanford, CA: Stanford University Press.

Thorndike, R. L., Hagen, E. P., & Sattler, J. M. (1986). *Stanford–Binet Intelligence Scale: Fourth Edition.* Chicago: Riverside.

Thurstone, L. L. (1938). *Primary mental abilities.* Chicago: University of Chicago Press.

Treffinger, D. J. (1995). Talent development: An emerging view. *Understanding Our Gifted, 7*(4), 3.

Tyler-Wood, R., & Carri, L. (1991). Identification of gifted children: The effectiveness of various measures of cognitive ability. *Roeper Review, 14,* 63–64.

U.S. Department of Education. (1993). *National excellence: A case for developing America's talent.* Washington, DC: U.S. Government Printing Office.

Watkins, M. W., Greenwalt, C. G., & Marcell, C. M. (2002). Factor structure of the Wechsler Intelligence Scale for Children—Third Edition among gifted students. *Educational and Psychological Measurement. 62,* 164–172.

Wechsler, D. (1974). *Wechsler Intelligence Scale for Children—Revised.* New York: Psychological Corporation.

Wechsler, D. (1991). *Wechsler Intelligence Scale for Children—Third Edition.* San Antonio, TX: Psychological Corporation.

Wechsler, D. (2003). *Wechsler Intelligence Scale for Children—Fourth Edition.* San Antonio, TX: Psychological Corporation.

White, W. L., & Renzulli, J. S. (1987). A forty year follow-up of students who attended Leta Hollingworth's School for Gifted Children. *Roeper Review, 10*(2), 89–94.

Woodcock, R. W., McGrew, K. S., & Mather, N. (2001). *Woodcock–Johnson III.* Itasca, IL: Riverside.

24

Psychoeducational Assessment and Learning Disability Diagnosis

DAWN P. FLANAGAN
JENNIFER T. MASCOLO

Evaluating an individual suspected of having a learning disability (LD) is a common activity for many psychologists and educators. Despite familiarity with this referral concern and the frequency with which LD assessments are conducted, reliable and valid diagnosis of LDs remains difficult. This is primarily due to the lack of (1) a guiding theoretical model from which to approach LD assessments; (2) a practical operational definition to aid in organizing assessments; and (3) a dependable assessment framework within which to evaluate assessment results. Without these factors, evaluators are left to search blindly through a vast array of vague conditions, unknown specifications, and inconsistent test results, in the hope that some sort of pattern might emerge from the data that could presumably establish the presence of an LD.

As stated above, one of the primary difficulties in assessing LD has been the lack of an operational definition that is based on an empirically supported theoretical perspective, and that offers reliable and valid specifications for assessment across a variety of disciplines. Without a consistently applied theoretical context and guidance concerning how the various components of LD evaluation relate to each other, let alone which ones are necessary or sufficient, reliable assess-

ment of LD cannot be established. The goal of this chapter is to present a comprehensive framework for assessment that follows established principles for reliable and valid assessment and that incorporates a modern, theory-based operational definition of LD. Specifically, this chapter illustrates how evaluators can use the proposed operational definition to (a) organize assessments of suspected LD using current cognitive and achievement batteries and (b) make decisions relevant to LD identification, particularly as they relate to the sufficiency of an evaluation (e.g., attributions of performance, potential mitigating factors, and reasons for underachievement). It is hoped that the information presented herein will aid in advancing the practice of LD evaluation.

PROBLEMS WITH TRADITIONAL OPERATIONAL DEFINITIONS OF LD

Operational definitions of LD have varied widely in the past and have not proven to be particularly accurate or useful. Traditional models used in diagnosing LD have been problematic because they often fail to discriminate adequately between students with LD and those without, who are better described as *low-achieving* (Aaron, 1995;

521

Brackett & McPherson, 1996; Kavale & Forness, 2000; Siegel, 1998, 1999; Stanovich, 1999). A review of the literature shows several possible reasons why traditional models have failed in this regard. Many of the reasons are related to a variety of misconceptions; most notable among these are misconceptions about the nature of IQ and intelligence, which seem to remain rather consistent and ubiquitous in virtually all conceptualizations of LD (Flanagan & Ortiz, 2001; Kavale & Forness, 2000; Siegel, 1998, 1999; Stanovich, 1999).

To develop a more valid method of LD assessment, it is necessary to derive proper methods based on operational definitions that are grounded in contemporary theory and research. Accordingly, the major aim of this chapter is to provide an extended discussion of the core elements that are essential to effectively operationalizing LD from a modern theoretical perspective. We propose that these elements, when used within the context of a comprehensive assessment and evaluation framework of learning difficulties, provide a substantive, consistent, and easily replicable means with which to reliably and validly evaluate LD. Discussion of the essential elements in LD assessment represents the integration of various ideologies and interdisciplinary concepts. Consequently, the resulting operationalization is one that we believe can be adopted by virtually all professionals involved in LD assessment, regardless of their particular training, education, or discipline.

ESSENTIAL ELEMENTS OF AN OPERATIONAL DEFINITION OF LD

A current operational definition of LD is presented in Figure 24.1. The essential elements in defining LD as illustrated in the figure include (1) academic ability analysis, (2) evaluation of exclusionary factors, (3) cognitive ability analysis, (4) reevaluation of exclusionary factors, (5) integrated ability analysis, and (6) evaluation of interference with functioning. These elements are depicted as levels and together form the complete operational definition of LD that we believe provides a means for accomplishing reliable and valid diagnosis. The levels depicted in Figure 24.1 represent an adaptation and ex-

tension of recommendations and/or concepts from many different researchers (e.g., Flanagan, McGrew, & Ortiz, 2000; Flanagan & Ortiz, 2001; Flanagan, Ortiz, Alfonso, & Mascolo, 2002; Kavale & Forness, 2000; McGrew & Flanagan, 1998; Siegel, 1999; Stanovich, 1999; Vellutino, Scanlon, & Lyon, 2000). Cognitive and academic assessment batteries can be used effectively to gather information and test hypotheses at each level of this operational definition. To this end, tables that include tests from the major psychoeducational assessment batteries are presented.

Before we discuss each level of the operational definition, it is important to note that the operational definition presented in this chapter differs from the ones presented by other researchers (e.g., Kavale & Forness, 2000) in four important ways. First, the current levels are firmly grounded in an established contemporary theory of the structure of abilities (i.e., Cattell–Horn–Carroll [CHC] theory). Second, traditional LD models consider an ability–achievement discrepancy to be a necessary but not a sufficient condition for an LD. In contrast, this type of discrepancy analysis occurs much later in the LD evaluation framework presented here (i.e., after sufficient evidence of an LD is established). This is because the proposed framework accommodates the notion that a significant ability–achievement discrepancy *need not be present* to establish an LD (Siegel, 1999; Stanovich, 1999), primarily because the finding of such a discrepancy is largely dependent upon the specific ability measure used in a discrepancy formula (Flanagan et al., 2000; Flanagan & Ortiz, 2001). That is, different ability measures will result in different discrepancies (either significant or nonsignificant) for different reasons.

Third, although most LD definitions include an exclusionary clause (and such a clause is also included in the present definition), we believe that evaluation of exclusionary criteria should occur earlier in the LD assessment process to prevent individuals from having to undergo needless and invasive testing. Therefore, it is represented at levels I-B and II-B in our definition. And fourth, although there is a somewhat logical progression from one level to the next, we seek to reinforce the notion that LD assessment is a recursive process. Information gen-

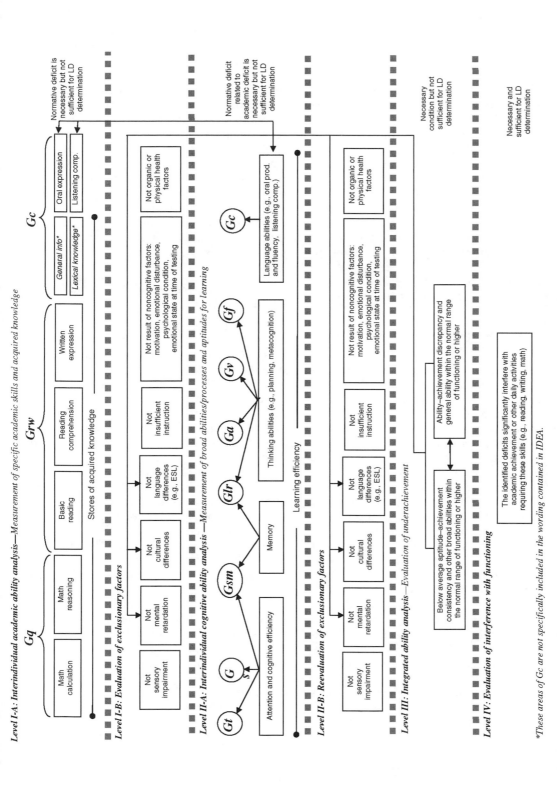

FIGURE 24.1. An operational definition of LD. From Flanagan et al. (2002). Published by Allyn and Bacon, Boston, MA. Copyright 2002 by Pearson Education. Reprinted by permission.

523

erated and evaluated at one level may inform decisions made at other levels, and specific circumstances unique to a case may warrant a return to prior levels. The recursive or iterative nature of LD assessment has not been included in traditional conceptualizations, but forms an important component of the present model. It is important to understand that despite the linear appearance of the levels illustrated in Figure 24.1, the operational definition is best conceptualized as cyclical or recursive in nature. This notion becomes particularly evident later in this chapter, when the operational definition is embedded within the presentation and discussion of a comprehensive framework for LD assessment. Readers may wish to refer to Figure 24.1 often for clarification of the descriptions of the essential elements of our operational definition of LD that follow.

Prereferral Activities and A Priori Hypotheses

It is assumed that the levels of evaluation depicted in Figure 24.1 are undertaken after prereferral assessment activities have been conducted and when a focused evaluation of specific abilities and processes through standardized testing is deemed necessary. Evaluation of the presence of an LD is based on the assumption that an individual has been referred for testing specifically because of observed learning difficulties, and that these difficulties have undergone an appropriate remedial prereferral intervention or accommodation process with little or no apparent success (i.e., failure to respond to intervention; see IDEA reauthorization). Moreover, prior to the beginning of LD assessment, other significant data sources could have (and probably should have) already been uncovered within the context of these intervention activities. These data may include results from informal testing, direct observation of behaviors, work samples, reports from people familiar with the individual's difficulties (e.g., teachers, parents), and information provided by the individual. In principle, level I-A assessment should begin only after the scope and nature of an individual's learning difficulties have been documented (Flanagan et al., 2002).

It is important to note that before begin-ning level I-A assessment, evaluators should also decide what type of analysis will be conducted at level III. For example, many educators and psychologists are constrained by school district or state department regulations that require an ability–achievement discrepancy analysis in the process of LD determination. Assessment batteries may offer numerous procedures for discrepancy analysis, only some of which may be relevant within the context of individual district and state criteria. An a priori selection of these analyses guards against the unsupported practice of running multiple discrepancy analyses in an attempt to find a significant discrepancy for the purpose of satisfying existing criteria.

Level I-A: Interindividual Academic Ability Analysis

Level I-A focuses on the basic concept of an LD: that learning is somehow disrupted from its typical course by some type of internal dysfunction. Although the specific mechanism that inhibits learning is not directly observable, one can proceed on the assumption that it manifests itself in observable phenomena, particularly academic achievement. Thus the first component of the operational definition of an LD involves documenting that some type of *learning* dysfunction exists. As we have noted elsewhere (Flanagan et al., 2002), the issue of an LD is moot in the absence of academic weaknesses or deficits because such dysfunction is a necessary component of the definition. Therefore, in our method, the presence of a *normative deficit*, established either through standardized testing or through other means (such as clinical observations of academic performance, work samples, or some combination thereof), is a necessary but insufficient condition for LD determination. Level I-A includes the first criterion of several necessary for determining the presence of an LD. When the criterion at each level is met, an evaluator can be reasonably confident that a diagnosis of LD is appropriate.

The process at Level I-A involves comprehensively measuring the academic achievement areas in which the individual is suspected of being deficient (e.g., reading, writing, math). The academic abilities represented at sented at this level are organized according to the seven achievement areas specified in the federal definition of LD as outlined in IDEA. These seven areas include math calculation, math reasoning, basic reading, reading comprehension, written expression, listening comprehension, and oral expression (see Figure 24.1). Our rationale for using the IDEA labels (Flanagan et al., 2002) is based primarily on the fact that most prevailing definitions of LDs include these learning domains. We argue, however, that such definitions are largely atheoretical and thus are generally vague and nonspecific. Also, the labels may not be practical or sufficient. For example, the category of basic writing skills is absent, even though this is an area in which an individual's LD can manifest. Therefore, for theoretical and psychometric reasons, the academic abilities depicted at level I-A in Figure 24.1 are also organized according to the CHC broad abilities that encompass these achievement domains (i.e., Gq, Grw, and Gc).

Figure 24.1 shows that level I-A abilities represent an individual's stores of acquired knowledge (Carroll, 1993; Woodcock, 1993). These specific knowledge bases (i.e., Gq, Grw, and Gc) primarily develop as a function of formal instruction, schooling, and educationally related experiences. We believe that an exception to this rule is Gc (Flanagan et al., 2002). That is, Gc abilities include examples not only of repositories of learned material (e.g., lexical knowledge, general information, information about culture, etc.) but also abilities that reflect more active information processing, such as oral production, oral fluency, and listening ability. As such, a minor distinction is made between the narrow Gc abilities represented at level I-A and those represented at level II-A (see Figure 24.1). We (Flanagan et al., 2002) have proposed that the Gc abilities representing the stores of acquired knowledge are those that are likely to be of interest at level I-A, whereas any assessment that proceeds to level II-A is likely to focus more on the process-oriented abilities included in Gc. The dual nature of Gc is illustrated by the bidirectional arrows in Figure 24.1 that connect Gc (and its corresponding narrow abilities) at levels I-A and II-A (see Flanagan et al., 2002, for a more detailed discussion).

It is important to note that our operational definition for LD evaluation is based on presumptions of typical functioning rather than on presumptions of dysfunction. As such, in the absence of any evidence of gross physiological trauma or developmental dysfunction, and given an appropriate and sufficient instructional history and adequate learning opportunities, the expectation is that an individual undergoing LD assessment will perform "within normal limits" (i.e., the low average to high average range of functioning) on standardized academic tests (i.e., standard scores of 85 to 115, inclusive[1]). This is true for each area depicted at level I-A in Figure 24.1 that may have been assessed. Testing this hypothesis requires comparing an examinee's standard score performance to that of the standardization sample.

Table 24.1 provides a structure of norm-referenced score performances that may be used to guide practitioners' interpretations of standard scores. The classifications appearing in Table 24.1 were introduced to the field recently (e.g., Flanagan & Kaufman, 2004; Kaufman & Kaufman, 2004). These classifications may be used to evaluate a priori and a posteriori hypotheses that guide the interpretation process (Flanagan & Ortiz, 2002; Lezak, 1995). In the operational definition presented in Figure 24.1, the rejection criterion for the null hypothesis (i.e., the hypothesis that performance is within normal limits) is set at a level of greater than ±1 standard deviation from the mean. When this range is adopted, performance is considered exceptional only when it falls either significantly above or below the mean—indicating

TABLE 24.1. Alternative Descriptive System of Score Classification

Standard score range	Alternative description of performance
131+	Upper extreme/Normative strength
116–130	Above average/Normative strength
85–115	Average range/Normal limits
70–84	Below average/Normative weakness
≤69	Lower extreme/Normative weakness

Note. From Flanagan and Kaufman (2004). Copyright © 2004 by John Wiley & Sons, Inc. Reprinted by permission.

either normative strengths or weaknesses in functioning, respectively.

Essentially, after assessment data have been gathered, the first test in the operational definition (level I-A in Figure 24.1) involves answering the following question: "Is the examinee's academic performance within normal limits, relative to that of same-age peers in the general population?" Figure 24.2 shows the decision process that is involved in assessment at level I-A (and subsequent levels). Note that such a comparison is based on the examinee's individual performance against other individuals included in the standardization sample (see Table 24.1), rather than being based on performance within the examinee. Person-relative (or intraindividual) discrepancies, no matter how large, should not be interpreted as indicators of dysfunction unless one or more of the examinee's scores falls below the typical range of functioning (e.g., standard score < 85).

The intraindividual ability analyses that are offered by some of the major assessment batteries reflect statistical rarity in score differences as compared to the general population (e.g., based on actual discrepancy norms). However, evaluators should recognize that statistical rarity, despite its common association with the term *abnormal*, is not synonymous with impairment or deficiency. In fact, some deviations from the norm are *valuable* deviations. As such, not all rarities are abnormal in the negative sense. In addition, test score differences may be statistically significant and rare, but this does not automatically imply that they are clinically meaningful. Evaluators should always seek to establish meaningful clinical significance as well as statistical significance. "The major weakness of the statistical rarity approach is that it has no values; it lacks any system for differentiating between desirable and undesirable behaviors. Of course, most users of the statistical rarity approach acknowledge that not all rarities should be identified as abnormal" (Alloy, Acocella, & Bootzin, 1996, p. 6).

Intraindividual achievement discrepancy analysis can be used most effectively to identify an individual's *relative* strengths and weaknesses. The data generated from this type of person-relative analysis can be used to assist in developing remedial strategies,

educational plans, and specific academic interventions, based on the data gathered at level I-A. In addition to intraindividual academic discrepancy procedures, some batteries (e.g., the Woodcock–Johnson III [WJ III]) offer criterion-referenced scores that may be used to develop educational plans and interventions. Despite these uses of person-relative data, population-relative data are necessary to compare an individual's performance in the domains assessed at level I-A to that of a representative sample of same-age peers from the general population. The population-relative information offered may include standard scores, percentiles, T scores, normal curve equivalents, and stanines. Information from these scores provides the data necessary to determine whether performance is within the average range (i.e., ±1 standard deviation from the normative mean) or any other ability range (e.g., above average, below average, etc.). Overall, the most assessment information can be derived when the results from both intra- and interindividual ability analyses are considered conjointly. The latter are more useful for diagnostic purposes, and the former are more useful for instructional purposes (see Flanagan & Ortiz, 2001; Flanagan et al., 2002; and Flanagan, Bernier, Keiser, & Ortiz, 2003, for more detailed discussions). Because certain batteries provide a range of criterion-referenced and norm-referenced scores, practitioners must understand their purposes and uses to realize fully the benefits and meaning of derived score information. Table 24.2 shows the tests of the major achievement batteries that correspond to the CHC abilities and LD areas listed in level I-A of the operational definition. This table shows the academic domains that can be assessed with several major achievement batteries (some more comprehensively than others).

It is important to distinguish between adequate assessment or representation of a CHC broad ability, such as Gf, Gc, or Gq, and adequate assessment of a federally specified academic achievement area, such as basic reading, math computation, or listening comprehension, within the context of LD determination. For example, Table 24.2 shows that some of the major achievement batteries measure many qualitatively different aspects of Grw. For instance, the WJ III Letter–Word

TABLE 24.2. Representation of CHC and Academic Abilities by LD Area on Select Comprehensive Achievement Batteries

LD areas listed in IDEA definition	CHC abilities listed at Level I of the operational definition of LD (Figure 24.1)				Other CHC abilities important in the assessment of LDs	
	Grw reading[a]	Grw writing[a]	Gq	Gc	Ga	Gs
Basic reading skills	WJ III Letter–Word Identif. (RD) WJ III Word Attack (RD, PC:A) WIAT-II Word Rdng. (RD) WIAT-II Pseudoword Decoding (RD, PC:A) KTEA-II Letter and Word Recog. (RD) KTEA-II Nonsense Word Decoding (RD, PC:A) WJ III Sound Awareness (PC:A, PC:S) KTEA-II Phonological Awareness (PC:A)				*WJ III Sound Awareness (PC:A, PC:S)* *KTEA-II Phonological Awareness (PC:A)*	WJ III Rdng. Fluency (RS, RC) KTEA-II Timed Nonsense Word Decoding (RS, RD, PC:A) *KTEA-II Timed Letter and Word Recog. (RS, RD)* *KTEA-II Fluency (Semantic and Phonological) (RS)* KTEA-II Rapid Automatized Naming (Glr-NA)[b]
Reading comprehension	WJ III Pass. Comp. (RC, CZ) WIAT-II Rdg. Comp. (RC) KTEA-II Rdg. Comp. (RC)					
Math calculation			WJ III Calculation (A3) WIAT-II Num. Op. (A3) KTEA-II Math Comp. (A3)			WJ III Math Fluency (N, A3)

(continued)

TABLE 24.2. (continued)

LD areas listed in IDEA definition	CHC abilities listed at Level I of the operational definition of LD (Figure 24.1)			Other CHC abilities important in the assessment of LDs		
	Grw reading[a]	Grw writing[a]	Gq	Gc	Ga	Gs
Math reasoning			WJ III App. Problems (A3, KM, Gf-RQ) WJ III Quant. Concepts (KM, Gf-RQ) WIAT-II Math Rsng. (Gf-RQ) KTEA-II Math Concepts and App. (Gf-RQ, A3)			
Written expression		WJ III Spelling (SG) WJ III Wrtg. Samples (WA) WJ III Editing (Gc-MY, EU) *WJ III Punct. and Cap. (EU)* *WJ III Spelling of Sounds (SG, PC:A, PC:S)* WIAT-II Spelling (SG) WIAT-II Writ. Exp. (WA) KTEA-II Writ. Exp. (WA) KTEA-II Spelling (SG)		WJ III Editing (MY, EU)	*WJ III Spelling of Sounds (SG, PC:A, PC:S)*	WJ III Writing Fluency (R9, WA)
Oral expression				WJ III Story Recall (LS, Glr-MM) WJ III Picture Vocab. (LD, VL) WIAT-II Oral Exp. (CM) KTEA-II Oral Exp. (CM)		

Listening comprehension

Other areas to consider at Level I:

General knowledge[c]

WJ III Undrstndng. Direct. (LS, Gsm-WM)
WJ III Oral Comp. (LS)
WIAT-II List. Comp (LS)
KTEA-II List. Comp. (LS)
WJ III Verb. Comp. (VL, LD)
WJ III Gen. Info. (K0)
WJ III Acad. Knwldg. (K0, K1, K2, A5)
Wech. Info. (K0)
Wech. Sim. (LD, VL; Gf-I)
Wech. Vocab. (VL)
Wech. Comp. (K0, LD)
SB5 V Knwldg. (VL; Gf-I)
SB5 NV Knwldg. (K0)
KABC-II Express. Vocab. (VL)
KABC-II Verbal Knowledge (VL, KO)

Note. Story Recall—Delayed (Glr-MM) and Handwriting Legibility are two supplemental measures on the WJ III ACH not included in this table. Test names appearing in italics are supplemental measures. Tests in boldface are from cognitive batteries; all other tests listed are from achievement batteries. CHC ability abbreviations: A3, math achievement; A5, geography achievement; CM, communication ability; EU, English usage knowledge; K0, general (verbal) information; K1, general science information; K2, information about culture; KM, math knowledge; LD, language development; LS, listening ability; MM, meaningful memory; MY, grammatical sensitivity; N, number facility; PC:A, phonetic coding:analysis; PC:S, phonetic coding: synthesis; RC, reading comprehension; RD, reading decoding; RQ, quantitative reasoning; RS, reading speed; SG, spelling ability; V, verbal (printed) language comprehension; VL, lexical knowledge; WA, writing ability; WM, working memory; WS, writing speed. Test battery abbreviations: WJ III, Woodcock–Johnson III; WIAT-II, Wechsler Individual Achievement Test—Second Edition; KTEA-II, Kaufman Test of Educational Achievement—Second Edition; Wech., all Wechsler scales; SB5, Stanford–Binet Intelligence Scales, Fifth Edition (V, Verbal; NV, Nonverbal); KABC-II, Kaufman Assessment Battery for Children—Second Edition.

[a]The reading and writing (Grw) factor has been split in this table. This semantic distinction is intended to be congruent with the federal definition, which treats these abilities as distinct academic areas (e.g., basic reading, reading comprehension, written expression). This distinction was made for practical reasons and is not supported by current theory and research.

[b]The KTEA-II Rapid Automatized Naming subtest is a measure of naming facility, a narrow ability subsumed by Glr. In the absence of a separate Glr column, it has been included in the Gs column in this table, primarily to denote the speeded nature of this measure.

[c]The list of cognitive measures in this portion of the table does not include mixed measures (i.e., tests measuring more than one broad CHC ability domain). From Flanagan, Ortiz, Alfonso, and Mascolo (2002). Published by Allyn and Bacon, Boston, MA. Copyright © 2002 by Pearson Education. Adapted by permission.

Identification and Passage Comprehension tests provide adequate representation of Grw, because they assess two qualitatively different CHC narrow abilities—namely, (1) reading decoding (RD) and (2) reading comprehension and cloze ability (CZ), respectively. This same fact holds true for the Wechsler Individual Achievement Test—Second Edition (WIAT-II) and Kaufman Test of Educational Achievement—Second Edition (KTEA-II) reading subtests listed in Table 24.2. However, using subtests in this manner (e.g., to represent CHC broad abilities) merely provides a *sampling* of functioning in broad ability domains, as opposed to an *in-depth* assessment (see McGrew, Woodcock, & Ford, 2002). This sampling of functioning provides important baseline information that can be used to draw inferences about performance within a broad ability domain.

For example, if performance on tests of reading decoding and cloze ability falls within the average range, it may be reasonable for the examiner to conclude that broad Grw ability is within normal limits, despite the fact that Grw encompasses more than these two abilities. However, a below average Grw cluster (e.g., Grw scores between 70 and 84 on these two tests) may be sufficient for the examiner to conclude that the individual is limited in the broad Grw domain, but may be insufficient for a conclusion that an individual is limited in either basic reading skills or reading comprehension, which are two of the seven areas listed in the federal definition of LD. This outcome is possible because a single test (1) may not be adequately reliable to serve as a basis for such conclusions, and (2) typically underrepresents the construct of interest (e.g., basic reading skills). Thus, although adequate (or in-depth) assessment of Grw and Gq may be accomplished by administering two or more tests listed in the Grw and Gq columns in Table 24.2, adequate or in-depth assessment of the LD areas (e.g., basic reading skills) requires that two or more tests in the rows of Table 24.2 be administered.

For example, to document that an individual has a deficit in basic reading skills, an evaluator will need to assess more than reading decoding via a single test. This is because several other CHC narrow abilities contribute to an understanding of basic reading skills. The first row in Table 24.2 shows that WJ III subtests such as Word Attack (a measure of reading decoding and phonetic coding: analysis), Sound Awareness (a measure of phonetic coding), and Reading Fluency (a measure of reading speed) may be administered in addition to Letter–Word Identification to achieve a comprehensive evaluation of this academic domain. Similarly, KTEA-II subtests such as Timed Nonsense Word Decoding, Phonological Awareness, Timed Letter and Word Recognition, Fluency, and Rapid Automatized Naming, can be used to augment information provided by the KTEA-II Letter and Word Recognition subtest. Therefore, when documentation of an individual's basic reading skills is warranted, a test of reading decoding should be augmented with one or more qualitatively different tests of other basic reading skills. The same holds true for each LD academic assessment area. That is, prior to concluding that an individual is deficient in one or more of the academic areas specified in the federal definition, examiners should ensure that the specific area in question is assessed adequately. At least two CHC narrow abilities that correspond to an LD area (see Table 24.2) should be included in an assessment of the academic area (see Flanagan et al., 2002, for an in-depth discussion). It is important to note that not all batteries provide measures that will permit an in-depth assessment of a particular LD area. In such cases, examiners may wish to augment their core battery with subtests from another battery via CHC cross-battery principles and procedures (see Flanagan et al., 2000; Flanagan & Ortiz, 2001; McGrew & Flanagan, 1998; for more in-depth discussions of the CHC cross-battery approach).

The specific purpose for using a battery to assess academic performance will determine whether the assessment should be organized in accordance with either the CHC broad academic abilities (e.g., Grw, Gq, etc.), or one or more of the seven academic ability areas listed in the federal definition. It is likely that assessment of the CHC broad academic abilities will remain focused on ensuring adequate or in-depth representation of these abilities for evaluators who are interested in directly comparing them with CHC broad cognitive abilities (e.g., Flanagan et al., 2002;

Flanagan & Ortiz, 2001). For example, the operational definition of LD presented in Figure 24.1 requires professionals to evaluate the relationship between specific academic skills functioning and underlying cognitive processes and abilities. Organizing assessments according to the CHC broad academic and cognitive ability domains will facilitate this process. Psychologists and educators who engage in the assessment of both academic and cognitive abilities, therefore, may benefit from organizing their assessment in accordance with the CHC broad domains (Flanagan et al., 2002).

Not all evaluators, however, are involved in the assessment of both academic and cognitive abilities; many focus exclusively on either one or the other. For those evaluators who focus mainly on assessing academic abilities, it is likely that a focus on the seven academic LD areas (as opposed to the CHC domains) will be desirable. For example, LD specialists, educational evaluators, reading specialists, and similar personnel may work as members of a multidisciplinary team in which their contributions involve the assessment and evaluation of one or more academic ability domains, particularly in referrals of individuals with learning difficulties. When the assessment focuses primarily on academic abilities, organizing tests according to commonly accepted academic ability domain labels, such as those listed in the federal definition of LD, may be more appropriate (see Table 24.2).

In addition to deciding on the organization of an academic assessment (i.e., by CHC abilities or LD areas), evaluators should decide whether a particular assessment initially warrants a sampling of functioning in a given area, or whether a more in-depth assessment of a particular academic skill domain is warranted. This decision will influence the initial organization of an assessment. As stated previously, sampling functioning in a given CHC broad ability domain (such as Grw or Gq) would require selecting two qualitatively different measures of the broad ability listed in the corresponding column in Table 24.2. In-depth assessment will require additional testing. The more qualitatively different aspects of the ability or academic skill that are measured, the better

the estimate of functioning in that area (Messick, 1995).

In summary, psychologists and educators may find it necessary either to sample functioning in a given domain (i.e., a CHC broad academic ability or an LD area) or to conduct more in-depth or comprehensive assessments in one or more domains, depending on the purpose of evaluation. When either method is deemed necessary, and evaluators are utilizing a comprehensive assessment battery, Table 24.2 is useful for identifying the most appropriate measures to assess academic functioning.

Level I-B: Evaluation of Mitigating or Exclusionary Hypotheses

Level I-B requires professionals to evaluate whether a documented academic skill or knowledge deficit identified through level I-A analysis is *primarily* the result of individual noncognitive factors (e.g., motivation) or other facilitating–inhibiting factors that are external to the individual (e.g., inadequate instruction). As we have noted elsewhere (Flanagan et al., 2002), because identified academic deficits do not immediately substantiate a true manifestation of an LD, evaluators should refrain from ascribing causal links to an LD, and should instead attempt to develop or consider alternative hypotheses related to other potential causes. For example, cultural or language differences are two common factors that can have a negative impact on test performance and result in data that appear to suggest an LD. In addition, lack of motivation, emotional disturbance, performance anxiety, psychiatric disorders, sensory impairments, medical conditions (e.g., hearing or vision problems), and so forth need to be ruled out as potential explanatory correlates to the deficiencies identified at level I-A. Evaluation at level I-B involves answering the following question: "Are one or more external factors the *primary* reason for the deficient academic performance uncovered at level I-A?" Results of test observations may be used, along with other data gathered at this level, to assist in answering this question.

If the answer to the question at Level I-B is "yes" (meaning that external factors are the primary cause of academic skill deficits), then the criterion for LD at this level of the operational definition is not met, and assessment should not proceed to the next level. In fact, assessment may proceed to level II-A only when the evaluator has gathered sufficient evidence and data to conclude confidently that the manifest pattern of learning difficulties is not due primarily to exclusionary factors, even if such factors are contributory (Flanagan & Ortiz, 2001).

We have noted (Flanagan et al., 2002) that a primary reason for placing the evaluation of exclusionary factors at an early point in the assessment process is to increase practitioners' efficiency in both time and effort, and to help prevent unnecessary test administration and other invasive and unnecessary evaluation procedures. Administering standardized tests should not be considered a benign process. The consequences that can result from their use demands that they be applied carefully and selectively. Of course, it may be impossible to completely and convincingly rule out all of the potential exclusionary factors at this early stage in the assessment process. Indeed, many possibilities may explain poor performance on any given achievement test. Therefore, evaluators should strive to uncover and evaluate as many possibilities as is practical or necessary (Brackett & McPherson, 1996; Flanagan & Ortiz, 2001; Wilson, 1992).

It is possible that some relevant and important factors may not become apparent until later stages of the assessment process (i.e., following level II-A assessment). For instance, it may not be possible to rule out mild mental retardation or low general ability, because identifying these conditions requires, to a large extent, the types of data gathered at level II-A of the operational definition (i.e., cognitive ability). Overall, evaluation of exclusionary factors should be considered as a recursive activity that occurs throughout the course of a given evaluation. The process of ruling out external factors that contribute significantly to poor academic achievement, including psychological conditions, pervasive low ability, and so forth, begins early in the evaluation process and continues through the final level of analysis (Flanagan et al., 2002).

Level II-A:
Interindividual Cognitive Ability Analysis

The assessment at level II-A in Figure 24.1 is similar to that at level I-A, except that it is conducted with mostly cognitive (as opposed to academic) ability tests. In general, the assessment process at level II-A, as at level I-A, proceeds with the assumption that an individual will perform within normal limits (i.e., standard scores of 85 to 115, inclusive) in each of the areas assessed at this level (see Figure 24.1). Therefore, one criterion for LD at this level is met when the following question can be answered "no": "Is the examinee's standard score performance on cognitive tests within normal limits, relative to that of same-age peers in the general population?" Establishing that one or more cognitive ability deficits exist and are either empirically or logically related to, and the presumptive cause of, the previously identified academic deficit(s) (e.g., from level I-A analysis and other data) are perhaps the most salient aspects of an operational definition of LD (Flanagan et al., 2002). The requirement of a link between cognitive and academic deficits has historically been ill-conceived and vague. The lack of a guiding theory to define this component may be a primary reason for the lack of clarity with regard to the *cognitive ability or processing disorder or deficiency* condition of LD definitions. Practitioners have long understood the need to identify some type of psychological dysfunction as an explanatory mechanism for academic performance deficiencies, but there has been minimal if any theoretical specification to guide or support this practice; hence illogical assumptions are often made (Flanagan et al., 2002).

The cognitive abilities illustrated at level II-A in the operational definition of LD (i.e., Gs, Gsm, Glr, Ga, Gv, Gf, and Gc; see Figure 24.1) are organized in Table 24.3 according to their representation on select major cognitive batteries. Figure 24.1 further organizes these CHC abilities according to the processes they represent within an information-processing perspective, including attention and cognitive efficiency, memory, thinking abilities, executive processes, and language abilities (e.g., Dean & Woodcock, 1999; Woodcock, 1993). The latter category represents the collection of Gc narrow abilities

TABLE 24.3. Representation of CHC Abilities on Select Cognitive Batteries

Broad	WISC-IV	WAIS-III	SB5	KABC-II	WJ III COG
Gf	Picture Concepts (I, Gc-K0) Matrix Reasoning (I, RG) Arithmetic (RQ, Gq-A3)[1]	Matrix Reasoning (I, RG)	Nonverbal Fluid Reasoning (I, Gv-Vz) Nonverbal Quantitative Reasoning (RQ, Gq-A3) Verbal Fluid Reasoning (RG) Verbal Quantitative Reasoning (RQ, Gq-A3)	Pattern Reasoning (I, Gv-Vz) Story Completion (I, RG, Gc-K0, Gv-Vz)	Concept Formation (I) Analysis Synthesis (RG)
Gc	Similarities (LD, VL, Gf-I) Vocabulary (VL) Comprehension (K0, LD) Information (K0) Word Reasoning (VL, Gf-I)	Vocabulary (VL) Similarities (LD, VL, Gf-I) Information (K0) Comprehension (K0, LD)	Nonverbal Knowledge (K0) Verbal Knowledge (VL, Gf-I)	Riddles (VL, LD, Gf-RG) Expressive Vocabulary (VL) Verbal Knowledge (VL, K0)	Verbal Comprehension (VL, LD) General Information (K0)
Ga	—	—	—	—	Incomplete Words (PC:A) Sound Blending (PC:S) Auditory Attention (US/UR)
Gv	Block Design (SR, Vz) Picture Completion (CF, Gc-K0)	Picture Completion (CF, Gc-K0) Block Design (SR, Vz) Picture Arrangement (Vz, Gc-K0) Object Assembly (CS, SR)	Nonverbal Visual-Spatial Processing (Vz, SR) Verbal Visual-Spatial Processing (Vz, Gc-LS, LD)	Conceptual Thinking (Vz, Gf-I) Block Counting (Vz, Gq-A3) Face Recognition (MV) Triangles (SR, Vz) Rover (SS, Gf-RG, Gq-A3) Gestalt Closure (CS)	Spatial Relations (Vz, SR) Picture Recognition (MV)
Gsm	Digit Span (MS, WM) Letter-Number Sequencing (WM)	Digit Span (MS, WM) Letter-Number Sequencing (WM)	Nonverbal Working Memory (WM, Gv-MV) Verbal Working Memory (WM, MS)	Word Order (MS, WM) Number Recall (MS) Hand Movements (MS, Gv-MV)	Memory for Words (MS) Numbers Reversed (WM) Auditory Working Memory (WM)
Glr	—	—	—	Atlantis (MA, L1) Rebus (MA) Atlantis Delayed (MA, L1) Rebus Delayed (MA, L1)	Visual Auditory Learning (MA) Visual Auditory Learning Delayed (MA) Retrieval Fluency (FI) Rapid Picture Naming (NA)
Gs	Symbol Search (P, R9) Coding (R9) Cancellation (P, R9)	Symbol Search (P, R9) Digit Symbol/Coding (R9)	—	—	Visual Matching (P, R9) Decision Speed (R4)
Gq	—	Arithmetic (A3, Gf-RQ)	—	—	—

Note. Narrow ability classifications are based on expert consensus (see Caltabiano & Flanagan, 2004) and information presented in the test manuals of each cognitive battery. WISC-IV, Wechsler Intelligence Scale for Children—Fourth Edition; WAIS-III, Wechsler Adult Intelligence Scale—Third Edition. A3, Math Achievement; CF, Flexibility of Closure; CS, Closure Speed; FI, Ideational Fluency; I, Inductive Reasoning; K0, General (Verbal) Information; L1, Learning Abilities; LD, Language Development; LS, Listening Ability; MA, Associative Memory; MS, Memory Span; MV, Visual Memory; NA, Naming Facility; P, Perceptual Speed; PC:A, Phonetic Coding: Analysis; PC:S, Phonetic Coding: Synthesis; R4, Semantic Processing Speed; R9, Rate-of-Test-Taking; RG, General Sequential Reasoning; RQ, Quantitative Reasoning; SR, Spatial Relations; SS, Spatial Scanning; UR, Resistance to Auditory Stimulus Distortion; US, Speech Sound Discrimination; VL, Lexical Knowledge; Vz, Visualization; WM, Working Memory. SB5, Stanford–Binet Intelligence Scale, Fifth Edition; KABC-II, Kaufman Assessment Battery for Children—Second Edition; WJ III COG, Woodcock–Johnson Tests of Cognitive Abilities—Third Edition.
[1]The primary classification of Arithmetic as Gf is based on the factor analyses of Keith and colleagues (2004).
From Flanagan and Kaufman (2004). Copyright 2004 by John Wiley & Sons, Inc. Reprinted by permission.

that we believe (Flanagan et al., 2002) more accurately reflect processing skills, as opposed to the Gc abilities that represent stores of acquired knowledge (which form the focus of evaluation at level I-A).

In general, the abilities depicted at level II-A provide important information about an individual's *learning efficiency*. Development of the cognitive abilities represented at this level tends to be less dependent on formal classroom instruction and schooling than development of the academic abilities represented at level I-A. Furthermore, specific or narrow abilities across many of the CHC areas listed in level II-A may be combined to yield specific aptitudes for learning in different areas (e.g., reading, math, writing). These aptitudes (e.g., reading aptitude) are expected to be consistent with their respective academic areas measured at level I-A (e.g., basic reading skills; Flanagan et al., 2002).

Table 24.4 summarizes the recent literature on the relationship between CHC cognitive abilities and specific academic ability domains (Flanagan et al., 2002). For example, narrow abilities subsumed by Gc (lexical knowledge, language development, listening ability), Gsm (working memory), Ga (phonetic coding), Glr (naming facility), and Gs (perceptual speed) have demonstrated significant relations to reading achievement. Similarly, narrow abilities within these CHC broad domains have been shown to be related to writing achievement. Narrow abilities within the areas of Gf, Gc, Gsm, and Gs (but not Glr, Ga, and Gv) have also demonstrated significant relationships with math achievement, and Gf (induction and general sequential reasoning) in particular has shown a stronger relationship to the math domain than to the reading and writing domains. Practitioners can use the information in Table 24.4 to identify those CHC abilities that should receive primary consideration in the design of assessments for individuals referred for reading, math, or writing difficulties. Once these areas are considered, Tables 24.2 and 24.3 may be used to help identify the tests that assess these abilities. The information in Table 24.4 can also be used to determine whether the assessment data support a relationship between academic and cognitive deficits that may have been uncovered at levels I-A and II-A.

It is important to note that a deficiency in cognitive ability or processing may be established through means other than standardized test performance. For example, deficient orthographic processing may not be apparent on standardized ability tests in the form of low score performance, simply because no existing valid measures have been designed specifically to assess this skill. However, orthographic processing difficulties may be documented through error analysis procedures and clinical observations, for example, that are consistent with current research.

Data generated from level II-A analyses, like those generated at level I-A, also provide input for level III analyses if the process should advance to this level. Typically, in addition to specific cognitive ability data (e.g., cluster scores, processing composites), a global ability score is often derived for use in ability–achievement discrepancy analysis, although the reauthorization of IDEA demonstrates that this type of analysis is not necessary in the LD determination process (see Flanagan et al., 2002). Regardless of the specific nature of the data gathered, the process advances beyond level II-A only when two specific criteria are met: (1) A deficiency in at least one area of cognitive ability or processing is identified reliably; and (2) empirical or logical links between at least one area of cognitive deficiency and the deficient academic skill(s) uncovered in level I-A is identified (see Table 24.4).

The first criterion is necessary to establish the presence of a psychological processing disorder or dysfunction as defined by the pertinent LD literature (see Flanagan et al., 2002, for a discussion). Poor academic performance that exists in the absence of any cognitive impairment does not meet most existing operational definition of LD, including the one proposed herein (Flanagan et al., 2002, 2003). In addition, as is true for level I-A, person-relative (i.e., intraindividual) discrepancies, no matter how substantial, should not be interpreted as reflecting dysfunction unless one or more of the examinee's scores in the discrepancy analysis falls outside and below the normal limits of functioning (i.e., standard score < 85). Because the results of individual intraindividual ability discrepancy analyses may or may not reveal dysfunction, it is essential to evaluate any and all scores used in intraindividual

TABLE 24.4. Relations between CHC Cognitive Abilities and Academic Achievement

CHC ability	Reading achievement	Math achievement	Writing achievement
Gf	Inductive (I) and general sequential reasoning (RG) abilities play a moderate role in reading comprehension.	Inductive (I) and general sequential reasoning (RG) abilities are consistently very important at all ages.	Inductive (I) and general sequential reasoning (RG) abilities are related to basic writing skills primarily during the elementary school years (e.g., ages 6–13) and consistently related to written expression at all ages.
Gc	Language development (LD), lexical knowledge (VL), and listening ability (LS) are important at all ages. These abilities become increasingly important with age.	Language development (LD), lexical knowledge (VL), and listening abilities (LS) are important at all ages. These abilities become increasingly important with age.	Language development (LD), lexical knowledge (VL), and general information (K0) are important primarily after age 7. These abilities become increasingly important with age.
Gsm	Memory span (MS) is important, especially when evaluated within the context of working memory.	Memory span (MS) is important especially when evaluated within the context of working memory.	Memory span (MS) is important to writing, especially spelling skills, whereas working memory has shown relations with advanced writing skills (e.g., written expression).
Gv		May be important primarily for higher-level or advanced mathematics (e.g., geometry, calculus).	
Ga	Phonetic coding (PC) or "phonological awareness/processing" is very important during the elementary school years.		Phonetic coding (PC) or "phonological awareness/processing" is very important during the elementary school years for both basic writing skills and written expression (primarily before age 11).
Glr	Naming facility (NA) or "rapid automatic naming" is very important during the elementary school years. Associative memory (MA) may be somewhat important at select ages (e.g., age 6).		Naming facility (NA) or "rapid automatic naming" has demonstrated relations with written expression, primarily the fluency aspect of writing.
Gs	Perceptual speed (P) abilities are important during all school years, particularly the elementary school years.	Perceptual speed (P) abilities are important during all school years, particularly the elementary school years.	Perceptual speed (P) abilities are important during all school years for basic writing and related to all ages for written expression.

Note. The absence of comments for a particular CHC ability and achievement area (e.g., Ga and mathematics) indicates either that the research reviewed did not report any significant relations between this CHC ability and achievement area, or that if significant findings were reported, they were weak and were for only a limited number of studies. Comments in boldface represent the CHC abilities that showed the strongest and most consistent relations with the respective achievement domains. Data from McGrew and Flanagan (1998), Flanagan, McGrew, and Ortiz (2000), and Flanagan, Ortiz, Alfonso, and Mascolo (2002).

ability analyses in terms of where they fall relative to the general population (see Flanagan & Ortiz, 2001).

The second criterion is needed to establish a valid basis for linking the identified cognitive deficiency with the identified academic deficiency. For instance, when an individual is referred for reading difficulties, it is reasonable to assume that observable reading difficulties will become apparent via level I-A assessment, and that if the reading difficulties are not primarily attributable to exclusionary factors (level I-B assessment), then one or more cognitive abilities or processes that underlie reading achievement may be manifested as weaknesses following level II-A assessment. Theory-based research supports this assumption (see Table 24.4).

Level II-B: Reevaluation of Mitigating or Exclusionary Factors

Establishing the existence of a cognitive deficit that is empirically or logically related to an academic deficiency identified at level I-A forms the core of the level II-A testing; however, it is not the only consideration. Although the absence of a defensible relationship between level I-A and level II-A deficiencies may preclude advancing to level III assessment, the process can also cease or be redirected through a reevaluation of mitigating or exclusionary hypotheses as identified in level II-B (see Figure 24.1). The presence of substantiated cognitive deficits that are directly related to academic performance difficulties is integral to the operational definition of LD. However, evaluators must determine yet again whether such deficiencies are primarily the result of mitigating or exclusionary factors. To do so, they must test hypotheses regarding reasonable explanations for observed cognitive deficiencies to ensure that the data accurately reflect examinees' true ability. The recursive and iterative nature of the LD evaluation process is illustrated by the reevaluation of these mitigating and exclusionary factors. Reliable and valid measurement of LD depends on the ability to exclude the numerous factors that could negatively affect standardized test performance. When such factors have been evaluated carefully and excluded as the primary reason for the observed cognitive deficits at this level, and when the two necessary crite-

ria for the test at level II-A have been satisfied, the process may advance to level III (Flanagan et al., 2002). Figure 24.2 shows the decision process that is involved in assessment at levels II-A and II-B.

Level III: Integrated Ability Analysis— Evaluation of Underachievement

Advancing to level III implies that three necessary conditions for LD determination have already been satisfied: (1) Performances on standardized tests (or data gathered through other means) support the presence of one or more interindividual academic ability deficits at level I-A; (2) performances on standardized tests (or data gathered through other means) support the presence of one or more interindividual cognitive ability or processing deficits at level II-A; and (3) the academic and cognitive deficits are empirically or logically related and have been determined not to result primarily from exclusionary factors (levels I-B and II-B). What has yet to be determined, however, is whether the pattern of level I-A and level II-A assessment results supports the notion of underachievement in the manner that might be reasonably expected in cases of suspected LDs. Thus the criterion at level III of the operational definition that must be met is as follows: The examinee has specific, circumscribed, and related academic and cognitive deficits that exist within an otherwise typical ability profile. As we have described (Flanagan et al., 2002), the process of determining whether this criterion of underachievement is met at level III can be undertaken via two methods: below average aptitude–achievement consistency analysis, or ability–achievement discrepancy analysis.

Our below average aptitude–achievement consistency analysis (Flanagan et al., 2002) is similar to certain intraindividual discrepancy analyses conducted with some of the major batteries (e.g., the WJ III). However, level III evaluation does not necessarily seek to find only statistically significant, person-relative (intraindividual) discrepancies within the context of an examinee's own pattern of cognitive or academic abilities (although this information is useful). Rather, the nature of intraindividual analysis (called *integrated ability analysis* in Figure 24.1) at this point is specifically concerned with evaluating whether a circumscribed set of related cognitive and academic deficiencies, relative to the performance of same-age peers in the general population, exists within an otherwise typical ability profile. To evaluate whether this condition of underachievement exists, evaluators must consider performance in all of the areas included in this analysis from a population-relative (interindividual) perspective.

Table 24.5 includes the results of an intraindividual discrepancy analysis conducted with WJ III data. It is used here to demonstrate how evaluators can integrate person-relative and population-relative data. A review of the last column in Table 24.5 shows that Working Memory and Math Calculation Skills emerge as significant intraindividual weaknesses (see dark gray bands in Table 24.5). The literature on the relationship between cognitive functions and math achievement supports this connection (see Table 24.4). However, a review of the second column in Table 24.5 (labeled "Actual") shows that, in addition to the actual standard scores for the Working Memory and Math Calculation Skills clusters (71 and 66, respectively), there are similar deficiencies in the areas of Basic Writing Skills (74) and Written Expression (78; see light gray band in Table 24.5). Not only are Basic Writing Skills and Written Expression considered deficient relative to those of same-age peers in the general population (Table 24.1), but the relationship between working memory and writing achievement is empirically supported (see Table 24.4). In addition, an examination of the actual standard scores in Table 24.5 shows that a number of cognitive and academic abilities are within normal limits relative to those of same-age peers (e.g., Gc, Gv, Ga, Gs, oral expression, listening comprehension). This example demonstrates that when person-relative and population-relative information are considered conjointly, a more complete picture of an individual's circumscribed (or domain-specific) levels of function and dysfunction emerges. In summary, the data presented in Table 24.5 demonstrate a performance *consistency* between a specific learning aptitude (i.e., working memory) and math and writing achievement. This consistency is circumscribed in the below average range of functioning and is present within an otherwise typical ability profile. Such a finding meets the level III criterion for an LD diagnosis.

When level II-A assessment activities are designed to allow for the calculation of CHC broad ability clusters and a global ability score, it is possible to conduct ability–achievement discrepancy analysis. If (1) the academic and cognitive deficits identified at levels I-A and II-A are empirically or logically related, and 2) the standard scores associated with the cognitive deficits are lower than the remaining CHC broad ability clusters, and (3) the measures of the specific ability deficiencies identified at level II-A are not included in the calculation of the global ability score, it would then be logical to expect that global ability will fall within normal limits and be significantly discrepant from the identified academic deficits. A discrepancy occurs in this case primarily because the global ability composite contains few, if any, tests on which the individual exhibits difficulties; therefore, expectation of consistency is unwarranted. If, on the other hand, the global ability score is obtained by using one or more measures in which the individual demonstrates a deficit, then the global ability estimate may be attenuated to such an extent that it is not significantly discrepant from the academic area(s) of deficiency. In this situation, consistency evaluation becomes salient, and the evaluator must examine functioning across the CHC broad ability clusters to determine whether some (but not necessarily all) broad abilities fall within or above the average range of functioning.

Although the criterion of *a below average aptitude–achievement consistency within an otherwise typical ability profile* represents a reasonable and research-based method for evaluating underachievement, the same is not true of discrepancy analysis. Practitioners should avoid using discrepancy analysis as the sole or primary criterion for LD determination (Flanagan et al., 2002, 2003; Fletcher et al., 1998; Heath & Kush, 1991; McGrew et al., 2002; Siegel, 1999; Stanovich, 1991). In our operational definition of LD (Flanagan et al., 2002), as well as in the recent reauthorization of IDEA, identification of an ability–achievement discrepancy is neither a necessary nor a sufficient condition for determination of an LD. Aptitude–achievement consistency analysis, however, when conducted within the context of the operational definition of LD presented here, may be used to diagnose LD because it

TABLE 24.5. Example of Intraindividual Discrepancy Analysis from the WJ III Compuscore and Profiles Program

Intraindividual discrepancies	Actual	Predicted	Difference	PR	SD	Significant at + or − 1.50 SD (SEE)
Comp. Knowledge (Gc)	93	85	+8	78	+0.77	No
L-T Retrieval (Glr)	86	88	−2	43	−0.17	No
Vis.-Spatial Think. (Gv)	96	93	+3	58	+0.19	No
Auditory Process (Ga)	95	91	+4	61	+0.28	No
Fluid Reasoning (Gf)	87	88	−1	47	−0.06	No
Process Speed (Gs)	106	91	+15	88	+1.15	No
Short-Term Mem. (Gsm)	86	90	−4	37	−0.33	No
Phonemic Aware	108	90	+18	91	+1.36	No
Working Memory	71	90	−19	5	−1.63	Yes
Basic Reading Skills	85	87	−2	41	−0.24	No
Reading Comp.	85	88	−3	40	−0.26	No
Math Calc. Skills	66	91	−25	2	−1.99	Yes
Math Reasoning	80	87	−7	21	−0.81	No
Basic Writing Skills	74	89	−15	9	−1.36	No
Written Expression	78	90	−12	17	−0.96	No
Oral Expression	100	88	+12	85	+1.05	No
Listening Comp.	98	87	+11	84	+0.99	No
Academic Knowledge	94	88	+6	73	+0.60	No

Note. From Schrank and Flanagan (2003). Copyright © 2003 by Elsevier Science. Reprinted by permission.

is both psychometrically and theoretically defensible (Flanagan et al., 2002).

Level IV: Evaluation of Interference with Learning

When the LD determination process reaches level IV, it is assumed that the criteria at each previous level were satisfied. Additional data gathering and analysis hardly seem necessary. But an operational definition of an LD based solely on the criteria of previous levels would be incomplete. This is primarily due to the fact that one of the basic eligibility requirements in both the legal and clinical prescriptions for LD diagnosis is that the suspected learning problem(s) must actually result in significant or substantial academic failure or other restrictions or limitations in daily life functioning.

This final criterion requires not only surveying the assessment data in their entirety, but also considering the real-world manifestations and practical implications of any presumed disability. Generally speaking, if evaluators carefully and completely follow the principles specified in levels I-A through III and adhere to the specified criteria, it is likely that in the vast majority of cases, level IV analysis will further substantiate the conclusions that have already been drawn. However, in cases where data may be equivocal or where procedures other than those specified in the comprehensive framework proposed herein have been used, level IV analysis serves as an important safety precaution: It ensures that any representations of LD that the data may suggest are indeed manifested in observable impairments in one or more areas of real-life functioning. Overall, level IV analysis assists practitioners in guarding against the tendency to identify LD on the basis of insufficient data or inappropriate criteria.

A COMPREHENSIVE FRAMEWORK FOR LD DETERMINATION

As is evident from the aforementioned presentation of the operational definition and Figure 24.2 in particular, assessment of LD is perhaps best thought of as an exercise in decision making. Relevant and pertinent data are collected at various stages of assessment and evaluated carefully to determine the next step and direction of the process. The best available evidence that fully support the actions taken and conclusions reached by the evaluator should guide the decisions. The entire process may therefore be characterized as a course that is charted on the basis of what the collected data and data patterns reveal. The LD assessment process described here is in keeping with these principles and may be used as a framework for the implementation of the LD definition in the reauthorization of IDEA. Whereas the operational definition illustrated in Figure 24.1 provides evaluators with the types of assessment information that should be collected and considered during LD assessment, Figure 24.2 offers a decision-based flowchart that expands upon the operational definition and focuses on the analysis of assessment results. This decision-based flowchart specifies particular assessment activities that proceed on the basis of responses to "yes" or "no" questions. A more comprehensive discussion of the major features and decision points involved in this process follows.

Perceived Academic Difficulties

The assessment process begins with the perception of academic difficulties as depicted in the uppermost box in Figure 24.2, but this does not imply that the assessment process has already begun. There is an inclination to view assessment as beginning at the point where standardized testing becomes central to the process (i.e., when the individual is referred for such testing). However, it is more appropriate to view assessment and evaluation as beginning at the point when the individual's behavior or performance becomes suspect and is examined with greater scrutiny than is usual. In many cases, attempts to ameliorate any identified difficulties may have (and should have) been undertaken before standardized testing begins, and specific interventions or modifications may have already been instituted and data or information collected. Thus the activities that constitute the assessment process should be viewed as including both pre- and postreferral activities.

Prereferral intervention activities are conducted for different reasons than the testing itself is. In the former case, the goal is to identify areas of need and to provide appro-

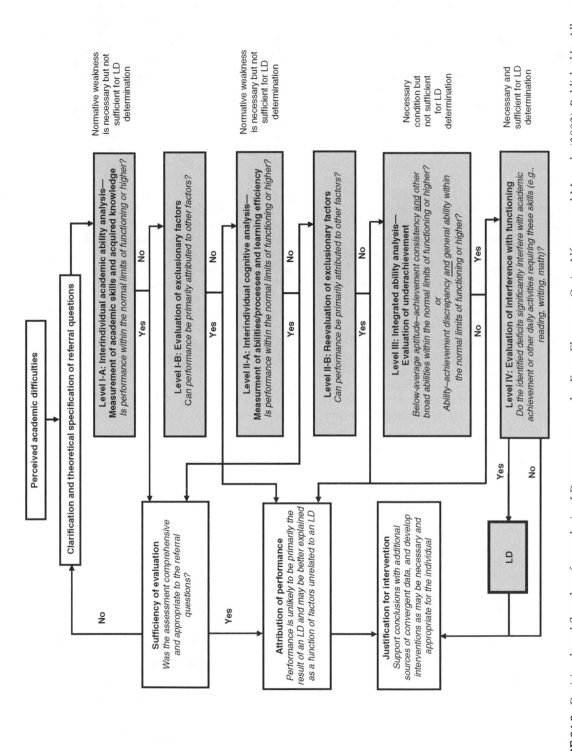

FIGURE 24.2. Decision-based flowchart for analyzing LD assessment results. From Flanagan, Ortiz, Alfonso, and Mascolo (2002). Published by Allyn and Bacon, Boston, MA. Copyright © 2002 by Pearson Education. Reprinted by permission.

priate modifications and interventions that may assist in improving the individual's success. Although the same is often said for the latter case, in many instances the focus of standardized testing is more on issues related to identification and diagnosis of intrinsic learning difficulties, and less on intervention. Assessment goals in the latter case often encompass a need for establishing a specific diagnosis, which may lead to additional services or accommodations. As such, the relationship between assessment and intervention is central to both pre- and postreferral activities (see Mather & Wendling, Chapter 13, this volume). It is clear that evaluations focused primarily or exclusively on diagnosis do not retain links to intervention. Psychologists and educators should recognize that the mere process of measuring an individual's functioning is not in and of itself an intervention, but only an attempt to sample the individual's behavior in such a way that it may improve understanding of the individual's difficulties. Professionals should also remain aware (as will be discussed) that implications for intervention exist, regardless of the success or failure of attempts to identify suspected cognitive deficits.

Clarification and Theoretical Specification of Referral Questions

Perception of difficulties (especially problems with academic skills) that have not been responsive to systematic and carefully planned intervention and remediation attempts very often lead to additional evaluation—in particular, the use of standardized tests. The second box in Figure 24.2 represents this stage in the process and reflects the need to operationalize the referral issues and questions, so that they may be answered by additional data to be generated from testing. Examiners should strive to measure the relevant abilities in a theoretically and empirically supported manner, so that the sufficiency of the evaluation is ensured. Doing so requires using valid and reliable ability measures and representing constructs in a psychometrically defensible manner. For example, the CHC cross-battery approach is designed specifically to create a scientifically and psychometrically defensible basis for identifying cognitive and academic deficits and integrities (see Alfonso, Flanagan, & Radwan, Chapter 9, this vol-

ume). Without theory-based clarification and specification of constructs and adequate representation, it may be difficult if not impossible for evaluators to determine whether the tests administered are sufficiently comprehensive and reliable to produce data that can assist in addressing the specific referral questions. This fact holds true for other types of data collection as well. Whatever the method used, the specific referral questions must be operationalized in a defensible and systematic manner.

The remaining boxes on the right side of Figure 24.2 represent the levels (I–IV) of the operational definition of LD, which have already been discussed (see Figure 24.1). Thus it is not necessary to present them again, except to highlight the fact that the decision-making process is based on establishing conditions at each point and following the next appropriate step. The following discussion focuses on the process and decisions that form the assessment activities represented by the boxes on the left side of Figure 24.2.

Sufficiency of Evaluation

If the process of operationalizing the specific referral questions is accomplished without benefit of theory, sufficiency of evaluation may become a significant problem for the evaluator. Any particular question or concern can be operationalized in many different ways, and the nature and manner of data collection can vary widely. As noted previously, CHC cross-battery assessment is one method that is very useful in this regard, particularly when standardized testing is deemed appropriate in LD assessment. However, even careful and deliberate selection of standardized tests according to this approach may not always result in direct or sufficient measurement of the exact areas of dysfunction that may be the underlying causes of an individual's difficulties. As such, it may be difficult to properly evaluate a priori hypotheses regarding particular areas of typical versus deficient performance.

In some cases, standardized test performance may reveal otherwise unremarkable and generally proficient functioning on both academic and cognitive ability tests. If other existing data appear to contradict this scenario, examiners may need to evaluate whether the scope of their assessment, as conducted, was sufficiently broad and comprehensive to adequately measure the suspected area of dysfunction. If it is determined that the assessment has either failed to evaluate the specific area of concern, or failed to evaluate it sufficiently, additional assessment based on the construction of a new set of tests is certainly one option. Alternatively, if examiners determine that the assessment provided sufficient and specific data to adequately evaluate the area of concern, if performance was found to be generally average, and if these findings are supported by other data, then observed performance problems may need to be attributed to factors that are noncognitive in nature. In either case, the professionals should review the referral information, case history, and current functioning more carefully to determine more precisely the nature of the individual's difficulties.

Attribution of Performance

Even when academic or cognitive ability evaluations pass the test of sufficiency and result in data that substantially indicate the presence of normative deficits, professionals must still evaluate the specific reasons why an individual's performance significantly deviates from the norm. This is because several factors may lead to deficient performance, many of which are not related to LD or other types of cognitive dysfunction. This analysis is closely related to evaluation of exclusionary and mitigating factors and is conducted after examiners reliably determine that external factors, as opposed to intrinsic factors, provide the most likely explanation of an examinee's deficient performance. Data collected from a variety of sources should be analyzed and evaluated within the context of the examinee's complete learning environment. In an evaluation of reasons for deficient performance (e.g., levels I-B and II-B in the operational definition), the core issue is determining whether deficient performance can be *primarily* attributed to other factors. When the answer to this question at level I-B and level II-B analysis is "yes," then performance must be attributed to the identified external causes (which generally revolve around factors unrelated to learning difficulties or LD). Exclusionary factors can include such things as poor motivation, anxiety, psychological disturbance, cultural and linguis-

tic differences, pervasive developmental dysfunction, and mental retardation. Indeed, there are many reasons why an examinee may exhibit deficient performance on any given test. When such performance is attributed to exclusionary factors, the course of the entire evaluation shifts, and a total reconceptualization may be needed.

Justification for Intervention

Regardless of the decisions that evaluators make and the conclusions they reach in the context of an assessment, identifying an individual's needs or learning problems involves corroborating such needs or problems with additional supporting and convergent evidence and data (from review of school records, work samples, observations, diagnostic interviews, etc.). This is particularly true when an LD is diagnosed. Reliable and valid LD determination is only accomplished by collecting a broad range of data that support specific conditions and that meet particular criteria, as specified in the operational definition. In most cases, collecting standardized test data is only one procedure within the entire scope of assessment-related activities and should not be relied upon as the sole basis for determining the presence or absence of an LD. Without sufficient and convincing corroborating data, making an LD diagnosis primarily on the basis of standardized test data is both poor practice and wholly indefensible. The comprehensive framework for LD determination described here specifies careful evaluation of case history information (e.g., educational records, medical records, prior evaluations, background information, developmental history), the inclusion of data from relevant sources (e.g., parents, teachers, employers), and the framing of an individual's difficulties within the context of modern theory and research. No matter how compelling its results may be, no single procedure or test should be used to make definitive interpretations or clinical decisions regarding LD identification.

Corroborating and convergent evidence is crucial regardless of whether or not an LD is identified, because in either case, it forms the basis for developing necessary and appropriate interventions. The mere act of evaluating an individual suspected of having an LD does not resolve his or her functional difficulties. Although those individuals identified as having an LD may be entitled to particular accommodations, those not identified as having an LD are equally in need of some type or form of appropriate intervention to resolve their particular issues. Interventions should therefore be justified on the basis of the collected data, and decisions regarding their format, schedule, or intensity should be guided by determining how all the data generated can be applied within the most appropriate context.

The arrows emanating from level IV analysis in Figure 24.2 represent this issue. In one instance, the criterion for level IV (evaluation of interference with functioning) is not met, and the arrow points directly to "Justification for intervention." In the other instance, the criterion for level IV is met; the arrow first points to the box labeled "Learning disability," but then also continues to "Justification for intervention," reinforcing the importance of this step regardless of the diagnosis or reason for deficient functioning.

CONCLUSIONS

Perhaps the most central point made in this chapter has been that the practice of LD assessment has remained difficult and problematic primarily because of the lack of a clear and practical operational definition. To this end, this chapter began with a discussion of the problems that exist with traditional operational definitions and models for determining LD. The three major reasons why current models are inadequate are lack of an empirically supportable guiding theory; vague and nonspecific operational definitions of LD; and lack of a systematic, comprehensive framework for LD assessment. This chapter has focused primarily on the latter two issues—providing a modern operationalization of LD, and specifying a practical and comprehensive framework for LD determination. More specifically, we have described an operational definition that incorporates essential elements for LD identification from the current literature and integrates these within a comprehensive framework for assessment that follows a straightforward decision-making process. Taken together, the definition and framework cir-

cumvent many of the errors and misconceptions about achievement and cognitive ability that continue to plague the practice of identifying LD, and outline a viable method for measurement and interpretation that can be applied by professionals in their attempts to implement the guidelines for LD identification in the reauthorization of IDEA. We believe that the operational definition presented here is the first attempt to integrate modern cognitive theory with the accepted notions of LD, including the current federal definition. It also represents a decreased emphasis on, if not outright rejection of, those LD concepts that are illogical and unsupportable, such as those focused almost exclusively on discrepancies between ability and achievement.

NOTE

1. The range of ±1 standard deviation of the normative mean (85–115, inclusive) for a test having a mean of 100 and a standard deviation of 15 is widely recognized as the range into which most people fall (i.e., 68% of the general population; see Lezak, 1995).

REFERENCES

Aaron, P. G. (1995). Differential diagnosis of reading disabilities. *School Psychology Review, 24*(3), 345–360.

Alloy, L. B., Acocella, J., & Bootzin, R. R. (1996). *Abnormal psychology: Current perspectives* (7th ed.). New York: McGraw-Hill.

Brackett, J., & McPherson, A. (1996). Learning disabilities diagnosis in postsecondary students: A comparison of discrepancy-based diagnostic models. In N. Gregg, C. Hoy, & A. F. Gay (Eds.), *Adults with learning disabilities: Theoretical and practical perspectives* (pp. 68–84). New York: Guilford Press.

Carroll, J. B. (1993). *Human cognitive abilities: A survey of factor-analytic studies.* New York: Cambridge University Press.

Dean, R., & Woodcock, R. (1999). *The WJ-R and Bateria-R in neuropsychological assessment* (Research Report No. 3). Itasca, IL: Riverside.

Flanagan, D. P., Bernier, J., Keiser, S., & Ortiz, S. O. (2003). *Diagnosing learning disability in adulthood.* Boston: Allyn & Bacon.

Flanagan, D. P., & Kaufman, A. S. (2004). *Essentials of WISC-IV assessment.* New York: Wiley.

Flanagan, D. P., McGrew, K. S., & Ortiz, S. O. (2000). *The Wechsler intelligence scales and Gf-Gc theory: A contemporary approach to interpretation.* Boston: Allyn & Bacon.

Flanagan, D. P., & Ortiz, S. O. (2001). *Essentials of cross-battery assessment.* New York: Wiley.

Flanagan, D. P., & Ortiz, S. O. (2002). Best practices in intellectual assessment: Future directions. In A. Thomas & J. Grimes (Eds.), *Best practices in school psychology IV* (pp. 1351–1372). Bethesda, MD: National Association of School Psychologists.

Flanagan, D. P., Ortiz, S. O., Alfonso, V., & Mascolo, J. (2002). *The achievement test desk reference (ATDR): Comprehensive assessment and learning disabilities.* Boston: Allyn & Bacon.

Fletcher, J. M., Francis, D. J., Shaywitz, S. E., Lyon, G. R., Foorman, B. R., Stuebing, K. K., et al. (1998). Intelligent testing and the discrepancy model for children with learning disabilities. *Learning Disabilities Research and Practice, 13*(4), 186–203.

Heath, C. P., & Kush, J. C. (1991). Use of discrepancy formulas in the assessment of learning disabilities. In J. E. Obrzut & G. W. Hynd (Eds.), *Neuropsychological foundations of learning disabilities: A handbook of issues, methods and practice* (pp. 287–307). San Diego, CA: Academic Press.

Individuals with Disabilities Education Act, Pub. L. 108-446 (2004).

Kaufman, A. S., & Kaufman, N. L. (2004). *Kaufman Assessment Battery for Children—Second Edition, technical manual.* Circle Pines, MN: American Guidance Service.

Kavale, K. A., & Forness, S. R. (2000). What definitions of learning disability say and don't say: A critical analysis. *Journal of Learning Disabilities, 33,* 239–256.

Lezak, M. D. (1995). *Neuropsychological assessment* (3rd ed.). New York: Oxford University Press.

McGrew, K. S., & Flanagan, D. P. (1998). *The intelligence test desk reference (ITDR): Gf-Gc cross-battery assessment.* Boston: Allyn & Bacon.

McGrew, K. S., Woodcock, R. W., & Ford, L. (2002). The Woodcock–Johnson—Third Edition (WJ III):

Description and application with adolescents and adults. In A. Kaufman, N. Kaufman, & E. Lichtenberg (Eds.), *Clinical assessment with adolescents and adults* (2nd ed.). New York: Wiley.

Messick, S. (1995). Validity of psychological assessment: Validation of inferences from persons' responses and performances as scientific inquiry into score meaning. In A. E. Kazdin (Ed.), *Methodological issues and strategies in clinical research* (2nd ed., pp. 241–261). Washington, DC: American Psychological Association.

Siegel, L. S. (1998). The discrepancy formula: Its use and abuse. In B. K. Shapiro, P. J. Accardo, & A. J. Capute (Eds.), *Specific reading disability: A view of the spectrum* (pp. 123–136). Timonium, MD: York Press.

Siegel, L. S. (1999). Issues in the definition and diagnosis of learning disabilities: A perspective on *Guckenberger v. Boston University. Journal of Learning Disabilities, 32,* 304–319.

Stanovich, K. E. (1991). Discrepancy definitions of reading disability: Has intelligence led us astray? *Reading Research Quarterly, 26,* 7–29.

Stanovich, K. E. (1999). The sociopsychometrics of learning disabilities. *Journal of Learning Disabilities, 32*(4), 350–361.

Vellutino, F. R., Scanlon, D. M., & Lyon, G. R. (2000). Differentiating between difficult-to-remediate and readily remediated poor readers. *Journal of Learning Disabilities, 33,* 223–238.

Wilson, B. C. (1992). The neuropsychological assessment of the preschool child: A branching model. In I. Rapin & S. J. Segalowitz (Vol. Eds.), *Handbook of neuropsychology: Vol. 6. Child neuropsychology* (pp. 377–394). Amsterdam: Elsevier.

Woodcock, R. W. (1993). An information processing view of Gf-Gc theory. *Journal of Psychoeducational Assessment Monograph Series: WJ-R Monograph,* pp. 80–102.

Woodcock, R. W., McGrew, K. S., & Mather, N. (2001). *Woodcock–Johnson III Tests of Achievement.* Itasca, IL: Riverside.

25

Use of Intelligence Tests with Culturally and Linguistically Diverse Populations

SAMUEL O. ORTIZ
AGNIESZKA M. DYNDA

The rapid expansion and the dramatic increase in ethnic composition of the population of the United States over the past few decades has brought issues of diversity to the forefront of psychological practice. Regardless of region or locale, practitioners are encountering more and more situations requiring evaluation of individuals whose cultural and linguistic backgrounds may differ significantly from their own. Many practitioners recognize that such evaluations require particular knowledge, experience, and competency that is not always a routine part of graduate training and that fair and equitable assessment of diverse individuals includes challenges to the very assumptions that underlie the psychometric foundations of testing. It is unfortunate, however, that limited training and vague, nonspecific legal prescriptions often lead practitioners to assume that the language barrier is either the only or most important variable in conducting intellectual evaluations of diverse individuals. Practitioners often fail to realize that it is culture that constitutes the defining variable in the process of assessment. Culture defines and shapes the individual, including their behavior as measured by standardized tests of intelligence or cognitive ability. Compounding this problem has been the tendency to equate culture with race or ethnic-

ity, particularly in the construction of norm samples and examinations of psychometric test bias. Although culture and race are often related, they are not the same thing and cannot be treated as interchangeable variables. Less biased or nondiscriminatory assessment requires paying considerable attention not to issues of race or even ethnicity, but to the profound and dynamic influence of culture and its attendant native language and how they interact to define behavior, especially during test situations. At the core of any evaluation, it is the issue of validity because above all else it provides the defensible foundation upon which meaning can be ascribed confidently to obtained results. In the measurement of cognitive abilities in individuals from culturally and linguistically diverse backgrounds, the question of validity remains tied directly to the extent to which the methods and procedures used in the evaluation were appropriate and successful in accounting for the known influence of culture and language on test performance.

The purpose of this chapter is to describe the most salient and relevant issues involved in the assessment and evaluation of individuals from culturally and linguistically diverse backgrounds. In particular, differences between the foundations and assumptions underlying general assessment versus

545

multilingual/multicultural assessment will be highlighted. Multicultural assessment issues included in graduate training are often brief and based primarily on examination of test bias. Such treatment is inadequate for the purposes of illuminating clearly the factors that must be considered and integrated into practice that involves assessment of diverse individuals. Without a clear understanding of the central differences and variables, assessment has little chance of being fair or equitable. It should be noted that this discussion by itself is not intended to serve as a guide to equitable evaluation of diverse individuals. Rather, the intent is to provide a discussion that may advance knowledge and understanding of issues that form the basis for selecting appropriate procedures and methods that practitioners may later choose to employ. Comprehensive nondiscriminatory assessment goes well beyond consideration of particular factors. Such assessment involves the collection of multiple sources of data within a broad, systematic framework and uses cultural and linguistic background as the appropriate context from which to derive meaning from obtained results. Such frameworks have been described elsewhere, including Chapter 11 of this volume, and the reader is referred to other sources for information and guidance on such methods (Flanagan & Ortiz, 2001; Ortiz, 2001, 2002, 2004).

BASIC ISSUES IN THE ASSESSMENT OF DIVERSE INDIVIDUALS

Ochoa, Powell, and Robles-Piña (1996) found that practitioners engaged in the assessment of diverse individuals utilized a variety of different instruments, with the most common being a combination that included a Wechsler Intelligence Scale (generally administered completely in English), a Bender Visual–Motor Gestalt Test, a Draw-A-Person test, and the Leiter. Interestingly, Ochoa and colleagues noted that this makeshift battery is not substantially different to the instruments employed in the evaluation of mainstream, monolingual English speakers. The similarity in test usage suggests that practitioners are effectively ignoring factors that differ markedly in the testing of one population as compared to the other, includ-

ing such things as inappropriate norms and comparison groups, linguistic and cultural confounds, and other threats to validity that make use of such an approach rather dubious. Even when practitioners turn to the use of native-language tests or utilize a translator/interpreter in assessment, the question of validity remains prominent and is not automatically or significantly resolved (Lopez, 1997, 2002; McCallum & Bracken, 1997). It is not, however, that practitioners are simply choosing the wrong tests or instruments. Were the issue of nondiscriminatory assessment only about what is the "right" test to administer, there would be little need for much discussion. The problem in conducting more equitable evaluations relates far more to the fact that whatever tests are chosen, they are often administered and interpreted in a manner that is neither systematic nor guided by research regarding the manner in which culture and language influence test performance. As a consequence, there is often no defensible or scientific basis for the types of interpretations and diagnoses so rendered. How and in what manner patterns of "bias" exist in the course of psychological evaluations, particularly when standardized tests are utilized, must be understood well if there is to be any validity to conclusions drawn by practitioners. These potential patterns of bias in testing arise primarily from issues related to a failure to: (1) acknowledge the cultural content embedded in any given test; (2) understand the linguistic demands inherent in any given test; (3) appreciate meaningful differences in norm sample representation for diverse individuals; and (4) recognize the limitations of "nonverbal" assessment. The rest of this chapter provides a discussion of these issues.

Acknowledging Cultural Influences: Bias versus Loading

Intelligence and intelligence tests are as "American" as baseball, apple pie, and Coca-Cola. Although Binet developed the initial scale upon which intelligence tests were subsequently founded, social scientists in the United States were never hesitant in usurping his instrument for much grander purposes (Gould, 1996). From Yerkes and Goddard to Terman and Thorndike, the very definition of intelligence and the newfound means with which to measure it so objectively began and remains largely a pursuit of the well-educated, white males descended from Western European roots. According to Kamphaus (1993), "the traditions of Galton, Binet, Wechsler, Cattell, and others underlie all modern tests of intelligence. These tests emanated from French, British, German, North American, and other similarly European cultures" (p. 441). Because culture defines the manner in which we view the world, including such socially constructed phenomena as the concept of intelligence or race, it is not surprising that intelligence tests became reflections of the values of the men who devised them. It could hardly have been otherwise. An excellent and humorous illustration of the degree to which the cultural values and beliefs of such men entered into the construction of early intelligence tests is provided by Kaufman (1994) in his description of his collaboration with David Wechsler on the revision of the Wechsler Intelligence Scale of Children (WISC). Recalling his discussions with Wechsler on issues involving the potential problem with an item on the WISC that involved who should be saved first in a shipwreck, Kaufman described Wechsler's response as vehemently against dropping the item and quoted him as having said, "Chivalry may be dying. Chivalry may be dead. *But it will not die on the WISC*" (p. x; emphasis in original). There can be little dispute that the personal beliefs and values of the individuals who formulate tests, even in the present day, influence heavily the very content of those tests-tests that are often purported or believed to be objective measures of universal constructs.

Fair and equitable assessment must begin with acceptance of the fact that all tests of intelligence and cognitive ability are reflections of both the individuals and the culture that created them. Performance on such tests is, therefore, an indication of the degree to which an individual has acquired the knowledge or learned those skills and abilities deemed important by the culture as manifest on the test and in its tasks. In an article authored by more than a dozen scientists involved in research on intelligence, it was acknowledged that "it is obvious that the cultural environment—how people live, what they value, what they do—has a significant effect on the intellectual skills developed by

individuals" (Neisser et al., 1996, p. 86). This notion has been echoed by Cole and Cole (1993), who stated that "intelligence cannot be tested independently of the culture that gives rise to the test" (p. 502), and by Scarr (1978), who emphasized that "intelligence tests are not tests of intelligence in some abstract, culture-free way. They are measures of the ability to function intellectually by virtue of knowledge and skills in the culture of which they sample" (p. 339). By acknowledging that tests have cultural content, not that they are necessarily culturally biased, practitioners can begin to appreciate why an individual from a different culture may not perform on a given test in a manner that would be expected, given their age or grade—their culture may not share the same knowledge or skills being sampled by the test.

The literature on cultural influences on testing can be traced back many decades even to the very birth of testing with individuals (Goddard, 1913) and groups (Yerkes, 1921). Early researchers appeared to completely discount the effect of culture and acculturation on test scores despite clear data to the contrary. As psychometric methods and test construction techniques advanced, the nature of bias related to cultural issues was investigated more directly and systematically. With few exceptions, studies that have examined test bias as a function of test items (including content and novelty), test structure (sequence, order, difficulty), test reliability (measurement error or accuracy), factor structure (theoretical structure, cluster or composite scores), and prediction (academic success or achievement), have failed to find much evidence of it (Cummins, 1984; Figueroa, 1983, 1990b; Jensen, 1980; Valdés & Figueroa, 1994). This has led some researchers to conclude that bias in testing simply does not exist (Jensen, 1976, 1980; Sattler, 1992). Others, however, believe that the reasons underlying the failure to find much evidence of bias has everything to do with the way in which it has been defined. For example, Figueroa (1990a, 1990b) and Valdés and Figueroa (1994) have argued that conceptualizations of culture, as well as subsequent definitions of cultural bias, have viewed the construct as something that influences test results in the same way as other potentially biasing variables—that is, that its presence somehow mitigates the predictive ability of the test, or that the results do not correlate in expected directions or magnitude. Because bias (cultural or otherwise) has generally been couched as an inherent defect or flaw of the test (i.e., susceptibility to the influence of factors that should not systematically affect the results), it has remained largely an issue related to reliability. And because cultural differences have never shown a strong tendency to change the nature of the typical indices of reliability (prediction, correlation, factor structure, etc.), it has been posited that bias does not exist. Valdès and Figueroa assert that defined as such, it would be surprising if cultural bias were found because culture simply does not operate in such fashion.

As long as definitions of bias remain rooted in problems with reliability, there will never be much evidence to indicate that tests are biased with respect to culture. The continued development and refinement of ever more sophisticated test construction methods and techniques (e.g., item response theory) has in effect rendered psychometric definitions of cultural bias nearly inviolate. Examination of the psychometric definition of cultural bias reveals that it is logically flawed and specified in such a manner that findings to the contrary are nearly impossible. To understand the flaw, it must be understood that intelligence tests and tests of cognitive ability have been constructed intentionally to measure the degree to which anyone, irrespective of cultural background, has acquired the knowledge and developed the skills valued by the culture that gave rise to the test in the first place. In other words, it is not cultural differences that create bias per se, but rather the difference between an individual's relative exposure (or lack thereof) to the tests' underlying cultural content as compared to age or grade-related peers (Cummins, 1984; Figueroa, 1990b; Gould, 1996; Matsumoto, 1994; Valdés & Figueroa, 1994).

Acculturation is the term that best describes an individual's general acquisition and learning of the cultural elements of the society in which he or she is being raised. The immediate family system is the primary means of transmission of cultural information and when the culture of the family matches the dominant community culture,

learning of the information is further reinforced. For various reasons, most notably immigration, individuals in the United States may find themselves in situations where the cultural background and experiences of their family does not match that which is generally referred to as the "mainstream." Even in cases of second-generation (those born in the United States to immigrant parents) and third-generation individuals, the powerful influence of the family cultural system creates circumstances where the usual pattern of mainstream cultural acquisition may not occur as it would for individuals whose family cultural milieu matches the mainstream. Much like physical maturation and language acquisition, acculturation is a process that is predictable and developmentally invariant. As children grow, not only do we have milestones regarding walking, talking, and toilet training, we also have expectations about behaviors and knowledge germane to mainstream culture. Also consistent with other developmental patterns, the more simple and common elements of culture are learned first and the more esoteric and complex elements are learned later. The process of acculturation and age-related growth along this dimension is both recognized and integrated into the construction of standardized tests and has been described as the *assumption of comparability*. Salvia and Ysseldyke (1991) describe this assumption in the following manner:

> When we test students using a standardized device and compare them to a set of norms to gain an index of their relative standing, we assume that the students we test are similar to those on whom the test was standardized; that is, we assume their acculturation is comparable, but not necessarily identical, to that of the students who made up the normative sample for the test. (p. 18)

This statement illustrates that the foundations of validity related to comparative evaluations of performance lie in the degree to which the level of acculturation between the individual being tested matches the level of acculturation of the individuals on whom the test was normed and standardized. In other words, for the same reasons that it is not developmentally appropriate to compare the cognitive abilities of 5-year-olds with that of

10-year-olds, it is not developmentally appropriate to compare the cognitive abilities of individuals with 5 years of acculturation to those with 10. The problem in testing lies in the fact that not all 5-year-olds have 5 years' worth of mainstream acculturation. Whereas there can be only one physical maturation process that always remains directly tied to age, individuals from diverse cultural backgrounds can begin the process of acculturation at any point in their life. Such individuals may well then have a significant difference in their level of acquired knowledge as compared to same-age peers who began the same process when they were born. Thus in the vast majority of cases involving the evaluation of culturally diverse individuals, the assumption of comparability that underpins age- or grade-related performance comparisons does not hold and makes interpretation of results highly questionable. This point is further articulated by Salvia and Ysseldyke (1991) to the extent that:

When a child's general background experiences differ from those of the children on whom a test was standardized, then the use of the norms of that test as an index for evaluating that child's current performance or for predicting future performances may be inappropriate. (p. 18)

It can be said then that cultural bias in testing is a function of the match between an individual's cultural background and experiences and that of his or her age- or grade-related peers who comprise the norm sample or comparison group. The greater the match, the more valid the comparison. The greater the difference, the less valid are such comparisons. Because individuals from diverse cultural backgrounds rarely have levels of acculturation comparable to the mainstream, such bias is likely to operate in nearly every case where testing is conducted. Test results and any attempts at interpretation thus become invalid because the test has in effect measured the individual's level of acculturation, not actual ability.

To further illustrate the previous point, one need only consider the difference that exists between the average 10-year-old raised in the United States cultural mainstream who possesses 10 full years in terms of direct learning and incidental cultural exposure

versus a 10-year-old immigrant who came to the United States at the age of 5. To hold the immigrant child to the same standard as other 10-year-olds who have been raised in the United States their entire lives is an inherently unfair comparison. In most cases, the immigrant child simply will not have the age-related level of acculturation that his or her mainstream peers do and it will be this that attenuates performance, not lack of ability (Valdés & Figueroa, 1994). Therefore, it is more appropriate to speak not of cultural bias in testing, as culture itself is not the issue, but rather *cultural loading* because it is level of acculturation that confounds measures of ability. Tests of cognitive ability may not be considered culturally *biased* per se, but there is little question that they are culturally *loaded* (Sattler, 1992; Valdés & Figueroa, 1994).

In order to engage in more fair and equitable assessment practices, evaluators will need to consider carefully the degree to which an individual's cultural background and experiences deviate from the mainstream and understand that even those born in the United States may not have comparable age- or grade-related levels of acculturation. In short, the acculturation level of 10-year-olds can vary considerably and will directly affect their performance on tests.

Understanding Linguistic Issues: Bias versus Demand

Language and culture are inextricably linked. Like culture, language is transmitted initially within the family system and if the same language is extant in the community, it is reinforced outside the home as well. Like physical maturation, language is a developmental process that generally begins at birth and remains directly correlated with age throughout an individual's lifetime. But, similar to the process of acculturation, an individual may begin a second developmental language process at any point after birth. That is, individuals may acquire or learn a second (or third, or fourth) language beginning at some point after they were born. Unlike the aging process, individuals are not limited to only one language process.

It should not be surprising then that the effect language differences have on test performance is quite similar to that described previously for cultural differences. Once again, the effect of being linguistically different does not in any way alter the reliability of a particular test. If a non-English-speaking individual who just arrived in the United States is administered some type of intelligence test in English, they are likely to score quite low. It would be obvious that their performance was reflective more of their English language proficiency (or lack thereof in this case) more so than any actual lack of ability. Nonetheless, the test would predict quite well the individual's future success in school and society in general where, rightly so, English language ability is an important and valuable commodity. Other indices of reliability (e.g., item difficulty levels, factor structure, etc.) are also unaffected by the fact that an individual is linguistically different. The test itself is simply not altered by this variable in this way and it will continue to perform, and perform well, as designed. On this point, Valdés and Figueroa (1994) have disscused at length that "empirically established difficulty levels in psychometric tests are not altered by cultural differences. Neither are they because of proficiencies in the societal language" (p. 101). As with acculturation, the problem in testing individuals who are linguistically different rests on the question of validity—that is, exactly what is being measured by the test being administered?

It is necessary for practitioners to understand that the acquisition of any language is a developmental process with all its attendant features—invariance, predictability, age-linked, and so forth. For example, the number of vocabulary words possessed by the average 5-year-old is expected to be greater than that of the average 2-year-old but less than the average 8-year-old. As we continue to mature physically each year, our language also matures and grows accordingly. Moreover, as with acculturation, progress in language is sequential and builds upon itself. The easy, more common, and frequent elements of the language are learned first and the more difficult, complex components are learned later.

Unlike the developmental sequence of acculturation, age-related patterns of language development are quite readily identified and indeed, this sequence is part of what constitutes the assumption of comparability and upon which test items are selected. Not all children are expected to know every vocabulary word on a given test, they are only expected to know about as many words as other children of the same age or grade. It is precisely because the sequence of items on standardized tests is developmentally arranged that examinations of bias generally fail to find any. If an individual knows very little English, his or her scores on tests that are based on or require age-appropriate English proficiency will be low would predict poor school performance. The prediction is not altered irrespective of the reasons for the lack of proficiency, which can be due to factors such as recent immigration or true language deficits.

Bias in testing, with respect to language differences, pertains to validity. In the previous example, the low score may have been due to limited English proficiency or it may have been due to an actual language-based disorder. If the true reason was the latter, and the individual was a native English speaker, there would be no reason to question the validity of the results and the findings could be accepted as evidence of impairment. But if the true reason was the former, validity would be compromised and the results could only be presumed to be a reflection of limited English language proficiency, not actual deficits in language. In other words, although the test may have been designed to detect cognitive ability (via vocabulary), what was actually measured was not the construct of cognitive ability but rather English language proficiency. It is interesting that when empirical examinations of construct concurrence have been done, they have indeed provided evidence of bias. When research studies have attempted to measure the same construct, say general intelligence, through different modalities (e.g., verbal vs. nonverbal tasks), the results have consistently indicated that some other factor is present and that it tends to depress verbal scores more so than nonverbal scores but only for certain groups— those who are bilingual and have less English language proficiency than those who are native English speakers (Cummins, 1984; Jensen, 1974, 1976; Valdés & Figueroa, 1994). But such studies are rare and the overwhelming examinations of bias focus on issues of reliability that overshadow the true effect of linguistic difference that relates to validity

Understanding that language differences do not interact with test performance relative to item difficulty, factor structure, pre-diction, and the like, is only part of the equation for engaging in fair and equitable assessment. Test construction and structure related to language development must also be understood. Despite the claims of tests that are nonverbal in nature (a topic that will be discussed later in this chapter), all tests actually require some level of communication and interaction between individuals. Other than in some special cases (e.g., completely pantomimed tests or tests administered in sign language), testing relies on the verbal or oral language interaction between the examiner and examinee. In addition, tests are sensitive to language development both in terms of language skills that may be assessed as well as the language expectations for different age levels, including the ability to formulate and verbalize responses, comprehension of task instructions, and understanding of basic concepts (Cummins, 1984; Figueroa, Delgado, & Ruiz, 1984). In short, tests accurately reflect age- and grade-related language development so that deviations from normal patterns of development will be manifest in the results. In cases where fully acculturated, native English speakers are being evaluated, this structure holds true and remains valid in the sense that what is being measured is indeed cognitive deficits that may be related to language development because all other potentially confounding variables have been held constant. But in the case of individuals who are linguistically different, this assumption of comparability again rarely holds true. Unless an individual has been raised by monolingual English speaking parents here in the United States and educated only in English, there is not likely to be sufficient comparability. Any exposure or experience with a language other than English can be enough to render the assumption of comparability invalid. Differences in language background occur for several reasons and when present, do not allow for valid interpretation of test performance. Such differences affect the validity of the testing process in the sense that linguistically different individuals will have: (1) begun to learn English at a different point in time as compared to the monolingual English speaker (i.e., at a later age, such as at entry to kindergarten vs. at birth); (2) had backgrounds that cannot be considered exclusively monolingual English speaking; and (3) had varying and often significantly less amount of exposure and experience with English as compared to their monolingual English-speaking peers. These factors may be seen as representing the differences in "linguistic age" that exist between individuals, although this is, admittedly, a gross oversimplification. For example, a 12-year-old child who began learning English upon entry into the public school system at the age of 5 would have a linguistic age of 7 and reasonable expectations of performance on tests administered in English would more likely mirror the linguistic age of 7 than would the actual chronological age of 12. Again, this is much too simplistic an analogy upon which to guide evaluation practices and is meant only to highlight the critical error in logic that leads to inappropriate comparisons and subsequent bias in the interpretation of test results.

Practitioners should not underestimate the influence that linguistic differences play in affecting test performance. Even seemingly minor differences can be significant enough to attenuate results. Moreover, practitioners are cautioned to avoid making assumptions on the basis of how well an individual appears to speak English or their language preferences. The ability to pronounce words with native-like accuracy (i.e., accent) and personal preference in the use of one language over another (i.e., dominance) are not indicators of proficiency. Rather, accent only reflects the point at which an individual first began to learn the language, not how proficient or age-appropriate they are in the language. If the initial point of introduction was within the acquisition period—before the age of 10 or so—no accent will be evident but language development may still be widely disparate from chronological age. In a similar vein, dominance is only an indication regarding what language an individual feels most comfortable using in most social situations. Dominance is mediated heavily by social and emotional factors and the natural desire of individuals to "fit" into their environment. Again, dominance provides negligible information regarding proficiency, let alone reasonable expectations of test performance.

Figueroa (1990a) has summarized the issue of language differences in testing to the effect that lack of understanding of the linguistic demands of test results in situations where tests tend to "degenerate in unknown degrees into tests of English-language proficiency" (p. 93). The issue is not one of proficiency in the language so much as it is development in the language. This means that knowledge regarding the developmental patterns of all language an individual has been exposed to or has experience with is essential in order to approach evaluations in a less discriminatory manner. In addition, knowledge regarding the type and nature of language demands embedded in any test that may be administered is also crucial in evaluating whether results are valid. Ultimately, it will be the degree of linguistic difference that exists between an individual and mainstream English speakers that sets the standard for what should be expected whenever standardized tests of cognitive ability are administered.

Appreciating Norm Sample Issues: Inclusion versus Representation

The great utility of standardized, norm-referenced tests is the ability to make comparisons of performance that are valid and provide information regarding relative standing among a peer group. This is accomplished through several means, notably the standardization of administration instructions, control over the testing conditions, and relatively objective scoring criteria. In essence, standardized testing represents an experimental situation where a sample of behavior is obtained and all other extraneous and confounding variables are controlled. Apart from these factors, tests often imply norms or a norming sample that represents the peer group against which an individual's performance will be evaluated. Norm samples control for other variables that may influence the ability under measurement and are constructed in a manner so as to be as representative and as descriptive of the individuals on whom the test is designed to be administered. The more representative the norm sample, the more valid are the indicators of relative standing. Tests developed in the United States are generally designed for use with individuals of a given age range and who reside in the United States. Their norm samples thus seek to be as representative of the general population as possible and better sampling techniques has led to better norming samples, particularly on the variables of interest, notably age, grade, gender, race, education level, socioeconomic status, geographic location, and so forth. The

basic issue for practitioners in appreciating norm sample issues rests with the concept of representation and the degree to which culturally and linguistically diverse individuals are so represented.

As noted previously, valid comparisons of performance are obtained only when the individual's background and experiences are comparable to those of the individuals that comprise the norm sample. Whenever the assumption is not met, conclusions regarding the meaning of test results becomes dubious at best. This notion has been described by Salvia and Ysseldyke:

> Incorrect educational decisions may well be made. It must be pointed out that acculturation is a matter of experiential background rather than of gender, skin color, race, or ethnic background. When we say that a child's acculturation differs from that of the group used as a norm, we are saying that the *experiential background* differs, not simply that the child is of different ethnic origin, for example, from the children on whom the test was standardized. (1991, p. 18, original emphasis)

The comment above not only emphasizes the importance of comparability as central to the issue of validity but also highlights the actual variable that creates incomparability—experiential background or acculturation, which presumably includes language experience and development. Perhaps more revealing is what Salvia and Ysseldyke (1991) specify are *not* variables that automatically lead to violations of the assumption of comparability, including gender, skin color, race, or ethnic background. This is an extremely important point, albeit not an intuitive one, that is too often misunderstood. Perhaps by our own general acculturation or inadequate training experiences, we have become extremely sensitized to issues of racial differences. The controversial aspects of race-based differences tend naturally to draw the lion's share of our attention so that acculturation and language differences appear unimportant by comparison. As a consequence, norm samples are often carefully constructed to reflect precisely the racial or ethnic composition of the United States, whereas virtually no attention is paid to level of acculturation or varying degrees of English language proficiency as a function of bilingualism. Not only have racial issues taken center stage, they also appear to have become the de facto control for culture. It is not uncommon to read sales literature for many tests that boast of "cultural fairness" when in fact the examination of bias was predicated on issues of reliability as a function of racial or ethnic differences, not cultural ones.

Race and ethnicity cannot be equated so casually with culture, let alone acculturation differences. Although they are related, use of race or ethnicity as measures of culture does not provide an adequate representation for the influence and variation that actually results from differences in level of acculturation. Differences in performance are a function of differences in cultural and linguistic experiences, not racial or ethnic differences. Thus for a test to be truly "culture fair" it would need to establish a norm sample that does not merely pay lip service to culture by the inclusion of racially or ethnically diverse individuals in accordance with their frequency in the general population, but rather seeks to control actual variation in cultural and linguistic experiences much as it does with variation in age (Valdés & Figueroa, 1994). Unfortunately, there are no current tests where variation in experiential background, specifically level of acculturation, has been systematically addressed (Cummins, 1984; Figueroa, 1990a; Samuda, Kong, Cummins, Pascual-Leone, & Lewis, 1991; Valdés & Figueroa, 1994). For practitioners, this has the practical implication that there are actually no tests available that are valid for use with individuals whose cultural experiences differ from the mainstream. To put it another way, when tests are used with individuals whose cultural backgrounds are different from the mainstream, practitioners will need to find systematic ways of addressing the degree of difference and its relative influence on performance.

Because differences in background experiences include differences in language development, and because differences in language development can attenuate test performance, variation in levels of English language proficiency deserves considerable attention in the construction of norm samples. Not only do linguistically different individuals differ from the mainstream on the basis of English language proficiency, but they also differ on a broader basis in the sense that their experiential backgrounds include more than one pattern of language development, that is, they are *bilingual*. A common misconception about bilingualism is that it is an either/or

proposition and there is some element of truth to this notion. Perhaps this is why some test publishers have trumpeted their inclusion of "bilinguals" in their norm samples. The influence of linguistic difference is hardly ameliorated by such a simple procedure. Being bilingual versus monolingual is not the same as being male or female. Rather, bilingualism implies possession of two different language patterns and each may be at substantially different levels across the developmental spectrum (Grosjean, 1989). An individual who is fluent in English and fluent in their native language is bilingual but not at all comparable to an individual who is just beginning to learn English and also limited in their own native language (Hakuta, 1986; Valdés & Figueroa, 1994). Even if language acquisition were distilled into its four most rudimentary stages (i.e., preproduction, early production, speech emergence, and intermediate fluency), bilinguals would differ among themselves in the sense that 16 different combinations of each level of proficiency in both languages would need to be created just to represent comparability in linguistic development. Beyond the combination of two-language proficiencies, other factors that significantly influence language development would also have to be considered: prior educational history, current language of instruction, and chronological age. The complexity of these issues is perhaps best illustrated in the U.S. public school system where debates and controversy surrounding bilingual education are often couched in rhetoric that stems from an inadequate understanding of language development and its parallel relationship to cognitive development and academic instruction (Krashen, 1985).

The complexity of linguistic issues related to norm sample representation for the wide range of bilinguals that exist is rather daunting and remains a task not yet undertaken by major test publishers. Efforts at addressing language and bilingual issues seem to have instead focused on a more simple solution—development of native-language tests. Although there is some intuitive logic to the idea, it tends to miss the basic point that the individuals being tested are in fact bilingual, not monolingual. For the most part, individuals who come to the United States, particularly children who enter the public school system, will need or may even be required to learn English in order to survive and succeed in general society. To one extent or another, they are bilingual and possess varying levels of proficiency in both languages. In addition, the fact that they are living in the United States and being educated in the United States makes them substantially different than individuals who are monolingual speakers of their native language, living in their native country, and being educated in their native language. Such differences should be reflected in the norm sample of any test, yet native-language tests tend to utilize the latter group of monolingual native speakers. For example, the norm sample for use with the Batería-R: Pruebas de Habilidad Cognitiva (Batería-R COG; Woodcock & Muñoz-Sandoval, 1996) consists primarily of monolingual Spanish speakers much the same as the norm sample for the Woodcock–Johnson Psycho-Education Battery—Revised Tests of Cognitive Abilities (WJ-R COG; Woodcock & Johnson, 1989) and the Woodcock–Johnson III Tests of Cognitive Abilities (WJ III COG; Woodcock, McGrew, & Mather, 2001) consists primarily of monolingual English speakers.

Appreciation of norm sample issues is important for practitioners in being able to evaluate test results on individuals who are culturally and linguistically different. Individuals who are bilingual, either by circumstance or choice, are significantly different and do not have background experiences that are comparable to the monolingual individuals who comprise existing norm samples. Bilinguals are different not only from monolingual English speakers but also from monolingual native-language speakers so that tests that utilize one group or the other for comparison purposes remain equally inadequate. Simple inclusion of bilinguals does not obviate the problem because of the many different levels and combinations of bilingual proficiency that exist as a function of two different developmental processes that may or may not have begun at the same time. Existing norm samples are not appropriate or representative of the great majority of individuals who would be classified as either culturally or linguistically different here in the United States (Bialystok, 1991; Figueroa, 1990a; Samuda et al., 1991). In sum, Figueroa (1990b) asserts that "tests developed without accounting for language differences are limited in their validity and on how they can be interpreted" (p. 94).

Recognizing the Limitations of Nonverbal Assessment

Discussions regarding intellectual assessment of individuals from diverse backgrounds often center around nonverbal assessment tools and approaches. There is immense intuitive appeal to the idea that a test that is "nonverbal" effectively addresses the potential bias that might exist in testing as a function of an individual being a non-English or limited-English speaker. Such tests are often purported to be "culture fair" in spite of the fact that many contain significant elements of mainstream culture. It is unfortunate that practitioners often succumb easily to the misconceptions regarding the true fairness of such tests. Although it is true that nonverbal tests may help in reducing the language demands inherent in the testing process (McCallum & Bracken, 1997), they are not the panacea for assessment that they are often made out to be. The reduction in linguistic demands tends to be somewhat illusory in the sense that test administration continues to require some form of communication between the examiner and examinee (Figueroa, 1990b). Tests, even nonverbal ones, are not administered without interaction or some type of interpersonal exchange. Whether by gesture, pantomime, or visual stimuli, examiners must always communicate to the examinee aspects of the testing process, such as what to do on a given task, what a correct response is, when to start, when to stop, the speed at which to work, and so forth. Despite the lack of any oral language, testing remains dependent on effective communication and understanding (Flanagan & Ortiz, 2001; Ortiz, 2001).

Practitioners would do well to recognize that tests that are nonverbal do not automatically or necessarily constitute the best option for assessment of culturally and linguistically diverse individuals for several reasons. First, the particular approach or modality that may be best or most suitable for one individual is not always the same as that for another individual. The same holds true for individuals from diverse backgrounds. There is no single battery or approach that is best for all and evaluations should always be tailored to the unique aspects of each case. Second, individuals differ in terms of their levels of proficiency in both languages. A nonverbal approach generally works best in cases where the individual is rather limited in the language to be assessed. Individuals who are bilingual and have developed moderate or higher levels of English proficiency may not need or require a nonverbal approach. Third, most nonverbal tests tend to measure a relatively narrow range of intellectual abilities, notably visual processing (Gv) (Flanagan, McGrew, & Ortiz, 2000; Flanagan & Ortiz, 2001; McGrew & Flanagan, 1998). Even tests with broader coverage in measurement tend to be limited to tests of fluid intelligence (Gf), short-term memory (Gsm), and processing speed (Gs). Thus the use of such tests may result in constructs that are quite restricted and that fail to capture the full range of intellectual functioning of the individual. Fourth, nonverbal tests may not include the need for expressive language skills from the examinee but may well require normal, native-like proficiency with respect to receptive language skills, particularly for comprehension of test instructions. Because testing requires communication of some sort, even the use of gestures or pantomime can be influenced by cultural and linguistic differences. Communication that may be required for proper administration of a particular test—physical gestures, facial nuances, subtle body movements, and so forth—may well carry more culturally based implications than does verbal communication and affect performance (Ehrman, 1996). And fifth, whereas nonverbal tests may well reduce language demands, they continue to suffer from many of the same shortcomings that plague more verbal tests, particularly inadequate norm sample representation.

SUMMARY

As noted at the outset, the purpose of this chapter was to present a discussion of the main issues facing practitioners seeking to evaluate the cognitive abilities of diverse individuals in a fair and equitable manner. The issues so discussed represent those of which practitioners must have a solid understanding in order to integrate them into current practice in a manner that is comprehensive and systematic. Nondiscriminatory assessment is accomplished via recognition of the nature and source of potential bias and by methods and procedures that are specifically designed to address such influences. Toward that end, fair and equitable cognitive assessment of culturally and linguistically diverse individuals is predicated on a clear understanding of the basic influences on test performance, including cultural differences, linguistic differences, norm sample representation, and nonverbal assessment. A common theme across these issues related to the fact that tests of cognitive ability (in both English and the native language) are limited in the extent to which results obtained from their use can be interpreted validly as measures or estimates of true ability. Differences in the cultural and linguistic backgrounds and experiences of diverse individuals pose serious threats to the validity and meaning of test results. Likewise, such differences between diverse individuals and the mainstream backgrounds of the norm sample also create unfair standards for comparison of performance or relative standing. It was noted that the type of bias that stems from such differences is not related to any technical or psychometric flaws within the tests themselves, but rather are related primarily to violations of the assumption of comparability. Individuals who are culturally and linguistically different cannot be held fairly to the same expectations of age-related performance as that for monolingual English speakers of the mainstream. Current test and norm sample construction simply do not provide any mechanism or substantive basis with which to make judgments about ability in a wholly equitable manner. The complex nature of bilingualism and level of acculturation are such that practitioners should not expect that nondiscriminatory assessment will ever boil down to what is the "right" test to use. In conclusion, Sattler (1992) notes:

> Probably no test can be created that will entirely eliminate the influence of learning and cultural experiences. The test content and materials, the language in which the questions are phrased, the test directions, the categories for classifying the responses, the scoring criteria, and the validity criteria are all culture bound. (p. 579)

REFERENCES

Bialystok, E. (1991). *Language processing in bilingual children.* New York: Cambridge University Press.

Cole, M., & Cole, S. R. (1993). *The development of children.* New York: Scientific American Books.

Cummins, J. C. (1984). *Bilingual and special education: Issues in assessment and pedagogy.* Austin, TX: PRO-ED.

Ehrman, M. E. (1996). *Understanding second language learning difficulties.* Thousand Oaks, CA: Sage.

Figueroa, R. A. (1990a). Assessment of linguistic minority group children. In C. R. Reynolds & R. W. Kamphaus (Eds.), *Handbook of psychological and educational assessment of children: Intelligence and achievement* (pp. 671–696). New York: Guilford Press.

Figueroa, R. A. (1990b). Best practices in the assessment of bilingual children. In A. Thomas & J. Grimes (Eds.), *Best practices in school psychology II* (pp. 93–106). Washington, DC: National Association of School Psychologists.

Figueroa, R. A., Delgado, G. L., & Ruiz, N. T. (1984). Assessment of Hispanic children: Implications for Hispanic hearing-impaired children. In G. L. Delgado (Ed.), *The Hispanic deaf: Issues and challenges for bilingual special education* (pp. 124–153)/ Washington, DC: Gallaudet College Press.

Flanagan, D. P., McGrew, K. S., & Ortiz, S. O. (2000). *The Wechsler intelligence scales and Gf-Gc theory: A contemporary approach to interpretation.* Boston: Allyn & Bacon.

Flanagan, D. P., & Ortiz, S. O. (2001). *Essentials of cross-battery assessment.* New York: Wiley.

Goddard, H. H. (1913). The Binet tests in relation to immigration. *Journal of Psycho-Asthenics, 18,* 105–107.

Gould, S. J. (1996). *The mismeasure of man.* New York: Norton

Grosjean, F. (1989). Neurolinguists beware!: The bilingual is not two monolinguals in one person. *Brain and Language, 36,* 3–15.

Hakuta, K. (1986). *Mirror of language: The debate on bilingualism.* New York: Basic Books.

Jensen, A. R. (1974). How biased are culture-loaded tests? *Genetic Psychology Monographs, 90,* 185–244.

Jensen, A. R. (1976). Construct validity and test bias. *Phi Delta Kappan, 58,* 340–346.

Jensen, A. R. (1980). *Bias in mental testing.* New York: Free Press.

Kamphaus, R. W. (1993). *Clinical assessment of children's intelligence.* Boston: Allyn & Bacon.

Kaufman, A. S. (1994). *Intelligent testing with the WISC-R.* New York: Wiley.

Krashen, S. D. (1985). *Inquiries and insights: second language teaching, immersion and bilingual education, literacy.* Englewood Cliffs, NJ: Alemany Press.

Lopez, E. C. (1997). The cognitive assessment of limited English proficient and bilingual children. In D. P. Flanagan, J. L. Genshaft, & P. L. Harrison (Eds.), *Contemporary intellectual assessment: Theories, tests, and issues* (pp. 503–516). New York: Guilford Press.

Lopez, E. C. (2002). Best practices in working with school interpreters to deliver psychological services to children and families. In A. Thomas & J. Grimes

(Eds.), *Best practices in school psychology IV* (pp. 1419–1432). Washington, DC: National Association of School Psychologists.

Matsumoto, D. (1994). *Cultural influences on research methods and statistics.* Pacific Grove, CA: Brooks/ Cole.

McCallum, R. S., & Bracken, B. A. (1997). The Universal Nonverbal Intelligence Test. In D. P. Flanagan, J. L. Genshaft, & P. L. Harrison (Eds.), *Contemporary intellectual assessment: Theories, tests, and issues* (pp. 268–280). New York: Guilford Press.

McGrew, K. S., & Flanagan, D. P. (1998). *The intelligence test desk reference (ITDR): Gf-Gc cross-battery assessment.* Boston: Allyn & Bacon.

Neisser, U., Boodoo, G. Bouchard, T. J., Boykin, A. W., Brody, N., Ceci, S. J., et al. (1996). Intelligence: Knowns and unknowns. *American Psychologist, 51,* 77–101.

Ochoa, S. H., Powell, M. P., & Robles-Piña, R. (1996). School psychologists' assessment practices with bilingual and limited-English proficient students. *Journal of Psychoeducational Assessment, 14,* 250–275.

Ortiz, S. O. (2001). Assessment of cognitive abilities in Hispanic children. *Seminars in Speech and Language,* 22(1), 17–37.

Ortiz, S. O. (2002). Best practices in nondiscriminatory assessment. In A. Thomas & J. Grimes (Eds.), *Best practices in school psychology IV* (pp. 1321–1336). Washington, DC: National Association of School Psychologists.

Ortiz, S. O. (2004). Use of the WISC-IV with culturally and linguistically diverse populations. In D. P. Flanagan & A. S. Kaufman (Eds.), *Essentials of WISC-IV assessment* (pp. 245–254). New York: Wiley.

Saliva, J., & Ysseldyke, J. E. (1991). *Assessment* (5th ed.). Boston: Houghton Mifflin.

Samuda, R. J., Kong, S. L., Cummins, J., Pascual-Leone, J., & Lewis, J. (1991). *Assessment and placement of minority students.* New York: Hogrefe/Intercultural Social Sciences.

Sattler, J. M. (1992). *Assessment of children* (3rd ed.). San Diego, CA: Author.

Scarr, S. (1978). From evolution to Larry P., or what shall we do about IQ tests? *Intelligence, 2,* 325–342.

Valdés, G., & Figueroa, R. A. (1994). *Bilingualism and testing: A special case of bias.* Norwood, NJ: Ablex.

Woodcock, R. W., & Johnson, M. B. (1989). *Woodcock–Johnson Psycho-Educational Battery—Revised Tests of Cognitive Abilities.* Chicago: Riverside.

Woodcock, R. W., McGrew, K. S., & Mather, N. (2001). Woodcock–Johnson III Tests of Cognitive Abilities. Itasca, IL: Riverside.

Woodcock, R. W., & Muñoz-Sandoval, A. F. (1996). Batería Woodcock-Muñoz: Pruebas de Habilidad Cognitiva—Revisada. Itasca, IL: Riverside.

Yerkes, R. M. (1921). Psychological examining in the United States Army. *Memoirs of the National Academy of Sciences, 15,* 1–890.

26

A Comparative Review
of Nonverbal Measures of Intelligence

JEFFERY P. BRADEN
MICHELLE S. ATHANASIOU

Nonverbal measures of intelligence are essential complements to verbally loaded measures of intelligence. Since the inception of intelligence testing, researchers and test developers have understood that verbal loading within intelligence tests may skew results for individuals whose backgrounds differ from the norm (e.g., Seguin, 1907). Because verbal (or, to be more precise, *language-loaded*) tests of intelligence presume that examinees have met a threshold of exposure to a standard form of the dominant language, the use of language-loaded tests of intelligence has been suspect when examinees do not meet these assumptions (e.g., they speak a foreign language, have deafness/hearing impairments, or come from families using nonstandard forms of spoken language) (Lopez, 1997). Likewise, the presumption that individuals have the ability to understand language, and to use it to reason and respond, may be inappropriate for examinees who have experienced traumatic brain injury, stroke, or degenerative neurological conditions that affect language comprehension and expression. Therefore, nonverbal (or, to be more precise, *language-reduced*) measures of intelligence are essential tools for clinicians who desire to measure intelligence.

This chapter is intended to help clinicians and researchers better understand and use

nonverbal tests of intelligence. We divide the chapter into three major parts: (1) a review of critical issues, (2) a review of contemporary nonverbal tests, and (3) conclusions regarding the current and future state of the art for nonverbal tests of intelligence.

CRITICAL ISSUES IN NONVERBAL MEASURES OF INTELLIGENCE

The use of nonverbal measures of intelligence raises a number of critical issues related to assessing intelligence. Some of these issues are common to all measures of intelligence (e.g., reliability, validity), but others are unique to the use of nonverbal measures. We focus primarily on those issues that are unique to nonverbal measures, or on issues that may be altered when viewed from the perspective of nonverbal measures. Table 26.1 lists these issues in the form of questions and answers, which are elaborated in the following discussion.

The first critical issue is "What is a nonverbal test?" Some tests that use oral language directions, have some linguistic item content, or require an oral response are nonetheless characterized as "nonverbal." Most tests of intelligence that claim to be nonverbal by their titles (e.g., the Com-

TABLE 26.1. Critical Issues for Nonverbal Measures of Intelligence

Issue	Response
What is a nonverbal test?	A test that reduces language loading in directions, items, or responses.
Do nonverbal tests measure intelligence nonverbally or nonverbal intelligence?	Most nonverbal tests intend to measure intelligence nonverbally, but some examiners use them to identify unique nonverbal cognitive abilities.
Should clinicians decide whether to use composite, nonverbal, or verbal scores to estimate intelligence a priori or a posteriori?	Best practices suggest that a priori decisions are most reliable; in cases where verbal and nonverbal scores differ unexpectedly, examiners should conduct additional testing to validate hypotheses regarding intelligence.
What processes do examinees use to respond to nonverbal intelligence test items?	Test developers and users assume that examinees employ nonverbal cognitive mediation strategies, but little evidence is provided to support this assumption.
Do nonverbal tests of intelligence adequately represent the range of abilities comprised by the term *intelligence*?	Unlikely, as many abilities (e.g., crystallized abilities, literacy) have few or no nonverbal methods to measure them; however, general intelligence (*g*) is robust and can be accurately estimated even from a few nonverbal tests.
How should results of nonverbal assessment be used to make appropriate inferences about clients?	Although examiners may use nonverbal tools to reveal intellectual abilities obscured by examinee characteristics, they should not underestimate the role of verbal abilities in contexts demanding verbal skills.
When should examiners use nonverbal tests of intelligence with examinees?	Conditions associated with language differences and disabilities indicate use of nonverbal tests, but unusual examiner–examinee interactions (e.g., exclusive use of gestures) may contraindicate use of nonverbal tests.

prehensive Test of Nonverbal Intelligence [CTONI; Hammill, Pearson, & Wiederholt, 1997]) or use (e.g., the Wechsler Performance scales) provide opportunities for examinees to comprehend directions with little or no language, have limited linguistic content, and allow examinees to respond nonverbally. Few tests completely eliminate language from directions, content, and responses (McCallum, 2003). Therefore, tests that reduce or altogether eliminate the need for examinees to use language when understanding, processing, and responding to test items are considered "nonverbal."

The second critical issue for nonverbal tests relates to the processes examinees use to respond to test items. This issue is phrased in terms of what nonverbal tests of intelligence elicit or measure: Do they measure nonverbal intelligence, or do they measure intelligence nonverbally? This is not merely a semantic issue. Some (e.g., Rourke, 2000; Rourke et al., 2002) argue that nonverbal cognitive processes are different from verbal cognitive processes, whereas others (e.g., McCallum, Bracken, & Wasserman, 2001)

argue that most nonverbal tests of intelligence measure general intellectual abilities. Indeed, some nonverbal tests of intelligence, such as the Nonverbal scale of the Stanford–Binet Intelligence Scales, Fifth Edition (SB5; Roid, 2003) and the Universal Nonverbal Intelligence Test (UNIT; Bracken & McCallum, 1998), invoke models of intelligence that minimize verbal versus nonverbal processing. The argument against describing intelligence as "verbal" or "nonverbal" is that the cognitive processes underlying intelligence are consistent, whether or not they are verbally mediated. For example, most spatial visualization tasks are predominantly nonverbal, because they use incomplete or rotated geometric figures to test spatial visualization. However, spatial visualization can also be assessed verbally by describing the location of one or more objects and then asking the examinee to answer questions related to the objects' orientation to each other.

The argument that processes are largely independent of their language loading has gained favor over time, in large part because factor-analytic evidence does not support a verbal–nonverbal dichotomy in intellectual abilities (e.g., Horn & Noll, 1997). However, the nature of the findings varies. When typical or nondisabled populations are examined, most evidence fails to distinguish verbal from nonverbal processing when tests do not confound language loading with tests of specific cognitive factors (e.g., Carroll, 1993). However, studies of exceptional populations (e.g., individuals with autism or neurological conditions) yield evidence that nonverbal processing deficits, or nonverbal learning disabilities, may occur and may be associated with neurological abnormalities such as reduced myelin (e.g., Petti, Voelker, Shore, & Hayman-Abello, 2003; Weber-Byars, McKellop, Gyato, Sullivan, & Franz, 2001). Therefore, the distinction between verbal and nonverbal intellectual processes may be irrelevant for many examinees, but may be essential for some examinees.

The third critical issue related to the use of nonverbal intelligence tests is whether clinicians use them in an a priori or a posteriori manner. In an a priori approach, clinicians use data other than test results (e.g., background information, an examinee's stated language preferences) to decide whether to use a language-reduced measure of intelligence, a language-loaded measure, or a combination of the two to estimate general intellectual ability. For example, many clinicians recommend using and reporting scores only from language-reduced tests of intelligence when assessing examinees with deafness/hearing impairments (e.g., Vernon & Andrews, 1990); scores from language-loaded measures are not included in the general estimate of cognitive abilities, and may be excluded entirely from the assessment.

In an a posteriori approach, clinicians use test results to decide whether a language-loaded, language-reduced, or combined estimate of general intelligence is the best indicator of cognitive abilities for the examinee. In this approach, clinicians use and compare the results from a variety of language-loaded and language-reduced estimates of intelligence. When language-loaded and language-reduced scores for the same examinee differ reliably (e.g., score differences of $p < .05$) and rarely (e.g., base rate in the normal population of <15%), clinicians may interpret the difference as evidence that the individual's intelligence is not accurately repre-

sented by a combined score (e.g., Roid, 2003). In addition, clinicians typically select and report the higher of the scores as the best estimate of the examinee's general intelligence.

The practice of a posteriori decision making is controversial. On the one hand, critics of the practice (e.g., Kamphaus, Petoskey, & Morgan, 1997; Kamphaus, Winsor, Rowe, & Kim, Chapter 2, this volume) note that after-the-fact selection of scores consistently biases error in favor of overestimating examinees' intelligence. In addition, there is some evidence (e.g., Kelly & Braden, 1990) that language-loaded scores are better predictors of academic performance than language-reduced scores, regardless of which score is higher. On the other hand, proponents of a posteriori approaches (e.g., Sattler, 2001; Kaufman, cited in Benson, 2003) note that test scores may reveal previously undiagnosed problems that could suggest a particular score is a less valid representation of intelligence than another score. However, the default assumption that higher scores are more valid is incorrect for theoretical and statistical reasons, and so clinicians should be cautious about a posteriori selection of scores as being more or less valid. Flanagan and Ortiz (2002) suggest a compromise position, in which clinicians generate a posteriori hypotheses, but then test those hypotheses with new assessment data (i.e., the a posteriori hypotheses become a priori hypotheses in subsequent assessment).

A fourth critical issue is the dearth of validity evidence regarding response processes. Current test standards (American Educational Research Association [AERA], American Psychological Association [APA], National Council on Measurement in Education [NCME], 1999, especially Ch. 1) identify *response processes* as the psychological activities that the examinee invokes in responding to a test. This is a particularly relevant concept for nonverbal measures of intelligence, because nonverbal measures intend to measure intelligence without the use of language. However, examinees may use verbal mediation strategies even when presented with nonverbal tests (e.g., Carpenter, Just, & Shell, 1990), raising the possibility that examinees use response processes other than those intended by the test developers. Forms of response process evidence (e.g., posttest interviews, measurement of electrical or chemical activity in various parts of the brain, eye movements) that could suggest or reveal the psychological processes underlying examinees' responses are rarely if ever reported for nonverbal intelligence tests, despite the relevance of such research.

A fifth critical issue is whether nonverbal tests can adequately represent the intended construct in the assessment—that is, whether they sufficiently capture the range of cognitive processes that compose intelligence. Messick (1995) has argued that construct underrepresentation can invalidate assessment results. In the context of nonverbal assessment of intelligence, construct underrepresentation is important, because reduction or omission of language-loaded tests may reduce the construct of interest (e.g., general intellectual ability or g). Much research on the structure of cognitive abilities (e.g., Carroll, 1993; Horn & Noll, 1997; McGrew & Flanagan, 1998; see also Horn & Blankson, Chapter 3, Carroll, Chapter 4, and McGrew, Chapter 8, this volume) suggests that cognitive abilities are hierarchically organized into three tiers: *general intelligence* (often denoted as *g*), second-order factors (e.g., *crystallized abilities*, *fluid abilities*, *visualization*, *long-term retrieval*), and a number of very specific abilities (e.g., *word knowledge*, *finger-tapping speed*). Two of the second-order factors clearly identified in the hierarchical model are strongly related to language: crystallized abilities, and *literacy* or *reading/writing ability*. Most nonverbal tests of intelligence exclude measures of these attributes (the language-reduced measures of crystallized abilities on the SB5 are an exception), and therefore reduce representation of the abilities when estimating general intelligence (*g*). Although clinicians are appropriately reluctant to use language-loaded indices to reflect cognitive abilities in examinees who may lack typical language exposure and/or skills, the omission of language-loaded instruments may lead to a narrower—and less representative—estimate of general intelligence (Braden, 2003; Braden & Elliott, 2003).

The sixth critical issue to consider involves the consequences and intended uses of verbal and nonverbal assessments of intelligence. On the one hand, nonverbal measures with examinees who have language differences or disorders helps to reduce the inappropriate characterization of the examinees' mental capacities. One particularly poignant example of test use is the case of a girl with deafness who was placed in an institution for individuals with mental retardation on the basis of a language-loaded IQ, but who later earned a college degree and pursued a professional career (Vernon & Andrews, 1990, p. 203). On the other hand, nonverbal estimates of intelligence may overestimate an individual's ability to function in language-oriented environments (e.g., school, work), and therefore lead to inappropriate recommendations for educational placement, career selection, and the like. Clinicians must consider carefully the consequences of assessment as they decide whether and how to use language-loaded and language-reduced estimates of intellectual abilities to estimate future performance.

The final issue related to nonverbal measures of intelligence is when to use nonverbal tests for particular examinees. For most examinees, there are no meaningful differences between verbal and nonverbal estimates of intelligence. For some examinees, however, language-loaded estimates of intelligence are quite different from language-reduced estimates, due to factors that are directly related to language issues (i.e., lack of fluency in the language of the assessment) or indirectly related to features of the assessment (e.g., visual impairments may impede performance on nonverbal tests). Table 26.2 lists examinee characteristics that may interact with language loading on tests; it is suggested that examiners should anticipate issues related to language-loaded testing when assessing examinees with these characteristics. Ways in which examinee characteristics may influence examinees' ability to comprehend task demands, process information, and produce a response are suggested in the table. Although the table includes some examinee features (e.g., motor or visual impairment) that might contraindicate nonverbal assessment, we include them because other features (e.g., hearing impairment, language difference) that would strongly indicate the use of nonverbal tests may co-occur with other characteristics.

However, the table fails to consider responses of examinees to novel test content and administration. Examinees from cul-

TABLE 26.2. Possible Influences on Assessment Processes by Client Characteristics

Client characteristic	Possible influences on assessment processes		
	Comprehension (input)	Processing (elaboration)	Response (output)
Hearing impairment/ deafness	Limited oral and written language; increased sensitivity to examiner's nonverbal cues; frustration with indirect communication mode.	Limited internal language, few or no subvocalization strategies; limited vocabulary reduces processing accuracy.	Limited oral and written language; increased likelihood of changing responses because of examiner's nonverbal reaction.
Native-language difference	Limited oral and written language.	Use of alternative language may facilitate or inhibit processing on some tasks.	Limited ability to express ideas held in other language.
Language impairment/ disability	Increased likelihood of misunderstanding; secondary emotional reactions (e.g., frustration).	Deficits in automaticity, accuracy, and fluency of language-mediated processes; secondary emotional reactions (e.g., frustration).	Errors due to problems of language expression; secondary emotional reactions (e.g., frustration).
Brain injury	Perceptual deficits may increase complexity of stimuli, interfere with ability to perceive details, or impair some senses; secondary emotional reactions (e.g., frustration).	Inconsistency in selection and elaboration of cognitive processes; inability to sustain complex behavior; secondary emotional reactions (e.g., frustration).	Errors due to problems of verbal and nonverbal expression, motor accuracy; secondary emotional reactions (e.g., frustration).
Nonverbal learning disability	Limitations in perception of nonverbal stimuli (e.g., inattention to detail); misunderstanding of nonverbal data (e.g., situations).	Decreased visualization abilities; reliance on verbal processing; avoidance of nonverbal processing.	Possible difficulties organizing complex motor responses.
Visual impairment	Limited ability to perceive visual stimuli and objects.	Limited visual–spatial processing skills, ability to orient in space.	Limited fine motor control for spatial productions (e.g., writing, drawing).
Motor impairment	Difficulties manipulating objects.	None.	Difficulties organizing and executing motor responses; oral language may be limited by articulation difficulties.
Nonstandard exposure to language	Difficulties comprehending linguistic directions.	Limited internal language; limited vocabulary reduces processing accuracy.	Difficulties expressing linguistic responses.

tures in which social interaction is traditionally oral and rarely nonverbal may find an examiner who gives a test via gestures unusual and potentially disconcerting. For example, examinees who have limited hearing, or who do not speak the majority language, often communicate with others via gestures, whereas examinees who rarely interact with others who do not speak the same language may find gestures strange. Examiners must also consider how the interaction of novelty

and cognitive ability may affect examinees. Examinees with limited cognitive ability may be more reactive to or distracted by gestures than those with higher abilities. For example, an examiner who uses a sign language interpreter may be unable to assess individuals with mental retardation, because those examinees are so distracted by the sign/voice interpreter that they do not attend to test content (Kostrubala, 1996, in Ford & Braden, 1996). Therefore, examiners should consider carefully the potential for misunderstanding or error when adopting novel or unusual procedures in assessment.

REVIEW OF NONVERBAL INSTRUMENTS

This section contains a review of seven instruments that use a nonverbal format to measure intelligence. Instruments were chosen on the bases of (1) their measurement of intelligence via what test authors described as a nonverbal format, and (2) their relatively recent publication. Although a few major tests of intelligence include the measurement of fluid abilities (e.g., the Wechsler Intelligence Scale for Children—Fourth Edition), only those instruments that explicitly

use the term *nonverbal* for the instrument or a portion thereof are included in this review. The reviewed tests include the CTONI (Hammill et al., 1997); the General Ability Measure for Adults (GAMA; Naglieri & Bardos, 1997); the Leiter International Performance Scale—Revised (Leiter-R; Roid & Miller, 1997); the Naglieri Nonverbal Ability Test—Individual Administration (NNAT-I; Naglieri, 2003); the Nonverbal Scale of the SB5 (Roid, 2003); the Test of Nonverbal Intelligence—Third Edition (TONI-3; Brown, Sherbenou, & Johnsen, 1997); and the UNIT (Bracken & McCallum, 1998). A brief description of each of the instruments reviewed is presented in Table 26.3. For more information about each instrument, the reader is referred to the respective test manuals. In this section, technical characteristics of the

TABLE 26.3. Instruments Used in Review

Instrument	Age range	Description of scales/subtests	Notes
CTONI	6 to 89 years	• Each of three domains (i.e., analogical reasoning, categorical classifications, sequential reasoning) assessed in contexts of pictorial designs and geometric objects, for total of six subtests. • Scores provided for subtests and for Pictorial Intelligence Quotient, Geometric Intelligence Quotient, and Nonverbal Intelligence Quotient.[a]	
GAMA	18+ years	• Scores provided for four subtests (i.e., Matching, Analogies, Sequences, and Construction) and a GAMA IQ.	Can be group-administered
Leiter-R	2 to 20 years, 11 months	• 20 subtests (10 Visualization/Reasoning [VR], 10 Attention/Memory [AM]) • Subtest scores and scores for Brief IQ Screener (4 VR subtests) and Full Scale IQ[b] (6 VR subtests) provided.	Includes rating scale.
NNAT-I	5 to 17 years	• Total test score provided.	Parallel forms available.
SB5	2 to 85+ years	• 10 subtests, 5 each contributing to Verbal IQ and Nonverbal IQ. • Scores provided for subtests, Verbal IQ, Nonverbal IQ,[c] Abbreviated Battery IQ, and Full Scale IQ.	
TONI-3	6 to 89 years	• Total test score provided.	Parallel forms available.
UNIT	5 to 17 years	• Six subtests, each measuring either symbolic or nonsymbolic processes and either memory or reasoning. • Scores provided for subtests, Abbreviated Battery, Full Battery, and Extended Battery.[d]	

[a]Nonverbal IQ was used in these analyses.
[b]Full Scale IQ was used in these analyses.
[c]Nonverbal IQ and the subtests contributing thereto were used in these analyses.
[d]Extended Battery was used in these analyses.

instruments are presented and critiqued, and evidence related to the instruments' test fairness is discussed.

Technical Characteristics

Nonverbal tests of intelligence cannot be considered appropriate for examinees on the basis of their nonverbal nature alone. Like other instruments, nonverbal tests must be evaluated on their merits as standardized instruments. Therefore, the first portion of this review is a comparison of the instruments' technical characteristics. With regard to reliability, the following are addressed: (1) subtest internal consistency, (2) total test internal consistency, and (3) total test stability. Various scale properties are also considered: (1) subtest floors and ceilings, and (2) median item difficulty gradients. Finally, validity evidence is presented and organized according to the framework used in the 1999 *Standards for Educational and Psychological Testing* (AERA et al., 1999). The framework includes evidence related to (1) test content, (2) response processes, (3) internal structure, (4) relations with other variables, and (5) consequences of testing. Where applicable, all characteristics were evaluated according to Bracken's (1987) standards for minimal technical adequacy.

Reliability

Median Subtest Internal Consistency

Bracken (1987) stated that subtest reliability should meet or exceed .80, which is consistent with that recommended for use of screening instruments (Salvia & Ysseldyke, 2001). Table 26.4 presents internal consistency by age groupings used in the test manual for the respective instruments, as well as median averages across ages. The Leiter-R Visualization/Reasoning (VR) and Attention/Memory (AM) subtests' reliability coefficients were calculated for disparate age groupings; hence their separation in Table 26.4.

The tests in general exhibit adequate subtest internal consistency. All instruments' average subtest reliability indices meet or exceed the .80 standard, with the exception of the GAMA, whose indices meet the criterion only at ages 35–54. The CTONI and SB5 evidence the strongest subtest internal consis-

tency, with all indices exceeding .80. Internal consistency appears to be slightly problematic for the Leiter-R VR subtests at ages 16–17, and the Leiter-R AM subtests at ages 8–10 and 16–20. It should be noted that reliabilities for the Attention Sustained and Attention Divided subtests of the Leiter-R AM battery are retest or stability indices, due to their timed nature (Roid & Miller, 1997). They are included in Table 26.4 because their removal does not significantly change the medians presented. Finally, at ages 6–7, 11, and 15, internal-consistency estimates for the UNIT approach, but do not meet, the .80 standard.

Total Test Internal Consistency

Total test internal consistency should be .90 or greater, especially if a test is used for diagnostic purposes (Bracken, 1987; Salvia & Ysseldyke, 2001). Table 26.5 presents total test reliability indices for each age grouping, and an average across ages. The average total test reliability indices for all the instruments reviewed meet or exceed the .90 standard. With regard to individual age groupings, the GAMA fails to meet the standard at ages 60–64 and 70–89+, and the NNAT-I falls short at age 11. Several indices approach but do not meet the criterion—namely, the NNAT-I at ages 5 and 7–9, the TONI-3 (Form A) at ages 6 and 9–10, and the TONI-3 (Form B) at age 10. With few exceptions, the instruments' total test scores are adequately internally consistent for diagnostic purposes.

Total Test Stability

The ability of a test of intelligence to produce similar results across short periods of time (i.e., 2–4 weeks) should also meet the standard of .90 described above (Bracken, 1987). Total test stability coefficients are presented in Table 26.6. Several instruments reviewed fail to show adequate stability. The GAMA and the NNAT-I appear to be the most problematic, and the UNIT indices approach the .90 standard for only one subsample (i.e., 11- to 13-year-olds). The CTONI, Leiter-R, SB5, and TONI-3 meet the standard, suggesting adequate stability. It should be noted that many of the stability investigations include small samples and lack representation of all ages covered by the instruments. For

TABLE 26.4. Median Subtest Internal-Consistency Coefficients by Age Groupings

Instrument	2	3	4	5	6	7	8	9	10	11	12	13	14	15	16	17	18	19	20	21–24	25–29	30–34	35–39	40–44	45–49	50–54	55–59	60–64	65–69	70–74	75–79	80–89+	Mdn. average
CTONI	N/A	N/A	N/A	N/A	.85	.87	.87	.90	.90	.90	.90	.90	.90	.91	.91	.92	.94			.90			.90		.90		.88		.93		.91		.90
GAMA	N/A	N/A	N/A	N/A	N/A	N/A	N/A	N/A	N/A	N/A	N/A	N/A	N/A	N/A	N/A	N/A	.76	.76		.78	.77		.82		.80		.78	.67	.76	.67	.61	.58	.73
Leiter-R (VR)[a]	.89	.85	.82	.81	.80	.74	.78	.79	.81	.82	.82		.83		.76			.74	N/A	N/A	N/A	N/A	N/A	N/A	N/A	N/A	N/A	N/A	N/A	N/A	N/A	N/A	.81
Leiter-R (AM)[b]	.83		.85		.80		.76				.82						.73		N/A	N/A	N/A	N/A	N/A	N/A	N/A	N/A	N/A	N/A	N/A	N/A	N/A	N/A	.81
NNAT-I[c]	N/A	N/A	N/A	N/A	N/A	N/A	N/A	N/A	N/A	N/A	N/A	N/A	N/A	N/A	N/A	N/A	N/A	N/A	N/A	N/A	N/A	N/A	N/A	N/A	N/A	N/A	N/A	N/A	N/A	N/A	N/A	N/A	N/A
SB5[d]	.87	.90	.87	.87	.81	.84	.83	.83	.81	.82	.86	.81	.86	.87	.86		.88	.88		.90		.89	.89	.88	.88	.89	.89	.87	.87	.89		.84	.86
TONI-3[c]	N/A	N/A	N/A	N/A	N/A	N/A	N/A	N/A	N/A	N/A	N/A	N/A	N/A	N/A	N/A	N/A	N/A	N/A	N/A	N/A	N/A	N/A	N/A	N/A	N/A	N/A	N/A	N/A	N/A	N/A	N/A	N/A	N/A
UNIT	N/A	N/A	N/A	.82	.79	.79	.83	.80	.82	.79	.82	.82	.81	.79	.81		N/A	N/A	N/A	N/A	N/A	N/A	N/A	N/A	N/A	N/A	N/A	N/A	N/A	N/A	N/A	N/A	.80

[a]VR, Visualization/Reasoning subtests.
[b]AM, Attention/Memory subtests.
[c]Only total test scores provided.
[d]Nonverbal subtests only.

TABLE 26.5. Total Test Internal-Consistency Coefficients by Age Groupings

Instrument	2	3	4	5	6	7	8	9	10	11	12	13	14	15	16	17	18	19	20	21–24	25–29	30–34	35–39	40–44	45–49	50–54	55–59	60–64	65–69	70–74	75–79	80–89+	Avg.
CTONI[a]	N/A	N/A	N/A	N/A	.95	.96	.96	.96	.97	.97	.97	.97	.97	.97	.97	.97	.97			.96		.96	.96	.96	.96	.96	.96	.97	.97		.97		.97
GAMA	N/A	N/A	N/A	N/A	N/A	N/A	N/A	N/A	N/A	N/A	N/A	N/A	N/A	N/A	N/A	N/A	.91	.91	.91	.91	.90	.90	.94	.94	.92	.92	.92	.88	.91	.86	.85	.79	.90
Leiter-R[b]	.92	.92	.92	.92	.91	.91	.91	.91	.91	.93	.93	.93	.93	.93	.93	.93	.93	.93	.93	N/A	N/A	N/A	N/A	N/A	N/A	N/A	N/A	N/A	N/A	N/A	N/A	N/A	.90
NNAT-I	N/A	N/A	N/A	.89	.90	.89	.89	.89	.90	.88	.92	.92	.94	.94	.95	.95	N/A	N/A	N/A	N/A	N/A	N/A	N/A	N/A	N/A	N/A	N/A	N/A	N/A	N/A	N/A	N/A	N/A
SB5[a]	.95	.96	.95	.95	.94	.94	.94	.95	.94	.94	.94	.93	.95	.96	.96	.96	.96	.96	.96	.96	.96	.95	.95	.97	.97	.97	.97	.97	.97	.97	.97	.96	.95
TONI-3 (Form A)	N/A	N/A	N/A	N/A	.89	.93	.90	.89	.89	.91	.93	.93	.93	.93	.93	.92	.91			.94		.95	.95	.93	.93	.90	.90	.95	.95	.95	.95	.97	.93
TONI-3 (Form B)	N/A	N/A	N/A	N/A	.91	.93	.91	.90	.89	.92	.93	.93	.94	.93	.93	.92	.91			.94		.95	.95	.93	.93	.90	.90	.95	.95	.95	.95	.91	.93
UNIT[c]	N/A	N/A	N/A	.92	.91	.91	.92	.91	.93	.92	.94	.94	.93	.93	.94	.94	N/A	N/A	N/A	N/A	N/A	N/A	N/A	N/A	N/A	N/A	N/A	N/A	N/A	N/A	N/A	N/A	.93

[a]Coefficients are based on Nonverbal IQ.
[b]Coefficients are based on Full Scale IQ.
[c]Coefficients are based on Extended Battery Full Scale IQ.

TABLE 26.6. Total Test Stability Coefficients

Instrument	Age of sample	N	Interval	r
CTONI[a]	3rd grade	33	4 weeks	.90
	11th grade	30	4 weeks	.94
GAMA	18–80+ years	86	2–6 weeks	.67
Leiter-R (Full Scale Battery)	2–5 years	57	2–4 weeks	.90
	6–10 years	48	2–4 weeks	.91
	11–20 years	58	2–4 weeks	.96
NNAT-I[b]	6–7 years	70	14–49 days	.69
	8–11 years	65	14–49 days	.68
	12, 14–17 years	65	14–49 days	.78
SB5[b]	2–5 years	96	1–39 days	.92
	6–20 years	87	1–27 days	.90
	21–59 years	81	2–32 days	.89
	60+ years	92	1–22 days	.93
TONI-3				
Form A	13 years	43	1 week	.92
	15 years	87	1 week	.92
	19–40 years	40	1 week	.90
Form B	13 years	43	1 week	.94
	15 years	87	1 week	.93
	19–40 years	40	1 week	.89
UNIT[b] (Extended Battery)	5–7 years	46	3 weeks	.78
	8–10 years	42	3 weeks	.85
	11–13 years	46	3 weeks	.89
	14–17 years	63	3 weeks	.87

[a]Pantomime instructions given on first administration; oral instructions given on second.
[b]Coefficients reported are corrected for variability in initial testing.

example, the stability coefficients from the CTONI are based on small samples of 3rd and 11th graders only, and the GAMA used one sample of persons spanning the entire age range of the test. Additional stability data are needed for these instruments before solid conclusions can be drawn.

Scale Properties

Floors and Ceilings

According to Bracken (1987), standard scores for measures of intelligence should be sensitive enough to discriminate the lowest and highest 2% from the remainder of the distribution (i.e., a z score of –2.00 for floors and 2.00 for ceilings). For this review, z scores associated with the lowest and highest standard scores possible were calculated for each age group. Several of the instruments, especially at lower ages, included multiple normative tables for each year of age. In those cases, an average of the subtests for each age interval was calculated.

With regard to subtest floors, the instruments by and large have sufficient floors, with subtests failing to meet the criterion in only a few instances. Floors for the CTONI at ages 6, 7, and 8 are –1.22, –1.56, and –1.83, respectively. Floors at age 2 for the Leiter-R and SB5, respectively, are –1.33 and –1.91. Floors for those over 65 and older on the GAMA also fall short of the standard—specifically, at ages 65–69 (–1.83), 70–74 (–1.75), 75–79 (–1.58), and 80–89+ (–1.58). For the remaining age groups, and for all ages on the UNIT, the criterion is met, suggesting that the lowest 2% of the population can be differentiated from the rest of the distribution.

Subtest ceilings indicate that with only two exceptions, the tests reviewed meet the criterion of a z score of 2.00 or greater. Specifically, at ages 30–39 and 40–49, the ceiling on the CTONI is +1.89. Overall, these results support the tests' ability to distinguish the top 2% of the population. With regard to total test scores, all the instruments reviewed are able to distinguish the top and bottom 2% of the population, with floors and ceilings that extend to 2 standard deviations (2 SDs) or more above and below the mean, respectively.

Difficulty Gradients

Difficulty gradients address the degree of standard score change for varying increases in raw scores. According to Bracken (1987), only those tests whose normative tables include 3 raw score points or more per SD are sensitive enough to discern small differences in ability. For this review, at each age interval, the total number of raw score points available was divided by the number of SDs spanned by the subtest. Multiple quotients within a 1-year age level were averaged. The median of quotients across subtests was then calculated. Any quotient greater than 3 meets Bracken's criterion. The results of this analysis suggest that all the instruments are sensitive to small ability differences. The median difficulty gradients obtained ranged from 3.18 (GAMA, ages 18–34) to 7.47 (Leiter-R, age 2).

Validity

As acceptable validity depends on the purpose for which a test is used, it is difficult to determine a numerical criterion for validity (Bracken, 1987). According to the *Standards for Educational and Psychological Testing* (AERA et al., 1999), the validation process "involves accumulating evidence to provide a sound scientific basis for the proposed score interpretations" (p. 9). As such, this review includes an accumulation of validity evidence presented in the respective tests' manuals (see Table 26.7), which is organized according to the framework presented in the *Standards*. A description of this framework follows.

According to the *Standards*, validity is a unitary concept. Therefore, tests can be described in terms of the types of evidence for validity included. Sources of evidence include these:

1. Evidence based on *test content* refers to evidence about the themes, wording, and format of test items, tasks, or questions, as well as procedures for administration and scoring. Test content information may include logical or empirical evidence about construct relevance, construct representation, and opinions of expert judges (with sufficient detail provided about the judges and procedures used).

2. Evidence based on *response processes* refers to information indicating that examinees use the hypothesized cognitive or psychological processes that the test purports to measure or elicit. Such information can be theoretical or empirical in nature.

3. Evidence based on *internal structure* indicates the extent to which test items and subparts are consistent with the construct that forms the basis for proposed test interpretation. Such evidence may include information about the behavior of individual items, within-test correlations, factor analysis, and so on.

4. Evidence based on *relations to other variables* includes convergent and discriminant evidence and test–criterion relationships that support proposed interpretation of scores.

5. Evidence based on *consequences of testing* involves demonstrating that intended benefits of test use are in fact realized. This may be shown through prediction analyses, but can include logical or theoretical arguments.

As seen in Table 26.7, the tests reviewed present a significant amount of evidence for validity. Table 26.7 differentiates the validity evidence to which the respective test manuals refer from the empirical evidence that they provide. This is an important distinction, because without the actual investigation results, readers do not have the opportunity to draw their own conclusions about the meaning of the results. The tests include ample evidence with regard to internal structure and relations to other variables, and the SB5 and UNIT, in particular, make a strong case for validity of test content. Nevertheless, much less information is provided about response processes and consequences of testing. With regard to response processes, several of the tests address operative processes by linking such processes to the theory on which the

TABLE 26.7. Evidence for Validity across Instruments

Category	Criterion	CTONI	GAMA	Leiter-R	NNAT-I	SB5	TONI-3	UNIT
Evidence based on test content	Item relevance	×	×	×	×	×	×	×
	Item adequacy or relevance					×		×
	Detailed content	×	×	×	×	×	×	×
	Expert judgment			×		×		×
	Expert judges and procedures used					×		×
Evidence based on response processes	Theoretical basis for operative cognitive processes	×		×		×	×	×
	Empirical basis for operative cognitive processes				D			
Evidence based on internal structure	Age trends	E	E	E		E	E	
	Group differentiation	E	E	E	E	E	E	E
	Item analysis	E	D	D	D	D	E	D
	Differential item functioning	E	D	E		E	E	D
	Factor analysis	E		E		E	E	E
	Item–subtest correlations		D		N/A		N/A	
	Item–total correlations		D	D		D	D	
	Subtest intercorrelations	E	E	E	N/A	E	N/A	E
	Subtest–total correlations		E	E	N/A	E	N/A	E
	Experimental intervention studies			E				
Evidence based on relations to other variables	Correlations with other measures of ability	E	E	E	E	E	E	E
	Correlations with other nonverbal measures of ability	E		E		E	E	E
	Correlations with achievement measures		E	E	E	E	E	E
	Cross-battery factor analysis			E		E		
Evidence based on consequences of testing	Prediction analyses							

Note. ×, instrument meets criterion; D, discussed in test manual; E, empirical evidence provided in test manual.

test is based. Because examinees may use cognitive processes that differ from those theorized by test authors, more empirical evidence is necessary to support test claims. Only the NNAT-I mentions empirically investigating processes used by examinees, but little detail about how this was studied is provided. None of the instruments provide empirical evidence that test results are linked to test consequences. This is especially problematic for those instruments that claim to relate to academic success. Although it is possible that such evidence exists in other sources, none is included in the test manuals. More evidence for validity related to testing consequences is sorely needed.

Test Fairness Indices

Nonverbal instruments need not only to demonstrate adequate technical characteristics. Developers of nonverbal tests must also demonstrate that tests can be used without bias with examinees from diverse backgrounds. Most nonverbal instruments, because they have fewer requirements for spoken language, are touted as useful for examinees who speak languages other than English, for example. Nevertheless, the lack of focus on verbal instructions or response requirements alone is insufficient for determining test fairness.

Test fairness is based both on development procedures and on specific test characteristics that minimize potential bias and statistical analyses designed to rule out bias. From a review of relevant literature, several criteria related to test development, test characteristics, and statistical analyses were identified and are the basis of this review (e.g., Athanasiou, 2000). Test development criteria reviewed include information related to (1) foundation, and (2) content review. Test characteristics reviewed include (1) mode of instructions, (2) response modes, (3) use of timed items, and (4) inclusion of practice items. Finally, statistical analyses reviewed include (1) group comparisons, (2) item characteristics, (3) reliability, (4) predictive validity, and (5) construct validity.

Test Development

Efforts to reduce bias begin at the test development stage. Each of the instruments reviewed was designed to be useful for those from various cultural backgrounds, as well as those who use a language other than English. Therefore, the instruments were reviewed according to criteria related to test development. Table 26.8 contains a summary of comparative information.

Foundation

This aspect of the review included an examination of measurement of multiple abilities, the degree of emphasis on fluid abilities, and the theoretical basis of the instruments. With regard to multiple abilities, Harris, Reynolds, and Koegel (1996) have stated that because of their effort to reduce language, nonverbal tests are able to measure only a limited number of abilities (i.e., nonverbal tests suffer from construct underrepresentation). Relatedly, Bracken and McCallum (2001) have differentiated *unidimensional* and *multidimensional* tests. The former are those that measure reasoning, usually through matrix analogies; the latter are more comprehensive, measuring a broader array of abilities (e.g., memory, attention, reasoning). Only three of the instruments reviewed are multidimensional (i.e., the Leiter-R, SB5, and UNIT). The remainder exclusively measure nonverbal or spatial reasoning abilities, and may therefore be more prone to construct underrepresentation.

With regard to theoretical basis, one weakness of nonverbal intelligence tests is that many are not model-based. Of the seven instruments reviewed here, only the manuals of the multidimensional instruments (i.e., the Leiter-R, SB5, and UNIT) include a comprehensive discussion of the theoretical model on which the instrument is based. The authors of the other instruments either report the use of an eclectic approach to the intelligence construct, or do not mention intelligence theory. The reader is referred to the tests' respective manuals for a more detailed description of theoretical foundations.

Finally, instruments that measure predominantly fluid abilities are typically preferred over those that measure abilities reliant upon prior learning, simply because people from certain cultures or from certain social strata may not have had the types of learning experiences that would prove useful on most tests of intelligence. Although focusing on fluid

TABLE 26.8. Indices of Fairness Related to Test Development across Instruments

Instrument	Foundation	Content review
CTONI	No specific theoretical model; unidimensional	No expert review
GAMA	No specific theoretical model; unidimensional	No expert review
Leiter-R	Carroll (1993) and Gustafsson (1988) models; multidimensional	No expert review
NNAT-I	No specific theoretical model; unidimensional	No expert review
SB5	Cattell–Horn–Carroll model; multidimensional	Eight expert reviewers examined items for potential bias; expert reviews conducted from perspectives of diverse groups
TONI-3	No specific theoretical model; unidimensional	No expert review
UNIT	Jensen's (1980) parsimonious two-factor model; multidimensional	Expert reviews from consultants representing diverse backgrounds reviewed items, artwork, manipulables

abilities limits the breadth of abilities measured, it may be more difficult on tests that stress abilities requiring prior learning to remove biased content or arrange test administration in a way that allows all participants to perform to their potential. Each of the reviewed instruments places primary emphasis on fluid abilities, with one exception. Two of the five abilities measured nonverbally on the SB5 are highly dependent on learning history. Specifically, the Knowledge subtest is intended to measure crystallized ability, and the Quantitative Reasoning subtest is intended to measure quantitative abilities, which are influenced by prior learning.

Content Review

Although expert review of item content for the detection of bias in and of itself is insufficient for eliminating it, the use of experts representing various groups can be useful for identifying potential bias in items or procedures, as well as identifying content that may be perceived as objectionable to some groups. Helms (1997) has stated that a group's performance on particular items is only one method of determining bias. In addition, items must have the same meaning and/or invoke similar response processes. Although response processes should be measured in a variety of ways, expert reviewers may lend insight into the meaning items or

procedures may hold for certain groups. The manuals of only two of the instruments (i.e., the SB5 and UNIT) describe in detail the incorporation of an expert review process into test development. The SB5 review appeared to be specifically related to item content, whereas the UNIT reviewers examined item content, artwork, and manipulables. Rules for decision making about item retention based on reviewer feedback are discussed in the respective tests' manuals.

Test Administration

All instruments were reviewed for a description of test administration procedures that have been shown or hypothesized to minimize bias. Table 26.9 summarizes the relevant administration procedures for the seven instruments reviewed.

Presentation of Instructions

A truly nonverbal test, according to Jensen (1980), does not include the use of spoken language on the part of either the examinee or the examiner. Spoken or written English puts any examinee who uses a different language at a disadvantage, thereby increasing the likelihood of test bias. Of the seven instruments reviewed, four can be administered in a language-free manner: the CTONI, Leiter-R, TONI-3, and UNIT. The SB5's and

NNAT-I's instructions are presented orally, and the GAMA's are in written English. These last three instruments, therefore, have the greatest potential for bias when used with examinees not fluent in English.

Response Modes

Varying response modes may increase motivation, thereby reducing the possibility of bias. Therefore, response modes for nonverbal instruments should be entirely nonverbal but varied. Varied response modes are included in the Leiter-R, SB5, and UNIT. Pointing is used on the CTONI, NNAT-I, and TONI-3. The GAMA is the instrument

with the most potential for bias, because responses consist of shading bubbles on an answer sheet. This activity may put those who have had less experience with paper-and-pencil tasks at a disadvantage.

Use of Time Limits

Although the use of timing procedures is common in many available tests of intelligence, it holds the potential for bias. Specifically, imposing time limits may unfairly penalize those for whom the concept of time is less closely equated with the concept of speed, or is only minimally important (Harris et al., 1996). Table 26.9 shows

TABLE 26.9. Indices of Test Fairness Related to Test Administration across Instruments

Instrument	Presentation of instructions	Response modes	Use of time limits	Practice/teaching items
CTONI	Pantomimed or verbal instructions	Pointing; clicking mouse if computerized version used	No time limits	Unscored sample items
GAMA	Directions written in English in test booklet and read aloud	Marking bubbles on answer sheet	No time limits on items; time limit of 25 minutes for entire test	Unscored sample items
Leiter-R	Pantomimed instructions, but examiner can supplement with spoken language if necessary	Pointing; placing/arranging cards; marking in test booklet	Bonus points for speed and accuracy on three subtests; pacing procedure for slow responders	Scored teaching items
NNAT-I	Spoken English; Spanish and French translations included in manual	Speaking or pointing	No time limits	Unscored sample items
SB5	Spoken English	Handing examiner items; pointing; completing puzzles; finding objects; pantomiming actions; tapping blocks; arranging geometric pieces	Time limits on one nonverbal subtest	Unscored sample items and scored teaching items
TONI-3	Pantomimed	Pointing	No time limits	Unscored teaching items
UNIT	Pantomimed	Pointing; placing chips on grid; arranging cards; completing drawn mazes; building cube designs	Time limits on one subtest; bonus points for speed on one subtest	Unscored demonstration items and scored sample items; scored checkpoint items

that the potential for bias related to timed administration is minimized in the CTONI, NNAT-I, and TONI-3. The GAMA imposes no time limits on individual items, but test takers are limited to 25 minutes to complete the test. The UNIT and SB5 include time limits on two and one subtests, respectively, and the Leiter-R gives bonus points for speed and accuracy on three subtests.

Practice/Teaching Items

For those tests whose instructions are presented nonverbally, it is important to determine whether test takers comprehend the nature of the tasks and how they are to respond. For that reason, the use of practice and teaching items is important for minimizing bias (Jensen, 1980). All tests reviewed include procedures for providing feedback on a limited number of items. The CTONI, NNAT-I, GAMA, and TONI-3 include sample or teaching items that are not scored. Avoiding scoring such items is fairer to those who need instruction before they understand how to proceed. Although the UNIT scores sample items, demonstration items are also included as a training procedure. The SB5 includes sample items on only two of its subtests; perhaps the use of verbally presented instructions minimizes the need for those who understand English for practice/sample items.

Statistical Analyses

The presence or absence of bias is considered by some (e.g., Jensen, 1980) to be statistically determined. Several statistical procedures are recommended to rule out bias and/or to detect bias during test development. Table 26.10 contains a comparison of the reviewed instruments on statistical bias analyses reported in the test manuals. Information in the table is differentiated on the basis of whether results of relevant studies are presented in the manual or whether relevant studies are mentioned without presentation of relevant statistics.

Group Comparisons

It has been argued that the presence of mean score differences across groups is not a valid indication of test bias, as long as the test is detecting differences solely related to the construct(s) in question (e.g., Ackerman, 1992). Still, group comparison studies are important to most test users, and are often presented in test manuals. The controversy centering around intergroup mean score differences is well documented and will not be repeated here (e.g., Brown, Reynolds, & Whitaker, 1999). The controversy does, however, indicate the potential for misinterpretation of such data. Because within-group differences are larger than differences between groups (Puente & Salazar, 1998), it is helpful for research to explore variables that are related to between-group variation. However, it is also useful for test publishers to include correlations among variables used for such statistical control, so that the reader can more fully understand the comparisons. Only the group comparisons described in the NNAT-I and UNIT included a matching procedure, but neither included correlations among matching and dependent variables. Comparisons provided for the CTONI, Leiter-R, and TONI-3 did not include a matched control group. Finally, the GAMA provides group comparison information for various disability groups, but not for racial/ethnic samples.

Item Characteristics

Examination of item characteristics allows researchers to determine how performance on items varies among groups of test takers, while controlling for overall performance on an instrument. To the extent that members of various groups who are matched for ability pass items at different rates, the item is considered biased. The majority of the reviewed tests' manuals mention investigating item curve characteristics, but only the CTONI and TONI-3 provide related evidence. Of the seven tests reviewed, only the GAMA does not describe item characteristics for diverse samples.

Reliability

For a test to be considered fair, it must have similar degrees of reliability for all who take the test. Internal-consistency estimates for various subgroups are reported for the CTONI, SB5, TONI-3, and UNIT. In all

TABLE 26.10. Indices of Fairness Related to Statistical Analyses across Instruments

Instrument	Group comparison	Item functioning	Reliability	Internal structure	Consequences of testing
CTONI	Comparisons included; no matched controls[b]	Three-parameter IRT and delta scores[b]	Internal consistency for sexes, three minority groups, one non-native group, and subjects with deafness and ESL status[b]	No information	Correlations only[b]
GAMA	No comparisons	No information	No information	No information	No information
Leiter-R	Minimal comparisons; no matched controls[b]	Rasch item analysis[a]	No information	No information	Regression analysis for European Americans and African American samples[a, c]
NNAT-I	Comparisons with matched controls[b]	"IRT bias analysis" (p. 34)[a]	No information	No information	No information
SB5	No comparisons	Mantel–Haenszel procedure[a]	Internal-consistency estimates for three minority groups[b]	Chi-square tests of significance on subtest correlation matrices[a]	Equivalence of regression slopes across sexes and racial/ethnic groups[a]
TONI-3	Comparisons included; no matched controls[b, d]	Three-parameter IRT and delta scores[b]	Internal-consistency estimates for sexes, two minority groups, and subjects with deafness[b]	No information	Correlations only (using TONI and TONI-2)[b]
UNIT	Comparisons with matched controls included[b]	Mantel–Haenszel procedure[a]	Internal-consistency estimates for sexes and two minority groups[b]	Confirmatory factor analyses on sexes and two minority samples[b]	Equivalence of regression slopes for sexes, races, and sex × race[a]

Note. IRT, item response theory; ESL, English as a second language.
[a]Information discussed in manual; no statistical evidence provided.
[b]Statistical evidence presented in manual.
[c]Reader is referred to Woodcock, McGrew, and Mather (2001).
[d]Descriptive statistics only.

cases, reliability estimates for the various subgroups included in analyses (see Table 26.10) are statistically similar to those for the overall normative sample.

Internal Structure

With regard to internal structure, test developers should demonstrate that the constructs measured by the test are similar for diverse groups of test takers (Reynolds & Kaiser, 1990). Typically, this is determined by demonstrating that factor structures are consistent across groups. Such information is provided in the UNIT manual only, and it indicates similar factor structures for both sexes, African Americans, and Hispanics. The SB5 manual (Roid, 2003) includes an examination of subtest correlation matrices, on which chi-square tests of significance were conducted to determine whether the pattern of correlations was consistent across groups. All analyses were nonsignificant, indicating the absence of bias related to construct validity.

Consequences of Testing

When test authors claim that use of an instrument will result in a particular outcome, it is incumbent upon them to demonstrate that such consequences occur. Furthermore, instruments should predict outcomes for various subgroups with a consistent degree of accuracy (Reynolds & Kaiser, 1990). In the case of intelligence testing, for example, scores on the instrument should predict the same academic achievement score, and with equal accuracy, for members of all subgroups sharing the same IQ. The Leiter-R and UNIT both provide information about testing consequences. The Leiter-R reports results of equivalence analyses across two groups of European Americans and African American children; the UNIT describes examinations of prediction equivalence for sex, race (African American sample), and the interaction of sex and race. Similar regression slopes were found for both instruments. Neither of these instruments present information related to standard error of estimation/prediction or intercept. Correlational data, which are less rigorous, are provided in the CTONI manual. Similar data in the TONI-3 manual are based on earlier versions of the instrument.

CONCLUSIONS

Nonverbal tests of intelligence provide an important avenue for assessing intelligence. Nonverbal tests can corroborate or disconfirm findings from language-loaded tests, which can help to differentially diagnose linguistic and intellectual differences and difficulties. When results concur across verbal and nonverbal tests, examiners can have more confidence in their estimates of an examinee's intellectual abilities. Differences between verbal and nonverbal estimates of intelligence reduce examiner confidence in any particular set of results, and may prompt additional assessment to explore the cause of the verbal–nonverbal difference (e.g., language issues, nonverbal learning disabilities).

There have been many advances in nonverbal tests of intelligence in recent decades. Unlike their predecessors, contemporary tests of nonverbal intelligence have strong technical characteristics, representative norms, appropriate items, and technical data to support their use. Some of the nonverbal tests we have reviewed provide explicit theoretical models and include specialized efforts to address specific issues (e.g., use in special populations, test bias). Today's examiners are fortunate to have a wide variety of nonverbal tests, and research evidence, available to them.

However, there are also problems with the use of nonverbal tests of intelligence. First and foremost is this question: What processes do nonverbal tests of intelligence test? Historically, test publishers, researchers, and users have not been clear or consistent in deciding whether nonverbal tests measure the same processes as verbal tests but do so nonverbally, or whether they measure distinct (i.e., nonverbal) cognitive processes. For example, intelligence test batteries separate verbal from nonverbal or performance scores, implying measurement of different constructs; yet most tests suggest that either score represents general intellectual ability. Although research on intelligence in typical populations that suggests there is no clear verbal–nonverbal ability dichotomy (see Wasserman & Lawhorn, 2003), research with exceptional groups suggests that at least some individuals may have unique nonverbal processing characteristics that influence their ability to adapt, particularly in social circumstances (e.g., Rourke, 2000). At the current time, researchers and clinicians do not have a common framework for resolving conflicting findings and claims regarding verbal and nonverbal intellectual abilities.

Another unresolved problem is how to integrate research and practice using nonverbal intelligence tests with broader theories of intellectual abilities. Wilhoit and McCallum (2003) provide an intriguing step in this direction, as they attempt to integrate nonverbal tests of intelligence into a cross-battery approach (McGrew & Flanagan, 1998). Their effort underscores the limited range of cognitive abilities currently assessed with nonverbal tools; for example, they list only two nonverbal tests of crystallized abilities, and no nonverbal tests of auditory processing, quantitative reasoning, or literacy. Although a nonverbal test of literacy may by definition be impossible to create (but see Frisby, 2003, on nonverbal methods to assess academic achievement), test developers may be able to expand the range of cognitive abilities assessed by nonverbal tests.

Another major limitation of nonverbal tests is the absence of evidence needed to understand the processes that nonverbal tests measure. For example, an examinee who has native-language fluency might use subvocal language to facilitate encoding ("That's a blue triangle"), processing ("Shapes get turned"), and responding ("It's the upside-down blue triangle, or option D") in responding to a figural matrix item. Another examinee with identical language fluency may encode, process, and respond visually, without invoking any linguistic strategies. Relatively little is known about the nature of the processes examinees invoke when approaching nonverbal tests, but available research indicates that examinees use a range of strategies when responding to nonverbal figural matrices (Carpenter et al., 1990). The available research hints at the importance of understanding the cognitive processes that examinees use in responding to nonverbal tests of intelligence, although we also note that the dearth of response process research applies to verbal intelligence tests, too (see Braden & Niebling, Chapter 28, this volume, for a discussion of response processes in intelligence test validity).

One of the tacit, but largely unexamined, justifications for nonverbal tests with indi-

viduals who speak different languages is that nonverbal tests place examinees on an equal footing (e.g., McCallum, 2003; McCallum et al., 2001). However, little is known about whether language differences may influence performance on nonverbal tests of intelligence. For example, different languages predispose individuals to adopt or avoid cognitive processes, such as drawing distinctions among stimuli (Whorf, 1956/2002). If so, linguistic and cultural differences among examinees may influence nonverbal test performance, despite the relative absence of specific cultural or linguistic content in the nonverbal test items. Although there is little evidence showing linguistic or cultural group differences on nonverbal tests, there is also little evidence to support equivalence of nonverbal tests of intelligence across linguistic and cultural groups (Maller, 2003).

Although we have identified a number of unresolved issues regarding nonverbal tests of intelligence, we also appreciate that, despite these limitations, nonverbal tests of intelligence are superior to alternative methods for assessing intelligence in many situations. For example, raters' opinions of examinees' intelligence may be strongly affected by disability-related, racial, cultural, and linguistic stereotyping. Language-loaded tests of intelligence are clearly inappropriate for many examinees, and although the evidence base for the use of tests is inadequate, it is not contradictory. Therefore, examiners should use nonverbal tests of intelligence in the same manner as they use other tests of intelligence: cautiously, in a manner that is sensitive to contextual issues, and with an emphasis on collecting a variety of data sources to corroborate conclusions. Test researchers and developers should continue efforts to understand the role of nonverbal assessment in cross-battery approaches, the responses processes examinees invoke when responding to nonverbal tests, and the consequential validity of using—and not using—nonverbal tests of intelligence.

REFERENCES

Ackerman, T. A. (1992). A didactic explanation of item bias, item impact, and item validity from a multidimensional serial perspective. *Journal of Educational Measurement, 1,* 67–91.

American Educational Research Association (AERA), American Psychological Association (APA), & National Council on Measurement in Education (NCME). (1999). *Standards for educational and psychological testing.* Washington, DC: AERA.

Athanasiou, M. S. (2000). Current nonverbal assessment instruments: A comparison of psychometric integrity and test fairness. *Journal of Psychoeducational Assessment, 18,* 211–229.

Benson, E. (2003). Intelligent intelligence testing. *Monitor on Psychology, 43*(2), 48–51.

Bracken, B. A. (1987). Limitations of preschool instruments and standards for minimal levels of technical adequacy. *Journal of Psychoeducational Assessment, 4,* 313–326.

Bracken, B. A., & McCallum, R. S. (1998). *Universal Nonverbal Intelligence Test.* Itasca, IL: Riverside.

Bracken, B. A., & McCallum, R. S. (2001). Assessing intelligence in a population that speaks more than two hundred languages: A nonverbal solution. In J. G. Ponterotto, P. A. Meller, & L. A. Suzuki (Eds.), *Handbook of multicultural assessment: Clinical, psychological, and educational applications* (2nd ed., pp. 405–431). San Francisco: Jossey-Bass.

Braden, J. P. (2003). Accommodating clients with disabilities on the WAIS-III/WMS. In D. Saklofske & D. Tulsky (Eds.), *Use of the WAIS-III/WMS in clinical practice* (pp. 451–486). Boston: Houghton Mifflin.

Braden, J. P., & Elliott, S. N. (2003). Accommodations on the Stanford–Binet Intelligence Scales, Fifth Edition. In G. Roid, *Interpretive manual for the Stanford–Binet Intelligence Scales, Fifth Edition* (pp. 135–143). Itasca, IL: Riverside.

Brown, L., Sherbenou, R. J., & Johnsen, S. K. (1997). *Test of Nonverbal Intelligence—Third Edition.* Austin, TX: Pro-Ed.

Brown, R. T., Reynolds, C. R., & Whitaker, J. S. (1999). Bias in mental testing since *Bias in Mental Testing. School Psychology Quarterly, 14,* 208–238.

Carpenter, P. A., Just, M. A., & Shell, P. (1990). What one intelligence test measures: A theoretical account of the processing in the Raven Progressive Matrices Test. *Psychological Review, 97*(3), 404–431.

Carroll, J. B. (1993). *Human cognitive abilities: A survey of factor-analytic studies.* New York: Cambridge University Press.

Flanagan, D. P., & Ortiz, S. O. (2002). Best practices in intellectual assessment: Future directions. In A. Thomas, & J. P. Grimes (Eds.), *Best practices in school psychology IV* (pp. 1351–1372). Bethesda, MD: National Association of School Psychologists.

Ford, L., & Braden, J. P. (1996, August). *Equitable psychological assessment for language-minority learners: Theory, research, and practice.* Symposium presented at the annual meeting of the American Psychological Association, Toronto.

Frisby, C. L. (2003). Nonverbal assessment of academic achievement with special populations. In R. S. McCallum (Ed.), *Handbook of nonverbal assessment* (pp. 241–258). New York: Kluwer Academic/Plenum.

Gustafsson, J. E. (1988). Hierarchical models of individual differences in cognitive abilities. In R. J. Sternberg (Ed.), *Advances in the psychology of human intelligence* (Vol. 4, pp. 35–71). Hillsdale, NJ: Erlbaum.

Hammill, D. D., Pearson, N. A., & Wiederholt, J. L. (1997). *Comprehensive Test of Nonverbal Intelligence.* Austin, TX: Pro-Ed.

Harris, A. M., Reynolds, M. A., & Koegel, H. M. (1996). Nonverbal assessment: Multicultural perspectives. In L. A. Suzuki, P. J. Meller, & J. G. Ponterotto (Eds.), *Handbook of multicultural assessment: Clinical, psychological, and educational applications* (pp. 223–252). San Francisco: Jossey-Bass.

Helms, J. E. (1997). The triple quandary of race, culture, and social class in standardized cognitive ability testing. In D. P. Flanagan, J. L. Genshaft, & P. L. Harrison (Eds.), *Contemporary intellectual assessment: Theories, tests, and issues* (pp. 517–532). New York: Guilford Press.

Horn, J. L., & Noll, J. (1997). Human cognitive capabilities: Theoretical perspectives. In D. P. Flanagan, J. L. Genshaft, & P. L. Harrison (Eds.), *Contemporary intellectual assessment: Theories, tests, and issues* (pp. 53–91). New York: Guilford Press.

Jensen, A. R. (1980). *Bias in mental testing.* New York: Free Press.

Kamphaus, R. W., Petoskey, M. D, & Morgan, A. W. (1997). A history of intelligence test interpretation. In D. P. Flanagan, J. L. Genshaft, & P. A. Harrison (Eds.), *Contemporary intellectual assessment: Theories, tests, and issues* (pp. 32–47). New York: Guilford Press.

Kelly, M., & Braden, J. P. (1990). Criterion-related validity of the WISC-R Performance scale with the Stanford Achievement Test—Hearing Impaired Edition. *Journal of School Psychology, 28,* 147–151.

Lopez, E. C. (1997). The cognitive assessment of limited English proficient and bilingual children. In D. P. Flanagan, J. L. Genshaft, & P. L. Harrison (Eds.), *Contemporary intellectual assessment: Theories, tests, and issues* (pp. 503–516). New York: Guilford Press.

Maller, S. J. (2003). Best practices in detecting bias in nonverbal tests. In R. S. McCallum (Ed.), *Handbook of nonverbal assessment* (pp. 23–62). New York: Kluwer Academic/Plenum.

McCallum, R. S. (2003). Context for nonverbal assessment of intelligence and related abilities. In R. S. McCallum (Ed.), *Handbook of nonverbal assessment* (pp. 3–22). New York: Kluwer Academic/Plenum.

McCallum, R. S., Bracken, B. A., & Wasserman, J. D. (2001). *Essentials of nonverbal assessment.* New York: Wiley.

McGrew, K. S., & Flanagan, D. P. (1998). *The intelligence test desk reference (ITDR): Gf-Gc cross-battery assessment.* Boston: Allyn & Bacon.

Messick, S. (1995). Validity of psychological assessment. *American Psychologist, 50*(9), 741–749.

Naglieri, J. A. (2003). *Naglieri Nonverbal Ability Test—*

Individual Administration. San Antonio, TX: Psychological Corporation.

Naglieri, J. A., & Bardos, A. N. (1997). *General Ability Measure for Adults.* Minneapolis, MN: National Computer Systems.

Petti, V. L., Voelker, S. L., Shore, D. L., & Hayman-Abello, S. E. (2003). Perception of nonverbal emotion cues by children with nonverbal learning disabilities. *Journal of Developmental and Physical Disabilities, 15*(1), 23–36.

Puente, A. E., & Salazar, G. D. (1998). Assessment of minority and culturally diverse children. In A. Prifitera & D. H. Saklofske (Eds.), *WISC-III clinical use and interpretation* (pp. 227–248). San Diego, CA: Academic Press.

Reynolds, C. R., & Kaiser, S. M. (1990). Test bias in psychological assessment. In C. R. Reynolds & T. B. Gutkin (Eds.), *Handbook of school psychology* (2nd ed., pp. 487–525). New York: Wiley.

Roid, G. H. (2003). *Stanford–Binet Intelligence Scales, Fifth Edition.* Itasca, IL: Riverside.

Roid, G. H., & Miller, L. J. (1997). *Leiter International Performance Scale—Revised.* Wood Dale, IL: Stoelting.

Rourke, B. P. (2000). Neuropsychological and psychosocial subtyping: A review of investigations within the University of Windsor laboratory. *Canadian Psychology, 41*(1), 34–51.

Rourke, B. P., Ahmad, S. A., Collins, D. W., Hayman-Abello, B. A., Hayman-Abello, S. E., & Warriner, E. M. (2002). Child clinical/pediatric neuropsychology: Some recent advances. *Annual Review of Psychology, 53*(1), 309–339.

Salvia, J., & Ysseldyke, J. E. (2001). *Assessment* (8th ed.). Boston: Houghton Mifflin.

Sattler, J. M. (2001). *Assessment of children: Cognitive applications* (4th ed.). San Diego, CA: Author

Seguin, E. (1907). *Idiocy and its treatment by the psychological method.* New York: Teachers College, Columbia University.

Vernon, M., & Andrews, J. F. (1990). *The psychology of deafness: Understanding deaf and hard-of-hearing people.* New York: Longman.

Wasserman, J. D., & Lawhorn, R. M. (2003). Nonverbal neuropsychological assessment. In R. S. McCallum (Ed.), *Handbook of nonverbal assessment* (pp. 315–360). New York: Kluwer Academic/Plenum.

Weber-Byars, A. M., McKellop, M., Gyato, K., Sullivan, T., & Franz, D. N. (2001). Metachromitic leukodystrophy and nonverbal learning disability: Neuropsychological and neuroradiological findings in heterozygous carriers. *Child Neuropsychology, 7*(1), 54–58.

Whorf, B. L. (2002). Languages and logic. In D. J. Levitin (Ed.), *Foundations of cognitive psychology: Core readings* (pp. 707–715). Cambridge, MA: MIT Press. (Original work published 1956)

Wilhoit, B. E., & McCallum, R. S. (2003). Cross-battery assessment of nonverbal cognitive ability. In R. S. McCallum (Ed.), *Handbook of nonverbal assessment* (pp. 63–86). New York: Kluwer Academic/Plenum.

Woodcock, R. W., McGrew, K. S., & Mather, N. (2001). *Woodcock–Johnson III Tests of Achievement.* Itasca, IL: Riverside.

VI

Emerging Issues
and New Directions
in Intellectual Assessment

The book concludes with a section devoted to emerging and future issues related to intelligence tests. In Chapter 27, "Using Confirmatory Factor Analysis to Aid in Understanding the Constructs Measured by Intelligence Tests," Timothy Z. Keith provides comprehensive information regarding the use of confirmatory factor analysis in development of intelligence tests and interpretation of their results. Jeffery P. Braden and Bradley C. Niebling are authors of Chapter 28, "Evaluating the Validity Evidence for Intelligence Tests Using the Joint Test Standards." This chapter provides a detailed and logical analysis of the latest *Standards for Educational and Psychological Testing*, as well as an evaluation of the extent to which major intelligence tests meet the 24 validity standards.

Rachel Brown-Chidsey wrote Chapter 29, "Intelligence Tests in an Era of Standards-Based Educational Reform." Her chapter concludes the book with a presentation of the use of cognitive ability tests within educational settings; it provides a method for understanding intelligence tests in settings that are now required to focus on accountability, outcomes, and achievement of learning standards.

27

Using Confirmatory Factor Analysis to Aid in Understanding the Constructs Measured by Intelligence Tests

TIMOTHY Z. KEITH

Factor analysis is inexorably linked with the development of intelligence theory and intelligence tests. Early intelligence theories and factor-analytic methods were developed in tandem, and the connection continues to this day. Carroll's (1993) three-stratum theory of intelligence was developed in part through the use of *exploratory factor analysis* (EFA).

Until recently, the term *factor analysis* has meant what is now called EFA. In its simplest form, EFA involves making a series of decisions about the method of factor extraction to use, the number of factors to retain, and the method of rotation to use. For researchers who do not wish to make these decisions, most computer programs will default to a common method if none is specified (not always a wise choice). The output from the analysis consists of factor loadings of each variable on each factor and, if an oblique rotation was used, correlations among the factors. The researcher then assigns names to the factors based on the loadings of the variables on the factors, along with relevant theory and previous research.

Of course, in the hands of an expert, EFA can be much more complex and elegant than the simple approach just described. A variety of extraction methods can be used, depending on the questions of interest; complex decision rules and expert judgment can be used to determine how many factors should be extracted; and a variety of graphic and mathematical methods can be used to rotate the extracted factors to simple structure. For example, Carroll (1993, Ch. 3) outlined an approach to EFA that was an elegant combination of consistency and judgment. Whether simple or complex, EFA involves judgment on the part of the researcher: judgment concerning the decisions required, and judgment concerning the meaning of the extracted factors. It is this aspect of EFA that can be disconcerting to those wanting yes–no answers to questions, but it is also this requirement for thought that makes the approach so alluring and so powerful.

In its simplest form, *confirmatory factor analysis* (CFA) requires the researcher to decide, in advance, the nature of the factor structure underlying the data. He or she must specify the number of factors and the variables that load on each factor. So, for example, the researcher may specify that variable 1 loads on factor 1, but not on factor 2. The researcher may specify that factors are correlated, or may specify that they are uncorrelated. The results of the analysis provide *fit statistics*, which provide feedback as to the adequacy of the specified factor structure, or the degree to which the *model* (factor structure) *fits* the data (reproduces the covariances among the data). In CFA, in other words, the researcher tests the adequacy of a particular factor structure by restricting the factor solution (thus the method is sometimes called *restricted factor analysis*; Allen & Thorndike, 1995) and seeing whether that restricted solution is consistent with the data. In contrast, in EFA, the researcher examines and imparts meaning to the best factor structure (given the decision rules used).

CFA is often described as a more theory-driven approach than EFA. This assertion probably involves some overstatement. It is possible, for example, to use EFA in a theory-driven, hypothesis-testing manner (see Thorndike, 1990), just as it is possible to use CFA in a very exploratory, theory-absent manner. Indeed, Jöreskog and Sörbom (1993, p. 115) have argued that a combination exploratory–confirmatory "model-generating" approach is probably the most common approach to structural equation modeling (SEM) and CFA. Nevertheless, the simple fact that CFA requires the specification of a model—and thus knowledge about the probable structure of the characteristic being measured—means that some sort of theory (formal or informal, strong or weak) is required. EFA can easily be conducted in the absence of theory, although theoretically driven analyses are almost invariably more complete and informative than atheoretical ones. EFA can be a valuable tool for *developing* theory, whereas CFA may be better suited for *testing* existing theory. A combination of the two methods can also be quite valuable (e.g., Carroll, 2003).

This chapter demonstrates the use of CFA, with particular attention to using CFA to understand the constructs measured by modern intelligence tests. It begins with a "simple" CFA model, and gradually moves to CFA methods that provide a more complete evaluation of the theories underlying tests (e.g., hierarchical analysis, the comparison of alternative models, multisample analyses). It demonstrates how the method can be used to test formal theories as well. The emphasis is on the use of CFA to *test hypotheses* about *theories*.

There are a number of computer programs available that conduct CFA. These programs are designed to conduct latent-variable SEM; SEM includes and subsumes CFA (the *measurement model*, in the jargon of SEM), and thus SEM programs also conduct CFA. The oldest and most widely known program is LISREL (LInear Structural RELations; Jöreskog & Sörbom, 1996); extensive information about the program is available at *http://www.ssicentral.com*. Other common programs include EQS (Bentler, 1995; Bentler & Wu, 1995; *http://www.mvsoft.com*) and Mplus (Muthén & Muthén, 1998; *http://www.statmodel.com*). The analyses presented in this chapter were conducted with Amos (Analysis of MOment Structures; Arbuckle, 2003; *http://www.spss.com/amos*). Amos uses a sophisticated drawing program and provides pictorial input and output of models. The figures in this chapter were drawn with Amos, and the graphic output shown was produced by the Amos program. The journal *Structural Equation Modeling* publishes reviews of these and other SEM/CFA programs (e.g., Hox, 1995).

A SAMPLE CONFIRMATORY ANALYSIS

The Kaufman Adult and Adolescent Intelligence Test (KAIT) is a measure of cognitive abilities for adolescents and adults ages 11 through adulthood (Kaufman & Kaufman, 1993). According to the manual, the KAIT is designed to measure intelligence according to the Cattell–Horn theory of intelligence, although only two of the Cattell–Horn factors are included in the KAIT model (*fluid intelligence*, also known as *novel reasoning*, and *crystallized intelligence*, also known as *comprehension–knowledge*). In addition, the KAIT is designed to measure *delayed recall*, or a person's memory for material learned earlier in the test. Thus the KAIT includes 10 subtests designed to measure three abilities: fluid intelligence (Gf), crystallized intelligence (Gc), and delayed recall.

Figure 27.1 shows this "theory" of the KAIT in figural form. The 10 subtests are shown in rectangles, and the abilities they are designed to measure are enclosed in ovals. Arrows or paths point from the abilities to the subtests, in recognition of the implicit assumption that the abilities residing within a person are what cause him or her to

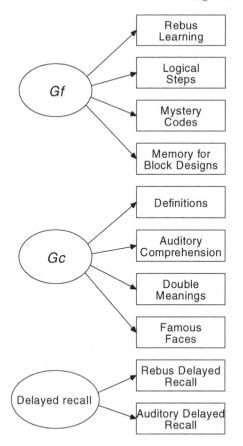

FIGURE 27.1. Theoretical structure of the KAIT.

tallized intelligence, as indicated by the path drawn from Gc to Double Meanings. At a practical level, the path from Gc to Double Meanings means that the factor loading will be estimated in the analysis, and the lack of the path from Gf to Double Meanings means that the factor loading of Double Meanings on Gf will be constrained to 0.

Figure 27.2 includes information beyond that included in Figure 27.1. The curved, two-headed arrows between factors represent covariances (or, in the standardized output, correlations). Although the KAIT manual does not say so explicitly, it is reasonable to expect that the abilities measured by the KAIT are not independent of (uncorrelated with) one another. Modern intelligence theories recognize this relation among factors (e.g., Carroll, 1993, Chs. 2–3), and CFAs of intelligence tests should generally specify correlated factors (unless the theory underlying the tests maintains that the factors are independent). The figure also includes small ovals, labeled u1 through u10, with paths drawn to each of the subtests. The factors are not the only cause of a person's scores on

score a certain way on a subtest. So, for example, examinees' levels of fluid intelligence are the primary determinant of their scores on the Mystery Codes subtest.

Figure 27.1 is also the beginning of a confirmatory factor model; a more complete CFA model is shown in Figure 27.2.[1] In the jargon of CFA, the variables enclosed in rectangles (the subtests) are the *measured variables*, whereas the variables enclosed in ovals (e.g., the KAIT abilities) are *unmeasured variables*, or *latent variables*, or *factors*. The paths from latent to measured variables represent the factor loadings. Notice that not all possible paths are drawn. Theoretically, the lack of a path from, say, Gf to Double Meanings means that the test authors believe that Double Meanings does not measure fluid intelligence, or that a person's level of fluid intelligence does not affect his or her scores on the Double Meanings subtest. Rather, scores on Double Meanings are a reflection of crys-

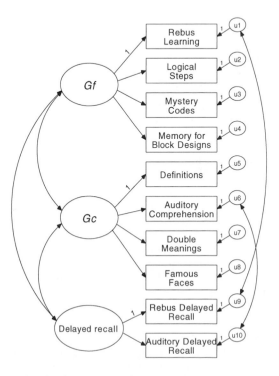

FIGURE 27.2. A confirmatory factor model of the structure of the KAIT.

the subtest; each subtest is also partially the result of other influences that are unique to each subtest, generally called *unique* or *specific variances* (see Keith & Reynolds, 2003). In addition, each subtest is also affected by errors of measurement (*error variance*). These unique and error variances, combined, are represented by u1 through u10; they are enclosed in ovals because they are unmeasured. These unique and error variances are hereafter termed *unique variances*, although they are referred to by a variety of names in the literature, including *errors* and *residuals*.

Several of the paths in Figure 27.2 have the value 1 beside them. The measured variables in the model have a defined scale, and that scale is whatever scale was used for each subtest (e.g., a raw score from 0 to 23). But none of the unmeasured variables (neither the factors nor the unique variances) have a predetermined scale. The 1's beside paths serve the purpose of setting the scales of the unmeasured variables by setting the path to 1.0. The path of 1.0 from Gf to Rebus Learning, for example, sets the scale of the Gf factor to be the same as the scale for Rebus Learning. Thus each factor includes one factor loading of 1.0, and the paths from each of the unique variances to the measured variables are set to 1.0 (to set the scale to be the same as the corresponding measured variable). The use of 1.0 is arbitrary—any value could be used—and once all of the parameters of the model are estimated with these constraints (called the *unstandardized* or *metric solution*), all values are restandardized (the *standardized solution*).

Finally, the model in Figure 27.2 includes a less common characteristic: correlations among the unique variances, as represented by the curved lines connecting several of the unique variances (e.g., u1 and u9). The Rebus Delayed Recall test on the KAIT requires examinees to remember rebuses learned earlier in the test for the Rebus Learning subtest. Since Rebus Delayed Recall builds on Rebus Learning, it seems likely that the unique variances affecting Rebus Delayed Recall will be related to those affecting Rebus Learning. Similarly, the *error* variances affecting Rebus Delayed Recall may well be related to those affecting Rebus Learning. These possibilities are built into the CFA model by specifying that the unique

variances of the Rebus Delayed Recall and Rebus Learning subtests are allowed to correlate.

The KAIT standardization data were used to estimate the model. The KAIT manual includes correlation matrices of subtests for the KAIT at each age level, along with an average correlation matrix for the entire sample (Kaufman & Kaufman, 1993, p. 136). The matrix and standard deviations for the entire standardization sample were used as input for the Amos computer program (Arbuckle, 2003). The average sample size ($N = 143$) for the different age groups was used as the sample size.

The results of the analysis are shown in Figure 27.3. First, notice the fit statistics for the model in the lower left of the figure. The model is *overidentified*, meaning that many more parameters could have been estimated in the model (e.g., the path from Gf to Definitions was set to 0, as were many other paths). In an overidentified model, the number of parameters estimated is less than the number of covariances used in estimation. As a result, the model has *degrees of free-*

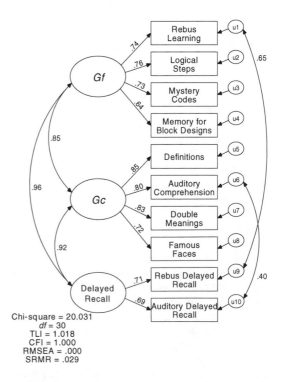

FIGURE 27.3. Results of a CFA of the structure of the KAIT.

dom. Degrees of freedom are an index of the degree of overidentification of a model; they are not, as in most other statistical analyses, related to the sample size. It is also possible to conduct the analysis in reverse: to estimate the correlation or covariance matrix from the solved model. But because the model is overidentified, the estimates of the covariances will not be identical to the covariance matrix used to estimate the model in the first place (see Kline, 1998, Ch. 5, for a discussion of overidentification). The fit statistics shown in the figure are all measures of the degree to which the matrix *implied* by the model differs from the *actual* matrix used to estimate the model.

Five fit statistics are shown in the figure, although there are dozens to choose from. Chi-square (χ^2) is the most commonly reported fit statistic. It has the advantage of allowing a statistical test of the fit of the model; it can be used with the degrees of freedom to determine the probability that the model is, in some sense, "correct." Thus a large χ^2 in comparison to the *df* (and a small probability—e.g., $p < .05$) suggests that the actual and implied covariance matrices are statistically significantly different, that the model provides a poor fit to the data, or that the model could not have produced the data. The model therefore is not a good representation of the "true" factor structure. In contrast, a small χ^2 in comparison to the *df* is statistically insignificant ($p > .05$), and suggests that the model does provide a reasonable explanation of the data.

Although χ^2 fits well within the tradition of significance testing in psychology, it also has well-known problems (as does the tradition of either–or significance testing itself; cf. Cohen, 1994). In particular, it is directly related to sample size, so that with large samples, virtually all χ^2s will be significant, even when the model is only trivially incorrect (see Tanaka, 1993, among others, for further discussion). With small samples, even inadequate models may have a good fit, as judged by χ^2. For this and other reasons, other fit statistics have been developed; the ones listed for this analysis were chosen because they highlight different dimensions of fit, and have shown promise in simulation studies (Fan, Thompson, & Wang, 1999; Hu & Bentler, 1998, 1999). The *Tucker–Lewis in-*

dex (TLI) and the *comparative fit index* (CFI) both compare the fit of the model with that of a "null" model, one in which the measured variables are assumed to be unrelated. The TLI appears to be relatively unrelated to sample size, whereas the CFI is designed to estimate the fit in the population. For both, values of .95 or greater suggest a good fit of the model to the data (Hu & Bentler, 1999), with values above .90 suggesting an adequate fit.

One criticism of χ^2 is that it is a measure of the exact fit of the model to the data, whereas at best, models are designed to *approximate* reality. The *root mean square error of approximation* (RMSEA) is therefore a measure of approximate fit. Smaller values suggest a better fit, with values of .06 or smaller suggesting a good fit (Hu & Bentler, 1999) and those of approximately .08 suggesting an adequate fit (Browne & Cudeck, 1993). Finally, the *standardized root mean square residual* (SRMR) may be one of the more intuitively appealing measures of fit. Recall that fit indices are derived from the similarity or dissimilarity between the actual covariance matrix used to estimate the model and the matrix implied by the model. The *root mean square residual* (RMR) represents the average of these differences, and the SRMR the *standardized* average of these differences. Because a standardized covariance is a correlation, the SRMR, therefore, represents the average difference in the actual *correlations* among the measured variables and those implied by the model. Values of .08 or less suggest little difference in the two matrices (Hu & Bentler, 1999).

Briefly, all of the fit statistics suggest that the KAIT model provides an excellent fit to the standardization data. χ^2 is small and statistically insignificant ($p = .668$); the TLI and CFI are large; and both the RMSEA and the SRMR are quite small. Thus the "theory" underlying the KAIT appears to fit the KAIT standardization data; the test appears to measure what the authors designed it to measure; and the structure of the KAIT appears valid. The next step, then, is to interpret the substantive results.

The paths from latent to measured variables show the factor loadings. They are all large, and examination of their standard errors and *t* values (shown in the detailed printout, but not included in the figure) shows that they are all statistically significant. Likewise, the factor correlations are large and statistically significant, ranging from .96 for the correlation between the latent delayed-recall and Gf factors to .85 between Gf and Gc. Finally, the correlations among unique variances suggests that there is a substantial correlation between the variance of the Rebus Learning test that is not accounted for by the Gf factor and the variance of the Rebus Delayed Recall subtest that is not accounted for by the delayed-recall factor (r = .65). Similarly, the unique and error variances of Auditory Comprehension and Auditory Delayed Recall are substantially correlated as well.

These substantive results are also generally supportive of the validity of the KAIT. One curious finding, however, is that the correlations between the delayed-recall factor and the Gf and Gc factors (.96 and .92, respectively) are higher than the correlation between the two more intellectual factors, Gf and Gc (.85). Such a finding could be investigated by comparing this model with alternative models, as shown below.

An Alternative Method of Specifying Factor Models

Before the comparison of competing alternative models is discussed, it is worth illustrating an alternative method of specifying factor models. The previous model set the scale of the latent factors by fixing a single factor loading from each factor to 1.0. An alternative is to fix the *factor variances* to 1.0, and then estimate all factor loadings; a KAIT model using this method is shown in Figure 27.4. This procedure has advantages over the method of fixing a factor loading. When the factor variances are set to 1, the factor covariances in the unstandardized solution are in fact correlations. Because constraints to models are made in the unstandardized metric, when one is using this method it is possible to set factor correlations to 1, or 0, or some other value to see what this constraint does to the fit of the model (this procedure is used in several subsequent examples). It is also often easier to make constraints in factor loadings when one is using this method. With hierarchical models (to be discussed below), however, only the highest factor level can use this alternative method.

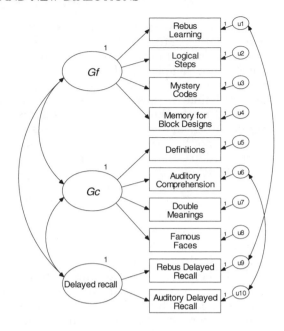

FIGURE 27.4. An alternative method of specifying factor models. Factor variances rather than factor loadings are set to 1 to set the scale of the factors.

The results of the analysis of the model shown in Figure 27.4 are identical to those shown in Figure 27.3, and will not be repeated here. It is worth noting, however, that this method can occasionally produce slightly different estimates than the set-factor-loading method (Millsap, 2001).

COMPARING ALTERNATIVE MODELS

The previous section has presented the basics of CFA, but has also presented a fairly sterile approach: the simple rejection of or support for a single model. Such an approach is problematic. The simple fact that a model does or does not fit the data provides only partial support for the validity of a test or theory. A model may fit the data well, but there may be other, competing models that fit the data as well or better. Or a given model may provide an inadequate fit to the data, but may be the best model among the alternatives. Formal or informal theory may suggest several possible models to explain the test scores we observe; if all fit the data well, how are we to decide which is the *best* model? What is needed is the ability to compare competing models, or to compare a target model with one or several alternative models. "At best, a given model represents a tentative explanation of the data. The confidence with which one accepts such an explanation depends, in part, on whether other, rival explanations have been tested and found wanting" (Loehlin, 1998, p. 63).

Fortunately, fit statistics can be used to compare competing models as well. If two models are *nested*—that is, if one model can be derived from another by placing additional constraints on the model—then the χ^2 for the two models can be compared. The χ^2 for the less constrained model (the model with smaller *df* and smaller χ^2) can be subtracted from the χ^2 for the more constrained model. The χ^2 difference ($\Delta\chi^2$) can then be compared to the change in degrees of freedom (Δdf) to determine whether the relaxation in the model results in a statistically significant decrease in χ^2. If the $\Delta\chi^2$ is not statistically significant—if one model is not significantly better than another—then, as scientists, we generally prefer the more *parsimonious* (more constrained) model. If the $\Delta\chi^2$ is statistically significant, then the less parsimonious model is preferred. Parsimony is reflected in CFA models by *df*; the larger the *df*, the more constraints in the model, and therefore the more parsimonious the model.

The *Akaike information criterion* (AIC) is another useful measure for comparing competing models, and does not require that the models be nested. The AIC is generally not interpreted in isolation; rather, the AICs for two or more competing models are compared, with the smaller AIC suggesting the better model. Other, related fit indices include the *Bayes information criterion* (BIC), and *Browne–Cudeck criterion* (BCC). Likewise, the other fit statistics already discussed may be compared across models, although such comparison is generally a subjective one rather than a test of significance. Finally, a highly constrained "baseline" model may be used instead of a null model in the calculation of fit indices such as TLI and CFI. For example, a one-factor *g* model may provide a useful baseline model in CFAs of intelligence tests (Humphreys, 1990). Of course, with these alternative baseline models, the resulting values will generally not approach the .95 cutoff recommended for these fit statistics when null models are used.

Comparing Alternative Models for the KAIT

Figure 27.3 displays the results of an initial CFA of the KAIT. The model fits the data well, and thus the model seems a good explanation of the KAIT standardization data. Nevertheless, questions concerning the structure, as displayed, are also reasonable. Since, for example, Rebus Delayed Recall asks examinees to recall material first learned in the Rebus Learning test, isn't Rebus Delayed Recall also a measure of Gf? Similarly, is Auditory Delayed Recall also a measure of Gc in addition to Delayed Recall? And why does the delayed-recall factor correlate so highly with Gf and Gc? If it is indeed a measure of delayed recall, shouldn't it correlate at a lower level with these highly intellectual factors than they do with each other?

Figure 27.5 shows a model that tests the first two of these questions: whether the Rebus and Auditory Delayed Recall subtests also measure Gf and Gc abilities. In addition to allowing RDR to load on the delayed-recall factor, it has also been allowed to load on the Gf factor; Auditory Delayed Recall loads on both the delayed recall and the Gc factors. Otherwise, the model shown in Figure 27.5 is the same as that shown in Figure 27.4, with one exception: For the model to be properly identified, some sort of additional constraint is required for the two Delayed Recall subtests. To allow estimation, the factor loadings for these two subtests on the delayed-recall factor have been constrained to be equal.[2]

The results of this analysis are also shown in the figure. Like the earlier model, this variation provides an excellent fit to the averaged standardization data. But does the model provide any better fit than the structure as intended by the authors? The χ^2 for the model is 15.779 for Figure 27.5 versus 20.031 for Figure 27.3. As shown in Table 27.1, the change in χ^2 is 4.232, which, given the change in *df* (Δdf = 1), is statistically significant ($p < .05$). Thus, specifying that the Rebus and Auditory Delayed Recall subtests measure Gf and Gc in addition to delayed recall leads to a statistically significant improvement in fit; Figure 27.5 may be a better explanation of the structure of the KAIT than Figures 27.3 and 27.4. The AIC shown in Figure 27.5 (67.799) is also smaller than

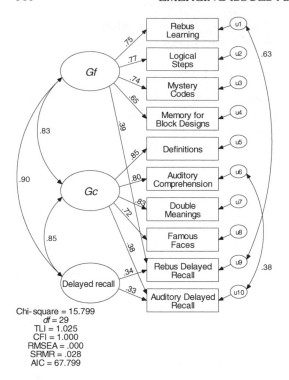

Chi-square = 15.799
df = 29
TLI = 1.025
CFI = 1.000
RMSEA = .000
SRMR = .028
AIC = 67.799

FIGURE 27.5. An alternative model of the structure of the KAIT. Rebus Delayed Recall and Auditory Delayed Recall are assumed to measure Gf and Gc, respectively, in addition to delayed recall ability.

the AIC for the models shown in Figures 27.3 and 27.4 (70.031); this also suggests that the model shown in Figure 27.5 is a better explanation of the structure of the KAIT than are the earlier models.

But what about substantive interpretation? With the changes in the model, it appears that Rebus Delayed Recall is a slightly better measure of Gf than it is of delayed recall, although it provides a strong measure of neither ability. Likewise, Auditory Delayed Recall appears as good, or slightly better, as

a measure of Gc as it is of delayed recall, but appears a strong measure of neither ability. As in Figure 27.3, the delayed-recall factor correlates with the Gf and Gc factors as highly as or more highly than they correlate with each other, suggesting that a more intellectually laden name might be more appropriate (e.g., Glr, or *long-term storage and retrieval*).

Given the small paths from delayed recall to the Rebus and Auditory Delayed Recall subtests in Figure 27.5, it is reasonable to ask whether these two subtests should be considered measures of fluid and crystallized ability only, and not measures of delayed recall. The results of the test of such a model are shown in Figure 27.6. This model is more constrained than the model shown in Figure 27.5, so the question of interest now becomes whether these constraints on the model result in a statistically significantly *worse* fit to the data over the model in Figure 27.5.[3]

The fit statistics suggest that the model in Figure 27.6 provides as good a fit to the data as does that in Figure 27.5: The change in χ^2 is not statistically significant (see Table 27.1). The model in Figure 27.6 is more parsimonious, but with an equivalent fit to Figure 27.5; the more parsimonious model is preferred. Likewise, the AIC suggests a better fit for the model in Figure 27.6.

The substantive interpretation of the model in Figure 27.6 is straightforward. The Rebus and Auditory Delayed Recall subtests provide measures of Gf and Gc abilities, respectively, that are almost as strong as the tests intended to measure those abilities.

The model shown in Figure 27.6 can also be compared to the one in Figure 27.3. Although the two models appear to fit the data equally well, the model in Figure 27.6 is a more parsimonious explanation of the data. Taken together, these comparisons of models

TABLE 27.1. Comparison of Various CFA Models of the KAIT

Model (Figure no.)	χ^2 (df)	$\Delta\chi^2(\Delta df)^a$	p	TLI	CFI	SRMR	AIC
Actual structure (Figure 27.3)	20.031(30)			1.018	1.000	.029	70.031
Delayed recall and Gf-Gc (Figure 27.5)	15.799 (29)	4.232(1)	.0397	1.025	1.000	.028	67.799
Gf-Gc (Figure 27.6)	19.158(32)	3.359(3)	.3395	1.022	1.000	.032	65.158
Subtests affect delayed recall (Figure 27.7)	15.833(30)			1.026	1.000	.028	65.833

^{a}All comparisons are with the preceding model.

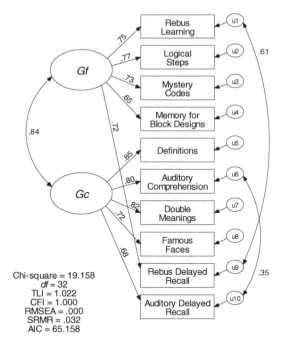

Chi-square = 19.158
df = 32
TLI = 1.022
CFI = 1.000
RMSEA = .000
SRMR = .032
AIC = 65.158

FIGURE 27.6. Another alternative model of the structure of the KAIT. The two Delayed Recall subtests (Rebus and Auditory) are assumed to measure Gf and Gc, not a separate delayed recall ability.

are not definitive, but do suggest that the Rebus and Auditory Delayed Recall subtests of the KAIT should be considered additional measures of the abilities measured by the two primary KAIT scales (Fluid and Crystallized), rather than measures of learning or delayed recall.

One final model is discussed before another topic is raised. In the models shown so far, the presumed overlap between the delayed recall tests and the nondelayed versions of the tests (i.e., Rebus Learning and Auditory Comprehension) was modeled using correlated error terms. This is a common method of dealing with such overlap, but is not the only way of doing so. It is not simply the case that performances on the two Delayed Recall subtests *share* unique and error variance with the tests from which they were derived. Rather, performances on these two tests should depend, in part, on how well the material was learned when first presented. Thus, in addition to being affected by delayed recall, Gf, and Gc, these two tests should also be *affected* by their original

versions. Figure 27.7 shows a model that embodies this reasoning, by having Rebus Learning affect Rebus Delayed Recall and having Auditory Comprehension affect Auditory Delayed Recall. As shown in this figure and in Table 27.1, this model fits the data quite well. The model is not nested with the other models, and thus the $\Delta\chi^2$ test is not appropriate (and is not shown). Judging by the AIC, this model fit better than most of the other models shown. Note the strong effect of Rebus Learning on Rebus Delayed Recall, and the moderate effect of Auditory Comprehension on Auditory Delayed Recall.

The only model that fits better than that shown in Figure 27.7 is the model in Figure 27.6. Although not shown, a version of Figure 27.7 in which Rebus and Auditory Delayed Recall load on Gf and Gc (with no delayed-recall factor) has the same fit and *df* as Figure 27.6. These, then, are equivalent models—models that cannot be evaluated on

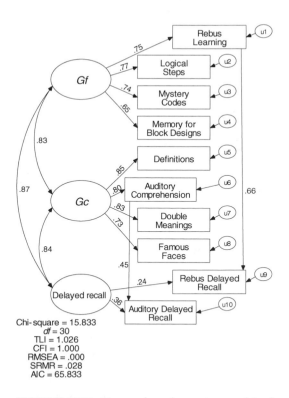

Chi-square = 15.833
df = 30
TLI = 1.026
CFI = 1.000
RMSEA = .000
SRMR = .028
AIC = 65.833

FIGURE 27.7. Yet another alternative model of the structure of the KAIT. The Rebus Learning and Auditory Comprehension tests are assumed to *affect* performance on the subsequent Rebus Delayed Recall and Auditory Delayed Recall tests.

the basis of fit. It is always worth considering alternative models to one's preferred model; other sources (Keith, in press; Kline, 1998) demonstrate rules for generating equivalent, alternative models. Before turning to the next topic, I simply note that these models are not an exhaustive examination of the structure of the KAIT; there are other plausible models from other perspectives (see, e.g., Cole & Randall, 2003; Flanagan & McGrew, 1998).

HIERARCHICAL CFA

Many modern theories of intelligence recognize an ability that is more general and broader than the specific abilities tested in first-order CFA. This ability is often considered to subsume, affect, or partially cause the more narrow abilities, and is often symbolized as g, for *general ability* or *general intelligence*. For example, Carroll's (1993) three-stratum theory of intelligence includes g as the most general, highest-order factor. Although it is conceptually similar to Spearman's g, most modern theories assume that g is a *hierarchical* ability (cf. Burt, 1949; Vernon, 1950). Most modern intelligence *tests* also tacitly recognize such a general, overall ability by summing subtests or subscales into an overall score. Although this general score may go by a variety of names—Full Scale IQ, General Cognitive Ability, or General Intellectual Ability—it generally represents an overall, general, summative ability.

If a general ability is recognized in formal theory and through the informal theory of the scoring of intelligence tests, it would also be valuable to test such a construct through CFA. One common approach has been to specify a single-factor model, such as the one shown in Figure 27.8 (a g-model version of the Wechsler Intelligence Scale for Children—Fourth Edition [WISC-IV]). Such a model suggests that scores on the individual subtests are a product of a general factor and of unique and error variances. Although such an approach is fairly common (see Psychological Corporation, 2003), and mirrors to some degree the common practice of isolating a g factor in EFA by examining the unrotated first factor in principal-components analysis, it is also an unsatisfying solu-

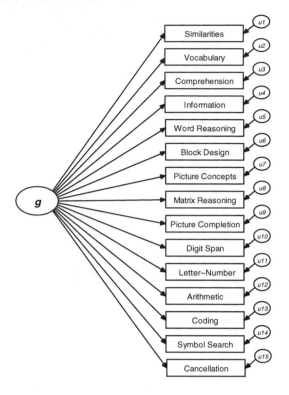

FIGURE 27.8. A general intelligence, or g, model of the structure of cognitive abilities as assessed by the WISC-IV. The model assumes that the WISC-IV tests are reflections of general intelligence only, rather than more specific, shared abilities, such as verbal or perceptual abilities.

tion for several reasons. First, g is generally recognized as a *hierarchical* factor; a more realistic structure for the tests from Figure 27.8 is shown in Figure 27.9, in which the subtests are explained (in part) by first-order factors (corresponding to the four Indexes of the WISC-IV), and the first-order factors are in turn partially explained by a second-order g factor.

Second, if Figure 27.9 represents the *true* structure of the abilities measured by the six hypothetical tests, then Figure 27.8 represents an inadequate test of the second-order g factor. The presence of first-order factors means that the WISC-IV Verbal Comprehension tests measure something in common other than general intelligence; the Perceptual Reasoning tests measure something in common other than g; and so on. To reiterate, Figure 27.8 represents an inadequate test of a higher-order g factor.

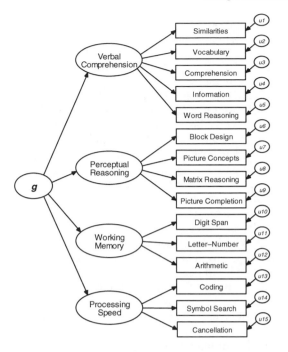

FIGURE 27.9. A hierarchical model of the structure of the WISC-IV. The model assumes that the subtests are explained in part by first-order abilities (e.g., Verbal Comprehension), and that these first-order factors are in turn partially explained by *g*.

Figure 27.10 shows a hierarchical model of the structure of the Differential Ability Scales (DAS; Elliott, 1990a).[4] In scoring the DAS, the "core" subtests (Word Definitions through Recall of Designs in the figure) are added together to form Verbal, Nonverbal Reasoning, and Spatial scores, and the Verbal, Nonverbal, and Spatial scores are added together to form a General Cognitive Ability score. Thus the core subtests are designed to measure both a *general* ability and more specific abilities. The informal theory underlying the test is clearly hierarchical in nature. Although Recall of Digits and Recall of Objects are not treated in the same manner, they could be classified as measuring memory skills, which also are affected by general intelligence. Thus a fourth first-order factor (Memory) is included in the figure. The Speed of Information Processing subtest is not included in these analyses.

The figure is quite similar to the general hierarchical model from Figure 27.9, except for the presence of small ovals (uf1 through uf4) pointing to the first-order factors. These represent the *unique* variances of each of the first-order factors. Just as the first-order factors are not the only causes of the scores on the subtests, *g* is not the only cause of a person's verbal or spatial ability; there is also something unique about verbal ability as opposed to spatial ability. This *unique factor* variance is recognized in the model through the presence of the latent variables uf1 through

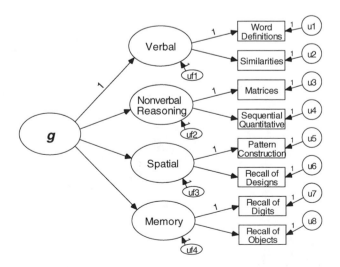

FIGURE 27.10. A hierarchical model of the structure of the DAS.

uf4.[5] As in earlier models, each latent variable (including the g and the unique factor variances) have their scales set by fixing one loading to 1.0.

The model was estimated using the *averaged* covariance matrix for ages 6–17 from the DAS standardization data (from Keith, 1990). The sample size was set to 200 for the analysis (the average sample size for each age level).

The results of the hierarchical CFA of the DAS are shown in Figure 27.11. The fit statistics suggest that the model provides an excellent fit to the data, and thus support the structure of the DAS. The first-order factor loadings suggest that the core subtests are all good measures of their corresponding factors, although Recall of Designs may not be as good a measure of spatial ability as is Pattern Construction. Although the loadings of Recall of Digits and Recall of Objects are statistically significant, they are not large, and thus these two tests do not form a strong Memory factor. This finding thus lends support to the test author's decision not to add these two subtests together to create a Memory ability score.

The second-order factor loadings are perhaps even more interesting. In scoring the DAS, the Verbal, Nonverbal Reasoning, and Spatial ability scores are combined to create an overall score, as noted above. The figure shows that the three corresponding latent factors are indeed strongly affected by g, thus supporting the hierarchical structure of the scale. Also of interest, the Nonverbal Reasoning factor has a very high loading, .98, on the second-order g factor. In fact, the 95% confidence interval of the factor loading (.72–1.24) includes 1.0, suggesting that this factor is statistically indistinguishable from the second-order g factor. This finding, in turn, lends support to the claim that the Nonverbal Reasoning scale of the DAS should be considered a measure of Gf (Keith, 1990; McGrew & Flanagan, 1998), given the evidence that Gf is often quite similar to, and sometimes indistinguishable from, g (e.g., Carroll, 1993, Ch. 15; Gustafsson, 1984).

Researchers and clinicians are often interested in the loading of subtests on g, or the relative strength or weakness of tests as measures of g. It is not necessary to resort to g-only models (Figure 27.8) or nested-factors models (discussed below) to get such estimates, however. In hierarchical models, the loadings of the subtests on hierarchical factors are calculated as the indirect effects of the hierarchical factors on the subtests, through the intermediate factors. So, for example, in Figure 27.11, the loading of the DAS Sequential and Quantitative Reasoning subtest on g is .784 (.98 × .80). SEM (and CFA) programs will easily calculate these indirect effects. The g loadings of the DAS subtests are shown in Table 27.2. Note that these g loadings are model-specific; the estimates shown in Table 27.2 apply to the model shown in Figure 27.11. If the model is correct, then the g loadings will be accurate.

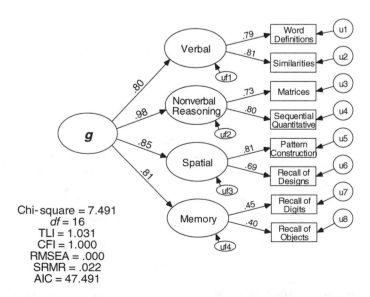

FIGURE 27.11. CFA solution for a hierarchical model of the structure of the DAS.

TABLE 27.2. Loadings of DAS Subtests on a Hierarchical *g* Factor

Subtest	Loading on *g*
Word Definitions	638
Similarities	.648
Matrices	.719
Sequential and Quantitative Reasoning	.782
Pattern Construction	.690
Recall of Designs	.589
Recall of Digits	.361
Recall of Objects	.325

Nested-Factors Models

An alternative method of testing hierarchical models is through what is called a *nested-factors model*, not to be confused with nested, competing models. In a nested-factors model, all subtests are loaded directly both on a *g* factor and on narrow factors, with the factors orthogonal or uncorrelated (cf. Carroll, 1995; Gustafsson & Balke, 1993).

Figure 27.12 shows the results of a hierarchical analysis of the WISC-IV. The model shown reflects the actual structure of the WISC-IV, and the analysis used the average covariance matrix from the WISC-IV standardization data (averaged via multisample CFA, discussed below; *N* was set to 1,000). As in several previous examples, I tested a model reflecting the actual structure of the WISC-IV rather than plausible alternative structures (some of which would be likely to

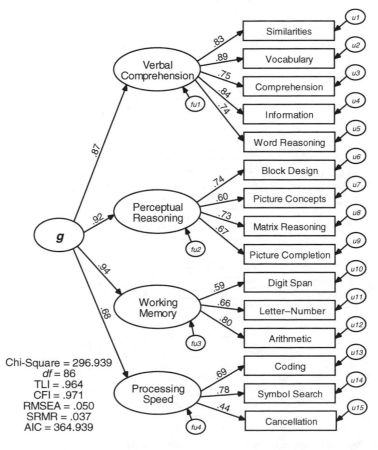

FIGURE 27.12. Possible hierarchical structure of the WISC-IV. The model tested is the actual structure of the test.

provide a better fit). As shown in the figure, the model provides a generally good fit to the standardization data.

A nested-factors version of the WISC-IV model is shown in Figure 27.13. (The ovals representing the unique variances of the subtests are not shown in the figure to help simplify it, but were included in the analysis.) This model also fits the data well—in fact, better than the hierarchical model does (the models are not nested, but the AICs suggest the superior fit of the nested-factors model). Many researchers treat nested-factors models as equivalent to hierarchical models, but clearly they are not. The nested-factor model makes no assumptions about the relation between g and the broad (first-order) factors, instead only specifying that the subtests measure both g and broad abilities.

Which model is better? The model analyzed should, at a minimum, reflect the theory underlying the test, or an alternative theoretical specification. Despite the advantages of the nested-models approach, it does not test an actual hierarchical model. And the model it does test is not consistent with any modern theoretical orientation with which I am familiar. Instead, users of this approach are usually more interested in a hierarchical model like that shown in Figure 27.12. For these reasons, I would argue that a hierarchical model should generally be preferred.

What are the perceived advantages, then, of the nested-models approach? The chief advantage is that the nested-models approach is quite similar to a Schmid–Leiman transformation in EFA, and, relatedly, gives direct estimates of loadings for the measured variables (subtests) on hierarchical factors. As

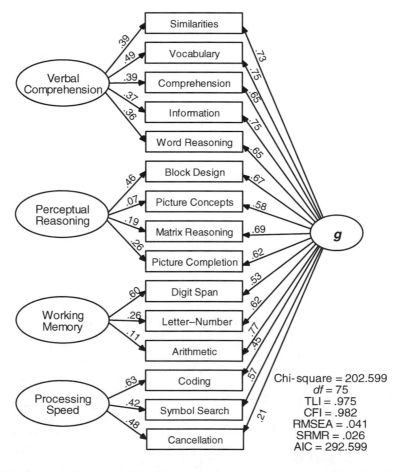

FIGURE 27.13. A nested-factors model. Although such a model may be considered an alternative to the hierarchical model, in that each test is assumed to be a product of both first-order factors shared abilities and g, the model makes no assumptions about the relation of the first-order factors to g.

already shown, however, it is quite simple to get such loadings in a true hierarchical model. Table 27.3 shows the *g* loadings of the WISC-IV subtests from the models shown in Figures 27.12 and 27.13. The *g* estimates are fairly similar; differences can probably be explained by the fact that all such estimates are model-specific.

The differences in the two methods may be smaller in practice than in theory. Although hierarchical models and nested-factors models differ considerably at a theoretical level, Mulaik and Quartetti (1997) have shown that they are rarely distinguishable on the basis of fit. Thus the illustration here is unusual. I suspect that the fact that the models used here have different levels of fit is an indication of problems with the model specification—that is, that the structure of the WISC-IV, as shown in Figure 27.12, is not the best structure. It may be, in fact, that comparison of the two methods can help illustrate problems with models. So, for example, the large differences in the loading of Arithmetic on Working Memory in the two models may suggest problems with placement of Arithmetic on the Working Memory factor. Further research will be needed to test this supposition. See Jensen and Weng (1993) for a more complete discussion of methods of estimating *g*, and Mulaik and Quartetti (1997) for additional comparison of hierarchical and nested models.

TABLE 27.3. Comparison of the *g* Loadings for WISC-IV Subtests from a Hierarchical versus a Nested-Factors Model

Subtest	Hierarchical *g*	Nested factors
Similarities	.726	.733
Vocabulary	.771	.751
Comprehension	.656	.646
Information	.729	.748
Word Reasoning	.648	.648
Block Design	.680	.672
Picture Concepts	.555	.582
Matrix Reasoning	.676	.687
Picture Completion	.615	.616
Digit Span	.558	.525
Letter–Number Sequencing	.626	.621
Arithmetic	.757	.768
Coding	.471	.454
Symbol Search	.534	.568
Cancellation	.297	.209

TESTING HYPOTHESES ABOUT THE SIMILARITY OF FACTORS

CFA is also a useful method for testing hypotheses about how factors or tests should be interpreted. Such research often involves testing the similarity of factors within a test or between two tests. CFA can be used to test whether two tests designed to measure the same factors (e.g., the Gf factors from the Woodcock–Johnson III [WJ III] and the KAIT) do, in fact, measure statistically indistinguishable factors. By the same token, the method can be used to test whether two tests designed to measure *different* abilities do, in fact, measure distinguishable factors.

What Types of Abilities Does the Cognitive Assessment System Measure?

The Cognitive Assessment System (CAS; Naglieri & Das, 1997) is a new measure of cognitive abilities based on the *planning, attention, simultaneous, and successive* (PASS) theory of intelligence. The PASS model is a neuropsychological and information-processing theory of cognition, and the CAS is the only test based entirely on this theory (see Naglieri & Das, Chapter 7, and Naglieri, Chapter 20, this volume, and Das, Naglieri, & Kirby, 1994, for more information).

Cattell–Horn–Carroll (CHC) theory is a combination of Carroll's three-stratum theory and Cattell and Horn's Gf-Gc theory—theories that have already overlapped considerably. (For more information about CHC theory, see McGrew, Chapter 8, this volume.) Although the CAS was designed to measure the PASS abilities, several authors have questioned whether the CAS in fact measures those abilities or whether it measures several abilities from CHC theory (Carroll, 1995; Kranzler & Keith, 1999). In particular, my colleagues and I (Kranzler & Keith, 1999; see also Keith & Kranzler, 1999, and Kranzler, Keith, & Flanagan, 2000) have argued that the Planning and Attention tests of the CAS measure components of processing speed (Gs); that the Simultaneous tests measure a mixture of visual processing and fluid reasoning (Gv and Gf); and that the Successive tests measure components of short-term memory (Gsm).

CFA across tests can be used to help settle this debate. The previous (Woodcock &

Johnson, 1989) and current (Woodcock, McGrew, & Mather, 2001) versions of the Woodcock–Johnson Tests of Cognitive Ability (the WJ-R COG and WJ III COG, respectively) are closely tied to and appear to provide strong measures of the CHC abilities (Bickley, Keith, & Wolfle, 1995; McGrew & Flanagan, 1998; McGrew & Woodcock, 2001; Taub & McGrew, 2004). If so, then joint CFA of the WJ III COG and the CAS could be used to test the similarity of the CAS factors and those from the WJ III COG.

We (Keith, Kranzler, & Flanagan, 2001) have reported a series of joint CFAs of these two instruments; a few of these are described briefly here to illustrate the CFA methodology. Figure 27.14 shows one of the initial models tested in this research. The model shows a CFA of the WJ III tests on the left, and a CFA of the CAS tests on the right. The CAS factors have been labeled with both the CHC theory-derived names and those from the PASS/CAS orientation.

If the CAS tests in fact measure the PASS abilities, the correlations of the CAS factors with the WJ III factors Gs, Gv, Gf, and Gsm should be of moderate magnitude, presumably close to the average correlation among the WJ III factors (average $r = .490$). In contrast, if the CAS tests measure CHC abilities, the corresponding correlations should be considerably higher. Figure 27.15 shows the results of a joint CFA in which the correlations among factors were unconstrained and freely estimated. To simplify the display, only the relevant correlations are shown, but all were estimated (for the complete factor correlation matrix, see Keith et al., 2001).

As shown in the figure, all of the relevant correlations are higher than the average factor correlation. The Simultaneous–Gf and Simultaneous–Gv correlations are .77 and .68, respectively; the Planning–Gs and Attention–Gs correlations are .98 and .88, respectively; and the correlation between Successive and Gsm is greater than 1 (1.06; this value is not statistically significantly different from 1.0, however). The overall fit of the model is adequate to good. These initial, unconstrained analyses support a CHC interpretation of the CAS abilities rather than a PASS interpretation.

It is possible to conduct a stronger test of the convergence or divergence of factors by constraining correlations among factors and comparing the fit of those models. Note that the initial model was specified by setting factor variances to 1.0 (rather than factor loadings), so that constraints to factor covariances are in fact made to factor correlations (because correlations are standardized covariances). Figure 27.16 shows the second step in these analyses, in which the correlations between the WJ III Gs factor and the CAS Planning and Attention factors were constrained to .49, the average correlation among WJ III factors. (All other factor correlations were allowed to vary, but are not shown so as to simplify the figure.) A comparison of the fit of this model with the initial model tests whether the correlations between Gs and Planning and Attention are no higher than would be expected for mental factors measuring distinct abilities. As shown in Table 27.4, these constraints to the model result in a statistically significant increase in $\Delta\chi^2$, however, suggesting the rejection of this hypothesis. In step 3, these same factor correlations were constrained to a value of 1.0, to test whether the Planning and Attention factors are instead statistically indistinguishable from processing speed (Gs). As shown in the table, these constraints result in a statistically insignificant increase in $\Delta\chi^2$, thus supporting the contention that the Planning and Attention tests of the CAS measure processing speed.

We (Keith et al., 2001) conducted numerous additional analyses to test whether the CAS measures PASS or CHC abilities. In addition to testing the similarity of factors, we tested a series of joint hierarchical, integrated, and PASS-derived models; for additional information, see the original article. I believe that the article is a good illustration of the use of CFA to test competing hypotheses about the nature of constructs measured by intelligence tests.

Testing Hypotheses about the Wechsler Scales

Despite their long clinical and research history, there are still questions about the constructs measured by the Wechsler scales. One is whether the Performance/Perceptual scales in general, and the Block Design subtest in particular, measure novel reasoning (Gf) or visual processing (Gv). Briefly, clinical lore and research suggest that these tests, and es-

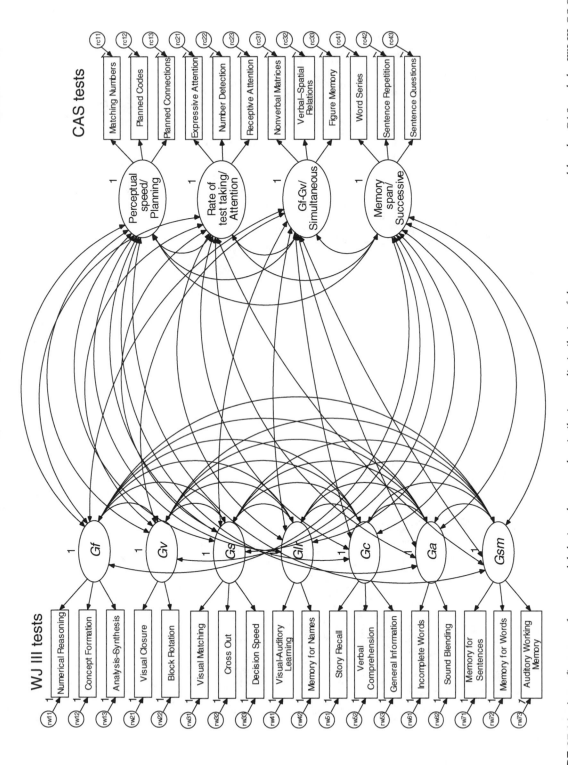

FIGURE 27.14. A confirmatory factor model designed to test the similarity or dissimilarity of the constructs measured by the CAS and the WJ III COG. From Keith, Kranzler, and Flanagan (2001). Copyright 2001 by the National Association of School Psychologists. Adapted by permission.

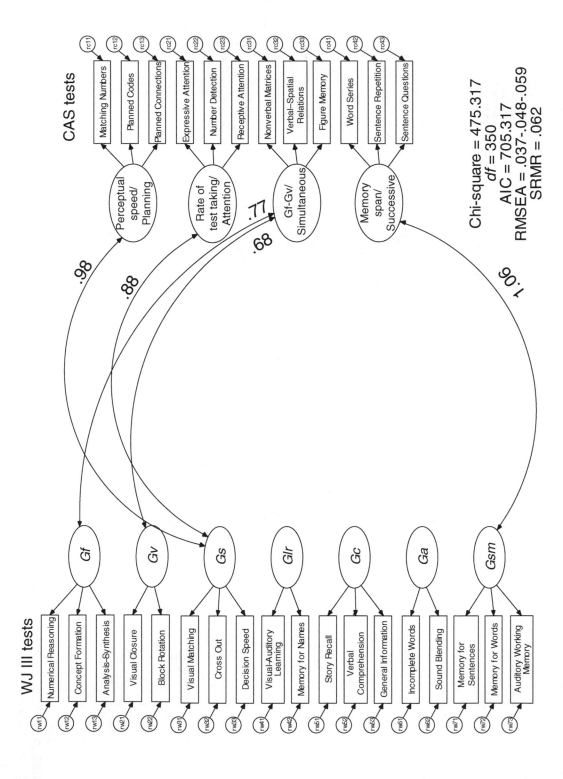

FIGURE 27.15. Correlations between selected factors from the WJ III COG and the CAS. The factor correlations suggest that the CAS tests overlap considerably with the WJ III CHC abilities.

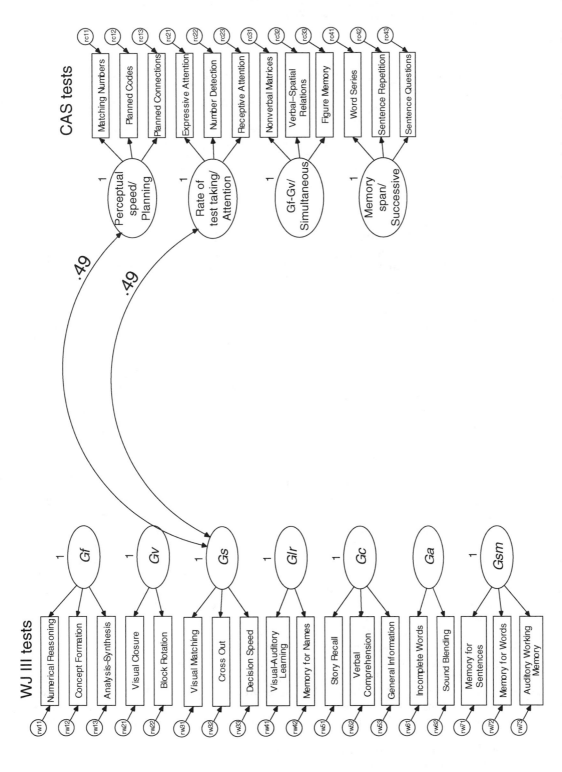

FIGURE 27.16. Testing hypotheses using the CAS/WJ III COG model. The correlations between WJ III Processing Speed and the CAS Planning and Attention factors were set to the average value for factor correlations. The fit degrades as a result of these model constraints.

TABLE 27.4. Comparison of the Competing Hypotheses about the Nature of the CAS Planning and Attention Tests

Model	$\Delta\chi^2$ (df)	p	AIC
Unconstrained conjoint model	475.317 (350)[a]		705.317
Factors are distinct; correlation of Planning, Attention with Gs = .49	43.259 (2)	<.001	744.576
Factors are indistinguishable; correlation of Planning, Attention with Gs = 1.00	4.902 (2)	.086	706.219

Note. Each model was compared to the unconstrained model. The $\Delta\chi^2$ value reported for the unconstrained model is the χ^2. From Keith, Kranzler, and Flanagan (2001). Copyright 2001 by the National Association of School Psychologists. Adapted by permission.

pecially Block Design, measure fluid intelligence (cf. Kaufman, 1994). Others contend—also with research backing—that these tests (including Block Design) are better considered measures of broad visualization (Carroll, 1993; McGrew & Flanagan, 1998; see Kaufman, 1996; McGrew & Flanagan, 1996; and Willis, 1996, for a summary of this debate). Another question is the nature of the Arithmetic test: Does it measure freedom from distractibility, working memory, quantitative reasoning, or some other ability (cf. Carroll, 1997; Kamphaus, 2001; Keith, 1997b; Keith & Witta, 1997; Kranzler, 1997)? These debates are likely to intensify with the recent publication of the WISC-IV, in which new Perceptual Reasoning tests have been added to improve the measurement of Gf, and the memory demands of Arithmetic have been increased so that it more clearly measures working memory.

CFA across tests can provide evidence to inform this debate as well. Here I illustrate one possible use of the method to answer questions about the abilities measured by the Block Design subtest. Stone (1992) conducted a joint CFA of the DAS and the WISC-R. His primary purpose was to compare models similar in structure to that guiding the WISC-R to those guiding the DAS (the DAS-type structure was more strongly supported). The data presented in Stone (1992), however, can also be used to test specific hypotheses about the abilities measured by the WISC. Although these data are from an earlier version of the WISC (the WISC-R vs. the WISC-IV), given the similarity in these tests across editions, the results should be very relevant concerning the abilities measured by Block Design.

There is considerable evidence that the Nonverbal Reasoning scale of the DAS provides a strong and useful measure of fluid reasoning (e.g., Elliott, 1990b; Keith, 1990; McGrew & Flanagan, 1998; Stone, 1992). The DAS Spatial scale, in turn, appears to measure primarily broad visualization (Gv). Thus, in an integrated CFA of the two tests, Block Design should behave differently if it measures Gf versus Gv. Figure 27.17 shows an initial model in a series of models designed to test the abilities measured by Block Design. In the figure, the WISC tests are listed on the left, and the DAS tests on the right. The factors shown in the center of the figure are the CHC abilities presumably measured by the two tests (cf. McGrew & Flanagan, 1998). In this initial model, Block Design is specified as loading on a Gv factor only. Figure 27.18 shows the results of this analysis; as shown in the figure, the model fits the data well, and factor loadings generally look reasonable. Although not shown in the figure, factor correlations range from .203 (between processing speed [Gs] and Gc) to .773 (between Gc and quantitative reasoning [Gq]); the correlations were all estimated, but are not shown in the figure to simplify presentation.

In Figure 27.19, the Block Design subtest has been allowed to load on both the Gv and the Gf factors. If Block Design in fact measures fluid reasoning rather than visual processing, then this model allowing a dual loading by Block Design should fit the data better than the initial model, and the factor loading for Block Design should be considerably larger on Gf than on Gv. As shown in Table 27.5, the relaxation of the initial model does not result in a statistically

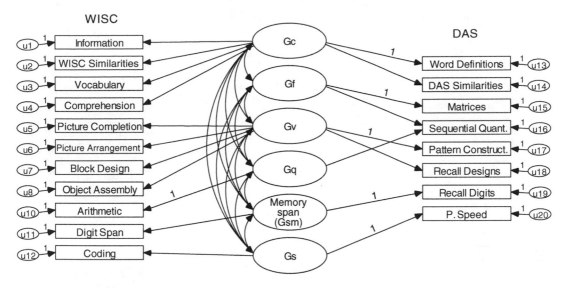

FIGURE 27.17. Understanding the ability measured by the WISC Block Design subtest.

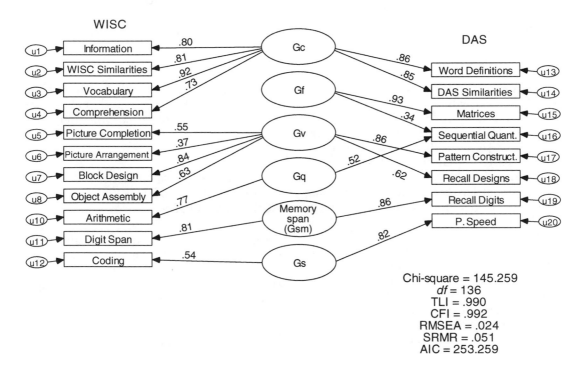

Chi-square = 145.259
df = 136
TLI = .990
CFI = .992
RMSEA = .024
SRMR = .051
AIC = 253.259

FIGURE 27.18. Results of the initial analysis probing the nature of Block Design.

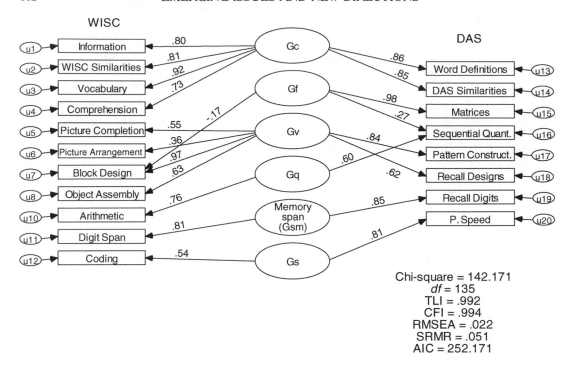

FIGURE 27.19. Block Design is allowed to load on both Gf and Gv factors. The fit of the model does not improve, and Block Design has a negative loading on Gf.

significant decrease in χ^2, suggesting that the initial model, with Block Design loading only on Gv, is a better model. The negative loading of Block Design on Gf in Figure 27.19 also suggests that Block Design is a better measure of Gv than of Gf.

In a third model (not shown in a figure), Block Design has been specified as loading only on Gf. This model results in a statistically significant increase in χ^2 (see Table 27.5) over the model in Figure 27.19, meaning that this model fits worse that the model allowing double loadings. Although the Gv-only and the Gf-only models cannot be compared via χ^2 (because the two models are not nested), they can be compared via the AIC. When this fit index is used, the initial, Gv-only model fits considerably better than the

Gf-only model. These analyses support the hypothesis that Block Design should be considered a measure of visual processing, not fluid/novel reasoning.

TESTING THE SIMILARITY OF FACTOR STRUCTURE ACROSS GROUPS

An important subset of questions about the constructs measured by intelligence tests involves questions about whether the test measures the same constructs across groups. Does a multiple-age battery, for example, measure the same set of constructs for 8-year-olds as it does for 18-year-olds? Does a new intelligence test measure Gf and Gc abil-

TABLE 27.5. Testing Hypotheses about the Abilities Measured by the WISC Block Design Subtest

Model/hypothesis tested	χ^2 (df)	Δ^2 (df)	p	AIC
Initial model: Block Design measures Gv	145.259 (136)			253.259
Block Design measures Gv and Gf	142.171 (135)	3.088 (1)	.079	252.171
Block Design measures Gf	168.799 (136)	26.628	<.001	276.799

ities for white students, but merely test-taking skills for minority students? These questions ask, in essence, whether the factor structure of the tests varies across groups. The method of *multisample CFA* (MCFA) provides an excellent method for answering such questions.

In MCFA, any of the parameters that are estimated or fixed in a model can be specified as being invariant across two or more groups. For example, suppose I wish to determine whether a set of tests measures the same constructs for boys and girls. I could specify that the factor loadings of that series of tests are the same for boys and girls, but I could also specify that the factor inter-correlations, the factor variances, and the unique and error variances are identical across groups. The resulting χ^2 and other fit statistics provide "a measure of the fit of all models in all groups," taking into account the constraints across the groups (Jöreskog & Sörbom, 1993, p. 54). That is, the fit statistics test the adequacy of both the imposed factor structure and the equivalence of the factor structures across groups. Various degrees of equivalence can also be compared. I could begin by specifying that all possible parameters—factor loadings, factor correlations, factor variances, and subtest unique and error variances—are identical across groups, and could then gradually free those restrictions and see whether the fit improves. It is even possible to compare the equivalence of measurement across groups independent of a factor structure by comparing the equivalence of the covariance matrices for the two groups. Since the factor structure is contained within and solved from the covariances, this comparison of matrices evaluates whether the test measures the same construct across groups without testing a particular factor structure. One important use of MCFA is to determine whether a test measures the same constructs across its full age span (e.g., Taub & McGrew, 2004). It is also useful as a method of testing for construct bias across groups; the second use is illustrated here.

Is There Construct Bias in the DAS?

MCFA is an excellent method for evaluating the presence and extent of construct bias in tests of intelligence. We (Keith, Quirk, Schartzer, & Elliott, 1999) used MCFA to determine whether the DAS measures the same constructs for African American, Hispanic, and European American students. A finding of differences across groups would suggest that different constructs are being measured, and thus that the DAS is biased against one group.

We (Keith et al., 1999) followed a six-step process for testing increasingly lenient models as a method of determining both the extent of the bias in the test and the "location" of that bias. In the first step, the covariance matrices are compared for the three groups (in this case, three ethnic groups). Since any factor structure is contained within the original covariance matrix, a test of the equality of the covariance matrices tests whether the instrument (in this case, the DAS) measures the same attributes across groups, without specifying the nature of those attributes. If the fit statistics lead to the rejection of this initial model, then a confirmatory factor model is developed and used in all subsequent steps. Second, a CFA is conducted across the groups with *all* aspects of the model—factor loadings, factor correlations (for first-order models), higher-order factor loadings (for hierarchical models), factor and factor unique variances, and unique and error variances—specified as invariant across the groups. This highly constrained CFA is no less constrained than the comparison of matrices (everything is invariant), but in addition to testing for equality across groups, it tests a *specific* factor model. Thus the fit statistics from this second analysis provide a baseline for further comparisons in which the model is relaxed. In the third through sixth steps, these constrained parameters are gradually relaxed (e.g., the unique and error variances are allowed to be different for the two groups, then the factor or factor unique variances, and so on). It is also possible to test the equivalence of latent means across groups (McArdle, 1998), but that step was not done in the analyses discussed here.

Table 27.6 shows the results of these comparisons for African American, Hispanic, and European American 6- to 11-year-olds from the DAS standardization and supplemental samples. The comparison of the covariance matrices for the three groups is shown in the first row of the table. Although most of the fit statistics (TLI = .978, CFI = .989, RMSEA = .023) suggested a good fit of

TABLE 27.6. Comparison of the Fit of Models Specifying Various Degrees of Equivalence of the DAS across Three Ethnic Groups for 6- to 11-Year-Olds

Model description	χ^2 (df)	$\Delta\chi^2$ (df)[a]	p
Step 1. Covariance matrices invariant	60.197 (42)		
Step 2. Factor model: All parameters invariant	69.620 (48)	9.423 (6)	.151
Step 3. Factor model: Unique/error variances vary	40.028 (36)	29.592 (12)	.003
Step 4. Factor model: Unique/error and factor variances vary across groups	38.419 (28)	1.609 (8)	.991
Step 5. Factor model: Unique/error and factor variances, second-order loadings vary	35.008 (24)	3.411 (4)	.492
Step 6. Factor model: All parameters vary across groups	31.890 (18)	3.118 (6)	.794

Note. From Keith, Quirk, Schartzer, and Elliott (1999). Copyright 1999 by The Psychoeducational Corporation. Adapted by permission.
[a]Compared to the previous model.

the model to the data, we decided to test additional models because the χ^2 was statistically significant (60.197 [42], $p = .034$), suggesting the rejection of the hypothesis that the DAS measures identical attributes for African American, Hispanic, and European American children. We argued that it seemed prudent to conduct further tests, despite the generally positive nature of the fit statistics.

We next tested the hierarchical structure of the DAS, as described in the DAS manual (Elliott, 1990a), across ethnic groups. Table 27.6 also shows the results of the gradual relaxation of the models from all parameters invariant across groups (step 2) to all parameters free to vary in magnitude across ethnic groups (step 6). The imposition of a factor model (step 2) led to a statistically insignificant increase in χ^2 over the test of the equality of covariance matrices, supporting the imposition of a hierarchical factor model underlying the DAS. The results of this step of the analyses are shown in Figure 27.20. Allowing the unique and error variances of the subtests (step 3) to vary across groups resulted in a statistically significant decrease in χ^2, suggesting that these parameters are not equivalent across the three ethnic groups. As we noted, unique and error variances are not expected to be equivalent across groups, so

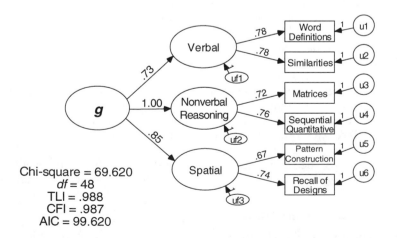

Chi-square = 69.620
df = 48
TLI = .988
CFI = .987
AIC = 99.620

FIGURE 27.20. Hierarchical MCFA of the DAS across ethnic groups. From Keith, Quirk, Schartzer, and Elliott (1999). Copyright 1999 by The Psychoeducational Corporation. Adapted by permission.

this finding of differences does not suggest construct bias in the DAS (steps 5 and 6, if statistically significant, would suggest bias). As shown in the table, allowing additional parameters to vary resulted in only statistically insignificant decreases in χ^2. Thus it appears that the differences in the matrices for the three groups seen in the first step of the analysis are due to differences in the unique variances of the subtests, which are in turn relatively unimportant differences (Marsh, 1993, p. 851). The other age levels also showed few, and minor, differences across groups.

We concluded that the MCFA approach has several advantages over more traditional methods for assessing construct bias (e.g., comparison of factor loadings). Specifically, MCFA provides a more organized, more direct, more objective, and more complete analysis of bias over more traditional methods (Keith et al., 1999).

TESTING THEORIES OF INTELLIGENCE

Most of the examples used in this chapter are examples of CFA used to understand the constructs measured by specific tests. The method is equally applicable, however, for asking and answering questions about *theories* of intelligence. Some analyses serve both functions; the joint CFA of the WJ III and CAS discussed earlier has implications for CHC and PASS theory, in addition to the tests derived from these theories. That is, the fact that the hypotheses derived from CHC theory are supported provides support for that theory.

CHC and Three-Stratum Theory

CHC theory is based in part on Carroll's three-stratum theory of cognitive abilities. Both theories posit a hierarchical model of intelligence, with narrow-order abilities at the bottom and the most general ability, *g*, at the apex. The three-stratum theory is described in detail in Carroll (1993 and Chapter 4, this volume), and CHC theory is described in McGrew (Chapter 8, this volume).

Carroll speculated that there might well be *intermediate* factors between his second-stratum (e.g., Gf, Gc, Gv) and third-stratum

abilities, but he left the task of describing this intermediate structure up to other researchers. Bickley and colleagues (1995) addressed the possibility of intermediate factors and tested one such model, and Keith (1997b) explored several such possible models, but neither study pursued the matter in depth. One difference between three-stratum theory and Gf-Gc theory (the other component of CHC theory) is the nature of quantitative reasoning. Gf-Gc theory has traditionally treated quantitative reasoning skills as a separate construct, Gq, whereas Carroll argued that quantitative reasoning (RQ in his theory) is in fact a part of fluid or novel reasoning (Gf). To complicate matters further, in current versions of CHC theory, Gq is often treated as a mathematics achievement factor (see McGrew, Chapter 8, this volume). To demonstrate CFA's applicability to testing theory, one model with intermediate factors is explored here, and several models exploring the nature of quantitative reasoning are tested.

The WJ III COG is based on CHC theory, and research suggests that it provides valid measures of CHC constructs (McGrew & Woodcock, 2001; Taub & McGrew, 2004), so it is a good tool for testing basic questions about CHC theory. A basic CHC model is shown in Figure 27.21 (cf. Floyd, Keith, Taub, & McGrew, 2003). The data used were the matrices of correlations and standard deviations for children ages 9–13 from the WJ III standardization data (McGrew & Woodcock, 2001). Not all WJ III tests were used; the model includes three good measures of each factor. The sample sizes for tests in this matrix varied, so an overall sample size of 1,000 was used in these analyses (the EM [expectation maximization] algorithm was used to deal with incomplete data in the calculation of the matrices).

Figure 27.22 shows the results of the analysis of this initial model for 9- to 13-year-olds in the WJ III standardization sample. As shown in the figure, the initial model provides a good fit to the WJ III data; the SRMR, RMSEA, TLI, and CFI all suggest an excellent fit to the data. The RMSEA information in the figure is a little different from that presented previously; the figure shows the point value of the RMSEA (.043) surrounded by the 90% confidence interval of the RMSEA (.039–.047).

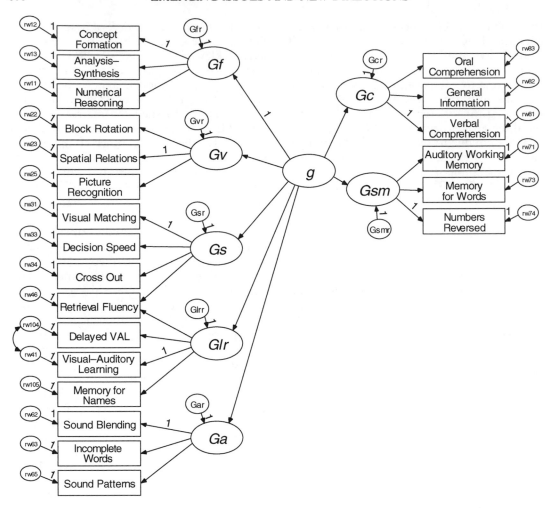

FIGURE 27.21. A three-stratum-theory-derived model of the WJ III COG.

The model shown in Figure 27.23 presents one possible set of intermediate factors between the second and third strata from CHC/three-stratum theory (in the model, these intermediate factors are second-order factors, and g is a third-order factor). Woodcock (1993) proposed a *cognitive performance model* (CPM) of abilities as a method of explaining how abilities work in concert to affect a person's overall functioning, and this model has been refined and built into the scoring of the WJ III COG. The CPM includes three intermediate factors between the broad abilities (*Gf, Gc,* etc.) and *g: verbal ability, thinking ability,* and *cognitive efficiency.* Two of these intermediate factors are included in the model; verbal ability and Gc are the same, so there was no need to build a verbal ability intermediate factor into the model (an intermediate factor could have been built into the model, but the fit would be the same as that of the simpler model shown).

As shown in the figure and in Table 27.7, this categorization of second-stratum abilities into thinking ability and cognitive efficiency leads to an improvement in the fit of the model. In particular, the intermediate CPM factors produce a statistically significant decrease in χ^2, thus suggesting the division of some of the second-stratum abilities into thinking ability and cognitive efficiency as a worthwhile addition to the three-stratum theory.

One interesting aspect of this model is the essential equivalence of g and thinking ability (the path from g to thinking ability is actually 1.02, but is not statistically significantly different from 1). This finding in turn suggests a more parsimonious model, in which the two factors are combined (Figure 27.24). As shown in the table, this model does not result in a statistically significant increase in χ^2, and thus is preferred as a more parsimonious version of the CPM model. This modified model supports the combination of the Gs and Gsm factors into a hierarchical cognitive efficiency factor, but suggests that g and thinking ability are interchangeable.

One final variation of this model is mentioned briefly. One could argue that the path

from cognitive efficiency to g should be reversed, so that efficiency affects g rather than the reverse. This modification could be based on the assumption that processing speed and short-term memory (and cognitive efficiency) are fundamental mental skills that influence one's level of general intelligence—essentially, gatekeepers of general cognitive ability (cf. McGrew, Chapter 8, this volume). Unfortunately, without further modification, this model is statistically equivalent to the modified CPM model, and the two cannot be distinguished on the basis of fit statistics.

The final two models (Figures 27.25 and 27.26) in this chapter test Carroll's contention that quantitative reasoning is a part of Gf rather than a separate second-stratum factor. (I here symbolize the quantitative fac-

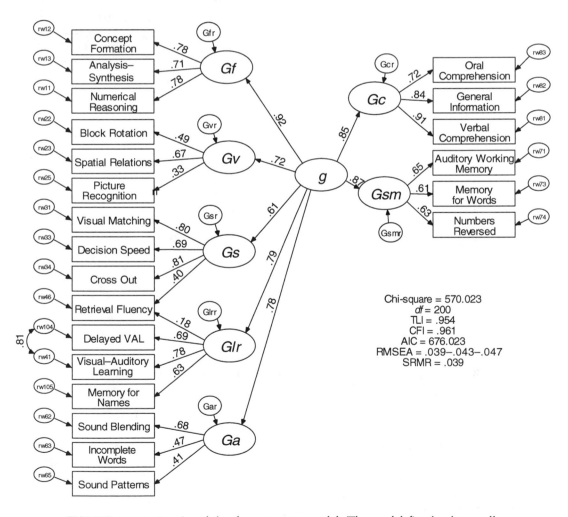

FIGURE 27.22. Results of the three-stratum model. The model fits the data well.

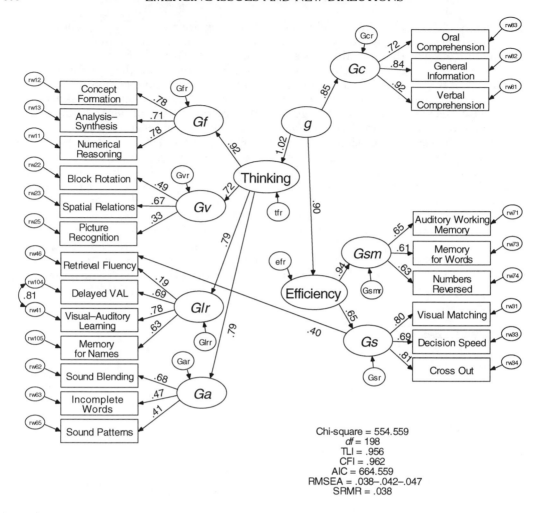

FIGURE 27.23. A test of possible intermediate factors between Carroll's stratum II and stratum III abilities. The model is based on Woodcock's cognitive performance model (CPM).

TABLE 27.7. Comparison of the Fit of Models Testing Different Intermediate-Level Factors in the Three-Stratum Theory

Model description	χ^2 (df)	$\Delta\chi^2$ (df)	p	AIC
1. Initial model: No intermediate factors	570.023 (200)			676.023
2. Cognitive performance model	554.559 (198)	15.464 (2)[a]	.001	664.559
3. Cognitive performance model 2	556.827 (199)	2.268 (1)[a]	.132	664.827
4. Initial Gf-Gq model: Separate factors	645.144 (220)			757.144
5. Gf subsumes Gf (narrow) and Gq	628.853 (219)	16.291 (1)[a]	.001	742.853

[a]Compared to the previous model.

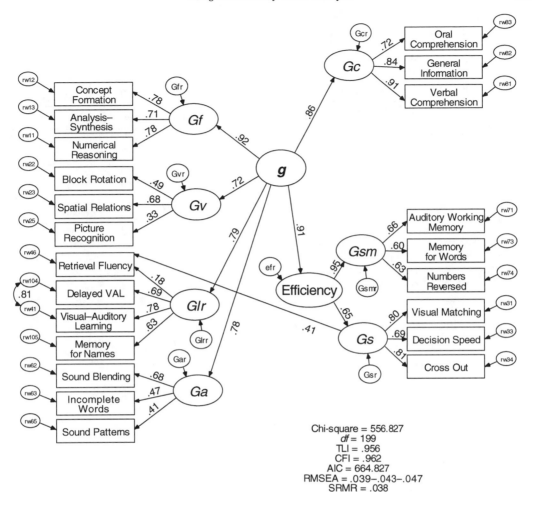

FIGURE 27.24. A simplified version of the CPM model in Figure 27.23.

tor as Gq, with the recognition that not everyone would equate quantitative reasoning and Gq.)

The initial quantitative model adds a further test (Quantitative Concepts) to allow for two subtests each measuring the Gq and Gf factors. This initial model with separate Gf and Gq factors (in the upper left of the figure) is shown in Figure 27.25, and the fit statistics for comparing models are shown in Table 27.7. As shown in the figure, the initial quantitative model provides a good fit to the data using common criteria. In contrast, Figure 27.26 shows a model in which the narrow Gf (symbolized as Gfn) and Gq factors are subsumed under a broader Gf factor. As shown in Table 27.7, this specification results in a considerable improvement in

model fit over the initial quantitative model. Said differently, the broad Gf factor may be considered an intermediate factor between the narrow Gf and Gq factors and g. This preliminary investigation supports the contention that quantitative reasoning is a part of fluid/novel reasoning (Gf).

SUMMARY

This chapter has provided an overview of and introduction to the method of CFA, with particular attention to the use of the method as an aid in understanding the constructs measured by modern tests of intelligence. The chapter has covered "simple" CFA—in other words, first-order CFA, a method that

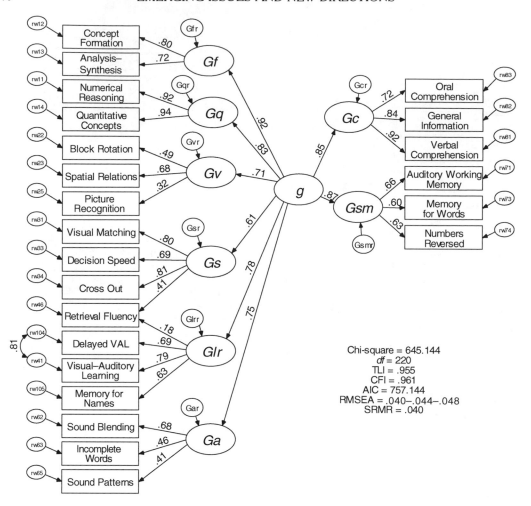

FIGURE 27.25. A model designed to probe the nature of the relation between Gf and Gq.

is becoming fairly common in the factor-analytic/intelligence literature.

I believe, however, that additional uses of CFA are needed if we are really interested in understanding the constructs we are measuring. Thus I encourage the comparison of meaningful alternative explanations to a researcher's pet theory through the testing and comparison of alternative factor models. This practice too is becoming more common, although alternative models are not always meaningful. For example, I argue that a single-factor model is generally not a meaningful alternative and does not represent modern thinking about the nature of g as a construct.

Many modern theories of intelligence are hierarchical in nature, with the most prominent example being the three-stratum theory,

a "metatheory" developed and tested by John Carroll (and incorporated into CHC theory). Most tests of intelligence tacitly recognize a hierarchical nature of intelligence as well. I strongly believe that our research should therefore test these hierarchical notions of intelligence if we are to fully understand the constructs we are measuring. Put another way, a test of a first-order version of a hierarchical theory/test is an incomplete test of that theory. Furthermore, hierarchical analysis provides a more thorough understanding of the first-order abilities (Carroll, 1993, Ch. 3). This chapter has demonstrated several variations of hierarchical CFA, using second- and even third-order factors.

This chapter has demonstrated several other important uses of CFA: to compare the constructs measured across different tests, and to compare the constructs measured by one test across different groups. Many of the most vexing problems in the intelligence field center around these issues, and CFA is an excellent method for answering these important questions. For example, MCFA provides an organized, effective method for testing for construct bias across groups. Finally, CFA provides a powerful method for testing theory, and especially for testing competing theories of intelligence.

I have not covered or tried to cover all possible uses of CFA; those uses are limited only by the imagination of the researcher. In addition, CFA is a subset of a more general approach, SEM—and this broader approach is also useful for understanding the nature of the constructs measured by tests of intelligence. To mention only two examples, SEM provides an excellent method for testing the stability over time of the *constructs* we measure, independent of the method of measurement; and multisample SEM provides an excellent method for evaluating the presence of *predictive* bias in our measurements (cf. McArdle, 1998). Nevertheless, I hope that this chapter has provided enough of an overview to stimulate thought and further study, and to fire the imaginations of future CFA readers and researchers. For those interested in additional study, there are numerous resources available (e.g., Byrne, 2001; Keith, in press; Kline, 1998; Loehlin, 1998).

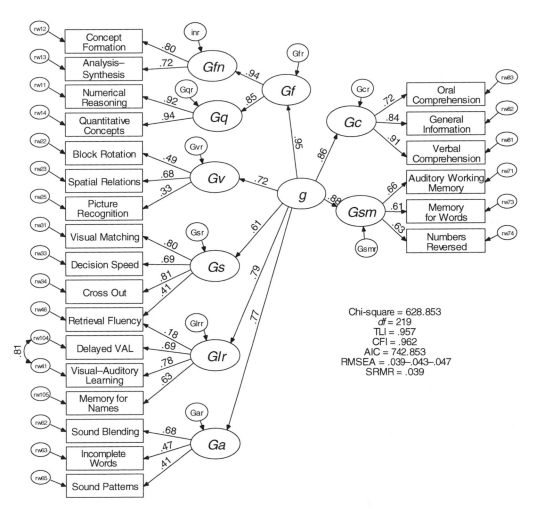

FIGURE 27.26. In this model, Gf subsumes Gq and a narrow Gf factor. The model shows an improvement in fit over the previous model.

ACKNOWLEDGMENTS

I am grateful to Patricia Keith for her assistance, and to Kevin McGrew for his comments on an earlier draft of this chapter.

NOTES

1. The factor model tested is one that matches the intended structure of the KAIT. Other models (e.g., Flanagan & McGrew, 1998; McGrew & Flanagan, 1998) are certainly plausible, but are not evaluated here.
2. Without this constraint, this portion of the model would have been underidentified.
3. More generally, if $\Delta\chi^2$ is statistically significant, the less constrained model (the model with the smaller df) is selected; if $\Delta\chi^2$ is not statistically significant, the more parsimonious model (the model with the larger df) is selected. It may not be immediately obvious why the model in Figure 10 is a constrained version of that in Figure 27.9. Figure 27.10 is statistically identical to Figure 27.9, with the paths from delayed recall to the two Delayed Recall subtests set to 0, and the correlations between delayed recall and the other two factors set to 0.
4. Again, I here test one possible structure that fits fairly closely with the test author's intended structure. For other possible structures, see Keith (1990), McGrew and Flanagan (1998), or Stone (1992).
5. In SEM, these are known as *disturbances* and represent all other causes not included in the model. Thus, for the DAS example, uf1 represents all causes of verbal ability other than g.

REFERENCES

Allen, S. R., & Thorndike, R. M. (1995). Stability of the WPPSI-R and WISC-III factor structure using cross-validation of covariance structure models. *Journal of Psychoeducational Assessment, 13,* 3–20.

Arbuckle, J. L. (2003). *Amos 5.0 update to the Amos user's guide.* Chicago: Smallwaters.

Bentler, P. M. (1995). *EQS structural equations program manual.* Encino, CA: Multivariate Software.

Bentler, P. M., & Wu, E. J. C. (1995). *EQS for Windows user's guide.* Encino, CA: Multivariate Software.

Bickley, P. G., Keith, T. Z., & Wolfle, L. M. (1995). The three-stratum theory of cognitive abilities: Test of the structure of intelligence across the life span. *Intelligence, 20,* 309–328.

Browne, M. W., & Cudeck, R. (1993). Alternative ways of assessing model fit. In K. A. Bollen & J. S. Long (Eds.), *Testing structural equation models* (pp. 136–162). Newbury Park, CA: Sage.

Burt, C. L. (1949). The structure of the mind: A review of the results of factor analysis. *British Journal of Educational Psychology, 19,* 100–111, 176–199.

Byrne, B. M. (2001). *Structural equation modeling with Amos: Basic concepts, applications, and programming.* Mahwah, NJ: Erlbaum.

Carroll, J. B. (1993). *Human cognitive abilities: A survey of factor-analytic studies.* New York: Cambridge University Press.

Carroll, J. B. (1995). [Review of the book *Assessment of cognitive processes: The PASS theory of intelligence*]. *Journal of Psychoeducational Assessment, 13,* 397–409.

Carroll, J. B. (1997). Commentary on Keith and Witta's hierarchical and cross-age confirmatory factor analysis of the WISC-III. *School Psychology Quarterly, 12,* 108–109.

Carroll, J. B. (2003). The higher-stratum structure of cognitive abilities: Current evidence supports g and about ten broad factors. In H. Nyborg (Ed.), *The scientific study of general intelligence: Tribute to Arthur R. Jensen* (pp. 5–21). Amsterdam: Pergamon Press.

Cohen, J. (1994). The earth is round (*p* < .05). *American Psychologist, 49,* 997–1003.

Cole, J. C., & Randall, M. K. (2003). Comparing cognitive ability models of Spearman, Horn and Cattell, and Carroll. *Journal of Psychoeducational Assessment, 21,* 160–179.

Das, J. P., Naglieri, J. A., & Kirby, J. R. (1994). *Assessment of cognitive processes: The PASS theory of intelligence.* Boston: Allyn & Bacon.

Elliott, C. D. (1990a). *Differential Ability Scales: Introductory and technical manual.* San Antonio, TX: Psychological Corporation.

Elliott, C. D. (1990b). The nature and structure of children's abilities: Evidence from the Differential Ability Scales. *Journal of Psychoeducational Assessment, 8,* 376–390.

Fan, X., Thompson, B., & Wang, L. (1999). Effects of sample size, estimation methods, and model specification on structural equation modeling fit indexes. *Structural Equation Modeling, 6,* 56–83.

Flanagan, D. P., & McGrew, K. S. (1998). Interpreting intelligence tests from modern Gf-Gc theory: Joint confirmatory factor analysis of the WJ-R and Kaufman Adolescent and Adult Intelligence Test (KAIT). *Journal of School Psychology, 36,* 151–182.

Floyd, R. G., Keith, T. Z., Taub, G. E., & McGrew, K. S. (2003). *Cattell–Horn–Carroll cognitive abilities and their effects on reading decoding skills: To g or not to g.* Manuscript submitted for publication.

Gustafsson, J.-E. (1984). A unifying model for the structure of intellectual abilities. *Intelligence, 8,* 179–203.

Gustafsson, J.-E., & Balke, G. (1993). General and specific abilities as predictors of school achievement. *Multivariate Behavioral Research, 28,* 407–434.

Humphreys, L. G. (1990). View of a supportive empiricist. *Psychological Inquiry, 1,* 153–155.

Hox, J. J. (1995). Amos, EQS, and LISREL for Windows: A comparative review. *Structural Equation Modeling, 2*, 79–91.

Hu, L., & Bentler, P. M. (1998). Fit indices in covariance structure modeling: Sensitivity to underparameterized model misspecification. *Psychological Methods, 3*, 424–453.

Hu, L., & Bentler, P. M. (1999). Cutoff criteria for fit indexes in covariance structure analysis: Conventional criteria versus new alternatives. *Structural Equation Modeling, 6*, 1–55.

Jensen, A. R., & Weng, L. (1993). What is a good *g? Intelligence, 18*, 231–258.

Jöreskog, K. G., & Sörbom, D. (1993). *LISREL 8: Structural equation modeling with the SIMPLIS command language.* Hillsdale, NJ: Erlbaum

Jöreskog, K. G., & Sörbom, D. (1996). *LISREL 8 user's reference guide.* Lincolnwood, IL: Scientific Software.

Kamphaus, R. W. (2001). *Clinical assessment of child and adolescent intelligence* (2nd ed.). Boston: Allyn & Bacon.

Kaufman, A. S. (1994). *Intelligent testing with the WISC-III.* New York: Wiley.

Kaufman, A. S. (1996). Wechsler and Horn: A reply to McGrew and Flanagan. *Communiqué, 24*(6), 15–17.

Kaufman, A. S., & Kaufman, N. L. (1993). *Manual: Kaufman Adolescent and Adult Intelligence Test.* Circle Pines, MN: American Guidance Service.

Keith, T. Z. (1990). Confirmatory and hierarchical confirmatory analysis of the Differential Ability Scales. *Journal of Psychoeducational Assessment, 8*, 391–405.

Keith, T. Z. (1997a). Using confirmatory factor analysis to aid in understanding the constructs measured by intelligence tests. In D. P. Flanagan, J. L. Genshaft, & P. L. Harrison (Eds.), *Contemporary intellectual assessment: Theories, tests, and issues* (pp. 373–402). New York: Guilford Press.

Keith, T. Z. (1997b). What does the WISC-III measure?: A reply to Carroll and Kranzler. *School Psychology Quarterly, 12*, 117–118.

Keith, T. Z. (in press). *Multiple regression and beyond: A conceptual introduction to multiple regression, confirmatory factor analysis, and structural equation modeling.* Boston: Allyn & Bacon.

Keith, T. Z., & Kranzler, J. H. (1999). The absence of structural fidelity precludes construct validity: Rejoinder to Naglieri on what the Cognitive Assessment System does and does not measure. *School Psychology Review, 28*, 303–321.

Keith, T. Z., Kranzler, J. H., & Flanagan, D. P. (2001). What does the Cognitive Assessment (CAS) measure? Joint confirmatory factor analysis of the CAS and the Woodcock–Johnson Tests of Cognitive Ability (3rd Edition). *School Psychology Review, 30*, 89–119.

Keith, T. Z., Quirk, K. J., Schartzer, C., & Elliott, C. D. (1999). Construct bias in the Differential Ability Scales? Confirmatory and hierarchical factor structure across three ethnic groups. *Journal of Psychoeducational Assessment, 17*, 249–268.

Keith, T. Z., & Reynolds, C. R. (2003). Measurement and design issues in research on the assessment of children. In C. R. Reynolds & R. W. Kamphaus (Eds.), *Handbook of psychological and educational assessment of children: Intelligence, aptitude, and achievement* (2nd ed., pp. 79–111). New York: Guilford Press.

Keith, T. Z., & Witta, L. (1997). Hierarchical and cross-age confirmatory factor analysis of the WISC-III: What does it measure? *School Psychology Quarterly, 12*, 89–107.

Kline, R. B. (1998). *Principles and practices of structural equation modeling.* New York: Guilford Press.

Kranzler, J. H. (1997). What does the WISC-III measure? Comments on the relationship between intelligence, working memory capacity, and information processing speed and efficiency, *School Psychology Quarterly, 12*, 110–116.

Kranzler, J. H., & Keith, T. Z. (1999). Independent confirmatory factor analysis of the Cognitive Assessment System (CAS): What does the CAS measure? *School Psychology Review, 28*, 117–144.

Kranzler, J. H., Keith, T. Z., & Flanagan, D. P. (2000). Independent examination of the factor structure of the cognitive assessment system (CAS): Further evidence challenging the construct validity of the CAS. *Journal of Psychoeducational Assessment, 18*, 143–159.

Loehlin, J. C. (1998). *Latent variable models: An introduction to factor, path, and structural analysis* (3rd ed.). Hillsdale, NJ: Erlbaum.

Marsh, H. W. (1993). The multidimensional structure of academic self-concept: Invariance over gender and age. *American Educational Research Journal, 30*, 841–860.

McArdle, J. J. (1998). Contemporary statistical models for examining test bias. In J. J. McArdle & R. W. Woodcock (Eds.), *Human cognitive abilities in theory practice* (pp. 157–195). Mahwah, NJ: Elbaum.

McGrew, K. S., & Flanagan, D. P. (1996, March). The Wechsler Performance Scale debate: Fluid intelligence (Gf) or visual processing (Gv). *Communiqué, 24*(6), 14, 16.

McGrew, K. S., & Flanagan, D. P. (1998). *The intelligence test desk reference (ITDR): Gf-Gc cross-battery assessment.* Needham Heights, MA: Allyn & Bacon.

McGrew, K. S., & Woodcock, R. W. (2001). *Woodcock–Johnson III technical manual.* Itasca, IL: Riverside.

Millsap, R. E. (2001). When trivial constraints are not trivial: The choice of uniqueness constraints in confirmatory factor analysis. *Structural Equation Modeling, 8*, 1–17.

Mulaik, S. A., & Quartetti, D. A. (1997). First-order or higher-order general factor? *Structural Equation Modeling, 4*, 193–211.

Muthén, L. K., & Muthén, B. O. (1998). *Mplus user's guide* (2nd ed.). Los Angeles: Muthén & Muthén.

Naglieri, J. A., & Das, J. P. (1997). *Das–Naglieri Cog-

nitive Assessment System: Interpretive handbook. Itasca, IL: Riverside.

Psychological Corporation. (2003). *Wechsler Intelligence Scale for Children—Fourth Edition: Technical manual.* San Antonio, TX: Author.

Stone, B. J. (1992). Joint confirmatory factor analyses of the DAS and WISC-R. *Journal of School Psychology, 30,* 185–195.

Taub, G. E., & McGrew, K. S. (2004). A confirmatory factor analysis of Cattell–Horn–Carroll theory and cross-age invariance of the Woodcock–Johnson Tests of Cognitive Abilities III. *School Psychology Quarterly, 19,* 72–87.

Tanaka, J. S. (1993). Multifaceted conceptions of fit in structural equation models. In K. S. Bollen & J. S. Long (Eds.), *Testing structural equation models* (pp. 10–39). Newbury Park, CA: Sage.

Thorndike, R. M. (1990). Would the real factors of the Stanford–Binet Fourth Edition please come forward? *Journal of Psychoeducational Assessment, 8,* 412–435.

Vernon, P. E. (1950). *The structure of human abilities.* New York: Wiley.

Willis, J. O. (1996). A practitioner's reaction to McGrew & Flanagan and Kaufman. *Communiqué, 24*(6), 15, 17.

Woodcock, R. W. (1993). An information processing view of Gf-Gc theory. *Journal of Psychoeducational Assessment, Monograph Series: Woodcock–Johnson Psycho-Educational Battery—Revised,* 80–102.

Woodcock, R. W., & Johnson, M. B. (1989). *Woodcock–Johnson Psycho-Educational Battery—Revised Tests of Cognitive Abilities.* Chicago: Riverside.

Woodcock, R. W., McGrew, K. S., & Mather, N. (2001). *Woodcock–Johnson III Tests of Cognitive Abilities.* Itasca, IL: Riverside.

28

Using the Joint Test Standards to Evaluate the Validity Evidence for Intelligence Tests

JEFFERY P. BRADEN
BRADLEY C. NIEBLING

The current edition of the *Standards for Educational and Psychological Testing* (American Educational Research Association [AERA], American Psychological Association [APA], & National Council on Measurement in Education [NCME], 1999) provides a framework for evaluating contemporary tests of intelligence. The *Standards* help test publishers and test users decide how to present, use, and evaluate tests, and help users to select and interpret tests as well. However, we believe that many users of intelligence tests are not familiar with the *Standards*, and may be uncertain how to apply them to such tests.

Therefore, we begin our chapter with a brief description of the *Standards*. In the next section of the chapter, we articulate a framework for judging the validity evidence provided by test developers. We then use the framework to evaluate the validity evidence presented for selected contemporary tests of intelligence at their time of publication. We conclude our discussion by assessing common strengths, weaknesses, and challenges confronting test developers and users in understanding the validity of intelligence tests.

DEVELOPMENT AND CONTENT OF THE *STANDARDS*

The *Standards* first appeared as a joint publication in 1974 (APA, AERA, & NCME, 1974). The joint publication combined three distinct sets of standards promulgated by different groups interested in educational and psychological tests (i.e., APA, 1954, 1966; AERA, 1955). The *Standards* were revised in 1985 (AERA, APA, & NCME, 1985), and were revised again in 1999.

Each edition of the *Standards* attempted to reflect professional consensus regarding expectations for the development and use of educational and psychological tests. As stated in the current version, "the purpose of publishing the *Standards* is to provide criteria for the evaluation of tests, testing practices, and the effects of test use" (AERA et al., 1999, p. 2). That is, the *Standards* are intended to apply both to those who produce tests (developers) and to those who use tests (examiners). Additional standards apply to test users (e.g., APA, 2002) and to test takers (e.g., APA, 1998), but the *Standards* are intended to reflect the contemporary and common consensus for the use of educational and psychological tests.

The current edition of the *Standards* contains three sections, covering the following topics: (1) test construction, evaluation, and documentation; (2) fairness in testing; and (3) testing applications. Although specific standards in all three sections apply to test publishers and users, the standards applying to test developers appear primarily in the first section.

The current edition differs from previous editions in a number of important ways. First, specific standards are no longer identified as either primary or secondary. Instead, the salience of any given standard is determined by its relevance for the intended uses of the test. Second, the new *Standards* volume specifies that standards cannot be applied in a literal or rote checklist. Rather, professional judgment, the degree to which the test developer and user satisfy each standard, availability of alternatives, and research must influence the degree to which a test is deemed acceptable.

Third, the *Standards* employ an important shift in the use of the term *construct*. Rather than meaning unobservable characteristics, this term is broadened to mean "the concept or characteristic that a test is designed to measure" (AERA et al., 1999, p. 5). This redefinition alters the understanding of *validity* from that of previous versions. Instead of describing three distinct types of validity (*content*, *construct*, and *criterion*), the new *Standards* regard validity as being "the degree to which evidence and theory support the interpretations of test scores entailed by proposed uses of tests" (p. 9). In other words, validity is the degree to which evidence supports the assumption that the test score reflects the construct the test claims to assess. Therefore, the distinctions among content, construct, and criterion validity in previous versions are replaced by the notion that multiple sources of evidence must support the claim that the test measures the construct.

The *Standards* identify five sources of evidence: (1) *test content*, (2) *response processes*, (3) *internal structure*, (4) *relations to other variables*, and (5) *consequences of testing*. Three of these sources appeared in previous editions: test content (content validity),

internal structure (construct validity), and relations to other variables (criterion validity). However, the other two sources of evidence are new. Response process evidence supports the contention that test takers use the intended psychological processes when responding to items (e.g., a reasoning test elicits reasoning rather than recall). Test consequence evidence should support the contention that testing and test outcomes actually fulfill the claims made for test use (e.g., a test demonstrates that results are useful for designing psychoeducational interventions).

In this chapter, we focus on the intersection of the new *Standards* and intelligence tests. We attempt to identify those standards that are more or less relevant to particular intelligence tests, based on the claims of those tests. Our primary focus is on validity claims and evidence, mainly because of the importance of these standards for intellectual assessment. Intelligence tests are more often criticized for failing to assess their intended construct (intelligence) than for lacking reliability, norms, and other attributes found in other parts of the *Standards*.

Although we appreciate that appropriate use of intelligence tests is a joint responsibility shared by test developers and test users, our primary focus is on evaluating the validity evidence provided by test developers to support tests of intelligence. Standard 11.1 states: "Prior to the adoption and use of a published test, the test user should study and evaluate the materials provided by the test developer" (AERA et al., 1999, p. 113). Although Standard 11.1 goes on to specify four areas of particular importance for test users to consider, our review focuses on two: (1) the purpose of the test, and (2) the validity data available to support score interpretations consistent with those purposes. We suggest a framework for evaluating the materials and information provided by a test developer to help test users fulfill their obligation to meet Standard 11.1, although we also appreciate that users should obtain and consider evidence from other sources as well (e.g., professional publications, test reviews). We focus primarily on those standards dealing with validity, which are found in Chapter 1 of the *Standards*.

VALIDITY EVIDENCE FRAMEWORK

We developed an organizational and conceptual framework for evaluating the importance and quality of validity evidence presented by test developers shortly after the publication of the *Standards*. The original draft of this framework was used to evaluate the validity evidence presented by the test developers of a wide variety of assessment instruments commonly used by school psychologists (Braden et al., 2001a, 2001b). Although the content of the new *Standards* was written to represent a shift in philosophy for establishing validity, the fact that no explicit guidance was provided for applying the new *Standards* prompted us to develop a framework for evaluating validity claims and evidence.

Our original framework assigned each of the 24 validity standards (AERA et al., 1999, Ch. 1) to one of the five evidence domain areas: content, response processes, internal structure, relation to other variables, and consequences. To increase the functionality and objectivity of these standards, and to help users meet the spirit of Standard 11.1, we created two Likert-type scales. The first Likert-type scale rates the *importance* of the validity evidence presented in each of the five domain areas for the claims made by the test developer. For example, evidence of test content is more important for tests claiming to measure specific content (e.g., tests of mathematics abilities that employ a state's math standards) than for tests not making such claims (e.g., projective tests). Ratings on this scale range from 1 = "not important" to 5 = "critical/very important." The second Likert-type scale asks test users to rate the *quality* of the validity evidence presented in each of the five domain areas by the test developer. Ratings on this scale range from 1 = "weak" to 5 = "strong," with a 0 rating for "no evidence present."

As we applied our framework to these psychological tests, we invited test developers and other experts to provide feedback to us about our efforts (see Braden et al., 2001a, 2001b). On the basis of that feedback, we realized that our framework was inadequate. Consequently, we updated the framework in two ways. First, we created an additional domain area called the *cross-cutting* domain. This domain was created for the standards dealing with validity issues that cut across, or serve as a type of umbrella for, the other five domain areas. For example, Standard 1.1 directs test developers to justify and support recommended interpretations, and does not clearly fall into a specified domain of evidence. Second, we decided that some standards fit into more than one of the five evidence domain areas. Third, we felt that standards in multiple domains serve either a **primary** (in bold) or *secondary* (in italics) role within each domain. For example, the primary emphasis of Standard 1.14 relates to a test's relations to other variables, but it is also related to internal test structure when test evidence includes factor-analytic evidence, such as the kind of evidence presented to support cross-battery analyses of cognitive processes.

Figure 28.1 graphically presents the allocation of standards to the six categories. Table 28.1 presents an organizational framework for jointly considering the importance of a body of evidence or standards, and the quality of available evidence to respond to the domain.

Once the framework was updated, we developed a set of coding procedures (Niebling & Braden, 2003) to evaluate validity claims and the evidence test developers provide to support those claims. The materials accompanying each assessment instrument (e.g., technical manuals, administration manuals, test publisher bulletins) formed the foundations for evaluating test claims and validity. The first step was to identify each of the claims listed by the test developer for use of the test. These claims guided the collection of validity evidence and determined the relative importance of evidence. For example, a test claiming to assess cognitive processes has a greater obligation to provide evidence of response processes than a test that does not make such a claim. Next, the validity evidence was identified and evaluated within each evidence domain area; the standards in those domain areas were used as the lens through which to examine that evidence. The next step was to rate the importance of the gathered evidence for the domain. We repeated the process for each of the six domain areas to provide a structured, but subjective,

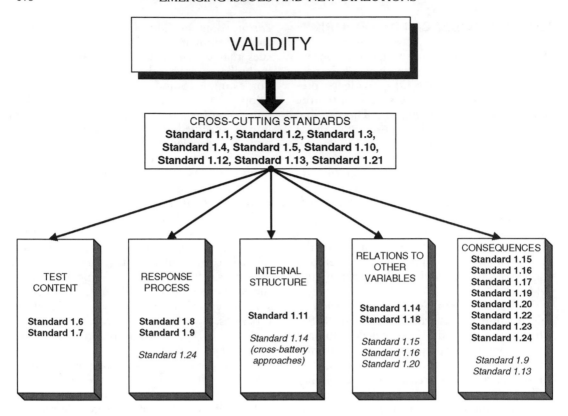

FIGURE 28.1. Conceptual framework for understanding and applying validity standards.

evaluation of evidence supporting the claims made for the test.

The framework described here was designed to increase the functionality and objectivity of the *Standards* for evaluating validity evidence presented by test developers. We note, however, that this framework is not intended to remove the importance of pro-

fessional judgment in using the *Standards* to examine validity evidence. Furthermore, our framework is not a checklist or test; rather, the framework describes the *process* of collecting and evaluating validity evidence. Ratings represent the importance and quality of evidence presented relative to *test claims*, and are not a rote application of the *Stan-*

TABLE 28.1. Validity Evidence Rating Grid

Standard domain	Importance					Quality						Evidence
Cross-cutting	1	2	3	4	5	0	1	2	3	4	5	
Test content	1	2	3	4	5	0	1	2	3	4	5	
Response processes	1	2	3	4	5	0	1	2	3	4	5	
Internal structure	1	2	3	4	5	0	1	2	3	4	5	
Relation to other variables	1	2	3	4	5	0	1	2	3	4	5	
Consequences	1	2	3	4	5	0	1	2	3	4	5	

dards. Our ratings should be viewed in this context.

ANALYSIS OF VALIDITY EVIDENCE FOR SELECTED TESTS OF INTELLIGENCE

In this section, we describe how we applied the framework we developed to tests of intelligence. We used three criteria to select tests for review: (1) The tests are described in other chapters of the present book; (2) the test was published after the publication of the *Standards* (so test developers had the opportunity to use the new *Standards*); and (3) publication data were available to us in time for inclusion in our chapter. These criteria identified the following tests for review: (1) the Wechsler Intelligence Scale for Children—Fourth Edition (WISC-IV; Wechsler, 2003); (2) the Stanford–Binet Intelligence Scales, Fifth Edition (SB5; Roid, 2003a); (3) the Woodcock–Johnson III Tests of Cognitive Abilities (WJ III COG; Woodcock, McGrew, & Mather, 2001); and (4) the Reynolds Intellectual Assessment Scales (RIAS; Reynolds & Kamphaus, 2003). Other tests included in this volume were excluded primarily because they were published prior to 1999, although one test (the Kaufman Assessment Battery for Children—Second Edition) was excluded because information about the test was not available at the time this chapter was written. Exclusion of other tests is in no way intended to convey judgments about those tests; our review is not exhaustive. Rather, our review is intended to illustrate one way that test users might respond to Standard 11.1 regarding review of test developer information, particularly as it applies to the purposes and validity of contemporary tests of intelligence.

Review of the WISC-IV

We reviewed the administration (Wechsler, 2003) and technical (Psychological Corporation, 2003) manuals for claims regarding the WISC-IV. The claims we identified are presented in Table 28.2. We then consulted these sources, as well as three technical bulletins provided by the test developers (Williams, Weiss, & Rolfhus, 2003a, 2003b,

2003c), for evidence to support test claims. Our ratings of importance for various domains, and the quality of evidence within those domains, are presented in Figure 28.2.

Review of the SB5

We reviewed the administrative (Roid, 2003a), interpretive (Roid, 2003b), and technical (Roid, 2003c) manuals for the SB5 to identify test claims and evidence. These three sources substantially overlap, and in some cases, replicate some sections in their entirety. In addition, we included three Assessment Services Bulletins distributed by the test developer (i.e., Becker, 2003; Braden & Elliott, 2003; Ruf, 2003) for additional evidence in support of test claims. The claims we identified for the test are presented in Table 28.3. Our ratings of importance for various domains, and the quality of evidence within those domains, are presented in Figure 28.3.

Review of the WJ III COG

We reviewed the examiner's (Woodcock et al., 2001) and technical (McGrew & Woodcock, 2001) manuals for the WJ III COG to identify test claims. We also consulted three technical bulletins provided by the test developers (Flanagan, 2001; Mather & Schrank, 2001; Schrank, McGrew, & Woodcock, 2001) for test claims and evidence to support test claims. The claims we identified are presented in Table 28.4. Our ratings of importance for various domains, and the quality of evidence within those domains, are presented in Figure 28.4.

Review of the RIAS

We reviewed the professional manual (Reynolds & Kamphaus, 2003) for the RIAS to identify test claims. The claims we identified are presented in Table 28.5. We then consulted this source, and information on the test publisher's web page (Psychological Assessment Resources, 2003), for evidence to support test claims. Our ratings of importance for various domains, and the quality of evidence within those domains, are presented in Figure 28.5.

TABLE 28.2. Claims Made for the WISC-IV by the Test Developer

Administration manual (Wechsler, 2003, pp. 7–8)

- The WISC-IV is for use with examinees 6 years, 0 months to 16 years, 11 months of age.
- It provides comprehensive assessment of general intellectual functioning.
- It identifies giftedness, mental retardation, and cognitive strengths and weaknesses.
- Specific suggestions for use with adaptive behavior, memory, and achievement measures are provided.
- Results can guide treatment planning and placement decisions.
- The WISC-IV provides invaluable clinical information for neuropsychological evaluation.
- It is also useful in research.

Technical manual (Psychological Corporation, 2003)

- The WISC-IV measures four major cognitive clusters loosely aligned with Cattell–Horn–Carroll (CHC) theory (Ch. 1, pp. 7–8):
  - Fluid Reasoning
  - Verbal Comprehension
  - Working Memory
  - Processing Speed
- Subtests measure specific cognitive processes (pp. 16–20).

Technical Bulletin No. 2 and other sources (in parentheses)

- Use for clients with the following special conditions is implied by directions and data:
  - Deafness and hearing impairments (Wechsler, 2003, pp. 12–18)
  - Physical/motor disabilities (Wechsler, 2003, p. 11; Psychological Corporation, 2003, pp. 100–101)
  - Language or speech disabilities (Wechsler, 2003, p. 11; Psychological Corporation, 2003, pp. 91–93)
  - Sensory disabilities (Wechsler, 2003, p. 11)
  - English-language learner status (Wechsler, 2003, p. 12)
  - Non-English-speaking status (Wechsler, 2003, p. 12)
  - Intellectual giftedness (Psychological Corporation, 2003, pp. 79–80)
  - Mild to moderate mental retardation (Psychological Corporation, 2003, pp. 80–84)
  - Learning disorders (Psychological Corporation, 2003, pp. 84–88)
  - Attention-deficit/hyperactivity disorder (Psychological Corporation, 2003, pp. 89–91)
  - Traumatic brain injury (Psychological Corporation, 2003, pp. 93–97)
  - Autistic disorder (Psychological Corporation, 2003, pp. 98–100)

FIGURE 28.2. Summary of validity evidence for the WISC-IV.

Cross-cutting standards	Importance	4
Standards **1.1, 1.2, 1.3, 1.4, 1.5, 1.10, 1.12, 1.13, 1.21**	Quality	3

- Clear statements are made regarding test user qualifications and responsibilities.
- Theoretical descriptions/rationales for claims regarding general intelligence are extensive and well documented.
- Little to no direct evidence is provided for specific claims regarding treatment planning or links to neuropsychological foundations.
- Clear statements help users distinguish between statistically reliable differences and unusual (base rate) differences among test scores.
- The norming sample is described in detail, including information regarding age, grade level, census region, community size, gender, race, type of school attended, and status of parents. The sample matches the target population very well.
- Collection procedures of the norming data are described in detail, as are procedures for test administration.
- Extensive discussion of how to identify intraindividual strengths and weaknesses by using Index, subtest, and within-subtest responses does not include discussion of contradictory findings available in the literature.

Test content	Importance	4
Standards **1.6, 1.7**	Quality	3

- Test content is described extensively, and inferences about the psychological processes they elicit are based in part on test content. Research findings on previous versions of the Wechsler scales are also cited to support the contention that subtests elicit specific processes.

(continued)

FIGURE 28.2. *(continued)*

- Test items were developed and reviewed by expert panels to ensure that they reflect their intended constructs. However, details regarding the selection and composition of the panels are lacking.

Response processes	Importance		5
Standards **1.8**, **1.9**, *1.24*	Quality	3	

- Research on previous versions of the Wechsler scales is cited as evidence that subtests and Index scores elicit specific processes; however, most of the cited evidence is inferential, because it relies on subjective identification of common item content and infers the psychological processes that would explain the correlation between the items. For example, factor loadings are explained by invoking common psychological processes, without direct evidence that examinees used those processes.
- Multiple-choice item errors were analyzed for common patterns that might suggest measurement of unintended processes.
- Interview evidence from examinees was obtained and analyzed for two new subtests, but not for other subtests.
- The use of the term *process score* implies scores reflect neuropsychological processes, although no direct evidence is provided to support this implication.

Internal structure	Importance		5
Standards **1.11**, *1.14*	Quality		5

- Ample evidence of correlations among items and subtests provides convergent and divergent validity evidence.
- Confirmatory and exploratory factor analyses concur in strongly supporting the four-factor model claimed by the test developers.
- Stability and reliability indices also provide evidence of internal consistency and the stability of the constructs measured within the battery.

Relationship to other variables	Importance		5
Standards **1.14**, **1.18**, *1.15*, *1.16*, *1.20*	Quality	4	

- Correlations among a variety of measures are provided; these generally support the notion that the test measures general intelligence, predicts academic achievement, is related to clinical diagnostic categories, and is consistent with previous versions of the test.
- Corrected correlations are provided; uncorrected correlations are not.
- A rationale for including unusual or unexpected measures is provided; although a rationale for expected measures (e.g., other tests of intelligence, achievement) is not provided, it is not needed. References to other measures allow test users to find and evaluate the quality of external measures.
- Extensive data are provided for a variety of clinical samples, supporting test performance across a range of relevant conditions.
- An extensive narrative review of research on previous editions, coupled with evidence that the new edition is highly related to older editions, provides unusually broad evidence linking the test to many attributes. However, the narrative review is selective, and could have been more powerful if it used contemporary methods to summarize research findings (e.g., meta-analysis).

Test consequences	Importance		5
Standards **1.15**, **1.16**, **1.17**, **1.19**, **1.20**, **1.22**, **1.23**, **1.24**, *1.9*, *1.13*	Quality	1	

- The technical manual (p. 101) addresses this issue in a single paragraph, arguing that it is the sole responsibility of the test user to supply evidence regarding test consequences.
- Extensive data from clinical groups imply support for claims of diagnostic utility; however, these data are not provided at the individual level, and therefore are difficult to evaluate.
- The omission of research on previous test editions that addresses test consequences stands in stark contrast to the extensive use of research on previous editions to support other claims.
- The extensive description of how users may use test results to identify cognitive strengths and weaknesses in the technical manual (Ch. 6) implies value for meeting claims regarding clinical and educational interventions; however, no evidence is cited or provided in direct support of these claims.
- Item bias indices were used to identify and eliminate or modify items indicating evidence of bias. However, no summary evidence is provided regarding means, variances, or item bias influence for groups.
- Unintended consequences (particularly as they relate to score differences between groups defined by ethnic, gender, and socioeconomic status) are not mentioned. This omission is puzzling, given the extensive research and debate that previous editions of the same test have sparked on this topic, as well as the substantial (but unreported) differences in means between some ethnic groups on this test.

TABLE 28.3. Claims Made for the SB5 by the Test Developer

Administration manual (Roid, 2003a)

- The SB5 is appropriate for examinees 2–85 years of age (p. 1).
- It is useful for clients with the following special conditions (pp. 1–2):
  - Deafness and hearing impairments
  - Communication disorders
  - Autism
  - Specific learning disabilities
  - Limited English-language background
  - Traumatic brain injury
  - Other conditions affecting language ability (e.g., aphasia, stroke)
  - Limited vision
  - Orthopedic impairment
  - Highest level of gifted performance
  - Low intellectual functioning or mental retardation
  - Various neuropsychological difficulties
- Appropriate uses include the following (pp. 4–5):
  - Diagnosis of developmental disabilities and exceptionalities, including mental retardation, learning disabilities, developmental cognitive delays, and intellectual giftedness.
  - Clinical and neuropsychological assessment
  - Research on abilities
  - Early childhood assessment
  - Psychoeducational evaluations for special education placements
  - Adult Social Security and workers' compensation evaluations
  - Provide information for interventions such as individual family plans, individual education plans, career assessment, employee selection and classification, and adult neuropsychological treatment.
  - Must be used with additional measures for diagnostic purposes (e.g., adaptive behavior for mental retardation diagnosis).
- The SB5 measures intelligence and five broad cognitive abilities or factors (Ch. 2):
  - Fluid Reasoning
  - Knowledge
  - Quantitative Reasoning
  - Visual–Spatial Processing
  - Working Memory
- Subtests measure unique, narrow cognitive abilities (pp. 138–143).
- Cognitive strengths and weaknesses are identified via score contrasts (pp. 147–150).
  - Abbreviated Battery IQ is useful for neuropsychological examinations when used with additional tests (p. 1).

Interpretive and technical manuals (Roid, 2003b, 2003c)

- Claims made in the administration manual are reiterated.

FIGURE 28.3. Summary of validity evidence for the SB5.

Cross-cutting standards	Importance	4
Standards **1.1, 1.2, 1.3, 1.4, 1.5, 1.10, 1.12, 1.13, 1.21**	Quality	5

- Clear statements are made regarding test user qualifications and responsibilities.
- Theoretical descriptions/rationales for claims regarding general intelligence are extensive and well documented.
- Little to no direct evidence is provided for specific claims regarding value for treatment planning.
- Clear statements help users distinguish between statistically reliable differences and unusual (base rate) differences among test scores.
- The norm sample is described in detail, including information regarding age, grade level, census region, gender, race, and education level. The sample matches the target population very well.
- Collection procedures for norms data are described in detail, as are procedures for test administration.
- Extensive discussion of how to identify intraindividual strengths and weaknesses by using index, subtest, and within-subtest responses includes some discussion of contradictory findings available in the literature, but no justification is provided for subtest-specific interpretations beyond content analyses.
- Extended discussion is provided of administration and interpretation issues for special populations, including detailed guides for test accommodations.

(continued)

FIGURE 28.3. *(continued)*

Test content	Importance	4
Standards **1.6, 1.7**	Quality	5

- Test content is described extensively, and inferences about the psychological processes they elicit are made in part based on test content. Research findings on previous versions of the SB are also cited to support the contention that subtests measure general intelligence.
- Test items were developed and reviewed by expert panels to ensure that they reflect their intended constructs. Explicit details about the processes, and names of expert consultants and review committee members, are provided.

Response processes	Importance	4
Standards **1.8, 1.9**, *1.24*	Quality	1

- Research on previous versions of the SB is cited as evidence to justify the realignment of factor structures and processes to CHC theory.
- Claims that subtests and index scores elicit specific processes rest exclusively on subjective identification of common item content and inferences about psychological processes that would explain correlations among items and scores. For example, factor loadings are explained by invoking common psychological processes, without direct evidence that examinees used those processes.
- Although the *Standards* volume is cited frequently in all manuals, the chapter on validity evidence (Roid, 2003c) omits response processes.
- Change-sensitive scores (i.e., Rasch item scores) are described and provide general evidence that the test measures processes that increase and change across the developmental spectrum.

Internal structure	Importance	5
Standards **1.11**, *1.14*	Quality	5

- Exploratory and confirmatory factor-analytic data strongly support test claims, and were replicated by dividing the norm sample in half. Comparisons of factor models support five-factor claim; internal fit statistics are strong, although residual mean squares are slightly higher than desired.
- Cross-battery factor analysis (with WJ III) statistics strongly support factor structure claims within and between tests.
- Stability and reliability indices also provide evidence of internal consistency and the stability of the constructs measured within the battery.
- Correlation tables reporting relationships among subtests are not provided.

Relationship to other variables	Importance	5
Standards **1.14, 1.18**, *1.15, 1.16, 1.20*	Quality	4

- Overall, correlations among a variety of measures are provided; these generally support the notion that the test measures general intelligence, predicts academic achievement, is related to clinical diagnostic categories, and is consistent with previous versions of the test.
- A rationale for expected measures (e.g., other tests of intelligence, achievement) is not provided, but it is not needed. References to other measures allow test users to find and evaluate the quality of external measures.
- Data are provided for a variety of clinical samples, supporting test performance across a range of relevant conditions.
- An extensive narrative review of research on previous editions, coupled with evidence that the new edition is highly related to older editions, provides unusually broad evidence linking the test to many attributes. However, the narrative review is selective; could have been more powerful if it used contemporary methods to summarize research findings (e.g., meta-analysis); and notes that research on previous versions of the test does not generalize well beyond broad measures of general intelligence (i.e., research on factor structures and processes in previous editions does not generalize to the new version).
- Relationships between test scores, abilities, and performance in important social contexts are theoretically justified (Roid, 2003b, Ch. 5), but no direct evidence is provided to support the rationale.
- Correlations with other intelligence tests (previous versions of the SB, two other contemporary intelligence tests) are inexplicably characterized as criterion validity. However, correlations are moderate and appropriate, with a few anomalies (e.g., the correlation between Visual–Spatial Processing scores and WISC-III Performance IQ are lower than the correlation with Verbal IQ).
- Correlations with two achievement batteries (the WJ-III Tests of Achievement [WJ III ACH] and the Wechsler Individual Achievement Test—Second Edition [WIAT-II]) are described as predictive, but are concurrent. Correlations are moderate and appropriate, with a few anomalies (e.g., the SB5 Knowledge score is more highly correlated with WJ III ACH Reading Comprehension than with Mathematics Reasoning, but the opposite pattern occurs on the WIAT-II).

(continued)

FIGURE 28.3. *(continued)*

Test consequences	Importance		5
Standards **1.15, 1.16, 1.17, 1.19, 1.20, 1.22, 1.23, 1.24**, *1.9*, *1.13*	Quality	2	

- Extensive data from clinical groups implies support for claims of diagnostic utility. Although the administration manual does not provide data at the individual level, the interpretive manual does so, and includes recommended cutoff scores.
- The extensive description of how users may use test results to identify cognitive strengths and weaknesses in all three manuals implies value for meeting claims regarding clinical and educational interventions; however, no direct evidence is cited nor provided in direct support of these claims.
- Case studies elaborate the recommended seven-step interpretive procedure. It is noteworthy that the first three steps intend to establish the validity of scores for the examinee; the last four steps are similar to profile interpretation recommended for other tests, and are not explicitly justified via treatment response studies or other direct evidence.
- Item bias indices were used to identify and eliminate or modify items indicating evidence of bias. Summary evidence of item bias statistics, correlations, and internal consistency for various groups are provided, but no summary evidence is provided regarding means and variances for groups.
- Unintended consequences and concerns with diagnosis (particularly as they relate to score differences between groups defined by ethnic, gender, disability, and socioeconomic status) are discussed often, and include references to critical research and appropriate ethical guidelines and cautions.
- Although the chapter on validity in the technical manual does not include a section on consequential validity (despite citing the *Standards*), the interpretive manual includes a chapter addressing consequential validity in the context of test bias and fairness for groups.
- Explicit directions to examiners to include data from other sources are provided for some diagnostic decisions (e.g., mental retardation, learning disability).

TABLE 28.4. Claims Made for the WJ III COG by the Test Developers

Examiner's manual (Woodcock, McGrew, & Mather, 2001)

- The WJ III COG is for use with preschool through geriatric levels.
- It measures intelligence according to the domains set forth in CHC theory.
- Appropriate uses include the following:
  - Diagnosis (p. 5)
  - Determination of intraindividual ability discrepancies (in conjunction with WJ III ACH; p. 5):
    - Understanding strengths and weaknesses
    - Diagnosing and documenting specific disabilities (however, multiple sources of information in addition to a discrepancy are needed for a learning disability diagnosis)
    - Acquiring *most* relevant information for educational and vocational planning
- Educational and vocational programming
- Planning individual programs
- Guidance
- Assessing growth
- Research and evaluation
- Psychometric training

FIGURE 28.4. Summary of validity evidence for the WJ III COG.

Cross-cutting standards	Importance	4
Standards **1.1, 1.2, 1.3, 1.4, 1.5, 1.10, 1.12, 1.13, 1.21**	Quality	3

- The test user is encouraged to integrate other, "nontest" information when making diagnostic and classification decisions.
- The test developers strongly discourage making interpretations based on subtests only, but rather when each score is interpreted within the context of all other scores and assessment data.
- Discussion of "strengths" and "weaknesses," and of using test and cluster scores to examine them, is ambiguous. Although warnings against the practice are provided, ample directions and case examples illustrate the practice. Little to no empirical support is provided for how these analyses are beneficial, despite abundant evidence regarding intraindividual differences.
- Several of the tests can be interpreted according to the executive functions required and the corresponding processes used to perform the tasks (e.g., attention, working memory, planning, and cognitive flexibility).
- The norming sample is described in detail, including information regarding age, grade level, census region, community size, gender, race, type of school/college attended, education of adults, employment status, and occupation.
- Collection procedures of the norming data are described in detail. Based on this information, test users should be able to judge the relevance of statistical findings in the technical manual to local conditions.
- The examiner's manual provides detailed and accessible information about administration, scoring, qualifications, and training suggestions.

Test content	Importance	4
Standards **1.6, 1.7**	Quality	4

- A detailed description is provided of the CHC theory of cognitive abilities, around which content was crafted.
- Multiple tests cover each domain of the CHC theory.
- The Rasch model was employed to ensure that all items in each test measure the same narrow ability or trait. This process of item selection also helped the test developers to avoid selecting items that measured processes extraneous to the intended construct.
- Cognitive items range from lower-level processing to high-level thinking and reasoning.
- An expert panel was utilized in decisions about test content, but no details are given regarding panel selection or membership.
- Nine reviewers examined all WJ III COG items to identify potentially sensitive issues for women, individuals with disabilities, and cultural or linguistic minorities. Again, details about panel selection and composition are lacking.

Response processes	Importance	4
Standards **1.8, 1.9**, *1.24*	Quality	1

- Again, an extensive description is provided of the CHC theory of cognitive abilities, and of the theoretical response processes associated with each test within this framework.
- Descriptions are given of the WJ III cognitive performance model and the WJ III information-processing model. These models provide additional information regarding the processes theorized to be necessary for answering the test items.
- The CHC broad and narrow abilities measured by each of the WJ III COG tests are outlined. Also, a brief description is given of the test content by defining the nature of the stimuli, test requirements, and response modalities.
- A description of each test with its relationship to the CHC theory is included in the examiner's manual. This description includes the type of responses required from the test taker and the theorized psychological processes necessary to answer the items.
- Evidence is primarily theoretical, not empirical.
- No evidence is provided to guide examiners how to select among the three different characterizations of response processes (i.e., the CHC, cognitive performance, and information-processing models); all three frameworks are implied to be potentially valid for understanding clients' cognitive processes, but no guidance or evidence is provided to help users decide which model is appropriate for a given client.

Internal structure	Importance	5
Standards **1.11**, *1.14*	Quality	5

- Fit statistics for all five age levels are lower for WJ III than for competing intelligence models; evidence supporting the WJ III CHC model of intelligence from age 6 to late adulthood is provided.
- Confirmatory factor analyses are provided at five different age levels; the CHC interpretation is generally stable across age levels, providing evidence for structural integrity of the measure across the lifespan.

(continued)

FIGURE 28.4. *(continued)*

- Items were selected to reflect an average difference in difficulty of 3–4 *W* scale points between items.
- Extensive statistical evidence is provided for developmental patterns of cognitive performance on the tests and for the CHC-based structure of the tests.
- Internal-structure data are provided in Appendices D and E, the technical manual, and technical bulletins.

Relationship to other variables	Importance	4
Standards **1.14, 1.18**, *1.15, 1.16, 1.20*	Quality	4

- Special study samples were employed to provide evidence for diagnostic utility and for use with a range of populations.
- The test developers provide convergent and divergent validity evidence in the form of correlations between the WJ III COG and other measures of cognitive abilities and achievement. They reference the measures they use, so that readers will be able to find additional information about those instruments. However, they do not provide a rationale for selecting the other measures.
- All evidence presented in the technical manual and technical bulletins is concurrent, with no predictive evidence presented.

Test consequences	Importance	5
Standards **1.15, 1.16, 1.17, 1.19, 1.20, 1.22, 1.23, 1.24**, *1.9, 1.13*	Quality	1

- Evidence for diagnosis of common learning and attention difficulties is provided for groups, but not for individuals.
- Theoretical and conceptual evidence to support claims that the test measures intelligence is provided, but no direct evidence to support claims of value for planning educational or psychological interventions is provided.

TABLE 28.5. Claims Made for the RIAS by the Test Developers

Professional manual (Reynolds & Kamphaus, 2003)

- The RIAS is for use with ages 3–94 years.
- It is a measure of verbal and nonverbal intelligence (p. 12).
- It can be used for diagnosis and educational placement of individuals with these conditions (pp. 11–13):
  - Learning disability
  - Mental retardation
  - Giftedness
  - Memory impairment/central nervous system disturbances
  - Various forms of childhood psychopathology where intellectual functioning is an issue
- It can also be used for individuals with these conditions (p. 13):
  - Visual impairment (verbal subtests only)
  - Hearing deficiency (professional judgment on case-by-case basis)
  - Physical/orthopedic impairment
  - Neuropsychological impairments (other than those noted above)
  - Emotional/psychotic disturbances (due to brevity of measure)
- Other uses include the following:
  - Informing evaluation recommendations and remediation strategies (p. 14)
  - Research (p. 14)
  - Predicting specific outcomes (e.g., academic success) (Table 1.5, p. 12)

FIGURE 28.5. Summary of validity evidence for the RIAS.

Cross-cutting standards	Importance	4
Standards **1.1, 1.2, 1.3, 1.4, 1.5, 1.10, 1.12, 1.13, 1.21**	Quality	4

- Theoretical descriptions/rationales for test developers' usage claims are clear.
- Little to no empirical evidence is provided to suggest treatment utility of assessment results.
- Theoretical and empirical evidence warning against profile analysis is provided.
- The norming sample is described in detail, including information regarding age, grade level, census region, community size, gender, race, type of school/college attended, education of adults, employment status, and occupation.
- Collection procedures for the norming data are described in detail. An appropriate description is given of statistical correction procedures used to account for regional overrepresentation.
- The examiner's manual provides detailed and accessible information about administration, scoring, qualifications, and training suggestions.

Test content	Importance	4
Standards **1.6, 1.7**	Quality	4

- A brief description is given of the qualifications of expert panel members, but details are omitted.
- Content evidence is primarily in the form of historical reference, theory, and logical argument.
- Final items were chosen based on the basis of item statistics derived from true-score theory.
- Carroll's three-stratum theory was the primary foundational theory for the content of this instrument.

Response processes	Importance	4
Standards **1.8, 1.9**, *1.24*	Quality	1

- The test developers place primary responsibility for gathering this evidence on the test user during test administration.
- The developers provide little to no direct evidence for this domain.
- Primary evidence is based on theory and logical argument, and this is limited.
- The developers spend some time describing the hypothesized types of response processes that should be invoked for each subtest, but do not provide evidence to support their hypotheses.

Internal structure	Importance	5
Standards **1.11**, *1.14*	Quality	5

- All items are correlated at least .40 with subtest total scores, with most at least .50.
- Extensive empirical evidence that individual subtest internal-consistency measures are high and significant is provided.
- Internal consistency of subtests across different age and other subgroups is above .90.
- Exploratory and confirmatory factor analyses support test structure.

Relationship to other variables	Importance	5
Standards **1.14, 1.18**, *1.15, 1.16, 1.20*	Quality	4

- The test developers provide convergent and divergent validity evidence via correlations between the RIAS and other measures of cognitive abilities and achievement. They reference the measures they use, so that readers will be able to find additional information about those instruments.
- The developers provide a rationale for selecting the other measures.
- A rationale and good validity evidence are provided for relations to variables besides other IQ tests, such as developmental trends and clinical status.
- A detailed description is given of clinical group performance relative to other groups.
- No evidence is presented on the individual level, only group-level data.

Test consequences	Importance	5
Standards **1.15, 1.16, 1.17, 1.19, 1.20, 1.22, 1.23, 1.24**, *1.9, 1.13*	Quality	1

- Group-level evidence of accurate diagnoses made with the RIAS is provided, but no individual-level data are given, and there is no differential comparison over other measures used for diagnosis.
- The test developers provide evidence indicating a minimization of item and cultural bias.
- No direct evidence is presented relating stated test purposes to test consequences.

CONCLUSIONS

In our reviews of these four test batteries, we have attempted to illustrate how test users might evaluate validity claims and evidence for tests claiming to measure intelligence. The degree to which tests make additional claims (e.g., value for selecting psychoeducational or psychological interventions, diagnosis) places greater burdens on the test developers to provide evidence showing that those claims are met. Not all forms of evidence are equal in supporting test claims; nor does an abundance of some forms of evidence compensate for a lack of other forms. Despite the differences in claims and evidence in the tests we reviewed, we note two clear strengths shared by most tests.

First, contemporary tests of intelligence provide a substantial amount of evidence to support their validity. Contemporary intelligence tests compare favorably to most other instruments used in psychology and education; for example, most of the tests we reviewed devote one or more volumes, such as a technical manual, to supporting evidence. This is also a substantial improvement over earlier versions of intelligence tests, which often failed to provide any meaningful validity evidence.

Second, test developers tend to provide an abundance of evidence in two primary forms: the internal structure of the test, and relationships to other variables. Extensive evidence regarding items (e.g., bias), scales or subtests (e.g., reliability, stability), and relationships among scales (e.g., correlations, exploratory and confirmatory factor analyses) help test users understand the internal structure of the test. Also, test developers provide a strong array of relationships between test scores and other variables. This evidence is primarily in the form of correlations with other tests, and secondarily in the form of relating test scores to diagnoses in clinical samples.

However, we have also noted some weaknesses in the validity evidence provided by test developers. We appreciate at the outset that test users are somewhat analogous to prosecuting attorneys, whose primary guiding principle is "One can never have too much evidence." Test developers are constrained by economic, ethical, and practical issues, and cannot be expected to provide all

the evidence that test users might want. Therefore, we limit our criticisms to those forms of validity evidence that are absent but are highly relevant, or absent but could be made available at little additional cost.

None of the tests we reviewed provides much direct evidence of response processes, and none provides much evidence for test consequences. This is not surprising, given that these domains are new to the *Standards*. However, intelligence tests claim to measure cognitive processes (e.g., rather than past learning or "test-wiseness"), and psychology's growing technology for identifying such processes provides ample opportunities to measure response processes. Evidence supporting claims (e.g., that a test elicits spatial processing or verbal reasoning) could be as simple as posttest interviews of test takers, or as complex as real-time magnetic resonance imagery or positron emission technology scans illuminating which parts of the brain are active during various test activities. We hope that future tests and test revisions will incorporate more direct and elaborated measures of response processes in the test development process.

Likewise, none of the tests we reviewed provides much evidence of testing consequences—although all tests claim beneficial test consequences as a purpose for using the test. We appreciate that test developers cannot be held accountable for all possible consequences of test scores; nor can they be responsible for the quality of educational, medical, or social programs to which examinees are often assigned in part on the basis of test scores. Instead, we believe that test developers should be held accountable to a standard similar to the one applied to drug companies. That is, test developers should provide some evidence that when the test is used as specified, some real benefit is conferred to the test taker that would not be conferred in the absence of testing (e.g., random assignment to a treatment or program vs. assignment guided by test results). This is particularly pertinent for claims that tests are helpful in selecting and planning psychoeducational interventions (a claim common to all the tests we reviewed). If a test developer claims that test results are valuable for this purpose, then we believe the test developer should demonstrate that test scores are more valuable than the psychological equivalent of a placebo or other tests currently available for similar purposes via response to treatment studies.

Finally, we argue that much of the evidence currently provided by test developers to support validity is inappropriately presented from the perspective of groups rather than individuals. For example, data for individuals in various clinical categories are typically represented by means, standard deviations, and statistical differences between typical (so-called "normal") and atypical (so-called "abnormal") groups. These data are usually congruent with the claims of the developer that the test is useful for diagnosis. However, testers who use individually administered intelligence tests are rarely if ever charged with deciding whether a group of clients is atypical; rather, test users must decide whether a specific client is atypical. Showing the proportion of individuals in typical and atypical groups who have particular scores would provide test users with a much better understanding of how test scores relate to diagnosis. Likewise, reporting means and standard deviations of test scores by demographic group would help examiners understand the degree to which test scores differ for groups. Reporting test bias statistics would help users understand that differences in score distributions between groups are not due to faulty measurement; conversely, failing to provide information about the degree to which test score distributions differ impairs test users' ability to understand the degree to which groups do or do not differ.

This information could be provided at little additional cost, because the data needed to generate such tables are already available to test developers. Furthermore, the information would help test users avoid errors in diagnosing individuals, and help users understand the probability of error associated with various score interpretations (see Watkins, Glutting, & Youngstrom, Chapter 12, this volume, for a discussion of these and related issues). Finally, although we appreciate that score differences between groups (particularly ethnic groups) are controversial, we believe that the controversy is not resolved simply by suppressing evidence that groups do in fact differ.

Test development and use constitute an evolving and symbiotic enterprise, with shared responsibilities for obtaining, providing, and using validity evidence. Clearly, test developers provide much more evidence for contemporary tests than was available for previous tests, and the evidence available generally supports the claims that contemporary intelligence tests are well aligned with the theoretical constructs that define intelligence. Evidence relating to the clinical application of tests to improve client welfare is more limited, or altogether absent. We appreciate that theory typically develops more rapidly than practical application, and we hope that by examining the strengths and weaknesses in the evidence regarding intelligence test validity through the lens of the new *Standards*, we will encourage test users and developers to continue the progress in developing validity evidence to support tests of intelligence.

ACKNOWLEDGMENTS

We would like to acknowledge the efforts of our colleagues Lori Bruno, Latrice Green, Ryan Kettler, Patricia Aleman, and Elisa Steele-Shernoff, for their assistance in developing and applying the validity standards framework. We also acknowledge feedback on our efforts from test developers James DiPerna, Stephen Elliott, Randy Kamphaus, Nancy Mather, Cecil Reynolds, Larry Weiss, and Richard Woodcock. We further thank David Goh for his assistance, which was instrumental in helping us conceptualize how to apply the *Standards*.

We also note that Jeffrey P. Braden received funds from Riverside Publishing, Inc., for preparing a guide to test accommodations for the SB5, and that he has accepted grants providing test materials to support test training from The Psychological Corporation, Riverside Publishing, and the Woodcock–Muñoz Foundation.

REFERENCES

American Educational Research Association (AERA) Committee on Test Standards. (1955). *Technical recommendations for achievement tests*. Washington, DC: Author.

American Educational Research Association (AERA), American Psychological Association (APA), & National Council on Measurement in Education (NCME). (1985). *Standards for educational and psychological testing* (2nd ed.). Washington, DC: American Psychological Association.

American Educational Research Association (AERA), American Psychological Association (APA), & National Council on Measurement in Education

(NCME). (1999). *Standards for educational and psychological testing* (3rd ed.). Washington, DC: AERA.

American Psychological Association (APA). (1954). *Technical recommendations for psychological tests and diagnostic techniques.* Washington, DC: Author.

American Psychological Association (APA). (1966). *Standards for educational and psychological tests and manuals.* Washington, DC: Author.

American Psychological Association (APA). (1998). *The rights and responsibilities of test takers: Guidelines and expectations.* Retrieved from http://www.apa.org/science/ttrr.html

American Psychological Association (APA), American Educational Research Association (AERA), & National Council on Measurement in Education (NCME). (1974). *Standards for educational and psychological tests.* Washington, DC: American Psychological Association.

Becker, K. A. (2003). *istory of the Stanford–Binet In-telligence Scales: Content and psychometrics* (Stanford–Binet Intelligence Scales, Fifth Edition, Assessment Services Bulletin No. 1). Itasca, IL: Riverside.

Braden, J. P., & Elliott, S. N. (2003). *Accommodations on the Stanford–Binet Intelligence Scales, Fifth Edition* (Stanford–Binet Intelligence Scales, Fifth Edition, Assessment Services Bulletin No. 2). Itasca, IL: Riverside.

Braden, J. P., Niebling, B. C., Bruno, L., Green, L. Y., Kettler, R. J., Aleman, P., et al. (2002, April). *New validity standards for educational and psychological tests: An overview and application.* Symposium conducted at the annual meeting of the National Association of School Psychologists, Washington, DC.

Braden, J. P., Niebling, B. C., Bruno, L., Green, L. Y., Kettler, R. J., Aleman, P., et al. (2001b, August). *New validity standards for educational and psychological tests: An overview and application.* Symposium conducted at the annual meeting of the American Psychological Association, San Francisco.

Flanagan, D. P. (2001). *Comparative features of the WJ III Tests of Cognitive Abilities* (Woodcock–Johnson III Assessment Service Bulletin No. 1). Itasca, IL: Riverside.

Mather, N., & Schrank, F. A. (2001). *Use of the WJ III discrepancy procedures for learning disabilities identification and diagnosis* (Woodcock–Johnson III Assessment Service Bulletin No. 3). Itasca, IL: Riverside.

McGrew, K. S., & Woodcock, R. W. (2001). *Woodcock–Johnson III technical manual.* Itasca, IL: Riverside.

Niebling, B. C., & Braden, J. P. (2003). *Coding procedures: Evaluating the validity of test instrument interpretation.* Unpublished manuscript.

Psychological Assessment Resources. (2003). *Reynolds Intellectual Assessment Scales.* Retrieved from http://www.parinc.com/RIAS.cfm

Psychological Corporation. (2003). *Wechsler Intelligence Scale for Children—Fourth Edition: Technical manual.* San Antonio, TX: Author.

Reynolds, C. R., & Kamphaus, R. W. (2003). *Reynolds Intellectual Assessment Scales and the Reynolds Intellectual Screening Test: Professional manual.* Lutz, FL: Psychological Assessment Resources.

Roid, G. H. (2003a). *Stanford–Binet Intelligence Scales, Fifth Edition: Examiner's manual.* Itasca, IL: Riverside.

Roid, G. H. (2003b). *Stanford–Binet Intelligence Scales, Fifth Edition: Interpretive manual.* Itasca, IL: Riverside.

Roid, G. H. (2003c). *Stanford–Binet Intelligence Scales, Fifth Edition: Technical manual.* Itasca, IL: Riverside.

Ruf, D. L. (2003). *Use of the SB5 in the assessment of high abilities* (Stanford–Binet Intelligence Scales, Fifth Edition, Assessment Services Bulletin No. 3). Itasca, IL: Riverside.

Schrank, F. A., McGrew, K. S., & Woodcock, R. W. (2001). *Technical abstract* (Woodcock–Johnson III Assessment Service Bulletin No. 2). Itasca, IL: Riverside.

Wechsler, D. (2003). *Wechsler Intelligence Scale for Children—Fourth Edition.* San Antonio, TX: Psychological Corporation.

Williams, P. E., Weiss, L. G., & Rolfhus, E. L. (2003a). *Wechsler Intelligence Scale for Children—Fourth Edition: Clinical validity* (Technical Report No. 3). Retrieved from http://www.wisc-iv.com

Williams, P. E., Weiss, L. G., & Rolfhus, E. L. (2003b). *Wechsler Intelligence Scale for Children—Fourth Edition: Psychometric properties* (Technical Report No. 2). Retrieved from http://www.wisc-iv.com

Williams, P. E., Weiss, L. G., & Rolfhus, E. L. (2003). *Wechsler Intelligence Scale for Children—Fourth Edition: Theoretical model and test blueprint* (Technical Report No. 1). San Antonio, TX: Psychological Corp. Available: www.wisc-iv.com/.

Woodcock, R. W., McGrew, K. S., & Mather, N. (2001). *Woodcock–Johnson III Tests of Cognitive Abilities.* Itasca, IL: Riverside.

29

Intelligence Tests in an Era of Standards-Based Educational Reform

RACHEL BROWN-CHIDSEY

It has become commonplace for U.S. students to be required to take tests at specified grades (e.g., grades 3, 8, and 11; Heubert & Hauser, 1999). Indeed, the No Child Left Behind Act (NCLB) of 2001 mandates such testing in all schools that receive federal aid (NCLB, 2001). These tests are often referred to as *high-stakes,* because they may determine whether a student is eligible to move on to the next grade or graduate from high school. As of August 2003, all 50 U.S. states required some form of statewide testing of students (Thurlow, Wiley, & Bielinski, 2003). Although NCLB does not mandate that a student take a test to be eligible for a high school diploma, it does require states to develop statewide school accountability programs (National Center on Educational Outcomes [NCEO], 2003).

Data related to student performance on selected statewide tests suggest that many students are not passing these tests. The passing rates on Florida's statewide test, the Florida Comprehensive Assessment Test, for 2003 revealed that fewer than half of the state's high school seniors passed the test in most counties (Florida Department of Education, 2003). Yet there are some indicators of improvement and growth, too. The 2002 *Iowa Annual Condition of Education Report* (Iowa Department of Education, 2002) included data to show that the reading scores

for students of different racial and cultural backgrounds had improved over a 3-year period. Still, the fact that many students are not passing high-stakes tests has led to recommendations for review of education policies. New York State Education Commissioner Richard Mills issued a report in October 2003 suggesting that New York State allow the passing rate on the Regents Exam to remain at 55, rather than require the higher passing rate of 65 (Mills, 2003). Mills's justification for retaining the lower passing rate was based on his concern that too many students would fail the exam if the passing score were raised. Mills also noted that additional alternatives for testing students with disabilities were needed.

One of the distinguishing features of the recent widespread use of high-stakes tests is that virtually all students are required to participate in such exams (Shriner, 2000; (Thurlow et al., 2003). In contrast to past practice, when students with disabilities were often exempted from state-mandated tests, the current high-stakes testing movement has focused on the importance of having all students—both those with and without disabilities—participate in large-scale, high-stakes tests. In fact, the 1997 amendments to the Individuals with Disabilities Education Act (IDEA) put a heavy emphasis on the participation of students with disabilities in all general education, state-mandated testing. The rationale behind the participation of students with disabilities in high-stakes tests is to provide indicators of the students' progress toward individualized education program goals, and to provide the students with greater access to postsecondary educational opportunities (Shriner, 2000; Thurlow et al., 2003).

Although the provisions of IDEA 1997 have been in place for several years now, there is still a paucity of data on implications of including students with disabilities in high-stakes tests. The staff of the NCEO has conducted a series of studies related to the effects of participation by students with disabilities in high-stakes tests (e.g., Thurlow et al., Bielinski, 2003). As yet these data are inconclusive, because not all states have implemented full participation of students with disabilities in such tests. Preliminary evaluation indicates that students in general are performing at levels lower than desired, and that students with disabilities generally perform lower than other students (Thurlow et al., 2003). In the most comprehensive review of the assessment data for students with disabilities yet conducted, Thurlow and colleagues (2003) found that although states have made gains in reporting the performance of students with disabilities in statewide assessments, not all states have complied with the requirements of IDEA 1997 regarding state-mandated testing. Based on 2000–2001 data, Thurlow and colleagues concluded that 28 states had reported the performance of students with disabilities on state-mandated tests, and that students with disabilities scored lower than other students in these tests.

The widespread use of high-stakes tests in U.S. schools has led to cautions about their use. The National Association of School Psychologists (NASP) has issued a position statement on the use of high-stakes tests in educational decision making (NASP, 2003); this stipulates that such a test should never be the sole criterion for determining a child's educational future, "including access to educational opportunity, retention or promotion, graduation or receipt of a diploma" (p. 1). The American Psychological Association (APA) has issued a position statement on the presence of high-stakes tests in schools as well (APA, 2003). The APA acknowledges the potential benefit of high-stakes tests for demonstrating the outcomes and efficacy of specific instructional programs. Like the NASP, the APA cautions against using a high-stakes test score as the only measure on which a critical decision about a child's educational future is based. The APA statement calls for additional research into the relationship between student performance on high-stakes tests and other indicators of learning. Despite these cautions from professional organizations, high-stakes tests are more widespread than ever, even with incomplete data from states as to the performance of students with disabilities.

One of the issues facing those who seek to make sense out of high-stakes test data is the extent to which predisposing characteristics of the learners influence their test scores. Specifically, high-stakes tests are designed in part to document the progress that students make in a given program of study or curriculum. The basic premise behind high-stakes testing is that those students who have mastered the curriculum should score high enough on the test(s) to move on to the next level of education. Essentially, this follows from the idea that all children can learn. Still, there is abundant evidence of the heterogeneity of learners, and some students have characteristics that prevent them from mastering the program of study.

In cases where a student's particular learning characteristics can be identified as the result of a specific disability, special education services are provided so that all students can have access to education. The 1997 version of IDEA included 14 specific disability categories. In the 1999–2000 school year, the majority of students receiving special education services (46%) were identified as having specific learning disabilities (LDs) (U.S. Department of Education, 2002). Importantly, under IDEA 1997 and its predecessors, both the definition of an LD and the process for identifying an LD have been interpreted to involve the administration of a test of cognitive abilities, such as an IQ test (Peterson & Shinn, 2002).

Many, if not most, of the students identified as having LDs were identified as such on the basis of discrepancies between their scores on an IQ test and a measure of academic achievement (Peterson & Shinn, 2002; U.S. Department of Education, 2002). This so-called "discrepancy method" is based on the idea that students with LDs have at least average intellectual ability but are under-performing in school because of some other learning deficit. Some students with LDs have taken high-stakes tests under typical conditions with good results, and the performance of these students is of little concern (Thurlow et al., 2003). Other students with LDs have done poorly on high-stakes tests under typical conditions, and therefore have been able to take these tests using accommodations. Anecdotal evidence suggests that some students using accommodations have improved their scores while others have not.

Interestingly, there are virtually no data on the relationship(s) between IQ scores and high-stakes tests. Despite the extensive use of IQ scores in the identification of the largest subgroup of students receiving special education services in the United States, there has been no systematic evaluation of the connection between the students' general cognitive abilities and their performance on the test(s) that determine whether they are allowed to move forward along the education continuum. Certainly, there are a number of barriers to collecting such data, including the need for parental permission and access to records. Nonetheless, recognition of issues related to IQ and high-stakes testing is important, because of the implications both types of tests have for U.S. education policies. This chapter includes a discussion of the use of IQ tests in U.S. education and of how, in many ways, the current widespread use of high-stakes tests was foreshadowed by previous assessment efforts such as IQ testing.

CONTEXT OF INTELLIGENCE TESTING IN EDUCATION POLICY

Intelligence (IQ) tests were initially created for the purpose of determining which students would benefit from school-based education and which would not (Gould, 1981; Sattler, 2001). Alfred Binet is credited with creating the first IQ test for use with a school-age population in France (see Wasserman & Tulsky, Chapter 1, this volume). His test was adapted and used in many settings, including U.S. schools. Although it was hoped that IQ tests would help educators make decisions about the best instruction for different stu-

dents, the tests have never met that expectation fully. Many studies have shown that all IQ tests have limited reliability (Gould, 1981; Reschly & Grimes, 2002). In addition, other research has shown that the original view of IQ as a fixed trait, immune to instruction, is not accurate (Reschly & Grimes, 2002).

The limits of the reliability of IQ tests have been documented repeatedly (Gould, 1981; Kranzler, 1997; Reschly & Grimes, 2002; Sattler, 2001). Although certain features of IQ appear to be more stable than others (Flanagan & Ortiz, 2002; Glutting, McDermott, Watkins, Kush, & Konold, 1997; Reschly & Grimes, 2002), there is much variability in even average performance on IQ tests. In addition to concerns about the instability of IQ scores, other problems with their use in educational decision making have been identified. The validity of such tests for students from diverse linguistic, cultural, ethnic, and ability backgrounds has been widely challenged (Helms, 1997; Lopez, 1997).

At one time, IQ test scores were widely used in the United States as the sole criteria for determining which students would be enrolled in general education programs and which ones would take remedial classes. This practice was found to be highly discriminatory against certain groups of students, including African American students, and was litigated (e.g., in the well-known case of *Larry P. v. Riles*). For this reason, other ways of identifying aptitude and skills were developed. Many different measures of academic and other skills are widely used in schools for both individualized and large-group assessment. The presence of these skills tests has allowed educators to identify students' levels of performance and then provide instruction to improve the skills of low-achieving students.

Importantly, the premise behind skills and achievement testing is that missing skills can be learned with appropriate instruction. The assumption that instruction can have an impact on academic skills is in contrast to the interpretation of intellectual abilities as fixed traits that vary little over a person's lifetime. What researchers have learned from the use of skills testing followed by teaching and retesting is that certain skills can be improved through instruction (Reschly & Grimes,

2002). A by-product of the test–teach–retest model has been the discovery that IQ scores also improve with certain types of instruction and environmental enrichment (Elliott & Fuchs, 1997; Reschly & Grimes, 2002). Over time, numerous reliable and valid assessment methods have been developed for the purpose of identifying which students need what type of instruction. Many researchers have put forward the case for the superiority of measures other than IQ, such as curriculum-based measurement (CBM), for this task (Brown-Chidsey, Davis, & Maya, 2003; Deno, 1985; Elliott & Fuchs, 1997; Shinn, 1989).

The Current Standards-Based Reform Movement

The current national trend toward the use of statewide high-stakes tests as part of standard educational practice is the next chapter in the unfolding story of using assessment to guide instructional decision making. Just as IQ tests were initially intended to help educators identify which students should be in school, high-stakes tests are designed to identify which students are meeting certain learning standards and which ones are not. The current standards-based reform movement is often associated with the publication of the report entitled *A Nation at Risk* (U.S. Department of Education, 1983). This report, which was commissioned and published by the Reagan administration, deeply criticized the state of U.S. public education. Following the publication of *A Nation at Risk*, a number of federal and state-level education reform initiatives were implemented with the goal of (re)establishing higher standards for what U.S. students learn.

The most recent of the federal reform initiatives is the 2001 NCLB, sponsored by the George W. Bush administration. This act goes farther than earlier federal efforts to achieve higher learning outcomes for all public school students, because it pins federal education money to the states' plans and success in achieving the NCLB objectives. According to NCLB, all U.S. states must submit plans for implementing and achieving the NCLB goals to the U.S. Department of Education. Those schools that do not meet certain standards may lose funding and/or be taken over by state departments of education

until the NCLB goals are met. The way that schools are evaluated in relation to achieving NCLB goals is through statewide high-stakes tests, which are, for the first time, mandated for students in grades 3 through 8 (NCLB, 2001).

The NCLB, and its corollary state programs and initiatives, have carried the practice of testing for instructional decision making forward into the 21st century. The current standards-based reform programs have essentially the same purpose as Binet's first IQ scale: determining which students receive access to which educational services. The current high-stakes tests come with far more levels of assessment and decision making than solitary IQ tests administered once, but in the end they are likely to yield similar results. Students who receive passing scores on the high-stakes tests will follow a stepwise progression through the educational system, while students who do not pass will get remedial instruction until or unless they pass the test(s) to earn a diploma or they drop out of school (Thurlow & Esler, 2000; *Special Education Report*, 2002). In either case, the educational future of all public school students is heavily influenced by the high-stakes tests, in the same way that IQ tests in the past determined students' educational futures.

Equality of Access to Education

Much of the debate surrounding the use of both IQ measures and high-stakes tests is related to equity. As noted above, IQ tests have been found to have lower reliability and limited validity when used with certain groups of students or under certain conditions (Ortiz, 2002). Similarly, many critics have argued that group-based high-stakes tests have similarly questionable reliability and validity for certain students. Although data for all U.S. states are incomplete, test scores reported in past years have revealed that students from high-income families tend to score higher on statewide tests than students from low-income families (U.S. Department of Education, 2002).

Given that a disproportionate number of students from diverse linguistic, cultural, racial, and ability backgrounds tend to live in poverty, high-stakes tests generally reveal that lower-income students are not making satisfactory educational progress. Although some of the students who do poorly on high-stakes tests may be receiving special education services, special education was not created to provide remedial services to all underperforming students. Thus students who do not pass statewide tests may not have recourse to specialized instruction. Although special education was designed to increase access to education for all students, regardless of ability, the use of high-stakes tests may have the effect of reducing educational access.

Shriner (2000) found that procedures for allowing students who receive special education services to have accommodations or take alternative forms of state-mandated tests have not been fully developed or implemented in many states. Similarly, Thurlow and Esler (2000) reported that the process for appealing a failed graduation test for all students, regardless of disability, is nonexistent in most states. Indeed, some states have chosen to lower the criterion for passing the state test rather than to deal with appeals (*Education USA*, 2001; Mills, 2003). These policy trends suggest the emergence of recognition that high-stakes tests may constitute a significant obstacle to educational access for some students—one that may be challenged through litigation in the future.

Unlike IQ tests, high-stakes tests are designed to reveal the skills that students lack and then to serve as a starting point for designing instruction by which the students can gain the skills. When joined with high-quality instruction and frequent assessment of progress, such methods have been shown to be very effective (Berninger, 2002; Elliott & Fuchs, 1997). Often, however, the results from statewide tests of student achievement are returned to schools after a considerable time delay. For example, scores for tests taken in winter or spring may not be sent to the schools until the summer, after the school year has ended (Brown-Chidsey et al., 2003). This time delay means that the students and their teachers do not get the chance to review the test results and adjust instruction during the school year.

When compared with the initial use of IQ tests over 100 years ago, the shift to wide-scale, large-group testing for the purpose of fine-tuning instruction to meet the needs of individual learners is an improvement.

Nonetheless, as currently implemented in many areas, state-mandated high-stakes tests may not be meeting the intended goal of improving instruction: The tests are not reliable and valid for all learners, and the results are provided to the students and teachers too late for change to occur. The common thread linking IQ and high-stakes tests is access to education. As noted, IQ tests have been used for many years as a cornerstone of individualized assessment of students to determine special education eligibility. More recently, IQ tests have been criticized as inappropriate indicators of students' aptitudes and other forms of assessment have been introduced, including statewide high-stakes tests of student achievement in targeted skills. In isolation, neither IQ tests nor once-a-year statewide tests are effective tools for evaluating student progress. Yet there is evidence that both IQ instruments and high-stakes tests may have unique roles in educational assessment, when used appropriately and in combination with other tools.

ROLE OF INTELLIGENCE TESTING IN ACCESS TO EDUCATION

From their creation, IQ tests were considered to offer unique insight into a student's potential as a learner (Gould, 1981). In time, however, researchers and educators realized that IQ tests were limited in the extent to which they could predict a student's learning potential. Instead, researchers into cognitive assessment turned their attention to understanding a learner's profile (Flanagan & Ortiz, 2001, 2002; McGrew, Flanagan, Keith, & Vanderwood, 1997). Focusing on cognitive pattern analysis, researchers such as Flanagan, Ortiz, McGrew, and others have suggested that the true usefulness of IQ tests is in their ability to show *how*, not *whether*, a person learns. Nonetheless, others have maintained a position that ipsative analysis and other forms of subtest evaluation are not helpful when it comes to designing instructional interventions for low-achieving students (McDermott & Glutting, 1997; Reschly & Grimes, 2002; Stage, Abbott, Jenkins, & Berninger, 2003). Such research has pointed to other methods for determining which students need additional instruction and what kind (e.g., CBM and performance assessment; Elliott & Fuchs, 1997; Howell & Nolet, 2000).

IQ and Access to Special Education Services

An important change was included in the 2004 reauthorization of IDEA. Instead of requiring an IQ score, as well as academic achievement information, IDEA 2004 allows schools to document how a student responds to instruction as partial evidence of a learning disability. The requirements for diagnosis of mental retardation still include an IQ score. These requirements are minimum criteria and do not preclude the use of additional assessment measures for the purpose of identifying which students are eligible and in need of special education services for these disability types. Still, the presence of the requirement of an IQ score in any of the federal special education disability subtypes suggests that such scores will continue to have a role in determining at least some of the students who are eligible for special education services.

Importantly, federal and state special education regulations all stipulate that an IQ score can never be the only basis on which a student's eligibility for special programming is based. Over 100 years of IQ research have shown that there is much more to human abilities than a single number or group of numbers. Still, IQ scores are likely to continue to be used for special education eligibility decisions. As required by law, IQ scores should always be used alongside a number of other indicators of a student's abilities. For example, in the case of diagnosis of mental retardation, the IQ score must be accompanied by an assessment of adaptive behavior, as well as other information about how an individual's characteristics fit with the diagnosis (Brown-Chidsey & Steege, 2004).

IQ and High-Stakes Testing

In many ways, high-stakes tests and IQ tests can be understood as the two endpoints of an assessment continuum. Figure 29.1 illustrates this continuum. The continuum includes four stages of assessment, moving from large-group assessment to individualized IQ tests. Of note, the "group" or "individualized" nature of the assessments repre-

sented in Figure 29.1 refers to which students participate in the tests, not the circumstances under which they are tested or what is contained in the tests. Several or many students may participate in CBM testing or other assessment sessions using published norm-referenced tests. These may be given during individualized or group sessions, but all the students interact with the same assessment materials.

Stage 1 of this model includes large-group (whole-class or whole-grade) testing and is shown at the far left of Figure 29.1. The large-group box is larger than the others and represents the largest grouping in which a student in K–12 education is likely to be tested. All students in a given class or grade participate in such testing. The next box represents a smaller group of students who participate in additional assessments as a result of concerns about their scores on the large-group tests. For example, if a subset of fourth graders perform poorly on a state's annual exam, they participate in follow-up testing in only the area(s) in which their statewide exam scores are problematic. CBM is one type of assessment tool that can be used for stage 2 testing. Those students who perform poorly on the stage 2 testing are represented in the box for stage 3. These students participate in additional assessments geared toward identifying the specific subskills that are interfering with their school progress. For example, if these students perform poorly on the CBM materials in the area of reading, additional reading assessment that incorporates specific reading subskill assessment (e.g., the Comprehensive Test of Phonological Processing) can be used.

Stage 4 of the continuum is IQ testing. IQ tests are the most individualized of any assessment tools. They must be individually administered, and they are designed to detect specific unique individual differences. As represented in Figure 29.1, IQ tests should be given only when other attempts to understand a student's learning needs have not resulted in improved student performance. The IQ data are used to evaluate whether a student's learning difficulties are the result of a specific cognitive feature. Importantly, there is a dynamic and continuous feature of the testing continuum presented in Figure 29.1. Each stage of the model is related to the other stages, and once results are obtained

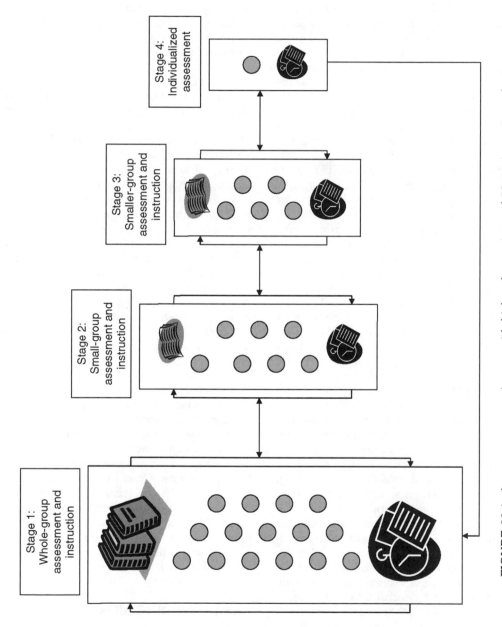

FIGURE 29.1. An assessment continuum, with high-stakes testing and IQ testing as its endpoints.

from a given stage, they should be used to provide related instructional changes designed to improve student performance on any subsequent tests. The interactive nature of the testing stages is seen in the bidirectional arrows between each pair of stages. Similarly, vertical arrows alongside stages 1, 2, and 3 represent how assessment data is used to inform instruction and how subsequent assessments follow from the instruction given. This dynamic instructional approach is true also of IQ tests, but in a more limited way. IQ tests may be used to create testing and instructional accommodations for certain students; however, it is not possible to determine the efficacy of specific instruction from an IQ test alone. The influence of IQ scores on large-group testing is represented by the arrow at the bottom of Figure 29.1 showing feedback from IQ results to large-group testing situations.

High-stakes tests are designed to be given to large groups of students at one time, and they are intended to measure those aspects of the students' knowledge and skills that are learned as a result of general school experiences. Used alone, neither IQ nor high-stakes test scores can provide adequate information about a student's learning progress. Even when an IQ score is coupled with a statewide test score, this coupling will not yield much information from which to design instruction. The many other measurement tools along the assessment continuum must also be used in order for an accurate description of a student's learning needs to be created. When used in conjunction with both formal and informal measures of skill and learning, IQ scores and/or high-stakes test scores may be useful for planning future instruction.

As noted, the assessment continuum needs to be understood as bidirectional. Again, this is reflected in Figure 29.1 by the double-headed arrows between each pair of stages. Ultimately, a student's scores on a statewide test may be part of a decision for that student to be given an IQ test. Similarly, a student's score and/or pattern of responses on an IQ test, as well as other measures of achievement, may be used to decide whether a student should participate in large-group testing and under what conditions. For some students with severe and profound disabilities, taking high-stakes tests serves no instructional or functional purpose. In these cases, the students' progress can best be documented through an alternate assessment process. For most students with disabilities, however, participation in statewide high-stakes testing not only is possible, but may provide useful information for instructional planning. Indeed, the courts have upheld the requirement that students with disabilities be required to take state-level graduation exams (*Special Education Report*, 2001).

For students with disabilities who are required to take high-stakes tests, it is important to determine whether accommodations or modifications need to be made (Wasburn-Moses, 2003). Most states have been very strict about the extent and nature of high-stakes test accommodations, but when these are documented and appropriate, alterations to standard testing conditions can be made. Such accommodations and/or modifications should be based on a variety of assessment and evaluation information about the student. It may be the case that information from an IQ test or other individually administered tests can help to document the basis for a student's high-stakes testing accommodations or modifications. For example, some students need extra time to complete the items on high-stakes tests in order to demonstrate their mastery of the learned material. The need for extra time as a result of slower-than-average processing can be documented by providing evidence from a psychological evaluation that included IQ measures. Similarly, a psychological evaluation with IQ information can provide evidence that a student is capable of processing and responding to questions on a test in the expected time, but needs assistive technology in order to produce a response. In both these cases, IQ scores or similar individualized assessment data are appropriate ways to indicate why a student needs accommodations for instruction and assessment.

AREAS NEEDING MORE RESEARCH

A number of details related to the use of IQ tests in an era of standards-based reform need to be addressed with future research. Given that all U.S. schools are now expected to participate fully in standards-based assessment activities, the nature of the questions needing to be addressed by researchers may continue to change over time. Three major lines of research that would serve as general starting points for understanding the general effects of standards-based reform on individual students are discussed below.

Relationship between IQ and High-stakes Tests

As noted at the beginning of the chapter, there is very little research on the actual relationship between IQ scores and students' scores on high-stakes tests. Without even small datasets documenting the relationship between IQ and high-stakes test scores, it is impossible to tell whether the hypothesized assessment continuum shown in Figure 29.1 is accurate. It may be the case that student performance on high-stakes tests has very little relationship with IQ scores, and the continuum model needs to be reexamined and changed. Alternatively, there may be a considerable degree of consistency between IQ scores and high-stakes test scores. If that is the case, then it seems pertinent to ask this question: How might students' scores on high-stakes tests and other achievement indicators be used to make instructional decisions? Such a practice could reduce the number of IQ tests given, potentially saving many hours of work and freeing up personnel for other activities—such as implementing and monitoring instruction, or conducting in-depth assessment of students with complex learning needs.

Accommodations and Alternative Assessment

There is a growing amount of information on the use and effects of accommodations, modifications, and alternative forms of assessment. The NCEO has conducted a number of reviews of states' data about the use of testing accommodations, modifications, and alternate assessments (Thurlow et al., 2003). Although it remains difficult to compare data between and among states, there is an increasing database of students' scores on high-stakes tests under a variety of testing conditions. These data should help to shed light on the extent to which students from diverse backgrounds and experiences are able to be successful on high-stakes tests over time. Similarly, the states themselves are now required to collect and report data on student performance on high-stakes tests according to population characteristics and subgroups (e.g., language, race, disability). These data may help policymakers to determine whether the use of high-stakes tests is any more useful than previous attempts to identify and address students' learning needs.

High-Stakes Test Data and Student Improvement

Similar to the need for disaggregated data about student performance on high-stakes tests, there is a need for longitudinal data about how students in a given testing pool (i.e., a particular state) perform on the newly required tests as instructional adjustments are made. Some states have such data already, and others are making adjustments to state testing requirements to facilitate better reporting and analysis of students' test scores. Over time, these data may help to show which instructional programs are most effective in meeting learning objectives. Once such data are obtained, a thorough review of the role and function of high-stakes tests in regard to state-specific educational standards will be necessary.

CONCLUSION

It is very clear that standards-based reform programs are part of the current and future landscape of U.S. public education. Such programs had their origins in criticisms of public education dating from the early 1980s, but have been added to by educators, policymakers, and members of the public who have sought to establish clearer and more challenging educational goals for all students. One of the prominent features of current reform initiatives is the use of high-stakes tests intended to identify which students have met the learning objectives and which have not. There is some evidence that high-stakes tests are related to improved student outcomes, but the data are inconsistent (Viadero, 2003).

The current focus on high-stakes tests has renewed awareness of the importance of access to education for all students. As noted by Thurlow and Esler (2000), access to a high-quality education has already been identified as a property right by some courts. If equal access to education remains part of U.S. education policy, then it should not be a question of whether IQ or high-stakes tests are used, but rather under what circumstances they are used and for what purposes. For a century now, researchers have argued both the benefits and limitations of IQ tests. With time, a similar body of research will exist for group-based, high-stakes tests. Regardless of the merits or drawbacks of either type of test, what really matter for individual students are how, when, and for what purpose they are used.

As suggested by Reschly and Grimes (2002), there should be a "Surgeon General's warning" on all tests to remind us that every test has limitations, and that no one test should ever be used in isolation to make "high-stakes" decisions about students' educational futures. Instead of expecting any one test to serve as a universal prescription for students' learning needs, educators, parents, policymakers, and the public need to recognize that high-quality assessment comes from the use of a range of evaluation tools over time. Those who are vexed by the current debate over high-stakes testing can learn from the history of IQ testing and research that no one test will yield all the answers, but over time a range of indicators can help provide information about what instruction may be most effective in the future.

REFERENCES

American Psychological Association (APA). (2003). *Appropriate use of high-stakes testing in our nation's schools*. Retrieved from *http://www.apa.org/pubinfo/testing.html*

Berninger, V. (2002). Best practices in reading, writing, and math assessment–intervention links: A systems approach for schools, classrooms, and individuals. In A. Thomas & J. Grimes (Eds.), *Best practices in school psychology IV* (pp. 851–866). Bethesda, MD: National Association of School Psychologists.

Brown-Chidsey, R., Davis, L., & Maya, C. (2003). Sources of variance in curriculum-based measures of silent reading. *Psychology in the Schools, 40,* 363–377.

Brown-Chidsey, R., & Steege, M. W. (2004). Adaptive behavior assessment. In T. S. Watson & C. H. Skinner (Eds.), *Encyclopedia of school psychology* (pp. 14–15). New York: Kluwer Academic/Plenum.

Deno, S. L. (1985). Curriculum-based measurement: The emerging alternative. *Exceptional Children, 52,* 219–232,

Education USA. (2001). Mass[achusetts] officials mull appeals process for exit exams. *Education USA: The Independent Biweekly News Digest for School Leaders, 43*(20), 1–2.

Elliott, S. N., & Fuchs, L. S. (1997). The utility of curriculum-based measurement and performance assessment as alternatives to traditional intelligence and achievement tests. *School Psychology Review, 26,* 224–233.

Flanagan, D. P., & Ortiz, S. (2001). *Essentials of cross-battery assessment*. New York: Wiley.

Flanagan, D. P., & Ortiz, S. (2002). Best practices in intellectual assessment: Future directions. In A. Thomas & J. Grimes (Eds.), *Best practices in school psychology IV* (pp. 1351–1372). Bethesda, MD: National Association of School Psychologists.

Florida Department of Education. (2003). *FCAT 2003 grade 12 passing percent by district*. Retrieved from *http://www.firn.edu/doe/sas/fcat/pdf/grade12pass03.pdf*

Glutting, J. J., McDermott, P. A., Watkins, M. M., Kush, J. C., & Konold, T. R. (1997). The base rate problem and its consequences for interpreting children's ability profiles. *School Psychology Review, 26,* 176–188.

Gould, S. J. (1981). *The mismeasure of man*. New York: Norton.

Helms, J. E. (1997). The triple quandary of race, cultures, and social class in standardized cognitive ability testing. In D. P. Flanagan, J. J. Genshaft, & P. L. Harrison (Eds.), *Contemporary intellectual assessment: Theories, tests, and issues* (pp. 517–532). New York: Guilford Press.

Howell, K. W., & Nolet, V. (2000). *Curriculum-based evaluation: Teaching and decision-making*. Belmont, CA: Thomson Learning.

Heubert, J. P., & Hauser, R. M. (Eds.). (1999). *High stakes: Testing for tracking, promotion, and graduation*. Washington, DC: National Academy Press.

Individuals with Disabilities Education Act Amendments of 1997, Pub. L. 105-17, 20 U.S.C. 33 §§ 1400 et seq. (1997).

Individuals with Disabilities Education Act, Pub. L. 108–446 (2004).

Iowa Department of Education. (2002). *Iowa annual condition of education report, 2002*. Retrieved from *http://www.state.ia.us/educate/fis/pre/coer/index.html*

Kranzler, J. H. (1997). Educational and policy issues related to the use and interpretation of intelligence tests in the schools. *School Psychology Review, 26,* 150–162.

Lopez, R. (1997). The practical impact of current research and issues in intelligence test interpretation and use for multicultural populations. *School Psychology Review, 26,* 249–254.

McDermott, P. A., & Glutting, J. J. (1997). Informing stylistic learning behavior, disposition, and achievement through ability subtests—or, more illusions or meaning? *School Psychology Review, 26*, 163–175.

McGrew, K. S., Flanagan, D. P., Keith, T. Z., & Vanderwood, M. (1997). Beyond *g*: The impact of Gf-Gc specific cognitive abilities research on the future use and interpretation of intelligence test batteries in the schools. *School Psychology Review, 26*, 189–210.

Mills, R. (2003). *Commissioner Mills recommends four major policies on testing to Board of Regents*. Retrieved from *http://www.oms.nysed.gov/press/testing_policy.htm*

National Association of School Psychologists (NASP). (2003). *Position statement on using large scale assessment for high stakes decisions*. Bethesda, MD: Author.

National Center on Educational Outcomes (NCEO). (2003). *Accountability for assessment results in the No Child Left Behind Act: What it means for children with disabilities*. Retrieved from *http://education.umn.edu/NCEO/OnlinePubs/NCLBaccountability.html*

No Child Left Behind Act (NCLB) of 2001, Pub. L. 107-115, 20 U.S.C. 6301 (2001).

Ortiz, S. O. (2002). Best practices in nondiscriminatory assessment. In A. Thomas & J. Grimes (Eds.), *Best practices in school psychology IV* (pp. 1321–1336). Bethesda, MD: National Association of School Psychologists.

Peterson, K. M. H., & Shinn, M. R. (2002). Severe discrepancy models: Which best explains school identification practices for learning disabilities. *School Psychology Review, 31*, 459–476.

Reschly, D. J., & Grimes, J. P. (2002). Best practices in intellectual assessment. In A. Thomas & J. Grimes (Eds.), *Best practices in school psychology IV* (pp. 1337–1350). Bethesda, MD: National Association of School Psychologists.

Sattler, J. M. (2001). *Assessment of children: Cognitive applications* (fourth ed.). San Diego, CA: Jerome M. Sattler.

Shinn, M. R. (Ed.). (1989). *Curriculum-based measurement: Assessing special children*. New York: Guilford Press.

Shriner, J. G. (2000). Legal perspectives on school outcomes assessment for students with disabilities. *Journal of Special Education, 33*, 232–239.

Special Education Report. (2001, July 4). Court: Disabled students must take Ind[iana] exit exam. *Special Education Report, 27*(14), 5–6.

Special Education Report. (2002, October 9). Lawyer: failing exam could lead disabled to drop out. *Special Education Report, 28*(21), 8.

Stage, S. A., Abbott, R. D., Jenkins, J. R., & Berninger, V. W. (2003). Predicting response to early reading intervention from Verbal IQ, reading-related language abilities, attention ratings, and Verbal IQ–word reading discrepancy: Failure to validate discrepancy method. *Journal of Learning Disabilities, 36*, 24–33.

Thurlow, M., & Esler, A. (2000). *Appeals process for students who fail graduation exams: How do they apply to students with disabilities?* (Synthesis Report No. 36). Retrieved from *http://education.umn.edu/NCEO/OnlinePubs/Synthesis36.html*

Thurlow, M., Wiley, H. I., & Bielinski, J. (2003). *Going public: What 2000–2001 reports tell us about the performance of students with disabilities* (Technical Report No. 35). Retrieved from *http://education.umn.edu/NCEO/OnlinePubs/Technical35.htm*

U.S. Department of Education, The National Commission on Excellence in Education. (1983). *A nation at risk: The imperative for educational reform*. Washington, DC: Author.

U.S. Department of Education, National Center for Education Statistics. (2002). *Digest of education statistics, 2001*. Retrieved from *http://nces.ed.gov/pubs2002/digest2001/tables/dt052.asp*

Viadero, D. (2003). Researchers debate impact of tests. *Education Week, 22*(21), 1–2.

Wasburn-Moses, L. (2003). What every special educator should know about high-stakes testing. *Teaching Exceptional Children, 35*, 12–15.

Ysseldyke, J. (2002). Intended and unintended consequences of high-stakes assessment systems. *Trainer's Forum: Periodical of the Trainers of School Psychologists, 22*, 1–3, 11.

Author Index

McDowd, J. M., 55
McFall, R. M., 256, 257
McFie, J., 297
McGhee, R., 139, 160, 174
McGrath, E. A., 261
McGrath, M., 258
McGregor, P., 12
McGrew, K. S., 32, 36, 40, 43,
  45, 48, 73, 81, 137, 139, 140,
  141, 145, 146, 147, 148, 157,
  158, 159, 160, 161, 162, 164,
  165, 169, 170, 171, 172, 174,
  175, 185, 186, 188, 189, 191,
  192, 193, 195, 197, 198, 200,
  204, 209, 210, 219, 221, 227,
  229, 235, 242, 261, 262, 273,
  275, 283, 284, 285, 326, 331,
  334, 337, 345, 347, 354, 371,
  377, 378, 379, 381, 384, 403,
  405, 411, 412, 427, 435, 436,
  449, 450, 490, 492, 497, 499,
  506, 518, 522, 530, 535, 537,
  554, 555, 560, 573, 575, 590,
  592, 595, 596, 600, 603, 605,
  607, 612, 619, 624, 635
McGue, M., 145
McIntosh, D. E., 413, 414, 416,
  508
McKellop, M., 559
McKenna, M. C., 302
McKenna, P., 314
McKeown, M. G., 277
McKinnon, M., 493
McLean, J. E., 353, 364, 365, 474
McLean, J. F., 284
McLean, M., 489, 490
McLeod, P., 205
McLloyd, V., 487
McNamara, D. S., 205
McNamee, G. D., 88, 93, 95
McNemar, Q., 169, 204, 253
McPherson, A., 522, 532
Mednitsky, S., 366
Meehl, P. E., 256
Meisels, S. J., 84, 88, 95, 487,
  488, 489, 493, 494
Melendez, L., 85, 93
Melnyk, L., 132
Melville, N. J., 11
Menchetti, B. M., 274
Mercer, J. R., 244, 249
Meredith, W., 45
Merikle, P. M., 172
Merino, B., 239
Merkel, C., 493
Merrill, M. A., 12, 24, 325, 419
Merritt, C. R., 17
Messick, S., 192, 193, 198, 269,
  450, 531, 560
Meyer, M. S., 272, 281

Michael, W. B., 74
Milgram, S., 113
Miller, A., 94, 499
Miller, G., 278
Miller, G. A., 57
Miller, L., 283
Miller, L. J., 332, 430, 494, 498,
  562, 563
Miller, L. S., 366
Miller, P. H., 82
Miller, S. A., 82
Mills, R., 631, 635
Millsap, R. E., 586
Milne, L., 258
Milone, M. N., 88
Minkoff, S. R. B., 164
Minskoff, E., 456
Minton, H. L., 11, 12
Mishra, R. K., 129, 130, 132,
  451
Mishra, S. P., 510, 511
Miyake, A., 172
Moats, L. C., 278
Mock, D., 272
Moffitt, T. E., 252
Mollner, N. R., 259
Molloy, G. N., 125
Monahan, J., 256
Moody, S. W., 270
Moore, D. D., 299
Morgan, A. W., 559
Morgan, J., 493
Morgan, P. L., 272
Morris, R. D., 224, 277, 313,
  314
Morrow, D., 57
Morse, D. T., 510, 511
Moses, J. A., Jr., 366
Moss, P., 84
Mueller, H. H., 30, 253
Mulaik, S. A., 595
Mulholland, T. M., 107
Mullen, E. M., 494, 495, 496
Muñoz-Sandoval, A. F., 238,
  384, 386, 429, 554
Munson, S. M., 490
Murphy, D. L., 366
Murphy, S., 411, 412
Murray, C., 64, 77, 80
Muter, V., 280
Muthén, B. O., 404, 582
Muthén, L. K., 582

N

Nagle, R. J., 258, 259, 489, 493
Naglieri, J. A., 34, 120, 122,
  123, 124, 125, 126, 128, 129,
  130, 131, 132, 133, 161, 191,

195, 222, 223, 273, 354, 360,
  367, 441, 442, 443, 445, 446,
  447, 448, 449, 450, 451, 453,
  454, 455, 456, 457, 458, 506,
  514, 562, 595
Nagoshi, C. T., 74
Nathan, J. S., 12
Naylor, G. F. K., 47
Nebes, R. D., 51
Neisser, U., 36, 80, 107, 137,
  185, 203, 204, 308, 547
Neisworth, J. T., 490, 493
Nellis, L., 495
Nelson, G., 404
Nelson, H. E., 314
Nelson-Goff, G., 149
Nesselroade, J. R., 63
Nettelbeck, T., 51, 156, 285
Neubauer, A. C., 308
Neuman, G. A., 159
Newell, A., 106, 204, 217
Newstead, S. E., 229, 302
Neyens, L. G. J., 254
Nicholson, J., 84
Nieberding, R., 297
Niebling, B. C., 617
Nimmo-Smith, I., 328
Nolet, V., 229, 636
Noll, J., 16, 18, 45, 48, 53, 54,
  55, 69, 74, 137, 138, 143,
  144, 150, 158, 162, 171, 173,
  175, 203, 299, 345, 347, 377,
  403, 499, 559, 560
Norman, D. A., 49
Norman, K. A., 388, 508
Novak, M. A., 299
Novick, M. R., 74
Nuttall, E. V., 488
Nyborg, H., 162, 163, 168

O

Oakland, T., 262
Oberauer, K., 164, 172
Ochoa, S. H., 236, 237, 238,
  239, 240, 241, 242, 546
O'Connell, A., 314
O'Connor, T. A., 141
Oden, M. H., 508
Oehler-Stinnett, J., 499
Ofiesh, N. S., 286
Oh, H. J., 261
Okagaki, L., 113
Olson, R., 276
O'Neal, M., 145
O'Neil, H. F., 95
Ormrod, J. E., 279
Ortiz, S. O., 140, 148, 183, 185,
  188, 189, 192, 199, 235, 236,

Subject Index

Ability, defined, 204
Academic performance
  ability testing to predict, 115,
    274–275
  assessment, 336–338
  Cognitive Assessment System
    scores and, 447–449
  component cognitive abilities
    in, 274–275
    fluid reasoning, 286–287
    long-term memory, 280–282
    phonological processing,
      277–278
    processing speed, 285–286
    short-term memory, 278–
      280
    verbal abilities and
      knowledge, 275–277
    visual-spatial thinking, 282–
      284
  g factor and, 168–170
  implications of triarchic
    theory, 115–116
  IQ score discrepancy, 272–
    273, 632–633
  language acquisition and, 238–
    239
  learning disability assessment,
    524–531
  PASS-based interventions,
    129–132
  PASS profiles and, 125, 126–
    128
  profile analysis to predict,
    261–262

Reynolds Intellectual
    Assessment Scales
    assessment and, 474
  Stanford–Binet assessment,
    336–338
  See also High-stakes tests
Access to education, 634–638,
  639–640
Accommodations in testing, 638,
  639
Accountability, 631
Acculturation knowledge, 43
  development, 46, 47
  Stanford–Binet test
    considerations, 328–329
Acculturation process, 548–549
Active information, 206
Activity as unit of analysis in
  assessment, 94–95
Adaptation
  in concept of successful
    intelligence, 104
  fluid intelligence for, 18
  in triarchic theory, 104, 111–
    112
Adaptive control of thought–
  rational theory, 207–208
Adjustment Scales for Children
  and Adolescents, 262–
  263
Age-graded norms, 7
Akaike information criterion,
  587
Analysis of Moment Structures,
  582

Aptitude, 172–173
Area under the curve, 257
Armed Services Vocational
  Aptitude Battery, 159
Articulatory rehearsal, 206
Association area, 120–121
Associative memory, 280
  Woodcock–Johnson III Tests of
    Cognitive Abilities
    assessment, 380
Assumption of comparability,
  548, 552
Attentional processes
  Cognitive Assessment System
    assessment, 443–444
  cognitive speed and, 54–55
  neurophysiology, 121
  PASS-based intervention, 132
  PASS theory, 121, 124, 441–
    442
  susceptibility to interference,
    55
  Woodcock–Johnson III Tests of
    Cognitive Abilities
    assessment, 388
Attention-deficit/hyperactivity
  disorder
  Cognitive Assessment System
    assessment, 451–452
  PASS profiles, 125, 128
  profile analysis to diagnose,
    259, 260
  Woodcock–Johnson III Tests of
    Cognitive Abilities
    assessment, 388